Diving and Subaquatic Medicine

FIFTH EDITION

Diving and Subaquatic Medicine

FIFTH EDITION

Carl Edmonds was the OIC of the Royal Australian Navy Diving Medical Unit, Foundation President of the South Pacific Underwater Medical Society and Director of the Australian Diving Medical Centre, Sydney, Australia

Michael Bennett is Academic Head, Wales Anaesthesia and Senior Staff Specialist, Diving and Hyperbaric Medicine, Prince of Wales Hospital and University of New South Wales, Sydney, Australia

John Lippmann is Founder and Chairman of Divers Alert Network Asia-Pacific, Ashburton, Australia

Simon J. Mitchell is a Consultant Anaesthesiologist and Diving Physician, and Head, Department of Anaesthesiology, University of Auckland, Auckland, New Zealand

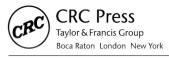

CRC Press
Taylor & Francis Group
Boca Raton London New York

CRC Press is an imprint of the
Taylor & Francis Group, an **informa** business

CRC Press
Taylor & Francis Group
6000 Broken Sound Parkway NW, Suite 300
Boca Raton, FL 33487-2742

First issued in paperback 2020

© 2016 by Taylor & Francis Group, LLC
CRC Press is an imprint of Taylor & Francis Group, an Informa business

No claim to original U.S. Government works

ISBN 13: 978-0-367-57555-7 (pbk)
ISBN 13: 978-1-4822-6012-0 (hbk)

This book contains information obtained from authentic and highly regarded sources. While all reasonable efforts have been made to publish reliable data and information, neither the author[s] nor the publisher can accept any legal responsibility or liability for any errors or omissions that may be made. The publishers wish to make clear that any views or opinions expressed in this book by individual editors, authors or contributors are personal to them and do not necessarily reflect the views/opinions of the publishers. The information or guidance contained in this book is intended for use by medical, scientific or health-care professionals and is provided strictly as a supplement to the medical or other professional's own judgement, their knowledge of the patient's medical history, relevant manufacturer's instruc-tions and the appropriate best practice guidelines. Because of the rapid advances in medical science, any information or advice on dosages, procedures or diagnoses should be independently verified. The reader is strongly urged to consult the relevant national drug formulary and the drug companies' and device or material manufacturers' printed instructions, and their websites, before administering or utilizing any of the drugs, devices or materials mentioned in this book. This book does not indicate whether a particular treatment is appropriate or suitable for a particular individual. Ultimately it is the sole responsibility of the medical professional to make his or her own profes-sional judgements, so as to advise and treat patients appropriately. The authors and publishers have also attempted to trace the copyright holders of all material reproduced in this publication and apologize to copyright holders if permission to publish in this form has not been obtained. If any copyright material has not been acknowledged please write and let us know so we may rectify in any future reprint.

Library of Congress Cataloging-in-Publication Data

Edmonds, Carl, author, editor.
  Diving and subaquatic medicine / Carl Edmonds, Michael Bennett, John Lippmann, Simon Mitchell. -- Fifth edition.
  p. ; cm.
  Preceded by: Diving and subaquatic medicine / Carl Edmonds ... [et. al.]. 4th ed. c2002.
  Includes bibliographical references and index.
  ISBN 978-1-4822-6012-0 (hardcover : alk. paper)
  I. Bennett, Michael (Michael H.) author, editor. II. Lippmann, John, 1951- , author, editor. III. Mitchell, Simon, Dr., author, editor. IV. Title.
  [DNLM: 1. Submarine Medicine. 2. Diving. WD 650]

RC1005
616.9'8022--dc23   2015021369

Visit the Taylor & Francis Web site at
http://www.taylorandfrancis.com

and the CRC Press Web site at
http://www.crcpress.com

Authors

Carl Edmonds, OAM, MB, BS (Sydney), MRCP (Lond.) FRACP, FAFOM, DPM, MRC Psych, MANZCP, Dip DHM

Director, Diving Medical Centre, Sydney, Australia (1970–2000)

Formerly, Officer in Charge Royal Australian Navy School of Underwater Medicine (1967–1975)

Formerly, President, South Pacific Underwater Medicine Society (1970–1975)

Consultant in Underwater Medicine to the Royal Australian Navy (1975–1991)

Consultant in Diving Medicine (1967 until retired in 2015)

Michael Bennett, MB, BS (UNSW), DA (Lond.), FFARCSI, FANZCA, MM (Clin Epi) (Syd.), MD (UNSW), Dip DHM, FUHM

Director, Department of Diving and Hyperbaric Medicine, Prince of Wales Hospital, Sydney, Australia (1993–2008)

Academic Head, Wales Anaesthesia, Sydney, Australia (2012–present)

Formerly, President, South Pacific Underwater Medicine Society (2008–2014)

Formerly, Vice-President, Undersea and Hyperbaric Medical Society (2006–2007 and 2011–2012)

Conjoint Associate Professor in Anaesthesia and Diving and Hyperbaric Medicine, University of New South Wales, Sydney, Australia (2010–present)

Simon Mitchell, MB ChB, PhD, Dip DHM, Dip Occ Med, Cert DHM (ANZCA), FUHM, FANZCA

Head of Department, Department of Anaesthesiology, University of Auckland, Auckland, New Zealand (2011–present)

Consultant in Diving and Hyperbaric Medicine, Slark Hyperbaric Unit, North Shore Hospital, Auckland, New Zealand (2012–present)

Formerly, Medical Director, Wesley Centre for Hyperbaric Medicine, Brisbane, Australia (1998–2002)

Formerly, Director, Slark Hyperbaric Unit, Royal New Zealand Navy Hospital, Auckland, New Zealand (1995–1998)

John Lippmann, OAM, BSc, Dip Ed, MAppSc

Founder, Chairman and Director of Research, DAN (Divers Alert Network) Asia-Pacific (1994–present)

Author or co-author of: *The DAN Emergency Handbook, Deeper Into Diving, The Essentials of Deeper Sport Diving, Scuba Safety in Australia, Oxygen First Aid, First Aid and Emergency Care, Automated External Defibrillators, Advanced Oxygen First Aid, Basic Life Support, Cardiopulmonary Resuscitation, Decompression Illness, Am I Fit to Dive?* and various incarnations of these books.

Contents

List of abbreviations

ADS	atmospheric diving suit	FEV_1	forced expiratory volume in 1 second
ADV	automatic diluent valve	FIO_2	fraction of inspired oxygen
AGE	arterial gas embolism	FVC	forced vital capacity
ALS	advanced life support	HBOT	hyperbaric oxygen therapy
ARDS	acute respiratory distress syndrome	HPNA	high-pressure neurological syndrome
ATA	atmosphere absolute	IBCD	isobaric counterdiffusion
ATG	atmosphere gauge	ICP	intracranial pressure
BCD	buoyancy compensator device	IDDM	insulin-dependent diabetes mellitus
BLS	basic life support	ILCOR	International Liaison Committee on Resuscitation
BOV	bail-out valve		
BSAC	British Sub-Aqua Club	IPE	immersion pulmonary oedema
CAD	coronary artery disease	IPPV	intermittent positive pressure ventilation
CAGE	cerebral arterial gas embolism		
CCR	closed-circuit rebreather	ISO	International Organization for Standardization
CMF	constant mass flow		
CPAP	continuous positive airway pressure	lpm	litres per minute
CPR	cardiopulmonary resuscitation	MOD	maximum operating depth
CSF	cerebrospinal fluid	msw	metres of sea water
CSL	Commonwealth Serum Laboratories	NEDU	Navy Experimental Diving Unit
DAN	Divers Alert Network	NOAA	National Oceanic and Atmospheric Administration
dB	decibel		
DCI	decompression illness	NUADC	National Underwater Accident Data Centre
DCIEM	(Canadian) Defence and Civil Institute of Environmental Medicine		
		OPV	over-pressure valve
DCS	decompression sickness	$PaCO_2$	alveolar pressure of carbon dioxide
DDC	deck decompression chamber	$PaCO_2$	arterial pressure of carbon dioxide
DPV	diver propulsion vehicle	PADI	Professional Association of Diving Instructors
EAD	equivalent air depth		
ECC	external cardiac compression	PaO_2	alveolar partial pressure of oxygen
ECG	electrocardiogram	PaO_2	arterial partial pressure of oxygen
ECMO	extracorporeal membrane oxygenation	PCO_2	partial pressure of carbon dioxide
ECoG	electrocochleography	PEEP	positive end-expiratory pressure
EEG	electroencephalogram	PEF	peak expiratory flow
ENG	electronystagmography	PFO	patent foramen ovale
EPIRB	electronic position-indicating radio beacon	$PICO_2$	inspired partial pressure of carbon dioxide

PIO_2	inspired partial pressure of oxygen	SDPE	scuba divers' pulmonary oedema
PMCT	post-mortem computed tomography	SMB	surface marker buoy
PMDA	post-mortem decompression artefact	SPUM	South Pacific Underwater Medicine Society
PMV	pressure maintaining valve		
PN_2	partial pressure of nitrogen	SSBA	surface-supply breathing apparatus
PO_2	partial pressure of oxygen	SWAS	salt water aspiration syndrome
PPV	positive pressure ventilation	UHMS	Undersea and Hyperbaric Medical Society
RAN	Royal Australian Navy		
RCC	recompression chamber	UPTD	unit of pulmonary toxic dose
RGBM	reduced gradient bubble model	USN	United States Navy
RMV	residual minute volume (also respiratory minute volume)	VC	vital capacity
		VER	visual evoked response
SCR	semi-closed-circuit rebreather	VGE	venous gas emboli
scuba	self-contained underwater breathing apparatus	VPM	varying permeability model
		V/Q	ventilation-perfusion

Preface and excerpts from earlier editions

This book is written for doctors and paramedics who are called on to minister to the medical needs of those divers who venture on or under the sea. It was based on our experience in dealing with a vast number of diving accidents and with troubleshooting many diving problems, and it is also an attempt to integrate the experience and more erudite research of others.

The very generous praise bestowed by reviewers on the first edition of *Diving and Subaquatic Medicine*, and its surprising acceptance outside the Australasian region, inspired us to prepare further editions of this text.

In the later editions, we attempted to be less insular. Instead of an Australian book about Australian experiences, we sought the advice and guidance of respected friends and colleagues from other countries, and from other disciplines, especially in the United Kingdom, the United States, Canada, Japan and mainland Europe. This has not prevented us from being judgemental and selective when we deemed it fit. This is still a very specialized field where evidence-based medicine is in its infancy. Truth is not always achieved by voting, and consensus is often a transitory state. We have documented what we believe to be current best practice. The future will judge this.

The extension of diving as a recreational and commercial activity has led to the bewildered medical practitioner's being confronted with diving problems about which he or she has received little or no formal training. Doctors interested in diving had previously found themselves without a comprehensive clinical text. We tried to remedy this. Our primary focus remains on the diving clinician, the physician responsible for scuba divers, the diving paramedic and the exceptional diving instructor who needs some guidance from a practical reference text.

Diving accidents are much better defined, investigated and treated than when we commenced writing on this subject, many years ago. It was our intent to present, as completely as possible, an advanced and informative book on clinical diving medicine. We have avoided the temptation to write either a simplistic text or a research-oriented tome.

This text encompasses the range of diving disorders experienced by divers. It presents all aspects of diving medicine from ancient history to the latest trends, in a concise and informative manner. Each disorder is dealt with from a historical, aetiological, clinical, pathological, preventive and therapeutic perspective. Summaries, case histories and revision aids are interspersed throughout. For the doctor who is not familiar with the world of diving, introductory chapters on physics and physiology, equipment and the diving environments have been included.

The inclusion of anecdotes and occasional humour may lessen the load on the reader, as it does on the authors. As in previous editions, each chapter is edited by one of the authors, with overview and peer review available from the others. This means that not always will there be exact agreement among authors, and there may be some variation among chapters. This is inevitable when evidence and consensus are not always complete. It is also healthy for the future.

Three of the four previous authors have departed from this scene, and the fourth is about to leave. The baton needs to be passed. Our legacy and intent are that our younger colleagues will experience as much excitement, fascination, achievement, camaraderie and fun from diving as we have.

Carl Edmonds, 2015
on behalf of all previous
and new authors of this text.

Dedication

This book is dedicated to the memory of Pluto, who died, even though he never left dry land.

I have often been asked who Pluto was. He was a much loved basset hound who strolled into our study when the original three authors were postulating about an appropriate dedicatee for their text. We could not decide between Paul Bert, Al Behnke, Jr., and J.B.S. Haldane. Pluto solved our dilemma.

Acknowledgements

Carl Edmonds, John Lippmann, Michael Bennett and Simon Mitchell would like to thank Christopher Lowry, John Pennefather and Robyn Walker for their invaluable contributions to previous editions, upon which material in this latest fifth edition is based.

We wish to acknowledge the assistance given by the Royal Australian Navy, the Royal Navy and the United States Navy for permission to reproduce excerpts from their diving manuals, and to the many pioneers on whose work we have so heavily drawn, our families who have suffered unfairly, and our clinical tutors – the divers.

Numerous experts have been consulted to review and advise on specific chapters of this or previous editions. Our gratitude is extended to these valued colleagues, but they are not to blame for the final text. They include the following:

Peter Bennett
Ralph Brauer
Greg Briggs
Ian Calder
Jim Caruso
Richard Chole
David Dennison
Chris Edge
Glen Egstrom
David Elliott
Des Gorman
John Hayman

Eric Kindwall
Clarrie Lawler
Christopher Lawrence
Dale Mole
Owen O'Neill
John Pearn
Peter Sullivan
Ed Thalmann
John Tonkin
John Williamson
David Yount

Originally published in 1976 by the Diving Medical Centre (Australia) ISBN 09597191-0-5.

PART 1

Diving

History of diving

BREATH-HOLD DIVING

The origins of breath-hold diving are lost in time. Archaeologists claim that the Neanderthal human, an extinct primitive human, dived for food, likely in the first instance gathering shell-fish by wading at low tide before diving from canoes. By 4500 BC, underwater exploration had advanced from the first timid dive to an industry that supplied the community with shells, food and pearls.

From the ancient Greek civilization until today, fishers have dived for sponges, which, in earlier days, were used by soldiers as water canteens and wound dressings, as well as for washing.

Breath-hold diving for sponges continued until the nineteenth century when helmet diving equipment was introduced, allowing the intrepid to gamble their lives in order to reach the deeper sponge beds. Greek divers still search the waters of the Mediterranean Sea as far afield as northern Africa for sponges.

The ancient Greeks laid down the first rules on the legal rights of divers in relation to salvaged goods. The diver's share of the cargo was increased with depth. Many divers would prefer this arrangement to that offered by modern governments and diving companies.

In other parts of the world, industries involving breath-hold diving persist, to some extent, to this time. Notable examples include the Ama, or diving women of Japan and Korea, and the pearl divers of the Tuamoto Archipelago.

The Ama has existed as a group for more than 2000 years. Originally the male divers were fisher-men, and the women collected shells and plants. The shells and seaweed are a prized part of Korean and Japanese cuisine. In more recent times, diving has been restricted to the women, with the men serving as tenders. Some attribute the change in pattern to better endurance of the women in cold water. Others pay homage to the folklore that diving reduces the virility of men, a point many divers seem keen to disprove.

There is a long history of the use of divers for strategic purposes. Divers were involved in operations during the Trojan Wars from 1194 to 1184 BC. They sabotaged enemy ships by boring holes in the hull or cutting the anchor ropes. Divers were also used to construct underwater defences designed to protect ports from the attacking fleets. The attackers in their turn used divers to remove the obstructions.

By Roman times, precautions were being taken against divers. Anchor cables were made of iron chain to make them difficult to cut, and special guards with diving experience were used to protect the fleet against underwater attackers.

An interesting early report indicated that some Roman divers were also involved in Mark Anthony's attempt to capture the heart of Cleopatra. Mark Antony participated in a fishing contest held in Cleopatra's presence and attempted to improve his standing by having his divers ensure a constant supply of fish on his line. The Queen showed her displeasure by having one of her divers fasten a salted fish to his hook.

Marco Polo and other travellers to India and Sri Lanka observed pearl diving on the Coromandel Coast. They reported that the most diving was to depths of 10 to 15 metres, but that the divers could reach 27 metres by using a weight on a rope to assist descent. They carried a net to put the oysters in and, when they wished to surface, were assisted by an attendant who hauled on a rope attached to the net. The divers were noted to hold their nose during descent.

The most skilled of the American native divers came from Margarita Island. Travellers who observed them during the sixteenth, seventeenth and eighteenth centuries reported that these divers could descend to 30 metres and remain submerged for 15 minutes. They could dive from sunrise to sunset, 7 days a week and attributed their endurance to tobacco! They also claimed to possess a secret chemical that they rubbed over their bodies to repel sharks. The Spaniards exploited these native divers for pearling, salvage and smuggling goods past customs. The demand for divers was indicated by their value on the slave market, fetching prices up to 150 gold pieces.

Free diving appears to have evolved as a modern sport in the mid-1940s, initially as a competition among Italian spearfishers. Currently the sport, which is steadily gaining popularity, encompasses a variety of disciplines. These include the following:

In 'no limits', a diver can use any means to travel down and up the line, as long as the line is used to measure the distance. Most divers descend down a line using a weighted sled and return to the surface aided by an inflatable balloon. Officially recorded depths in excess of 210 metres have been achieved using this method.

'Constant weight apnoea' diving is where descent and ascent occur along a line, although the diver is not permitted to pull on this line to assist movement. No weights can be removed during the dive. Monofins or bi-fins can be used.

'Constant weight without fins' is the same as constant weight apnoea but without the use of fins.

With 'variable weights', the diver again descends with the aid of a weighted sled, but this weight is limited. Ascent is achieved by finning or pulling up the cable, or both.

'Free immersion', which emerged in places where equipment was difficult to obtain, involves a finless diver (with optional suit, mask or weights) who pulls himself or herself down and then up a weighted line.

'Static apnoea' involves resting breath-holding (usually lying in a pool) with the face submerged. Officially recorded times in excess of 11 minutes have been achieved using this method.

'Dynamic apnoea' measures the distance covered in a pool during a single breath-hold.

EARLY EQUIPMENT

The history of diving with equipment is long and complex, and in the early stages it is mixed with legend. The exploits of Jonah are described with conviction in one text, but there is a shortage of supporting evidence. Further reference is made to him later, on the technicality that he was more a submariner than a diver. Because his descent was involuntary, Jonah was at best a reluctant pioneer diver. The history of submarine escape, when the submariner may become a diver, is discussed in Chapter 64.

Some claim that Alexander the Great descended in a diving bell during the third century BC. Details of the event are vague, and some of the fish stories attributed to him were spectacular. One fish was said to have taken 3 days to swim past him! It is most unlikely that the artisans of the time could make glass as depicted in most of the illustrations of the 'event'. This may have been a product of artistic licence or evidence that the incident is based more in fable than in fact.

Snorkels, breathing tubes made from reeds and bamboo (now plastic, rubber or silicone), were developed in many parts of the world. They allow a diver to breathe with the head underwater. Aristotle inferred that the Greeks used them. Columbus reported that the North American Indians would swim toward wild fowl while breathing through a reed and keeping their bodies submerged. They were able to capture the birds with nets, spears or even their bare hands. The Australian aborigines used a similar approach to hunt wild duck. Various people have 'invented' long hose snorkels. The one designed by Vegetius, dated 1511, blocked the diver's vision and imposed impossible loads on the breathing muscles.

Some have interpreted an Assyrian drawing dated 900 BC as an early diving set. The drawing shows a man with a tube in his mouth. The tube is connected to some sort of bladder or bag. It is more likely a float or life jacket. The tube length was a metre or more and so impossible to breathe through.

Leonardo da Vinci sketched diving sets and fins. One set was really a snorkel that had the disadvantage of a large dead space. Another of his ideas was for the diver to have a 'wine skin to contain the breath'. This was probably the first recorded design of a self-contained breathing apparatus. His drawings appear tentative, so it is probably safe to assume that there was no practical diving equipment in Europe at that time.

Another Italian, Borelli, in 1680, realized that Leonardo was in error and that the diver's air would have to be purified before he breathed it again. Borelli suggested that the air could be purified and breathed again by passing it through a copper tube cooled by sea water. With this concept, he had the basic idea of a rebreathing set. It could also be claimed that he had the basis of the experimental cryogenic diving set in which gas is carried in liquid form and purified by freezing out carbon dioxide.

Diving bells were the first successful method of increasing endurance underwater, apart from snorkels. These consist of a weighted chamber, open at the bottom, in which one or more people could be lowered under water. The early use of bells was limited to short periods in shallow water. Later, a method of supplying fresh air was developed. The first fully documented use of diving bells dates from the sixteenth century.

In 1691, Edmond Halley, the English astronomer who predicted the orbit of the comet that bears his name, patented a diving bell that was supplied with air in barrels (Figure 1.1). With this development diving bells became more widespread. They were used for salvage, treasure recovery and general construction work. Halley's bell was supplied with air from weighted barrels, which were hauled from the surface. Dives to 20 metres for up to 1 1/2 hours were recorded. Halley also devised a method of supplying air to a diver from a hose connected to the bell. The length of hose restricted the diver to the area close to the bell. It is not known whether this was successful. Halley was one of the earliest recorded sufferers of middle ear barotrauma.

Swedish divers had devised a small bell, occupied by one person and with no air supply to it. Between 1659 and 1665, 50 bronze cannons, each weighing more than 1000 kg, were salvaged from the *Vasa*. This Swedish warship had sunk in 30 metres of water in Stockholm harbour.

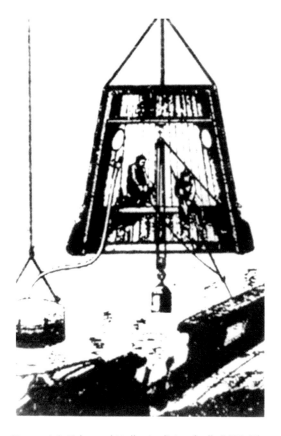

Figure 1.1 Edmond Halley's diving bell, 1691. The weighted barrels of air that were used to replenish the air can be clearly seen.

The guns were recovered by divers working from a bell, assisted by ropes from the surface. This task would not be easy for divers, even with the best of modern equipment.

MODERN DIVING EQUIPMENT

The first people to be exposed to a pressure change in a vessel on the surface were patients exposed to higher or lower pressure as a therapy for various conditions – the start of hyperbaric medicine. The origins of diving medical research can also be traced to these experiments.

During the second half of the nineteenth century, reliable air pumps were developed. These were able to supply air against the pressures experienced by divers. Several people had the idea of using these pumps for diving and developed what are now called open helmets, which cover the head and shoulders. Air was pumped down to the diver, and the excess air escaped from the bottom of the helmet. The diver could breathe because the head and neck were in air, or at least they were until the diver bent over or fell. If this happened, or if the hose or pump leaked, the helmet flooded and the diver was likely to drown. The Deane brothers were the inventors and among the major users of this equipment, and John Deane continued to use it up to the time of the Crimean War.

Standard rig, or **standard diving dress,** was first produced in 1840 by Augustus Siebe (a Russian immigrant engineer who later became a naturalized British citizen). This equipment consisted of a rigid helmet sealed to a flexible waterproof suit (Figure 1.2). Air was pumped down from the surface into the helmet, and excess air bled off through an outlet valve. The diver could control buoyancy by adjusting the flow through the outlet valve and thus the volume of air in the suit. This type of equipment, with a few refinements, is still in use.

Siebe's firm came to be the major manufacturer, but his role in the design may have been overstated, possibly for the marketing advantages gained by his firm, which marketed the first acceptable equipment of this type. The origins and evolution from open helmet and standard dress were the subject of a study by Bevan, who discussed several designs that were developed at

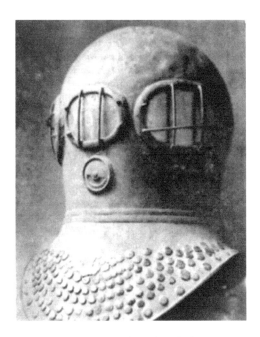

Figure 1.2 Augustus Siebe's first helmet.

the same time, with borrowing and stealing of ideas from each other.

By the mid-nineteenth century, several types of diving suits and a bell were used by the Royal Engineers on dives on the wreck of the *Royal George,* which obstructed the anchorage at Spithead. The Siebe suit was found to be greatly superior to the other designs. Siebe's apparatus allowed the diver to bend over or even lie down without the risk of flooding the helmet. Also, the diver could control his depth easily. A diver in an open helmet had to climb a ladder or rely on his tenders to do this.

In more modern versions, the helmet is fitted with communications to allow the diver to confer with another diver or the surface. One of the developments from the Siebe closed helmet was the US Navy Mark 5 helmet. It probably set a record by being in service for 75 years.

The Royal Engineers were taught to dive by civilian divers in 1939–40 while on the *Royal George.* They then established a training facility at Gillingham in 1844 where they reintroduced diving to the Royal Navy, which set up their first diving school on HMS *Excellent* later that year.

Decompression sickness was noted, albeit not recognized in divers, following the development of these diving suits. Divers were given fresh dry undergarments because the 'rheumatic' pains they suffered were attributed to damp and cold. Other divers suffered paralysis that was attributed to fatigue from zeal and overexertion. Most of these men would have been suffering from decompression sickness because they were diving for up to three times the accepted limits for dives without decompression stops.

Decompression sickness was also observed in workers employed in pressurized caissons and tunnels. In these operations, the working area is pressurized to keep the water out. The history of decompression sickness is discussed in Chapter 10.

Paul Bert and J. S. Haldane are the fathers of diving medicine. Paul Bert published a text book *La pression barométrique* based on his studies of the physiological effect of changes in pressure. His book is still used as a reference text even though it was first published in 1878. Bert showed that decompression sickness was caused by the formation of gas bubbles in the body and suggested that it could be prevented by gradual ascent. He also showed that pain could be relieved by a return to higher pressures. Such cases were initially managed by the diver's returning to the pressure of the caisson. However, specially designed recompression chambers were introduced and utilized at some job sites within a few years.

J.S. Haldane, a Scottish scientist, was appointed to a Royal Navy committee to investigate the problem of decompression sickness in divers. At that time the Royal Navy had a diving depth limit of 30 metres, but deeper dives had been recorded. Greek and Swedish divers had reached 58 metres in 1904, and Alexander Lambert had recovered gold bullion from a wreck in 50 metres of water in 1885, but he had developed partial paralysis from decompression sickness.

Haldane concluded from Paul Bert's results that a diver could be hauled safely to the surface from 10 metres with no evidence of decompression sickness. He deduced from this that a diver could be surfaced from greater than 10 metres in stages, provided that time was spent at each stage to allow absorbed nitrogen to pass out of the body in a controlled manner. This theory was tested on goats and then on men in chambers. Haldane's work culminated in an open water dive to 64 metres in 1906 and the publication of the first acceptable set of decompression tables.

Haldane also developed several improvements to the diving equipment used.

In 1914, US Navy divers reached 84 metres. The next year they raised a submarine near Hawaii from a depth of 93 metres. This was a remarkable feat considering that the salvage techniques had to be evolved by trial and error. The divers used air, so they were exposed to a dangerous degree of nitrogen narcosis, as well as decompression sickness.

SELF-CONTAINED EQUIPMENT

Self-contained underwater breathing apparatus (scuba) is used to describe any diving set that allows the diver to carry the breathing gas supply with him or her. There are several claims to its invention, based on old drawings. The first workable form probably dates from the early nineteenth century. There is a brief report of an American engineer, Charles Condert, who made a scuba in which the compressed air was stored in a copper pipe worn around his body. The gas was released into a hood that covered the upper half of his body. Accumulation of carbon dioxide was controlled by allowing the respired gas to escape through a small hole. It was then replaced by fresh gas from the storage pipe. Condert died while diving with his equipment in the East River in New York in 1831.

In 1838, Dr Manuel Guillaumet filed a patent in France for a back-mounted, twin-hose demand regulator that was supplied with air from hoses to the surface. A patent for a similar device was also filed in England earlier that year by William Newton, but it seems likely that this was done on behalf of Guillaumet.

Another early development was the Rouquayrol and Denayrouze device of 1865 (Figure 1.3). This set was supplied with air from the surface that was breathed on demand via a mouthpiece. It was fitted with a compressed air reservoir so that the diver could detach himself or herself from the air hose for a few minutes. The endurance, as a scuba, was limited by the amount of air in the reservoir.

The first successful scuba with an air supply appears to have been developed and patented in 1918 by Ohgushi, who was Japanese. His system could be operated with a supply of air from the surface or as a scuba with an air supply cylinder carried on the back. The diver controlled the air

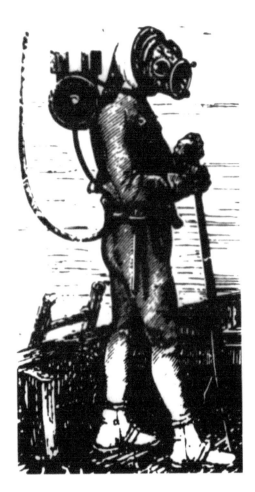

Figure 1.3 The aerophore, devised by Rouquayrol and Denayrouze, 1865. This device was widely used and was an important milestone in the development of the modern scuba.

supply by triggering air flow into the mask with the diver's teeth. Another scuba was devised by Le Prieur in 1933. In this set, the diver carried a compressed air bottle on the chest and released air into the face mask by opening a tap.

In 1943, Cousteau and Gagnan developed the first popular scuba as we know it today. It was an adaptation of a reducing valve that Gagnan had evaluated for use in gas-powered cars and was far smaller than the Rouquayrol-Denayrouze device.

Closed-circuit oxygen sets were developed during the same period as the modern scuba. In these rebreathing sets, the diver is supplied with oxygen and the carbon dioxide is removed by absorbent.

These sets are often called scuba, but they may be considered separately because of the difference in principles involved. The patent for the first known prototype of an oxygen rebreather was given to Pierre Sicard, who was French, in 1849. The first known successful rebreathing set was designed by English engineer H. A. Fleuss in 1878. This was an oxygen set in which carbon dioxide was absorbed by rope soaked in caustic potash.

Because of the absence of lines and hoses from the diver to the surface, the set was used in flooded mines and tunnels where the extra mobility, compared with the standard rig, was needed. Great risks were taken with this set and its successors when used underwater because the work of Paul Bert on oxygen toxicity was not widely known. This equipment was the precursor of oxygen sets used in clandestine operations in both world wars and of other sets used in submarine escape, firefighting and mine rescue.

MODERN MILITARY DIVING

The military use of divers in warfare was, until 1918, largely restricted to the salvage of damaged ships, clearing of channels blocked by wrecks, and assorted ships' husbandry duties. One significant clandestine operation conducted during the First World War was the recovery of code books and minefield charts from a sunken German submarine. This was of more significance as an intelligence operation, although the diving activity was also kept secret.

During the First World War, Italy developed a human torpedo or chariot that was used in 1918 to attack an Austrian battleship in Pola Harbour in what is now Croatia. The attack was a success in that the ship was sunk, but, unfortunately, it coincided with the fall of the Austro-Hungarian Empire, and the ship was already in friendly hands! The potential of this method of attack was noted by the Italian Navy. They put it to use in the Second World War with divers wearing oxygen rebreathing sets as underwater pilots. In passing, it is interesting to note that the idea of the chariot was suggested to the British Admiralty in 1909, and Davis took out patents on a small submarine and human torpedo controlled by divers in 1914. This was pre-dated by a one-person submarine designed by J.P. Holland in 1875.

Diving played a greater part in offensive operations during the Second World War. Exploits of note include those of the Italian Navy. They used divers riding modified torpedoes to attack ships in Gibraltar and Alexandria. After a series of unsuccessful attempts with loss of life, they succeeded in sinking several ships in Gibraltar harbour in mid-1941. Later that year, three teams managed to enter Alexandria harbour and damage two battleships and a tanker. Even Sir Winston Churchill, who did not often praise his enemies, said they showed 'extraordinary courage and ingenuity'. Churchill had previously been responsible for rejecting suggestions that the Royal Navy use similar weapons.

In Gibraltar, a special type of underwater war evolved. The Italians had a secret base in neutral Spain, only 10 kilometres away, and launched several attacks that were opposed by British divers who tried to remove the Italian mines before they exploded.

Divers from the allied nations made several successful attacks on enemy ships, but their most important offensive roles were in the field of reconnaissance and beach clearance. In most operations, the divers worked from submarines or small boats. They first surveyed the approaches to several potential landing sites. After a choice had been made, they cleared the obstructions that could impede the landing craft. One of the more famous exploits of an American diving group was to land unofficially and leave a 'Welcome' sign on the beach to greet the US Marines, spearheading the invasion of Guam. The British Clearance Divers and the US Navy Sea, Air, Land Teams (SEALs) evolved from these groups. The Clearance Divers get their name from their work in clearing mines and other obstructions, a role they repeated during and after the Gulf War.

The research back-up to these exploits was largely devoted to improvement of equipment and the investigation of the nature and onset of oxygen toxicity (Chapter 17). This work was important because most of these offensive operations were conducted by divers wearing oxygen breathing apparatus. The subjects were the unsung heroes of the work. This group of scientists, sailors and conscientious objectors deliberately and repeatedly suffered oxygen toxicity in attempts to understand the condition.

Oxygen-nitrogen mixtures were first used for diving by the Royal Navy in conjunction with a standard diving rig. This approach was based on an idea proposed by Sir Leonard Hill and developed by Siebe Gorman and Co. Ltd. The advantage of this equipment is that, by increasing the ratio of oxygen to nitrogen in the breathing gas, one can reduce or eliminate decompression requirements. It is normally used with equipment in which most of the gas is breathed again after the carbon dioxide has been removed. This allows reduction of the total gas volume required by the diver.

During the Second World War, this idea was adapted to a self-contained semi-closed rebreathing apparatus that was first used extensively by divers clearing mines. This development was conducted by the British Admiralty Experimental Diving Unit in conjunction with Siebe Gorman and Co. Ltd. The change to a self-contained set was needed to reduce the number of people at risk from accidental explosions in mine-clearing operations. The reduction, or elimination, of decompression time was desirable in increasing the diver's chances of survival if something went wrong. The equipment was constructed from non-magnetic materials to reduce the likelihood of activating magnetic mines and was silent during operation for work on acoustically triggered mines.

DEEP DIVING

The search for means to allow humans to descend deeper has been a continuing process. By the early twentieth century, deep diving research had enabled divers to reach depths in excess of 90 metres; at which depth the narcosis induced by nitrogen incapacitated most humans.

After the First World War, the Royal Navy diving research tried to extend its depth capability beyond 60 metres. Equipment was improved, the submersible decompression chamber was introduced and new decompression schedules were developed that used periods of oxygen breathing to reduce decompression time. Dives were made to 107 metres, but nitrogen narcosis at these depths made such dives both unrewarding and dangerous.

Helium diving resulted from a series of American developments. In 1919, a scientist, Professor Elihu Thompson, suggested that nitrogen narcosis could be avoided by replacing the nitrogen in the diver's gas supply with helium. At that stage, the idea was not practical because helium cost more than US $2000 per cubic foot. Later, following the exploitation of natural gas supplies that contained helium, the price dropped to about 3 cents per cubic foot.

Research into the use of helium was conducted during the 1920s and 1930s. By the end of the 1930s, divers in a compression chamber had reached a pressure equal to a depth of 150 metres, and a dive to 128 metres was made in Lake Michigan. Between the two world wars, the United States had a virtual monopoly on the supply of helium and thus dominated research into deep diving.

For **hydrogen diving,** the use of hydrogen in gas mixtures for deep diving was first tried by Arne Zetterstrom, a Swedish engineer. He demonstrated that hypoxia and risks of explosion could be avoided if the diver used air from the surface to 30 metres, changed to 4 per cent oxygen in nitrogen and then changed to 4 per cent or less oxygen in hydrogen. In this manner, the diver received adequate oxygen, and the formation of an explosive mixture of oxygen and hydrogen was prevented.

In 1945, Zetterstrom dived to 160 metres in open water. Unfortunately, an error was made by the operators controlling his ascent, and they hauled him up too fast, omitting his planned gas transition and decompression stops. He died of hypoxia and decompression sickness shortly after reaching the surface.

Hydrogen has been used successfully both for decreasing the density of the breathing gas mixture and ameliorating the signs and symptoms of high-pressure neurological syndrome. The cheapness of hydrogen compared with helium, and the probability of a helium shortage in the future, may mean that hydrogen will be more widely used in deep dives.

Other European workers followed Zetterstrom with radical approaches to deep diving. The Swiss worker Keller performed an incredible 305-metre dive in the open sea in December 1962 (Figure 1.4). He was assisted by Bühlmann, who developed and tested several sets of decompression tables and whose decompression algorithm has been adapted and used in many of the early and current generations of diving computers.

Modern gas mixture sets have evolved as the result of several forces. The price of helium has become a significant cost. This, combined with a desire to increase the diver's mobility, has

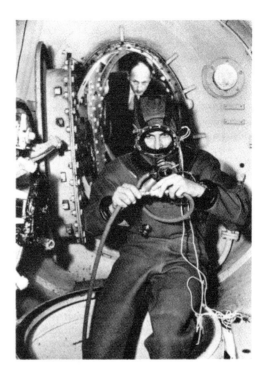

Figure 1.4 Prof Bühlmann (rear) and Hannes Keller prepare for the first simulated dive to 3000 m (1000 ft) on 25 April 1961.

encouraged the development of more sophisticated mixed gas sets. The most complex of these have separate cylinders of oxygen and diluting gas. The composition of the diver's inspired gas is maintained by the action of electronic control systems that regulate the release of gas from each cylinder. The first of these sets was developed in the 1950s, but they have been continually refined and improved.

Modern air or gas mixture helmets have several advantages compared with the older equipment. A demand system reduces the amount of gas used, compared with the standard rig. The gas-tight sealing system reduces the chance of a diver's drowning by preventing water inhalation. The primary gas supply normally comes to the diver from the surface or a diving bell and may be combined with heating and communications. A second gas supply is available from a cylinder on the diver's back. Americans Bob Kirby and Bev Morgan led the way with a series of helmet systems. A model, used for both compressed air and

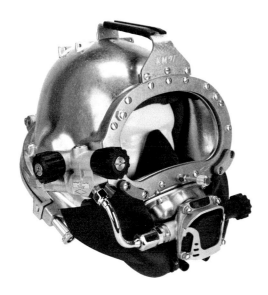

Figure 1.5 A Kirby-Morgan 97 helmet.

gas mixtures, is shown in Figure 1.5. These helmets have been used to depths of around 400 metres.

Saturation diving is probably the most important development in commercial diving since the Second World War. Behnke, an American diving researcher, suggested that caisson workers could be kept under pressure for long periods and decompressed slowly at the end of their job, rather than undertake a series of compressions and risk decompression sickness after each.

A US Navy Medical Officer, George Bond, among others, adopted this idea for diving. The first of these dives involved tests on animals and men in chambers. In 1962, Robert Stenuit spent 24 hours at 60 metres in the Mediterranean Sea off the coast of France.

Despite the credit given to Behnke and Bond, it could be noted that the first people to spend long periods in an elevated pressure environment were patients treated in a hyperbaric chamber. Between 1921 and 1934 an American, Dr Orval Cunningham, pressurized people to 3 ATA for up to 5 days and decompressed them in 2 days.

Progress in saturation diving was rapid, with the French-inspired Conshelf experiments and the American Sealab experiments seeking greater depths and durations of exposure. In 1965, the former astronaut Scott Carpenter spent a month at 60 metres, and two divers spent 2 days at a depth equivalent to almost 200 metres. Unfortunately, people paid for this progress. Lives were lost, and there has been a significant incidence of bone necrosis induced by these experiments.

In saturation diving systems, the divers live either in an underwater habitat or in a chamber on the surface. In the second case, another chamber is used to transfer the divers under pressure to and from their work sites. Operations can also be conducted from small submarines or submersibles with the divers operating from a compartment that can be opened to the sea. They can either transfer to a separate chamber on the submarine's surface support vessel or remain in the submarine for their period of decompression. The use of this equipment offers several advantages. The submarine speeds the diver's movement around the work site, provides better lighting and carries extra equipment. Additionally, a technical expert who is not a diver can observe and control the operation from within the submarine.

Operations involving saturation dives have become routine for work in deep water. The stimulus for this work is partly military and partly commercial. Divers work on the rigs and pipelines needed to exploit oil and natural gas fields. The needs of the oil companies have resulted in strenuous efforts to extend the depth and efficiency of the associated diving activities.

Atmospheric diving suits (ADSs) are small, one-person, articulated submersibles resembling a suit of armour (Figure 1.6). These suits are fitted with pressure joints to enable articulation, and they maintain an internal pressure of 1 ATA, so avoiding the hazards of increased and changing pressures. In effect, the diver becomes a small submarine.

The mobility and dexterity of divers wearing early armoured suits were limited, and these suits were not widely used. The well-known British 'JIM' suit, first used in 1972, enabled divers to spend long periods at substantial depths. However, these were never fitted with propulsion units and were replaced by the Canadian 'Newtsuit' and the WASP, which have propellers to aid movement and can be fitted with claws for manipulating equipment.

In 1997, the ADS 2000 was developed in conjunction with the US Navy. This evolution of the Newtsuit was designed to meet the Navy's needs.

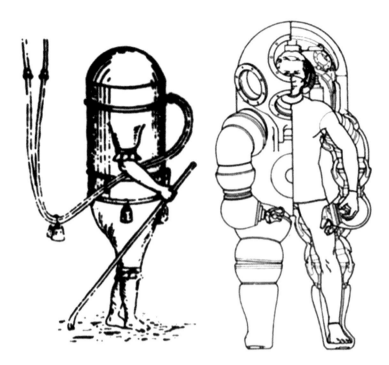

Figure 1.6 Armoured diving suits, past and present (JIM).

It was designed to enable a diver to descend to 610 metres (2000 ft) and had an integrated dual-thruster system to allow the pilot to navigate easily underwater. The ADS 2000 became fully operational and certified by the US Navy in 2006 when it was used successfully on a dive to 610 metres.

Liquid breathing trials, in which the lungs are flooded with a perfluorocarbon emulsion and the body is supplied with oxygen in solution, have been reported to have been conducted in laboratories. The potential advantages of breathing liquids are the elimination of decompression sickness as a problem, freedom to descend to virtually any depth and the possibility of the diver's extracting the oxygen dissolved in the water.

RECREATIONAL DIVING

Amateur diving started with breath-hold diving, mainly by enthusiasts in Italy and the south coast of France who were keen spearfishers. This was also the area where compressed air scuba diving developed as a result of the work of Hass, Cousteau and others. As a sport, diving rapidly spread to Britain and the United States and the rest of the world.

From this beginning, diving has become a recreational activity that is often combined with tourism and photography. Others explore caves and wrecks and seek the excitement that deeper and further penetrations provide. Special interest groups such as cave and technical divers have developed and in some areas are the modern pathfinders. These groups and their problems are discussed in greater detail in later chapters.

FURTHER READING

Bert P. *Barometric Pressure* (1878). Translated by Hitchcock MA, Hitchcock FA. Columbus, Ohio: College Book Co.; 1943.

Bevan J. *The Infernal Diver*. London: Submex; 1996.

Bevan J. *Another Whitstable Trade*. London: Submex; 2009.

Davis RH. *Deep Diving and Submarine Operations*. 6th ed. London: Siebe, Gorman & Co. Ltd.; 1955.

Dugan J. *Man Explores the Sea*. London: Hamish Hamilton; 1956.

Dugan J. *World Beneath the Sea*. Washington, DC: National Geographic Society; 1967.

Marx RF. *Into the Deep*. New York: Van Nostrand Reinhold; 1978.

Ohrelius B. *Vasa, the King's Ship*. Translated by Michael M. London: Cassell; 1962.

Rahn H. *Breathhold Diving and the Ama of Japan*. Pub. 1341, National Academy of Sciences. Washington, DC: National Academy Press; 1965.

Shelford WO. Ohgushi's Peerless Respirator. *Skin Diver* 1972;(Nov):32–34.

US Navy Diving Manual Revision 6 SS521-AG-PRO-010 (2008). Washington, DC: Naval Sea Systems Command; 2008.

This chapter was reviewed for this fifth edition by John Lippmann.

2

Physics and physiology

INTRODUCTION

A basic knowledge of the physics and physiology of diving is essential to understand most of the medical problems encountered. Aspects of physics and physiology that have a wide application to diving are discussed in this chapter.

Some of the basic physiological implications are also mentioned, but most aspects of diving physiology and pathophysiology are relegated to the relevant chapters on specific diving disorders.

PRESSURE, GASES AND DIVING

On the surface of the Earth, we are exposed to the pressure exerted by the atmosphere. This is called the atmospheric or barometric pressure. Most people regard this pressure as caused by the mass of the atmosphere pressing down on them. A flaw in this argument is that the pressure remains in a bottle after it is sealed, although its contents are contained and are no longer exposed to the column of air above. The physically correct explanation is that atmospheric pressure is generated by collisions of the molecules of gas in accordance with the kinetic theory of gases. Either explanation is acceptable for the following discussion.

The pressure decreases as we move upward through the atmosphere and increases as we move down into a mine or into the sea. At the top of Mount Everest the atmospheric pressure is about 40 per cent of that at sea level. Because water is much heavier than air, the pressure changes experienced by divers over a particular depth change are much greater than those encountered by climbers or aviators as they change altitude.

Pressure is measured in a variety of units from either of two reference points. It can be expressed with respect to a vacuum, i.e. zero pressure. This reading is called an **absolute pressure.** The second method measures pressures above or below local pressure. These readings are called **gauge pressures.** At sea level, the absolute pressure is 1 atmosphere (1 ATA) and the gauge pressure is 0. These units are commonly abbreviated to ATA and ATG.

Common examples are the barometric pressure used by weather forecasters, which is an absolute pressure, and the blood pressure, which is a gauge pressure reading.

With descent in water, pressure increases. For each 10 metres of depth in sea water, the pressure increases by 1 atmosphere, starting from 1 ATA or 0 ATG at the surface. The gauge pressure remains 1 atmosphere less than the absolute pressure. For example, at 10 metres, the pressure is 2 ATA and 1 ATG. At 90 metres, the pressure is 10 ATA and 9 ATG.

Table 2.1 Pressure conversion factors (commonly used approximations shown in brackets)

1 atmosphere = 10.08 (10) metres sea water
= 33.07 (33) feet sea water
= 33.90 (34) feet fresh water
= 101.3 kilopascals (kPa)
= 0.1013 megapascals (MPa)
= 1.033 kg/cm^2
= 14.696 (14.7) lbs/in^2
= 1.013 bars
= 760 millimetres mercury (mm Hg)
= 760 torr
= 1 ATA

Note: Actual conversions from sea water depth to ATA depend on salinity and temperature. A complete conversion matrix is provided in Table 2.2.

Pressure units

Because diving involves facets of engineering and science, it is plagued with many units of pressure. These include absolute and gauge atmospheres, pascals and multiples such as the kilopascal, metres or feet of sea water, bars, pounds per square inch, torr and several other rarer units. Table 2.1 lists conversions for the more commonly used units.

Pressure and the diver's body

Many people have difficulty in understanding why the pressure of the water does not crush the diver. The answer to this problem may be considered in two parts:

The solid and liquid parts of the body are virtually incompressible, so a pressure applied to them does not cause any change in volume and is transmitted through them. After immersion, the increased pressure pushes on the skin, which in turn pushes on the tissues underneath, and so the pressure is transferred through the body until the skin on the other side is pushed back against the water pressure. Therefore, the system remains in balance. This is in accordance with **Pascal's Principle,** which states: *'A pressure exerted anywhere in a confined incompressible fluid is transmitted equally in all directions throughout the fluid such that the pressure ratio remains the same'.*

Table 2.2 Pressure conversions

	atm	n/m^2 or Pa	bars	mb	kg/cm^2	gm/cm^2 (cm H$_2$O)	mm Hg	lb/in^2 (psi)
1 atmosphere	1	1.013 x 10^5	1.013	1013	1.033	1033	760	14.70
1 Newton (N)/m^2 or Pascal (Pa)	0.9869 x 10^{-5}	1	10^{-5}	0.01	1.02 x 10^{-5}	0.0102	0.0075	0.1451 x 10^{-3}
1 bar	0.987	10^5	1	1000	1.02	1020	750.2	14.51
1 millibar (mb)	0.9869 x 10^{-3}	100	0.001	1	0.00102	1.02	0.7502	0.01451
1 kg/cm^2	0.9681	0.9806 x 10^5	0.9806	980.6	1	1000	736	14.22
1 gm/cm^2 (1 cm H$_2$O)	968.1	98.06	0.9806 x 10^{-3}	0.9806	0.001	1	0.736	0.01422
1 mmHg	0.001316	133.3	0.001333	1.333	0.00136	1.36	1	0.01934
1 lb/in^2 (psi)	0.06804	6895	0.06895	68.95	0.0703	70.3	51.70	1

However, the effect of pressure on the gas spaces in the diver's body is more complex. The applied pressure does not cause any problems if the pressure in the gas space is close to that of the surrounding water. There is, for example, no physical damage to a diver's lungs if the air space was exposed to an internal pressure of 100 metres of water, provided that this pressure is balanced by the pressure exerted by surrounding water acting on the walls of the lung to balance any tendency of the lungs to expand. If the lungs were exposed to an internal pressure sufficiently more than the surrounding atmospheric tissue, they would overexpand and burst.

Water pressure and lung inflation

Immersion up to the neck in water reduces vital capacity by about 10 per cent (Figure 2.1 shows lung volumes). This is caused in part by the hydrostatic pressure of the water compressing the thorax. With immersion, there is also a loss of gravitational effects. This reduces the volume of blood in lower, mainly leg, veins and increases thoracic blood volume. This change in turn reduces the compliance of the lungs.

When a diver is using breathing equipment, pressure at the point from which the gas is inhaled can be different from the pressure at the chest. If upright in the water, a scuba diver is inhaling air released at the pressure at the level of the mouth. A snorkel diver is inhaling air from the surface, and this is at surface pressure. In both these cases, the air is at a lower pressure than the diver's lungs. This reduces the amount of air the diver can inhale because part of the inhalation force is used in overcoming this pressure difference.

Conversely, when descending, face-down, a diver whose air is released at mouth pressure can inhale to greater than normal vital capacity but could not exhale to the normal residual volume. This is because in this orientation, the water pressure is helping to inflate the lungs.

Pressure and volume changes

When a diver descends, the increased pressure of the surrounding water compresses gas in the gas spaces within the diver's body. These spaces include the lungs, middle ears, sinuses and intestines.

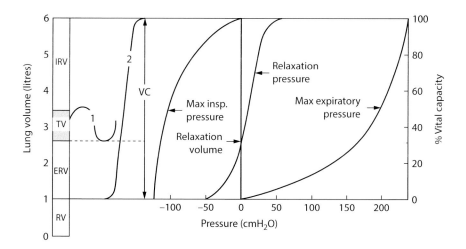

Figure 2.1 Lung volumes and intrapulmonary pressure. The various components of lung volumes are labelled on the left. On the right, the relationships among lung volume, airway pressure and the maximum effort that can be made for inhalation and exhalation of air are plotted. Curve 1 is the volume change during quiet breathing, and curve 2 is the volume change during a maximum inhalation starting at the residual volume. ERV, expiratory reserve volume; insp., inspiratory; IRV, inspiratory reserve volume; RV, residual volume; TV, tidal volume; VC, vital capacity. (Redrawn from Lamphier EH, Camporesi EM. Respiration and exertion. In: Bennett PB, Elliott DH. The phyisology & medicine of diving, 4th edn. London:WB Saunders Co Ltd; 1993, with permission).

This is one of the many aspects of diving medicine that is concerned with the relationship between pressure change and change of gas volume. The relationship between changes in volume of a gas and the pressure applied to it is described by **Boyle's Law.** This states: *'if the temperature remains constant, the volume of a given mass of gas is inversely proportional to the absolute pressure'.* This means that the absolute pressure multiplied by volume has a constant value, and this constant changes with the mass of gas considered. To a mathematician, this means that $P \times V = K$ or $P_1 \times V_1 = P_2 \times V_2$, where P and V are pressure and volume. For example, 10 litres of gas at sea level pressure (1 ATA) will be compressed to:

5 litres at 2 ATA (10 metres).
2 litres at 5 ATA (40 metres).
1 litre at 10 ATA (90 metres).

During ascent into the atmosphere, the reverse happens and the gas expands. This means that the 10 litres of air would expand to 20 litres at 0.5 ATA (an altitude of about 5000 metres or 18 000 feet) and to 40 litres at 0.25 ATA (an altitude of about 10 300 metres or 33 400 feet).

> Gas volumes expand when pressure decreases and contract when pressure increases.

The volume of a mass of gas in a flexible container decreases with pressure or depth increase and expands during ascent or pressure reduction (Figure 2.2). It should be noted that volume changes are greatest near the surface. Conversely, gas has to be added if the volume of a container or gas space is to remain constant as the pressure is increased. The effects of this law are important in many aspects of diving medicine.

During descent, the increasing pressure in the water is transmitted through the body fluids to the tissue surrounding the gas spaces and to the gas spaces themselves. The pressure in any gas space in the body should increase to equal the surrounding pressure. In the lungs, during descent on breath-hold dives, this is accompanied by a decrease in lung volume. Air should enter cavities with rigid walls,

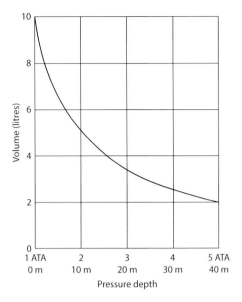

Figure 2.2 Effect of Boyle's Law: While breathing underwater, the diver's respiratory volume is about the same as it would be if he or she worked at the same rate on the surface. Because of the increase in density of this breathing gas under increased pressure, the diver must move a greater mass of gas with each breath. In some situations, this physical effect can limit the diver's capacity to do work.

such as the sinuses or the middle ear. If air entry does not take place to equalize pressures, then a pressure difference between the space and the surrounding tissue will develop, with the pressure in the gas space being less than in the surrounding tissue. The results are tissue distortion and damage, such as congestion, oedema or haemorrhage.

During ascent, as the pressure decreases, gas within body spaces will expand. Unless gas is vented from the space, the expanding gas will exert pressure on the surrounding tissue and will eventually damage it. Pressure changes in the middle ear can also result in rupture of the tympanic membrane.

The same volume changes with pressure occur in bubbles in tissue or blood. Again, the volume changes are greatest close to the surface. An injury caused by pressure change is called barotrauma.

> Barotrauma is the general name for an injury caused by pressure change.

Respiration in water and under pressure

While breathing air underwater, the diver's respiratory volume is about the same as it would be if he or she worked at the same rate on the surface. A consequence of this is that a cylinder that contains enough air for 100 minutes at 1 ATA would last about 50 minutes at 2 ATA (10 metres) or 20 minutes at 5 ATA (40 metres) for dives with the same energy expenditure. This is because the gas in the cylinder expands to a smaller volume when it is released against the ambient pressure at depth than it would if used at the surface. A cylinder that contains 5000 litres of gas if it is released at the sea surface would yield only 1000 litres of gas if it is released at 5 ATA, or 40 metres. A diving physician needs to keep this in mind when estimating the amount of gas needed for any task or therapy.

With depth, gas is compressed and there is an increase in density of the gas because there are more molecules in a given space. So, at depth, a diver must move a greater mass of gas with each breath. This requires greater effort and involves an increase in the work of breathing. In some situations, this can limit the capacity to do work.

The density of the breathing gas can be reduced by replacing nitrogen with a lighter gas such as helium. For example, the density of air at 1 ATA is about 1.3 kg/cubic metre. At 10 ATA, the density of air would be about 13 kg/cubic metre. The use of lighter gas helps to reduce density. For example, at 40 ATA, the density of a 1 per cent oxygen and helium mixture is 6.7 kg/cubic metre.

As the density of a gas increases, there is an increased tendency for the flow to become turbulent. This causes a further increase in the energy used in breathing. These factors can lead to fatigue of the inspiratory muscles and reduce maximum breathing capacity and the work output. To minimize this load, the body responds by using less gas for a given workload. This can result in the development of hypercapnia. Continued exposure to dense gas, as is encountered in deep dives, may cause an adaptive response.

Temperature and volume changes

Charles' Law states: *'If the pressure is constant, the volume of a mass of gas is proportional to the absolute temperature'.*

The absolute temperature (A°) is always 273° more than the centigrade temperature. A more useful expression of the law is as follows:

$$\frac{V_1}{T_1} = \frac{V_2}{T_2} \text{ or } \frac{V}{T} = K$$

Where V_1 is the volume of a mass of gas at temperatures T_1°A and V_2 is its volume after the temperature has changed to T_2°A.

This law has much less relevance to diving medicine than Boyle's Law. However, it should be remembered when considering gas volumes and how they may change.

Boyle's and Charles' Laws may be combined and used if temperature and pressure both change – from P_1 and T_1 to P_2 and T_2 with a volume change from V_1 to V_2. The combined laws can be expressed as the **universal gas equation:**

$$\frac{P_1 \times V_1}{T_1} = \frac{P_2 \times V_2}{T_2}$$

A temperature-pressure problem that often causes discord can be used to illustrate the use of this equation. This is the effect of temperature on the pressure in a gas cylinder.

A diver may ask to have the compressed air cylinder filled to 200 ATA. The gas compressor heats the gas so the cylinder may be charged with gas at 47°C. When the diver gets in the water at 7°C, the diver may find that he or she has only 175 ATA in the cylinder. In this case $V_1 = V_2$ because the cylinder is rigid and the pressure falls as the gas cools.

$$47°C = 320°A, 7°C = 280°A, V_1 = V_2$$

$$\frac{200 \times V_1}{320} = \frac{P_2 \times V_2}{280}$$

$$P_2 = 175 \text{ ATA.}$$

So the reduced pressure is a result of temperature change, not a leaking valve or fraud by the air supplier.

Partial pressures in gas mixtures

Dalton's Law states: *'the total pressure exerted by a mixture of gases is the sum of the pressures that would be exerted by each of the gases if it alone occupied the total volume'.* The pressure of each constituent in a mixture is called the partial pressure (Figure 2.3). In air, which is approximately 80 per cent nitrogen and 20 per cent oxygen, the total pressure at sea level (1 ATA) is the sum of the partial pressures of nitrogen, 0.8 ATA, and oxygen, 0.2 ATA. At 2 ATA (10 metres) these partial pressures will rise to 1.6 and 0.4 ATA, respectively.

The partial pressures of breathing gases can be manipulated to the diver's advantage. For example, the composition of the gas breathed may be modified to reduce the chance of decompression sickness (DCS) by decreasing the percentage of inert gas in the mixture.

Undesirable effects can also occur. Air from an industrial area may contain more than 0.3 per cent carbon dioxide and 0.002 per cent carbon monoxide. If incorporated in compressed breathing gas and delivered at high partial pressures, both constituents could be toxic unless measures were taken to remove these contaminants before use.

It may be necessary to combine Boyle's and Dalton's Laws in calculations. For example, it may be decided that a diver should be given a mixture with a partial pressure of 0.8 ATA oxygen and 1.2 ATA nitrogen in a recompression chamber pressurized to 2 ATA. If oxygen and air are the only gases available, the gas laws can be used to calculate how to prepare a cylinder charged with the right gas mixture.

The mixture will need to be 40 per cent oxygen and 60 per cent nitrogen (Dalton's Law). If the gas is to be prepared in a cylinder charged to 200 ATA, it should contain 120 ATA of nitrogen (60 per cent of 200). If this is to be obtained from compressed air (assumed to be 80 per cent nitrogen in this exercise), it will be necessary to put 150 ATA of compressed air into the cylinder (30 ATA of oxygen and 120 ATA of nitrogen) with 50 ATA of oxygen.

This simple mixing process cannot be used as successfully with helium mixtures. At high pressures, helium does not follow the predictions of Boyle's Law accurately. It is less compressible than the ideal gas described by Boyle's Law. Mixing can be conducted with allowance for this or by putting a calculated weight of each gas in the cylinder.

Solution of gases in liquids

Henry's Law states: *'at a constant temperature, the amount of a gas that will dissolve in a liquid is proportional to the partial pressure of the gas over the liquid'.* This law implies that an equilibrium is established with each gas passing into and out of any solution in contact with it (Figure 2.4). At sea level (1 ATA), an individual's body tissues contain about 1 litre of gaseous nitrogen in solution. If the diver dived to 10 metres and breathed

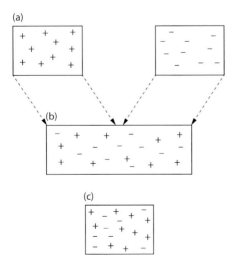

Figure 2.3 Dalton's Law: **(a)** two spaces each at 1 ATA; **(b)** total pressure 1 ATA, 0.5 ATA each component of the mixture; **(c)** total pressure 2 ATA, 1 ATA of each component of the mixture.

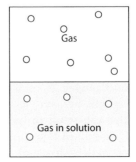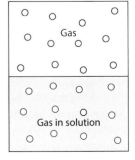

Figure 2.4 Henry's Law.

air at 2 ATA, more gas would dissolve and he or she would eventually reach equilibrium again and have twice as much nitrogen in solution in the body. The time taken for any inert gas to reach a new equilibrium depends on the solubility of the gas in the tissues and the rate of gas supplied to each tissue.

When the total pressure, or the partial pressure of a particular gas, is reduced, gas must pass out of solution. If a rapid total pressure drop occurs, a tissue may contain more gas than it can hold in solution. In this situation, bubbles may form and may cause DCS.

The physiological effects of the solubility of gases are also relevant in nitrogen narcosis and oxygen toxicity.

It should be noted that each gas has a different solubility and the amount of any gas that will dissolve in a liquid depends on the liquid. For example, carbon dioxide is very soluble in water compared with other common gases. Beer aerated with compressed air instead of carbon dioxide would have far fewer bubbles. Nitrogen is more soluble in fats and oils than in aqueous solutions.

Henry's Law is also time dependent. It takes time for gases to enter and leave solution or form bubbles. If this was not so, champagne would go flat as soon as the cork was popped.

At depth, a diver breathing air absorbs nitrogen in accord with Henry's Law. The amount depends on depth and time of exposure. When the diver surfaces, the excess nitrogen must pass from the body. If it is eliminated from solution through the lungs, there will not be any complications. In some cases, the nitrogen comes out of solution in the blood or tissues, thus forming bubbles that may lead to DCS.

Gas movement in body tissues

Gas transfer from the lungs to the tissues is dependent on the cardiovascular circulation, and the gas supplied to a portion of tissue depends on the blood perfusing it. In a permeable substance such as body tissues, gas molecules can migrate by diffusion. That is, gas molecules dissolve in the tissue fluids and tend to move from areas of high to low partial pressure until the partial pressure of the dissolved gas is uniform. This can take hours.

It is the dissolved gas pressures that tend to equilibrate, not the number of gas molecules. If a gas is twice as soluble in one tissue compared with another, then twice as many molecules will be in the first tissue to produce the same partial pressure in the tissue. This information can be estimated from the solubility coefficients of the gas in the components of the tissue.

The rate of gas movement between two points depends on several factors. The difference in partial pressure and the distance between the two points may be combined into a concentration gradient. The other major factor is the permeability of the tissue, an expression of the ease of gas movement. A large partial pressure between two points that are close together (a steep gradient) and a greater permeability both increase the rate of gas transfer.

Metabolic gas exchange

In divers, gas exchange mechanisms are basically the same as at normal pressure. Oxygen diffuses down a concentration gradient from the lungs to the tissues. The carbon dioxide gradient is normally in the opposite direction. The exchange of inert gases becomes important and there are changes in the finer details of metabolic gas exchange.

With increasing depth, there is an increase in the partial pressures of the constituents of the breathing mixture in accordance with Dalton's Law. This causes higher alveolar pressures and arterial pressures of the inhaled gases.

Elevated pressures of oxygen facilitate oxygen transport, but they may interfere with the elimination of carbon dioxide in two ways: first, by the depression of respiration induced by high arterial oxygen tensions; and second, by direct interference with the transport of carbon dioxide. When the inspired oxygen partial pressure is elevated, there is an increase in oxygen transport in solution in the plasma (Henry's Law). When one is inhaling oxygen at a partial pressure above 3 ATA, the total oxygen requirement may be carried in solution. If this happens, the haemoglobin may be still saturated with oxygen in the venous blood, and this can prevent the transport of carbon dioxide in the form of carbaminohaemoglobin.

The result is an increased tissue carbon dioxide level. In some situations, there may also be an increase in the inspired carbon dioxide pressure. Causes include contamination of the breathing gas supply, the external dead space of the equipment, inadequate ventilation or failure of the absorbent system.

There is a tendency for experienced divers to be less sensitive to elevated carbon dioxide partial pressures. This reduces the total ventilation requirement during working dives. Elevated arterial carbon dioxide levels increase susceptibility to oxygen toxicity, DCS and inert gas narcosis. For these reasons, it is desirable to control the factors that cause carbon dioxide retention.

> Diving is associated with a tendency to retain carbon dioxide.

Inert gas exchange

The topic if inert gas exchange is considered in the chapters on DCS. Therefore, to avoid duplication, the topic is not considered in detail here. As indicated earlier, increased total pressure is usually accompanied by an increase in nitrogen (and/or other inert gas) pressure (Dalton's Law). This causes gas transfer to the body tissues. When pressure is reduced at the end of the dive, the transfer is reversed. If there is an excess of gas, then it can come out of solution as bubbles. These bubbles are the cause of DCS. If bubbles do occur, they are also subject to the same physical laws. Their size decreases if the pressure is increased, and gas enters or leaves them depending on the concentration gradients of gases.

BUOYANCY

Archimedes' Principle states: *'any object, wholly or partially immersed in liquid, is buoyed up by a force equal to the weight of liquid displaced'.* A diver is an object immersed in water and is therefore affected by this principle. It determines the effort the diver must make to dive. If a diver weighs less than the weight of water he or she displaces, the diver will tend to float to the surface – i.e. he or she has positive buoyancy, which makes descent difficult. If the diver weighs more than the weight of water he or she displaces, the diver has negative buoyancy, which will assist descent and make ascent more difficult.

A diver can change buoyancy in several ways. If the diver wears a weight belt, he or she increases weight by a significant amount and displaces only a little more water and, as a result, will decrease buoyancy. If the diver displaces more water, he or she will increase buoyancy. This can be achieved by retaining more air in the lungs. It can also be achieved by inflating the diver's buoyancy compensator device (BCD) – a device used to control buoyancy. It has an air space that the diver can inflate or deflate to make him positively, negatively or neutrally buoyant, as needed.

An interesting combination of the effects of Boyle's Law and Archimedes' Principle is shown by the changes in buoyancy experienced by a diver wearing BCD or a compressible suit. If slightly positively buoyant at the surface with air in the BCD, the diver will experience some difficulty in descending. As the diver descends he or she will pass through a zone where he or she is neutrally buoyant and, if the diver descends further, he or she will become negatively buoyant. The increased pressure reduces the volume of gas in the BCD or suit, the volume of fluid displaced and, consequently, the diver's buoyancy.

The weight of a scuba cylinder decreases as gas is consumed from it, and this will lead to an increase in buoyancy. An empty cylinder can weigh 1 to 2 kg less than a full one, depending on the initial pressure and the size and type of the cylinder (e.g. steel, alloy).

Immersion creates a condition resembling the gravity-free state experienced by astronauts. In air, a standing person has a pressure gradient in the circulation where the hydrostatic pressure is greatest at the feet and least at the head. For an immersed diver, the hydrostatic gradients in the circulatory system are almost exactly counterbalanced by the ambient water pressure. This reduces the volume of pooled blood in the leg veins. In addition, peripheral vasoconstriction will occur in response to any cold stress. These changes result in an increase in central blood volume, leading to diuresis and subsequent haemoconcentration and decreased plasma volume.

The effect of haemoconcentration on normal dives is not major except that it gives divers a physiological excuse for well-developed thirst and sometimes the need to urinate. Urine production rates of more than 300 mL/hour cause problems for divers trying to keep their dry suit dry, unless it is fitted with a relief outlet.

The other effect of increased central blood volume is on cardiac performance. There is an increase in cardiac output as a result of increased stroke volume. Immersion alone, or in combination with various other factors associated with the diving environment, can precipitate cardiovascular dysfunction in susceptible individuals. This is discussed in Chapter 39.

ENERGY EXPENDITURE

Measurements of energy expenditure, while swimming on the surface and underwater, have been made using indirect calorimetry and by prediction from heart rate. These results show that oxygen consumption underwater of more than 3 litres/minute (lpm) is possible, and values greater than 2 lpm are quite common. The diver's energy expenditure when inactive may be lower than found on land, presumably because the absence of gravitational effects reduces the energy required to maintain posture underwater.

Typical gas consumption and energy expenditure levels are as follows:

For a slow swim, 0.5 knots, the diver would have an air consumption of 20 lpm and an oxygen consumption of 0.8 lpm. A swim of 0.8 knots would cause an air consumption of almost 40 lpm and an oxygen consumption of 1.4 lpm. A fast swim of 1.2 knots would cause an oxygen consumption of about 2.5 lpm and an air consumption of 60 lpm (air consumption measured at the depth the diver was swimming and oxygen consumption at 1 ATA).

Increased gas density increases the work of breathing. This increases the resistance to gas flow through the diver's airways and breathing apparatus, increases the work of breathing and reduces ventilatory capacity. A maximum breathing gas density (helium) of around 8 g/litre appears to be realistic for practical purposes, thus limiting diving to around 400 to 500 metres for useful work.

> Gas density may prove to be the limiting factor for deep diving.

It may be expected that the higher oxygen partial pressures in hyperbaric environments could improve physical performance. However, chamber experiments, in which the subjects exercised while breathing oxygen at 3 ATA, showed that the maximum aerobic work performance was not significantly increased.

ALTITUDE AND SATURATION DIVING

Our normal idea of diving is that a diver descends from sea level, 1 ATA, and returns when the dive has finished. There is a series of variations from this situation. A diver may have to dive in a mountain lake where the pressure on the surface is less than 1 ATA. Another variation occurs when a diver starts from an environment where the pressure is greater than 1 ATA. This happens when divers operate from a pressurized compartment or underwater habitat. These conditions introduce complexities that require understanding of the physics involved.

A diver operating in a high mountain lake is returning to a lower surface pressure than a diver at sea level. This decreases the pressure at which the diver is while releasing inert gas after a dive and so increases the tendency to form bubbles. Therefore, the diver may need to modify the decompression plan. Another minor correction will be required if it is a fresh water lake. Fresh water is less dense than salt water, so the diver is exposed to a slightly lower pressure change per unit depth.

In addition, this diver will have to exhale faster during ascent. A diver who ascends from 10 metres (2 ATA) to the surface (1 ATA) without exhaling would find that the volume of gas in the lungs has doubled. Most divers realize this and exhale at an adequate rate during ascent. However, they may not realize that a similar doubling in gas volume occurs during the last 5 metres of ascent to the surface, if the pressure at the surface was 0.5 ATA.

High-altitude diving may require that the depth or duration of dive and the rate of ascent be reduced to allow for the lower than normal surface pressure at the end of the dive. Tables are available for diving at higher altitudes, and many dive computers are programmed to compensate for this.

A diver living in a human-made environment where the pressure is high can operate to deeper than normal depths. This system is used in saturation diving, where the diver operates from a base at increased pressure and becomes equilibrated with it. The eventual return to the surface can take many days. The use of such environments has proved to be invaluable where deep or long dives are required (see Chapter 67).

Another pressure-related problem can occur when a diver dives and then flies or ascends into mountains. Some dives and ascents will require the diver to ensure that adequate time is spent at the surface before ascending to high altitude, to avoid DCS. This problem is encountered by a diver tourist who wants to fly home after diving or one who needs to pass over hills or mountains when returning from a dive. It is also encountered when it is necessary to transport a diver with DCS. There may be an increase in manifestations of DCS when the pressure is decreased, even by a relatively small amount.

PHYSICAL ASPECTS OF THE MARINE ENVIRONMENT

Heat

Diving and exposure to high pressures change the heat transfer from a diver's body. In air, there is some insulation from the air trapped near the body, either by the clothes or the hair and the boundary layer. In water this is lost. The water adjacent to the skin is heated, expands slightly, and causes a convection current that tends to remove the layer of warmed water. This process is accelerated by movement of the diver or the water. The net result is that a diver cools or heats up much more quickly than he or she would in air of the same temperature.

Heat loss is also increased in warming the cooler inhaled air or gas. For a diver breathing air, most of this heat is used to humidify the dry air used for diving and is not sufficient to cause concern in most circumstances. However, the heat lost in a helium dive is more significant. Helium has a greater specific heat than nitrogen. The problem is compounded because at depth, the mass of gas inhaled is increased.

The heat transfer by conduction is also increased in a helium environment. The result is that a helium diver may need external heating to maintain body warmth at a water, or gas, temperature where external warming would not be required if the diver was in an air environment.

In warm environments, it is possible for a diver to suffer heat stress. A diver who is wearing a protective suit cannot lose heat by sweating because the sweat cannot evaporate. In a pressure chamber, the atmosphere can become saturated with water, and evaporative cooling is prevented. The heat stress for a given temperature is also increased if there is helium in the mixture.

Despite wearing thermal insulation in warm tropical waters, divers can continue to lose heat over several days of repetitive diving, and 'silent' hypothermia can develop, somewhat insidiously.

> A diver in water or a helium-rich environment can cool or heat up at a temperature that would be comfortable in an air environment.

Light

Even in the cleanest ocean water, only about 20 per cent of the incident light reaches a depth of 10 metres and only 1 per cent reaches 85 metres. Clean water has a maximum transparency to light with a wave length of 480 millimicrometres (blue). This variation of absorption with wave length causes distortion of colours and is responsible for the blue-green hues seen at depth. Red and orange light is absorbed most. Because of the absorption of light, the deep ocean appears black, and lights are needed for observation or photography. Because of the greater absorption of reds by water, some illumination is needed to see the true colours, even at shallow depths. Part of the appeal of diving at night is that objects that have a blue-green colour in natural light have a new brightness when they are illuminated with a torch.

Coastal water, with more suspended material, has a maximum transparency in the yellow-green band, about 530 millimicrometres. Absorption and scattering of light by suspended particles restrict vision and can tend to even out illumination.

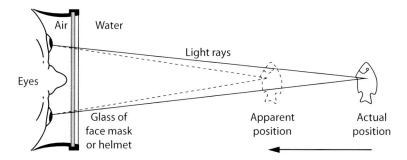

Figure 2.5 Displacement of image in water.

This can make the light intensity the same in all directions and is an important factor in causing loss of orientation.

When the eye focusses on an object in air, most of the refraction of light rays occurs at the air–cornea interface. In water, this refractive power is lost and the eye is incapable of focussing. A face mask provides an air-cornea boundary, which restores refraction at the cornea surface to normal. Refraction also occurs at the face mask surface, mainly at the glass–air boundary. This results in an apparent size increase of about 30 per cent and this makes objects appear closer than they are. Practice and adaption of the hand–eye co-ordination system allow the diver to compensate for this distortion, except when describing the size of fish (Figure 2.5).

Masks also restrict vision by narrowing the peripheral fields, and they distort objects that subtend large visual angles. Both absorption of light by water, which reduces apparent contrast, and scattering by suspended particles reduce visual acuity. Attempts have been made to improve the diver's vision by modification of the face mask, the use of coloured filters, ground mask lenses and contact lenses. These can be relatively successful but can also impose their own problems.

Sound

Sound in water is transmitted as waves with a longitudinal mode of vibration. The speed of sound is about 1530 metres/second in sea water and 1470 metres/second in fresh water at 15°C. Water is a better transmitter of sound than air, so sounds travel greater distances under water. Low-pitched sounds travel farther than higher-pitched sounds. Transmission of sound is enhanced by reflection from the surface. This reflection also enhances the transmission of sound in air over water but reduces the transmission of sounds from air to water and from water to air.

Both high-pressure air and helium-oxygen mixtures cause speech distortion. This is greater when breathing helium mixtures and can render speech unintelligible. Distortion in air causes the voice to become more nasal and crisp as the pressure increases.

It is often thought that divers cannot talk underwater. This is not so if the diver has an air space to speak into. Helmet divers can communicate easily by touching their helmets together and using the air-metal-air pathway. Some scuba divers have mastered the art of talking by taking their demand valve from their mouth and speaking into an air space created by cupping their hands.

DIVING GASES

Most diving is based on the use of compressed air and other oxygen–nitrogen mixtures as a breathing gas. Commercial, military, technical and experimental diving may involve the use of other gas mixtures. For this reason, it is desirable to give the reader some salient points on the gases mentioned in this text and related literature.

Oxygen (atomic weight 16, molecular weight 32) is the essential constituent of all breathing mixtures. At high altitude people survive with less than 0.1 ATA in their inspired air. However, for diving, oxygen should be present at a partial pressure of at least 0.2 ATA to avoid hypoxia. At higher partial pressures oxygen causes oxygen toxicity. Prolonged exposure to more than 0.55 ATA causes pulmonary oxygen toxicity, and shorter exposure to more than about 1.5 ATA results in central nervous system effects. The risk of these problems may be acceptable in a recompression chamber, where oxygen may be used at partial pressures of up to 2.8 ATA. Oxygen toxicity is discussed in Chapter 17.

In the range 0.2 to 2.8 ATA, oxygen has little effect on the respiratory centre and minute volume will remain close to normal. Oxygen is vasoactive; high oxygen tensions cause vasoconstriction.

Nitrogen (atomic weight 14, molecular weight 28) is the major component of air – about 79 per cent. Nitrogen is often considered to be physiologically inert. Bubbles, composed mainly of nitrogen, can cause DCS if a diver who has been breathing air or an oxygen–nitrogen mixture ascends too rapidly. In solution, it may cause nitrogen narcosis at depth (see Chapter 15). At partial pressures of nitrogen greater than about 3 ATA, there is a demonstrable decrement in the diver's performance. At higher partial pressures, the effect is likely to cause the diver to make mistakes. The other problem that restricts the use of nitrogen is that its density at increased pressure increases the work of breathing.

Despite these disadvantages, nitrogen is of major importance in diving, at depths less than 50 metres and as a part of more complex mixtures at greater depths.

Helium (atomic weight 4) is a light, inert gas. It is found in natural gas wells in several countries. Helium is used to dilute oxygen for dives to depths greater than 50 metres, where nitrogen should not be used alone. The two major advantages of helium are that it does not cause narcosis and, because of its lightness, helium-oxygen mixtures are easier to breathe than most alternatives. Helium-oxygen mixtures can allow a shorter decompression time (albeit often with a different profile) than an equivalent saturation dive with the diver breathing air because helium diffuses more rapidly than nitrogen.

The use of helium can cause several problems. The speech of a diver at depth may need electronic processing to make it understandable because of the distortion. A diver in a helium atmosphere is more susceptible to heat and cold because the high thermal conductivity speeds the transfer of heat to and from the diver. The other problem with the use of helium is that it is associated with a disorder called the high-pressure neurological syndrome (HPNS) (see Chapter 20).

Hydrogen (atomic weight 1, molecular weight 2) has the advantage of being readily available at low cost. Because of its lightness it is the easiest gas to breathe. These factors may lead to its use as a replacement for helium. The reluctance to use stems from fears of explosion. Explosions can be prevented if the oxygen level does not exceed 4 per cent, and such a mixture is breathable at depths in excess of 30 metres. Hypoxia can be prevented by changing to another gas near the surface. Hydrogen causes thermal and speech distortion problems similar to those encountered with helium.

FURTHER READING

Brubakk AO, Neuman TS (eds). *Bennett and Elliot's Physiology and Medicine of Diving.* 5th ed. Philadelphia: Saunders; 2004.

Doolette DJ, Mitchell SJ. Hyperbaric conditions. In: Pollock DM (ed). *Comprehensive Physiology.* Vol 1. New York: Wiley; 2011. http://www.comprehensivephysiology.com/WileyCDA/

US Navy Diving Manual Revision 6 SS521-AG-PRO-010 (2008). Washington, DC: Naval Sea Systems Command; 2008. (Vol. 1, Chapters 2 and 3 deal with these topics in a manner that assumes no previous knowledge.)

Schilling CW, Werts MF, Schandelmeier NR (eds). *The Underwater Handbook: A Guide to Physiology and Performance for the Engineer.* New York: Plenum Press; 1976.

This chapter was reviewed for this fifth edition by John Lippmann.

3

Free diving

INTRODUCTION

Free diving refers to dives made from surface to surface during voluntary apnoea on a single breath. No underwater breathing apparatus is used. Free diving (also often referred to as 'breath-hold diving' or 'snorkel diving') is regarded as the purest and most natural form of diving. Unencumbered by bulky equipment, the diver is free to move weightlessly and silently in the underwater world. Practised in some societies for thousands of years, free diving in its simplest form requires no equipment at all. The introduction of various performance-enhancing apparatus such as face masks, fins, weight belts, buoyancy vests and thermal protection suits may present new problems. For example, the addition of goggles or face masks allows for clear vision but introduces a gas space that must be 'equalized' to prevent barotrauma. Near the surface, wetsuits generate positive buoyancy that decreases as they are compressed during descent. If a weight belt is used to offset the initial positive buoyancy of the wetsuit, this will render the diver negatively buoyant as he or she begins the ascent. Nevertheless, recreational free divers and spearfishers often wear a mask, snorkel, fins, wetsuit and weights and carry a spear gun, knife and bag. Competitive free divers may also employ specialized devices such as weighted sleds for descent and inflatable lift bags for ascent to achieve remarkable depths. Even with such modern specialized equipment, human diving capabilities are paltry in comparison with those of marine mammals and other sea animals (Table 3.1).

HUMANS AS FREE DIVERS

> You're running on reserve tank and there's no warning before you hit empty!
>
> *Record-holding free diver*

There are two principal (and somewhat interrelated) challenges in free diving:

1. The challenge of increasing depth, with its attendant risk of pressure-related injury to gas-containing spaces.
2. The challenge of increasing duration, with its attendant risk of exhaustion of oxygen (O_2) stores.

Table 3.1 Depth penetrations of human divers and marine animals

Comparative depth penetrations	Depth (m)
Human free (breath-hold) diver	
• 'Constant ballast no fins'	101
• 'No limits'	214
Human diver using underwater breathing apparatus	
• Bounce dive (surface to surface)	318
• Saturation diving lockout from bell	>400
Sperm whale	1150
Northern elephant seal	1500
Wreck of *Titanic*	3810
Octopus species	5639
Deepest known fish	7703
Amphipod crab	9789
Deepest manned submersible dive	10911
Deepest part of ocean	~11000

A third challenge that is most relevant to the more extreme exponents of free diving is the related exposure to markedly elevated gas partial pressures with related risks such gas toxicities and decompression sickness.

The challenge of increasing depth

Any anatomical or equipment gas spaces are subject to compression during descent, and their volumes may need to be compensated if barotrauma is to be avoided. Obvious examples, which are discussed elsewhere in this text, include the middle ear (see Chapter 7), sinuses (see Chapter 8) and mask. The lung is of particular relevance to free divers because, unlike divers using underwater breathing apparatus who compensate intrapulmonary pressure and volume with each breath of compressed gas, the lung volume of a free diver is progressively compressed as depth increases.

It was long believed that the limiting factor on depth in free diving would be the point at which lung volume was compressed to residual volume because compression to smaller volumes could, logically, result in trauma to the chest wall or lung itself. Thus, a diver with a total lung capacity of 6 litres and a residual volume of 1.5 litres should theoretically be able to breath-hold dive to 30 metres (4 ATA) where the total lung volume

would be compressed to the residual volume (1.5 litres), a simple application of Boyle's Law. A corollary was that divers with a larger total lung capacity and/or a smaller residual volume would be capable of greater depths before injury occurred.

The fallacy of the 'residual volume limit' is immediately clear when it is considered that a human has descended to 214 metres (22.4 atmospheres absolute [ATA]) without suffering obvious lung barotrauma and that free divers regularly descend to depths greater than a theoretical maximum calculated in this way. The factors that were missing from these early attempts to predict maximum depth were the distensibility of the pulmonary vasculature and the concomitant potential for intrapulmonary blood pooling to compensate for compression of lung volume, effectively allowing for compressions below predicted residual volume. The beginnings of such compensation can be seen with simple head-out immersion in an upright subject. The negative transthoracic pressure generated by having the airway open to a pressure of 1 ATA while the thorax is exposed to greater pressure (because of the surrounding water pressure) results in a shift of about 0.7 litre of blood into the thorax. A greater engorgement of the pulmonary circulation is likely if the transthoracic pressure increases further.

Notwithstanding this remarkable and fortunate mechanism for compensation, there will nevertheless come a point where pulmonary vascular capacitance is maximized and further descent will cause the lung's remaining gas volume to develop an increasingly negative pressure relative to the environment and surrounding tissue. If this becomes excessive, then both fluid extravasation from capillaries to the alveolar space and frank haemorrhage are possible, and there is evidence from competitive free diving that both occur. This problem is referred to as pulmonary barotrauma of descent or 'lung squeeze'. Although it is interesting and potentially of increasing importance as free diving depths are extended, this is currently a minor contributor to free diving accidents in comparison with the challenges of increasing duration underwater.

The challenge of increasing duration

It is self-evident that oxygenation is maintained from steadily dwindling O_2 stores during a free dive. In contrast to marine mammals, a human's stores are relatively small. The total O_2 stores in a 70-kilogram man at resting lung volume (functional residual capacity) have been calculated to be approximately 1.5 litres. This store would be increased at total lung capacity whose value is variable among individuals. If nearly all this O_2 can be extracted, one could predict that a resting man who has an O_2 consumption of 300 mL per minute would completely deplete his O_2 stores in 5 minutes. In reality, most untrained humans can only breath-hold for approximately 1 minute because the drive to breathe is dependent largely on rising pressures of carbon dioxide (CO_2) rather than falling levels of O_2 (although the two are synergistic). This inherent inability to breath-hold voluntarily to the point of critical hypoxia (an arterial partial pressure of O_2 [Po_2] above approximately 25 mm Hg must be maintained to avoid loss of consciousness) is clearly protective in free diving. However, it can be confounded in two important ways: by the use of hyperventilation before breath-holding and through the effects of changing ambient pressure during descent and ascent from a free dive.

Hyperventilation refers to taking a series of rapid deep breaths before breath-holding. This is often done in the mistaken belief that it significantly enhances O_2 stores. Although hyperventilation does increase the alveolar O_2 content to a small extent, the volume of O_2 involved is effectively inconsequential. What hyperventilation can achieve is a marked lowering of arterial CO_2 levels. Competitive breath-hold divers have had end-tidal CO_2 pressures as low as 20 mm Hg measured at the end of their typical pre-apnoea routine. This has the effect of prolonging the breath-hold duration before the onset of a strong urge to breathe.

The obvious danger associated with hyperventilation is that it will extend the breath-hold duration closer to the point where the arterial Po_2 falls below that required to maintain consciousness. There is little doubt that hyperventilation has been a contributory factor in many free diving deaths. There is also some evidence that well-practised free divers can induce a decrease in sensitivity of the medullary respiratory control centre to CO_2, or they can learn to resist the uncomfortable urges to breathe that CO_2 generates as its arterial pressure rises, or both. Interestingly, however, although competitors in static apnoea events (effectively breath-holding competitions without pressure change) aggressively employ hyperventilation and are highly motivated not to breathe for as long as possible, symptomatic hypoxia is not frequent as would be expected. This brings the discussion to changing ambient pressure during a free dive as an added and significant risk factor for critical hypoxia.

Arterial gas tensions during breath-hold dives change with the partial pressure of the gases in the lungs. When the breath-hold diver descends, the partial pressures of the gases in the lungs increase as their volume is decreased and gas inside is compressed. The reverse takes place during ascent back toward the surface. This leads to concomitant rises and falls in alveolar and arterial Po_2.

Figure 3.1 shows alveolar pressures of the metabolic gases during (a) a breath-hold period without ambient pressure change, (b) a breath-hold dive to 10 metres and (c) a breath-hold dive to 10 metres with prior hyperventilation. In Figure 3.1 (b) and 3.1 (c), ambient and thus alveolar gas partial pressures rise during descent according to Boyle's Law. The rise in O_2 is somewhat reduced because of continued consumption. Because of the high alveolar

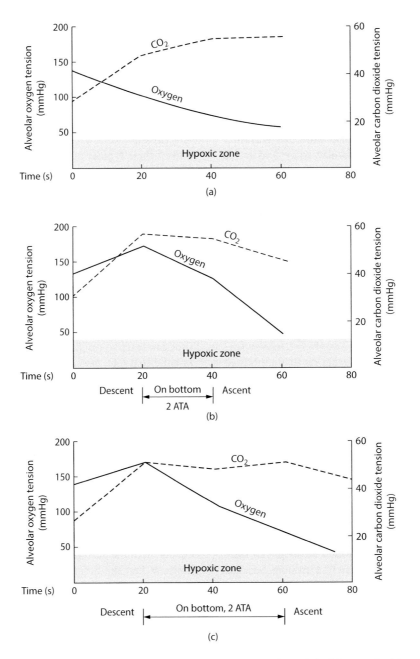

Figure 3.1 Alveolar pressures of the metabolic gases during **(a)** a breath-hold period without ambient pressure change, **(b)** a breath-hold dive to 10 metres and **(c)** a breath-hold dive to 10 metres with prior hyperventilation.

Po_2 at depth, there is a sufficient alveolar-arterial gradient to allow continuing O_2 uptake for a considerable time.

In contrast, during ascent there is a rapid fall in alveolar Po_2 as the lung re-expands and the volume of the alveolar gas increases. This is greater than expected from gas laws alone, thus reflecting ongoing oxygen metabolism. The dive with prior hyperventilation depicted in Figure 3.1 (c) had a longer bottom time as would be expected when prior lowering of the arterial CO_2 makes the diver more comfortable remaining at depth for longer. It can be seen that a lower alveolar partial pressure of O_2 develops by the time the diver reaches the surface, and such falls in alveolar and arterial Po_2 during ascent would be even more dramatic on deeper dives. The obvious risk is that the diver could experience critical arterial hypoxaemia as the alveolar Po_2 is rapidly falling in the latter stages of the ascent. Indeed, loss of consciousness during either the final phase of ascent or on arrival at the surface is a recurring event at free diving competitions. The dangers of breath-hold diving and hyperventilation are discussed further in Chapter 16.

In addition to hyperventilation, there are two other strategies, both controversial, that elite free divers use or manipulate in order to extend their duration underwater.

The first of these is an attempt to expedite the so-called diving reflex that can be observed in all air breathing vertebrates but that is highly developed in marine mammals (see later). This reflex is initiated by apnoea and also by facial cooling. Its principal effector arm is a marked sympathetically mediated increase in peripheral vascular resistance that increases blood pressure and in turn elicits a vagally mediated bradycardia. At the same time, there is some evidence that the sympathetic activation induces splenic contraction, increasing circulating red blood cells. Peripheral vasoconstriction has the effect of reducing the circulation of blood to the peripheries, and the bradycardia reduces O_2 consumption by the heart. Central redistribution of blood makes more O_2 available to vital organs. A concurrent and unwanted side effect of these processes is a predisposition to arrhythmias. This probably arises from vagal inhibition of nodal conduction combined with sympathetic sensitization of ectopic pacemakers. Not surprisingly, ventricular ectopic beats are common.

Although these are autonomically mediated phenomena, there is a strong belief among free divers that they can manipulate the process through conditioning, relaxation techniques and practice. Given that there is considerable inter-subject variability in the potency of the diving reflex, and that it tends to wane with age, it does seem plausible that it is 'open' to manipulation by skilled divers. In a 2014

interview William Trubridge, holder of the constant ballast no fins world depth record of 101 metres, articulated it thus:

> The training I do is targeted at creating a physiology that conserves oxygen as much as possible. Whereas someone who is extremely fit would be able to supply a high amount of oxygen to their muscles very quickly, I need to shut down that oxygen flow to the muscles so that they can work anaerobically and that conserves the oxygen for the heart and the brain. Physiology for freediving is such a different set of effects to what is found in any other sport that we're still discovering exactly what they consist of.

> *New Zealand Listener Magazine,*
> *4 January 2014*

Similarly, on his website Francesco "Pippin" Ferreras, a previous world record holder, described his approach in more detail:

> My heart, under direct control of the Central Nervous System, begins a rapid slowdown. This diminution of my cardiac output is a result of the body's decreasing needs for oxygen and energy consumption. This efficiency in energy conservation is of vital importance for survival in the undersea environment while in a state of apnea. As an example, when I begin my pre-immersion preparations my resting heart rate is 75 bpm, 10 minutes after entering a stare of deep relaxation it drops, to 55 bpm. As I begin my descent, in a matter of seconds it has slowed to 30 bpm. My cardiovascular performance is influenced by other factors, foremost being my physical conditioning, and mental preparation.... Once I have reached a depth of 110 m., I institute one last command to my heart to slow down. At this point my heart is down to a mere 10 to 14 bpm. On several immersions when all of the above mentioned factors are

ideal I have obtained readings of an incredible 7 bpm! Obviously these findings are augmented by the power of mind over body that I have developed over the years, through the study and practice of Yoga.

The second controversial strategy used by elite free divers to extend both depth and duration underwater is so-called 'lung packing', more correctly referred to as glossopharyngeal insufflation. This technique involves using the glossopharyngeal muscles to pump air into the lungs, thus enabling an increase in the total lung capacity by up to 20 per cent. This extra volume potentially increases the depth at which lung compression becomes hazardous (as described earlier) and also represents an increase in the O_2 stores. Adept exponents of lung packing can increase the volume of air carried by several litres, although this does not translate directly into an increase in lung volume because the gas is held in the lungs under positive pressure and is therefore compressed. Therein lies the potential problem with this strategy. There are sporadic reports of excessive packing leading to pulmonary barotrauma because of the high positive transpulmonary pressures that can reach 60 mm Hg or even more. There are also reports of hypotensive loss of consciousness resulting from profound reduction in venous return associated with high intrathoracic pressure during the act of packing. In view of these potential hazards the technique cannot be recommended. Nevertheless, it is unlikely that packing will be abandoned by extreme free divers looking for any possible edge.

Largely for completeness (and for curious interest value), there are some extreme free divers who have developed the technique of glossopharyngeal exsufflation, that is, packing in the opposite direction. This is used in those situations near terminal depth when the lungs are compressed at or below residual volume, and it is therefore impossible to generate a Valsalva manoeuvre to clear the ears or sinuses. An alternative approach to avoiding barotrauma under these conditions, and one that has been proven radiologically, is to let the sinuses (and to some extent the middle ears) flood with water!

The challenge of avoiding gas toxicities and decompression sickness

The combination of increasing depth and duration (particularly the former) during free diving opens up the possibility that extreme exponents will suffer gas toxicities and decompression sickness, complications usually associated with compressed gas diving. Neurological decompression sickness in breath-hold divers has been reported. Although some cases may be caused by arterial gas embolism following pulmonary barotrauma, predictions of inert gas tensions following repeated and closely spaced deep breath-hold dives do suggest that pathological bubble formation from dissolved inert gas is certainly possible (see Chapter 10).

Despite the extreme depths reached by free divers, overt effects of nitrogen narcosis are only rarely reported, although there may be a strong reporting bias operant here. It may also be that narcosis is not as likely as predicted on the basis of depth alone simply because the partial pressure of nitrogen in the relevant tissues takes time to equilibrate with the partial pressure of nitrogen in the lungs, and the short duration of the dives therefore limits any effect. Nevertheless, as extreme free divers are pushing deeper, there are increasing numbers of stories of strange sensations and 'funny turns' during these dives. It is impossible to know their exact cause, but potential explanations include nitrogen narcosis (see Chapter 15), high-pressure neurological syndrome (see Chapter 20) and cerebral O_2 toxicity (see Chapter 17). Cerebral O_2 toxicity seems an unlikely explanation given the very short exposures, the starting fraction of inspired O_2 of 0.21 and the fact that O_2 is being consumed from the moment apnoea begins. However, some reported events (e.g. facial or diaphragmatic twitching) are very typical of O_2 toxicity. These sorts of problems are likely to become more common as record depths are pushed further.

Record diving

Trained free divers have been able to achieve remarkable underwater feats, and in certain societies these divers are accorded celebrity status.

Records are attempted for various categories of diving involving depth, duration and underwater distance. Because of the potential risks involved, dedicated competitions sanctioned by an umbrella society are run according to strict protocols. Physiologists and physicians need to be aware of these remarkable achievements. The records cited here are valid for January 2015 but may have been superseded at the time of reading. A complete list of current records is available at: http://www.aidainternational.org/competitive/worlds-records.

The purest form of depth record is referred to as *constant weight apnoea without fins* and involves return to the surface with the same weights carried down (if any) and, as the name implies, no use of fins. The record is currently 101 metres for male divers and 69 metres for female divers.

At the opposite end of the spectrum is so-called *no limits* free diving. This is the most extreme category in respect of depth and requires no swimming at all. Divers hold onto a weighted, rope-guided sled for descent. On reaching the target depth, they detach themselves from the sled and pull a pin that releases compressed air from a cylinder into a lift bag, which tows them back to the surface. The current record depths are 214 metres for male divers and 160 metres for female divers. The latter is the longest-standing free diving record at the present time, set by Tanya Streeter in 2002.

The absolute limit of these hazardous 'experiments' remains unknown, but it seems likely that depth record increments will become smaller and smaller as immutable physiological barriers are approached. Death may be precipitated at depth by pulmonary haemorrhage, pulmonary oedema or cardiac dysrhythmias. Cerebral hypoxia is an invariable development during the latter stages of ascent. Quite often these divers require rescue by standby divers because they become unconscious as a result of rapidly developing hypoxia as they approach the surface.

Records are also held for *static apnoea,* which is a motionless, energy-conserving head immersion exposure. The current records are a mind-boggling 11 minutes 35 seconds for male participants and 9 minutes 2 seconds for female participants.

Underwater breath-hold horizontal distances (*dynamic apnoea with fins*) of 281 metres (male swimmers) and 234 metres (female swimmers) have been achieved in 50-metre swimming pools with swimmers using fins for propulsion.

DIVING MARINE MAMMALS

The study of diving animals offers the scientist an ideal opportunity to study the physiological consequences and defence mechanisms required to survive extended breath-holding. It is also of great interest to diving physicians to see how diving animals avoid the perils induced by exposure to pressure and hypothermia.

The northern elephant seal and the sperm whale can dive to 1500 metres. The southern elephant seal can stay submerged for 2 hours, although usual dives are 20 to 30 minutes in duration. The Weddell seal regularly dives for food to greater than 100 metres and can remain submerged for up to 60 minutes. Typical humans, with some practice, can breath-hold underwater for 1 to 2 minutes and descend to 10 to 15 metres.

How are marine mammals able to achieve these remarkable underwater depth and/or duration exposures that appear to defy conventional wisdom with respect to limits of hypoxia? How also do they achieve these feats without developing some of the disorders (e.g. hypoxic blackouts, barotrauma, decompression sickness, nitrogen narcosis, O_2 toxicity or high-pressure neurological syndrome) that are the subjects of subsequent chapters in this book?

Obvious anatomical adaptations include a streamlined shape, low-friction body surface (skin or fur) and the development of flippers or fins. Dolphins can reach speeds of 20 knots with remarkably low energy consumption. A dorsal blowhole in whales and dolphins also aids energy efficient respiration. Of more interest to the diving physician and physiologist are the mechanisms to cope with prolonged apnoea. The adaptations that allow diving animals to achieve long periods underwater are both physiological and biochemical.

Oxygen stores

All diving mammals have an increased total body O_2 store. The relative contribution of the lungs, blood and muscles storage areas depends on the diving pattern of the animal.

Deep diving mammals do not dive at full lung capacity and may exhibit reduced lung perfusion during dives for reasons discussed later, so the bulk of O_2 is stored in blood and muscle. Such animals have increased blood volume (~15 per cent of body mass versus ~5 to 7 per cent for humans), and the blood has a higher haemoglobin concentration. About 70 per cent of the total O_2 store is found in the blood. They also have a markedly increased myoglobin concentration (5 to 12 times that found in a human), especially in the swim muscles, and this myoglobin increase is proportional to the diving capacity of the animal. Myoglobin carries approximately 25 per cent of the total O_2 sore. Only a tiny proportion (~5 per cent) is found in the lungs (versus ~25 per cent in humans).

An intriguing and controversial mechanism for augmenting O_2 storage and delivery during a dive is the pre-dive sequestration of oxygenated red cells in the spleen followed by the release of these cells by splenic contracture during a dive. The time course of release into the systemic circulation may be further regulated by a valve-like sphincter in the vena cava. The fact that this occurs is not disputed, but its role in marine mammal diving adaptation is uncertain. It has been noted that re-sequestration after release on one dive typically takes far longer than the typical surface interval between subsequent dives during a dive series. Thus, any benefit may be restricted to the initial dive. It is possible that this adaptation is more important for keeping blood haematocrit (and viscosity) at optimal levels when the animal is not diving than for improving oxygenation during dives.

Oxygen consumption and the diving response

The increases in blood volume, haemoglobin and myoglobin described earlier all contribute to the seal's impressive O_2 supply, but O_2 still needs to be conserved. Indeed, it can be readily calculated that if the submerged seal continued to metabolize at the same rate as before diving, its O_2 stores would not be sufficient during long dives. Not surprisingly, these animals exhibit multiple strategies aimed at conserving O_2 and ensuring that it is supplied preferentially to vital organs during the period of a dive.

The term *diving response* refers to a sequence of physiological events, including apnoea, bradycardia and redistribution of cardiac output, which are under the control of multiple reflexes. O_2 conservation is thus partly accomplished by selective redistribution of circulating blood. Blood may be preferentially distributed to swimming rather than non-swimming muscles. Studies indicate that pinniped skeletal muscles have an enhanced oxidative capacity to maintain aerobic metabolism under the relatively hypoxic conditions associated with diving and that these adaptations are more pronounced in swimming than in non-swimming muscles. Other tissues that are most critical for survival (e.g. retina, brain, spinal cord, adrenal glands and, in pregnant seals, the placenta) are also selectively perfused. The seal essentially shuts off the flow of blood to non-essential tissues and organs, such as the kidneys, until it resurfaces.

Rapid onset of bradycardia (to as low as 10 per cent of baseline rate) at the start of a dive may be seen in diving species. This reduces cardiac work and O_2 consumption. A substantial reduction in cardiac output has been shown in Weddell seals. Because stroke volume falls by only about 30 per cent, the predominant effector of this reduction is the bradycardia.

Arterial blood pressure is reasonably well preserved despite this reduction in cardiac output, and this is important to maintain perfusion of vital organs. Maintenance of arterial pressure is facilitated by the stretching of the elastic walls of large arteries during systole and their recoil during diastole. This function is augmented in many species of marine mammals by a bulbous enlargement of the root of the aorta, the aortic bulb. The aortic bulb approximately doubles the diameter of the ascending aorta in harbour and Weddell seals, thus providing an elastic capacitance for maintaining pressure and flow into the constricted arterial tree during the long diastolic intervals characteristic of diving. The entire human aorta contains less volume than the aortic bulb alone in seals of a similar body weight. The increase in left ventricular afterload that would be expected as a consequence of elevated peripheral resistance and decreased large artery compliance is reduced by this unique anatomy. The net result is a diminished peak systolic pressure, which reduces cardiac work and O_2 consumption while at the same time maintaining stroke volume.

The *electrocardiogram* of the diving animal shows some progressive changes during prolonged apnoeic dives. In addition to bradycardia, these changes may include the gradual diminution or even abolition of the P wave. Cardiac rhythm is then apparently set independently of the sino-atrial node by a ventricular pacemaker site. Other cardiac dysrhythmias occasionally appear.

Anaerobic metabolism

With prolonged dives certain tissues switch to anaerobic metabolism, which produces lactic acid as a by-product. There is an increased tolerance to lactic acid in the muscles through increased buffering capacity. High levels of lactic acid, however, lower the pH of the blood and can lead to acidosis, causing a weakening of the heart's ability to contract. Acidosis is avoided by confining anaerobic metabolism to the skeletal muscles and other tissues isolated from the blood supply. When the animals resurface, these tissues release the lactic acid into the blood for metabolism by the liver.

Diving technique

Modified diving behaviour to limit muscle activity and thus O_2 consumption has been demonstrated in Weddell seals. Prolonged downward gliding, with minimal muscular effort, as a result of reducing buoyancy with lung compression at depth can result in up to a 60 per cent reduction in energy costs. Gliding is used during dives exceeding 18 metres in depth and occupies approximately 75 per cent of the descent.

Pressure changes

Structural adaptations to accommodate thoracic compression during deep dives include a flexible rib cage, stiffened alveolar ducts and attachments of the diaphragm such as to permit some shifting of abdominal contents into the thorax. These changes help the animal avoid pulmonary barotrauma of descent. Quarantining of pulmonary gas from perfusing blood minimizes accumulation of nitrogen (decompression sickness), which may occur in repetitive diving. It likely also reduces nitrogen narcosis.

Deep diving mammals do not dive on a full lung volume. As well as limiting nitrogen uptake, this means that the animal is not exposed to O_2 toxicity because the partial pressures never reach dangerous levels.

How the elephant seal and sperm whale avoid the high-pressure neurological syndrome during their impressive diving feats is not yet understood.

Hypothermia

A thick layer of blubber and a relatively low surface area to reduce heat loss maintain core temperature. A reduction of blood flow to the skin increases insulation of the fat layer and allows surface cooling, which is not transmitted to the internal core. Well-developed countercurrent heat exchange systems also aid in conserving heat by cooling arterial blood and heating venous blood as it returns to the core. Examples can be found in the fins and flippers of whales and seals. Working muscles are close to the surface and have little fat insulation. Also, many animals, when not diving, have a raised metabolic rate to produce heat.

FURTHER READING

Kooyman GL, Ponganis PJ. The physiological basis of diving to depth: birds and mammals. *Annual Review of Physiology* 1998;**60**:19–32.

Lindholm P, Lundgren CEG. The physiology and pathophysiology of human breath hold diving. *Journal of Applied Physiology* 2009;**106**:284–292.

Thornton SJ, Hochoachka PW. Oxygen and the diving seal. *Undersea and Hyperbaric Medicine* 2004;**31**:81–95.

This chapter was reviewed for this fifth edition by Simon Mitchell.

Diving equipment

INTRODUCTION

The first part of this chapter deals with the equipment used by most recreational divers. The more complex and unusual types of diving equipment that are used by technical, commercial or military diving operations are dealt with in the second part of the chapter. Attention is paid to the problems the equipment can cause, particularly for the student or novice. This is of importance in understanding the medical problems that are related to diving equipment. It may also help the reader to understand the stresses experienced by the novice diver.

EQUIPMENT FOR RECREATIONAL DIVING

Snorkeling/breath-hold diving equipment

The simplest assembly of diving equipment is that used by snorkelers – a mask, snorkel and a pair of fins. In colder climates, a wetsuit may be added for thermal insulation and a weight belt to compensate for the buoyancy of the suit. In tropical waters, a 'stinger suit' provides not only a little thermal comfort but also some protection from box jelly-fish and other stings.

MASK

A mask is needed to give the diver adequate vision underwater. The mask usually covers the eyes and nose. Traditionally, masks were made from rubber, although now most are made from silicone. The mask seals by pressing on the cheeks, forehead and under the nose with a soft silicone edge to prevent entry of water. Swimming goggles, which do not cover the nose, are not suitable for diving. The nose must be enclosed in the mask so that the diver can exhale into it to allow equalization of the pressure between the face and mask with the water environment. It should be possible to block the nostrils without disturbing the mask seal to enable the wearer to perform a Valsalva manoeuvre. Full-face masks that cover the mouth as well as the eyes and nose, or helmets that cover the entire head, are more commonly used by professional divers and are considered in the section on professional diving equipment.

The faceplate of the mask should be made from hardened glass. A diver with visual problems can choose from a selection of corrective lenses that are commercially available. These are designed to attach directly to certain masks. Alternatively, prescription lenses can be ground and glued to a variety of masks. Ocular damage can occur if hard corneal lenses are used for diving (see Chapter 42). Certain contact lenses may be lost if the mask floods and the diver fails to, or is unable to, take preventive action. Some people with allergy problems react to the rubber of the mask, although this is rarely an issue with silicone.

All masks cause a restriction in vision. With most masks, the diver can see about one third of his or her normal visual field. The restriction is most marked when the diver tries to look down toward the feet. This restriction can be a danger if the diver becomes entangled. However, there are some masks available with a tilted lens to provide a better downward field of vision.

The more nervous beginner may find the visual restriction worrying and may possibly fear that there is a lurking predator just outside the field of vision. The visual field varies with the style of mask. Experimentation is also needed to find which mask gives a good seal, to minimize water entry. The diver needs to master a technique to expel water from the mask. If it is not learned and mastered, a leaking mask can become a major problem, sometimes leading to panic.

SNORKEL

The typical snorkel is a tube, about 40 cm long and 2 cm in diameter, with a pre-moulded or creatable U-bend near the mouth end. A mouthpiece is fitted to allow the diver to grip the tube with the teeth and lips. The tube is positioned to pass upward near the wearer's ear to enable him or her to breathe through the tube while floating on the surface and looking down. Any water in the snorkel should be expelled by forceful exhalation before the diver inhales through the snorkel.

Many attempts have been made to 'improve' the snorkel by lengthening it, adding valves, modifying its shape and some other means. There is little evidence of the success of most of these attempts.

All snorkels impose a restriction to breathing. A typical snorkel restricts the maximum breathing capacity to about 70 per cent of normal. The volume of the snorkel also increases the diver's anatomical dead space. Because of this, increasing the diameter substantially to reduce the resistance is not a viable option. These problems add to the

difficulties of a diver who may be struggling to cope with waves breaking over him or her (and into the snorkel) and a current that may force the diver to swim hard. There have also been anecdotal reports of divers inhaling foreign bodies that have previously lodged in the snorkel.

FINS

Fins (or flippers) are mechanical extensions of the feet. Fins allow the diver to swim faster and more efficiently, and they free the diver's arms for other tasks. The fins are normally secured to the feet by straps or are moulded to fit the feet. Various attempts have been made to develop fins that give greater thrust with special shapes, valves, controlled flex, springs and materials, all competing for the diver's dollar. Some of these fins can improve the thrust, but the wearer needs to become accustomed to them. Others have little effect.

Divers often get cramps, either in the foot or calf, if fins are the wrong size, if the diver has poor technique or if the diver has not used fins for an extended period. The loss of a fin may also cause problems for a diver, especially if he or she has to a swim against a current, or fails to attain appropriate orientation underwater or buoyancy on the surface.

WEIGHTS

Even without the buoyancy of a wetsuit, some divers require extra weights to submerge easily. The weights are made from lead, and most are moulded to thread onto a belt. Some weights are designed to fit into pouches, either on a belt or, for scuba divers, attached to a buoyancy compensator device (BCD). Whatever weighting mechanism is used needs to be fitted with a quick-release buckle or other mechanism to allow a diver to drop the weights quickly and so aid his or her return to, or enable the diver to remain on, the surface. The situations in which a quick-release buckle may not be fitted (or may be de-activated) are those where it would be dangerous to ascend, such as in caves where there is no air space above the water.

In some circumstances, it is necessary for a diver to ditch the weight belt to reach, or remain on, the surface in an emergency. Such situations include an emergency in which the scuba diver cannot inflate the BCD, for example, if the diver is out of breathing gas. Unfortunately, divers often fail to release the belt if they are in difficulty. The reason for this omission is not clear, but it is likely often the result of stress or panic. Adequate initial training and practice help to reinforce the skill so that it will become more automatic when required. It also needs to be reinforced periodically. Unfortunately, much of the current training fails to focus adequately on this important emergency drill.

An alternative drill of taking the belt off and holding it in one hand (preferably away from the body) is useful in some situations in which the diver is likely to become unconscious and inflating the BCD is not an option or may not be sufficient (e.g. when deep). In the event of unconsciousness, the belt will hopefully fall away, causing the diver to rise to the surface. Holding the belt away from the body should reduce the chance of entanglement with the diver if it is dropped.

In many fatal diving accidents the diver did not release his or her weights.

This basic free diving equipment is adequate for diving in shallow, relatively warm water. Experience with this gear is excellent training for a potential scuba diver. The diver can gain the basic skills without the extra complications caused by scuba gear. It allows a more realistic self-assessment of the desire to scuba dive and the subsequent rewards. With the confidence gained in snorkeling and breath-hold diving and the associated aquatic skills, the diver is also less likely to become as dependent on the breathing apparatus. In cold climates, a snorkel diver needs a suit to keep warm. Suits are discussed in Chapter 27.

Self-contained underwater breathing apparatus – scuba

The simplest form of breathing apparatus consisted of a gas source and a tap that the diver turned on to obtain each breath of air. This system was in use until the 1930s, but much of the diver's time and concentration were taken up in operating the tap. In the most common breathing apparatus, the **Aqualung** or **self-contained**

underwater breathing apparatus (scuba), the tap is replaced by a two-stage valve system. The flow of gas to the diver is triggered by the diver's inspiratory effort and is closed by expiration or cessation of inspiration.

Figure 4.1 and Figure 4.2 (a) and (b) show the operating principles of a simple regulator and demand valve system. The air is stored in a cylinder at a maximum pressure that is determined by the design of the cylinder. For most cylinders this pressure, called the working pressure, is 160 to 300 bar (2300 to 4350 psi).

The first stage of the valve system (see Figure 4.1) reduces the pressure from cylinder pressure to the equivalent of about 10 ATA greater than the pressure surrounding the diver, and it regulates its outlet pressure at this value. The valve is held open by the force of a spring until the pressure above the first stage piston builds up and forces the valve seal down on the seat, thus shutting off the gas. The first-stage

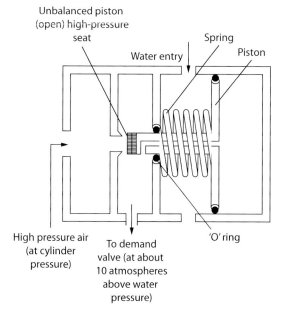

Figure 4.1 First stage reducer valve: the gas escapes from the cylinder until the pressure above the piston increases to a level where the force on the piston can compress the spring, pushing the first stage valve seat down and shutting the gas flow off. The valve opens again when the pressure above the piston (and in the hose to the second stage valve) falls. This is normally because the diver has taken another breath.

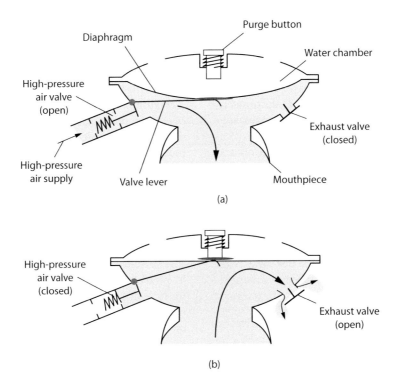

Figure 4.2 SCUBA demand valve **(a)** during inspiration and **(b)** exhalation. The arrows indicate air flow. During inspiration the diver decreases the pressure in the mouthpiece. This causes the diaphragm to curve in and tilt the air supply valve open. At the end of inspiration air continues to flow until the pressure in the mouthpiece equals the pressure in the water chamber, at this stage the diaphragm will return to the position shown in 4.2(b), and the air supply valve shuts. During exhalation the pressure in the mouthpiece is greater than that in the surrounding water. This pressure difference forces the exhaust valve open and allows exhaled air to escape. The purge button is used to trigger a flow of gas from the supply without the need to inhale from the regulator.

valve opens and closes as gas is drawn from the system by the diver. In some regulators, the water can enter the water chamber and helps the spring to hold the valve open. In others, the ambient water pressure is transmitted indirectly. This adjustment of the supply pressure with water pressure is designed to prevent the flow decreasing as the diver descends.

When the diver inhales, he or she reduces the pressure in the mouthpiece chamber, or second-stage valve. As the diver does so, the diaphragm curves inward and depresses the lever (see Figure 4.2 (a)). The inlet valve opens and remains open until inhalation ceases. At this stage, the diaphragm moves back into the position shown in Figure 4.2 (b). The second-stage valve is usually called the demand valve.

Expired gas passes out of the second stage through an exhaust valve. In the demand valve, gas flow increases with respiratory effort because the valve opens more, allowing the diver to breathe normally. The purge button allows the diver to open the inlet valve to force any water out of the regulator. The diver may need to do this if he or she takes the regulator from the mouth while underwater or if the seal around the mouthpiece is poor.

> The scuba regulator is designed to provide the diver with a gas supply matched to his or her respiratory needs.

Most divers have little difficulty using scuba. However, when they first don it, the weight and bulk will make them awkward, and may aggravate back problems. In the water, the buoyancy of the set offsets its weight.

The diver's lips should be sealed around the mouthpiece to prevent the entry of water. Water can enter through a hole in the mouthpiece if the mouthpiece is poorly attached or through the diaphragm or exhaust valve if either is faulty. A leak can generate an aerosol if the water reaches the inlet valve of the second-stage valve. The aerosol can cause distress to the diver and may sometimes cause a syndrome called *salt water aspiration syndrome,* or it may trigger other medical conditions such as asthma or possibly a cardiac dysrhythmia.

Another problem associated with demand valves is that they may cause pain in the temporomandibular joint. This condition is considered in Chapter 42.

In very cold water, the first stage of the regulator may 'freeze up'. This occurs because the air cools as it passes through the first stage and can ice up with the piston frozen in the open position. The problem can be reduced by using a first stage that is designed for operation in cold water.

Because the first stage regulates the pressure to the second stage, the inspiratory effort required to cause a flow does not vary until the cylinder is almost empty. Then the pressure in the hose to the second stage falls and the flow decreases. The diver's first warning that the cylinder is almost empty is increased resistance on inhalation. However, this warning may be minimal or absent with modern regulators.

Most divers have a console that includes a pressure gauge connected to the cylinder by a hose. Some modern systems transmit the cylinder pressure via radiofrequency signals rather than via a hose. The pressure gauge provides the diver with a measure of the remaining air supply. The contents of the cylinder are proportional to the pressure, so the gauge is often called the 'contents gauge'. Divers tend to say they have 50 bar left, rather than the volume this represents. A major problem is that a diver who is entranced by the scenery, concentrating on a task or distracted may run out of air because he or she forgets to check the gauge. An audible low-air warning is incorporated into some systems and is valuable. A diver needs to ensure

that he or she has a cylinder or cylinders with adequate gas supply for the planned dive, and an additional reserve.

A traditional and almost obsolete system to prevent divers from running out of air is a reserve valve. In operation it resembles a boiler safety valve; the air escapes to the diver until the cylinder pressure falls to the level at which the reserve valve seats. The remainder of the air can be released by pulling a lever that opens the reserve valve. One problem with this is that the valve lever may be inadvertently put into the 'on' position, causing the diver to use the reserve of gas without being aware of this. Another common problem is valve failure.

Surface-supply breathing apparatus

A diver can also use a demand valve with air supplied by a hose from the surface. This equipment, **surface-supply breathing apparatus (SSBA),** restricts the diver's range and depth to the length of the air supply hose. Its advantages are that the diver is freed from the cumbersome air cylinders and the air supply can be as large as needed, instead of being restricted by the diver's carrying capacity and need for mobility. The air for SSBA may be stored in large tanks or compressed as required. The use of a compressor, often called a '*hookah*' system, is economically attractive because the air is compressed to a lower pressure than that required for storage tanks. However, the compressor needs to be reliable and there needs to be an observer to monitor the compressor during operation.

Two modified forms of SSBA have found support in some circles. In one, a small motor and air compressor are supported on a float on the surface. This apparatus supplies air to one or two divers. In the other, the divers tow a float that supports an air cylinder. An advantage of these systems is that, if the hoses are short, the divers are unable to reach the depth needed to develop decompression sickness (DCS). A significant problem is that the user has no indication of when the gas supply will fail. Therefore, it is prudent for the diver to carry a small bail-out cylinder and regulator. Also, some novice users may forget that they are still exposed to the other hazards of scuba diving, such as pulmonary barotrauma.

In some resort areas, these devices are hired by novices who have had no training and who may be medically unfit to dive. Such use should be controlled and monitored in a similar manner to normal scuba instruction and equipment hires.

Safety and protective equipment

The best safety measures available to a diver are adequate health and fitness, proper training, appropriate and functional equipment and common sense. Almost all accidents are preventable, and the authors do not ascribe the popularly held belief that these accidents are attributable to an 'act of God'. Many accidents involve human, often predictable and thus correctable, mistakes. This point is developed in Chapter 46, in which deaths and accidents are considered. Several items of equipment that reduce the hazards of diving, or assist with coping with them, are discussed here.

EMERGENCY AIR SUPPLIES

Emergency air supplies can take a variety of forms. In the early days it was common to rely on *buddy-breathing,* a procedure in which two divers shared an air supply in the event one of them had an air supply failure. Both anecdote and analysis of diving accident statistics showed that this procedure often did not work in an emergency. The use of a second regulator attached to the scuba set, often called an **octopus rig,** has now become standard fare, and its introduction and widespread use have helped to avoid many serious diving accidents. However, neither buddy-breathing nor an octopus rig will be of use if the diver with gas is not available or is unwilling to cooperate. For this reason, a second source of air (redundant supply) that is available to each diver without external assistance is now favoured. For cave divers this may essentially be a second scuba set. For technical divers with substantial mandatory decompression obligations, a redundant gas supply is also essential, and they often carry what is known as a **stage cylinder**.

For most divers, who have relatively ready access to the surface, a smaller cylinder with an independent regulator can be used. One commercially available device, known as *Spare Air* (Submersible Systems, Inc.), is carried by some divers. However, the air supply is very small, enabling only a few breaths for ascent. For this reason, these devices are not commonly used and are not sufficient for deep dives or dives requiring decompression. It is important that a redundant supply provides adequate gas for a relatively safe ascent.

It is also sometimes possible for a diver to breathe air from the BCD for a short period of ascent. However, this has potential hazards, including aspiration of water, infection and buoyancy control problems. A BCD with an independent air supply is available but not commonly used.

THERMAL PROTECTION

Thermal protection is needed in cold water or on prolonged dives to minimize the risk of hypothermia. This protection is normally provided by insulated clothing, which reduces heat loss. The most common protection is a **wetsuit,** made from air-foamed Neoprene rubber. The water that leaks into spaces between the suit and the diver soon warms to skin temperature. Foamed Neoprene has insulation properties similar to those of woollen felt. Its effectiveness is reduced by loss of heat with water movement and increasing depth. Pressure decreases insulation by reducing the size of the air cells in the foam. At 30 metres of depth, the insulation of a wetsuit is about one third of that on the surface (see Figure 27.1). The compression of the gas in the foam also means that the diver's buoyancy decreases as he or she goes deeper. The diver can compensate for this by wearing a BCD. If the diver does not, he or she needs to limit the weights, but this will mean that the diver is too buoyant when closer to the surface. The buoyancy and insulation of a wetsuit decrease with repeated use.

Another other common form of thermal protection is the **drysuit.** This is watertight and has seals round the head, feet and hand openings. There is an opening with a waterproof seal to allow the diver to get into the suit. The drysuit allows the diver to wear an insulating layer of warm clothes. A gas supply and exhaust valve are needed to allow the diver to compensate for the effect of pressure changes on the gas in the suit. The gas can be supplied from the scuba cylinder or a separate supply.

The diver needs training in the operation of a drysuit or he or she may lose control of buoyancy by excessive addition of air into the suit. This can lead to an uncontrolled ascent, sometimes inverted, when the excess of gas expands, speeding the ascent. If the diver tries to swim downward, or otherwise becomes inverted in the water, the excess gas may accumulate around the legs, from where it cannot be vented through the exhaust valve. The excess gas can also expand the feet of the suit and cause the diver's fins to pop off. The diver can find himself or herself floating on the surface with the suit grossly overinflated, a most undignified and potentially dangerous posture.

Heat can also be supplied to a diver to help him or her keep warm. The commonly used systems include hot water pumped down to the diver through hoses. Various chemical and electrical heaters are also available. External heat supplies are more often used by commercial divers.

Semi-drysuits are essentially wetsuits with enhanced seals at the neck, hands, feet and zippers. These seals help to reduce the amount of water entering and leaving the suit and so reduce heat loss. They are not as effective as drysuits in keeping the diver warm, but they can provide thermal protection similar to that of a significantly thicker wetsuit and so increase the level of comfort for the wearer, as well as reducing the amount of weight carried.

BUOYANCY COMPENSATOR DEVICES

BCDs consist of an inflatable vest (or back-mounted bags [wings]) worn by the diver and attached to a gas supply from the regulator. The BCD allows the diver to adjust buoyancy underwater or helps bring the diver to the surface and/or support him or her there. The ability to change buoyancy allows the diver to hover in the water and adjust for any factor that causes density to increase (e.g. wetsuit compression, picking up a heavy object on the bottom).

Most BCDs can be inflated via a hose from the regulator. Some have a small separate air bottle that can also be used as an emergency air supply, although these are now rare. Several valves to release gas are fitted so the diver can reduce buoyancy by venting gas from the compensator.

Divers can lose control of their buoyancy while ascending. As the diver starts to ascend, the expanding gas in the BCD increases its lift and in turn increases the rate of ascent. Such a rapid, uncontrolled ascent can lead to a variety of diving medical problems including pulmonary barotrauma and DCS.

In the past, BCDs were also designed to float an unconscious diver face-up on the surface. However, with the current designs this useful benefit has been largely foregone.

DEPTH GAUGES

A depth gauge, timer and a means of calculating decompression are needed if an unsupervised diver is operating in a depth or time zone where decompression stops may be needed. Electronic, mechanical and capillary gauges have been used as depth gauges by divers. Capillary gauges, although now rarely used, measure pressure by the reduction in volume of a gas bubble in a graduated capillary tube and were useful only at shallower depths. Most gauges record the maximum depth reached by the diver during the dive, an important feature for tracking decompression status if using tables. Although the modern digital gauges are relatively accurate, there can occasionally be problems (as there often were with mechanical gauges), and the need to check the accuracy of gauges is often overlooked. Faulty gauges have caused divers to develop DCS.

DIVE COMPUTERS

Dive computers use a depth (pressure) sensor, timer, microprocessor, display and various other features. They are encoded with a decompression algorithm – a set of mathematical equations designed to simulate the uptake and elimination of inert gas within a diver's body. By sampling the depth and recalculating every few seconds, these computers enable dive times well beyond those permitted by tables on most dives, especially on multi-level and repetitive dives. Some of the more sophisticated models take into account ambient temperature and/or gas consumption, and some even measure heart rate (Figure 4.3). However, they can still only 'guesstimate' a diver's actual saturation, and DCS remains a significant concern with computer users. In fact, most people diagnosed with DCS these days have been diving within the limits indicated as theoretically safe by their devices. Users are well advised to use more conservative limits than the 'factory settings'. Some models enable the user to adjust the computer to more conservative modes.

Despite this, dive computers have revolutionized diving because of their flexibility and

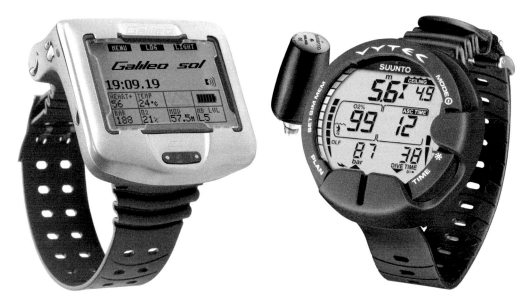

Figure 4.3 Two of the more sophisticated current model recreational dive computers **(a)** Galileo Sol (Scubapro, USA); and **(b)** Vytec (Suunto, Finland).

the vastly increased underwater times enabled. Possibly their greatest contribution to diving safety is the incorporation of ascent rate warnings to caution the wearer when he or she ascends faster than the recommended rate, which is usually substantially slower than traditional rates used with most decompression tables.

CONTENTS GAUGE

The role of this gauge is discussed earlier. The contents gauge indicates the pressure and, by extrapolation, the amount of gas remaining in the supply cylinder.

COMMUNICATION

Because of the risks in diving, it is generally considered foolhardy to dive without some method of summoning assistance. Most commercial divers do this with an underwater telephone or signal line. Divers who do not want the encumbrance of a link to the surface can dive in pairs, commonly called a 'buddy pair'. Each diver has the duty to aid the other if one gets into difficulty. The common problem in the use of the buddy system is attracting the attention of the buddy if he or she is looking elsewhere or if separation has occurred, whether intentional or otherwise.

Underwater audible signalling devices are commercially available and are useful in such circumstances. These are generally driven by breathing gas and are attached to the low-pressure hose in series with the BCD inflator.

DIVER LOCATION DEVICES

Sometimes divers can be difficult to sight on the surface after a dive because of the sea conditions and/or divers surfacing distant from the boat, often swept away by current. This can lead to stranding of divers at sea for extended periods, with some lost forever.

Various devices are available to try to prevent this problem. Commonly used location devices include horns, whistles, mirrors, safety sausages and other surface marker buoys (SMBs). There are also commercially available electronic diver location devices. Some consist of a receiver and a number of transmitters. The receiver is located on the boat (or can be elsewhere), and individual transmitters are issued to divers. This system enables a charter operator to track its divers continuously. Suitable electronic position-indicating radio beacons (EPIRBs) have been developed or adapted for use by divers, and these are becoming more frequently used. One such device is

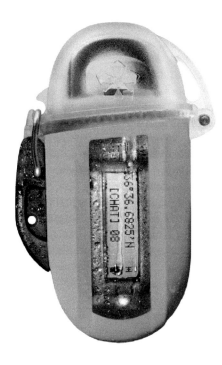

Figure 4.4 Nautilus Lifeline, BC, Canada.

shown in Figure 4.4. They can be especially helpful when diving in remote locations. However, rescue depends on adequate monitoring of distress signals, as well as the willingness and ability of local authorities to perform a search and rescue. This can be a problem in some developing countries.

LINES

A **'mermaid' line** is attached to the stern of the boat and extends down-current. It aids recovery of divers when they surface downstream. (Some call this the 'Jesus line' as it saves sinners – i.e. divers who have erred and surfaced down-current from the dive boat!) This is not needed if a lifeline or pickup boat is being used, or if the current is insignificant.

A **shot line** is a weighted line that hangs down from the dive boat or from a buoy. It is often used to mark the dive site and as a descent and ascent line. It can also be the centre for a circular pattern search. It can be marked with depth markers that can be used to show the decompression stop depths. The diver can hold onto the line at the depth mark. A **lazy shot** line is a weighted line that does not reach the bottom and is used for decompression stops.

A **lead line** is often used to assist the diver on the surface. It leads from the stern of the boat to the anchor chain. It allows the diver, who has entered the water at the stern of the boat, to reach the anchor when the current is too strong to swim to it.

When diving in caves or some wrecks, a 'guide line' should be use. This is a continuous line to the entrance is needed so that it can be followed if the divers become disorientated or when visibility is lost because of torch failure or formation of an opaque cloud by disturbed silt. Each diver should be within arms reach of the main line.

Dive boats

Boats used for diving range from kayaks and canoes to large, specialized vessels that support deep and saturation diving. The facilities required depend on the nature of the diving, but there are minimum requirements. In some conditions, a second safety boat or tender may be needed. Divers may need to be picked up after drifting away from the main vessel.

Propellor guards, or a safe propulsion system such as a water jet, is desirable if there is any chance that the engine will be engaged during diving operations.

A **diving platform** or **ladder** is needed on most boats to facilitate the diver's return from the water. Consideration should be given to the recovery of an unconscious or incapacitated diver, which is ideally done with the diver positioned horizontally. This can be very difficult with both large and small boats, and an appropriate system should be established and practised. Recovery into an inflatable craft is often an easier alternative because the diver can be dragged, rather than lifted, into the boat. Also, the softer air-filled hull is less likely than a rigid hull to injure a diver.

Diving flags, lights or other signals as required by the local maritime regulations should be available. These are designed to warn boat operators to slow down or keep clear. In some places they can offer legal, if not physical, protection from the antics of other craft. Unfortunately, in many places the flag is not recognized or is ignored, and in most areas 'boat propeller attacks' cause more deaths than shark attacks.

The **first aid kit** and **emergency medical equipment** (see Chapter 48) should be chosen depending on local hazards and the distance from assistance.

PROFESSIONAL OR TECHNICAL DIVING EQUIPMENT

This section deals with the more specialized equipment used by professional and military divers, as well as some recreational technical divers. Many of the military diver's tasks, and some of those of the professional diver, involve comparatively shallow depths. Such tasks could be conducted with scuba gear of the type described earlier. Equipment fitted with communication devices allows the diver to confer with the surface support. Communication devices operate better in air, so they are commonly fitted into a helmet or full-face mask. In these devices, the airflow may either be continuous or on demand.

More specialized equipment is used for some military diving where an element of stealth is required. For these tasks, an oxygen rebreathing system that can be operated with no telltale bubbles may be used. In dealing with explosive mines, stealth is again required to avoid activating the noise- or magnetically triggered circuits. If the mine may be too deep for an oxygen set, a rebreathing system with an oxygen-nitrogen mixture may be used.

For even deeper tasks, for which oxygen-helium mixtures are used, some method of reducing the gas loss gives cost and logistical savings. This can be achieved by the diver's using a rebreathing system or returning the exhaled gas to the surface for reprocessing.

Breathing systems

OPEN-CIRCUIT BREATHING SYSTEMS

For most tasks, the professional diver is working in a small area for long periods. Because of this, he or she does not need the mobility of the scuba diver. The breathing gas normally comes from the surface in a hose, either supplied from storage cylinders or compressed as needed by a motor-driven compressor. The cable for the communication system and a hose connected to a depth measuring system are often bound to the gas supply hose. Another hose

with a flow of hot water may also be used to warm the diver. It is normal for the diver to have an alternative supply of breathing gas in a cylinder on his or her back. This supplies the diver with breathing gas if the main supply should fail.

Free-flow systems were used in the first commercial air diving apparatus. The diver was supplied with a continuous flow of air that was pumped down a hose by assistants turning a hand-operated pump. The hand-operated pumps have long gone, but the same principle is still in use. In the most common system, called **standard rig,** the diver's head is in a rigid helmet, joined onto a flexible suit that covers the body. The diver can control buoyancy by controlling the amount of air in the suit. The main problem with the system is that the flow of fresh breathing gas must be sufficient to flush carbon dioxide from the helmet. The flow required to do this is about 50 litres/minute (lpm), measured at the operating depth; this is well in excess of that needed with a demand system.

The other problem associated with free-flow systems and the high gas flow is the noise this generates. In the early days, the diver was also exposed to the risk of a particularly unpleasant form of barotrauma. If the pump or air supply hose breaks, the pressure of the water tends to squeeze the diver's soft tissues up into the helmet. This is prevented by fitting a one-way valve that stops flow back up the hose. For deep dives, where oxygen-helium mixtures are used, the cost of gas becomes excessive. A method of reducing the gas consumed may be fitted. For example, some units incorporate a canister of carbon dioxide absorbent to purify the gas. The gas flow round the circuit is generated by a Venturi system that does away with the need for valves to control gas flow. The rig is converted into a rebreathing system, which has a separate set of problems that are considered in a later section.

Demand systems were developed to gain a reduction in gas consumption compared with free-flow systems. They also enable the diver to talk underwater. Several types of equipment are in common use. One type uses a full-face mask that seals round the forehead, cheeks and under the chin. The back of the diver's head may be exposed to the water or covered with a wetsuit hood that is joined onto the face mask.

Another type is fitted in a full helmet. An oro-nasal mask in the helmet reduces rebreathing of exhaled air. The helmets are often less comfortable than the face masks, but they give better thermal and impact protection.

These helmets may also be used at greater depths, where helium mixtures are used. A return hose may be used to allow collection of the exhaled gas at the surface for reprocessing.

When compared with a demand valve held in the mouth, all the systems mentioned earlier have the major advantage of reducing the chance of the diver's drowning. This is important if the diver becomes unconscious and/or has a convulsion while breathing high partial pressures of oxygen (PO_2). The increased safety and the advantages of a clear verbal communication system have led to the adoption of helmets by most diving firms.

Sets that use a helmet and a full-face mask reduce the risk of drowning and can allow the diver to converse with people on the surface.

REBREATHING SYSTEMS

Respiration is designed to provide our tissues with oxygen and to eliminate carbon dioxide produced by metabolism. When we breathe on the surface, we consume about 25 per cent of the oxygen that we inhale with each breath. Thus, if our respiratory minute volume (RMV) were to be 20 lpm, we would breathe in 4 litres of oxygen each minute, of which 1 litre would be consumed and 3 litres would be exhaled back into the surrounding atmosphere. Although this may not seem very efficient, the situation becomes substantially worse when we descend on open-circuit scuba equipment.

As the depth and pressure increase, the amount of gas we inhale with each breath must also increase to compensate. Thus, at 40 metres (5 ATA), we would need to breathe 100 lpm from our cylinder to achieve the same 20 lpm surface RMV. This 100 litres of air would contain about 20 litres of oxygen, of which 19 litres are being exhaled into the ocean unused!

One solution to this inefficiency of gas consumption is to recirculate the gas, removing the carbon dioxide and adding only the oxygen that is consumed by the diver back into the circuit. This is called a 'rebreather', and such breathing apparatus can offer substantial reductions in gas consumption over open-circuit systems. The following is a summary of some advantages and disadvantages of rebreather systems, which are expanded upon in the following paragraphs:

Advantages

- Vastly reduced gas consumption, especially during deep diving.
- Reduction of cold stress and dehydration by the breathing of warm, humidified gas.
- Lack of bubbles good for photography, covert operations, fragile environments such as caves.
- Improved decompression efficiency because of maintenance of 'optimal PO_2'.
- Excellent duration in relatively small unit.

Disadvantages

- Significant initial cost.
- Greater complexity and vastly increased need for training, vigilance and maintenance.
- Different hazards to diver, higher overall risk.

Rebreathers fall into one of two main types – closed-circuit rebreathers (CCRs) and semi-closed-circuit rebreathers (SCRs). Although both types recirculate all, or part, of the breathing gas, the main difference lies in the way that the oxygen level is controlled and added into the circuit.

In general, SCRs are less complex but less efficient and have depth limitations dependent on the gas selection. CCRs are the most complex but also the most efficient and most capable with regard to depth and duration.

Because of the similarity between SCR and CCR sets, their common features are discussed first, and features peculiar to each type are then highlighted separately.

The usual gas flow pattern found in a rebreathing set is shown in Figure 4.5. The movement of inhaled and exhaled gas is controlled by one-way valves at the mouthpiece as the gas flows round the circuit. For largely historical reasons, rebreathers of UK or European origin usually have a clockwise gas flow pattern, whereas those of US origin have an anticlockwise pattern. However, this is not universally so.

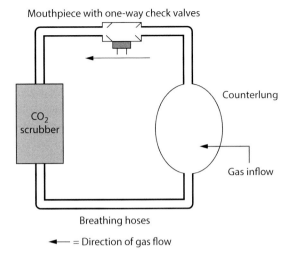

Mouthpiece with one-way check valves

CO₂ scrubber

Counterlung

Gas inflow

Breathing hoses

← = Direction of gas flow

Figure 4.5 A stylised rebreather layout.

As the diver descends, gas must be added from a high-pressure cylinder into the breathing loop so that a constant volume is maintained within the system. In most units, the gas is automatically added via a regulator-type valve (automatic diluent valve [ADV]). A manually controlled valve allows the diver to add extra gas if it is required. This addition of gas will affect buoyancy.

The counterlung acts as a gas storage bag that expands and contracts as the diver breathes. It normally incorporates a relief valve (over-pressure valve [OPV]) that releases surplus gas into the water and prevents excess pressure building up. Venting of excess gas is needed in CCR sets when the diver ascends and the gas in the counterlung expands. In SCR sets, excess gas vents regularly through the relief valve.

The carbon dioxide absorbent is usually a mixture of calcium and sodium hydroxides. These chemicals react with carbon dioxide to form carbonates and water, as shown:

$$M(OH)_2 + CO_2 \rightarrow MCO_3 + H_2O$$

Closed-circuit oxygen systems are the simplest CCR sets. The counterlung is filled with oxygen from the cylinder. As oxygen is consumed, the volume of the bag decreases. In some units, a trigger mechanism that operates like a demand valve releases more gas into the bag. In other units, there is a mechanism that releases

a continuous flow of oxygen into the circuit. A manually operated method of adding oxygen to the breathing bag is also usually fitted. This will be needed when the diver puts the unit on, when he or she goes deeper and the gas in the breathing bag is compressed, or when the diver needs to increase buoyancy.

The unit can be operated as a closed system because, unless something goes wrong, the gas in the breathing bag will contain a high concentration of oxygen, diluted with nitrogen that was in the lungs and body of the diver when he or she put the unit on. It is standard practice to flush the counterlung with oxygen at set intervals to 'denitrogenate' before starting the dive to prevent a build-up of diluting gases.

Possible problems with these units include carbon dioxide toxicity if the absorbent fails, dilution hypoxia if the oxygen is impure or the diver neglects to flush nitrogen from the lungs and the counterlung and oxygen toxicity if the diver descends too deep.

To reduce the risk of oxygen toxicity, a depth limit of about 6 to 8 metres is often imposed on the use of these units to limit the PO_2 to 1.6 to 1.8 ATA, a range generally deemed acceptable for military operations, although too high for recreational technical diving, where a lower risk is appropriate and consequently a PO_2 significantly lower than 1.6 ATA is usually maintained.

Closed oxygen rebreathing apparatus has the particular advantage that a small unit may give a long endurance. A unit weighing less than 15 kg can allow dives of more than 2 hours. The lack of bubbles and quietness of this unit are also important in some specialized roles such as clandestine operations.

> Rebreathing units are quieter and have a greater endurance than scuba units. The extra hazards and costs involved restrict their use and demand significant extra training, maintenance and vigilance.

In **closed-circuit mixed gas systems,** oxygen and a diluting gas are fed into the breathing loop at rates required to keep the PO_2 within safe limits and to provide an adequate volume of the mixture.

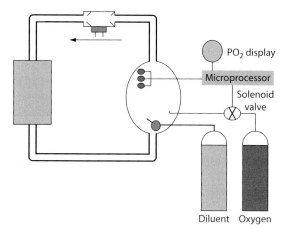

Figure 4.6 Electronic closed-circuit mixed gas rebreather layout.

Figure 4.6 shows the fundamental features of this system.

As with the closed-circuit oxygen unit, the diver inhales breathing gas from the counterlung and exhales through the carbon dioxide absorber back into the counterlung. As the diver consumes oxygen, the PO_2 in the counterlung falls, and this fall is detected by oxygen sensors. At a certain level, a valve injects more oxygen into the circuit. Both mechanically and electronically controlled units are commonly seen in recreational diving, and there has been much controversy as to which arrangement is safer.

Although all rebreather divers should know their PO_2 at all times, the above argument hinges on the requirement for the diver in the manual system to be forced to know his or her PO_2 at all times (although in most systems a basal flow of oxygen is continually bled into the unit). However, the requirement to manage the PO_2 in this system can create problems during times of high task loading. In contrast, there is less obvious compulsion for the diver using an electronic rebreather to know the PO_2 at all times, and should the controlling computer fail, the diver would be at risk, although the chances that the computer will fail in an electronic rebreather are very low. The reality is that, to date, neither system has been shown to offer a survival advantage and all rebreather divers should make a habit of knowing their PO_2 at all times.

Most modern mixed gas CCRs use a series of three redundant oxygen sensors (galvanic fuel cells)

to track the PO_2 in the loop. This allows for the comparison of the outputs of the sensors because they are relatively fragile and prone to failure, as well as having a limited life (usually ~18 months).

If the volume of gas in the bag falls, this triggers a second valve that adds diluting gas (diluent) from a separate cylinder. Air, trimix (helium, nitrogen and oxygen) or heliox (helium and oxygen) may be used as the diluent depending on the planned depth and profile of the dive. The selection of the gas is determined largely by oxygen toxicity and work of breathing issues. For the former, the diluent gas should not have a PO_2 greater than a predetermined set-point at depth (preferably a little lower so that an 'oxygen spike' does not happen during descent when diluent is added to the loop). To manage the latter, the diver should calculate the density of the gas at the proposed maximum depth, such that it does not exceed the manufacturer's recommendation and maintains the work of breathing within the specifications of the unit.

Manual controls and displays indicating the oxygen concentration are often fitted to allow the diver to override the controls if the automatic control fails. In many cases, divers also either raise the 'set-point' or flush the unit with oxygen during the final decompression stop at 6 metres to shorten decompression time.

This system would appear to be the most efficient breathing system. It is more economical in terms of gas usage than any other gear apart from the oxygen-breathing apparatus. It enables a diver to go deeper for longer and with fewer encumbrances than other equipment.

As an example of the efficiency of this type of equipment, it has been estimated that in a helium saturation dive program involving a prolonged series of dives to 180 metres, the cost of helium for a CCR apparatus was about 2.5 per cent of the cost of an SCR diving apparatus. These advantages must be balanced against the greater initial cost and complexity of the system. This complexity can lead to fatal malfunctions.

SCRs offer some of the saving in gas obtained in the closed systems while avoiding the depth limitations of the oxygen sets and the greater complexity of the closed mixed gas sets. The basic system is shown in Figure 4.7.

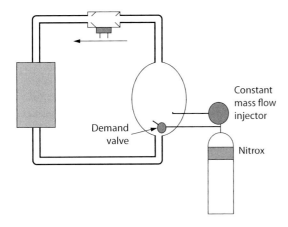

Figure 4.7 Semi-closed rebreathing system.

SCRs typically use oxygen-enriched air (nitrox) as the breathing mix instead of oxygen. Two major types of SCR are in common use. The most common is the constant mass flow (CMF) type, but the keyed respiratory minute volume (RMV keyed) type has some advocates, especially with US cave divers.

In a typical CMF SCR system, the gas flow and composition are chosen for maximum efficiency for the proposed dive. First, the composition of the gas is chosen, with as high an oxygen concentration as possible without creating an unacceptable risk of oxygen toxicity at the planned maximum depth. This level may be changed depending on the duration of exposure. The flow is then chosen so that the diver will receive sufficient oxygen while working on the surface.

The oxygen concentration in the diver's inspired gas is determined by the flow into the system, the diver's consumption and loss through the relief valve. It ranges from close to that in the supply bottle when the diver is resting down to about 20 per cent when the diver is working at the maximum expected rate.

In the RMV keyed sets, a fixed volume of gas is dumped from the circuit with each breath, with 'new' gas added via a demand valve.

As a safety precaution with an SCR, almost invariably an excess of gas is added to the loop and is vented through the relief valve, thus making these devices less efficient on gas than CCRs. However, an SCR system with a flow of 12 lpm gives an eightfold saving of gas compared with a demand system when the diver is consuming 1 lpm of oxygen. This saving would increase if the scuba diver was working harder and consuming more air.

The high oxygen concentrations in both SCR and CCR systems mean that the diver may not absorb as much nitrogen as he or she would if breathing air. This can give a decrease in the decompression needed, but unless the PO_2 in the loop is actually measured, the diver must 'guess-timate' the PO_2 for decompression purposes. On occasion, this has resulted in problems.

Military divers have traditionally been the main users of SCR sets, although they have become increasingly popular in recreational diving. The reduced gas flow with these sets means that they can be designed to make little noise. If they are constructed from non-magnetic materials, they can be used for dives near mines, although CCRs are now more often used for mine countermeasures.

Problems with rebreathers

Both CCR and SCR systems introduce a variety of potential hazards (see Chapter 62):

Carbon dioxide accumulation can occur if the scrubber fails. This can occur if the scrubber material is used for too long, if the scrubber is incorrectly attached or if the scrubber's instantaneous capacity to remove carbon dioxide is exceeded because of a diver's high demand, such as with exertion.

Oxygen toxicity can occur if the diver exceeds his or her depth limit, descends too quickly when diving at a particular PO_2 (set-point) or uses a mixture with too much oxygen in it. This can occur if an excessively oxygen-rich mix was added to the diluent cylinder or if the solenoid or manual oxygen injection valves jam open.

Hypoxia may result if the gas flow decreases. This can be caused by omitting to turn on the gas supply before descending, exhausting the oxygen supply, solenoid or electronics failure, and ascending too rapidly to enable the solenoid to add sufficient oxygen to the loop. Hypoxia can also occur if the diver works harder than expected or if a mix with too little oxygen is used.

A review of the 181 reported recreational CCR-related deaths that occurred between 1998 and 2010 estimated that the fatality rate for CCR users was about 10 times that of recreational open-circuit divers. The author also suggested that CCRs have a 25-fold increased risk of component failure compared with manifolded twin-cylinder open-circuit systems. It was suggested that this risk could be partly offset by carrying a redundant bail-out system.

Chambers, habitats and underwater vehicles

Divers may use several special types of vehicles and living facilities. These include vehicles that are hoisted and lowered to transport divers to and from deep dive sites, propelled vehicles to increase the diver's range and endurance (i.e. diver propulsion vehicles [DPVs], often used by technical divers) and machines to carry underwater equipment. The accommodations to be considered include underwater houses and pressurized houses at the surface.

Submersible decompression chambers (SDCs), often called personnel transfer capsules, are used to transport divers and any attendants from the surface to the work site, and they may also be used as a relay station and store for gas and equipment. The most complex SDC may carry the diver at constant pressure from a deck decompression chamber (DDC) to the work site and back. The simplest SDC consists of a bell chamber that is open at the bottom and allows the diver to decompress in a dry environment, exposed to the same pressure as the surrounding water.

Habitats are underwater houses that accommodate divers in air- or gas-filled environments. They are used by divers to rest between excursions. Divers have lived in some of these habitats for weeks at a time.

Deck decompression chambers (DDCs) can be small and used for surface decompression, a procedure that allows a diver to be decompressed in a dry chamber instead of in the water. Larger chambers can be used to treat divers with decompression illness and other diseases that respond to compression, in which case the chamber may be called a **recompression chamber.**

DDCs are also used to house divers for prolonged periods under elevated pressure. In this case, divers are carried to their work by an SDC or a small submarine that keeps the diver in a pressurized environment. At the end of the job, possibly after several weeks, the pressure in the DDC is lowered slowly to return the diver to atmospheric pressure.

Transport vehicles can carry the divers at normal atmospheric pressure, at ambient pressure in a dry environment or in a wet environment. These include vehicles towed by a boat. A small motor and propeller that pulls the diver along gives increased speed with reduced effort. Some submarines have a lock system to allow divers to leave and enter underwater.

One atmosphere diving equipment, such as the **JIM suit,** seals the diver in a pressure-resistant compartment. It has flexible arms with tools on the 'hands' for the diver to work underwater. The early types of suit had legs that gave the diver the ability to walk on firm surfaces if there was little current. The diver had no control in mid-water and had to be lowered and hoisted from the surface. In other designs, such as the **Newtsuit** and **WASP** system, the diver controls a set of propellers that make him or her a cross between a diver and a one-person submarine.

Life support systems are required to provide the occupants of all these vehicles, habitats and chambers with a respirable atmosphere. These work on the same principles as a diver's breathing apparatus, and in some vehicles the diver may even be wearing a breathing apparatus. The system must be self-contained for transport vehicles, but for habitats and SDCs the gas is generally supplied from the surface.

Gas from the surface can be supplied in a free flow and escape out the bottom or be recirculated through a purifying system. Simple gas purifying systems can involve a hand-powered pump to force gas through a carbon dioxide absorption canister with a manually operated system for adding oxygen. The most complex systems are those found on large submersibles, nuclear submarines and chambers used for deep saturation dives. These have automatic closed systems with provision for removing trace contaminants and odours, and they also regulate temperature, pressure and humidity.

Gas reclaimers are mainly used to recover helium to be used again. They help to lower costs by reducing the amount of gas used. One type cools the gas until the other gases are liquefied, leaving pure helium to be stored and used again. Other types use a chromatographic technique to separate the gases.

FURTHER READING

Bozanic JE. *Mastering Rebreathers*. Flagstaff, Arizona: Best Publishing Company; 2002.

Fock A. Analysis of recreational closed-circuit rebreather deaths 1998–2010. *Diving and Hyperbaric Medicine* 2010;**43**(2):78–85.

Mitchell SJ, Cronjé FJ, Meintjes J, Britz HC. Fatal respiratory failure during a technical rebreather dive at extreme pressure. *Aviation, Space and Environmental Medicine* 2007;**78**(2):81–86.

Rebreather Forum 3. http://www.rf30.org/presentation/

US Navy Diving Manual Revision 6 SS521-AG-PRO-010 (2008). Washington, DC: Naval Sea Systems Command; 2008.

This chapter was reviewed for this fifth edition by John Lippmann.

5

Undersea environments

INTRODUCTION

For the diver who is adequately trained and physically fit, who is aware of the limitations of the equipment and who appreciates the specific requirements of different environmental diving conditions, the sea is rarely dangerous. Nevertheless, it can be hazardous and unforgiving if attention is not paid to all these factors.

Diver training is specific to the environment in which the diver is trained. Specialized techniques are recommended to cope with different environments. They cannot be automatically extrapolated to other diving environments. The induction of fear in the inexperienced diver and of physical stress in the more skilled diver is appreciated only when one examines each specific environmental threat. These environmental stresses are mentioned in this and other chapters. The reason for including them in a medical text is that unless the physician comprehends the problems and dangers, the medical examinations for diving fitness and the assessments of diving accidents will be less than adequate.

Some aspects of the environments have physiological and pathological sequelae and therefore have specific chapters devoted to them. They include

the effects of cold (see Chapters 27 and 28), altitude and fresh water diving (see Chapter 2), explosives (see Chapter 34), depth (see Chapters 2, 15, 20, 46 and 68) and marine animal injuries (see Chapters 31 and 32). Other environmental topics that are covered more comprehensively in diving texts are summarized in this chapter.

Being kept underwater and exceeding the limited air supply will result in drowning. This is a situation common to many of the hazardous environments, including caves and wrecks and under ice, overhangs, water flows and so forth. A variety of materials can trap the diver, including kelp, lines (even 'safety' lines), fishing nets and fishing lines. If the diver does not have a compromised air supply, then knowledge of the environment, a buddy, a communication facility, a calm state of mind and a diving knife or scissors will cope with most of these circumstances.

ALTITUDE DIVING

The term *altitude diving* refers to diving at an altitude of 300 metres or more above sea level. Non-diving disorders should be considered, such as the dyspnoea and hypoxia induced by high altitude and the altitude sickness that frequently develops above 3000 metres. Diving at altitudes higher than this is strongly discouraged.

The following numerical examples do not represent actual diving conditions and are used to explain the problems as simply as possible, thus avoiding complicated mathematics. The conventional idea of diving is that a diver descends with the sea surface (1 ATA) as the reference point and returns there when he or she has finished the dive. A diver may have to dive at altitude, in a mountain lake or dam, where the pressure on the surface is less than 1 ATA. Problems stem from the physics at this altitude.

For simplicity's sake, the following description is based on the useful, but not strictly correct, traditional theory that the ratio between the pressure reached during the dive and the final pressure determines the decompression required. If this ratio is less than 2:1, then a diver can ascend safely without pausing during ascent. This means that a diver from the sea surface (1 ATA) can dive to 10 metres (2 ATA) and ascend safely, as regards decompression requirements. A diver operating in a high mountain lake, with a surface pressure of 0.5 ATA, could dive only to 5 metres (1 ATA) before he or she had to worry about decompression. This statement ignores the minor correction required with fresh water. Fresh water is less dense than salt water.

Another pressure problem occurs when a diver, who dives at sea level, then flies or ascends into the mountains after the dive. For example, a 5-metre dive (1.5 ATA) from sea level could be followed by an immediate ascent to a pressure (altitude) of 0.75 ATA, with little theoretical risk. Deeper dives or greater ascents may require the diver to pause at sea level if the diver is to avoid decompression sickness. If the diver ascends, in a motor vehicle or an airplane, the reduced pressure will expand 'silent' bubbles or increase the gas gradient to produce larger bubbles, thereby aggravating the diseases of pulmonary barotrauma and decompression sickness.

Thus, exposure to altitude after diving, or diving at altitude, increases the danger of decompression sickness, compared with identical dives and exposures at sea level. It influences the decompression obligations, the depths and durations of decompression stops, the nitrogen load in tissues afterward, the safe durations before flying or repetitive diving, the ascent rates recommended during diving and so forth. Formulae are available to convert the equivalent altitude decompressions to sea level decompressions.

Another problem of diving in a high-altitude lake is the rate at which a diver may have to exhale during ascent. A diver who ascends from 10 metres (2 ATA) to the ocean surface (1 ATA) would find that the volume of gas in the lungs has doubled. Most divers realize this and exhale at a controlled rate during ascent. They may not realize that an equivalent doubling in gas volume occurs in only 5 metres of ascent to the surface, if the dive was carried out at an altitude (pressure) of 0.5 ATA. Equivalent effects are encountered with buoyancy, which can more rapidly get out of control at altitude.

The diver's equipment can also be affected or damaged by high-altitude exposure. Some pressure gauges start to register only when the pressure is greater than 1 ATA. These gauges (oil-filled, analogue and mechanical types) may try to indicate a negative depth, perhaps bending the needle, until the diver reaches 1 ATA pressure. Thus, the dive depth would have to reach more than 5 metres before it even started measuring, if the dive had commenced at an altitude of 0.5 ATA.

The other common depth gauge, a capillary tube, indicates the depth by an air-water boundary. It automatically adjusts to the extent that it always reads zero depth on the surface. The volume of gas trapped in the capillary decreases with depth (Boyle's Law). For a diver starting from 0.5 ATA altitude, this gauge would read zero, but it would show that the diver had reached 10 metres when he or she was only at 5 metres depth. Theoretically, the diver could plan the dive and decompression according to this 'gauge' depth, but only if he or she was very courageous.

Many electronic dive computers do permit correction for altitude, and some need to be 're-zoned' at the dive site. Other decompression meters are damaged by exposure to altitude (e.g. as in aircraft travel), and the applicability of other dive computers to altitude diving or saturation excursions is questionable.

Divers who fly from sea level to dive at altitude, as in high mountain lakes, may commence the dive with an already existing nitrogen load in excess of that of the local divers, who have equilibrated at the lower pressures. Thus, the 'sea level' divers are in effect doing a repetitive dive, and 'residual nitrogen' tables must be employed.

Decompression tables that supply acceptable modifications for altitude exposure include the Buhlmann and Canadian Defence and Civil Institute of Environmental Medicine (DCIEM) tables (see Appendix A).

Altitude exposure and altitude diving are more hazardous extensions of conventional diving. They are not as well researched, and the greater the altitude, the more applicable is this statement. It includes not only the problems already mentioned, but also the complication of diving in fresh, often very cold, water. This water may contain debris that has not decomposed as it would in the ocean and may therefore threaten entrapment. The sites are often distant from diving medical facilities. Undertaking a specialized course in altitude diving is a basic prerequisite.

CAVE AND WRECK DIVING

These enclosed environments are hazardous to open water divers. Cave diving and wreck diving are more complex than they first appear. Completion of the open water scuba training course is inadequate preparation for cave and wreck diving. Planning involves not only the setting of goal-oriented objectives, but the delineation of maximum limits (depths, distances). The main problems are as follows:

- No direct ascent to the surface (i.e. safety).
- Disorientation and entrapment.
- Loss of visibility.
- Enclosed spaces and panic.

Cave diving

The techniques of cave diving are very rigidly delineated. Specialized training includes dive planning, the use of reels and lines and the lost diver protocols. Most people who have difficulties with cave diving have not followed the recommended rules, and unfortunately cave diving problems tend to cause multiple fatalities.

The diver descends, often through a small access, passes down a shaft, goes around a few bends and is faced with multiple passages, in total darkness. Under these conditions, and to make this particular type of diving safe, it is necessary to be accompanied by a diver who has considerable cave experience – in that cave – and whose judgement is trustworthy. It is equally important that the equipment is both suited to cave diving and totally replaceable with spares during the dive. Apart from the obvious environmental difficulties inherent in diving through a labyrinth of passageways, there are added specific problems.

Safety in cave diving is not usually achievable by immediate surfacing. Thus, all necessary equipment must be duplicated for a long return swim, at depth, and possibly while rescuing a disabled companion.

Air pockets found in the top of caves are sometimes non-respirable because of low oxygen and high carbon dioxide levels (especially in limestone caves), so when entering this pocket, breathing should be continued from the scuba equipment. Sometimes the roof of the cave is supported by the water, and when this water is replaced by air from the diver's tanks, the roof can collapse. The common claim that 'the diver was so unlucky for the roof to collapse while he was there' is incorrect. It collapsed because he was there.

The minimum extra safety equipment includes a compass, powerful lights and a safety reel and line. It is a diving axiom that entry into a cave is based on the presumption that the return will have to be carried out in zero visibility.

For visibility, each diver takes at least two lights; however, other factors can interfere with the function of these lights. A great danger is the silt that can be stirred up if the diver swims along the lower part of the cave or in a head-up position (as when negatively buoyant). If there is little natural water movement, clay silts can be very fine and easily stirred up. It is for this reason that fins should be small, and the diver should be neutrally buoyant and should swim more than a metre above the bottom of the cave. Visibility can be totally lost in a few seconds as the silt curtain ascends, and it may remain that way for weeks. Sometimes it is inevitable, as exhaled bubbles dislodge silt from the ceiling. Layering of salt and fresh waters also causes visual distortion and blurring.

The usual equipment includes double tanks manifolded together, making a common air supply, but offering two regulator outlets. With the failure of one regulator, the second one may be used for the air supply – or as an octopus rig. The second regulator must have a long hose, given that often divers cannot swim alongside each other. Because of space limitations, buddy breathing is often impractical under cave conditions. An extra air supply ('pony' bottle) is advisable.

For recreational divers to explore caves, the ideal equipment is a reliable compressed air surface supply, with a complete scuba back-up rig.

All the instruments should be standardized; e.g. the watch goes on the left wrist, the depth gauge above it, the compass on the right wrist and the dive computer (this can include a contents gauge, decompression meter, dive profile display, compass) attached to the harness under the left arm. The gauges and decompression must be modified for fresh water and altitude, if these are applicable. The knife is strapped to the inside of the left leg, to prevent entanglement on any safety lines.

The buoyancy compensator is often bound down at the top, to move the buoyancy centre more toward the centre of gravity (cave divers do not need to be vertical with the head out of water). There is no requirement for excess buoyancy because safety in cave diving is not usually equated with a direct ascent; thus, any carbon dioxide cylinders should be removed and replaced with exhausted ones to prevent accidental inflation of vests. A principle of cave diving is that safety lies in retracing the entry path by the use of lines and not by ascent, as in the normal open ocean diving.

Preferably no more than three divers should undertake a single dive, and on completion of the dive each should have a minimum of one third of the initial air supply. If there is water flow within the cave, and the penetration is with the flow, this reserve air supply may not be adequate because the air consumption is greater when returning against the current.

Vertical penetrations need a heavy shot line moored or buoyed at the surface and weighted or fixed at the bottom. The reel is used for horizontal penetrations, not vertical. Otherwise, entanglement is likely with rapid ascents, especially if divers precede the lead diver. Thin, non-floating lines especially cause entanglement if they are allowed to slacken.

Specialized cave diving training is a prerequisite for this diving environment.

Wreck diving

Wreck diving has potentially similar problems to some cave and ice diving. In addition, it has the hazards of instability of the structure and the dangers of unexploded ordnance, sharp objects, toxic cargo and fuel. Exhausted gas from scuba may cause air pockets and disrupt the wreck's stability.

Silt in wrecks is usually heavier than that in still water caves. Thus, the sudden loss of visibility that can occur when silt is stirred up may be less persistent. The diver should ascend as far as is safe and wait until the silt cloud settles down.

COLD/ICE DIVING

The obvious problems are those of cold and hypothermia. They are so obvious that most people will avoid them by the use of heating systems, drysuits or efficient wetsuits. See Chapters 27 and 28 for the effects of a cold environment on physiological performance.

A major difficulty with cold and ice diving is the tendency of many single hose regulators to freeze, usually in the free-flow position, after about 20 to 30 minutes of exposure to very cold water (less than 5°C). This situation is aggravated if there is water vapour (potential ice crystals) in the compressed air and if there is a rapid expansion of air, which produces further cooling in both first and second stages. The first stage or the second stage may then freeze internally.

Expansion of air as it passes from the high tank pressure to the lower pressure demand valve and then to environmental pressures (adiabatic expansion) results in a drop in temperature. It is therefore not advisable to purge regulators if exposed to very cold temperatures. The freezing from increased air flow follows exertion, hyperventilation or panic. Octopus rigs become more problematic to use under these conditions, or at great depth, because of this increased air flow. An emergency air source (pony bottle) has replaced buddy breathing and octopus rigs.

'External' ice is formed in and around the first (depth compensated) stage of the regulator, thus blocking the orifice and interfering with the spring. Moisture from the diver's breath or water in the exhalation chamber of the second stage may also freeze the demand mechanism, causing free flow of gas or 'internal' freezing with no flow.

Modifications designed to reduce freezing of the water in the first stage include the use of very dry air and the replacement of first-stage water-containing areas with silicone, oils or alcohols (which require lower temperatures to freeze) or with an air flow from the regulator. The newer, non-metallic second stages are less susceptible to freezing. Despite all this, regulator freezing is common in polar and ice diving. Surface supply with an emergency scuba, or twin tank–twin regulator diving, as with cave diving, is probably safer. It must be presumed in under-ice diving that the regulator will freeze and induce an out-of-air situation, and this must be planned for.

Under ice there is little use for snorkels, and so these should be removed to reduce the likelihood of snagging. Rubber suits can become sharp and brittle. Zippers are best avoided because they freeze and may also allow water and heat exchange. Buoyancy compensators should be small and with an independent air supply.

As a general rule, and if well-fitting drysuits are unavailable, the minimum thickness of the Neoprene should increase with decreased water temperatures, as in the following examples:

<5°C – 9-mm-thick wetsuit
<10°C – 7-mm-thick wetsuit
<20°C – 5-mm-thick wetsuit
<30°C – 3-mm-thick wetsuit

Hood, gloves and booties should be of a considerable thickness, or heat pads can be used. Heat pads must not be in contact with high-oxygen gases because overheating can result.

Unheated wetsuits do not give sufficient insulation at depth (beyond 18 metres) when the Neoprene becomes too compressed and loses much of its insulating ability. In that case, non-compressible wetsuits, inflatable drysuits or heated suits are required. In Antarctic diving, to gain greater duration, we had to employ a wetsuit or other thick clothing under a drysuit.

Ice diving is in many ways similar to cave diving. It is essential that direct contact must always be maintained with the entry-exit area. This should be by a heavy-duty line attached to the diver via a bowline knot. The line must also be securely fastened at the surface, as well as on the diver. The dive should be terminated as soon as there is a reduced gas supply or any suggestion of cold exposure with shivering, diminished manual dexterity and so forth.

The entry hole through the ice should be at least two divers wide. Allowing room for only one diver to enter ignores two facts. First, the hole tends to close over by freezing. Second, in an emergency two divers may need to exit simultaneously. There should be a surface tender with at least one standby diver. A bright light, hanging below the surface at the entry-exit hole, is also of value in identifying the opening. If large diving mammals contest the opening in the ice, they should be given right of way.

If the penetration under the ice is in excess of a distance equated with a breath-hold swim, then a back-up scuba system is a requirement, as with cave diving.

DEEP DIVING

'Divers do it deeper' represents a problem with ego trippers and a challenge to adventure seekers. Unfortunately, the competitive element sometimes overrides logic, and divers become enraptured, literally, with the desire to dive deeper. They then move into a dark, eerie world where colours do not penetrate, where small difficulties expand, where safety is farther away and where the leisure of recreational diving is replaced with an intense time urgency.

Beyond the 30-metre limit the effect of narcosis becomes obvious, at least to observers. The gas supply is more rapidly exhausted and the regulator is less efficient. Buoyancy, resulting from wetsuit compression, has become negative, with an inevitable reliance on problematic equipment, such as the buoyancy compensator. The reserve air supply does not last as long, and the buoyancy compensator inflation takes longer and uses more air. Emergency procedures, especially free and buoyant ascents, are more difficult. The decompression tables are less reliable, and ascent rates become more critical.

Overcoming some problems leads to unintended consequences. Heliox (helium-oxygen mixtures) reduces the narcosis of nitrogen, but at the expense of thermal stress, communication and altered decompression obligations. Inadequate gas supplies can be compensated by larger and heavier cylinders, or even by rebreathing equipment, but with many adverse sequelae (see Chapter 62).

Many of the older, independent instructors would qualify recreational divers only to 30 metres. Now, with instructor organizations seeking other ways of separating divers from their dollars, specialty courses may be devised to entice divers to 'go deep' before they have adequately mastered the shallows.

FRESH WATER DIVING

The main problem with fresh water is that it is not the medium in which most divers were trained. Thus, their buoyancy appreciation is distorted. Acceptable weights in sea water may be excessive in fresh water. Depth gauges are calibrated for sea water, and so they need to be corrected for diving in dams, lakes, quarries and so forth. Because these waters are often stationary, there may be dramatic thermoclines, requiring adjustments for thermal protection and buoyancy, as one descends.

There are also many organisms that are destroyed by sea water but that thrive in warm fresh water. Some of these, such as *Naegleria,* are fatal.

KELP DIVING

Kelp beds are the equivalent of underwater forests. Kelp can be useful in many ways to the diver. It allows a good estimate of clarity of the water by assessing the length of plant seen from the surface. The kelp blades indicate the direction of the prevailing current. In kelp beds there is usually an abundance of marine life, and the kelp offers other benefits such as dampening wave action both in the area and the adjacent beach. Kelp can be used

as an anchor chain for people to use when they are equalizing their ears, as well as to attach other objects such as floats, diver's flags, surf mats, specimen bags and so forth.

Giant members of this large brown algae or seaweed may grow in clear water to depths of 30 metres. The growth is less in turbid or unclear water. Kelp usually grows on hard surfaces, e.g. a rocky bottom, a reef or, for more romantic divers, a Spanish galleon. It is of interest commercially because it is harvested to produce alginates, which are useful as thickening, suspending and emulsifying agents, as well as in stabilizing the froth on the diver's glass of beer (*après dive,* of course).

Kelp has caused many diving accidents, often with the diver totally bound up into a 'kelp ball' that becomes a coffin. The danger of entanglement is related to panic actions and/or increased speed and activity of the diver while in the kelp bed. Twisting and turning produce entanglement.

Divers who are accustomed to kelp diving usually take precautions to ensure that there is no equipment that can snag the strands of kelp; i.e. they tend to wear knives on the inside of the leg, tape the buckles on the fin straps, have snug quick-release buckles and not use lines. Divers descend vertically feet first to where the stems are thicker and there is less foliage to cause entanglement. The epitome of bad practice in kelp diving is to perform a head first roll or back roll because it tends to result in a 'kelp sandwich with a diver filling'.

The kelp is pushed away by divers as they slowly descend and ascend; i.e. they produce a clear area within the kelp, into which they then move. They ensure that they do not run out of air because this situation will produce more rapid activity. If they do become snagged, divers should avoid unnecessary hand and fin movements. Kelp can be separated either by the use of a knife or by bending it to 180 degrees, when it will often snap (this is more difficult to achieve while wearing gloves). It is unwise to cut kelp from the regulator with a knife without first clearly differentiating it from the regulator hose. Some divers have suggested biting the strands with one's teeth. This may be excellent as regards dietary supplementation, kelp being high in both B vitamins and iodine, but it does seem overly dramatic.

Kelp does float, and it can often be traversed on the surface by a very slow form of dog paddling or 'kelp crawl', in which one actually crawls along the surface of the water, over the kelp. This can be done only if the body and legs are kept flat on the surface, thus using the buoyancy of both the body and the kelp, and by using the palms of the hands to push the kelp below and behind as one proceeds forward. Any kicking that is performed must be very shallow and slow.

NIGHT DIVING

Because of the impaired visibility, extra care is needed for night diving. Emergency procedures are not as easy to perform without vision. There is a greater fear at night. For inexperienced divers it is advisable to remain close to the surface, the bottom or some object (e.g. anchor, lines). Free swimming mid-water and without objects to focus on causes apprehension to many divers.

Preferably the site should be familiar, at least in daylight, without excessive currents or water movements and with easy beach access – diving between the boat and the shore. On entry the diver sometimes encounters surface debris that was not obvious from the surface.

Any navigational aid needs to be independently lighted. This includes the boat, the exit, buoys, buddies and so forth. A chemoluminescent glow stick (Cyalume light) should be attached firmly to the tank valve, and at least two reliable torches should be carried. The snorkel should have a fluorescent tip. A compass is usually required. A whistle and a day-night distress flare are sometimes of great value in summoning the boat operator, who has not the same capabilities of detecting divers at night.

Marine creatures are sometimes more difficult to see. Accidents involving submerged stingrays and needle spine sea urchins are more likely.

Signals include a circular torch motion ('I am OK, how about you?') or rapid up and down movements ('something is wrong'). The light should never be shone at a diver's face because it blinds him or her momentarily. Traditional signals can be given by shining the light onto the signaling hand. Waving a light in an arc, on the surface, is a sign requesting pickup.

WATER MOVEMENTS

Because of the force of water movement, a diver can become a hostage to the sea.

White water

This water is white because of the foaming effect of air bubbles. This dramatically interferes with both visibility and buoyancy, as well as implying strong currents or turbulent surface conditions. A diver in white water is a diver in trouble. Under these conditions, the recommendation is usually to dive deeper.

Surge

The to-and-fro movement of water produces disorientation and panic in inexperienced divers, who often try to swim against it. Other divers use the surge by swimming with it, then hold onto rocks or corals when the surge moves in the opposite direction. This approach may be detrimental to the ecology, but good for survival.

Inlets and outlets

Occasionally, there is a continuous water flow, because of a **pressure gradient** through a restricted opening, which can siphon and hold (or even extrude) the diver. It is encountered in some *caves, blue holes* or *rock areas near surf* (an underwater 'blow hole'), in human-made structures such as the water inlets in *ships' hulls* and in outlets in *dams* and water cocks (taps). The pressure gradient may slowly draw the diver into its source and then seal him or her in, like a bath plug. Protection is by not occluding these inlets and by avoiding the area or covering it with a large grating.

Tidal currents

These currents are very important to the diver. If used correctly, they take the diver where he or she wants to go. Otherwise, they are likely to take the diver where he or she does not want to go. The latter event can be both embarrassing and terrifying, and it can also be very physically demanding.

Frequently, divers are lost at sea because of currents. Sometimes these currents can be vertical and cannot be combated by swimming or buoyancy. Certain popular diving areas, such as at Palau (especially Pelalu), Ras Muhammad, the Great Barrier Reef and Cozumel, are famous for their currents, and multiple fatalities are not uncommon.

Divers sometimes relate their successful swims against 4- to 5-knot currents. In fact, the average fast swim approximates 1.2 knots. For brief periods, it may be possible to reach up to 1.5 knots. The average swimmer can make very slow progress or none at all against a 1-knot current. A half-knot current is tolerable, but most divers experience this as a significant problem, and so it is. They tend to exaggerate the speed of the current as the hours go by, and especially during the *après-dive* euphoria (1 knot = approximately 2 km/hour).

Tidal currents are usually much faster on the surface than they are on the sea bed because of friction effects. A helpful observation is that the boat will usually face the current with its anchor upstream and the stern of the boat downstream. Any diver worth his or her salt knows that it is safer to swim against the current for the first half of the usable air and allow the current to bring the diver back to the boat for the second half of the dive. The '**half-tank rule**' is worked out by taking the initial pressure, say 200 ATA, subtract the 'reserve' pressure (the pressure needed to charge the regulator), say 40 ATA, i.e. 160 ATA, and divide this by 2, i.e. 80 ATA. Thus, for this example, 80 ATA is used on the outward trip, and then the return is made with ample air to allow for misadventure (e.g. navigational error).

Untrained divers tend to make unplanned dives. They submerge and 'just have a look around'. While they are having their look around they are being transported by the current, away from the boat, at a rate of 30 metres every minute in a 1-knot current. When they consider terminating the dive, after they have used most of their air, they have a very hard return swim against the current. They surface, because of their diminished air supply, well downstream from the boat and have to cope with a faster, surface current. This is a very difficult situation and far more hazardous, than that of the experienced diver who used the half-tank rule, who surfaced upstream from the boat and floated back to it, but who also had enough air to descend

underwater and return with ease if desired or to rescue a companion.

The **lines** attached to the boat are of extreme importance when there are currents. First, there is the *anchor line,* and this is the recommended way to reach the sea bed upstream from the boat. The anchor chain should not be followed right down to the anchor because this may occasionally move if the boat moves, and it can cause damage to the adjacent divers. More than one diver has lost an eye from this 'freak accident'. How may the diver reach the anchor line? A line may be attached to the top of the anchor line, with the other end to the stern of the boat. It should have enough play in it to allow divers to sit on the side of the boat and to hold it with one hand – the hand nearest the bow of the boat – while using the other hand to keep the face mask and demand valve in place. On entry, the diver ensures that he or she does not let go the line. The diver then pulls himself or herself forward to the anchor line and descends.

Perhaps the most important line, if there is a current, is a *float line* or *'Jesus' line*. This line drags 100 metres or more behind the boat, in the direction of the current, and it has some floats to ensure that it is always visible to divers on the surface. It is often of value to have one diver on this line while the others are entering the water. The diver on the line virtually acts as a backstop to catch the odd stray diver who has not followed instructions and is now floating away with the current. The Jesus line is also of immense value at the end of the dive when divers have, incorrectly, exhausted their air supply or when they come to the surface for some other reason and find themselves behind the boat. This would not have happened had a dive plan been constructed and followed correctly. Occasionally, however, it does happen to the best divers, and it is of great solace to realize that the Jesus line is there and ready to save the sinner – irrespective of religious persuasion.

Even divers who surface only a short way behind the boat in a strong surface current may find that it is impossible to make headway without a Jesus line. If this is not available, they can descend and use their compass to navigate back to the anchor line or inflate the buoyancy compensator, attract the attention of the boat lookout and hope to be rescued.

Buddy breathing while swimming against a strong current is often impossible. Even the octopus (spare) regulator is problematic at depth or when two people are simultaneously demanding large volumes of air, typical of divers swimming against a current. An alternative air supply (a reserve or pony bottle) is of value, if it has an adequate capacity.

In dive planning, there should be at least one accessible fixed diving exit, easily identifiable, that serves as a safe haven. This may be an anchored boat, in areas with tidal currents. The safety boat is a second craft – not anchored – and this, like any boat that is driven among divers, needs a guard on its propeller. To attract the safety boat, various rescue options include the following:

- A towed buoy.
- An inflatable 2-metre-long bag, called the 'safety sausage', to attract attention.
- Pressure tested distress flare (smoke/light).
- Personal floatation devices.
- Personal electronic, sonic or luminous location devices.

Divers can now carry a personal location beacon or emergency position-indicating radio beacon (EPIRB), especially of value if diving in fast currents. These devices need to be pressure protected and are of value only once on the surface.

There are other problems with currents, and these are especially related to general boat safety and ensuring that there is a stable anchorage.

When the current is too strong or the depth or sea bed is not suited to an anchored boat, a float or **drift dive** may be planned. This requires extreme care in boat handling. Divers remain together and carry a float to inform the safety boat of their position. It allows the surface craft to maintain its position behind the divers as they drift.

The concept of 'hanging' an anchor, with divers drifting in the water near it and the boat being at the mercy of the elements, has little to commend it. The raising of the diver's flag under such conditions, although it may appease some local authorities, is often not recognized by the elements, reefs or other navigational hazards, including moored boats.

Some currents are continuous, e.g. the standing currents of the Gulf of Mexico, the Gulf Stream off Florida and the Torres Strait, but tidal currents are likely to give an hour or more of slack water with the change of tide. At these times diving is usually safer and more pleasant because the sediment settles and enhances visibility. To ascertain the correct time for slack water, reference has to be made to the tidal charts for that area. The speed of the current can be predicted by the tidal height.

Surf

Entry of a diver through the surf is loads of fun to an experienced surf diver. Otherwise, it can be a tumultuous moving experience and is a salutary reminder of the adage 'he who hesitates is lost'. The major problem is that people tend to delay their entry at about the line of the breaking surf. The diver, with all his or her equipment, is a far more vulnerable target for the wave's momentum than is any swimmer.

The warning given to surfers, referring to water colour, is that 'White is right but green is mean and blue is too'. This ensures that the surfer enters the surf and avoids rips. For the diver, it is the opposite. The diver may use the apparently calmer water to ride the rip into the ocean.

When the surf is unavoidable, the recommendation is that the diver should be fully equipped before entry and not re-adjust face masks and fins until he or she is well through the surf line. The fins and face mask must be firmly attached beforehand because it is very easy to lose equipment in the surf. The diver walks backward into the surf while looking over his or her shoulder at the breakers and also toward a buddy. The face mask and snorkel have to be held on during the exposure to breaking waves. The regulator must be attached firmly to the jacket, with a clip, so that it is easily recoverable at all times.

When a wave does break, the standing diver presents the smallest possible surface area to it; i.e. he or she braces against the wave, sideways, with feet well separated, and he or she crouches and leans, shoulder forward, into the wave. As soon as possible, the diver submerges and swims (in preference to walking) through the wave area. If the diver has a float, then this is towed behind. It should never be placed between the diver and the wave.

Exit should be based on the same principle as entry, except then the surf is of value. The wave may be used to speed the exit by swimming immediately behind it or after it has broken. The float then goes in front of the diver and is carried by the wave.

FURTHER READING

Australian Antarctic (ANARE) Diving Manual, Australian Antarctic Division, Kingston, Tasmania, Current edition.

British Sub-Aqua Club Diving Manual. ISBN: 9781905492220. Hutchinson, U.K. Current edition.

Lippmann J, Mitchell S. *Deeper Into Diving.* 2nd ed. Melbourne: Submariner Publications; 2005.

Exley S. *Basic Cave Diving.* Jacksonville, Florida: National Speleological Society; 1981.

National Oceanographic and Atmospheric Administration. *NOAA Diving Manual.* 5th ed. Washington, DC: US Government Printing Office; 2013.

Royal Australian Navy Diving Manual, ABR 155. Dept of Defence, Royal Australian Navy, Canberra, ACT, Australia Current edition.

US Navy Diving Manual Revision 6 SS521-AG-PRO-010 (2008). Washington, DC: Naval Sea Systems Command; 2008.

This chapter was reviewed for this fifth edition by Carl Edmonds.

PART 2

Dysbaric Diseases: Barotraumas

6

Pulmonary barotrauma

INTRODUCTION

Pulmonary barotrauma (PBT) of ascent is the most serious of the barotraumas, and it causes concern in all types of diving operations. It is a clinical manifestation of Boyle's Law because it affects the lungs and results from overdistension and rupture of the pulmonary tissue by expanding gases during ascent. It can occur in compressed air divers, submariners undertaking escape ascent training, hyperbaric patients during decompression and airline passengers during ascent to altitude (though the last two situations are rare and invariably associated with gas-trapping disease in the lung).

A 1988 review[1] of submarine escape training from 11 nations showed that despite careful selection procedures and extremely high standards of training and supervision, hooded buoyant ascent (in which the trainees head is enclosed by a hood providing a breathable air space) had an incident rate for PBT between 0.1 and 0.6 per 1000 escapes and a fatality rate 10 to 50 times lower than that.

In non-hooded ascents (in which the trainee must breathe out continually during the ascent), the incident range was 1 to 19 per 1000 escapes. The incidence in recreational diving is unknown.

PATHOPHYSIOLOGY

All gas-filled spaces within the body are potentially subject to volume change as ambient pressure changes. For highly compliant organs such as those of gastrointestinal tract, the contraction and expansion of gases with descent and ascent are accommodated with ease. The lungs are less compliant, however, and if gas breathed at depth is not adequately vented during ascent, transmural pressure gradients sufficient to cause injury may result. This disorder is known as PBT of ascent.

The pathophysiology of PBT is complex and poorly understood. Injury appears dependent to some extent on both volume distension of lung tissue and development of a harmful transmural pressure gradient. Thus, not surprisingly, there is evidence that the degree of overpressure required to cause lung tissue injury depends on the extent to which the lung is splinted by its surrounding structures[2]. Experimentally, cadaver lungs have been shown to rupture with a positive inflation pressure of 70 mm Hg, but if the thorax is prevented from expanding (e.g. by thoracic binding), pressures up to 110 mm Hg are tolerated before rupture occurs. It seems that a distended lung is damaged by a lower transmural pressure, whereas a higher transmural pressure is required to cause injury when the lung is prevented from distending[2]. It is notable that a transmural pressure of 70 mm Hg, shown to be harmful in cadaver studies, can be generated by an ascent from only 1 metre if the lungs are near total lung capacity (TLC) before ascent.

It is also possible that lung 'injuries' that are benign, unnoticed and possibly frequent at the surface may be unmasked and clinically relevant in diving. Denison[3] reported cases of pulmonary rupture occurring with deep inspiration and suggested that this may be an asymptomatic yet frequent event. In addition, he postulated that when the lungs are close to TLC, sneezing or coughing generates enough pressure to exceed the elastic limits of the lung, thus possibly resulting in damage. Although this damage may remain asymptomatic and go unreported at 1 ATA, the leakage of gas from the lung into the mediastinum or chest cavity and its subsequent expansion with ascent in a diver may be symptomatic or even life-threatening. Novice divers, because of inexperience with their equipment and the environment, tend to swim with lung volumes close to TLC. Skip breathing, a procedure used by many divers in an attempt to conserve air, is a voluntary reduction in breathing rate, but it is usually associated with close to maximal lung volumes. Both these situations, in which the lungs are held close to TLC, may predispose the individual to PBT.

Scarring within the lung parenchyma has long been considered to increase risk of PBT. However, Calder[4] reported that the site of injury was inconsistently related to the site of the scar. This finding may be explained by differing compliance in the scar and surrounding tissue. If gas begins to expand in both sites, the more compliant healthy tissue will expand more, creating a shear stress between the two zones. This shear stress may result in an injury to the adjacent healthy tissue.

When alveoli rupture, the escaping gas can either enter any blood vessels that are injured simultaneously or escape into the lung interstitium. The former process will cause alveolar gas to enter the arterial circulation, commonly referred to as 'arterial gas embolism'. Escape into the interstitium allows gas to track along the outside of the pulmonary airways and blood vessels toward the hilum of the lung where the pleura is discontinuous. Its subsequent escape into the mediastinum gives rise to mediastinal emphysema. From there, gas can track upward along the trachea to lie subcutaneously at the base of the neck, thus giving rise to 'subcutaneous emphysema'. Finally, if there is rupture of alveoli adjacent to the visceral pleura, then gas may enter the pleural cavity and produce a pneumothorax (Figure 6.1).

These events may occur singly or in combination. In a Royal Navy series[5] of 109 non-fatal cases of PBT submarine escape training accidents, the disorder in the majority of the cases was cerebral arterial gas embolus (CAGE). However, 15 divers with arterial gas emboli also had mediastinal emphysema, 7 with arterial gas embolism also had pneumothorax (3 bilateral, 4 unilateral), 4 had only mediastinal and cervical subcutaneous emphysema, and 1 had only unilateral pneumothorax.

The most feared (and probably the most common) of these events is arterial gas embolism. During overdistension of the lung, the capillaries and small vessels are stretched and may tear, along with other lung tissue. Because these vessels are small and often compressed by distended air sacs, air embolism may not result until overdistension is relieved by exhalation. Gas from ruptured alveoli is introduced to the pulmonary veins and carried back to the heart. Rarely, the volumes of gas are so great that the left ventricle can become air-locked and the diver will die instantly. More commonly, smaller and variable amounts of gas are entrained into the arterial circulation. The bubbles tend to distribute with flow; thus, those organs receiving a significant proportion of the cardiac output, particularly the brain, are likely to suffer the greatest exposure to bubbles. There is also some evidence that the distribution of bubbles in large blood vessels, particularly larger bubbles, can also be influenced by buoyancy. Therefore, in an upright diver (e.g. during ascent, when PBT is most likely to

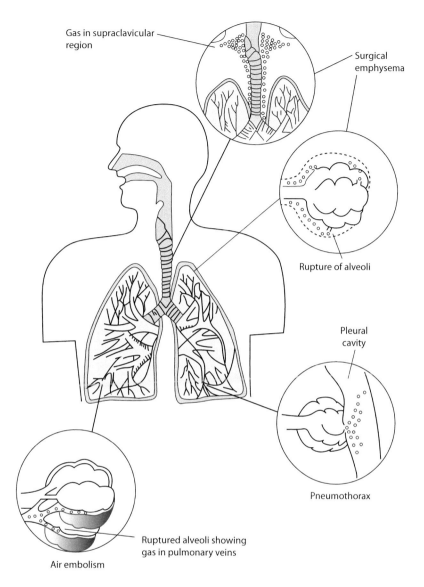

Figure 6.1 Pulmonary barotrauma of ascent.

occur), larger bubbles tend to track around the roof of the aortic arch and are more likely to enter the vessels supplying the upper body and brain.

Passage of these bubbles through the circulation is interrupted by the systemic capillary beds. Bubble behaviour and effects at this point are largely influenced by their size. Bubbles that are large enough that their leading end occupies several generations of branching arterioles may stick and cause obstruction to flow. Smaller bubbles can redistribute through the microcirculation and thus cause minimal obstruction. Even larger bubbles redistribute in this way as the gas inside them is absorbed and they shrink. Clearly, however, even transient obstruction to flow in a tissue sensitive to hypoxia (e.g. the brain) may result in damage before bubble redistribution occurs. Loss of oxygen supply impairs neuronal ability to regulate intracellular ionic homeostasis because of breakdown in the sodium-potassium pump. Uncorrected inward leak of sodium is followed by cellular oedema and depolarization, the latter resulting in release

Table 6.1 Presenting signs and symptoms in 114 Royal Navy submarine escape training accidents and 74 scuba diving accidents involving arterial gas embolism

Signs and symptoms	Percentage incidence	
	Submarine escape training	Scuba diving
Coma with convulsions	7	18
Coma without convulsions	29	22
Stupor and convulsion	14	24
Collapse	8	4
Vertigo	14	8
Visual disturbance	6	9
Headache	2	1
Unilateral motor changes	17	14
Unilateral sensory changes	10	8
Unilateral motor and sensory changes	6	1
Bilateral motor changes	1	8
Bilateral sensory changes	1	1

Source: From Pearson RR. Diagnosis and treatment of gas embolism. In: Schilling CW, Carlston CB, Mathias RA, eds. *The Physician's Guide to Diving Medicine.* New York: Plenum Press; 1984.

Note: Data were compiled from case histories and records of initial post-accident examinations. In the case of submarine escape training accidents, the examinations were always carried out within 5 minutes of onset of symptoms.

of excitotoxins (e.g. glutamate) and a cascade of injurious events that may lead to early neuronal death or delayed apoptosis. The resulting cerebral dysfunction manifests most commonly as sudden-onset unconsciousness and/or multifocal stroke-like events (see later).

Even the redistribution of bubbles is not a benign event. Bubbles may cause endothelial disruption as they pass through small arterioles and capillaries, and white blood cells adhere to the damaged vessel walls. Their activation leads to release of inflammatory cytokines which can also cause tissue oedema and other forms of secondary damage. There is clear evidence from animal studies that shows a secondary decline in blood flow and neuronal function in cerebral tissue following redistribution of small aliquots of gas; this decline is caused by these processes and does not take place if the animal is depleted of white blood cells before the bubble exposure. This sort of inflammatory sequel to arterial gas embolism is thought to explain the frequent observation of initial improvement in early symptoms (which

may reflect bubble redistribution) followed by a secondary deterioration (caused by the inflammatory events).

Secondary deterioration may also be caused by re-embolization by further bubbles that have been trapped in the pulmonary veins and heart chambers. Although there is little proof that this process is materially affected by postural changes, this possibility underpins the frequent advice to keep an apparent victim of arterial gas embolism in a supine position, even in the presence of apparent recovery, until the diver is seen at a hyperbaric chamber.

The understandable focus on cerebral effects of arterial gas embolism should not be allowed to obscure the potential for effects on other organs. It has already been suggested that large amounts of gas can cause early cardiac arrest by air locking the heart. It is also possible for bubbles to enter the coronary arteries and cause myocardial ischaemia and arrhythmias. The heart may also be affected indirectly by disturbance in function of the brainstem cardiovascular centres by cerebral arterial emboli. It is likely that many other tissues are affected by arterial bubbles without necessarily producing symptoms. For example, creatinine kinase levels (skeletal muscle fraction) and some liver enzymes are commonly elevated after arterial gas embolism, a finding suggesting that subclinical injury has occurred in these organs.

PREDISPOSING FACTORS

Predisposing disorders include lesions that may result in local compliance changes, gas trapping or airway obstruction. These include sub-pleural blebs of the type associated with spontaneous pneumothorax, asthma, sarcoidosis, cysts and bullae, tumors, pleural adhesions, pulmonary fibrosis, infection and inflammation.

Precipitating factors include inadequate exhalation or outright breath-holding during ascent (often in association with panic), rapid ascent, faulty breathing apparatus or water inhalation.

Although many cases of PBT may be caused by voluntary breath-holding during ascent or by the pathological lesions mentioned earlier, it is clear that these risk factors are not present in all cases. About half the submarine escape ascent trainees who develop PBT have been observed to carry out correct exhalation techniques. These divers were also passed as medically fit before the dive and exhibited none of the contributory pathological features afterward. A frequent finding with some of these subjects is a reduction of compliance at maximum inspiratory pressures, i.e. the lungs are less distensible (stiffer) and are exposed to more stress than normal diver's lungs, when distended. Brooks and colleagues[6] demonstrated that a lower than predicted forced vital capacity (FVC) was associated with PBT in submarine escape trainees, and this finding further supports the suggestion that reduced pulmonary compliance is a predisposing factor. Interestingly, many medical standards refer to the requirement for the ratio of forced expiratory volume in 1 second (FEV_1) to FVC (FEV_1/FVC ratio) to be greater than 75 to 80 per cent of predicted levels, yet this spirometric parameter has not been shown to be causally related to PBT in trainees who have no evidence of lung disease.

CLINICAL FEATURES

Pulmonary tissue damage

At the point of surfacing in a panic ascent situation, an explosive exhalation of expanded gases may be accompanied by a characteristic sudden, high-pitched cry. Although lung damage resulting from barotrauma can produce respiratory symptoms in the absence of any of the other associated complications, this seems rare in practice. Nevertheless, symptoms that may be seen include dyspnoea, cough and haemoptysis. Clearly, these symptoms may occur in association with any of the complications of PBT discussed later, but the symptoms of pulmonary tissue damage are not invariably present, and their absence should never be used to rule out any of the following diagnoses.

Mediastinal emphysema

As previously described, after alveolar rupture gas may escape into the interstitial pulmonary tissues and track along the loose tissue planes surrounding the airways and blood vessels into the hilar regions and thence into the mediastinum and neck (subcutaneous emphysema). It may also extend into the abdomen as a pneumoperitoneum. When the pleura is stripped off the heart and mediastinum, a pneumoprecordium may be misdiagnosed as a pneumopericardium (Figure 6.2).

Symptoms may appear rapidly in severe cases, or they may be delayed for several hours in lesser cases (Case Report 6.1 and Case Report 6.2). Delay may reflect that the symptoms are often 'mild' or that it takes time for gas to migrate to the sites where it provokes symptoms. Symptoms may include a voice change including hoarseness or a brassy monotone, a feeling of fullness in the throat, dyspnoea, dysphagia and retrosternal discomfort. In very rare severe cases syncope and shock are possible. The voice changes are described as 'tinny' and have been attributed to 'submucosal emphysema' of the upper airways and/or recurrent laryngeal nerve damage, although it is difficult to see how bubbles external to the nerve in a relatively compliant tissue space would achieve nerve damage.

Clinical signs include subcutaneous emphysema of neck and upper chest wall, i.e. crepitus

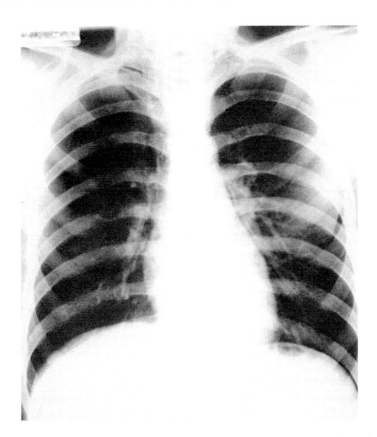

Figure 6.2 Pulmonary barotrauma of ascent: chest x-ray film showing mediastinal emphysema causing the 'tram track' sign, from air stripping the pleura from the edge of the cardiac shadow.

CASE REPORT 6.1

RJN, a 19-year-old, was having his second dive in scuba equipment at a depth of 5 metres when he noted a slight pain in his chest. He then noted a restriction in his air supply and thought he had exhausted his gas. He opened his reserve valve and ascended to the surface. He was asymptomatic after the dive, but later, during physical training, he noted that he was breathing heavily and felt weak. A few minutes later he noted slight retrosternal chest pain. During lunch, he developed a fullness in his neck (a 'tightness') and dysphagia.

An hour and a half after the dive, he decided to see the doctor because he was not feeling well. It was then noted that his voice was altered in quality and that he had subcutaneous emphysema in both supraclavicular fossae, bilateral generalized crepitus over the chest and positive Hamman's sign. Chest x-ray study showed gas in the upper mediastinum and neck. An electrocardiogram showed ischaemic changes in leads II, III and aVF.

He was treated with 100 per cent oxygen and improved rapidly.

Chest x-ray study and electrocardiogram were normal 6 days later. Subsequent lung function studies showed that pulmonary compliance was reduced below predicted values.

Diagnosis: Pulmonary barotrauma with mediastinal emphysema and coronary artery embolism.

CASE REPORT 6.2

TC, an experienced Navy clearance diver, developed epigastric discomfort toward the end of a 90-minute, 11-metre scuba work dive. The dive was otherwise unremarkable, although he had at times worked hard, and he made four controlled ascents during the dive to change his tools.

Approximately 15 minutes after leaving the water, he developed retrosternal chest pain, which increased in intensity over the next few hours. The pain extended from the epigastrium to the base of the throat. The pain was pleuritic in nature and aggravated by inspiration, coughing and movement. He was not dyspnoeic, and there was no associated cough or haemoptysis.

Examination was unremarkable; in particular there were no palpable subcutaneous emphysema and no positive neurological signs. He had no clinical evidence of pneumothorax.

Chest x-ray study revealed the presence of surgical emphysema in the neck and superior mediastinum. No pneumothorax was seen and the lung fields were clear. A computed tomography (CT) scan of the chest was reported as showing 'air in the mediastinum. Inferiorly, this is seen around the oesophagus in the retrocardiac recess. Superiorly, it is seen surrounding the descending aorta at the level of the carina. It also extends along the major branches of the aortic arch adjacent to the trachea and oesophagus superiorly into the base of the neck on both sides. The spread of air appears to be mainly along the major vessels of the aortic arch into the base of the neck'.

He was treated with 100 per cent oxygen and bed rest, with complete resolution of his symptoms. He was considered permanently medically unfit to dive.

Diagnosis: Pulmonary barotrauma with mediastinal emphysema.

---

under the skin (described as the sensation of eggshell crackling, by divers), decreased cardiac dullness to percussion, faint heart sounds, left recurrent laryngeal nerve paresis and in severe cases cyanosis, tachycardia and hypotension. Precordial emphysema may be palpable and produce Hamman's sign – crepitus related to heart sounds that can sometimes be heard at a distance from the patient. An extension of the mediastinal gas into the tissues between the pleura and the pericardium, rather than gas in the pericardial sac, has occasionally produced cardiac tamponade with its classic clinical signs. There may be radiological evidence of an enlarged mediastinum with air tracking along the cardiac border or in the neck.

Pneumothorax

If the visceral pleura ruptures, air enters the pleural cavity and expands during any subsequent ascent. It may be accompanied by haemorrhage, forming a haemopneumothorax. The pneumothorax may be unilateral or bilateral, the latter being more common following dramatic emergency ascents.

> Pneumothorax from diving has the same clinical features and management as pneumothorax from other causes.

Symptoms usually have a rapid onset and include sudden retrosternal or unilateral (sometimes pleuritic) pain, with dyspnoea and tachypnoea. Clinical signs may be absent, or they may include diminished chest wall movements, diminished breath sounds and hyper-resonance on the affected side, tracheal deviation toward the unaffected side with a tension pneumothorax, signs of shock and x-ray evidence of pneumothorax (Figure 6.3).

Arterial gas embolism

This dangerous condition is the result of gas passing from the ruptured alveoli into the pulmonary veins and thence into the systemic circulation, where it can cause vascular damage or obstruction, hypoxia, infarction and activation of an inflammatory cascade (see earlier).

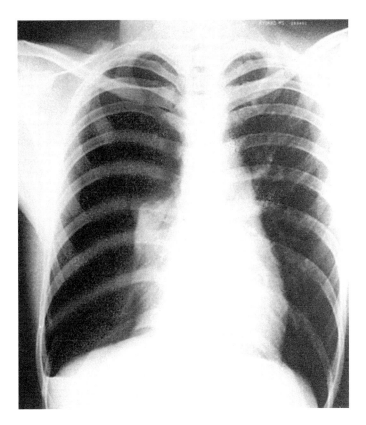

Figure 6.3 Pulmonary barotrauma of ascent causing a large, right-sided pneumothorax with a slight hemothorax.

Most of the clinical series refer to the brain (CAGE) as the dominant site of disease. Onset typically occurs immediately on surfacing or very soon afterward. In one large series[5] of CAGE, the longest interval to onset of symptoms and signs was 8 minutes in a single case, with all other divers showing evidence of CAGE within 5 minutes of completing the dive. There were no cases occurring in excess of 10 minutes.

> Serious neurological symptoms consistent with cerebral involvement, which develop immediately after ascent, must be regarded as air embolism and treated accordingly until a definitive diagnosis has been made.

MANIFESTATIONS

The manifestations of CAGE may include the following:

- Loss of consciousness and other neurological abnormalities such as confusion, aphasia, visual disturbances, paraesthesiae or sensory abnormalities, vertigo, convulsions and varying degrees of paresis, which is usually lateralized (Case Report 6.3). Paraplegia with a sensory level is more likely to be caused by spinal decompression sickness (DCS) (see Chapter 10) than by CAGE.
- Cardiac-type chest pain and/or abnormal electrocardiograms (ischaemic myocardium, dysrhythmias).

In a series of 88 cases of CAGE[7], mainly from free ascent practices, 34 per cent of the divers suffered loss of consciousness within seconds of surfacing, 23 per cent had become confused, disoriented or uncoordinated after emerging from the water, and 17 per cent had presented with paresis (6 cases with upper monoparesis and 6 with hemiparesis).

CASE REPORT 6.3

Al was a relatively inexperienced diver, 19 years old and in good health. He was performing a free ascent from 10 metres. On reaching the surface, he gave a gasp, his eyes rolled upward and then he floated motionless. While he was being rescued from the water it was noted that blood and mucus were coming from his mouth and that he was unconscious. Resuscitation was commenced immediately, using oxygen. He was noted to be groaning at this time but soon after appeared dead. Resuscitation was continued while he was rushed to the nearest recompression chamber. Thirty minutes after the dive he was compressed to 50 metres but with no response. Autopsy verified the presence of pulmonary barotrauma (PBT).

Diagnosis: air embolism resulting from PBT of ascent.

In another series presented by Pearson[5] that included scuba divers without access to immediate recompression, 15 per cent had complete spontaneous remission within 4 hours, and 53 per cent had some spontaneous improvement before therapy; 77 per cent with coma improved to some degree before treatment. These spontaneous improvements were not always sustained, and 15 per cent of the divers died. It seems clear that divers who exhibit symptoms of CAGE may show partial or even complete recovery within minutes or hours of the incident. As discussed earlier, this may reflect redistribution of the embolus through the cerebral vasculature. Even those divers who become comatose may improve to a variable degree after the initial episode. Unfortunately, such recovery is unreliable. It may not occur or it may not be sustained. Recurrence of symptoms has an ominous prognostic significance.

DIFFERENTIAL DIAGNOSIS

Focal cerebral symptoms and signs (including unconsciousness) arising immediately after ascent from a compressed gas dive should always be considered most likely caused by PBT and CAGE, especially where the time and depth exposure would normally be considered 'unprovocative' for DCS (see Chapters 10 and 11). As previously mentioned, an absence of signs of the presumed barotraumatic injury to the lung (e.g. haemoptysis) is surprisingly common and should not influence the diagnosis.

The differential diagnosis for rapid-onset neurological symptoms after a dive that could be considered provocative for DCS is more problematic, but there are several relevant points. First, the principal competing diagnoses are CAGE and DCS, and distinguishing between them is unimportant from a management point of view. The management is virtually identical (see later). Second, it remains uncertain whether the venous bubbles formed from dissolved gas after decompression and 'arterialized' across a right-to-left shunt (see Chapter 10) are large enough to cause the stroke-like syndromes seen after PBT and CAGE. In addition, bubbles are unlikely to form from dissolved gas in the brain tissue itself (see Chapter 10). Third, for the purposes of diagnosis, emphasis should be placed on the putative organ involvement. Manifestations best explained by cerebral involvement (unconsciousness, lateralizing signs, loss of vision, aphasia) are most likely to result from PBT and CAGE (especially if there are concomitant symptoms of PBT), and manifestations best explained by spinal involvement (paraplegia, quadriplegia, loss of anal or bladder tone) are most likely caused by DCS. Confusingly, the two diagnoses may coexist and even interact. Thus, arterial bubbles from PBT may enter tissue micro-vessels and grow as a result of inward diffusion of supersaturated tissue inert gas (see Chapter 10). This mechanism has sometimes been referred to as type III DCS.

Another diagnosis that may cause confusion with CAGE is a haemorrhagic or thromboembolic cerebrovascular accident (CVA) occurring coincidentally with ascent from diving. Such events do occur but are extremely rare, and it is far more likely that cerebral symptoms occurring after a dive are the result of a diving disorder. Indeed, the principal reason for mentioning this differential diagnosis is the frequent inappropriate attribution of CAGE to a CVA when divers are taken to peripheral hospitals staffed by doctors unfamiliar with diving medicine. The same problem arises in cases of DCS.

Previously it was considered important to differentiate between CAGE and DCS because the recommended recompression regimen was different. DCS was treated with a 2.8-ATA oxygen table, e.g. US Navy (USN) Table 6, whereas CAGE was treated using USN Table 6A (which includes an initial deep excursion to 6 ATA). Several animal studies were not able to show an advantage in the initial deep excursion, and most centres now manage patients with CAGE and those with DCS identically (see Chapter 13). Consequently, recompression has become the priority rather than establishing the 'correct' diagnosis. It is still considered relevant subsequently to assess the likelihood of whether PBT occurred because this diagnosis has implications for future risk in diving.

TREATMENT

Aggravation of pulmonary barotrauma

As a general principle, at all stages of managing a diver with PBT it should be remembered that further decompression (e.g. ascent to altitude during air evacuation or decompression from hyperbaric treatment) can aggravate the problem. In particular, a diver with pneumothorax should always have a chest drain inserted before any air evacuation, or before recompression if there is another problem such as CAGE or DCS that justifies recompression in the presence of a pneumothorax. Failure to do this risks development of a tension pneumothorax during a reduction in ambient pressure.

Similarly, physical exertion, increased respiratory activity, breathing against a resistance, coughing, Valsalva's maneuver and mechanical ventilation may also result in further pulmonary damage or in more extra-alveolar gas passing into the mediastinum or into the pulmonary veins.

If a victim of PBT requires mechanical ventilation, a pressure-control mode should be used, employing the lowest inflation pressures required to achieve adequate tidal volumes. Higher rates may be appropriate to allow lower tidal volumes and minimal inflation pressures, although care must be taken not to cause 'breath stacking' or 'auto-peeping' with excessively high rates. Positive end-expiratory pressure should probably be avoided unless clinically indicated to treat hypoxia, and the diver should be kept well sedated and relaxed to minimize both inflation pressures and the possibility of coughing on the endotracheal tube.

Pulmonary tissue damage

Treatment involves the maintenance of adequate oxygenation by administration of sufficient oxygen. The treatment is similar to that of near drowning or the acute respiratory distress syndrome. Positive-pressure respiration could increase the extent of lung damage and should be used only if necessary (see earlier). Cardiovascular support may be required.

Mediastinal emphysema

The need for therapy may not be urgent in mediastinal emphysema. However, exclusion of air embolism or pneumothorax is necessary, and, if in doubt, treatment for these disorders should take precedence. Management of mediastinal emphysema varies according to the clinical severity. If the patient is asymptomatic, observation and rest may be all that is necessary. With mild symptoms, 100 per cent oxygen administered by mask without positive pressure will increase the gradient for removal of nitrogen from the emphysematous areas. This may take 4 to 6 hours.

If symptoms are severe, cardiovascular support and therapeutic recompression using oxygen may be useful.

Pneumothorax

The treatment of a pneumothorax follows the standard principles used in treating a pneumothorax from any other cause.

Small pneumothoraces may resolve with the administration of 100 per cent oxygen. This will often appreciably reduce the size of the pneumothorax within a few hours. Larger pneumothoraces justify the insertion of an intercostal catheter.

The presence of a pneumothorax is not a contraindication to recompression if other sequelae of PBT such as CAGE are present. However, because the pneumothorax may re-expand during decompression, the placement of an intercostal catheter is mandatory before recompression. Staff managing a chest drain in a hyperbaric chamber must be experienced in this procedure; particularly in the management of underwater seal drains in the hyperbaric environment.

Pneumothorax must always be considered if a diver develops respiratory symptoms such as chest pain or dyspnea during decompression from a hyperbaric treatment (Case Report 6.4). The decompression should be halted and careful clinical examination undertaken, which is often difficult in the noisy confines of a recompression chamber. If a pneumothorax is found, then it must be vented before resumption of decompression. Ideally, this would be achieved with a standard intercostal drain, which could be connected to a Heimlich valve for expediency. If this is not possible, then insertion of a smaller catheter (e.g. a large intravenous angiocatheter) in the second interspace, mid-clavicular line, could be used as a temporizing measure.

Cerebral arterial gas embolism

Treatment of CAGE is urgent. The effect of delay on treatment outcome is to increase mortality and morbidity.

POSITIONING

The 'modified Trendelenburg' position or the head-down left lateral position was recommended in the past. Some authorities even recommended a 45-degree angle, which is virtually impossible to maintain even in a conscious cooperative patient, let alone a seriously ill victim requiring resuscitation. This position was recommended to discourage bubbles passing into the aorta from entering the cerebral vessels. However, this is no longer recommended because of its impracticality and the possibility of compounding the embolic brain injury by increasing central venous pressure, reducing cerebral perfusion pressure and promoting cerebral oedema.

The current advice is that the patient should be nursed horizontally, on his or her back if conscious and/or the airway is not threatened, or lying on the side in the 'coma' position (preventing the tongue from causing airway obstruction, or if there is a possibility of aspiration of stomach contents or sea water).

A similar position should be maintained in transit to the chamber, while the chamber is being compressed and for an uncertain period of time (usually one to two oxygen periods) while breathing oxygen. This advice recognizes the potential for further gas to be trapped in places such as the heart chambers and pulmonary veins and that this gas could be released from those locations by postural change. The patient is initially allowed to sit or stand once recompressed to the initial treatment depth and after a period of oxygen breathing. A sudden deterioration in the clinical state may (rarely) follow the resumption of an erect position. This would suggest the continued existence of gas emboli.

OXYGEN

Oxygen (100 per cent), via a close-fitting mask, should be administered in transit to the chamber:

- To improve oxygenation of hypoxic tissues.
- To help dissolve bubbles.
- To ensure that any subsequent bubbles introduced through injured lungs are composed of oxygen, instead of nitrogen.

RECOMPRESSION

Recompression should be instituted as soon as possible. The patient is kept horizontal for at least the first 30 minutes of 100 per cent oxygen breathing in the recompression chamber before being allowed to move and possibly redistribute emboli. Most treatment facilities use a conventional 2.8-ATA oxygen table such as the USN Table 6 (see Chapter 13). Compression reduces bubble size, and this may assist redistribution through the arterial

CASE REPORT 6.4

This case was described by a diver/doctor, in his incident report.

On day 1 the diver, using a helium-oxygen system, carried out a bounce dive to 492 feet. The dive job was carried out successfully and was completed without incident in 13 minutes. During decompression upon reaching 90 feet, the diver reported tightness in his chest, some shortness of breath and discomfort while breathing.

The diver was recompressed to 100 feet, where he had complete relief and felt normal. The chamber atmosphere was at this point changed over to a saturation atmosphere, and the diver was decompressed at a saturation decompression rate. The diving superintendent at this point informed Mr A (a senior diving supervisor). on shore that a treatment procedure was being carried out.

When the diver reached 85 feet, the symptoms redeveloped and other treatment procedures were instituted. The diver was recompressed to 185 feet and a treatment schedule was implemented.

Decompression was uneventful, with the diver feeling fine until day 2 at 02:53 hours, where, at 105 feet, the diver had recurrence of symptoms. The diver was recompressed according to the treatment schedules and then decompressed. He experienced a second recurrence of the symptoms at 85 feet during decompression, and he was once more recompressed to 185 feet for therapeutic decompression at 14:33 hours. At this point a special treatment was instituted at Mr A's instructions. He had now diagnosed the case as a burst lung problem and discounted any kind of bend.

On day 3 at 13:00 hours, upon reaching 75 feet during his decompression, the diver complained of restriction to his breathing, whereupon he was recompressed to 125 feet, where he obtained complete relief. It was decided to attempt decompression once more to see whether the diver could be decompressed all the way or whether there would be a further recurrence of symptoms. At 23:25 hours while reaching 83 feet in the decompression, the diver again complained of breathing difficulties. Recompression to 135 feet relieved all symptoms.

At this point Mr A. decided that the problem could not be an ordinary decompression problem and was reasonably certain that the symptoms were the result of a pneumothorax. A doctor was called, and arrangements were made to go to the rig in the morning of day 4. The doctor was informed of the treatment to date and of the diagnosis and was asked to bring the necessary needles with him to vent a pneumothorax.

On day 4 at 10:49 hours Mr A. and the doctor arrived at the rig. At 13:49 hours while the diver was at 80 feet, the doctor made a cursory examination of the diver without taking his temperature and diagnosed the diver's condition as 'full blown pneumonia and pleurisy of the left lung' and ruled out the possibility of a pneumothorax. The doctor was challenged on the fact that the diver obtained relief by recompression; however, the doctor stated that this would be the case with pneumonia and that he had previously treated a very similar case.

At this point the doctor took over the treatment and instructed the diver to be decompressed at the rate of 3 feet per hour and emphasized the fact that the diver would experience severe chest pains during decompression as a result of the pneumonia. By the afternoon of day 4 the diver was treated with penicillin injections, and, because of severe pain, the rig medic administered an injection of painkiller at 22:45 hours of day 4.

The doctor left the rig by evening of day 4. He stated that it was a routine case and that he would be available ashore for consultation. By the morning of day 5, the diver had been decompressed to a depth of 60 feet, and his condition had steadily deteriorated. Mr A. at this point requested the opinion of a second doctor regarding the diver's treatment and condition. Attempts were unsuccessfully made to obtain another doctor to go to the rig.

The attending doctor was notified of these attempts and of the worsening of the diver's condition. During day 5 the diver received injections of penicillin and painkiller, with little apparent effect. During the early hours of day 6, further drugs were administered, and the diver's condition was worsening. The doctor had been summoned and examined the patient at 03:40 hours while the diver was at 39 feet.

The doctor stated that the diver's condition had improved, that the pneumonia was disappearing and that the decompression rate was to be increased so that the diver could be transferred to a hospital as soon as possible.

At 09:00 hours the diver's pulse had stopped, and by 09:15 he was pronounced dead by the doctor.

CAUSE OF DEATH

1. Death resulted from a tension pneumothorax of the left lung (postmortem finding).
2. The cause of the pneumothorax was unknown; however, it was learned that the diver had a slight chest cough on the day before the incident and complained to the rig medic of some pain on the left side of his chest and over the central area.

and micro-circulation into the veins. The denitrogenated state of the blood assists in rapid bubble resolution. Oxygenation of damaged tissues and a reduction of cerebral oedema may be contributory to benefit. As discussed elsewhere, hyperbaric oxygen helps to suppress white blood cell activation and some of the related inflammatory consequences.

A variation in this technique is to expose the patient to an initial short 6-ATA compression during air breathing (e.g. USN Table 6A), to enhance the redistribution of obstructing arterial emboli before continuation with an oxygen table. This is becoming progressively less popular because it is logistically challenging, exposes chamber attendants to increased risk and seems unnecessary. The 4-ATA 50 per cent oxygen-nitrogen Comex tables may be an acceptable compromise between these opposing concepts. Repetitive hyperbaric oxygen treatment may be of value in those neurologically impaired patients who do not recover fully on the first compression. These treatments are continued until there is full recovery or no sustained improvement over two consecutive treatments (see Chapter 13).

ADJUVANT AND SUPPORTIVE THERAPY

Coronary artery gas embolism may cause cardiac arrest, and cardiopulmonary resuscitation may be necessary.

Rehydration may be crucial if there is hypotension or haemoconcentration. Intravenous fluid resuscitation with a non–glucose-containing balanced electrolyte crystalloid should be titrated to signs of vascular filling, urine output, haemodynamics and haematocrit.

There are no drugs with proven efficacy in the treatment of CAGE. There has been interest in the use of lignocaine (lidocaine) as a neuroprotective agent in this acute setting, and there are some supportive data from animal models of CAGE and human studies in cardiac surgery[8]. In an environment conducive to its safe administration, lignocaine could still be considered in cases strongly suggestive of CAGE. A loading dose in combination with an infusion regimen designed to produce a therapeutic antiarrhythmic level is appropriate. In a healthy adult male patient, this would usually be achieved with a 1 mg/kg loading dose given over 5 minutes, followed by 240 mg administered over 1 hour, 120 mg administered over the second hour, and 60 mg/hour administered thereafter for the duration of the infusion (usually 24 to 48 hours). Lignocaine is not, however, considered a standard of care in this setting.

Radiological investigations such as CT, magnetic resonance imaging and single photon emission CT may assist in the diagnosis and management of DCS and CAGE. These investigations are most helpful in post-recompression diagnosis and evaluation of treatment. These studies may show areas of infarction and oedema, and occasionally gas in acute cases, but they should take second place to recompression therapy in the acute phases.

DIVING AFTER PULMONARY BAROTRAUMA

It is widely considered that an incident of PBT is a contraindication for further scuba diving. The reasons are two-fold: first, the diver may have demonstrated a pulmonary abnormality or predisposition; and, second, pulmonary damage has been sustained and may produce local scarring on healing, thus predisposing to further problems by alteration of lung compliance.

It must be acknowledged that these considerations are largely based on first principles rather than hard outcome data, and some degree of uncertainty over the validity of considering prior PBT an automatic contraindication to further diving must be acknowledged. This becomes most problematic when there is doubt over the diagnosis of PBT itself, and the diver is highly motivated to continue diving. In the recreational diving setting this is often resolved by fully informing the diver of all the relevant issues and leaving the diver to make a decision about continued diving as an informed risk acceptor.

PREVENTION

Attempts to prevent PBT, or reduce its incidence, have centered on standards of fitness for divers and modification of training and diving techniques.

Dive training

Entry level recreational divers are taught that the most important rule in scuba diving is to breathe normally at all times and never hold your breath. Considerable effort goes into instilling this mantra. In addition, dangerous diving practices to be avoided include skip breathing, buddy breathing at depth and during ascent, ditch and recovery training, and emergency free ascent training when there are no experienced medical staff and

full recompression facilities on site. In recent years major dive training agencies have abandoned free ascent training from bottom to surface, and instead simulate it in a horizontal orientation.

Medical selection

Predisposing disease includes previous spontaneous pneumothorax, asthma, sarcoidosis, cysts, tumors, pleural adhesions, intrapulmonary fibrosis, infection, previous penetrating chest wounds and inflammation. These disorders may result in local compliance changes or airway obstructions. Some (spontaneous pneumothorax and known gas trapping lesions in particular) merit automatic exclusion from diving, whereas others (e.g. 'asthma') imply an increase in the magnitude of risk that is very context sensitive, and determinations about diving are made for each case based on its own merits. Pleurodesis for spontaneous pneumothorax may protect from pneumothorax but does not mitigate the risk of other barotraumatic injuries arising from the same predisposing lesions that led to the pneumothorax.

Medical standards are dealt with in Chapters 53 and 54 and involve the exclusion of candidates with significant pulmonary disorders as described earlier. Diver evaluation may involve the performance of respiratory function tests and a pre-diving chest x-ray study. In most cases, a single full-plate chest x-ray film is acceptable. However, some groups insist upon inspiratory and expiratory x-ray studies to demonstrate air trapping in the latter view. If there is a high index of suspicion for gas trapping, more sophisticated lung function tests are indicated. High-resolution or spiral CT scans of the lungs are useful in demonstrating emphysematous cyst and pleural thickening but also frequently reveal lung changes whose significance is uncertain.

SYNCOPE OF ASCENT

The so-called syncope of ascent is a cause of a transitory state of confusion, often described as either disorientation or lightheadedness and associated with a sensation of imminent loss of consciousness. It is caused by inadequate exhalation of the expanding lung gases during ascent, with resultant distension of the lungs and an increase in intrathoracic pressure causing an impairment of venous return. It is analogous to cough syncope.

Syncope of ascent most commonly occurs during rapid ascents, when the pressure gradients are magnified, and also when the diver attempts to retain the air in the lungs instead of exhaling it. In the past, free ascent training from 18 to 30 metres was carried out by divers and submariners, and this was a typical situation in which this disorder occurred – it caused considerable problems with differential diagnosis.

Because there is no actual lung disease, it is technically incorrect to describe this as PBT, but it could sometimes be a step in the progression to this disease.

REFERENCES

1. Weathersby PK, Ryder SJ, Francis TJR, Stepke BK. Assessment of medical risk in pressurized submarine escape training. *Undersea and Hyperbaric Medicine* 1988;**25(suppl)**:39.
2. Francis TJR, Denison DM. Pulmonary barotrauma. In: Lundgren CEG, Miller JN, eds. *The Lung at Depth*. New York: Marcel Dekker; 1999.
3. Denison DM. Pulmonary function: long term effects of diving on the lung. In: Hope A, Lund T, Elliott DH, Halsey MJ, Wiig H, eds. *Long Term Health Effects of Diving*. Bergen, Norway: Norwegian Underwater Technology Centre; 1994.
4. Calder IM. Autopsy and experimental observations on factors leading to barotrauma in man. *Undersea Biomedical Research* 1985;**12**(2):165–182.
5. Pearson RR. Diagnosis and treatment of gas embolism. In: Schilling CW, Carlston CB, Mathias RA, eds. *The Physician's Guide to Diving Medicine*. New York: Plenum Press; 1984.
6. Brooks GJ, Pethybridge RJ, Pearson RR. Lung function reference values for FEV(1), FVC, FEV(1)/FVC ratio and FEF(75-85) derived from the results of screening 3788 Royal Navy submariners and submariner candidates by spirometry. In: *Proceedings of XIV Annual Meeting of EUBS*. Aberdeen: European Underwater and Baromedical Society; 1988.
7. Elliott DH, Harrison JAB, Barnard EEP. Clinical and radiological features of 88 cases of decompression barotrauma. *Proceedings of the Sixth Underwater Physiology Symposium*. Bethesda MD: Federation of American Societies for Experimental Biology; 1978.
8. Mitchell SJ, Pellett O, Gorman DF. Cerebral protection by lidocaine during cardiac operations. *Annals of Thoracic Surgery* 1999;**67**:1117–1124.

FURTHER READING

Colebach HJH, Smith MM, Ng CKY. (1976). Increased elastic recoil as a determinant of pulmonary barotrauma in divers. *Respiratory Physiology* 1976;**26**:55–64.
Gorman DF, Browning DM. Cerebral vasoreactivity and arterial gas embolism. *Undersea Biomedical Research* 1986;**13**(3):317–335.
Leitch DR, Green RD. Pulmonary barotrauma in divers and the treatment of cerebral arterial gas embolism. *Aviation, Space and Environmental Medicine* 1986;**57**:931–938.
Macklin MT, Macklin CC. Malignant interstitial emphysema of the lungs and mediastinum. *Medicine* 1944;**23**:281–358.

This chapter was reviewed for this fifth edition by Simon Mitchell.

7

Ear barotrauma

INTRODUCTION

Barotrauma is defined as the tissue damage caused by expansion or contraction of enclosed gas spaces, according to Boyle's Law and its pressure-volume changes.

The volume change in gas spaces with depth is proportionally greatest near the surface, and so it is in this zone that ear barotrauma is more frequently experienced. It is probably the most common occupational disease of divers, experienced to some degree by most.

Ear (also called otological or aural) barotrauma may affect any of the following:

- External ear (when a sealed gas space exists).
- Middle ear (which incorporates an enclosed gas space).
- Inner ear (which adjoins a gas space) (Figure 7.1).

Middle ear barotrauma is the most common form. Barotrauma problems may contribute to panic and diving deaths in novice divers or to permanent disability – tinnitus, balance and hearing loss.

In the earlier literature on caisson workers' and divers' disorders, otological barotrauma symptoms were hopelessly confused with decompression sickness symptoms. This confusion still exists in many clinical reports today.

> Barotrauma refers to damage to tissues resulting from changes in volume of gas spaces, which in turn are caused by the changes in environmental pressure with descent and ascent (Boyle's Law).

Barotrauma of descent is a result of a failure or an inability to equalize pressures within the ear cavities as the volume of contained gas decreases. Because enclosed cavities are surrounded by cartilage and bone, tissue distortion is limited, and the contracting space may be taken up by engorgement of the mucous membrane, oedema and haemorrhage. This, together with the enclosed compressed gas, assists in equalizing the pressure imbalance. It is commonly called a 'squeeze' by divers.

Barotrauma of ascent is the result of the distension of tissues around the expanding gas within the ear, when environmental pressures are reduced, i.e. on ascent. Divers use the misnomer 'reverse squeeze' to describe it.

> Middle ear barotrauma of descent is the most common disorder encountered by divers.

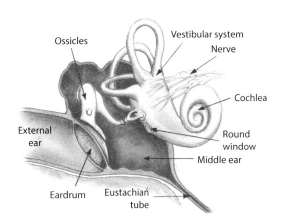

Figure 7.1 Basic anatomy of the ear.

Similar problems are encountered with aviation and space exposure, in hypobaric or hyperbaric chambers and by caisson workers (who work under increased pressure).

Barotrauma is classified according to its anatomical sites and whether it is caused by ascent or descent. It may occur in any combination in the external, middle, or inner ear.

Breathing helium-oxygen gases when diving makes equalization of pressures ('autoinflation') in middle ear and sinus cavities easier, and so barotrauma is less.

General information on the ear in diving, including many references to barotrauma, is included in Chapters 35 to 38.

EXTERNAL EAR BAROTRAUMA OF DESCENT (EXTERNAL EAR SQUEEZE, REVERSED EAR)

Because the external auditory canal is usually open to the environment, water enters and replaces the air in the canal during descent, equalizing the pressures.

If the external ear is occluded, water entry is prevented. Contraction of the contained gas is then compensated by tissue collapse, outward bulging of the tympanic membrane, local congestion and haemorrhage. This is observed when a pressure gradient between the environment and the blocked external auditory canal is +150 mm Hg or more, i.e. 2 metres descent in water (Figure 7.2).

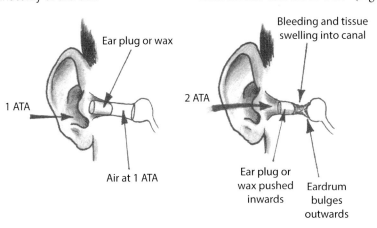

Figure 7.2 External ear barotrauma, when the diver descends from the surface (1 ATA pressure) to 10-metre depth (2 ATA pressure) with an occluded external ear.

The common causes of blockage of the external auditory canal include wax or cerumen, large exostoses, foreign bodies such as mask straps, tight-fitting hoods and mechanical ear plugs.

Clinical symptoms are usually mild. Occasionally, a slight difficulty in equalizing the middle ear is experienced. Following ascent there may be an ache in the affected ear and/or a bloody discharge.

Examination of the external auditory canal may reveal petechial haemorrhages and blood-filled cutaneous blebs that may extend onto the tympanic membrane. Perforation of this membrane is uncommon.

Treatment for this condition includes maintenance of a dry canal, removal of any occlusion, possibly cleansing of the canal with an antiseptic solution warmed to body temperature and prohibition of diving until all epithelial surfaces appear normal. Secondary infection may result in a recurrence of the pain and may require antibiotics and local treatment (see Chapter 29).

This condition is easily *prevented* by ensuring patency of external auditory canals and avoiding ear plugs or tight-fitting hoods that do not have apertures over the ear to permit water entry.

External ear barotrauma of ascent is theoretically possible.

MIDDLE EAR BAROTRAUMA OF DESCENT (MIDDLE EAR SQUEEZE)

Middle ear barotrauma of descent is by far the most common organic medical disorder experienced by divers and patients undergoing hyperbaric medical treatment. It follows the failure to equilibrate middle ear and environmental pressures (auto-inflation) via the Eustachian tubes during descent. An abnormal pressure difference (gradient) causes the tissue damage (Figure 7.3).

> Any condition that blocks the Eustachian tube predisposes the diver to middle ear barotrauma. More commonly, it is caused by faulty technique during attempted voluntary middle ear autoinflation.

Diving marine animals avoid this disorder by having an arterio-venous plexus in the middle ear that responds to the pressure changes. It fills during descent and empties on ascent, accommodating the volume changes.

Pathophysiology

The Eustachian tubes may open when the pressure gradient between the pharynx and middle ear cavity reaches 10 to 30 mm Hg. These figures theoretically equate to an underwater depth of about 25 cm. Equalization of pressure occurs when the Eustachian tubes open. This can be achieved normally by yawning, moving the jaw or swallowing or by voluntarily inflating the middle ear cavity by the Valsalva manoeuvre. The procedure is termed 'equalizing' or 'clearing the ears' by divers and 'middle ear autoinflation' by otologists.

If the Eustachian tubes are closed during descent, a subjective sensation of pressure will develop when the environmental pressure (external

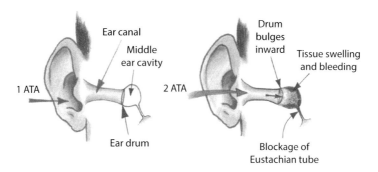

Figure 7.3 Middle ear barotrauma of descent. A diver moving from the surface (1 ATA) to 10-metre depth (2 ATA) with a blocked Eustachian tube, which causes failure to equalize the middle ear cavity and consequent middle ear barotrauma of descent.

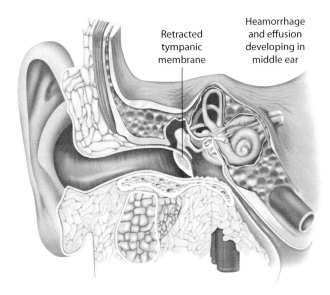

Figure 7.4 Middle ear barotrauma of descent, showing greater anatomical detail.

to the tympanic membrane) exceeds that in the middle ear cavity by 20 mm Hg, or after about 25 to 30 cm descent in water (Figure 7.4).

> **Note:** Extrapolations from physiological pressure gradients to sea water depths are not strictly appropriate because the tympanic membrane is partly moveable and can offset some pressure change.

Discomfort or pain may be noted with a descent from the surface to 2 metres, a 150 mm Hg pressure change and causing a volume reduction of less than 20 per cent in the middle ear cavity. If the middle ear pressure is then equalized, for another 20 per cent middle ear volume reduction (and its associated ear pain to occur) the diver must descend to 4.4 metres, then to 7.3 metres, then to 10.8 metres, and so forth. Thus, the deeper the diver goes, the fewer autoinflation manoeuvres are required per unit depth to prevent symptoms. For this reason, barotrauma is more evident near the surface than at greater depths.

If equalization is delayed, a locking effect may develop on the Eustachian tube and prevent successful autoinflation. This effect results when the tubal mucosa is drawn into the middle ear,

thereby becoming congested and obstructing the Eustachian tube.

If a diver continues descent without equalizing, mucosal congestion, oedema and haemorrhage within the middle ear cavity are associated with inward bulging of the tympanic membrane. This partly compensates for the contraction of air within the otherwise rigid cavity. The tympanic membrane will become haemorrhagic (the 'traumatic tympanum' of older texts). Eventually it may rupture.

It is commonly inferred that perforation is the ultimate damage from not equalizing the pressure in the middle ear cavity, and perforation follows the extreme degrees of haemorrhage described in gradings of middle ear barotrauma of descent. Many tympanic membrane perforations caused by diving are not associated with gross haemorrhages in the tympanic membrane. It is likely that perforation competes with middle ear effusion and haemorrhage as a pressure-equalizing process – the former demonstrating tympanic membrane fragility and the latter demonstrating vascular capillary fragility. Perforation is more likely with rapid descents or from old perforations and scarring.

There is a time factor in the development of middle ear congestion and haemorrhage, with greater degrees resulting from longer exposure to unequalized middle ear pressures.

Middle ear barotrauma of descent has two major causes:

- Pathological processes of the upper respiratory tract obstructing the Eustachian tube.
- Inadequate autoinflation techniques.

Blockage of the Eustachian tubes may be caused by mucosal congestion as a manifestation of upper respiratory tract infections, allergies, otitis media, effects of some drugs, respiratory irritants, venous congestion, mechanical obstructions such as mucosal polyps or individual variations in size, shape and patency of the tube.

Aviation exposure may also cause middle ear barotrauma of descent, and it is similar to diving exposure. It also may be countered by training the flier in the correct 'equalizing ahead of the descent' technique (see later).

For some divers, with very patent Eustachian tubes, attention to autoinflation is not of much import. For others, especially novice divers and those with less patent Eustachian tubes, early and positive middle ear autoinflation techniques are needed.

Opening of the Eustachian tubes is more difficult in the inverted position, when the diver swims downward. This has been attributed to increased venous pressure. It is easier if the diver descends feet first, when air flows more readily upward into the vertical tubes.

Factors leading to blockage of the Eustachian tube include the following:

- Upper respiratory infections and allergies.
- Premenstrual mucosal congestion.
- Gross nasal disorders, septal deviation, mucosal polyps and so forth.
- Delay in autoinflation during descent (flying or diving).
- Descent to the point of 'locking'.
- Horizontal or head-down position.
- Alcohol ingestion.
- Cigarette or marijuana smoking, respiratory irritants.
- Drugs – cocaine, beta blockers, parasympathomimetics.

The incidence of middle ear barotrauma of descent varies with the foregoing factors as well as with the speed of descent and the adequacy of autoinflation techniques. Risk factors have been proposed, based on surveys of dive masters and instructors, indicating ear problems in 4.3 and 11.9 per 1000 dives for male and female divers, respectively. Higher numbers are reported in patients receiving hyperbaric medical treatment and in aviation exposures.

Symptoms

Symptoms consist initially of a sensation of pressure or discomfort in the ear, followed by increasing pain if descent continues. This pain may be sufficiently severe to prevent further descent.

Occasionally, a diver may have few or no symptoms despite significant barotrauma. This occurs in some divers who seem particularly insensitive to the barotrauma effects and also when a small pressure gradient is allowed to act over a prolonged time, e.g. when using scuba in a swimming pool or when not autoinflating the ears at maximum depth following the final metre or so of descent.

Some divers reduce the symptoms (but not the disorder) by slowing the descent or engaging in repeated short ascents after they notice discomfort (the 'yo-yo' descent).

Difficulties are more frequently encountered within the first 10 metres because of the greater volume changes occurring down to this depth.

Eventually, rupture of the ear drum may occur, usually after a descent of 1.5 to 10 metres (100 to 760 mm Hg pressure) from the surface. This causes instant equalization of pressures by allowing water entry into the middle ear cavity. After an initial shock, pain is automatically relieved; however, nausea and vertigo may follow the caloric stimulation by the cold water (depending on the spacial position of the head – see Chapter 38). Unless associated with vomiting or panic, this condition is seldom dangerous because it quickly settles when the water temperature within the middle ear cavity warms to that of the body.

Occasionally, there is a sensation of vertigo during the descent, but this not as common as in middle ear barotrauma of ascent or inner ear barotrauma (see later), both of which can follow and

---

CASE REPORT 7.1

JQ performed three scuba dives, to a depth of 5 metres. He was not able to equalize the pressure in his middle ears during descent, but in the first dive he did manage to achieve this after he had reached 5 metres. Following this first dive his ears felt 'full' or 'blocked'. He then went down to 3 metres 'to see if I could clear them' for his second dive, with the same result. On the third dive he felt pressure in his ears during descent and again could equalize them only after he had reached the bottom; considerable pressure was used in attempted autoinflation. After ascent he again noted that his ears felt blocked and he again attempted to equalize them, this time using considerable pressure. Suddenly pain developed in the right ear, and it gave way with a 'hissing out'. On otoscopic examination of the left ear there was a grade III aural barotrauma with a very dark tympanic membrane, haemorrhage over the handle of the malleus and the membrana flaccida and a small haemorrhage anterior to the handle of the malleus. The right ear had similar features, but with a large perforation (which caused the hissing sound as air escaped) posterior to the tip of the handle of the malleus. Daily audiograms revealed a 15-dB loss in this ear throughout the 150- to 4000-Hz range. This hearing loss disappeared after 2 weeks when the perforation had almost healed over.

The reason for the disorder in the middle ears was that they had 'equalized' by haemorrhaging and perforation.

Diagnosis: middle ear barotrauma of descent.

---

be caused by middle ear barotrauma of descent. It may also result from the Valsalva manoeuvre.

Blood or blood-stained fluid may be expelled from the middle ear during ascent and run into the nasopharynx (to be spat out or swallowed) or appear from the nostril on the affected side (epistaxis). Blood is occasionally seen in the external ear, near a haemorrhagic tympanic membrane.

Following a dive that caused middle ear barotrauma of descent, there may be a mild residual pain in the affected ear. A full or blocked sensation may be felt. This is sometimes associated with a mild conductive deafness involving low frequencies and is the result of haemotympanum, fluid in the middle ear or some dampening effect on the ossicles. It is usually only temporary (hours or days). In severe cases, fluid may be felt in the middle ear for longer periods, possibly with crackling or bubbling sounds as it becomes aerated, before it resolves.

Tympanic membrane perforation, if it occurs, is usually either an oval or crescent-shaped opening below and behind the handle of the malleus or adjacent to previous scarring.

Middle ear barotrauma is classified into six grades based on the otoscopic appearance of the tympanic membrane. The grades are shown in Table 7.1.

The foregoing classification was based on Lieutenant Commander R. W. Teed's observations on submariners, modified by Macfie and subsequently including a symptomatic grade 0 by Edmonds – where there is no obvious tympanic membrane disorder but a clear description of middle ear discomfort on descent and relief on ascent. The tympanic membrane appearance of the higher grades (1 to 5) is simple enough to be identifiable by diving paramedics. Nevertheless, more variable and complex pathologies may be observed, as are illustrated on the front of Plate 1.

A specialized otological classification was presented by O'Neill and is shown on the back of Plate 1. It is especially appropriate for hyperbaric units where specialist otologists are available and may eventually supersede traditional classifications (Table 7.2). The main difficulty with O'Neill's classification is that tympanic membrane photography must precede diving, an impractical situation in the recreational setting at this stage.

Damage and disease involve the whole of the middle ear cleft (middle ear space and mastoid) and not just the tympanic membrane.

Recent overt or sub-clinical middle ear barotrauma of descent results in congestion of the middle ear spaces and subsequent Eustachian

Table 7.1 Middle ear barotrauma of descent – tympanic membrane grading

Grade 0 – Symptoms without signs.
Grade I – Injection of the tympanic membrane, especially along the handle of the malleus.
Grade II – Injection plus slight haemorrhage within the substance of the tympanic membrane.
Grade III – Gross haemorrhage within the substance of the tympanic membrane.
Grade IV – Free blood in the middle ear as evidenced by blueness and bulging.
Grade V – Perforation of the tympanic membrane.

Source: Compiled from Teed, Macfie and Edmonds.

Table 7.2 O'Neill's classification of middle ear barotrauma

O'Neill grade	Potential intervention/treatment
Grade 0 Eustachian tube dysfunction	**Grade 0**
Baseline photograph depicting anatomical appearance of the tympanic membrane	Encourage frequest equalization maneuvers on descent
Symptoms despite no change (injury) from *baseline* photo	Slow/non-linear/controlled descent
	Consider medical therapy on 2 or more failed attempts at equalization
Grade 1 Barotrauma	**Grade 1**
Erythema increase from *baseline*	Encourage frequest equalization/
Increased fluid or air trapping noted in the middle ear space	Slow/non-linear/controlled descent
	Consider medical therapy
Grade 2 Barotrauma	**Grade 2**
Any bleeding noted in the tympanic membrane-middle ear space	ENT referral
Perforation	Restrict diving until tympanic membrane returns to *baseline*

Source: Supplied by Owen J. O'Neill. Clinical Assistant Professor of Medicine, New York Medical College. Medical Director, Dept. of Hyperbaric Medicine. Phelps Memorial Hospital Center.

tube blocking. Autoinflation becomes progressively more difficult with repeated descents, possibly preventing further attempts. Alternately, if the middle ear is almost totally full of fluid, then there is little problem with further descents, but at the cost of middle or inner ear disease.

Sometimes the Eustachian tube may be narrowed and produce a 'hissing' sound during autoinflation, as opposed to the normal 'popping' sound of the Eustachian tube opening or the tympanic membrane movement.

A patulous Eustachian tube can also follow either descent barotrauma or forceful attempts at Valsalva techniques (see Chapter 37).

Treatment

Clinical management consists of the following:

- Avoiding all pressure changes such as diving, flying and forceful autoinflation techniques, until resolution.
- Systemic or local decongestants occasionally (very rarely).
- Systemic antibiotics, but only where there is evidence of a pre-existing or developing infection, gross haemorrhage or perforation, and possibly with culture and sensitivity tests.

In treating many thousands of middle ear barotrauma cases, the authors of this text rarely use decongestants or antibiotics. Investigations are of value (see Chapter 36).

Serial audiometric examination should be undertaken to exclude any hearing loss and to assist in other diagnoses (especially inner ear barotrauma) and management if such a hearing loss is present.

Impedance audiometry (tympanometry) may be used to follow the middle ear pathological changes. If there is a perforation, this investigation can aggravate it. Occasionally, this test is needed to verify a tympanic membrane perforation that is difficult to visualize.

> Serial audiograms should be performed on all but the most minor cases of middle ear barotrauma.

Diving can be resumed when resolution is complete and voluntary autoinflation of the middle ear has been demonstrated during otoscopy. If there is no perforation (grades 0 to 4), recovery may take from 1 day up to 2 weeks.

With perforation (grade 5), recovery may take 1 to 2 months, if the condition is uncomplicated and managed conservatively. Although the tympanic membrane may appear normal much earlier, recurrent perforation frequently results from premature return to diving. There is rarely an indication for such surgical procedures as tympanoplasty, unless healing is incomplete or if the lesion recurs with minimal provocation.

It is important to clearly identify and correct the contributing factors (pathological processes and autoinflation technique) in each case before diving or flying is resumed.

Prevention

Prevention of this disorder consists of ensuring patency of the Eustachian tubes before diving and appropriate training in autoinflation techniques to be used while diving.

Autoinflation is best checked by otoscopic examination of the tympanic membrane during a Valsalva manoeuvre, when the tympanic membrane will be seen to move outward. The degree of force needed to autoinflate, and the degree of movement of the ear drum, will provide an estimation of the probable ease of pressure equalization when diving.

If either tympanic membrane appears to move sluggishly or if much force is necessary, then decongestant nasal drops or sprays may marginally improve the patency of the Eustachian tubes. These agents are of value to trainees who can use them to facilitate middle ear autoinflation techniques and improve this skill on land before diving. Pseudoephedrine may reduce aviation-induced barotrauma problems to some degree, more so than nasopharyngeal sprays.

The use of *decongestants* to improve Eustachian tube patency while diving is to be discouraged. In a prospective comparison of topical decongestants, these drugs did not seem to be of value in preventing middle ear barotrauma.

The rebound congestion of the mucosa is cited by otologists as a reason for avoidance of decongestants, but the diving clinician is also concerned with the systemic problems of sympathomimetic agents and the increased incidence of middle ear barotrauma of ascent encountered with these medications. The reason for this may be that decongestants are more effective in improving nasal airflow and thereby affecting the pharyngeal cushions of the Eustachian tube than in influencing the tubal mucosa or middle ear orifice, which may be affected by the same pathological process. Decongestants, both local and general, are effective only in the marginally obstructed tube, thus permitting a slow descent and some descent barotrauma with resultant congestion of the middle ear orifices of the tube – which then block on ascent and cause middle ear distension and ascent barotrauma (see later).

From the safety aspect, difficulties with descent are less dangerous than with ascent.

In most cases, and especially in the novice diver, practice and instruction in middle ear autoinflation and the use of correct diving techniques are much more effective than drugs in ensuring Eustachian tube patency and reducing barotrauma.

It is possible to measure the force or pressure necessary to open the Eustachian tubes. Eustachian tube patency and middle ear pressure changes can be measured if specialized impedance audiometers are employed clinically. See Chapter 36 for more information.

When dealing with divers who have not adequately autoinflated their middle ears during descent – despite the ability to perform this in the clinic – the following errors are commonly encountered.

1. Not autoinflating early enough, i.e. waiting until the sensation of pressure is felt. This indicates a negative middle ear pressure. Commonly the novice diver, instead of performing a Valsalva manoeuvre before descent, will concentrate on his or her struggle to descend and will often be 2 to 3 metres underwater before remembering to clear the ears. This situation is referred to as 'equalizing behind the dive (exposure)' and is overcome by autoinflating on the surface before descent and with each metre of descent. Alternately, the diver may employ autoinflation after each breath during descent. Open water diving, without use of a descent line or anchor line, disrupts control of the descent and thus contributes to this barotrauma.
2. Attempting to autoinflate while in the horizontal or, even worse, head-down position. If only one ear causes difficulty, it is advisable to tilt that ear toward the surface while attempting autoinflation. This manoeuvre stretches the pharyngeal muscles and puts the offending tube in a more vertical position, thus capitalizing on the pressure gradient of the water.
3. Diving with problems that cause Eustachian tube obstruction, such as mucosal congestion from such factors as infections, irritants such as cigarette smoke, drugs or allergies. After an upper respiratory tract infection has cleared, another week or two is necessary before diving is resumed safely. Divers who have an allergic diathesis should avoid the allergens (e.g. avoid dairy products for 12 to 24 hours before diving). Divers should be advised of the dangers of delaying middle ear autoinflation and of using excessive force in achieving it.

Correct middle ear autoinflation for divers: **'equalizing ahead of the dive'**

- Practice and ensure reliable middle ear autoinflation on land. Only then, consider diving.
- Autoinflate the middle ear on the surface immediately before descent.
- Autoinflate every 1 metre of descent. Use a descent line.
- Autoinflate with the head upright.
- Do not descend if pressure is felt on the ears. Abort the dive.
- Do not use multiple ascents (yo-yo) or waiting at depth, to equalize.
- Do not dive if you have upper respiratory disorders.

Some physicians have claimed the use of local proteolytic or allegedly mucus-softening enzymes to be of value. Even if they did work, they would have the same complications as decongestants.

HYPERBARIC EAR PLUGS

There are repeated promotions of ear plugs to reduce the symptoms of middle ear barotrauma in both divers and aviators. The principle on which these ear plugs are employed is as follows: A small malleable, plastic, compressible and porous plug is fitted with an airtight seal into the external ear. This allows for air to move more slowly into the external ear space during pressurization (descent) in a chamber.

The use of these 'hyperbaric plugs' will delay the inward distortion of the tympanic membrane (being pulled into the middle ear) given that the membrane tends to move in the opposite direction, i.e. outward, because of the external ear obstruction. Thus, the discomfort and pain of the 'negative' pressure in the middle ear are less, and the barotrauma may be slower in developing.

Nevertheless, use of these ear plugs does not change the pathological features of middle ear barotrauma, other than the effect on the tympanic membrane. Thus, the damage to the middle ear mucosa, the oval and round windows and the inner ear all remain (being dependent on the pressure gradient between the middle ear space and its surrounding body tissues). The only thing that has really changed is that the symptom of pain with middle ear barotrauma has been lessened.

The potential costs of reducing the symptoms of middle ear barotrauma are as follows: the production of mild external ear barotrauma of descent; the persistence of pathological features of ear barotrauma affecting the middle ear mucosa and inner ear; possible aggravation of ascent barotraumas affecting the ear because of the disorder induced in the middle ear during descent; and vertigo from unequal middle ear pressures when the plugs are not inserted equally into both sides.

It is doubtful that the masking of middle ear disease by reducing the symptoms is a wise move.

An alternative to the hyperbaric ear plugs is to pressurize more slowly (i.e. the same effect on the middle ear without inducing external ear barotrauma to achieve it).

'Diving' ear plugs, in which a restricted opening replaces the ceramic filter, slow the barotrauma disorder as described earlier and increase the possibility of ascent barotrauma.

Gadgets that connect the oral cavity with the external ear have been used in the false belief that they overcome the effect of impaired middle ear autoinflation. This could happen only if there is a tympanic membrane perforation, in which case the diver should not be diving.

In patients who are unconscious and need hyperbaric treatment (in a recompression chamber), middle ear barotrauma is particularly frequent, and *myringotomy* is often required.

Professor Joe Farmer stated that myringotomies are required for hyperbaric exposure in patients who are comatose or who have a tracheostomy or orotracheal or nasotracheal tubes. If repeated treatments are considered likely, tympanostomy tubes can be inserted.

As an alternative for divers in recompression chambers, who should need only one such treatment, an alternative to myringotomy in conscious patients is to have repeated pauses or a very slow descent, accepting slower barotrauma and giving more opportunity for autoinflation.

MIDDLE EAR AUTOINFLATION TECHNIQUES

Passive opening of the Eustachian tubes is the ideal and natural way to equalize pressure between the middle ear and the nasopharynx, although it is not always possible. Most amateur divers need to use an active technique, under their voluntary control, which will inflate the middle ears and prevent the pain and discomfort of barotrauma during descent. During ascent, passive equalization of ear pressures is more common, and active techniques are rarely needed.

Sometimes reluctant trainees use the failure to autoinflate ears as an acceptable excuse to avoid diving. Other times they are scared to use sufficient nasopharyngeal pressure for fear of causing damage.

It is part of the routine diving medical examination to ensure that the diving candidate can autoinflate the middle ear actively. This is achieved by using a positive pressure manoeuvre described to the diver while the examiner is observing the tympanic membrane and its movement with an otoscope. The latter is employed either by focusing on the light reflex or on another part of the tympanic membrane that reflects light (either the membrane flaccida or the circumference). As the candidate autoinflates the middle ear, the tympanic membrane moves outward.

Investigations using otoscopy and modified diving tympanometry (see Chapter 36) are reasonably reliable in predicting which candidates will have trouble resulting from Eustachian tube disorders. However, many divers fail because of an inadequate autoinflation and diving technique.

The following techniques for autoinflation are recommended. Different candidates perform them with varied ease. In each case, practice of the technique is recommended on land, before subjecting the novice to hyperbaric and aquatic conditions that interfere with the application of this new skill.

The **Valsalva manoeuvre** is probably the most easily understood. It involves occluding the nostrils, closing the mouth and exhaling so that the pressure in the nasopharynx is increased. This separates the cushions of the Eustachian tube and forces air up this tube into the middle ear. The pressure required to achieve this is usually 20 to 100 cm H_2O.

Middle ear equalization answers to clients' problems

Client:
1. I descend a bit slower than my buddies. Or,
2. If there is any pressure, I halt my descent and wait a bit. Or,
3. I may ascend until the ear clears (yo-yo technique).

Answer: Why? If you are not equalizing the middle ear promptly or sufficiently, then these procedures merely allow the middle ear to fill with blood or tissue fluids and thus allow further descent with less pain or discomfort. This is not a sensible way to equalize the middle ear. It results in middle ear congestion, Eustachian tube obstruction and other disorders that may be temporary or permanent.

Client: I am trying to use swallowing to equalize the middle ear.

Answer: If you have any difficulty with middle ear equalization, then employing techniques that result in relatively negative middle ear pressures, cause middle ear congestion and Eustachian tube blockage. Use the positive pressure Valsalva technique (or Lowry or Edmonds techniques) before and during descents.

Client: I have middle ear equalization problems when I swim down the shot line.

Answer: This requires greater force to autoinflate the middle ear because you are trying to force air down the Eustachian tube. Descend feet first and you can blow air up the Eustachian tube. Air travels more easily up than down in the water. Remember bubbles? They rise.

Client: If there is any water in my ears (fullness, crackling) after the dive, I use alcohol ear drops to dry them out.

Answer: It is likely that the 'water' is really fluid in your middle ear from barotrauma. See earlier.

Client: I sometimes have a bit of blood from my nostril (or in my throat).

Answer: Although the blood may be from your sinus, following expansion of air with ascent, it is more likely from the middle ear on that side. In either case, correct middle ear equalization ('ahead of the dive') may well fix both. See earlier.

Client: When I dive and equalize the middle ear, I hear a squeaking sound in my ear.

Answer: This suggests a narrowed Eustachian tube, possibly from inadequate middle ear equalization and barotrauma. The sound you should hear when you equalize the middle ear and the ear drum moves outward is a click or pop. It takes a split second to achieve. It is not a long, drawn-out sound.

Client: I can often dive once, without problems, but cannot equalize the middle ear on other dives.

Answer: You have probably produced some middle ear congestion (barotrauma) in the first dive but continued the dive. By the second dive, you start off with significant middle ear congestion, and so middle ear equalization is more difficult.

Client: One ear equalizes before the other.

Answer: Not a problem. It is normal. You may wish to assist the slow ear by pointing it toward the surface as you equalize the middle ear.

The force necessary for successful autoinflation will vary with the diver's body position. Using the Valsalva technique, novice divers average 40 cm H_2O in the head-up, vertical position and in the horizontal 'ear-up' position. In the horizontal 'ear-down' position they need 50 cm H_2O. In the vertical, swimming-down position they average about 60 cm H_2O.

The Valsalva manoeuvre used by divers is modified from that employed originally by Antonio Valsalva to increase intrathoracic pressure. Trials performed on divers indicate that they do not produce the prolonged high thoracic pressures often encouraged by cardio-thoracic physiologists. With the latter, the problems induced by prolonged high Valsalva pressures include cardiac arrhythmias, hypertension and hypotension, arterial and venous haemorrhages, pulmonary and otological barotrauma, gastric reflux, stress incontinence and the possible shunting of blood through right-to-left vascular shunts (atrial septal defects and patent foramen ovale) thus increasing the possibility of paradoxical gas embolism with diving.

The **Frenzel manoeuvre** involves closing the mouth and nose, both externally and internally (this is achieved by closing of the glottis), and then contracting the muscles of the mouth and pharynx upward ('lifting the Adam's apple'). Thus, the nose, mouth and glottis are closed, and the elevated tongue can be used as a piston to compress the air trapped in the nasopharynx and force it up the Eustachian tube. Pressure of less than 10 cm H_2O may accompany this manoeuvre.

As divers become more experienced, they tend to use such techniques as jaw movements, commencing a yawn, swallowing, lifting the soft palate and so forth, which allow for equalization of the middle ear without pressurizing the nasopharynx.

The **Toynbee manoeuvre** involves swallowing with the mouth and nose closed, and it is of value in relieving the overpressure in the middle ear during ascent. It is also of value during descent when movement of the Eustachian cushions produces a nasopharyngeal opening of the Eustachian tube, with an equalization of pressures between the nasopharynx and the middle ear. Thus, the final pressure in the middle ear with the Toynbee manoeuvre may be negative (less than environmental).

A combination of techniques has also been proposed. A very successful one is the combination of the Toynbee and Valsalva techniques, known as the **Lowry technique.** This involves occlusion of the nostrils, then a swallowing movement that is made continuous with a Valsalva manoeuvre. The diver is thus advised to 'hold your nose, swallow and blow at the same time'. Despite the rather confusing (and impossible to achieve) instruction, the technique is extremely valuable in resistant cases. It is easily learned with practice, on land.

The **Edmonds technique** is rather similar and involves the opening of the Eustachian cushions by rocking the lower jaw forward and downward (similar to the start of a yawn) so that the lower teeth project well in advance of the upper teeth and performing the Valsalva manoeuvre at the same time.

The **Edmonds number 2 technique** is to advise the diver to 'block your nose, close your mouth then suck your cheeks in, then puff them out – quickly'.

Soft palate contraction is a technique whereby the diver contracts and raises the soft palate, thereby moving the Eustachian cushions, occluding the nasopharynx and causing minimal elevation of the pressure within this space, opening the Eustachian tube and forcing air up the tube. It is sometimes called the *béance tubaire voluntaire* or **BTV**, and it is usually employed by experienced divers who have relatively patent Eustachian tubes and who, over the years, have developed this muscular skill. An interesting variation of the BTV is the **Roydhouse technique**. Here the diver is asked to identify the uvula hanging down from the posterior of the hard palate, then raising it as he or she moves the back of the tongue downward. This opens the Eustachian tubes, and the diver can verify it by hearing his or her own humming sounds reverberate in the ears.

When examining potential divers, attempts to demonstrate either the Frenzel technique or the BTV are not usually successful. In the author's practice, during otoscopy, the Valsalva manoeuvre is tried first, followed by the Toynbee, the Lowry and then the Edmonds techniques. If there is any difficulty remaining with equalization, then the candidate is advised to repeat the most effective procedure a few times a day and achieve success, determined by hearing both ears click, before commencing diving.

Academic arguments abound as to which is the best technique. Whichever works is the best. The major problem is not the danger of middle ear autoinflation, but the dangers of not autoinflating.

Some techniques (Valsalva, Lowry, Edmonds) have the disadvantage of a transitory pressure that may extend into the thorax, but this is not usual with divers. These techniques have the advantage of distending the middle ear and thus allow further descent without the problems of a negative middle ear pressure developing and producing middle ear congestion and Eustachian tube obstruction. These techniques are therefore better for novice divers and for those who have trouble with middle ear autoinflation. They also assist in equalizing sinus pressures and avoiding sinus barotraumas.

Other techniques (Toynbee, BTV) are effective if there is easy and frequent middle ear autoinflation. They either equalize the pressures passively or produce negative middle ear pressures. Wave action or descent can also cause a negative middle ear pressure with resultant congestion and Eustachian tube obstruction, and these techniques may aggravate this condition.

Experienced divers, who have mobile tympanic membranes, resembling small spinnakers, can often descend to great depths before they need to equalize their middle ear pressures. They also autoinflate their ears by using less pressure.

Most patients with an inability to autoinflate their middle ears who have been referred to the authors of this text have suffered more from inadequate diver instruction than from Eustachian tube obstruction. To ascertain the extent of this problem, 200 consecutive otoscopic examinations were recorded on potential diving candidates. Autoinflation was successful using the Valsalva, Toynbee, Lowry or Edmonds technique in 96 per cent of subjects, with 4 per cent unsuccessful in one or both ears.

Decongestants probably do work on the mucosal membranes and do improve nasal air flow, but their effect on the Eustachian tube is greater at the nasopharyngeal orifice. Thus, these drugs may be more effective in reducing descent than ascent middle ear barotrauma.

Some otologists have recommended the use of the *pneumatic otoscope* to demonstrate passive tympanic membrane movement. This instrument is certainly of value in assessing middle ear disease, but it is inadequate for diving assessment because it fails to demonstrate the procedure that is required, i.e. *voluntary* autoinflation of the middle ear.

Other investigations of more value in assessing middle ear autoinflation include the modified tympanogram (see Chapter 36) and examination of the Eustachian cushions with a fibre optic nasopharyngoscope.

MIDDLE EAR BAROTRAUMA OF ASCENT (REVERSE SQUEEZE, ALTERNOBARIC VERTIGO)

This disorder is caused by distension of enclosed gases within the middle ear, expanding with ascent. Because it may prevent ascent, it is usually more serious than middle ear barotrauma of descent, which allows an uncomplicated return to safety.

During ascent, the middle ear opens passively, with a pressure gradient of less than 50 cm H_2O. If the Eustachian tube restricts release, symptoms may include sensations of pressure or pain in the affected ear *(reverse squeeze)* or vertigo resulting from increased middle ear pressure difference *(alternobaric vertigo)*. Occasionally, these conditions coexist.

Middle ear barotrauma of ascent usually follows recent, but sometimes mild, middle ear barotrauma of descent and/or the use of nasal decongestants. In each case the common factor is probably congestion and therefore blockage of the Eustachian tube.

The mild vertigo is often rectified by further ascent, which may force open the less patent Eustachian tube. When the pressures in both middle ears are equalized with the ambient pressure, the stimulus to vertigo ceases. Also, subsequent opening of the tube is easier. Other divers may reach the surface while still having an asymmetry of pressure within the middle ear cavities, or residual damage from excessive middle ear pressure, and so experience vertigo following the ascent.

Most cases of vertigo from middle ear barotrauma of ascent are mild, lasting seconds or minutes. This is not always so, however, and there have been instances of temporary or permanent inner ear damage, seventh nerve palsy, severe pain during ascent and/or perforation of the tympanic membrane.

The vertigo is most pronounced when the diver assumes the vertical position and is least pronounced in the horizontal position. The spinning is toward the ear with the higher pressure. It tends to develop when the middle ear pressures differ by 60 cm H_2O or more.

Otoscopic examination often reveals evidence of tympanic membrane injection or haemorrhage. Congestion of blood vessels is common but is less than with descent barotrauma. It is more pronounced around the circumference of the tympanic membrane than along the handle of the malleus. The tympanic membrane may appear to be bulging.

Hearing loss in the affected ear, if present, may be conductive and follow damage to the tympanic membrane or the middle ear structures. The tympanic membrane may rupture occasionally. Inner ear barotrauma with sensorineural hearing loss is a possible complication (see Chapter 37). Seventh nerve palsy is another possible complication.

For *first aid,* the diver may be able to take remedial action. A short descent may relieve symptoms and allow middle ear equalization. Occasionally, the Valsalva technique, jaw movements or performing a Toynbee manoeuvre (see earlier) will relieve the discomfort, as may sudden pressure applied to the external ear (by occluding the external ear with the tragus or middle lobe, then pushing on it and thus exerting external pressure on the water column in the external ear). Equalization may be easier if the affected ear is facing the sea bed, thereby using the pressure gradient along the now vertical Eustachian tube.

Treatment

Fortunately, most effects are short-lived, and treatment should consist of prohibition of diving until clinical resolution has occurred, normal hearing and vestibular function are demonstrated and prevention of future episodes is addressed.

Rarely the diver is seen soon after the event, and if the middle ear is still distended, the first aid procedures described earlier may be satisfactory. Otherwise, the use of oxygen inhalation or minimal recompression is effective.

Antibiotics are used if there is evidence of infection, and decongestants are sometimes recommended to improve Eustachian tube patency. Usually, neither type of drugs is needed.

Decongestants, especially topical ones, are rarely of use in preventing this disorder, unless they prevent a causal middle ear barotrauma of descent. Usually, they have the opposite effect. Systemic decongestants are more effective, but they have other disadvantages, permitting the diver to descend with marginal improvement in Eustachian tube patency and inadequate autoinflation of middle ear.

Prevention is best achieved by avoiding nasal decongestants and by training the diver in correct middle ear equalization techniques during descent (see earlier). Unless descent barotrauma is prevented, ascent barotrauma is likely to recur.

Once middle ear barotrauma of ascent has been experienced, particular care should be taken to ensure that if it does recur the diver will always have adequate air to descend briefly, use the techniques described earlier and then gradually ascend. A low-on-air situation could cause extreme discomfort or danger if the diver's ascent is restricted by symptoms.

Vestibular function has been tested experimentally during pressure changes in a recompression chamber, to replicate the sequence of events and verify the aetiology and diagnosis (see Chapter 38). This testing is not generally required.

INNER EAR BAROTRAUMA

Overview

There is always the possibility of inner ear damage in divers who have any of the following:

- A history of ear barotrauma of any type.
- Previous difficulty in equalizing middle ear pressures.
- Subsequent application of excessive force to achieve this equalization.
- Structural abnormalities that make the divers susceptible to this damage.

In these cases, sensorineural hearing loss may immediately follow the dive, or it may develop over the next few hours or days. Tinnitus is a common association. Some patients may complain of vertigo, nausea and vomiting. Vertigo is often increased with exercise, altitude changes and head movements.

Combined cochlear and vestibular injury is experienced in 50 per cent.
Only cochlear injury occurs in 40 per cent.
Only vestibular injury occurs in 10 per cent.

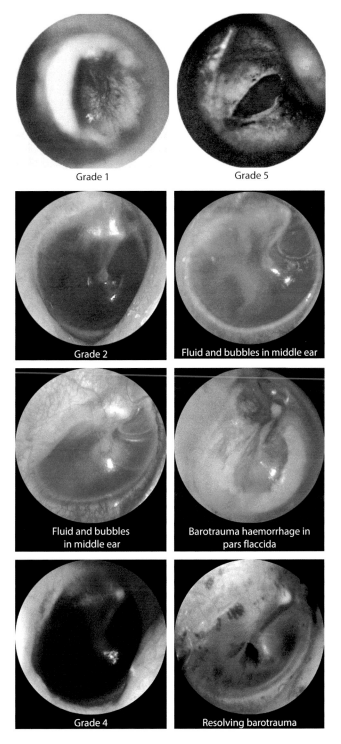

Grade 1

Grade 5

Grade 2

Fluid and bubbles in middle ear

Fluid and bubbles in middle ear

Barotrauma haemorrhage in pars flaccida

Grade 4

Resolving barotrauma

Plate 1, front. Middle ear barotrauma from diving. Tympanic membrane pathologies. Photos courtesy of Richard A. Chole, MD, PhD, Professor and Chairman, Department of Otolaryngology, Washington University in St. Louis and Frank Blackwood, Royal Australian Navy, School of Underwater Medicine.

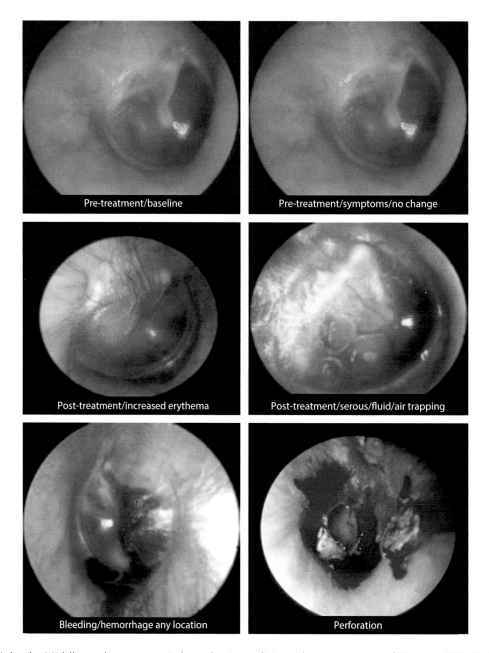

Plate 1, back. Middle ear barotrauma in hyperbaric medicine. Photos courtesy of Owen J O'Neill, Clinical Assistant Professor of Medicine, New York Medical College; Medical Director, Department of Hyperbaric Medicine, Phelps Memorial Hospital Center. See also Table 7.2.

There may be no otoscopic signs. This disorder has been reported from dives as shallow as 2 metres and has been observed in a surfer who dived under a wave. Animal experiments reproduce the pathological features with equivalent depths of 1 to 6 metres.

> In the event of otological barotrauma, a sensorineural or combined hearing loss, tinnitus or demonstrable vestibular damage implies inner ear barotrauma.

In a series of 50 cases of inner ear barotrauma, most occurred in experienced divers, 10 per cent were in free divers, ear, nose and throat disease was present beforehand in 48 per cent, previous diving middle ear barotrauma occurred in 62 per cent, aviation middle ear barotrauma occurred in 24 per cent and inner ear barotrauma occurred in 12 per cent. In the eventful dive, 98 per cent experienced middle ear barotrauma (88 per cent descent, 10 per cent ascent). The incidence of symptoms was as follows: tinnitus, 86 per cent; hearing loss, 80 per cent; vertigo, 38 per cent; and dysacusis, 10 per cent. Sixty two per cent noted symptoms during the dive, and 38 per cent had symptoms within some hours. Both conservative and surgical treatments had a two thirds success rate, but most divers were treated conservatively. Tinnitus and vertigo often responded to early treatment.

Pathophysiology

Middle ear barotrauma is the most common cause of inner ear damage in diving. Various inner ear disorders have been demonstrated. For anatomical background, see Chapter 35 (Figure 7.5). Inner ear damage is also reported in aviators and flight attendants.

A *perilymph fistula* is a common pathological entity of inner ear disease. The perilymph leak is variable in volume and may come from the round window (most often), the oval window or a membrane rupture within the labyrinth.

Perilymph fistulae from the labyrinthine windows are now well recognized and result in a leakage of perilymph into the mastoid or middle ear space. In general medical practice, the disorder may be related to congenital syphilis, other infections, cholesteatoma or any sudden increase in intracranial or labyrinthine pressure. It can develop spontaneously or may be caused by trauma, especially with head injury, weight lifting and physical straining. The intracranial pressure wave so produced can be transmitted into the inner ear by the cochlea and possibly the vestibular aqueducts. An increased pressure of 120 mm H_2O in the cerebrospinal fluid (CSF) is sufficient to induce this disorder in some patients.

Any procedure that involves manipulation of the ossicular chain can cause an oval window

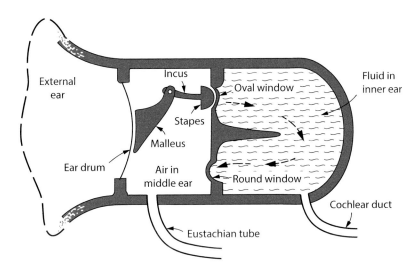

Figure 7.5 Diagrammatic representation of the ear anatomy.

perilymphatic fistula, and this disorder occurs in up to 7 per cent of patients after stapedectomy.

The hearing may fluctuate, depending on the replacement of perilymph, or hearing loss may progress slowly or suddenly as the perilymph leaks out. The more quickly the ear replenishes its perilymph, the less likely it is to sustain permanent damage. The prognosis is better when only the low or middle frequencies are affected. The loss of pressure within the perilymphatic system, the relative endolymph hydrops (similar to Ménière's disease) and the possible electrolyte imbalances affect the dynamics of the hearing and vestibular systems, and the damage may become permanent if it is not corrected.

The initial presentations with verified perilymph fistulae are sudden or fluctuating sensorineural hearing loss in 83 per cent, vertigo in 77 per cent, tinnitus in 63 per cent and aural fullness in 25 per cent.

Exposure to environmental pressure change is possibly one of the most common causes, and this includes ear barotrauma of diving or aviation exposure.

There are two postulated mechanisms for this disorder in diving. If the middle ear pressure is not equalized during descent, the tympanic membrane moves inward because of the pressure gradient; as a result, the foot plate of the stapes is pushed inward. This causes a displacement of perilymph through the helicotrema, so that the round window membrane bulges outward. If at this stage a forceful Valsalva manoeuvre is performed, there is a sudden increase in the pressure within the middle ear cleft that causes the tympanic membrane to be very rapidly returned to its normal position, the stapes to move outward and the round window to be pushed inward. The reversed flow of perilymph may not be sufficiently rapid to avoid damage to the inner ear structures that results in haemorrhages or rupture of the round window membrane.

The other explanation involves a pressure wave transmitted from the CSF through a patent cochlear aqueduct during the Valsalva manoeuvre and 'blowing out' the round window into the middle ear. This has been demonstrated in animal experiments, with a rise of CSF pressure. The aqueduct constricts with age, and this may explain why children are more susceptible.

Inner ear barotrauma has occurred in unconscious patients and guinea pigs, thus indicating that a forceful Valsalva manoeuvre is not a necessary prerequisite.

Animal experiments suggest *multiple pathological processes* for the inner ear damage, mainly labyrinthine window ruptures, intralabyrinthine membrane ruptures, haemorrhage and acoustic trauma. Stretching of the round window, thus permitting the entry of air into the cochlea and causing sensorineural hearing loss, has been demonstrated. Increasing the CSF pressures by 120 to 300 mm Hg can also transmit pressure through the cochlear aqueduct and increase the perilymph pressure in the inner ear, thereby rupturing the round window. Rupture of the round window membrane can develop in water as shallow as 1.3 metres.

It is likely that cochlear and vestibular haemorrhages and internal inner ear membrane ruptures are common, but they are not so amenable to treatment.

End artery spasm, thrombosis and gas or lipid embolism are aetiological proposals that have little experimental or clinical support.

Post-mortem histological examination of temporal bones after inner ear barotrauma, or at autopsy, may indicate an occasional association with enlarged vestibular and/or cochlear aqueducts that allows for a greater CSF-perilymph communication. These anomalies may be detected on high-resolution computed tomography (CT) scans. Other anomalies or malformations are sometimes detected that may indicate a predilection for inner ear barotrauma. These anomalies may be detected by high-resolution CT scans.

A tear of Reissner's membrane results in an isolated loss in one or two frequencies (tested In 100-Hz increments between 400 and 1300 Hz).

A progressive sensorineural loss or vertigo that develops hours or days after a barotrauma incident is most likely the result of a **fistula of the round window** with leakage of the perilymph into the middle ear and/or air into the perilymph. This can develop at any stage of the dive or afterward.

Symptoms

Many of these divers develop the first symptoms after the completion of the dive while performing energetic tasks, e.g. pulling up the anchor. This may be because the middle ear (including the round window) has been damaged by the earlier barotrauma. The subsequent fistula follows a rise of pressure in the CSF, the cochlear aqueduct and the perilymph, as a result of exertion.

Sudden tinnitus and hearing loss may be more frequent in patients with inner ear haemorrhages.

Progressive deterioration of sensorineural hearing, over hours or days, fluctuating hearing loss and position-induced hearing loss indicate a perilymph fistula. Persistence of vestibular symptoms may indicate perilymph fistula.

Deafness is of the sensorineural type, either a total loss (all frequencies) or a selectively high-frequency loss (4000 to 8000 Hz). It also may be variable and altered by changing head positions, possibly because of the buoyancy of air in the perilymph or increased leakage into the middle ear. If left untreated, the sensorineural hearing loss may become total and/or permanent.

Tinnitus, with a roaring, popping or running water sound, is frequent. Aural fullness and hyperacusis are described.

Impairment of speech discrimination may precede or overshadow the delayed and progressive hearing loss.

There is often an associated conductive or lower-frequency hearing loss that resolves over the subsequent 1 to 3 weeks and may be mistakenly interpreted as a therapeutic success. Bone conduction audiograms are indicated to identify this condition.

Oval window fistulae, probably caused by damage from the stapes foot plate, have been observed, often with a severe vestibular lesion that may persist until surgical repair. This fistula is more likely in divers who have had surgical treatment of otosclerosis.

The symptoms of inner ear barotrauma may include those of vestibular origin such as vertigo, nausea, vomiting and ataxia. Vestibular symptoms vary from almost unnoticeable to incapacitating.

In the cases that initially, predominantly or solely involve vestibular function, the symptoms may progressively diminish as adaptation occurs. Even though the symptoms may diminish, the disorder may progress to destruction of the vestibular system. In other cases, vertigo may persist or recur while the fistula persists or recurs.

Symptoms associated with inner ear barotrauma may include the following:

- Sensation of blockage or fluid in the affected ear.
- Tinnitus of variable duration.
- High-frequency or total hearing loss, hyperacusis.
- Vestibular disturbances such as nausea, vomiting, vertigo, disorientation and ataxia.
- Clinical features of an associated middle ear barotrauma (with or without conductive hearing loss).

Unfortunately, the clinical differential diagnosis of cochlear or vestibular trauma, haemorrhage and perilymph fistula, based on the foregoing criteria, is by no means certain.

Once inner ear barotrauma has been experienced, the diver is more predisposed to similar incidents, which further aggravate both the tinnitus and the hearing loss.

Cochlear injury is permanent in more than half the cases, whereas vestibular symptoms are usually temporary.

Meningitis is a possible complication of perilymph fistulae.

Inner ear barotrauma is suspected in the presence of hearing loss, tinnitus, vertigo or ataxia.

Investigations

To demonstrate inner ear barotrauma, serial investigations may be necessary. Any combination of middle ear barotrauma symptoms, nausea, vertigo, tinnitus and hearing loss should be immediately and fully investigated by serial measurements of clinical function, daily audiometry up to 8000 Hz (with bone conduction if the loss is in the <4000 Hz range) and positional electronystagmography. Caloric testing is indicated only if the tympanic membrane is intact or if the technique guards against pressure or fluid transmission into the middle ear.

A test proposed to support the diagnosis of perilymphatic fistula, as opposed to other causes of inner ear damage, is positional pure tone audiometry. The patient lies horizontal with the affected ear uppermost, for 30 minutes, and the hearing improves more than 10 dB in at least two frequencies when the patient lies supine. The theoretical explanation for this improvement is that air is displaced from the perilymph-leaking windows.

Hennebert showed that an increase in pressure in the ear canal could produce nystagmus in patients who were known to have perilymph leakage. Tullio described a similar response with loud sounds. In patients with perilymph fistula, the vertigo is induced by any activity that increases the pressure in the ear canal (ascent and/or descent, loud sounds of low frequency, the Valsalva manoeuvre, tragus pressure, pneumatic otoscopy or tympanometry).

Other investigations are sometimes thought to be even more sensitive than the basic electro-nystagmogram. In diagnosing perilymph fistulas, Kohut suggested that the presence of Hennebert's sign, or its equivalent the Tullio phenomenon, is required before vestibular symptoms are attributed to a perilymph fistula. Other tests being investigated to verify this disorder include dynamic posturography, vestibulo-spinal response (body sway) reactions to stress (Hennebert's or the Tullio phenomenon) and electrocochleography.

Investigations that may be of value include temporal bone polytomography and high-resolution and contrast imaging techniques. Until now they have not been particularly helpful in diagnosis or treatment of diving induced perilymph fistulae, but their discrimination is improving. Objective testing becomes especially important when the history of antecedent trauma is vague or remote. A perilymphatic fistula test or elevated SP/AP ratio (cochlear summating potential and auditory nerve action potential) on electrocochleography significantly raises the likelihood of perilymphatic fistula.

There is no agreed upon diagnostic test with enough sensitivity and specificity to identify the presence or absence of perilymph fistula reliably.

Treatment

Treatment should be initiated promptly.

1. Avoid any increase in CSF pressure, such as from the Valsalva manoeuvre, sneezing, nose blowing, straining with defecation, sexual activity, coughing, lifting weights, fast movement or physical exertion. Loud noises should be avoided; some clinicians recommend ear plugs or other devices to reduce the external ear pressure changes. Divers very commonly perform middle ear autoinflation, almost as a matter of habit. Advise the patient that under no circumstances should autoinflation be attempted. Otherwise, the already damaged round window may not withstand the pressure wave.

2. Almost total bed rest with the head elevated to 30 degrees and careful monitoring of otological changes are indicated. This instruction is given irrespective of which of the other treatment procedures are followed.

3. Bed rest should continue until all improvement has ceased and for a week or more, to allow the inner ear membranes to heal and the haemorrhages to resolve.

4. If there is no improvement within 24 to 48 hours in cases of severe hearing loss, or if there is progressive deterioration in hearing, operative intervention should be considered. It may be delayed for 1 to 2 weeks in less severe cases, to allow the associated middle ear disorder to heal, but this may be at the expense of more permanent sensorineural hearing loss. This is a judgement call without a great deal of experimental evidence to assist.

5. Reconstructive micro-aural surgery is indicated when there is deterioration or no improvement with bed rest, with severe hearing loss or incapacitating vertigo. In patients with developing hearing loss, repair to the round or oval window will prevent the further leakage of perilymph and has proved curative in some cases, sometimes restoring hearing acuity. It may stop vertigo and may reduce tinnitus, both of which may be disabling. In a survey of 197 cases of presumed perilymphatic fistula (not necessarily related to diving), Fitzgerald reported that 87 per cent of patients with vestibular symptoms had complete or nearly complete relief. With hearing loss, 40 per cent had improvement. If a fistula is

not visualized during middle ear exploration, a graft should still be applied to the window because sometimes the fistula is intermittent. Some surgeons use colour dyes to make the leakage more obvious. Others employ techniques to increase the CSF pressure. Surgery, which was employed in most cases in earlier years, is rarely needed now if conservative treatment is given conscientiously. After 2 weeks' delay, it will rarely improve hearing. Middle ear surgical exploration is not indicated in cases of inner ear haemorrhage because it is not a harmless procedure, and in rare cases it can induce further or complete hearing loss.

6. Prohibition of diving and flying is essential for the first few weeks following a perilymph fistula. If medical evacuation by air is required, an aircraft with the cabin pressurized to ground level is necessary. For most cases, but especially those precipitated by minimal provocation and in patients who have poor Eustachian tube function or nasal disease, it is prudent to advise against any further hyperbaric (scuba or free diving) exposure. The same applies if permanent hearing loss, tinnitus or vestibular asymmetry persists.

7. Treatment of vertigo is based on routine medical principles. Vertigo is usually suppressed by cerebral inhibition within a few weeks, but may be precipitated by sudden movement or other vestibular stimulation (caloric or alternobaric). It may persist if the fistula remains patent.

8. Other regimens. Vasodilators (e.g. nicotinic acid, carbogen) have been recommended by some investigators, but little evidence exists to show any favourable effect. Aspirin is to be avoided because of its anticoagulant effects. Steroids have no verified place in treatment of this type of hearing loss.

9. Air entry into the perilymph, as a cause of the disorder, has yet to be quantified. As a relatively harmless procedure, the authors sometimes add 100 per cent oxygen breathing to the conservative treatment regimen for 4 to 6 hours a day for 3 days.

10. Hyperbaric oxygen therapy has been used and recommended by some experienced hyperbaric therapists, and so it warrants further consideration and investigation. There is no reason to believe that recompression therapy *per se*, employing air or normoxic gases, is of value. Hyperbaric oxygen therapy may be of value in other forms of sudden hearing loss, with or without steroids. The authors of this text have tried it in patients with inner ear barotrauma, but had to proceed to surgery subsequently. Hyperbaric oxygen therapy has the potential to aggravate the fistula and increase the perilymph flow into the middle ear during descent – both from the relatively negative middle ear pressures and the need for the Valsalva manoeuvre. It has been responsible for apparent 'cures' in some cases of middle ear barotrauma with conductive generalized hearing loss, misdiagnosed and reported as inner ear barotrauma. In these cases, if the middle ear is autoinflated with descent, the gas expansion removes middle ear fluid on ascent.

An excellent review of the various approaches to this disorder in divers is given by Elliott and Smart.

Prognosis

After inner ear barotrauma there may be an apparent complete cure or persisting residue. The cochlear acuity (especially lower-frequency hearing) may improve for a few weeks, and then the remaining high-frequency loss is usually permanent, to be aggravated by the influence of ageing.

Tinnitus often improves over the next 6 to 12 months, possibly the effect of repair or death of damaged sensory endings.

If the vestibular system is damaged and asymmetry persists, the patient will never be able to dive or fly safely, because of alternobaric vertigo. He or she may continue to have occasional vertigo, aggravated by sudden head movement, which is then a hazard in all occupations that involve balance, exposure to heights or driving.

The authors of this text would advise against piloting aircraft because of the danger of alternobaric vertigo, which has followed some cases of unilateral inner ear damage.

Too many cases of inner ear barotrauma have recurred for these authors to propose a resumption of diving – either free or with equipment – once permanent inner ear damage has been demonstrated.

MIDDLE EAR BAROTRAUMA COMPLICATIONS

Seventh nerve palsy

The seventh or facial cranial nerve may be affected, causing 'facial baroparesis'. Recorded in both aviators and divers, this disorder sometimes follows middle ear barotrauma. It manifests as a unilateral facial weakness similar to Bell's palsy, and it tends to recur in the same patient if the cause is not corrected.

The reason for this disorder is explained by the anatomy of the facial canal. This is open to the middle ear in some people and so shares its barotraumatic pathology. Also, middle ear air expands during ascent and could force its way into this seventh nerve canal.

Paralysis of the facial nerve makes frowning impossible, prevents the eye from closing on that side and causes drooping of the lower eyelid (which may result in tears running down the face because they do not drain into the nasolacrimal duct). The cheek is smooth, and the mouth is pulled to the normal side. Whistling becomes impossible, and food collects between the cheek and gum.

A metallic taste may be noticed at the start of the illness, as may impaired taste in the anterior part of the tongue on the same side, from chorda tympani involvement. Hyperacusis may result from paralysis of the stapedius muscle.

Early treatment could include inhalation of 100 per cent oxygen for some hours, based on the theoretical pathophysiology involved, to remove air from the seventh nerve canal.

Both physicians and otologists frequently omit to interrogate patients with Bell's palsy regarding their swimming, diving and aviation exposure.

Otitis media

Although not frequent, otitis media is an occasional complication of middle ear barotrauma, with the middle ear collecting fluid that forms a medium for growth of organisms (see Chapter 29). Thus, ear pain developing hours or days after middle ear barotrauma should be considered to indicate a middle ear infection. This not only is a serious illness in its own right, but is also a possible cause of narrowing of the Eustachian tube and further middle ear barotraumas.

Mastoiditis

The mastoid, being part of the middle ear cleft, responds in the same way as the middle ear to a negative pressure situation. Thus, the production of fluid and blood in the mastoid, especially during

---

CASE REPORT 7.2

This diver, who had been exposed to gunfire in the past, experienced considerable pain and difficulty in equalizing both middle ears during a dive to 10 metres. He continued to dive despite the pain and performed forceful autoinflations. He noted tinnitus, and he also experienced ear pain and vertigo during ascent. Otoscopic examination of the tympanic membrane revealed the effects of barotrauma. The diver became progressively more deaf, with a sensorineural pattern in both ears, over the next few days. Transient episodes of vertigo were noted. Exploratory surgery was performed. A fistula of the round window was observed, together with a frequent drip of perilymph fluid into the middle ear. The round window was packed. A similar procedure was performed 5 days later in the other ear, with the same result. Subsequent audiograms over the following month revealed a considerable improvement in hearing.

Diagnosis: inner ear barotrauma (with perilymph fistula of the round window) caused by middle ear barotrauma of descent and forceful autoinflation, resulting in sensorineural hearing loss.

descent, can develop and produce the conditions conducive to bacterial growth.

Under these circumstances, the patient usually has pain and tenderness over the mastoid, and the pathological features can be demonstrated by CT scans of the temporal bone.

Meningitis

Although rare, meningitis is a possible extension of otitis media, mastoiditis, sinusitis and so forth and a complication of both labyrinthine fistula and pneumocephalus.

Pneumocephalus/intracranial haemorrhage

Another rare complication from the middle ear cleft and mastoid air cells is pneumocephalus, resulting from the expansion of gas in a space that is now occupied by blood and fluid from descent barotrauma. A rupture into the cranial cavity, with air and/or fluids, produces a sudden and excruciating headache, with the pathological features demonstrated by CT brain scans and magnetic resonance imaging (see Chapter 8). The bony roof over the middle ear–mastoid space, the tegmen tympani of the petrous temporal bone, is frequently very thin or incomplete, allowing for the contents of this space (air, blood) to rupture into the middle cranial fossa, into the epidural or sub-dural areas.

REFERENCE

1. Elliott E, Smart DR. A literature review of the assessment and management of inner ear barotrauma in divers and recommendations for returning to diving. *Diving and Hyperbaric Medicine Journal* 2014 (in press).

FURTHER READING

Alexsson A, Miller J, Silverman M. Anatomical effects of sudden middle ear pressure changes. *Annals of Otology* 1979:**88**:368–376.

Antonellip J, Parell GJ, Becker GD, Paparella MM. Temporal bone pathology in scuba diving deaths. *Otolaryngology and Head and Neck Surgery* 1993;**109**:514–521.

Becker GD, Parell GJ. Otolaryngologic aspects of scuba diving. *Otolaryngology and Head and Neck Surgery* 1979;**87**(5):569–572.

Carlson S, Jones J, Brown M, Hess C. Prevention of hyperbaric associated middle ear barotrauma. *Annals of Emergency Medicine* 1992;**21**(12):1468–1471.

Conde JF. Auricular and sinus barotrauma. *Acta oto-rino-laringológica ibero-americana* 1970;**21**(3):309–315.

Demard F. Les accidents labyrinthiques aigus au cours de la plongée sous-marine. *Forsvarsmedicin* 1973;**9**(3):416–422.

Edmonds C. Round window rupture in diving. *Forsvarsmedicin* 1973;**9**(3):404–405.

Edmonds C. Dysbaric peripheral nerve involvement. *South Pacific Underwater Medicine Society Journal* 1991;**21**(4):190–197.

Edmonds C. Inner ear barotrauma: a retrospective clinical series of 50 cases. *South Pacific Underwater Medicine Society Journal* **44**(4):243–245.

Edmonds C, Freeman P, Thomas R, Tonkin J, Blackwood FA. *Otological Aspects of Diving.* Sydney: Australian Medical Publishing Co.; 1973.

Edmonds C, Lowry C, Pennefather J. *Diving and Subaquatic Medicine.* Sydney: Diving Medical Centre; 1973.

Edmonds C, McKenzie B, Thomas R. Pennefather J. *Diving Medicine for SCUBA Divers.* 5th ed. www.divingmedicine.info; 2013.

Elliott E, Smart DR. A literature review of the assessment and management of inner ear barotrauma in divers and recommendations for returning to diving. *Diving and Hyperbaric Medicine Journal* 2014;**44**(4):243–245

Farmer JC. Otological and paranasal sinus problems in diving. In: Bennett P, Elliott H, eds. *The Physiology and Medicine of Diving.* 4th ed. London: Saunders; 1993.

Fitzgerald DC, Getson P, Brasseux CO. Perilymphatic fistula: Washington DC experience. *Annals of Otology and Laryngology* 1997;**106**:830–837.

Freeman P, Edmonds C. Inner ear barotrauma. *Archives of Otolaryngology* 1972;**95**:556–563.

Goldmann RW. Pneumocephalus as a consequence of diving. *JAMA* 1986;**255**:3154–3156.

Hagberg M. Ornhagen H. Incidence and risk factors for symptoms of ear and sinus among male and female dive masters and instructors: a retrospective cohort study. *Undersea and Hyperbaric Medicine* 2003;**30**(2):93–102.

Hunter ES, Farmer JC. Ear and sinus problems in diving. In: Bove A, Davis J, eds. *Bove and Davis' Diving Medicine.* 4th ed. Philadelphia: Saunders; 2004.

Kitajima N, Sugita-Kitajima A, Kitajima S. Altered Eustachian tube function in SCUBA divers with alternobaric vertigo. *Otol Neurotol*; 2014; **35**(5):850–856.

Klokker M, Vesterhauge S, Jansen EC. Pressure equalizing earplugs do not prevent baro-trauma on descent from 8000 ft cabin altitude. *Aviation, Space, and Environmental Medicine* 2005;**76**(11):1079–1082.

Lehm JP, Bennett MH. Predictors of middle ear barotrauma associated with hyperbaric oxygen therapy. *South Pacific Underwater Medicine Society Journal* 2003;**33**:127–133.

Lundgren GEC. Alternobaric vertigo: a diving hazard. *British Medical Journal* 1965;**1**:511.

Macfie DD. ENT problems of diving. *Medical Services Journal Canada* 1964;**20**:845–861.

Markham JW. The clinical features of pneumo-cephalus based on a survey of 284 cases with a report of 11 additional cases. *Acta Neurochirurgica* 1967;**16**(1–2):1–78.

Molvaer OI. Otorhinological aspects of diving. In: Brubakk AO, Neuman TS, eds. *Bennett and Elliott's Physiology and Medicine of Diving.* 5th ed. Philadelphia: Saunders; 2003.

Molvaer OI, Albrektsen G. Alternobaric vertigo in professional divers. *Undersea Biomedical Research* 1988;**15**(4):271–282.

Money KE, Buckingham IP, Calder IM. et al. Damage to the middle ear and the inner ear in underwater divers. *Undersea Biomedical Research* 1985;**12**(1):77–84.

Neblett LM. Otolaryngology and sport scuba diving: update and guidelines. *Annals of Otology, Rhinology, and Laryngology Supplement* 1985;**115**:1–12.

O'Neill OJ. The O'Neill grading system for the evaluation of the tympanic membrane. 2015. in Undersea and Hyperbaric Medicine journal, in press.

Parell GJ, Becker GD. Inner ear barotrauma in scuba divers. *Archives of Otolaryngology* 1993;**119**:455–457.

Pulec JG, Hahn FW. The abnormally patulous Eustachian tube. *Otological Clinics of North America* 1970;**3**(1):131–140.

Pullen FW. Perilymphatic fistula induced by barotrauma. *American Journal of Otology* 1992;**13**(3):270–272.

Roland PS, Meyers AD. Inner ear, perilymph fistula. Medscape Reference, emedicine. medscape.com/article/856806 updated April 26, 2010.

Roydhouse N. 1001 disorders of the ear, nose and sinuses in scuba divers. *Canadian Journal of Applied Sport Sciences* 1985;**10**(2):99–103.

Simmons FB. Theory of membrane breaks in sudden hearing loss. *Archives of Otolaryngology* 1968;**88**:41–48.

Taylor D. The Valsalva manoeuvre: a critical review. *South Pacific Underwater Medicine Society Journal* 1996;**26**(1):8–13.

Teed RW. Factors producing obstruction of the auditory tube in submarine personnel. *US Naval Medical Bulletin.* 1944;**42**:293–306.

Tjernstrom O. Alternobaric vertigo. Proceedings of the First European Undersea Biomedical Symposium, Stockholm. *Forsvarsmedicin* 1973;**9**(3):410–415.

Vorosmarti J, Bradley ME. Alternobaric vertigo in military divers. *Military Medicine* 1970;**135**:182–185.

Yanagit N, Miyake H, Sakakibara K, Sakakibara B, Takahashi H. Sudden deafness and hyperbaric oxygen therapy: clinical reports of 25 patients. In: *Fifth International Hyperbaric Conference. IHC publication, Vancouver, Canada* 973:389–401.

This chapter was reviewed for this fifth edition by Carl Edmonds.

8

Sinus barotrauma

AVIATION EXPERIENCE

In the 1940s, sinus barotrauma from aviation exposure was well described by Campbell[1,2]. Although sinus barotrauma is the second most common disease in diving medicine, there has been very little detailed documentation, apart from individual case reports. The injury results from the changes in volume of the gas spaces within the paranasal sinuses during ascent or descent – when those changes could not be compensated for by the passage of air between the sinus and the nasopharynx. It is the clinical manifestation of Boyle's Law as it affects the paranasal sinuses (Figure 8.1).

The **pathological** changes found within the sinuses included: Mucosal detachment; submucosal haematoma; blood clots in membranous sacs; small haemorrhages within the mucosa; and swelling of the mucous membrane.

Weissman and associates[3] described a series of 15 cases of **frontal sinus barotrauma** in aviators. Most of these cases were grade III. These investigators used the following grading system:

- Grade I – a transient discomfort that cleared promptly and had only slight mucosal oedema, but no x-ray changes.
- Grade II – characterized by pain over the affected sinus for up to 24 hours. There was thickening of the mucosa seen on x-ray studies. If such a sinus was opened, small amounts of blood-tinged fluid were found. Serosanguineous fluid sometimes drained from the sinus, with or without the use of decongestants.
- Grade III – a severe pain or a 'bee sting' or 'being shot' sensation. If the pain was not quickly relieved by the Valsalva manoeuvre, the pilot had to descend rapidly to relieve symptoms.

Usually, aviators with grade I and II barotrauma did not seek medical aid, and symptoms usually cleared spontaneously. Grade III cases resulted in oedema and congestion of the sinus mucosa with submucosal haemorrhages. As the sinus mucous membrane was pulled away from

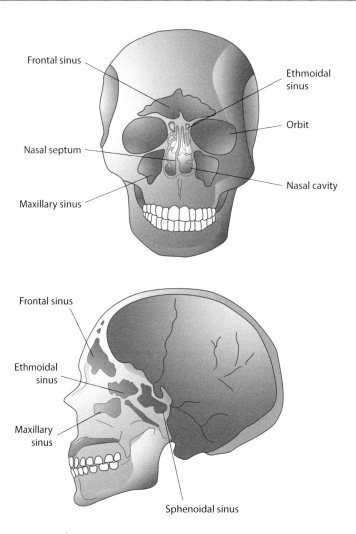

Figure 8.1 Accessory para-nasal sinuses.

the periosteum by the negative intrasinus pressure, a haematoma formed. Sinus x-ray studies showed an air-fluid level or a polypoidal mass. Incising this mass brought forth a spurt of old blood, with clots.

DIVING EXPERIENCE

Comprehensive reviews of **diving-related sinus barotraumas** were not easy to find. Flottes[4], in 1965, described sinus barotrauma in divers.

Sinus barotrauma has been described in various texts on diving medicine[5], but initially without specific clinical series being documented. A reasonably large clinical series of divers with sinus barotrauma was first described in Australia by Fagan, McKenzie and Edmonds in 1976[6] and was quoted widely thereafter. This series described minor and acute cases and was complemented by another series of 50 more serious cases in patients who were referred for definitive treatment[7].

The first Australian series

The cases in this series were equivalent to Campbell's aviation sinus barotrauma grades 1 and 2. This series included 50 consecutive cases of sinus barotrauma as they were observed in a Navy environment, where all such cases were referred for medical opinion irrespective of severity[6]. It included many cases that might otherwise have not attended for treatment.

In this series, 68 per cent of the presenting symptoms developed during or on descent, and they developed in 32 per cent during or after ascent.

In the majority, the divers were undergoing their first open water diver training course. **Pain** was the predominant symptom in all the cases on descent and in 75 per cent of those on ascent. Pain was referred to the frontal area in 68 per cent, the ethmoid in 16 per cent and the maxillary in 6 per cent. In one case it was referred to the upper dental area.

Epistaxis was the second most common symptom, occurring in 58 per cent of cases. It was rarely more than an incidental observation, perhaps of concern to the diver but not usually of great severity. It was the sole symptom in 25 per cent of the cases of ascent barotrauma.

Even though these were inexperienced divers, 32 per cent had a history of **previous sinus barotrauma,** produced by scuba diving, aviation exposure or free diving. Half had a history of recent **upper respiratory tract inflammation,** and others gave a history of intermittent or long-term symptoms referable to the upper respiratory tract, e.g. nasal and sinus disorders, recurrent infections or hay fever.

In 48 per cent of cases, otoscopy showed evidence of middle ear barotrauma on the tympanic membrane.

Radiologically, the affected sinuses did not replicate the clinical sites and manifestations. Either mucosal thickening or a fluid level was observed in the maxillary sinus in 74 per cent of the cases, in the frontal sinus in 24 per cent and in the ethmoid in 15 per cent. These findings contrast with the clinical manifestations. A fluid level was present in 12 per cent of the maxillary sinus cases.

Most of these divers required no treatment or responded to short-term use of nasal decongestants. Antibiotics were prescribed if there was pre-existing or subsequent sinusitis. Neither sinus exploration nor surgery was required in any case. This series has inappropriately been used to imply that such intervention is never applicable in the treatment of sinus barotrauma.

This prospective Australian series, by its design, included relatively minor cases of sinus barotrauma.

It has, by default, been used as being typical of all sinus barotrauma cases, even those that manifest in patients with recurrent or delayed symptoms, or complications, in emergency wards or ear, nose and throat consulting rooms. That extrapolation is not necessarily valid. Also, this study was done more than 4 decades ago, before computer imaging techniques became commonplace and when sphenoidal disease was not easily detected.

> Sinus barotrauma and its complications remain common medical problems of diving. The importance has been stressed by many workers including Edmonds, Freeman, Thomas and colleagues[8], Becker and Parell[9], Neblett[10] and Roydhouse[11].

The second Australian series

The cases in this series were equivalent to Campbell's aviation sinus barotrauma grade 3. A series of 50 more severe cases, i.e. in patients referred for medical treatment of sinus barotrauma, was reported in 1994[7]. These patients were seen within 1 month of the latest incident.

The cases were self-selecting because the divers with repetitive or more significant problems were more likely to present for treatment. The investigations frequently involved computed tomography (CT) scans of the sinuses, sinus endoscopy and occasionally magnetic resonance imaging (MRI).

These cases were in more experienced divers – 88 per cent had in excess of 50 dives. The distribution was skewed strongly to the extremely experienced, with 70 per cent of the divers having more than 5 years of experience, and many being dive masters, dive instructors or professional divers. Because of the extreme amount of diving exposure in this group, it is presumed that the sinus ostia or ducts may have become scarred and narrowed from the repeated insults they sustained.

In 12 per cent of the patients, the presenting **headache** developed and progressed while at depth. It could usually be made worse with subsequent ascents or descents, but the initial development of the headache during a time in which there was no substantial change in depth did cause some confusion in the initial physician's assessment.

From the aviation literature, it is believed that a small degree of negative pressure is sustainable within the sinuses, without symptoms[12]. Exceeding this pressure may be sufficient to cause a gradual effusion to develop, and the full or heavy sensation within the sinus may take some time to develop. Extrapolation would suggest that diving-related barotrauma could occur with a reduction in sinus air volume of 5 to 10 per cent, i.e. at a depth of 0.5 to 1 metre below the surface.

In 8 per cent of the patients there was a very clear-cut and dramatic sensation of a bursting or popping during depth changes. Of these, half were on descent and half on ascent. It has been described in aviation medicine as the 'popping of a champagne cork', a 'gunshot', 'like a bee sting over the eye' and 'like being struck on the head with a club or bat'. It is presumed, from the observations of Campbell[1,2] and of Mann and Beck[12], as well as from this series, that the sensation results from a haemorrhage stripping up the mucosa of the sinus, produced by the negative intrasinus pressure with descent.

A similar sudden sensation can also occur from the rupture of an air sac or release of pressure from a distended sinus during ascent. This may be followed by a 'hissing' sensation of air movement, which may then relieve discomfort and pain. One of the cases involved the ethmoidal area, and the patient had a subsequent small, oval haematoma noted over the ethmoid region within hours (Figure 8.2).

In 10 per cent, repetitive incidents of sinus barotrauma appeared to be provoked by inappropriate diving and equalization techniques. In these cases there would frequently be a head first descent, and/or swallowing as a method of middle ear equalization. The substitution of the feet first descent (preferably down a shot line), together with frequent positive-pressure middle ear equalization manoeuvres, appeared to rectify the situation. These are now described in medical texts used by divers[13].

A similar problem developed if descents were slow, because of discomfort noted in the sinus. The blood or effusion gradually accumulating in the sinus equalizes the pressure and reduces the

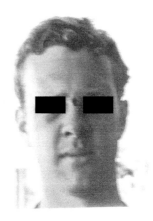

Figure 8.2 Ethmoidal haemorrhage. Following ethmoidal sinus barotrauma of descent, the sinus burst during ascent, with sudden excruciating pain, then bruising and haemorrhage into the adjoining skin, between the eyes.

degree of pain and discomfort. This may be appropriate for an emergency dive, but it is not prudent if disease is to be avoided. On the contrary, divers inappropriately used this development of the disorder (e.g. blood or effusion, mucosal congestion) as a measure to replace a contracting air space in the sinus during descent, to allow the dive to continue.

Divers in these categories were advised of the correct methods of descent and to use positive pressure middle ear equalization (e.g. the Valsalva manoeuvre; see Chapter 7). This may have an effect of aerating the sinuses before major disease and haemorrhage develop.

Previous radiological descriptions included haematomas, mucous cysts, mucocoeles, polyps or polypoid masses, opacification and, most commonly, a thickening of the mucosa. The series reported by the authors was no different in the various radiological descriptions; however, the CT scans showed more identifiable and definitive pathological features (Figure 8.3). MRI using T1- and T2-weighted imaging was more diagnostic in differentiating blood from mucosal thickening[14]. Sphenoidal involvement was common.

The current use of MRI and CT scans of the sinuses made diagnosis and treatment more definitive in most of these cases. Sinus endoscopy, sinus surgery or nasal surgery was needed in 12 per cent, often with excellent results.

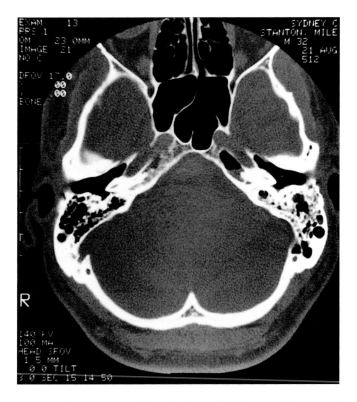

Figure 8.3 Sinus barotrauma affecting mastoid and sphenoidal sinuses. Computed tomography scan and magnetic resonance imaging have replaced x-ray studies in identifying sinus disorders. Left fluid level in petrous bone and loss of pneumatization of mastoid air cells.

SINUS BAROTRAUMA OF DESCENT (SINUS SQUEEZE)

If a sinus ostium is blocked during descent, muco-sal congestion and haemorrhage compensate for the contraction of the air within the sinus cav-ity. During ascent, expansion of the enclosed air expels blood and mucus from the sinus ostium. Ostia blockage may be the result of sinusitis with mucosal hypertrophy and congestion, rhinitis, redundant mucosal folds in the nose, nasal polyps and so forth.

As described with ear barotraumas, sinus baro-traumas are more frequently noted in female divers and in the young; however, chronic sinus problems are an increasing problem with age and excessive diving frequency (more in dive instructors than in dive masters[15]).

Symptoms include pain over the sinus during descent. It may be preceded by a sensation of tight-ness or pressure. The pain usually subsides with

ascent but may continue as a persistent dull ache for several hours. On ascent, blood or mucus may be extruded into the nose or pharynx, on the same side as the sinus disease.

Headache developing during the dive, with the diver neither ascending nor descending, should not exclude the diagnosis of sinus barotrauma. When this develops at considerable depth, the sedative effects of narcosis may distort the clinical features. Also, small changes of depth may not be particularly noticeable but produce a misleading history.

The pain is usually over the frontal sinus; less frequently it is retro-orbital and probably sphe-noidal. Maxillary pain is not common but may be referred to the upper teeth on the same side. Although the teeth may feel hypersensitive, abnor-mal or loose, they are not painful on movement. Coughing, sneezing or holding the head down may aggravate the pain and make it throb. Numbness over the maxillary division of the fifth nerve is pos-sible (see later).

The superficial ethmoidal sinuses near the root of the nose occasionally rupture and cause a small haematoma or discolouration of the skin between the eyes (see Figure 8.2).

Discomfort persisting after the dive may result from fluid within the sinus (continuous from the dive), infection (usually starts a few hours after the dive) or the development of chronic sinusitis or mucocoeles.

Investigations

Sinus x-ray examination, CT or MRI scan may disclose thickened mucosa, opacity or fluid levels. The opacities produced by the barotrauma may be haemorrhagic, serous or mucous cysts. The maxillary and frontal sinuses are commonly involved. The ethmoid and sphenoidal sinuses may also be affected. The newer imaging techniques can clearly demonstrate these features (Case Report 8.1).

SINUS BAROTRAUMA OF ASCENT

This disorder may follow the occlusion of sinus openings by mucosal congestion, folds or sinus polyps, preventing escape of expanding gases (Figure 8.4). The ostium or its mucosa will then blow out into the nasal cavity, with or without pain, and haemorrhage commonly follows. Bleeding from the nostril on the same side as the sinus disorder is sometimes the only manifestation. This disease is aggravated by rapid ascent, as in free ascent training, emergency ascents, submarine escape and so forth.

Uncommonly, other manifestations may develop. If the expanding air cannot escape through the sinuses, it may fracture the walls and track along the soft tissues and cause surgical emphysema. Rupture of air cells may cause severe and sudden pain, often affecting the ethmoidal or mastoid sinuses, on ascent. Occasionally, the air may rupture into the cranial cavity and cause a pneumocephalus or a small intracranial haemorrhage.

OTHER MANIFESTATIONS

General symptoms

In a small number of the cases (8 per cent), some additional symptoms did not appear to be easily explicable on the basis of local sinus disease. These included nausea or vomiting, a sensation of impending syncope and disorientation at the time of injury. These occurred in the more dramatic cases of sinus barotrauma.

CASE REPORT 8.1

DN, a 22-year-old sports diver, occasionally noticed a trace of blood from his face mask following ascent. He had often complained of nasal blockage and had various treatments for this, including cautery. His first dive to 12 metres for 10 minutes was uneventful. After a brief surface interval he again descended, but he was unable to proceed beyond 6 metres because of a severe tearing headache in the frontal region. He equalized his face mask, and this provided some relief. He then continued the descent feet first but still had some slight pain. On reaching the bottom, the severe sharp pain recurred. During ascent it lessened in severity, but on reaching the surface he noted mucus and blood in his face mask. A dull frontal headache persisted for 3 hours after the dive. Examination revealed a deviated nasal septum to both right and left, with hyperaemic nasal mucosa. X-ray studies showed gross mucosal thickening in both maxillary sinuses, the right being completely opaque. There was also some slight shadowing on the right frontal sinus. The radiological signs cleared over the next 2 weeks. Because the airways were patent on both sides of the nasal septum, operative intervention was not indicated. The patient's nasal mucosa returned to normal after he abstained from cigarette smoking.

Diagnosis: sinus barotrauma of descent.

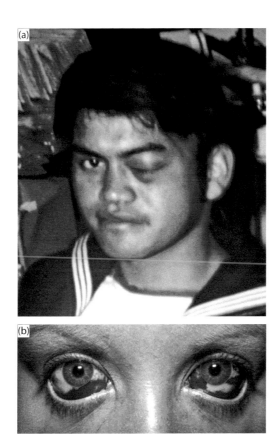

Plate 2, front. Orbital surgical emphysema and facial barotrauma of descent. **(a)** Orbital surgical emphysema. Orbital swelling following a Valsalva manoeuvre at 10 metres. The swelling expanded during ascent and resolved with 100 per cent oxygen breathing. Following a fracture of the lamina papyracea from a recent football injury, the Valsalva manoeuvre allowed gas to enter the orbit, thereby causing surgical emphysema and haemorrhage. **(b)** Facial barotrauma of descent ('mask squeeze') causing subconjunctival haemorrhages and facial oedema, following failure to equalize mask pressures during a descent to 15 metres.

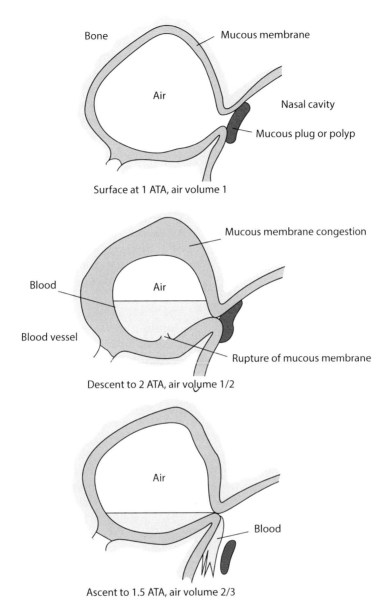

Figure 8.4 Diagrammatic changes of sinus barotrauma from obstruction of sinus ostia on the surface (top), then descent to 10 metres (2 ATA), halving the sinus air volume and replacing this with fluid and mucosal swelling (middle). During ascent, the gas expands and discharges fluid (blood, effusion).

Maxillary nerve involvement

In 4 per cent of the cases the pain was referred to the upper teeth, on the same side as the affected maxillary sinus. This is presumably an involvement of the posterior superior alveolar nerve.

In another 4 per cent there was involvement of the infraorbital nerve, with numbness over the skin of the cheek on the same side.

Two separate branches of the maxillary division of trigeminal nerve can thus be affected as they traverse the maxillary sinus[16,17]: the infraorbital nerve as it runs along the wall of the maxillary sinus and the posterior superior alveolar nerve as it runs along the lateral or inferior wall of the maxillary sinus. The former produces a numbness or paraesthesia over the cheek and the latter a numbness over the upper teeth, gums and mucosa on the same side. In some cases pain and hypersensitivity are observed. Problems with neurapraxia are more common with ascent than descent, a finding suggesting that impaired circulation is more frequent than congestion or haemorrhage of the nerve as a basis of the presentation.

There is a possibility of involvement of any division of the trigeminal nerve, including its maxillary division, with involvement of the sphenoidal sinus[18].

Acute sinusitis

Campbell[1] stated that infection occurs only rarely, and his series may be equitable, in terms of selection, with the initial Australian survey[6]. If, however, one considers the second Australian survey, with its more serious cases, then the infection complications are more frequent.

Acute sinusitis developed some hours after the dive and extended into subsequent days, in 28 per cent of the severe cases, usually with an exacerbation of pain over the affected area, a purulent nasal discharge and generalized systemic symptoms.

The patients with sinus barotrauma who subsequently developed a sinus infection possibly did so because of the haemorrhage and effusion in the sinus. This condition becomes a culture medium for organisms introduced by the flow of air into the sinus during descent. An occasional case of orbital cellulitis may extend from the ethmoidal or maxillary sinusitis, and it is a medical emergency. One case proceeded to blindness (Case Report 8.2). It is for this reason that the authors of this text now vigorously treat with antibiotics any persistence of symptoms following sinus barotrauma, i.e. commencing hours after the dive or continuing into the following day.

Chronic sinusitis

The criteria for this diagnosis included a continuation of sinus symptoms in excess of 1 month. In 18 per cent of the severe cases there was a continuation of the initial barotrauma episode and acute sinusitis into a syndrome of chronic sinusitis.

In another 14 per cent the chronic sinusitis was pre-existent, with recurrent barotraumas developing over it.

Chronic sinusitis is a long-term effect of diving, especially if the diver has experienced repeated barotrauma episodes. Thus, it often affects commercial divers near the end of their professional career. Then micro-surgery to open the scarred and narrowed ostia may be of great value in both prolonging their diving career and improving their life style from detrimental chronic sinusitis.

CASE REPORT 8.2

A 24-year-old professional trainee diver descended to 40 msw for 30 minutes despite an upper respiratory tract infection and descent-induced pain over his right maxilla and orbit. He slowed his descent to reduce these symptoms, but re-developed a sudden severe pain over his right cheek on ascent. Bleeding was evident after ascent, in his face mask. Three days later he complained of persistent right facial pain, blocked nose and epistaxis. The next day he had swollen right eyelids, mucopurulent nasal discharge and mild pyrexia. X-ray studies confirmed right maxillary and ethmoidal sinusitis. Antral washout and antibiotics were administered but did not prevent an extension of the orbital cellulitis and retinal artery thrombosis with permanent and total right-sided blindness. (From Bellini MJ. Blindness in a diver following sinus barotrauma. *Journal of Laryngology and Otology* 1987;**101**:386–389.)

Pneumocephalus/haemorrhage/ neurological involvement

The presence of pneumocephalus, in association with sinus injury in general medicine, has been well recorded by Markham[19], and it is one of the dangers associated with sinus barotrauma[5]. It has been well demonstrated by Goldmann[20] (see Figure 9.3).

Pneumocephalus results from the expansion during ascent of gas in a space (mastoid, ethmoidal and sphenoidal sinus) that has been partly occupied by blood and fluid from the descent barotrauma. A rupture into the cranial cavity, with air and/or fluids, produces an excruciating and sudden headache, with the pathological features demonstrated by radiology, CT brain scans or MRI. The temporal bony roof over the sinuses is frequently very thin or incomplete, allowing for the contents of this (air, blood) to rupture into the middle cranial fossa, into the epidural areas[21]. This condition is not infrequently observed at autopsy when the diver has descended while alive but unconscious, inducing para-nasal sinus barotrauma, and then being brought to the surface, where the gas space has expanded, even though the diver may have died.

Extension of infections following sinus barotrauma and subsequent sinusitis may result in orbital cellulitis, meningitis and other neurological problems[21-25].

Orbital haemorrhage may also result from the pressure gradient, with potential vision-threatening ocular complications. Sinus mucocoeles, produced during barotrauma, can also cause space-occupying lesions with neurological sequelae, including optic neuropathy and blindness. Demonstrable on MRI, these disorders require referral of the patient to an ophthalmic surgeon[21-25].

Surgical emphysema

This disorder has been seen on a number of occasions and was described previously[5]. The tracking of air expanding in the sinuses and erupting into the surrounding tissues can manifest as orbital surgical emphysema (usually from the ethmoidal sinus though a fracture of the egg-shell–thin lamina papyracea; see Plate 2). In other instances, the air has passed from other sinuses, and the disorder can first occur as a localized manifestation in the facial tissues.

DIFFERENTIAL DIAGNOSIS

In 6 per cent of the 'serious' cases, an initial diagnosis of **decompression sickness** was made, with the case subsequently demonstrated to be sinus barotrauma, often with complicating sinus infection. At the time of presentation, which could be some hours after the dive, the clinical pattern was confused with cerebral decompression sickness and treated as such. These were understandable mistakes, and there should be no hesitation in administering hyperbaric therapy if there is any doubt regarding the diagnosis. It would be preferable to miss and mistreat a case of sinus barotrauma than miss and mistreat a case of cerebral decompression sickness.

The only other case of incorrect diagnosis was one subsequently attributed to a **dental** aetiology (barotrauma associated with pneumatization around a carious tooth), and this case was therefore not included in the series.

Lew and his colleagues[18] referred not only to the symptoms of **sphenoidal sinusitis**, but also to its association with 'deep sea diving'. Sphenoidal sinus involvement occurred in 6 per cent of the 'serious' cases. It is important because of the failure of clinicians to recognize it and to not appreciate its potentially serious complications (Case Report 8.3).

Sphenoidal sinusitis is not easy to demonstrate with plain x-ray films, but it is often obvious on MRI or CT scans.

TREATMENT

Most of the effects of sinus barotrauma are minor and rapidly regress if diving is suspended and the underlying or consequential inflammatory disorder of the sinus is treated. Patients with a sinus or upper respiratory tract infection may require antibiotics and decongestants. Surgical drainage of acute lesions is rarely indicated, unless there are neurological or other sequelae. Attention is best paid to prevention.

Even mucoceles and chronic sinus disease usually resolve without intervention, if diving is suspended.

CASE REPORT 8.3

ID was not part of the 'serious' case series, but he sustained clinically obvious sphenoidal sinus barotrauma of descent. This caused some concern because of the proximity to other important structures around this sinus and the possibility that the computed tomographically verified space-occupying lesion was neoplastic. Although operative intervention was contemplated in this case, the lesion (a mucocele or haematoma) cleared up within 2 weeks, following abstinence from diving.

In the 'serious' cases (the second Australian series), the treatment could be divided into groups of patients:

1. Those whose disorder cleared up spontaneously and who were advised to not dive until this had happened.
2. Those who were using inappropriate diving techniques. These have been described previously. These patients usually responded to appropriate regimens of:
   a. Feet-first descent.
   b. Positive pressure manoeuvres to autoinflate both middle ears and sinuses, on the surface (immediately before descent) and then at regular intervals of half to 1 metre or so during descent. This is equalization ahead of the dive (see Chapter 7).
   c. Avoidance of diving exposure during respiratory tract inflammations.
3. Those who responded to medical treatment of the nasal disorders. This included the topical use of steroid nasal sprays, cromoglycate, topical or generalized decongestants, avoidance of nasal irritants and allergens and cessation of smoking (tobacco or marihuana).
4. Patients with infective sinusitis, who required treatment of the infections, usually by decongestants and antibiotics. The authors of this text so treat any persistence of symptoms following sinus barotrauma, i.e. symptoms commencing hours after the dive or persisting into the following day.
5. The intractable group, who required sinus exploration, usually with endoscopy and reconstruction, or nasal surgery. In some cases surgery was required to produce patency of the ostia and to remove polyps, mucocoeles or redundant mucosa that caused obstruction to the ostia. Other times it was needed to improve nasal air flow. Reference in the literature, by Bolger, Parsons and Matson[26] in 1990, has been made to the value of surgery in aviators with sinus barotrauma. The guarded enthusiasm of these investigators for functional endoscopic sinus surgery was tempered by the possible complications of this procedure. Nevertheless, endoscopic sinus surgery is advancing rapidly and may offer value to patients with the more serious and chronic cases. With current endoscopic surgical procedures[22], the maxillary, ethmoid and sphenoid sinuses can be treated to widen the sinus ostia, thus preventing sinus barotrauma. It is considered the treatment of choice in military aviators in the United States. The frontal sinus is less amenable to this treatment but may be explored in some cases.
6. The sixth group continued to have difficulties and usually ceased diving.

All patients were strongly advised to not dive during times of upper respiratory tract inflammation (e.g. infections, allergic or vasomotor rhinitis). As with the original series, more than 50 per cent of the divers in the second series had a history of diving with such conditions at the time of the barotrauma.

Some clients were moved between treatments because various measures failed to resolve or prevent problems completely.

Our general impression was that approximately equal numbers fell into each 'treatment' group. Various attitudes to the current treatments are discussed in the previously cited references and diving medical texts[6,7,13,24,26].

PREVENTION

Prevention of sinus barotrauma is achieved by refraining from diving with upper respiratory tract infections, sinusitis or rhinitis. Cessation of smoking will reduce the likelihood of mucosal irritation and sinus barotrauma. Avoidance of allergens may assist in persons so predisposed, as may treatment with local steroid nasal preparations. Correction of nasal abnormalities may be needed.

Systemic decongestants such as pseudoephedrine (Sudafed) are often used, as are topical nasal decongestants. Neither drug type is as effective as using the correct equalizing techniques. Positive pressure techniques during descent, such as the Valsalva manoeuvre, assist in aeration of the sinuses as well as the middle ears (as opposed to the passive equalization methods). Feet-first descents are preferable (i.e. head upright), and the techniques used for middle ear equalization ('equalizing ahead of the dive'; see Chapter 7) are advised. Slow descents and ascents will reduce the sinus damage where there is only marginal patency of the sinus ostia.

Some physicians have found the use of proteolytic or allegedly mucus-softening enzymes to be of value. Well-controlled experimental trials are required to demonstrate any efficacy of these drugs.

REFERENCES

1. Campbell PA. Aerosinusitis: its causes, course and treatment. *Annals of Otology* 1944;**53**:291–301.
2. Campbell PA. Aerosinusitis: a resume. *Annals of Otology* 1945;**54**:69–83.
3. Weissman D, Green RS, Roberts PT. Frontal sinus barotrauma. *Laryngoscope* 1972;**82**(2):160–162.
4. Flottes L. Barotrauma of the ear and sinuses caused by underwater immersion. *Acta oto-rino-laringológica ibero-americana* 1965;**16**(4):453–483.
5. Edmonds C, Lowry C, Pennefather J. *Diving and Subaquatic Medicine.* Sydney. Diving Medical Centre; 1971.
6. Fagan P, McKenzie B, Edmonds C. Sinus barotrauma in divers. *Annals of Otology, Rhinology, and Laryngology* 1976;**85**:61–64.
7. Edmonds C. Sinus barotrauma: a bigger picture. *South Pacific Underwater Medicine Society Journal* 1994;**24**(1):13–19.
8. Edmonds C, Freeman P, Thomas R, Tonkin J, Blackwood F. *Otological Aspects of Diving.* Sydney: Australian Medical Publishing Co.; 1974.
9. Becker GD, Parell GJ. Otolaryngologic aspects of scuba diving. *Otolaryngology and Head and Neck Surgery* 1979;**87**(5):569–572.
10. Neblett LM. Otolaryngology and sport scuba diving: update and guidelines. *Annals of Otology, Rhinology, and Laryngology Supplement* 1985;**115**:1–12.
11. Roydhouse N. 1001 disorders of the ear, nose and sinuses in scuba divers. *Canadian Journal of Applied Sport Sciences* 1985;**10**(2):99–103.
12. Mann W, Beck C. Aerosinusitis. *Archives of Otorhinolaryngology* 1976;**214**(2):167–173.
13. Edmonds C, McKenzie B, Thomas R, Pennefather J. *Diving Medicine for Scuba Divers.* 5th ed. www.divingmedicine.info; 2013.
14. Zimmerman RA, Bilaniuk LT, Hackney DB, et al. Paranasal sinus haemorrhages: evaluation with MR imaging. *Radiology* 1987;**162**(2):499–503.
15. Hagberg M, Ornhagen H. Incidence and risk factors for symptoms of ear and sinus among male and female dive masters and instructors: a retrospective cohort study. *Undersea and Hyperbaric Medicine* 2003;**30**(2):93–102.
16. Garges LM. Maxillary sinus barotrauma: case report and review. *Aviation, Space and Environmental Medicine* 1985;**56**(8):796–802.
17. Edmonds C. Dysbaric peripheral nerve involvement. *South Pacific Underwater Medicine Society Journal* 1991;**21**(4):190–197.
18. Lew D, Southwick FS, Montgomery WW, Webber AL, Baker AS. Sphenoid sinusitis. *New England Journal of Medicine* 1983;**309**:1149–1154.
19. Markham JW. The clinical features of pneumocephalus based on a survey of 284 cases with a report of 11 additional cases. *Acta Neurochirurgica* 1967;**16**(1–2):1–78.

20. Goldmann RW. Pneumocephalus as a consequence of diving. *JAMA* 1986;**255**:3154–3156.
21. Cortes MDP, Longridge MS, Lepawsky M, Nugent RA. Barotrauma presenting as temporal lobe injury secondary to temporal bone rupture. *AJNR American Journal of Neuroradiology* 2005;**26**:1218–1219.
22. Parell GJ, Becker GD. Neurological consequences of scuba diving with chronic sinusitis. *Laryngoscope* 2000;**110**:1358–1360.
23. Butler FK, Gurney N. Orbital hemorrhage following face-mask barotrauma. *Undersea and Hyperbaric Medicine* 2001;**28**(1):31–34.
24. Hunter ES, Farmer JC. Ear and sinus problems in diving. In: Bove A, Davis J, eds. *Bove and Davis' Diving Medicine.* 4th ed. Philadelphia: Saunders; 2004.
25. Mowatt L, Foster T. Sphenoidal sinus mucocoele presenting with acute visual loss in a scuba diver. *BMJ Case Reports* 2013;**Aug 20.** pii: bcr2013010309. doi: 10.1136/bcr-2013-010309.
26. Bolger WE, Parsons DS, Matson RE. Functional endoscopic sinus surgery in aviators with recurrent sinus barotrauma. *Aviation, Space and Environmental Medicine* 1990;**61**(2):148–156.

This chapter was reviewed for this fifth edition by Carl Edmonds.

Other barotraumas

DENTAL BAROTRAUMA

Dental barotrauma has been called *aerodontalgia* or *barodontalgia* when it is applied to altitude exposure. There are three common presentations of dental barotrauma.

In the first presentation, gas spaces may exist in the roots of infected teeth, along dying nerves, in necrotic or inflammatory areas of the pulp, alongside or associated with fillings that were poorly inserted or have undergone secondary erosion, jawbone cysts, impacted teeth or other oral maxillofacial disease. The gas may enter around the edge of the filling, adjacent to the tooth or through microfractures of the enamel and dentine (Figure 9.1).

Teeth with full cast crowns may be susceptible to air being forced into the cemented material between the crown and the tooth – especially with a zinc phosphate cement or, to a lesser extent, glass ionomer cement. Micro-leakage of gas is not as evident with resin cement.

During descent, the contracting gas space is replaced with the soft tissue of the gum or with blood and effusion. Pain may prevent further descent. If, because of slowed descent, symptoms are not noticed, then gas expansion on ascent may be restricted by the blood in these spaces, thus resulting in distension and pain.

Divers sometimes experience dental barotrauma reliably at a certain depth, but often without the gas space able to be readily visualized on dental x-ray films. Transillumination with a high-intensity light may reveal the micro-fractures. Because of the aetiologies described earlier, the barotrauma is often encountered in older divers.

A second type of presentation of dental barotrauma occurs in cases involving a carious tooth with a cavity and very thin cementum. As pressure differences across the cementum develop, the tooth may cave in (implode) on descent or explode on ascent, causing considerable pain. Fast rates of ascent or descent will precipitate this. Pressure applied to individual teeth may cause pain and identify the affected tooth. Sensitivity to cold may also localize the tooth.

A third form of dental barotrauma involves the tracking of gas into tissues (surgical emphysema), through interruptions of the mucosa, e.g. diving

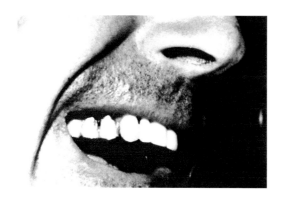

Figure 9.1 Dental barotrauma, showing collapse of the first right bicuspid during a dive to 20 metres. Dental treatment had converted an open cavity into one covered by a silver amalgam filling.

after oral surgery, dental extractions or manipulations. Scuba regulators produce a positive oral pressure, forcing gas into tissues.

Preventive measures include biannual dental checks (including x-ray examinations if indicated), avoidance of all diving after dental extractions and surgery until complete tissue resolution has occurred (i.e. intact mucosal surface) and slow descent and ascent.

Treatment consists of analgesia and dental repair. The differential diagnosis of sporadic or constant pain in the upper bicuspids or the first and second molars, but not localized in one tooth, must include other dental disorders (see Chapter 42), as well as referred pain from the maxillary sinus or the maxillary nerve (see Chapter 8). This may also manifest as a burning sensation along the mucobuccal fold.

EQUIPMENT BAROTRAUMA

Facial barotrauma of descent (mask squeeze)

A face mask creates an additional gas space external to, but in contact with, the face. Unless pressure is equalized by exhaling gas into the mask, facial tissues will be forced into this space during descent.

In some diving masks, such as with swim goggles, there is no way of equalizing the pressures during descent, so that facial barotrauma is almost inevitable with descent (limited to the

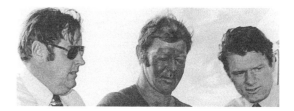

Figure 9.2 Facial barotrauma of descent (central figure). This severe 'mask squeeze' developed with a failure of surface supply of compressed air to a full-face mask. It did not have a non-return valve. Facial haemorrhage and gross swelling delineate the mask area.

eyes and surrounds, with goggles). Barotrauma is avoided in these situations by employing very flexible masks or adding flexible gas containers to the eye space.

Clinical features of mask barotrauma include puffy oedematous facial tissues especially around the eyes, purpuric haemorrhages, conjunctival haemorrhages, orbital haemorrhages and haematoma and generalized bruising of the skin underlying the mask (Figure 9.2 and Plate 2).

This condition is rarely serious, although orbital haemorrhage may be. Prevention involves exhaling into the face mask during descent. Treatment involves avoidance of diving until all tissue damage is healed.

Skin barotrauma of descent (suit squeeze)

This condition is encountered mainly with drysuits (especially if the air inlet hose is not functional) or poorly fitting wetsuits. During descent the air spaces are reduced in volume and trapped in folds in the suit. The skin tends to be sucked into these folds, leaving linear weal marks or bruises. The condition is usually painless and clears within a few days.

Genito-urinary barotrauma

A variant of suit barotrauma is the genital 'squeeze' from the P-valve, used to assist male divers to urinate out of the drysuit during long-duration dive exposures. The condom catheter is exposed to the same pressure gradients as the drysuit, as may be the female equivalent (the 'she-P collecting system'). A squeeze (a descent barotrauma equivalent) and a pneumatization of the urine (an ascent barotrauma equivalent) are possible, as is a subsequent urinary infection from organisms incubated in the drysuit tubing, usually *Pseudomonas* species. These problems may be reduced, but not eliminated, by use of a balanced P-valve, which adds a one-way valve into the system. Adequate equalization of the drysuit pressure during descent may also assist. Another problem with this equipment is flooding of the drysuit from tubing disconnection.

Head and body barotrauma of descent (diver's squeeze)

A rigid helmet, as used in standard diving, may permit this trauma (Figure 9.3). If extra gas is not added during descent to compensate for the effects of Boyle's Law, the suit and occupant may be forced into the helmet, thus causing fractured clavicles, bizarre injuries and death. The sequence of events may occur dramatically if the heavily weighted diver falls off his or her stage. There is a similar result when the diver loses compressed air pressure, e.g. as a result of a compressor or supply line failure. To prevent this, a non-return valve is inserted in the air supply line.

The clinical features include the following: dyspnoea and a heavy sensation in the chest; a bulging sensation in the head and eyes; swelling in the areas associated with rigid walls, e.g. the helmet, and then oedema and haemorrhages within the skin of the face, conjunctiva, neck and shoulders; and bleeding from the lungs, gastrointestinal tract, nose, ears and sinuses. These pathological changes are caused by the effects of barotrauma on the enclosed gas spaces and by a pressure gradient forcing blood from the abdomen and lower extremities into the thorax, head and neck because of the negative pressure differential in the helmet. Similarly induced haemorrhages occur in the brain, heart, respiratory mucosa and other soft tissues.

Suit barotrauma of ascent ('blow up')

During ascent in a standard diving ('hard hat') suit, the expanding gas must be able to escape. If it does not, then the whole suit will expand like a balloon and cause increased buoyancy and a rapid and uncontrolled ascent to the surface (Figure 9.4). This may result in barotrauma of ascent, decompression sickness, imprisonment of the diver and physical trauma.

With the decreasing use of standard diving suits, this emergency is now not often encountered,

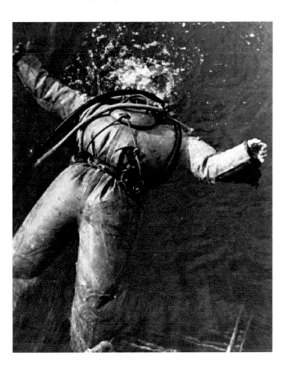

Figure 9.4 'Blow up'. Suit barotrauma of ascent.

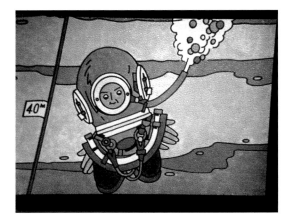

Figure 9.3 Barotrauma of descent. Total body squeeze. Diagrammatic representation.

but a variant is likely with divers who use a drysuit. It also can occur with other inflatable objects, such as a buoyancy vest or salvage/lift bag if inflated excessively or from failure to deflate during ascent.

A clinically dissimilar and relatively minor manifestation is noticed by divers in an upright position who are using rebreathing equipment that has a counterlung, or breathing bag, positioned below the head and neck. The pressure gradient from the bag to the diver's head results in a sensation of head and neck distension and bulging of the eyes.

GASTROINTESTINAL BAROTRAUMA

Gas expansion occurs within the intestines on ascent and may result in eructation, vomiting, flatus, abdominal discomfort and colicky pains. It is rarely severe, but can occasionally cause syncopal and shock-like states, stomach rupture and even death.

Inexperienced divers are more prone to aerophagia, predisposing to this condition. Swallowing to equalize middle ear pressures is one cause of aerophagia. Performing the Valsalva manoeuvre while in the head-down position may also cause air to pass into the stomach. Carbonated beverages and heavy meals can contribute and are best avoided before and during exposure to hyperbaric conditions.

Treatment involves slowing the rate of ascent, stopping ascent or even recompression. The simple procedure of releasing tight-fitting restrictions such as belts, girdles and so forth may give considerable symptomatic relief.

Although not common, notable examples of gastrointestinal barotrauma are recorded. Two Norwegian divers were badly affected during 122-metre dives using helium-oxygen, on *H.M.S. Reclaim* in 1961. An Australian lad, responding very well to hyperbaric oxygen therapy for gas gangrene, drank a 'flat' celebratory lemonade at 2.5 ATA and deteriorated into a shock state with abdominal distension and pains before ascent was terminated. A group of officials celebrating the successful construction of a caisson in the United Kingdom experienced a similar embarrassing fate, from imbibing flat champagne.

Stomach rupture

Rarely, with a large and rapid expansion of gas in the stomach, this organ may rupture with ascent. A review was conducted of 12 cases associated with relatively deep dives, more than 30 metres, with rapid ascents. The abdominal pain and distension were constant, with various other symptoms including vomiting (25 per cent), belching (16 per cent), haematemesis (33 per cent) and dyspnoea (50 per cent). Guarding of the abdomen and shock occasionally developed.

On x-ray examination, pneumoperitoneum was present in all cases, but sometimes this extended to include a pneumomediastinum and even pneumothorax. These radiological abnormalities can, of course, also be produced by pulmonary barotrauma.

Gastroscopy allowed identification and localization of the lesions, and laparoscopy usually showed these to be full thickness, usually on the lesser curvature of the stomach.

Treatment of rupture of the stomach is essentially a surgical procedure; however, breathing 100 per cent oxygen as a first aid measure and even hyperbaric oxygen as an initial treatment may have some value under some circumstances. As a general rule, decompression of the pneumoperitoneum is best achieved using surgical techniques.

If there has been a full-thickness tear, then gastric contents are likely to be present in the peritoneal cavity, and the treatment must then be on general medical and surgical grounds.

In the patients reviewed, an amount of approximately 4 litres or more of gas was necessary before rupture of the stomach would develop, and it usually required a pressure of 96 to 155 mm Hg. The reason given for the localization to the lesser curvature is that there the gastric wall is composed of only one muscular layer, compared with the three layers elsewhere.

It is postulated that rapid distension of the stomach will increase the angle of His and compress the cardia against the right diaphragmatic pillar, thus making the oesophageal-gastric junction act like a one-way valve, obstructing eructation.

MISCELLANEOUS BAROTRAUMA

Localized surgical emphysema

This disorder may result from the entry of gas into any area where the integument, skin or mucosa is broken and in contact with a gas space. Although the classical site involves the supraclavicular areas in association with tracking mediastinal emphysema from pulmonary barotrauma, other sites are possible.

Orbital surgical emphysema, severe enough to occlude the palpebral fissure completely, may result from diving with facial skin, intranasal or sinus injuries. The most common cause is a fracture of the naso-ethmoid bones. The lamina papyracea, which separates the nasal cavity and the orbit, is of egg-shell thickness. When these bones are fractured, any increase in pressure in the nasal cavity or ethmoidal sinus from ascent or a Valsalva manoeuvre may force air into the orbit (see Chapter 8 and Plate 3).

Surgical emphysema over the mandibular area is common with buccal and dental lesions. The surgical emphysema, with its associated physical sign of crepitus, can be verified radiologically as it tracks into loose subcutaneous tissue.

Treatment is by administration of 100 per cent oxygen with a non-pressurized technique, and complete resolution occurs within hours. Otherwise, resolution may take many days. Recompression is rarely indicated, but diving should be avoided until this resolution is complete and the damaged integument has completely healed.

Pneumoperitoneum

This disorder has been observed with pulmonary barotrauma, with movement of air from a ruptured pulmonary bulla dissecting along the mediastinum to the retroperitoneal area, and then released into the peritoneum, to track under the diaphragm. It is also possible that previous injury to the lung or diaphragm, producing adhesions, could permit the direct passage of air from the lung to the subdiaphragmatic area.

Another possible cause of pneumoperitoneum is, as described earlier, a rupture of a gastrointestinal viscus, especially with barotrauma of ascent or underwater explosions.

The condition may be detected by chest x-ray study or positional abdominal x-ray study (gas under the diaphragm, in the erect position).

Treatment is by administration of 100 per cent oxygen with a non-pressurized technique. Usually, complete resolution occurs within hours. Management of the cause (pulmonary or gastrointestinal) is required, and surgical management of a ruptured gastrointestinal viscus may be needed.

Pneumocephalus

Occasionally, the cranial gas spaces (mastoid, para-nasal sinuses) are affected by ascent barotrauma, when the expanding gas ruptures into the cranial cavity. This may follow descent barotrauma, when haemorrhage occupies the gas space and its orifice is blocked. The sudden bursting of gas and/or blood into the cranial cavity, usually through the tegmen tympani and the thinned petrous temporal bone into the epidural space, could cause significant brain damage.

The clinical presentation may have all the clinical features of a catastrophic intracerebral event, such as a subarachnoid haemorrhage. Excruciating headache immediately on ascent is probable, although the effects of a space-occupying lesion may supervene. Neurological signs may follow brain injury or cranial nerve lesions.

It is likely that the condition could be aggravated by excessive Valsalva manoeuvres ('equalizing the ears') or ascent to altitude (air travel). Diagnosis can be verified by positional skull x-ray study or computed tomography scan (Figure 9.5).

Treatment includes the following: bed rest, sitting upright; avoidance of the Valsalva manoeuvre, sneezing, nose blowing, altitude exposure, or other manoeuvres that increase nasopharyngeal pressures; 100 per cent oxygen inhalation for many hours; and follow-up radiology or scans to verify a reduction of the air volume. If untreated, the disorder may last a week or so, and subsequent infection is possible. On theoretical grounds, recompression or craniotomy could be considered in dire circumstances.

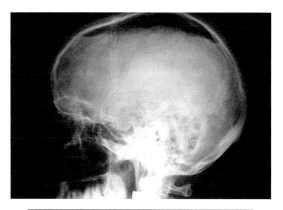

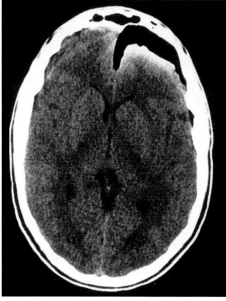

Figure 9.5 Pneumocephalus from sinus barotrauma of ascent. **(a)** The x-ray lateral view, showing gas at the vertex. **(b)** A computed tomography section showing gas anteriorly. (Courtesy of Dr R. W. Goldman.)

Bone cyst barotrauma

Occasionally, pain may develop from an intraosseous bone cyst, probably with haemorrhage into the area, during descent or ascent, and may last for hours after the dive. The pelvic bones are most often involved, in the ileum and near the sacroiliac joints. An x-ray study, computed tomography or magnetic resonance imaging scan may demonstrate the lesions (Figure 9.6). This disorder has been confused clinically with decompression

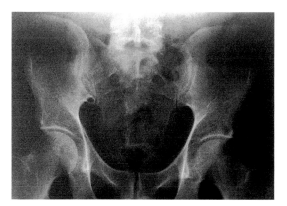

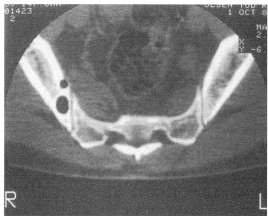

Figure 9.6 Bone cysts causing pain during ascent and or descent. **(a)** An x-ray study showing a translucent cyst in the right ilium, next to the sacro-iliac joint. **(b)** A computed tomography scan showing two air cysts in the right ilium. (Courtesy of Dr B. L. Hart.)

sickness, but it does not respond to recompression therapy and is sometimes aggravated by it.

Cranial nerve palsies

Patients occasionally present with cranial nerve lesions (fifth or seventh) attributed to neurapraxia. These lesions can be caused by the implosive tissue-damaging barotraumatic effects during descent, the distension in enclosed gas spaces during ascent or both. It is possible that air could be forced into the nerve canals as the gas expands with ascent. The nerve damage varies greatly, often transitory but occasionally long-lasting. These presentations are usually associated with barotrauma symptoms and signs, as described earlier (see Chapters 7 and 8).

With the cranial nerve palsies produced by ascent, there may be a delay of many minutes after the dive, and the diver may be aware of the feeling of distension of the gas space. The relief as gas escapes may coincide with improvement in the neurapraxia. This infers that the cause may be ischaemic, with a middle ear or sinus pressure in excess of the mean capillary perfusion pressure. Oxygen inhalation may assist, or even recompression may be indicated.

Other disorders

Other gas spaces have been observed in the body (e.g. in the kidneys, the intervertebral disc and nucleus pulposus), but these have not yet been identified as having dysbaric manifestations.

FURTHER READING

Edmonds C. Dysbaric peripheral nerve involvement. *South Pacific Underwater Medicine Society Journal* 1991;**21**(4):190–197.

Eidsvik S, Molvaer OI. Facial baroparesis. *Undersea Biomedical Research* 1985;**12**(4):495–463.

Fortes-Rego J. Etiologia de paralisia facial periferica. *Arquivos de neuro-psiquiatria* 1974;**32**:131–139.

Goldmann RW. Pneumocephalus as a consequence of diving. *JAMA* 1986;**255**: 3154–3156.

Harris R. Genito-urinary infection and barotrauma as complications of "P-valve" use in drysuit divers. *Diving and Hyperbaric Medicine* 2009;**39**(4):210–212.

Hart B, Brantly PN, Lubbers PR, Zell BK, Flynn ET. Compression pain in a diver with intraosseous pneumatocysts. *Undersea Biomedical Research* 1986;**13**(4):465–468.

Lyons KM, Rodda JC, Hood JA. Barodontalgia. *Military Medicine* 1999;**164**(3):221–227.

Markham JW. The clinical features of pneumocephalus based on a survey of 284 cases with a report of 11 additional cases. *Acta Neurochirurgica* 1967;**16**(1-2):1–78.

Molenat FA, Boussuges AH. Rupture of the stomach complicating diving accidents. *Undersea and Hyperbaric Medicine* 1995;**22**(1):87–96.

Molvaer OI. Otorhinological aspects of diving. In: Brubakk AO, Neuman TS, eds. *Bennett and Elliott's Physiology and Medicine of Diving.* 5th ed. Philadelphia: Saunders; 2003.

Neuman T, Settle H, Beaver G, Linaweaver PG. Maxillary sinus barotrauma with cranial nerve involvement. *Aviation, Space and Environmental Medicine* 1974;**46**:314–315.

Plattner T, Thali MJ, Yen K, et al. Virtopsy: postmortem multislice computed tomography (MSCT) and MRI in a fatal scuba diving incident. *Journal of Forensic Science* 2003;**48**(6):1–9.

Rose DM, Jarczyk PA. Spontaneous pneumoperitoneum after scuba diving. *JAMA* 1978;**239**(3):223.

Stein L. Dental distress. *Alert Diver SEAP* 2008;**July**:8–12.

Zadik Y, Drucker S. Diving dentistry: a review of the dental implications of scuba diving. *Australian Dental Journal* 2011;**56**(3):265–271.

This chapter was reviewed for this fifth edition by Carl Edmonds.

PART 3

Decompression Sickness

10

Decompression sickness: pathophysiology

INTRODUCTION

Decompression sickness (DCS) is a disease caused primarily by bubbles formed from dissolved gas in blood and/or tissue following a reduction in ambient pressure. It is most commonly seen in divers after surfacing, but it may also occur in aviators ascending to altitude in unpressurized or semi-pressurized aircraft or in astronauts decompressing for space walks. DCS is a puzzling, variable and to some extent unpredictable disorder with a wide range of potential presentations. At one extreme it may be rapidly fatal, whereas at the other it may manifest with mild, non-specific symptoms. Perhaps not surprisingly, it is the most widely recognized medical complication of diving and the subject of much interest among divers and diving physicians alike.

HISTORICAL PERSPECTIVE

Von Guericke developed the first effective air pump in 1650. This permitted pressurization of gas for respiration at elevated ambient pressure.

Shortly afterward, in 1670, Robert Boyle exposed experimental animals to the effects of increased and decreased pressures. His reports of these experiments included the first description of the presumed pathological vector of DCS, a bubble, in this case moving to and fro in the aqueous humour of the eye of a viper. The snake was 'tortured furiously' by the formation of bubbles in the 'blood, juices and soft parts of the body'.

There was a long hiatus before related effects were recognized in humans. In the 1840s Colonel **Pasley** noted rheumatism and excessive fatigue in divers employed on the wreck of the *Royal George*. The divers were presumably suffering from DCS, not surprising because their bottom times exceeded the accepted limits by a factor of three.

A French mining engineer, **Jean Triger,** described cases of DCS in humans in 1841. He designed and constructed what came to be known as a 'caisson'; a pressurized vertical shaft sunk into sites that would otherwise be flooded such as pylon sites in bridge construction or mine shafts extending below the water table. The air pressure excluded water from the shaft, and men could work at the bottom, albeit under whatever pressure was required to maintain a dry environment. Triger himself suffered knee pain on several occasions after pressure exposure in caissons, and as their use expanded there were fatalities and episodes of paralysis. There were almost certainly manifestations of DCS. Two physicians, **Pol** and **Watelle,** in 1854, published a report indicating the nature of the disease, together with case histories to demonstrate the relationship between decompression and onset of symptoms.

Hoppe-Seyler repeated the almost 200-year-old Boyle experiments, and in 1857 he described the obstruction of pulmonary vessels by bubbles and the inability of the heart to function adequately under those conditions. He suggested that some of the cases of sudden death in compressed air workers were the result of this intravascular liberation of gas. He also recommended recompression to remedy this.

Le Roy de Mericourt, in 1869, and **Gal,** in 1872, described an occupational illness of sponge divers that was attributed to the breathing of compressed air and equated this with the caisson workers' disease. Although some informed physicians were postulating a role for bubbles, a host of other imaginative theories were proposed during the nineteenth century to explain the aetiology of this disorder.

In 1872, **Freidburg** reviewed the development of compressed air work and collected descriptions of symptoms of workers given insufficient decompression after exposure to high pressure. He compared the clinical course of severe and fatal cases of DCS with that of the venous air embolism occasionally seen in obstetrics and surgery. He believed that rapid decompression would be responsible for a rapid release of the gas that had been taken up by the tissues under increased pressure. He suggested that the blood was filled with gas bubbles that interfered with circulation in the heart and lungs.

Smith described 'caisson disease' or 'compressed air illness' in 1873 as a disease dependent on increased atmospheric pressure, but always developing after reduction of the pressure. It was characterized, he noted, by moderate or severe pain in one or more of the extremities and sometimes in the trunk as well. There may or may not be epigastric pain and vomiting. In some cases, there may be elements of paralysis that, when they appear, are most frequently confined to the lower half of the body. Cerebral symptoms, such as headache, vertigo, convulsions and loss of consciousness, may be present.

Paul Bert, in 1878, demonstrated in a most conclusive manner that DCS is primarily the result of inert gas (nitrogen in the case of compressed air divers and caisson workers) dissolved in blood and tissues during pressure exposure and then released into the gas phase during or following decompression. He used various oxygen concentrations to hasten decompression, demonstrated the value of oxygen inhalation once experimental animals developed DCS and proposed the concept of oxygen recompression therapy.

Andrew Smith, a surgeon from the Manhattan Eye and Ear Hospital in New York, noted in the 1870s the origin of the term 'bends'. Because pain in the hips and lower extremities was generally aggravated by an erect position, the victims often assumed a stooping posture. Sufferers among the workers on the Brooklyn Bridge caissons in New York were the objects of good-natured ridicule by their comrades, who likened their angular postures to a fashionable stoop in walking, termed the 'Grecian bend', which was practiced by sophisticated metropolitan women at the time. He was aware of the value of recompression, but this was unacceptable to some of his patients. Instead he used hot poultices, ice packs, hot baths, ergot, atropine, whiskey and ginger – or morphine if the others failed. He constructed the first specialized treatment chamber.

Moir, in the early 1890s, working on the Hudson River caisson tunnel in New York, reduced the DCS death rate from 25 per cent of the work force *per annum* to less than 2 per cent by the use of more careful decompression from caisson exposures and by recompression therapy for symptomatic cases. However, problems were not eliminated, and in projects requiring exposure to relatively high pressures to construct tunnels under New York's East River in the early 1900s there remained a significant problem with mortality and morbidity, as reported by **Keays** in 1909.

Not surprisingly, during the early part of the twentieth century there was considerable controversy regarding the speed and manner in which divers and caisson workers should be decompressed.

An English physiologist, **John Scott Haldane,** proposed equations to describe tissue inert gas kinetics and proposed that limiting inert gas supersaturation (see later) during decompression was the key to preventing DCS. His decompression tables, first published in 1908, resulted in a remarkable reduction in the incidence of DCS in both diving and caisson work, and variants of Haldane's methodology are still in use for planning decompression today. These issues are discussed in Chapter 12.

UPTAKE AND ELIMINATION OF INERT GAS

Because it is believed that DCS is primarily caused by bubble formation from dissolved gas taken up into tissues during a dive, it is appropriate to examine process of gas uptake and elimination in some detail.

Most diving is performed using air as the respired gas. Dives to depths beyond the recreational diving range are performed using mixed gases that contain helium (see Chapter 62). The key point is that one or more inert gases are breathed in all but very shallow dives, where oxygen rebreathers may be used. For the general purpose of this discussion, the assumption is that the breathing gas is air and therefore that the relevant inert gas is nitrogen.

Underwater breathing apparatus supplies the diver with air at ambient pressure. Thus, the inspired (and alveolar) pressure of nitrogen (PN_2) is directly proportional to depth. Exposure to an elevated alveolar pressure of nitrogen will result in its uptake into the arterial blood, as predicted by Henry's Law, and its distribution to the tissues. Unlike highly soluble anaesthetic vapours, the equilibration of alveolar and arterial PN_2 occurs very quickly, and this process can largely be ignored in consideration of inert gas kinetics. In contrast, the exchange of dissolved nitrogen between blood and tissues is influenced by several factors.

There are multiple ways in which blood-tissue gas exchange can be conceived, but the simplest and most common approach in decompression modelling is to consider a tissue to be a well-stirred perfusion-limited compartment (Figure 10.1).

Within such a model, the arterial-tissue PN_2 difference declines mono-exponentially (Figure 10.2),

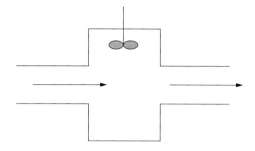

Figure 10.1 A tissue depicted as a single well-stirred perfusion-limited 'compartment'.

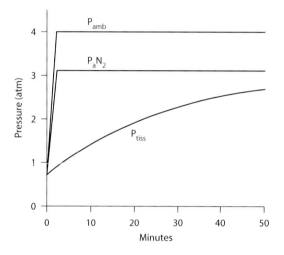

Figure 10.2 Nitrogen uptake in a hypothetical perfusion-limited tissue compartment during a dive to 30 metres (4 ATA) using air. P_{amb} is the ambient pressure in atmospheres (atm). The inspired pressure of nitrogen and the alveolar pressure of nitrogen rise to ~3.1 atm (not depicted in the figure), and the arterial pressure of nitrogen (PaN_2) 'immediately' equilibrates. In contrast, the pressure of nitrogen in the tissue (P_{tiss}) is slower to equilibrate. The arterial-tissue difference decays in a mono-exponential fashion. (Adapted with permission from a figure by Dr David Doolette.)

at a rate determined substantially by tissue perfusion, but also by the blood-tissue partition coefficient for nitrogen. Tissues with luxurious perfusion will take up inert gas quickly, whereas poorly perfused tissues will take up gas slowly. Similarly, tissues in which nitrogen is less soluble than blood will equilibrate quickly, whereas tissues with high solubility for nitrogen will equilibrate slowly. Thus, for the purposes of conceptualizing nitrogen kinetics (and for decompression modelling), the body is often regarded as a set of parallel compartments with differing kinetic properties for nitrogen exchange (Figure 10.3).

A notional depiction of differing nitrogen kinetics for each of the five hypothetical tissues in Figure 10.3 is illustrated in Figure 10.4. It can be seen that by the end of the period at depth the inert gas tension in the 'faster' tissues has equilibrated with arterial blood, whereas tensions in the slower tissues have not. Those tissues in which equilibration occurs are said to be 'saturated' with inert gas for that depth. If sufficient time were spent at depth, then all tissues would eventually saturate, a principle used in so-called saturation diving in which divers live under pressure for extended periods in the knowledge that no further inert gas uptake can occur (unless they venture deeper), and after becoming 'saturated' there is no increment in their decompression obligation if they remain under pressure longer. In contrast, the pattern of tissue equilibration with inert gas at the end of the period at depth on a typical recreational dive will look more like that depicted in Figure 10.4. Some of the faster tissues may be saturated and the slower tissues will not be. It should be self-apparent that the deeper the dive, the higher the tissue nitrogen pressures will be when

the tissue comes into equilibrium with the arterial tension. Similarly, the longer the diver remains at depth, the further toward saturation the various tissues will progress.

The principles discussed earlier in relation to nitrogen uptake remain relevant to nitrogen elimination during and after ascent from a dive. Ambient pressure decreases as the diver ascends. As ascent begins, the alveolar and arterial pressures of nitrogen will decline, and this will immediately create a diffusion gradient for nitrogen elimination from those tissues that equilibrated with arterial PN_2 at the bottom. As the ascent proceeds, similar outward diffusion gradients will be established in increasing numbers of slower tissues that had absorbed less nitrogen during the bottom time. Because the kinetics of nitrogen elimination in these tissues is slower and the ascent is relatively fast, the tissues will tend to develop a state of 'supersaturation' in which the sum of

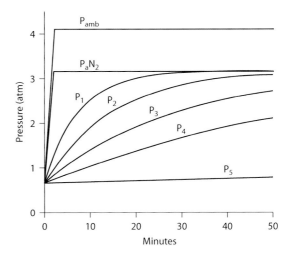

Figure 10.4 Nitrogen uptake in five hypothetical perfusion-limited tissue compartments during a dive to 30 metres (4 ATA) using air. P_{amb} is the ambient pressure in atmospheres (atm). The inspired pressure of nitrogen and the alveolar pressure of nitrogen rise to ~3.1 atm (not depicted in the figure), and the arterial pressure of nitrogen (PaN_2) immediately equilibrates. The tissue pressures of nitrogen are slower to equilibrate, with only tissues 1 and 2 approaching saturation within the duration of the exposure depicted. (Adapted with permission from a figure by Dr David Doolette.)

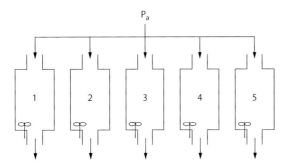

Figure 10.3 Conceptual depiction of body tissues as parallel compartments with differing kinetic properties (1 'fastest' to 5 'slowest' – see Figure 10.4) determined largely by perfusion and tissue composition. Pa, arterial pressure of inert gas. (Adapted with permission from a Figure by Dr David Doolette.)

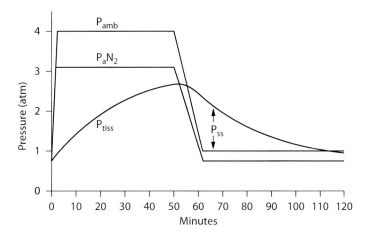

Figure 10.5 Nitrogen uptake and elimination in a hypothetical tissue compartment during and after a dive to 30 metres (4 ATA) using air. The tissue does not equilibrate with the arterial nitrogen pressure (PaN$_2$) (become saturated) during the bottom time, but because nitrogen elimination does not match the rapidly declining ambient pressure (P$_{amb}$) early in the ascent, the tissue becomes supersaturated; that is, the sum of dissolved gas in the tissue (of which most is nitrogen under these circumstances) exceeds the ambient pressure. The supersaturation pressure (P$_{ss}$) is represented by the vertical distance between the tissue pressure (Ptiss) and ambient pressure. (Adapted with permission from a figure by Dr David Doolette.)

dissolved gas pressures in the tissue exceeds the ambient pressure. This is depicted for a single tissue in Figure 10.5. Depending on the rate of ascent, the very fastest tissues may avoid this condition because they eliminate nitrogen extremely quickly, but tissues with slower kinetics are likely to become supersaturated at some point in the ascent.

Supersaturation of a tissue establishes a diffusion gradient for gas to pass from tissue to blood to alveolus, thus facilitating inert gas elimination. However, it is also the pivotal condition required for dissolved gas to separate into the gas phase, that is, to form bubbles.

These bubbles are generally accepted to be the pathological vectors in DCS, and the means by which they cause harm are discussed in detail in the following section. In general terms, a greater degree of supersaturation will drive more bubble formation with a correspondingly higher risk of developing DCS symptoms. Not surprisingly, most dive planning algorithms, used by divers to control their time/depth exposures and decompression procedures, invoke some means of calculating and controlling supersaturation during decompression as a core function. This is also discussed in more detail later.

BUBBLE FORMATION

Gas micronuclei

It is noteworthy that relatively small gas supersaturations seem capable of provoking bubble formation *in vivo* yet huge supersaturations are required to provoke bubble formation in pure solutions. This is almost certainly because of massive pressures caused by surface tension forces at the fluid-gas interface of an evolving bubble. These are inversely proportional to bubble radius, and a small bubble nucleating *de novo* from supersaturated dissolved gas would need to overcome them. The most popular and widely accepted explanation for *in vivo* bubble formation from relatively small supersaturations is the postulated presence of tiny gas micronuclei in blood and possibly tissues. These micronuclei are hypothesized to act as seeds for the inward diffusion of supersaturated gas after ascent from a dive, thus causing them to grow into bubbles.

Both the source and nature of these micronuclei are uncertain, but one suggestion is that they are created by tribonucleation in tissues where movement creates momentary areas of depressurization within

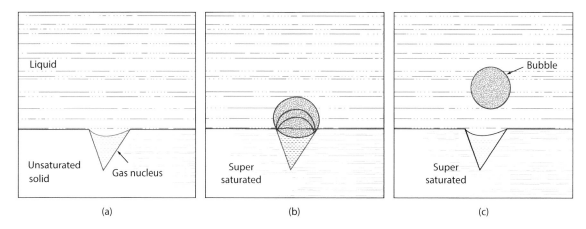

Figure 10.6 Depiction of a gas micronucleus resident in a crevice on a blood vessel wall. In the unsaturated state **(a)**, the nucleus is quiescent. When the underlying tissue becomes supersaturated **(b)**, gas diffuses into the nucleus and causes it to grow until such time that a bubble breaks off **(c)**, after which the cycle will be repeated.

the tissue fluid or blood. Bubbles created under such circumstances are usually tiny and rapidly involute in response to the high pressures caused by surface tension mentioned earlier that force the gas back into solution. However, micronuclei theory holds that some of these bubbles acquire a stabilizing outer layer of surface active molecules (these being extremely common *in vivo*) that reduce surface tension and increase the life span of the bubble, which now becomes a micronucleus.

Evidence supporting the existence of micronuclei is largely circumstantial, beginning (as described earlier) with the mere fact that bubbles can form *in vivo* following relatively small supersaturations. In addition, *in vivo* experiments in which a short 'spike' to particularly high pressure was imposed before a decompression demonstrated less bubble formation than expected; a finding implying that at least some micronuclei had been crushed out of existence during the high-pressure spike. Consistent with the notion (mentioned earlier) that tissue movement may result in regeneration of micronuclei, one famous experiment using shrimps showed that 'exercise' following the high-pressure spike partially reversed the spike's prevention of subsequent bubble formation.

Variations and parallel theories exist. For example, it has been proposed that micronuclei could reside in imperfections or crevices in capillary walls and that when the underlying tissue becomes supersaturated, nitrogen molecules will

diffuse into the micronucleus, thus causing it to grow and bud off bubbles in an analogous manner to the steady stream of bubbles that can be seen issuing from specific points on the wall of a glass containing a carbonated beverage. The essential features of this notion are illustrated in Figure 10.6.

Another theory invoked to explain bubble formation within tissues themselves is that if tribonucleation on movement or impact creates tiny bubbles in a tissue that is supersaturated at the time, the supersaturated gas will diffuse into the bubbles and not only prevent their early involution, but also cause them to grow. This is analogous the act of shaking an open soda bottle and could explain bubble formation even in the absence of persistent gas nuclei.

Venous bubbles

Of all the sites where bubbles form from supersaturated dissolved gas, most is known about bubbles in the veins. This reason in no small part is that Doppler technology has made it relatively simple to detect bubbles moving in the venous system. Doppler ultrasound systems can detect flow in blood vessels and generate an audible flow signal. The passage of a bubble through the ultrasound beam causes a characteristic 'chirp' over and above the background 'whooshing' sound of the flowing blood. More recently, high-quality echocardiography has become feasible with the use of small portable devices. This allows direct visualization of bubbles as they arrive in the right side of the heart. Much research about the quality of decompression has been conducted using quantitative estimates of venous bubble 'grades' as the outcome measure.

It has become clear that when bubbles form from supersaturated dissolved gas in blood they first appear in the veins (as opposed to the arteries, which are discussed later). This is logical because these bubbles almost certainly develop in the capillary beds of supersaturated tissues, and they can be expected to distribute with the flow of blood into the venous system. Bubbles may be present minutes after a dive, but their detection typically peaks around 30 minutes after surfacing and then may be sustained for several hours. Studies in animals suggest that these bubbles vary in size between 19 and 700 micrometres. This variability is difficult to interpret because once formed, bubbles may coalesce to create larger bubbles. Nevertheless, when it is considered that capillary diameter is somewhere around 5 to 10 micrometres, it is clear that even the smallest of these bubbles are likely to interact physically with any tissue bed that they enter.

Bubbles forming in the veins, often referred to as 'venous gas emboli' (VGE), pass to the right side of the heart and thence to the lungs, where they encounter a capillary network for the first time. Given that the pulmonary circulation is a low-pressure system, it is perhaps not surprising that the lungs are an efficient filter for VGE. Removal of most incoming VGE by the lungs has been documented in numerous experiments in both animals and humans. In most cases this does not appear to be associated with obvious harm, although harm can occur (see later) and this is probably dependent on the number of bubbles and their rate of arrival.

The formation of VGE after diving has been extensively studied. These studies have required a standardized means of quantifying the detected bubbles. There are two bubble classification and scoring systems commonly in use: the methods described by Spencer, and by Kisman and Masurel.

Spencer's grading system monitors the precordium for bubbles with the subject sitting quietly:

Grade 0 – No bubble signals on Doppler.
Grade I – An occasional bubble but with most cardiac periods free.
Grade 2 – With many, but less than half, of the cardiac periods containing Doppler signals.
Grade 3 – Most of the cardiac periods containing showers or single bubble signals, but not dominating or overriding the cardiac motion signals.
Grade 4 – The maximal detectable bubble signals sounding continuously throughout the heart cycle and overriding the amplitude of the normal cardiac signal.

The **Kisman-Masurel classification** system was designed with the aim of easily incorporating the bubble signal into a computer program. The bubble signal is divided into three separate categories – frequency, percentage of cardiac cycles with bubbles/duration of bubbles and amplitude. Each component is graded separately and then a single-digit bubble grade is awarded. The primary site for monitoring is the precordium over the right side of the heart. Monitoring is conducted at rest and after a specified movement, typically a deep knee bend (squatting up and down in a continuous fashion). Although this system appears more complicated than the Spencer system, it is the preference of many researchers and is easily learned.

Both systems suffer from interobserver error with some difficulties in subjectivity. Although computer-based counting programs are being developed, human observers are still more accurate than the automated models.

Most studies of VGE formation have had one or both of two interrelated goals in mind – first, to establish the relationship between appearance of VGE and DCS; and second, refining decompression strategies. In regard to the first goal, it has become abundantly clear that VGE are commonly detectable after recreational dives that do not result in DCS. Indeed, even the presence of high-grade bubbles is often not associated with the appearance of symptoms, and the positive predictive value of VGE grades for DCS is thus poor. Large studies do report a correlation between VGE grade and risk

Table 10.1 The incidence of decompression sickness associated with venous gas emboli grades (Kisman-Masurel system) following human dive trials at the Canadian Defence and Civil Institute of Environmental Medicine

Bubble grade	All grades	0	I	II	III	IV
Subjects	1726	819	287	183	365	72
DCS	35	0	3	2	23	7
Incidence (%)	2.03	0	1.1	1.1	6.3	9.7

DCS, decompression sickness.

Source: Data reported by Nishi R, Brubakk AO, Eftedal OS. Bubble detection. In: Brubakk AO, Neuman TS, eds. Bennett and Elliott's Physiology and Medicine of Diving. 5th ed. London: Harcourt Publishers; 2003:501–529.

(Table 10.1), but this is not precise enough for VGE grades to be used in diagnosis of DCS.

The lack of a 'diagnostic correlation' between VGE and DCS symptoms is perhaps not surprising when it is considered that some manifestations of DCS are almost certainly not directly caused by VGE (see later). However, even the weak correlation demonstrated in Table 10.1 suggests that numbers of VGE are at least indicative of the probability of significant bubble disorders in other sites, and this has encouraged the use of VGE grading as an admittedly imperfect tool for assessing and refining decompression strategies. The ongoing use of VGE grading in this regard is also influenced by the lack of readily acceptable alternative outcome measures. For example, performing manned dive trials using DCS as the outcome requires extremely large studies and may encounter ethical objections. It should be obvious from this discussion that although VGE counts are a useful tool in decompression research, great care must be taken over the conclusions that are drawn in relation to the risk of DCS.

Arterial bubbles

Bubbles almost certainly do not form from dissolved nitrogen in the arterial circulation because once the venous blood passes through the lungs, the dissolved PN_2 in the blood and alveoli should have equilibrated, and the arterial blood leaving the lungs will no longer be supersaturated. Bubbles can be introduced into the arterial circulation by pulmonary barotrauma (see Chapter 6) and also by left-to-right

(venous-to-arterial) transfer of VGE. This can occur via several recognized 'shunt' pathways.

The lesser known and least researched of these pathways are pulmonary 'shunts'. The existence of such shunts has been known for some time. They can be detected in some subjects at rest and in many subjects during exercise. Indeed, their physiological role may be to unload the right side of the heart to some extent during heavy exercise. The increasing use of echocardiography in the observation of bubble behaviour after diving, and also in saline contrast tests for patent foramen ovale (PFO; see later), has revealed that VGE can sometimes be seen emerging from the pulmonary veins into the left side of the heart. Thus, these bubbles have crossed the pulmonary circulation rather than an intracardiac shunt. It is notable that one small study failed to detect pulmonary shunting of VGE in divers exercising after a dive. Nevertheless, pulmonary shunts may contribute to the development of the DCS syndromes known to be associated with right-to-left shunting of VGE (see later), especially where there is no PFO to explain the mechanism.

The better known and most widely researched pathway is an intracardiac shunt, usually a PFO. The foramen ovale is a communication through the atrial septum that during fetal life allows blood arriving at the right side of the heart in the inferior vena cava to be directed straight across the septum into the left atrium, thereby by-passing the right ventricle and pulmonary circulation. With the haemodynamic changes that occur at birth, the foramen ovale closes in a valve-like manner, with the higher left atrial pressures tending to keep it shut. In the majority of people, the tissue pads that close the foramen ovale become 'healed' in the shut position, but in a minority (some 25 to 30 per cent), the foramen ovale remains open, or at least able to open should pressures in the right atrium exceed those on the left for any reason. This is referred to as a 'patent' foramen ovale (PFO).

As implied earlier, a PFO can be found in 25 to 30 per cent of adults who are unaware they have one, and most go through life suffering no ill effects. However, there are now multiple case-control studies that collectively demonstrate associations between the presence of a PFO and DCS involving the brain, spinal cord, inner ear and skin. In the various relevant studies, these associations are established by a substantially higher prevalence of PFO among cases of DCS than found among control divers who have not suffered DCS. If we cautiously accept that causation can be inferred from this association, the clear implication is that VGE that become 'arterialized' across a PFO are important in the pathophysiology of these forms of DCS. The way these small arterial bubbles may cause harm is discussed in more detail later. Another unsurprising and consistent finding among the relevant studies is that the size, or more correctly the shunting behaviour, of the PFO seems important. Thus, a grade 1 (see later) or 'small' PFO is likely to represent little if any risk, whereas a grade 3 or spontaneously shunting PFO almost certainly imparts extra risk for the relevant forms of DCS.

Not surprisingly, divers may request testing for the presence of a PFO. The issues of which divers should be tested for a PFO and what should be done when a PFO is found are discussed later in Chapter 12; however, the testing process is described briefly here because some of the terminology that arises is relevant to discussion of the pathogenicity of arterial bubbles. The process involves performing echocardiography while introducing agitated saline (which somewhat paradoxically contains many small bubbles) into a peripheral vein. The arrival of the bubbles in the right side of the heart often causes its virtual opacification on echocardiography, and the left side of the heart is then monitored to see whether bubbles cross the interatrial septum. Release of a Valsalva manoeuvre causes a temporary rise in right atrial pressure and is used to unmask a PFO that remains closed most of the time but that can open if right atrial pressure rises. The results are often crudely graded as follows: 0 = no bubble shunting; 1 = few bubbles shunted even during a Valsalva manoeuvre; 2 = moderate numbers of bubbles shunted during a Valsalva manoeuvre; 3 = spontaneous shunting of bubbles without a Valsalva manoeuvre.

There has been debate about whether echocardiography should be transthoracic (less expensive and less invasive) or transoesophageal (better-quality imaging) for these tests. In general, it is agreed that in expert hands and provided good views can be obtained, transthoracic echocardiography is ideal for this purpose. In fact, it is more likely to result in accurate studies because patients are typically better able to cooperate with provocative manoeuvres such as Valsalva manoeuvres than during transoesophageal echocardiography, when patients may be uncomfortable or sedated. If transthoracic views are poor, then a transoesophageal investigation should be considered. Another variant of the 'PFO test' is the use of carotid or transcranial Doppler imaging to detect bubbles in the respective arteries after injection of saline contrast and a Valsalva manoeuvre. These tests detect a right-to-left shunt, but they do not definitively distinguish among the lesions that are potentially permitting it (e.g. PFO, pulmonary shunt, atrial septal defect).

Tissue bubbles

Bubble formation from dissolved nitrogen in tissues is plausible wherever the supersaturation conditions are favourable. However, this is the least understood and documented of the processes likely to contribute to DCS mainly because, unlike bubbles moving in blood, tiny bubbles in tissue are difficult to detect with current technology, and studying small pathological bubbles in tissue post mortem is notoriously difficult.

The spinal cord is the most scrutinized organ in this regard. The 1990s saw a number of studies published that demonstrated 'non-staining space-occupying lesions' 20 to 200 micrometres in diameter and presumed to be bubbles in the spinal cord white matter after provocative decompressions. These experiments determined that the supersaturation threshold was moderately high for formation of these bubbles and that significant bubbling in the spinal cord white matter was unlikely unless dives were deeper than 25 metres. They also determined that tissue bubbles tend to form in the spinal cord early, because as supersaturation declines quickly after surfacing the probability of bubble formation also rapidly declines.

The brain tissue is not considered a likely site for bubble formation because of its luxurious perfusion, which prevents significant or prolonged supersaturation after most plausible decompressions. However, nitrogen is eliminated more slowly from the inner ear than the brain, and there is some experimental evidence for bubble formation in inner ear tissue itself. The inner ear is also uniquely vulnerable to enhancement of local tissue supersaturation by a process frequently referred to as 'isobaric counterdiffusion' (IBCD). This can arise during decompression from deep dives in which the diver makes a switch from a breathing mix containing helium to one containing nitrogen (see Chapter 62). Such switches are undertaken in the belief that they accelerate decompression because helium in the tissues will diffuse into blood faster than the nitrogen in the blood will diffuse into the tissue. The inner ear has a unique and relevant anatomy. There are relatively large unperfused reservoirs of helium (in the perilymph and endolymph) that can eliminate accumulated helium only via the vascularized labyrinthine tissue. This maintains an elevated partial pressure of helium in the vascular labyrinth after the switch to a nitrogen-based mix, while at the same time this tissue is also exposed to high pressures of nitrogen diffusing inward from the blood stream. This 'counterdiffusion' process may transiently enhance any pre-existing supersaturation of helium and result in bubble formation.

In addition to clinically relevant and largely proven tissue bubble formation in the spinal cord and inner ear, there is strong circumstantial evidence that tissue bubble formation is the cause of musculoskeletal pain in DCS. Specifically, the lack of any association between the presence of PFO and musculoskeletal pain in DCS suggests that *in situ* bubble formation is the most likely cause, rather than bubbles arriving in the arterial blood. The exact location of tissue bubbles responsible for musculoskeletal pain is unknown, but there are multiple possibilities including tendons, ligaments,

periosteum and marrow. Similar reasoning has led to the hypothesis that bubbles may form in peripheral nerve tissues. Patchy paraesthesiae in a non-dermatomal distribution are common symptoms that have not been linked to the presence of a right-to-left shunt, and it follows that tissue bubble formation is the likely cause. It is plausible that bubbles could form in the myelin of a peripheral nerve, or elsewhere within the perineurium, and cause neurapraxia through a mass effect. However, this mechanism is not substantively proven.

Finally, one presumed location for bubble formation most appropriately categorized as 'tissue' is the lymphatic system. The infrequent occurrence of discrete regional areas of oedematous soft tissue swelling, often accompanied by other symptoms of DCS, has led to the assumption that bubbles may form in lymphatic drainage channels and cause stasis.

Fate of bubbles after formation

The pathogenicity of bubbles is described later, but it is interesting to reflect on what happens to a notional bubble in tissue over time if only to discuss the concept of the so-called oxygen window because this will arise again in several subject areas.

We must begin by assuming that when a diver surfaces from a dive, a bubble forms from dissolved supersaturated nitrogen in a tissue. While the tissue remains supersaturated with nitrogen the bubble will grow, but eventually the PN_2 in the tissue will come to equilibrium with that in the blood and alveoli for an air breathing subject at 1 atm. The bubble will not grow any more, and one may then ask 'What is to stop the bubble, once formed, from simply sitting in the tissue unresolved for long periods?' There are two reasons.

First, the pressure inside a spherical bubble is always likely to be greater than 1 atm, creating a driving force for the inert gas contained therein to diffuse into tissue, thence to blood and alveolus. This is because some pressure will be generated by surface tension at the bubble–tissue fluid interface and because some pressure will be generated by surrounding tissue that has been displaced by the bubble. These factors are summarized by the following equation, whose middle term describes pressure resulting from surface tension and whose final term describes pressure resulting from tissue displacement:

$$P_{bub} = P_{amb} + \frac{2\sigma}{r} + \frac{4\pi r^3 B}{3V_{tis}}$$

where P_{bub} is the pressure inside the bubble, P_{amb} is the ambient pressure, σ is the surface tension of the fluid, r is the bubble radius, V_{tis} is the volume of tissue affected by bubble displacement, and B is a term describing the bulk modulus of elasticity of the tissue.

Second, even during air breathing, there is a small partial pressure gradient for nitrogen diffusion from bubble to tissue created by the oxygen window. This arises primarily because of the solubility difference between the oxygen consumed and the carbon dioxide (CO_2) produced by metabolism. The partial pressure of oxygen (PO_2) in alveolar gas during air breathing is approximately 100 mm Hg, and after exchange with the blood, the PO_2 in arterial blood is about 95 mm Hg. Oxygen is carried to the tissues, where a given number of molecules are consumed through metabolism and replaced with a similar number of molecules of CO_2. Removal of these oxygen molecules drops the PO_2 from 95 mm Hg in arterial blood to 40 mm Hg in venous blood. However, because CO_2 is much more soluble, the addition of the same number of molecules of CO_2 to the venous blood only raises its partial pressure to 46 mm Hg (from 40 mm Hg in arterial blood). The PO_2 in the tissues where the oxygen is actually being consumed is slightly lower than the venous

PO_2, but this is difficult to measure, so we have to speculate a little. Relevant data are summarized in Table 10.2.

Note from Table 10.2 that for the purposes of this discussion it is assumed that a tissue bubble has an internal pressure equivalent to ambient (760 mm Hg). As discussed earlier, the typical internal pressure of a bubble in tissue is probably higher, which would actually enhance the effect described here, but for the purposes of illustrating the oxygen window, we will assume that the internal pressure is same as ambient. The gas contained within the bubble will be composed of water vapour at a pressure equivalent to the saturated vapour pressure for water at 37°C (47 mm Hg), and oxygen and CO_2 in equilibrium with the tissue pressures of those gases. The balance of the bubble gas must be nitrogen, and by Dalton's Law of partial pressures, the $P_{bub}N_2$ must be given by this equation:

$$P_{bub}N_2 = P_{bub} - (P_{bub}O_2 + P_{bub}CO_2 + PH_2O)$$

where $P_{bub}N_2$ is the pressure of nitrogen inside the bubble, P_{bub} is the pressure inside the bubble that in this example we are considering to be the same as ambient pressure (760 mm Hg), $P_{bub}O_2$ is the partial pressure of oxygen in the bubble, $P_{bub}CO_2$ is the partial pressure of CO_2 in the bubble, and PH_2O is the saturated vapour pressure for water at 37°C.

Table 10.2 shows that this resolves to a PN_2 of approximately 637 mm Hg which is about 64 mm Hg greater than the PN_2 in the tissue, venous blood and alveoli (573 mm Hg). This difference, which

Table 10.2 Approximate gas partial pressures in millimetres of mercury at various sites during air breathing at a surface pressure of 1 ATA

Sample	Gas partial pressure				
	O_2 (mm Hg)	CO_2 (mm Hg)	N_2 (mm Hg)	H_2O (mm Hg)	Total (mm Hg)
Alveolar gas	100	40	573	47	760
Arterial blood	95	40	573	47	755
Venous blood	40	46	573	47	706
Tissues	~30	~46	573	47	696
Tissue bubble	~30	~46	637	47	760

Note: The data for nitrogen assume that sufficient time has passed since a dive for nitrogen partial pressures (PN_2) in blood and tissues to have equilibrated with alveolar pressures. The different PN_2 in the bubble is explained in the text.

creates a gradient for diffusion of nitrogen from the bubble to the tissue, is referred to as the 'oxygen window'. We reiterate that it is created by the dissolved gas partial pressure difference that arises from removing relatively insoluble oxygen from solution and replacing it with very soluble CO_2.

As discussed again later, the oxygen window could be further enhanced by breathing oxygen. Although this markedly elevates the alveolar and arterial PO_2, it has a much smaller effect on venous and tissue PO_2 because the small amount of extra oxygen dissolved in the arterial blood will be preferentially removed and metabolized, thereby dramatically dropping the PO_2 back down to near normal levels. The venous PO_2 (and therefore the venous oxygen saturation) may be marginally elevated. Because the same amount of oxygen is consumed and the same number of molecules of CO_2 is produced, there will be virtually no effect on tissue or venous PCO_2. Thus, the $P_{bub}N_2$ as calculated earlier will change very little, while at the same time the alveolar, arterial and tissue PN_2 will fall markedly; potentially to zero if 100 per cent oxygen is breathed for long enough. The difference in PN_2 between bubble and surrounding tissue will be correspondingly exaggerated, and nitrogen will diffuse out of the bubble more quickly. The same is true if the bubble is compressed. In this case, the P_{bub} in the foregoing equation is elevated, whereas bubble oxygen, CO_2 and water vapour are little affected, even if oxygen is breathed during the compression.

The existence of the oxygen window, even during air breathing at 1 atm, at least partly explains why bubbles of nitrogen cannot exist in a stable condition in tissues. It also explains why bubbles involute even more quickly during oxygen breathing, especially when combined with recompression.

PATHOLOGICAL EFFECTS OF BUBBLES

Having reviewed the processes that give rise to bubble formation after decompression, the discussion now turns to consideration of the potential pathological effects of those bubbles. As discussed earlier, bubbles may form from dissolved gas in blood and/or tissue, and this section considers their potential pathological effects within those broad 'anatomical' categories. The discussion further subdivides the consequences of bubbles forming in blood into those effects arising primarily because of the presence of bubbles in blood and those arising from their distribution in blood via the circulatory system.

Presence of bubbles in blood

The presence of bubbles in blood appears capable of activating reactive formed elements such as platelets and white blood cells, as well as inflammatory cascades such as the kinin, complement and coagulation systems. The means by which this occurs are not clearly established, but there are several possibilities for interactive activations involving known mechanisms. For example, platelet and coagulation activation can occur through exposure to foreign surfaces such as glass or to collagen beneath damaged endothelium. Bubbles may act in a similar way by acting as a foreign surface or by damaging endothelium, the latter having been demonstrated experimentally. Similarly, white blood cells can be activated by damage to endothelium.

There is rarely any obvious evidence of a role for these inflammatory activations in the pathogenesis of milder forms of DCS, although it has been suggested that constitutional symptoms such as fatigue and malaise may occur as a result. These processes may be important in producing specific serious manifestations. For example, one hypothesis for spinal cord injury that has been substantially demonstrated in an animal model holds that bubbles initiate coagulation in the epidural veins, thereby leading to venous stasis and a venous infarction in the spinal cord. Inflammatory responses may also be important contributors in severe or fulminant DCS. For example, disseminated intravascular coagulation can lead to a coagulopathy, and such patients may also develop severe haemoconcentration and shock secondary to the endothelial 'leakiness' that can follow inflammatory activations.

Distribution of bubbles in blood

It has been previously noted that bubbles forming from supersaturated dissolved gas first appear in the veins. In addition to any inflammatory responses and resulting harm that this may elicit (described earlier), these bubbles can be transported in the circulatory system to sites distant from their point of origin.

The most obvious target organ in the distribution of VGE is the lungs. As previously discussed, it seems that for the most part the lungs can tolerate and efficiently remove even grade IV VGE without obvious harm. However, on relatively rare occasions divers may develop symptoms caused by the arrival of VGE in large numbers over a sufficiently short space of time to exceed a poorly understood clinical threshold. The trapping of copious bubbles in the pulmonary vasculature can cause a significant rise in pulmonary artery pressure, a ventilation-perfusion mismatch and the various inflammatory changes described earlier. These events manifest as dyspnea, retrosternal chest pain and cough, a constellation of symptoms sometimes referred to as the 'chokes', but more correctly called cardiopulmonary DCS. Symptoms typically occur within the first 30 minutes after surfacing, but the natural history is variable. There may be rapid progression to hypotension, collapse and occasionally death, probably as a result of acute right-sided heart failure. There are also many stories of these symptoms resolving spontaneously, especially if oxygen is breathed, because this would markedly enhance the rate at which bubbles are eliminated from the pulmonary circulation. Not surprisingly, because the substantial numbers of VGE required to produce cardiopulmonary symptoms are predictive of a potential for distribution of VGE in to the arterial system (see later) and also of a strong provocation for bubble formation in tissues, it is not surprising that cardiopulmonary DCS is often followed by symptoms of other organ involvement.

VGE may also distribute into the arterial circulation via pulmonary shunts or a PFO as previously described. Little is known about the factors that promote pulmonary shunting of VGE, although formation of large numbers of VGE appears important, and experiments in non-diving situations suggest that exercise is a likely risk factor. One small study in animals also suggested that use of theophylline (a bronchodilator) reduced the efficacy of the lungs as a filter for VGE; however, whether this effect was via recruitment of shunts or another mechanism is unknown. Because these shunts appear to be dynamic and cannot be investigated easily, our knowledge of their role in DCS is poor, although they are potentially very significant.

The behaviour of PFOs is better characterized. As described earlier, some PFOs shunt spontaneously, and there are data suggesting that such lesions are the most significant in causation of DCS. Other PFOs require provocation to raise right atrial pressure sufficiently to open the communication. This can be provided by something as simple as bending and straightening, straining to lift something or possibly even coughing. Along with the Valsalva manoeuvre, all these provocations have in common the tendency transiently to impede venous return to the right side of the heart, thereby causing a brief exaggerated 'rush' of blood into the right atrium on termination of the impediment. This transiently increases the right atrial pressure and may open a PFO that is normally kept closed by the prevalent positive left-to-right pressure gradient.

The previously mentioned association between the presence of a PFO and cerebral, spinal, inner ear, and cutaneous DCS implies that the passage of small VGE into the arteries can injure these organs. How these small bubbles cause injury is uncertain, although there are several possibilities.

BRAIN

It is known that a large bubble or bubbles embolizing the arterial supply to the brain can interrupt flow sufficiently to cause ischaemic injury. Patients embolized by large aliquots of gas in iatrogenic accidents and pulmonary barotrauma events can develop stroke-like syndromes that are often multifocal (see Chapter 6). However, it is uncertain that bubbles in the size range that typically arise in the veins after decompression would cause such injuries. Unlike solid emboli, bubbles are known to redistribute through the microcirculation, and small bubbles are likely to do so very quickly. Therefore, it seems implausible that small VGE passing to the arterial system would cause large cerebral infarctions. When such lesions are seen after diving, there should be a high index of suspicion for arterial gas embolism secondary to pulmonary barotrauma.

Nevertheless, it is plausible that sufficient numbers of these small bubbles entering the cerebral circulation may result in dysexecutive symptoms such as cognitive impairment, memory impairment and confusion, which are often labelled 'cerebral DCS'. Exactly how small bubbles do this, however, is not certain. One possibility that has some experimental providence is that the passage of small bubbles through the microcirculation causes endothelial disruption with consequent inflammatory changes such as the activation and accumulation of white blood cells (see Chapter 6). This can cause a secondary decline in blood flow with a consequent degree of hypoxia, perivascular infiltration by the formed elements of blood, the release of inflammatory mediators and the development of tissue oedema; all of which may inhibit or injure nearby neurons. The widespread occurrence of this sort of event in the cerebral circulation could explain the 'global' cerebral impairment typically seen in cerebral DCS.

OTHER VULNERABLE NEUROLOGICAL ORGANS

Neurological organs other than the brain, such as the inner ear and spinal cord, are almost certainly exposed to fewer arterial bubbles than the brain because of their markedly poorer perfusion, meaning that fewer bubbles will be carried to these organs. Paradoxically, these organs may be more vulnerable to ischaemic injury caused by small bubbles for the same reason.

Modelling studies have demonstrated that after a dive the inner ear, for example, remains supersaturated with nitrogen for much longer than the brain, which washes out excess nitrogen within minutes. Thus, if VGE cross a PFO 15 minutes after a dive and enter the basilar artery, most of them will distribute to the brain, and perhaps a few will find their way into the tiny labyrinthine artery. However, whereas those VGE distributing to the brain will distribute through tissues that are not supersaturated, those entering the inner ear microcirculation will be exposed to supersaturated nitrogen and will likely grow as this gas diffuses into the bubble. Thus, despite being exposed to smaller numbers of bubbles, the inner ear may be selectively vulnerable to ischaemic injury because enlarging bubbles will be more likely to cause flow stasis. This mechanism may help explain the repeated reports of an association between PFO and inner ear DCS

(implying that arterialized VGE play a role) and the finding that these patients often present with only inner ear symptoms even though a much larger number of VGE must have distributed to the brain. Although less well studied, it is likely that similar mechanisms can be responsible for spinal DCS, which probably has inert gas kinetics similar to those of the inner ear. Moreover, irrespective of whether the bubbles grow from inward diffusion of supersaturated nitrogen, the spinal cord and inner ear circulations are almost certainly vulnerable to the same pro-inflammatory effects of bubble passage as described earlier for the brain.

SKIN

Other than the finding that arterialized VGE are implicated, exactly how the arrival of small bubbles in the arterial supply to the skin precipitates rash and itch is uncertain, although it could conceivably involve all the mechanisms (ischaemic and inflammatory) mentioned earlier in relation to the brain and other neurological organs. Indeed, one histopathological study of the cutis marmorata form of skin DCS reported endothelial disruption and perivascular inflammatory infiltrates entirely consistent with bubble-induced vasculitis. Questions remain, however, such as the reason for the typical finding of a localized lesion (often on the trunk) when arterialized VGE must distribute widely to cutaneous vascular territories. As with the selective vulnerability of the inner ear to vascular bubbles, the answer may lie in differing levels of post-dive inert gas supersaturation making some areas of skin more vulnerable than others.

Tissue bubbles

As discussed earlier, bubbles may form in tissues where the supersaturation conditions are favourable. Once formed these bubbles could cause harm through the following mechanisms: direct damage to immediately adjacent tissue; indirect trauma within any tissue displaced by the bubble (e.g. stretching or compression of axons in the spinal cord or a peripheral nerve); ischaemia caused by pressing externally on blood vessels; haemorrhage through disruption of nearby blood vessels; stimulation of pain receptors; and

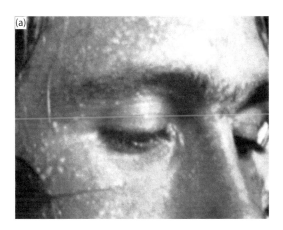

Plate 3, front. Decompression sickness. **(a)** Skin lesions from counterdiffusion. The subject breathed a neon-oxygen mixture at 360 metres (1200 feet) while exposed to a chamber of helium and oxygen. Gross itching accompanied the intradermal bubbles. (Courtesy of Professor C.J. Lambertsen.)

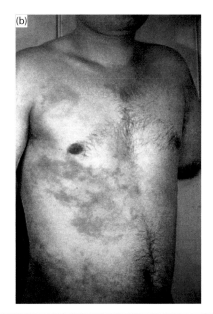

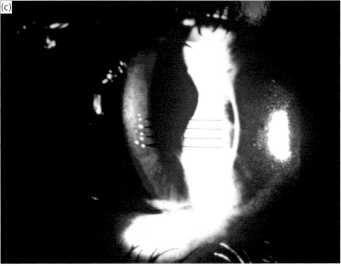

Plate 3, back. Decompression sickness. **(b)** A florid example of the truncal scarlatiniform rash seen in decompression sickness. This diver, who had had an upper limb amputation, developed 'bends' pain in the phantom limb and skin bends over the body. Both conditions responded to recompression therapy. (Courtesy of Dr Ramsay Pearson.) **(c)** Bubbles developing between the hard contact lens and the cornea as a result of decompression. These bubbles caused corneal injury and symptoms. (Courtesy of Drs Mark E. Bradley and David Simon.)

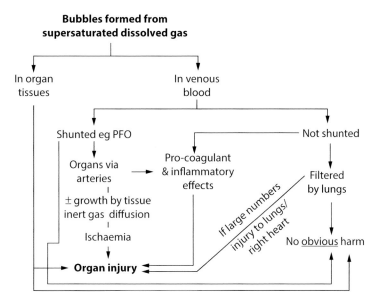

Figure 10.7 Summary of key pathophysiological processes in decompression sickness. PFO, patent foramen ovale.

incitement of inflammatory reactions initiated by tissue injury.

The pathophysiological paradigm for DCS described earlier is summarized in Figure 10.7.

Multiple disorders in single organ systems

It will not have escaped the astute reader's attention that in the case of some organs this discussion has proposed more than one way in which they can be injured by bubbles in DCS.

The most conspicuous example is the spinal cord, in which injury may be caused by: bubbles forming in the spinal tissue itself, by bubbles inciting coagulation in the epidural vertebral venous plexus and by bubbles formed in the veins distributing to the cord via a right-to-left shunt and the arterial circulation. It is emphasized that this is not self-contradictory and that in fact the spinal cord may be injured by all these mechanisms under various circumstances. The existence of these various forms of bubble pathology may help explain inconsistent results when divers with spinal DCS are recompressed. For example, failure to elicit any improvement may be explained by coagulation in the epidural veins that would not be expected to resolve during recompression even if the inciting bubbles were removed. In contrast, a brisk improvement soon after recompression could suggest that tissue bubbles pressing on surrounding structures were the main culprit because in this case bubble resolution could be expected to elicit some benefit.

The other important example is the inner ear, which, as previously described, may be injured either by bubbles forming within the tissues or by bubbles that have shunted from the veins and arrive in the arterial system. As explained, if these arterial bubbles arrive while the inner ear remains supersaturated with nitrogen, then they may expand as tissue nitrogen diffuses into the bubble. It is generally presumed that cases of inner ear injury arising during decompression from deep dives are most likely to be caused by bubbles forming within the inner ear tissue itself, particularly if symptom onset is temporally related to a switch from a helium-based breathing mix to air or nitrox. It is impossible to distinguish among disorders in cases arising after surfacing, but the strong association between such cases and the presence of a large PFO suggests that a significant proportion of them are caused by arterial bubbles.

ALTERNATIVE HYPOTHESES AND FUTURE DIRECTIONS

One newer avenue of research in relation to DCS pathophysiology that is very active but not concluded as this book goes to press relates to the role of so-called intravascular 'microparticles'. Microparticles are small fragments of membrane material that are shed from the surface of some formed elements of blood and also endothelium. Their presence in the circulation appears to activate or amplify inflammatory processes and coagulation, and as a result they appear capable of initiating or at least exacerbating vascular injury. Microparticles are increased in a variety of disease states including sepsis, myocardial infarction and vasculitis.

Microparticle numbers also appear to be increased by decompression stress, that is, in the presence of tissue supersaturation with inert gas. This raises the possibility that some of the pathophysiological events in DCS that are currently attributed to circulating bubbles may in fact be caused or exacerbated by microparticles. However, many questions remain unanswered. For example, is microparticle generation in decompression stress secondary to bubble formation, or is there some other unknown consequence of inert gas supersaturation that is responsible? How can the invariably wide distribution of harmful microparticles be reconciled against the selective vulnerability of certain organs such as the spinal cord and inner ear in DCS? Similarly, why does the brain seem relatively resistant to harm when in fact its luxurious perfusion would render it at highest risk of exposure to microparticles?

The answers to such questions are unlikely to be simple. The more effort that goes into researching the microparticle phenomenon, the more complex it seems to become. For example, it seems clear that microparticles are not homogeneous; they have different origins, some appear to have mixed origins and they seem to have variable inflammatory potential. Some larger microparticles even appear to have characteristics of gas micronuclei and may contain a core of gas.

This is an exciting line of research that is in its infancy but that has the potential to modify our pathophysiological paradigm for DCS significantly. Alternatively, it may transpire that microparticles are little more than an interesting epiphenomenon. It is a subject for those interested in the detail of this matter to watch closely.

FURTHER READING

Carraway MS, Key NS. The microbubble or the microparticle? *Journal of Applied Physiology* 2011;**110**:307–308.

Doolette DJ, Mitchell SJ. Hyperbaric conditions. *Comprehensive Physiology* 2011;**1**:163–201.

Francis TJR, Mitchell SJ. The pathophysiology of decompression sickness. In: Brubakk AO, Neuman TS, eds. *Bennett and Elliott's Physiology and Medicine of Diving*. 5th ed. London: Harcourt Publishers; 2003:530–556.

Mitchell SJ, Doolette DJ. Selective vulnerability of the inner ear to decompression sickness in divers with right to left shunt: the role of tissue gas supersaturation. *Journal of Applied Physiology* 2009;**106**:298–301.

Nishi R, Brubakk AO, Eftedal OS. Bubble detection. In: Brubakk AO, Neuman TS, eds. *Bennett and Elliott's Physiology and Medicine of Diving*. 5th ed. London: Harcourt Publishers; 2003:501–529.

This chapter was reviewed for this fifth edition by Simon Mitchell.

11

Decompression sickness: manifestations

INTRODUCTION

Decompression sickness (DCS) is an extremely variable disease with multiple possible symptoms, many of which are non-specific. There are no laboratory tests or other investigations that confirm the diagnosis, and diving physicians frequently have to integrate knowledge of diving, diver behaviour, DCS pathophysiology, DCS presentation and other competing diagnoses in formulating an appropriate response to reports of symptoms after diving. Not surprisingly, there are frequent diagnostic conundrums. This often occurs in the context of situations where the implications of the diagnosis are profound, such as when the victim is aboard a charter boat in a remote location and evacuation will cause a major disruption to multiple high-paying customers. These situations can be very challenging for the diving physician.

This chapter outlines the known patterns of presentation and manifestations of DCS based largely around effects by organ system. Before proceeding to that discussion, however, the discussion attempts to clarify some confusing issues in relation to terminology and classification of the dysbaric diseases.

TERMINOLOGY AND CLASSIFICATION

The pathophysiology of cerebral arterial gas embolism (CAGE) and decompression sickness (DCS) is described in Chapters 6 and 10, respectively. Although both CAGE and DCS are bubble-induced disorders and they share some commonality in pathophysiology and manifestations, the traditional approach to terminology (and the one largely used in this book) was to treat them as separate entities. Thus, symptoms presumed to be caused by formation of bubbles from supersaturated inert gas after diving were labelled DCS. Symptoms considered likely the result of the introduction of gas into the pulmonary veins after pulmonary barotrauma were most commonly labelled arterial gas embolism (AGE), or CAGE, given that cerebral involvement usually dominated the clinical picture. DCS was further subdivided into type 1 and type II categories. Type I was initially a designation for cases with musculoskeletal pain as the only symptom, and it is still sometimes referred to as 'pain only DCS'. However the definition has subsequently been inconsistently modified and may variously include rash, lymphatic symptoms and some mild neurological symptoms. Type II indicated the presence of neurological symptoms, but the unintended consequence of this was to give equal weight to symptoms with disparate prognostic significance such as patchy paraesthesiae and gross motor dysfunction, hence the shifting of the former into the type I definition. The authors of this text consider the type I and type II classification to be ambiguous and largely without value and do not recommend its use.

The separation of CAGE and DCS as clinical diagnoses was predicated on the perceived contrast between the stereotypical ultra-short latency of focal cerebral symptoms in CAGE and the typically longer latency, broader symptom range and tendency to spinal rather than cerebral involvement in DCS. This diagnostic paradigm was challenged after publication (in 1989) of two studies associating patent foramen ovale (PFO) with neurological DCS. As discussed in Chapter 10, the only plausible explanation for an association between PFO and neurological DCS was that the PFO allowed venous gas emboli (VGE) to enter the arterial circulation and to thence be carried to vulnerable organs. Although diving physicians had been aware of the possibility for right-to-left shunting of VGE before this, these studies brought the issue into sharper focus and fuelled speculation on whether right-to-left shunting of VGE could, in at least some cases, be responsible for short-latency focal cerebral symptoms typically labelled

'CAGE' and presumed secondary to pulmonary barotrauma. Although (as mentioned in Chapter 10) there is some doubt about whether 'arterialized' VGE are large enough to produce the gross focal cerebral lesions that can occur when air enters the circulation after pulmonary barotrauma, these concerns resonated in the diving medicine community. In particular, uncertainty developed about using diagnostic labels such as DCS and CAGE that implied the underlying pathophysiology.

This matter came to a head in 1991 with the hosting of a consensus meeting to debate the matter in the United Kingdom[1]. The meeting generated a system for characterizing dysbaric disease in descriptive terms as an alternative to diagnostic labels implying a particular underlying pathophysiology. Thus, the clinical syndromes previously labelled as either DCS or CAGE were amalgamated under the 'umbrella term' 'decompression illness' (DCI), with a descriptive paradigm in which an evolutionary term and an organ system term would be applied to each symptom. A simplified interpretation appears in Table 11.1.

Thus, a diver presenting with worsening musculoskeletal pain after a dive is said to have 'progressive musculoskeletal DCI'. A diver presenting with sudden loss of consciousness immediately after a rapid ascent and who is subsequently recovering is said to have 'remitting neurological (cerebral) DCI'. Under the more traditional pathophysiology-based nomenclature, these divers would likely be diagnosed with 'type I DCS' and 'CAGE', respectively.

Although this system conveys useful information and avoids implying pathophysiological interpretations that may be wrong, there are problems with it. First, it is imprecise when the

Table 11.1 Descriptive classification system for decompression disorders

Evolutionary term	Organ system term	
Static	Musculoskeletal	
Remitting	Cutaneous	
Progressive	Neurological (appended with cerebral, spinal, peripheral)	DCI
Relapsing	Vestibulocochlear	
	Lymphatic	
	Cardiopulmonary	

Note: Each symptom is given an evolutionary term, an organ system term and the diagnosis of DCI (decompression illness).

nature of the pathophysiological insult is known and inadequate when there is intent to imply a specific underlying mechanism. Clearly, the authors of this text encounter this situation in the pathophysiology chapters of this book where the DCS/CAGE terminology is used (while avoiding the terms type I and type II in relation to DCS). Second, the umbrella term 'decompression illness' is too similar to 'decompression sickness', and the two are often used interchangeably by commentators who do not appreciate the different meanings described here. Finally, the descriptive terminology has become a significant source of conflict in the field, with frequently polarized views on its utility. A compromise proposed in the last edition of another major diving medicine text published in 2003 was to retain the DCS/CAGE terms in discussion of pathophysiological mechanisms, but to use the descriptive terminology in clinical discussions. Albeit sensible, this policy has not been consistently applied. It is fair to say that the classification of decompression disorders remains 'messy' and inconsistent in the modern literature.

CLINICAL MANIFESTATIONS: GENERAL CONSIDERATIONS

DCS is precipitated by a decrease in environmental pressure. Although seemingly obvious, this means that any symptoms arising during descent or during the period at depth (before ascent) will not be caused by DCS (unless the symptoms have been 'carried over' from a previous decompression). Most cases arise after arrival of the diver at the surface, although there may rarely be onset of symptoms during the ascent; particularly on a dive with long decompression stops. This should be considered an ominous sign that more serious symptoms are likely after surfacing. If cases across the entire range of severity are considered, more than 50 per cent of patients develop symptoms within 1 hour of surfacing, and 90 per cent have symptoms within 6 hours. If severe manifestations such as motor weakness are considered alone, most will begin to manifest within the first hour.

Notwithstanding these estimates, there is frequently a significant latency between symptom onset and the victim's reporting the problem, particularly when mild symptoms are involved. Sometimes there are obvious reasons why this may be so, such as an asymptomatic diver retiring for the night several hours after the last dive and waking with symptoms in the morning. However, 'denial' and seeking alternative explanations for symptoms on the part of the diver are often contributory. This stems in part from a long-standing stigma about the diagnosis that has its roots in the entrenched notion that if someone has DCS then he or she must have done something incompetent or wrong. The way in which this belief can affect the behaviour of divers needs to be understood by any physician assessing a possible DCS case. Thus, not only do divers have a tendency to denial of symptoms and consequent late presentation, they may also then misrepresent timing of onset to avoid criticism for late reporting. This needs to be borne in mind when applying the typical symptom latencies described earlier to a diagnostic paradigm. Another reason for symptom denial among divers is the understanding that early reporting of symptoms may result in termination of a dive trip and/or a logistically difficult (and potentially expensive) evacuation for recompression treatment. Given such motivation to downplay problems, it is hardly surprising that physicians who eventually see evacuated divers at receiving units frequently find more serious symptoms than were reported in initial discussions by telephone.

Divers learn that for any depth, a period of 'bottom time' can be spent there that, when not exceeded and when followed by direct ascent to the surface at the correct rate, is associated with an acceptably small level of tissue nitrogen supersaturation (see Chapter 10) and a correspondingly small risk of DCS. These acceptable bottom times are often referred to as 'no decompression limits'. More advanced exponents (see Chapter 62) learn how to stage their ascent appropriately using 'decompression stops' to maintain a small level of risk if the no decompression limit is exceeded. Some divers inappropriately come to see adherence (or not) to no decompression limits or to decompression stop prescriptions as the threshold for a binary outcome. Thus, they may believe 'exceed the limits and you will get DCS' and 'stay within the limits and you can't get DCS'. Such beliefs are clearly false, but they can contribute to strange conduct such as symptom denial if a dive was within the limits or, at the other extreme, high anxiety and illness behaviour because a no decompression limit was slightly exceeded.

An appreciation of no decompression limits and how they are calculated or monitored by divers is important for the diving physician evaluating a potential DCS case because, notwithstanding the previous comments, it remains true that a dive is likely to carry a higher risk if there are events such as exceeding a no decompression limit, omitting recommended decompression stops or ascending too rapidly. Such events are often characterized as representing a 'provocation' for DCS. Similarly, but at the opposite end of the risk spectrum, a dive well inside the no decompression limit with a perfect controlled ascent would be considered 'unprovocative', and this could influence the way a physician interprets mild non-specific symptoms arising after the dive. Dive planning algorithms are discussed further in Chapter 12.

SPECIFIC CLINICAL MANIFESTATIONS

With the exception of the constellations of symptoms designated 'mild', 'combined', and 'fulminant', this section considers the clinical manifestations of DCS categorized by organ system. This corresponds to commonly used clinical terminology in which reference is often made to 'spinal DCS', 'cerebral DCS' and so forth in preference to the older type 1 and type II designations. A schema for classifying the clinical manifestations in this way is shown in Figure 11.1, which, for completeness, also puts DCS into the broader context of 'decompression illness' as described earlier.

Mild decompression sickness

It is logical first to discuss the constellation of symptoms that were defined as constituting 'mild DCS' by a consensus workshop hosted by Divers Alert Network (DAN) and the Undersea and Hyperbaric Medical Society (UHMS) in 2004[2]. Presentations with one or more of the mild symptoms are the most common. Indeed, of 520 patients with cases treated at Auckland, New Zealand between 1995 and 2012, only 36 per cent had objective signs found on examination[3]. This is clinically significant because if the diver meets the agreed criteria for the mild designation, then the workshop consensus holds that he or she would not be disadvantaged in the long term if not recompressed. This, in turn, has important implications for decision making about evacuation and treatment for divers in remote locations; an issue that is discussed further later.

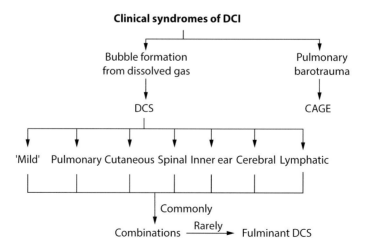

Figure 11.1 A schema for classification of the clinical manifestations of DCS.

The symptoms in the mild category are as follows:

1. Musculoskeletal pain.
2. Subjective sensory changes in a non-dermatomal distribution.
3. Constitutional symptoms such as fatigue and malaise.
4. Itch and rash of the superficial erythematous type.

Musculoskeletal pain is the most frequent symptom in DCS (Figure 11.2). It is often described by patients as a 'deep, boring ache', and it may be severe. Various references characterize the typical location as 'joint pain', and indeed, it is commonly reported in hips, knees, shoulders and elbows. However, the localization is often poor, and extra-articular pain (e.g. the whole 'upper arm') is also well recorded. It is common for pain to exist in more than one location, and it may migrate. Affected divers often remark that unlike musculoskeletal pain they have suffered in other circumstances, there seems little they can do (e.g. adopting different positions and rubbing) to effect relief. In that regard, the use of a sphygmomanometer cuff as a diagnostic aid (inflating the cuff over the affected area allegedly compresses bubbles and provides relief) is not a valid strategy. It is notable that new back pain or abdominal pain following diving must never be automatically assumed to be musculoskeletal in origin. These symptoms may be indicative of spinal involvement that is yet to declare itself in a more obvious way. Similarly, if a diver presents with bilateral and symmetrical shoulder or hip pain, a high index of suspicion must be maintained for spinal involvement, and other spinal manifestations (e.g. motor and sensory change) must be diligently excluded by competent examination.

Subjective sensory change is most commonly described as 'patchy tingling', and it is surprisingly common (see Figure 11.2). It may occur in multiple non-dermatomal distributions and may migrate. Sensory changes that lie in a dermatomal distribution are likely related to spinal involvement and do not meet the definition of mild.

Constitutional symptoms such as fatigue and a general sense of unwellness (malaise) are also common but very non-specific and difficult to interpret. Indeed, fatigue is an almost invariable consequence of a long day of diving. It would be most unusual to base a diagnosis of DCS solely on the presence of constitutional symptoms.

Itches and light erythematous or 'scarlatiniform' rashes, often with poorly defined boundaries,

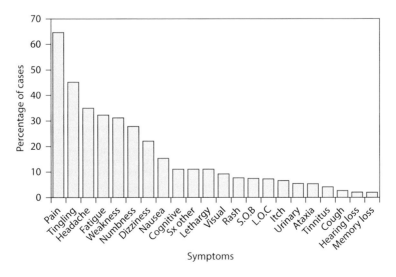

Figure 11.2 Percentage of 520 DCS and CAGE cases complaining of various symptoms. Note fatigue and lethargy appeared as separate entries in the database and so are shown separately here even though they likely represent the same phenomenon. SOB = shortness of breath, LOC = loss of consciousness.

are less common than pain but still relatively frequent (Plate 3). They are usually proximal in distribution, with the trunk being the most common involved site. However, they can effectively occur anywhere. The cutis marmorata form of cutaneous DCS (see later) is not considered mild because it is often associated with neurological DCS, and that is why there is a separate 'box' for cutaneous DCS in Figure 11.1 even though most skin manifestations fit within the mild category.

The symptoms of the mild DCS syndrome are summarized in Figure 11.3. Another symptom that many physicians have retrospectively suggested should have been included in the mild category is headache. Headache is a very non-specific symptom and has many potential causes in diving. Although it is often reported by divers presenting with other symptoms of DCS, it would be extremely unusual to make the diagnosis of DCS based on a post-dive headache alone. At the present time headache sits outside the mild categorization laid down by the workshop[2], but if a diver presented with mild symptoms (strictly as defined here) and a headache, then it would be reasonable to continue to designate the case as mild provided the other criteria outlined later are met.

In addition to fitting the qualitative symptom definitions described previously, the 2004 workshop also required compliance with a number of other conditions to designate a case as 'mild'. First, the mild designation could not be applied

while any of the symptoms were clearly worsening because this could herald the imminent appearance of new (and non-mild) symptoms. Second, the mild designation could not be applied unless the patient had undergone a competent neurological examination (which does not include '5-minute neuros' by divers with no medical training). This stipulation recognized the potential for undetected objective neurological manifestations even when the obvious symptoms appeared mild. Third, in recognition of the potential for (rare) delayed deterioration, the mild designation should not be 'signed off' for 24 hours, and the patient should be periodically reviewed during this time.

The natural history of mild DCS symptoms (as defined earlier) is for spontaneous resolution even in the absence of therapy. There is little doubt that surface oxygen therapy will often accelerate recovery, and in respect of pain in particular, recompression and hyperbaric oxygen are likely to accelerate resolution markedly. Despite this potential for accelerated symptom resolution by recompression, the 2004 consensus workshop[2] concluded that provided the presentation met the criteria for mild DCS, there was little or no evidence for any long-term disadvantage if the patient was not recompressed. It must be emphasized that the workshop was not advocating withholding of recompression for all patients with mild cases. Indeed, if recompression is readily available, then the best course of action is to treat the diver. However, the workshop did

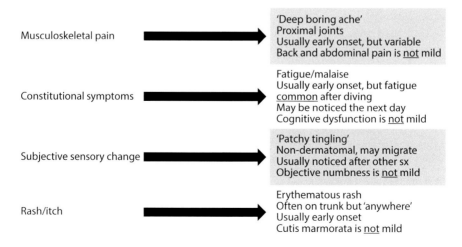

Figure 11.3 Symptoms of DCS that were designated "mild" by the 2004 remote DCS workshop[2].

identify surface oxygen and other adjuvants (see Chapter 13) as acceptable alternatives to recompression in mild cases where recompression would be difficult or hazardous to access (e.g. in a very remote location).

Pulmonary decompression sickness

Often referred to as cardiopulmonary DCS, this manifestation is rare and potentially fatal. The onset is usually early after diving and is more likely following a provocative profile (e.g. where decompression stops have been omitted for some reason). The diver may complain of cough and shortness of breath, which give rise to the colloquial name 'the chokes'. There may also be retrosternal chest pain and a progression from confusion to loss of consciousness and collapse, the latter most likely reflecting rapidly progressive hypotension. Cardiac arrest and death may rapidly follow. Alternatively, the symptoms may spontaneously resolve; especially if oxygen breathing is quickly commenced because this almost certainly accelerates the resolution of VGE affecting the lungs. Because large numbers of VGE are required to produce pulmonary symptoms, it is not surprising that symptoms of involvement of other organs often accompany or follow pulmonary DCS. Thus, even if pulmonary symptoms begin to resolve, there should be a high index of suspicion for other manifestations.

Cutaneous decompression sickness

The designation of superficial erythematous rash and itch as part of the mild constellation of DCS symptoms has already been discussed. The skin manifestation known as cutis marmorata sits outside the mild definition because of its frequent association with more serious manifestations. Cutis marmorata has a marbled, blotchy appearance in which areas of deep erythema and sometimes cyanotic change are interrupted and bounded by areas of pallor. The rash can evolve quite quickly and can even change appearance over a short period of observation. The rash can be itchy at first, but as it progresses it becomes less irritating or sometimes painful. Despite its often dramatic appearance, the rash almost invariably resolves with no obvious injury to the cutaneous tissues. The significance of cutis marmorata is its moderately frequent association with other more serious manifestations such as spinal DCS.

Spinal decompression sickness

All levels of the spinal cord may be involved, although a thoracolumbar distribution is most common. This disorder typically produces symptoms within the first 30 minutes after diving, and the first symptom is usually bilateral sensory change, which often ascends from distal to proximal, shortly followed by weakness producing ascending paraplegia. This is usually associated with a loss of bladder sensation and tone and a loss of anal tone. Cervical involvement may also produce sensory change and weakness in the upper limb. Examination findings are typically consistent with loss of upper motor neuron function under any circumstances, but in DCS there may be patchy involvement of different regions of the spinal cord, and detailed examination to delineate the location and extent of lesions is usually not necessary or helpful, especially at first presentation. Once the approximate extent of spinal involvement is understood, timely instigation of recompression treatment is the priority.

The natural history of spinal DCS is variable. In cases that progress to weakness, spontaneous recovery is possible, especially with surface oxygen administration. However, permanent sequelae are common even after treatment with recompression and hyperbaric oxygen. This makes spinal DCS the most feared and debilitating of the dysbaric diseases.

Inner ear decompression sickness

Inner ear DCS manifests with vestibular symptoms (vertigo, nausea, vomiting, ataxia) or cochlear symptoms (tinnitus, deafness) or both. Two distinct patterns of evolution are recognized. The first occurs during decompression from deep dives while the diver is still submerged, and it may be aggravated by a switch from a helium-based breathing gas to a nitrogen-based breathing gas. This is particularly dangerous because it can incapacitate the diver at a time when he or she still has hours of decompression to complete, thus forcing an early ascent with substantial missed decompression. The second occurs after arrival at the surface from more typical recreational air dives, although usually involving moderate depth exposure (greater than 25 metres). In this setting the onset is typically seen within the first 30 minutes of the dive. These different presentations probably have a different pathophysiological basis (see Chapter 10). Both may resolve spontaneously, but they are responsive to recompression and hyperbaric oxygen. Whether treated or untreated, it is certainly possible that long-term injury can follow inner ear DCS. In particular, permanent loss of hearing may occur. Although the vestibular apparatus may be permanently damaged, this does not usually result in long-term symptoms. There is a well-recognized ability for the brain to accommodate asymmetrical vestibular function that takes place over weeks to months and usually results in spontaneous resolution of vertigo and ataxia.

Cerebral decompression sickness

DCS can manifest with dysexecutive syndromes in which the diver complains of difficulties with concentration, memory, mood and other cognitive functions. These manifestations are frequently noticed 'late' when the diver returns home or to work. As described in Chapter 10, it seems most likely that such symptoms arise from exposure of the brain to VGE that have arterialized across a right-to-left shunt such as a PFO. It seems unlikely that these small VGE can cause the focal stroke-like manifestations typically associated with larger bubbles that may be introduced to the cerebral arterial circulation after pulmonary barotrauma. The latter type of presentation is described in Chapter 6. The natural history of cerebral DCS is poorly characterized, although the authors are aware of cases in which permanent cognitive sequelae have been reported.

Lymphatic decompression sickness

Lymphatic symptoms are among the more curious manifestations. Lymphatic DCS appears as subcutaneous swelling that is often surprisingly localized. It may lie over sites where there is musculoskeletal pain (which may be coincidental) or at other locations. The upper thorax and shoulder area appear selectively vulnerable. The disorder usually develops over a period of hours after diving and will eventually resolve whether the diver is recompressed or not. It is not usually painful, but it can create a conspicuously odd appearance (e.g. enlarging the breast area in a male patient). The natural history is to complete resolution, and there do not appear to be any long-term sequelae.

Combined presentations

The previously described manifestations can all appear in isolation, but combinations of symptoms are very common, particularly the constellation of symptoms described as constituting the mild DCS syndrome. Such combinations can be useful in helping to formulate the diagnosis. For example, whereas an isolated monoarthropathy after diving always raises suspicion of an alternative diagnosis such as a muscular strain, a monoarthropathy combined with patchy paraesthesiae and an erythematous rash would be a much more convincing basis for the diagnosis of DCS. Other common combinations include mild symptoms and any of the other forms of DCS, pulmonary DCS and spinal DCS, and cutis marmorata and spinal DCS.

Fulminant decompression sickness

Fulminant DCS is a poorly defined entity, but the term is sometimes used to describe those cases in which, in addition to combinations of the foregoing symptoms, there is clear evidence of widespread systemic effects of bubbles such as haemoconcentration, shock and coagulopathy. This form of the disease is frequently fatal unless there is expert and comprehensive intervention. In this regard, it is notable that access to supportive therapy such as sedation, appropriate airway management, fluid resuscitation, and pharmacologic support of haemodynamics may be a more pressing priority than recompression *per se*. If patients with fulminant DCS are recompressed without appropriate supportive therapy in place, the outcome is likely to be poor (Case Report 11.1).

CASE REPORT 11.1

A rebreather diver suffered an equipment malfunction after 9 minutes at 110-metre depth and made an uncontrolled ascent to the surface. He was sighted arriving at the surface and retrieved onto the boat, where he was found to be unconscious and apnoeic. He quickly resumed breathing and regained consciousness when cardiopulmonary resuscitation was initiated. A helicopter evacuation was extremely expeditious, and he arrived at a major tertiary hospital with a hyperbaric unit less than 1 hour after surfacing, having been treated with oxygen by a non-rebreather mask. He was complaining of dyspnoea and severe back pain. He had marked widespread cutis marmorata and quadriplegia. The pulse was 152, and peripheral pulses were unpalpable. The initial blood tests revealed marked haemoconcentration (haemoglobin, 254g/l), coagulopathy (activated partial thromboplastin time, 105; international normalized ratio, 2.0) and metabolic evidence of shock (pH, 7.24; lactate, 5; base excess, −12). He was diagnosed with fulminant DCS and catheterized, had large-bore intravenous access established, arterial and central venous lines placed and was aggressively fluid resuscitated and supported with vasopressors as the chamber was prepared for recompression. After sedation and intubation he was recompressed on a maximally extended US Navy Table 6. When sedation was withdrawn after 24 hours, he had recovered almost all motor function. After two further recompressions he, somewhat remarkably, made an essentially complete recovery.

DIFFERENTIAL DIAGNOSIS

The attribution of symptoms following diving to DCS is contingent on the symptoms being qualitatively consistent with one or more of those described. In addition, an evaluation of the 'provocation' of the dive is useful but not definitive. Thus, a dive that breached no decompression limits without adequate decompression (see Chapter 12), involved rapid ascent or involved risk factors (see Chapter 12) would be considered more provocative than one that, for example, was well inside the no decompression limits with no untoward events. The timing of symptom onset (discussed previously in this chapter) is also contributory to diagnosis, with DCS becoming less likely with greater symptom latencies after diving. Unfortunately, there is no formula in which these various factors can be integrated to give a definitive answer on diagnosis. There is no substitute for knowledge and experience in this regard. Diagnostic uncertainty and the non-specific nature of many DCS symptoms will inevitably result in recompression of divers with consistent symptoms caused by another disorder from time to time. Other disorders that may mimic DCS are briefly considered here. Although the authors of this text emphasize the fact that a temporal relationship between diving and symptom onset is compelling evidence of a diving-related problem, DCS has many non-specific symptoms, and there are often several differential diagnoses that should be considered, especially in respect of some of the mild symptoms. Some of the more common or important differential diagnoses for DCS symptoms are outlined in this section.

Musculoskeletal pain is the most common single symptom of DCS, and it may also be caused by many other problems. Muscular and soft tissue injuries are common events in the diving environment, where there is heavy lifting and ample opportunity for minor trauma. This should be considered, especially where the diver has a non-migratory monoarthropathy with a history consistent with a non-DCS cause. Examination findings such as bruising may help, although cutis marmorata can look a little like bruising, so care is needed in interpreting skin change. There have been a few cases of myocardial ischaemia manifesting after diving with left shoulder and arm pain and being diagnosed as musculoskeletal DCS.

Fatigue is extremely common after diving, and the diagnosis of DCS would never be made on the presence of fatigue alone. Malaise can occur in many systemic illnesses, and in particular, viral illness can induce significant malaise. Such illnesses are common on diving trips, especially where participants have travelled long distances on airplanes and have been exposed to many other travellers. The presence of other viral illness symptoms such as fever and coryza, which are not usually seen in DCS, can help with accurate diagnosis.

Patchy paraesthesiae and rash can occur as a result of contact exposures with irritants such as marine stingers (see Chapter 32) and soaps used to clean wetsuits. Other allergies can cause rash, and some toxic ingestions that may occur on dive trips (e.g. ciguatera fish poisoning) (see Chapter 33) can cause marked widespread paraesthesiae, as well as myalgias and malaise.

Pulmonary symptoms, such as chest pain and cough, can occur in many settings. The main clue to DCS as a cause would be early onset (usually within minutes) after diving. Nevertheless, this does not rule out other causes of diving-induced pulmonary irritation such as pulmonary barotrauma (rare) (see Chapter 6), immersion pulmonary oedema (rare) (see Chapter 30), oxygen toxicity (very rare) (see Chapter 17), near drowning (see Chapter 22) or salt water aspiration syndrome (see Chapter 24). Pulmonary barotrauma could be suspected if there was a history of rapid or panicked ascent, if the dive was unprovocative for DCS or if there were clear signs of pulmonary barotrauma such as haemoptysis, pneumothorax or subcutaneous emphysema in the supraclavicular area. Immersion pulmonary oedema can be a difficult differential diagnosis, although the symptoms often first appear at depth and force termination of the dive. Symptoms that appear at depth are not DCS. In addition, although some descriptions of pulmonary DCS refer to the possibility of pulmonary oedema, these may represent misdiagnoses. Pulmonary oedema has not been a feature of definite pulmonary DCS seen by these authors. Oxygen toxicity symptoms would be expected only at the end of very long periods of oxygen exposure in technical diving (see Chapter 62). Near drowning would almost certainly be indicated by a clear history of some sort of distress event and inhalation of water. Salt water aspiration syndrome usually has a longer latency than pulmonary DCS. Moreover, in all these differential diagnoses, the symptoms would be limited to pulmonary involvement.

The appearance of other DCS manifestations would point strongly to DCS as the diagnosis.

Spinal symptoms following diving are almost invariably the result of DCS. It is possible that degenerative spinal disease (e.g. 'sciatica') could manifest for the first time early after diving, but the symptoms would be unilateral and frequently preceded by a history of previous problems. The abdominal and back pain that may be a feature of spinal DCS can also occur in the Irukandji syndrome (see Chapter 32). Nevertheless, spinal symptoms arising early after diving should never be rationalized to an alternative diagnosis without an extremely good reason.

The diagnosis of inner ear DCS involves one of the most difficult and troublesome differential diagnoses in diving medicine – the separation between DCS and inner ear barotrauma (IEBT) (see Chapter 7). Both disorders may manifest with vestibular and/or cochlear symptoms early after diving, but the diagnoses have significantly different implications for subsequent management. DCS mandates recompression therapy, whereas recompression is relatively contraindicated in IEBT and these patients may warrant referral for round window surgery. A key point that frequently resolves the problem is that IEBT often manifests first during descent, and frequently in association with difficulty equalizing pressures in the middle ears. Manifestation before decompression rules out DCS, and a clear history of difficulty with ear 'clearing' increases suspicion of IEBT. A dive that is very non-provocative for DCS would also tip the diagnostic suspicion toward IEBT, whereas a more provocative dive would tip suspicion the other way, particularly if the dive involved a gas switch from a high-helium to a high-nitrogen mix, or if other manifestations of DCS emerged. Nevertheless, not infrequently there is ambiguity around the diagnosis, and difficult decisions about treatment have to be made.

Transient vertigo (usually lasting seconds) can also occur during ascent if there is a difference in the rates at which the middle ears vent expanding gas through the Eustachian tubes. This is known as 'alternobaric vertigo'. This phenomenon is relatively common, transitory and self-limiting. Alternobaric vertigo should never be used as an explanation for persistent vestibular symptoms after a dive.

As previously discussed in relation to classification of the bubble-induced dysbaric disorders, there is often diagnostic ambiguity around the appearance cerebral symptoms after diving where the competing diagnoses are CAGE secondary to pulmonary barotrauma or cerebral DCS caused by the left-to-right shunting of VGE across a PFO or pulmonary shunts. The circumstances of the dive may provide definitive clues. For example, CAGE would be plausible and cerebral DCS highly implausible as an explanation for the rapid onset of focal cerebral symptoms after a panic ascent during training in a swimming pool. In addition, irrespective of the circumstances of the dive, it is likely that gross focal symptoms are more compatible with a CAGE event, whereas dysexecutive symptoms are more likely to be caused by DCS. However, in respect of cerebral DCS *versus* CAGE, the diagnosis is almost irrelevant because recompression according to the same regimen is now the prevalent response to either diagnosis (see Chapter 13).

Another possible cause of gross focal symptoms is a cerebrovascular event coincident with completion of a dive. Such events have occurred, and on occasion, divers suffering cerebrovascular accidents have been recompressed before the misdiagnosis has been discovered. This is unlikely to be harmful, although it will delay access to therapies such as thrombolysis or clot retrieval. Equally, because most cerebral symptoms appearing early after diving are caused by either DCS or CAGE, the prioritization of recompression as first-line therapy without detailed investigation to exclude cerebrovascular accident is appropriate for most cases.

Dysexecutive symptoms arising after diving may also be caused by a gas toxicity such as carbon monoxide exposure. The related symptoms are often initially noticed at depth, and this provides a clue that something other than DCS is responsible. There may also be a history of foul-tasting breathing gas or multiple divers affected if they breathed gas from a common source.

REFERENCES

1. Francis TJR, Smith DH, eds. *Describing Decompression Illness: The Forty Second Undersea and Hyperbaric Medical Society Workshop.* Bethesda, Maryland: Undersea and Hyperbaric Medical Society; 1991.
2. Mitchell SJ, Doolette DJ, Wachholz C, Vann RD, eds. *Management of Mild or Marginal Decompression Illness in Remote Locations – Workshop Proceedings.* Washington, DC: Undersea and Hyperbaric Medical Society; 2005.
3. Haas RM, Hannam JA, Sames C, et al. Decompression illness in divers treated in Auckland, New Zealand 1996–2013. *Diving and Hyperbaric Medicine* 2014;**44**:20–25.

FURTHER READING

Francis TJR, Mitchell SJ. Manifestations of decompression disorders. In: Brubakk AO, Neuman TS, eds. *Bennett and Elliott's Physiology and Medicine of Diving.* 5th ed. London: Harcourt Publishers; 2003:578–599.

This chapter was reviewed for this fifth edition by Simon Mitchell.

12

Decompression sickness: prevention

INTRODUCTION

Given the potentially serious consequences of decompression sickness (DCS), it is not surprising that divers pay great heed to means of preventing it. These preventive measures can be broadly classified into two categories: the appropriate control of depth and time exposures using dive tables or computers and the amelioration of putative risk factors for DCS. Both are discussed in this chapter.

DECOMPRESSION PLANNING

As discussed in Chapter 10, DCS occurs when supersaturation of inert gas during decompression causes bubbles to form in sufficient numbers or size (and in the right location) such that some poorly defined clinical threshold is exceeded and symptoms occur. Decompression planning is the process of controlling depth, time and the ascent ('decompression') to reduce the probability of DCS.

Because tissue gas supersaturation is the fundamental condition required for bubbles to form, it is not surprising that all decompression planning approaches have, at their core, a means of

calculating the pressure of dissolved inert gasses in a range of tissues throughout a dive. These dissolved gas pressures can then be compared with ambient pressure to establish the degree of supersaturation, and adjustments to the dive profile can be made to prevent supersaturation from exceeding safe thresholds. With the intended audience in mind, it is the express intent of this account to discuss the broad principles of adapting tissue supersaturation calculations into decompression planning tools, rather than the related mathematics. Those wishing to study the mathematical principles and methods can find relevant accounts elsewhere[1,2].

Basic principles

As mentioned earlier, virtually any approach to decompression planning assumes that the inert gas tensions within tissues can be calculated and thereby tracked throughout a dive. As could be anticipated from the discussion of gas uptake and elimination in Chapter 10, the mathematical models that allow such calculations include tissue perfusion and the blood-tissue partition coefficient for the relevant gas(es) as inputs. It is also pertinent to reiterate that the 'tissues' considered in these models are not real or identifiable tissues *per se*. The models merely consider a range of hypothetical tissues with different inert gas kinetics and assume that the relevant real tissues behave in a manner analogous to one of the hypothetical compartments used in decompression calculations.

To illustrate the incorporation of tissue gas supersaturation data into decompression planning, the relevant events during a dive are depicted using the format introduced in Figure 12.1. It is important to appreciate that this and subsequent figures in this chapter are illustrating principles and do not purport to be scaled correctly or to –represent any particular tissue accurately.

In Figure 12.1, ambient pressure (depth) is shown on the horizontal axis, and tissue gas pressure is shown on the vertical axis. Time is not illustrated in the diagram but requires assumptions to be made about its passage, as will be described. Line A represents descent at the start of a dive. The descent occurs over a short space of time, and so there is little time for inert gas uptake and little increase in tissue gas pressure. The bottom depth is reached at the point indicated; therefore, there is no further change in ambient pressure until the ascent begins (see later). During time spent at the bottom depth, inert gas will dissolve into the tissue and the tissue

inert gas tension will increase, as depicted by line B. The other notable feature in Figure 12.1 is the line labelled 'Tissue pressure = ambient pressure'. This represents the point, for all depths, where the pressure of dissolved gas in tissue is equal to the ambient pressure and is often referred to as the 'ambient pressure line'. It should be clear that while remaining at any particular depth, the tissue gas pressure cannot rise above this line because once tissue gas pressure equals ambient pressure, there can be no further pressure gradient to drive diffusion of gas into the tissue unless the diver descends deeper. Depending on the kinetics of individual tissues and the time spent at depth, at the end of a period at the bottom depth, tissue gas pressure may have equilibrated with ambient pressure in some 'fast' tissues, whereas in other 'slower tissues' it may not (Figure 12.2).

Figure 12.2 illustrates a hypothetical situation that could prevail at the end of a period at depth in respect of tissue gas pressures in a range of tissues (represented by the grey dots) with differing kinetic properties. Depending on the duration of the bottom time, the tissue gas pressure in one or more tissues may have reached equilibrium with ambient pressure (thus having reached the ambient pressure line), and these tissues can be described as 'saturated' with inert gas for that depth. Other tissues with slower kinetics will have absorbed less inert gas and will have lower tissue gas pressures.

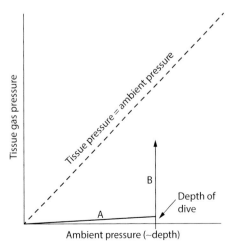

Figure 12.1 Depiction of changes in inert gas tension in a hypothetical single tissue during the early part of a dive. See text for explanation.

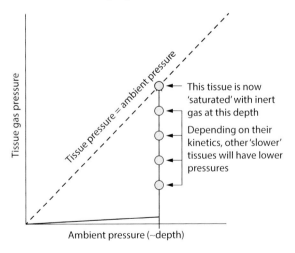

Figure 12.2 Gas pressures in a range of hypothetical tissues at the end of a period at depth. See text for further explanation.

For the purposes of illustrating the principles of decompression, this discussion temporarily ignores the fact that multiple tissues are involved and focusses on the behaviour of a single tissue. For the sake of simplicity, it is assumed that this tissue has reached the ambient pressure line (and is thus saturated with inert gas) at the end of a long bottom time. This is illustrated in Figure 12.3.

In Figure 12.3 (as in Figure 12.1), line A represents descent to the depth indicated at point 1 at the start of the dive, and line B represents the increase in tissue gas pressure as inert gas is absorbed during the time at depth. This tissue has reached the ambient pressure line (grey dot at point 2) and is thus saturated with inert gas. Line C represents the changes in tissue gas pressure and ambient pressure during the early part of the ascent. Ambient pressure decreases quickly as depth changes, whereas in this tissue the accumulated inert gas is not washed out at a rate that matches the fall in ambient pressure. In a tissue with very fast kinetics, the fall in tissue gas pressure could more closely match the falling ambient pressure, but in this tissue it can be seen that by point 3 on the ascent, the tissue gas pressure (point 4) markedly exceeds the ambient pressure (point 5) and the tissue is thus

'supersaturated'. The supersaturation pressure is indicted by the double-ended arrow in Figure 12.3.

It should be clear at this point that the key question when modelling decompression in this way is 'How much supersaturation is acceptable?' The means of deriving an answer to this question introduces a controversial dichotomy in decompression science between the so-called 'gas content models' and 'bubble models'. For the moment, the focus of this discussion is on the more traditional gas content models, and this approach is contrasted with bubble models later.

The original gas content model proposed by Haldane held that ascent could proceed until such time as the tissue gas pressure in any tissue reached twice the ambient pressure. This was Haldane's often-cited 2:1 ratio. At this point a decompression stop was imposed to allow the tissue gas pressure to fall while the ambient pressure remained constant. This approach was moderately successful, but it evolved over time, and the fixed ratio concept was eventually dropped in favour of ascent rules that prescribed maximum allowable supersaturations (sometimes referred to as 'M-values') for different tissues across a range of depths. The most famous of these sets of rules were the Zurich Limits for 16 hypothetical tissues (the ZH-L16 limits) prescribed by A. A. Buhlmann and based on physiological predictions with subsequent empirical modifications. The principles by which these work are illustrated for a single tissue in Figure 12.4.

As in Figure 12.3, line A in Figure 12.4 represents descent to the bottom depth indicted at point 1 at the start of the dive, and line B represents the increase in tissue gas pressure as inert gas is absorbed during the time spent at that depth (bottom time). By the end of the bottom time the illustrated tissue has reached the ambient pressure line (grey dot at point 2) and is thus saturated with inert gas. As in Figure 12.3, line C in Figure 12.4 represents the changes in tissue gas pressure and ambient pressure during the early part of the ascent. In Figure 12.4, the ascent rule is shown as a series of values for maximum allowable tissue gas pressures plotted against depth and is labelled 'supersaturation limit' for simplicity. As is typical, especially for tissues with fast kinetics, the rule allows greater supersaturation at deeper depths. Direct ascent (line C), at a rate not exceeding

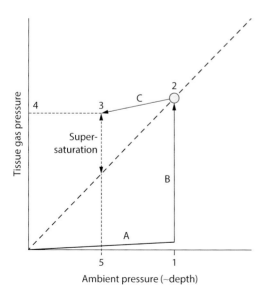

Figure 12.3 Development of supersaturation in a hypothetical single tissue during ascent. See text for further explanation.

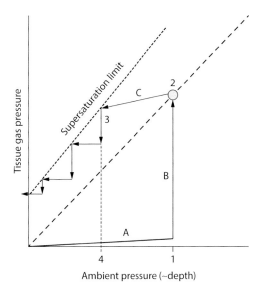

Figure 12.4 Representation of a decompression protocol determined by a gas content model ascent rule for a hypothetical single tissue. See text for further explanation.

a maximum prescribed by the model, proceeds until the tissue gas pressure equals the maximum allowed (point 3), at which time the first 'decompression stop' is imposed at a depth corresponding to point 4. After the tissue has 'off-gassed' sufficiently, the ascent is resumed with stops imposed each time the supersaturation limit is approached as depicted in Figure 12.4. Eventually, there is sufficient outgassing in the tissue to allow direct ascent to the surface while remaining just under the supersaturation limit.

Although diagrams such as Figure 12.4 are useful for illustrating some of the basic concepts underlying decompression planning, the process is much more complex in reality. In 'real' decompression modelling, we are usually not considering only one tissue but multiple tissues simultaneously. Whichever tissue is closest to its maximum supersaturation limit at any stage of the ascent becomes the 'controlling tissue'. Typically, this will be one of the tissues with faster kinetics early in the ascent (because these tissues are likely to have accumulated higher levels of inert gas during the bottom time). This means that the early decompression stops are shorter because the faster tissues that are controlling at that point will outgas quickly. Similarly, the

tissues with slower kinetics tend to be controlling later in the ascent for the shallower stops. These stops tend to be longer because the slower tissues take longer to outgas. The involvement of multiple tissues and the effect of tissue gas kinetics on decompression stop durations are not captured in diagrams such as Figure 12.4.

It is appropriate to acknowledge at this point that recreational divers undertaking entry level courses are taught 'no decompression diving'. This means that dives are planned to be of modest depth and duration so that a direct ascent to the surface (at the correct rate) can be made at any point in the dive without the gas pressure in any tissues crossing the supersaturation limit. Because tissue inert gas pressures will reach higher levels more quickly at greater depths (where the inspired inert gas pressures are higher), the permitted duration for a no decompression dive (referred to as a 'no decompression limit') becomes progressively shorter as the depth increases. For example, for many years the US Navy air diving table prescribed no decompression limits for 18-, 30- and 40-metre dives as 60, 25 and 5 minutes, respectively. Dives requiring decompression stops are routinely undertaken by recreational divers who refer to themselves as 'technical divers' (see Chapter 62).

Gas content versus bubble models

As described earlier, gas content models regulate ascent and impose decompression stops to maintain tissue supersaturation below empirically derived thresholds across the range of tissues with different kinetic behaviour. Such models have been very successful, but are not invariably so; that is, DCS can certainly still occur even when divers decompress according to the model. The occurrence of such events always results in interest in alternative approaches that may (potentially) be more successful. Moreover, as discussed in Chapter 10, it has long been known that even decompressions performed in accordance with established guidelines frequently result in the formation of venous gas emboli (VGE), whose numbers can be correlated (albeit imprecisely) with the risk of DCS. Much of the early research that revealed this VGE phenomenon took place when the use of gas content models to control decompression was almost ubiquitous.

Thus, the emerging recreational technical diving world of the late 1990s and early 2000s was fertile ground for well-meaning advocates of alternative approaches to decompression.

A school of thought that had been around for some time, but came to prominence during this period, was the so-called 'bubble-model' approach. Bubble model advocates had taken note of the frequently high VGE counts after decompression conducted according to gas content models and advanced the notion that, at least in part, the failure of these models to control bubble formation effectively could increase the risk of DCS even when the diver did everything right. Moreover, they proposed that initiation of bubble formation probably occurred during exposure to the relatively large supersaturations allowed by gas content models during the long ascent to the first decompression stop. Using advanced physics, bubble modellers purported to be able to quantify bubble formation from micronuclei (see Chapter 10) of a given size for a given level of supersaturation, and their calculations suggested that shorter initial ascents (and therefore smaller initial supersaturations) than allowed by gas content models would result in 'excitation' of smaller populations of micronuclei and therefore help prevent initiation of bubble formation. It was even suggested that by imposing deeper initial decompression stops a diver could reduce the requirement for the shallow decompression stops later in the ascent because initiation of bubble formation would have been controlled earlier. A stylized comparison between these two approaches to decompression using the same format as previous figures is shown in Figure 12.5.

As in Figures 12.3 and 12.4, line A in Figure 12.5 represents descent to the bottom depth indicted at point 1, and line B represents the increase in tissue gas pressure as inert gas is absorbed during the time spent at that depth (bottom time). By the end of the bottom time the illustrated tissue has reached the ambient pressure line (grey dot at point 2) and is thus saturated with inert gas. As in Figure 12.4, the supersaturation limit or M-value line as prescribed by a gas content model is depicted, and if the diver was following such a model, then direct ascent (line C) would proceed until the tissue gas pressure equalled the maximum allowed (point 3), at which time the first

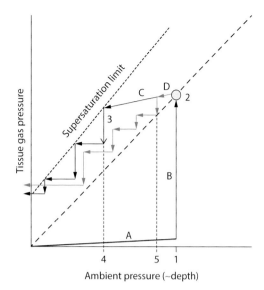

Figure 12.5 Stylized depiction of differences between decompression of a hypothetical single tissue prescribed by a gas content model (black line) and a bubble model (grey line). See text for further explanation.

decompression stop would be imposed at a depth corresponding to point 4. After the tissue has off-gassed sufficiently, the ascent would be resumed with stops imposed each time the maximum supersaturation is approached.

In contrast, the ascent prescribed by a typical bubble model (depicted by the grey arrows) involves shorter initial ascents, deeper initial decompression stops and smaller initial supersaturations. A bubble model could also (as depicted) allow surfacing with a tissue gas supersaturation greater than the maximum allowed by the gas content model, based on the belief that the process of bubble initiation had been controlled earlier and that this allowed exposure to greater supersaturation later in the ascent.

There was a compelling theoretical attraction to the concept of using 'deep stops' to 'control bubble formation early in the ascent'. There were also some widely discussed anecdotal observations from several prominent divers that insertion of deep stops into their ascents seemed to result in feeling less fatigued after dives. In the early 2000s these factors, combined with the burgeoning influence of Internet communication, became an article of faith among deep recreational technical divers that bubble model approaches to decompression were superior even though no formal testing of the algorithms had been undertaken. There was widespread adoption of the two most readily available bubble model algorithms (the varying permeability model [VPM] and the reduced gradient bubble model [RGBM]). It largely went unnoticed when VPM was revised into VPM-B to increase shallow stop time after reports of DCS began to emerge. Gas content models with their relatively rapid early ascents and longer shallow stops were derided as being a recipe for 'bending and mending' (an allusion to causing bubble formation with supersaturation of fast tissues early in the ascent and then fixing the problem with long shallow stops late in the ascent).

The use of gas content models did persist, perhaps because they were easier to understand or to program for use in computers, but even users of these algorithms began to manipulate them to make them behave more like bubble models. One technique for such a manipulation that became and remains popular is the use of so-called 'gradient factors'. This involves limiting supersaturation to less than permitted by the conventional supersaturation limit by redefining maximal permissible supersaturation as a fraction of the difference between ambient pressure and the limit. These fractions have come to be known as gradient factors. Thus, if a diver elects to limit supersaturation to 80 per cent of the usual difference between ambient pressure and the supersaturation limit, this is referred to as 'gradient factor 80' or 'GF 80'. Typical implementations of the gradient factor method require the diver to select two gradient factors: the first (often referred to as GF-Low) notionally controls supersaturation in the fast tissues early in the ascent, and the second (often referred to as GF-High) controls supersaturation in the slower tissues at the point of surfacing. The algorithm then interpolates a series of modified M-values in between these two user-specified points. Not surprisingly, lowering the first gradient factor limits supersaturation in the fast tissues early in the ascent by imposing deeper decompression stops, and lowering the second will produce longer shallower stops to reduce supersaturation in the slower tissues at the point of surfacing. Choosing a low

GF-Low and a higher GF-High produces a decompression profile that resembles a bubble model decompression. This is illustrated in Figure 12.6 for a GF-Low of 20 per cent and a GF-High of 90 per cent (in common use this terminology would be abbreviated to 'GF 20/90').

As in previous figures, line A in Figure 12.6 represents descent to the bottom depth indicted at point 1, and line B represents the increase in tissue gas pressure as inert gas is absorbed during the time spent at that depth (bottom time). By the end of the bottom time the illustrated tissue has reached the ambient pressure line (grey dot at point 2) and is thus saturated with inert gas. At the start of decompression, the initial ascent (line C) is allowed to proceed until the tissue reaches 20 per cent of the supersaturation limit, at which point a stop is imposed at the depth corresponding to point 3. The ascent then continues with further stops imposed when the tissue supersaturation approaches the modified supersaturation limit defined by a line joining the chosen GF-Low (black dot labelled 20 per cent) and the chosen GF-High (black dot labelled 90 per cent). If this approach is compared with the two profiles shown in Figure 12.5, it is clear that it is now very different

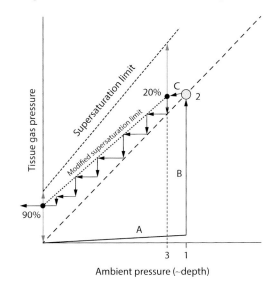

Figure 12.6 The stylized effect of imposing gradient factors GF 20/90 on the decompression prescribed by a gas content model for a single hypothetical tissue. See text for further explanation.

from the unmodified gas content model decompression and substantially similar to the bubble model decompression. For obvious reasons, the use of gradient factors with a low GF-Low and bubble model decompressions are collectively referred to as 'deep stop' approaches to decompression.

The ZH-L Buhlmann gas content model that forms the basis for most tables and computers designed to guide decompression diving by recreational divers was subjected to some human testing; albeit minimal for the trimix diving and depth range for which it is now implemented. The bubble models and gradient factor manipulations of gas content models have had essentially no testing. It is acknowledged that the preceding discussion of bubble model theory represents a gross oversimplification of a complicated matter, but the fact remains, no matter how attractive the theory, it has never been tested in a practical sense. Advocates frequently cite the ubiquitous nature of deep stop approaches as some sort of proof that they are optimal, but this is an invalid argument in the absence of comparative outcome data. These approaches clearly work in the majority of dives, but whether they are optimal is an unresolved question.

Debate over this issue has been rekindled with the publication of several studies that have suggested that the emphasis on deep stop approaches to decompression may need to be reconsidered. Several of these studies have focussed on measuring VGE after diving and suggest that deep stops may not reduce the appearance of VGE as previously widely assumed. However, by far the most significant development has been the 2011 publication of a study performed by the US Navy Experimental Diving Unit (NEDU) at Panama City in Florida[3]. The investigators compared outcomes after air dives to 170 feet for 30 minutes with same-duration decompression on air prescribed by either a gas content model or a bubble model. Both decompression protocols are US Navy models that are not used by recreational divers, but they nevertheless have characteristics that reflect the respective approaches; the gas content model allows greater supersaturation in faster tissues early in the ascent and distributes decompression time shallower, and the bubble model imposes deeper stops early in the ascent and thereby distributes decompression time deeper. The remarkable feature of

this study was that the primary outcome measure was DCS in human subjects. The divers performed a standardized workload during the bottom time, and temperature effects were standardized across the groups by having all divers wear no thermal protection in water at a temperature of 30°C. There were 11 cases of DCS in 198 dives in the deep stops group and 3 cases in 192 dives in the shallow stops group. The trial was ceased at this point because the difference became significant on sequential analysis.

This result was not the outcome expected or hypothesized by the investigators. Attempts to explain it have focussed on the likelihood that protection of fast tissues from supersaturation early in the ascent does not seem to be as effective as thought, and it comes at the expense of increased supersaturation in the slow tissues later in the ascent because they are continuing to absorb gas during deep stops. This principle is illustrated in Figure 12.7. As in previous figures, line A in Figure 12.7 represents descent to the bottom depth (indicted at point 1), and line B represents the increase in tissue gas pressure as

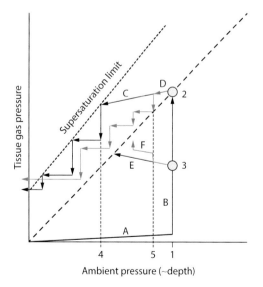

Figure 12.7 The stylized effect of a gas content model decompression (solid black arrows) and a bubble model decompression (grey arrows) on tissue gas pressure in a hypothetical fast tissue (arrows originating at point 2) and a hypothetical slower tissue (arrows originating at point 3). See text for further explanation.

inert gas is absorbed during the time spent at that depth (bottom time). By the end of the bottom time the tissue represented by the grey dot at point 2 has reached the ambient pressure line and is thus saturated with inert gas, whereas the slower tissue represented by the grey dot at point 3 is still absorbing inert gas. At the start of decompression, gas content model decompression allows an the initial ascent (line C) to proceed until the faster controlling tissue reaches the maximum supersaturation limit, where the first decompression stop is imposed at a depth indicated by point 4. In contrast, the bubble model allows a shorter ascent (line D) to the first stop at a depth indicated by point 5. In the slower tissue, whose tissue gas pressure at the beginning of ascent is indicated by point 3, the gas content model decompression gives the tissue little more time to absorb inert gas as illustrated by line E because absorption ceases and outgassing begins once the tissue reaches then crosses the ambient pressure line. In contrast, the deep stops prescribed by the bubble model will result in further inert gas absorption by this tissue (line F).

The NEDU study forces us to question whether the proposed benefit of using a bubble model (protection of fast tissues early in the ascent) is worth the disadvantage of the increased gas loading that occurs in slower tissues as a result. Bubble model advocates have tried to portray the study as irrelevant because the experiments involved air diving and used a deep stop profile that is not exactly the same as that prescribed by VPM-B. Nevertheless, analyses of 'real-world' VPM-B profiles prescribed for dives using accelerated decompression on oxygen (such as are typically undertaken by technical divers) suggest that the same disadvantageous pattern of protecting fast tissue from supersaturation early in the ascent at the expense of slower tissue supersaturation later still occurs.

It is clear that the optimal approach to decompression from the deep bounce dives undertaken by recreational technical divers is not established; however, it seems plausible to suggest that we have evolved an approach that risks overemphasizing deep stops. One trend that is emerging as this book goes to press is the use of gradient factors to reduce the emphasis on deep stops (by increasing the GF-Low) and re-emphasizing shallow stops (by decreasing the GF-High). Thus, whereas gradient factor combinations such as 10/90 were popular during the height of belief in deep stops, it is increasingly common to see combinations such as 40/70 or 50/70 now.

Dive tables, planning software and dive computers

Dive tables are pre-calculated and pre-printed implementations of a decompression algorithm that divers can use to plan their dives. These were most popular before the 1990s among recreational scuba air divers wanting to plan simple dives, and their use was taught as part of all recreational scuba diving courses. The most frequently used items of information were the no decompression limits (see earlier) provided by these tables. Thus, divers could look up the allowable bottom time they could spend at any particular depth and still make a direct ascent to the surface without decompression stops. Even though no decompression was prescribed for dives 'inside' the no decompression limits, most training agencies advocated the use of a 3- to 5-minute 'safety stop' at 3 to 5 metres during the final part of the ascent, as an added precaution. Such stops are probably useful in reducing the incidence of DCS on routine no decompression dives.

The dive tables also provided a series of steps (with minimal calculation) for divers to account for the effect of inert gas accumulated but not yet eliminated after previous dives when planning further 'repetitive' dives. In air diving, this is referred to as 'residual nitrogen', and its presence, not surprisingly, has the effect of reducing the no decompression limit for subsequent dives.

The use of dive tables has declined dramatically with the rise in use of dive computers (see later), and some entry level diving courses no longer teach their use. Whether this is a good or bad thing is impossible to say. Tables were inexpensive and readily available, whereas in the early days this was not true of computers. More recently, however, entry level dive computers have become much more reasonably priced and have the advantages of avoiding calculation errors, thus ensuring that the diver who carries one is receiving accurate time and depth information, and most of these computers provide ascent rate alarms.

Planning software that runs a decompression algorithm (and often multiple decompression algorithms) can be purchased for use on desktop, laptop and tablet computers, as well as telephones. Such software is effectively an electronic dive table and is often used to generate tables that are transcribed onto underwater slates for specific missions. The advantage of such software is that the decompression plan can be tailored specifically to the diver's equipment, gas mixes and decompression preferences (e.g. gas content model, bubble model, gradient factors). The multitude of combinations and permutations of circumstances that can be 'run' by such software would be very difficult, if not impossible, to replicate on pre-printed tables.

Dive computers that the diver carries underwater have become increasingly popular since the early 1990s and are now almost ubiquitous. These computers run software with one or more decompression algorithms programmed into them and with various levels of adaptability for decompression planning. They track time and depth exposures in real time and provide a constant display of parameters such as depth, dive duration, decompression ceiling and expected time to surfacing. These parameters are continuously updated as the depth varies and the dive duration lengthens, all with little or no effort on the part of the diver. Advanced computers allow the diver to choose the equipment being used (e.g. open-circuit or rebreather systems) and the gas mixes being breathed and to adjust decompression preferences such as gradient factors. Some computers can connect to the oxygen cells in a rebreather (see Chapter 62) so that they 'know' the inspired partial pressure of oxygen used by the diver and can incorporate this information in calculating decompression. Advanced computers that perform these functions and provide all relevant information in a head-up display constantly visible to the diver are now available.

AMELIORATION OF RISK FACTORS

Appropriate manipulation of the depth-time profile as discussed in the preceding section on decompression planning is obviously important in managing the risk of DCS. In addition, certain known or suspected risk factors for DCS, some of which have already been mentioned, can be manipulated or managed to reduce risk further.

Patent foramen ovale

The role of the patent foramen ovale (PFO) in the pathophysiology of DCS is discussed in Chapter 10, in which it was pointed out that PFO appears associated with an increased risk of cerebral, spinal, vestibulocochlear and cutaneous DCS. The most plausible explanation for this increase in risk is that a right-to-left shunt allows VGE to enter the arterial circulation, and these small bubbles can then distribute widely in the body and cause harm, as previously described. The degree of shunt facilitated by the PFO has consistently been found to be significant; with large and spontaneous shunts being important and very small shunts seemingly unimportant. The crucial question is this: 'How should this knowledge be applied to reducing risk of DCS?'

One obvious strategy would be to screen divers for PFO after an episode of neurological, inner ear or cutaneous DCS and, possibly, to repair large PFOs in divers who wish to continue diving. Another more radical strategy would be to screen all prospective divers before entry to the sport. Many divers have enthusiastically embraced such ideas. When participants on Internet diving discussion forums report an episode of DCS, a chorus of advice to check for a PFO inevitably follows, even if the event involved a form of DCS that has never been associated with a PFO (e.g. musculoskeletal DCS). However, decisions to screen divers for PFO or to repair any lesion that is discovered are not straightforward.

As pointed out in Chapter 10, PFO is very common (around 30 per cent of divers or diving candidates can be expected to have one) and so is the formation of VGE after diving; yet cerebral, spinal and inner ear DCS cases remain rare. There are clearly factors beyond merely having a PFO and producing venous bubbles that are involved in the chain of events leading to the relevant forms of DCS, and at this time we are not certain what they are. Screening all prospective divers by using an expensive invasive test (see Chapter 10), which would detect the target lesion in about 30 per cent of subjects (and potentially exclude them from diving), with the aim of preventing an event that occurs perhaps once in 10 000 dives (even in an unscreened population), is neither sensible nor justified.

In contrast, it may be appropriate to test divers who have had one of the relevant forms of DCS, particularly if there have been multiple events or if the event(s) followed dives that seem unprovocative in terms of decompression stress. It is also inevitable that the diving physician will be approached by enthusiasts who have never had DCS but who are aware of the association of serious DCS with PFO and who wish to be tested for this heart condition. Referring for testing may be appropriate under these circumstances, but the following points should always be explained to the diver before testing is undertaken.

1. The bubble contrast echocardiographic test is relatively safe, but there are some risks. Transient symptoms of cerebral arterial gas embolism have been reported following tests with strongly positive results for right-to-left shunt.
2. The test result is likely to be positive in at least 30 per cent of cases (or more depending on the context), and the diver may then have some difficult options to choose from (see later). If the diver does not intend to take one of those options, then there is little practical point in having the test.
3. A positive test result after an episode of DCS does not guarantee that the PFO was the cause of the DCS.
4. As a corollary to point 3, repairing a PFO discovered after an episode of DCS does not guarantee that another event will not occur.
5. A negative test result does not mean that the diver is 'resistant' to DCS, as many seem to believe.

If screening for a PFO is undertaken and the result is positive, the response should take account of the size or shunting behaviour of the lesion. There are data suggesting that a grade 1 PFO (see Chapter 10) is of little or no consequence and can be ignored. In contrast, a spontaneously shunting (grade 3) PFO is likely to confer increased risk and merits a response.

To mitigate the risk implied by a large PFO, the diver effectively has three options: cease diving, modify diving practice in an attempt to reduce VGE production or have the PFO repaired. The option to cease diving is self-explanatory and unpalatable to many. Modification of diving practice to reduce VGE production is an imprecise business, but the general aim is to reduce the provocation for bubble formation on arrival at the surface. Options for achieving this include diving well within no decompression limits, ensuring that safety stops are completed, using nitrox (see Chapter 62) but planning the dive as though using air and, if decompression diving using gradient factors, lowering the GF-High to force longer shallow decompression stops at the end of the dive. Breathing oxygen during those stops would also help. In a related vein, advice could also include avoidance of any heavy exercise that could open a pulmonary shunt, or manoeuvres that could encourage right-to-left shunting across a PFO (e.g. lifting or straining), over the typical 2-hour period of maximum VGE formation after a dive.

Having a PFO repaired involves the use of a transvenous catheter technique that leaves an occluder device across the atrial septum. It is an effective treatment, although repair may be incomplete in up to 10 per cent of cases. It is also an invasive procedure, and like many medical procedures considered 'safe', it nevertheless has significant risks, some of which are life-threatening. These risks include formation of blood clots on the device, loosening of the occluder from its position, the appearance of new heart rhythm disturbances and new mild aortic regurgitation. Patients are routinely required to take a potent antiplatelet agent for 6 months after placement. Occasionally, open heart surgery is required for explantation of devices that are causing complications. Despite these concerns, most procedures have satisfactory results, and the PFO is closed without complications. It is not known how many divers have taken this option to mitigate the risk of PFO in diving, but anecdotally the numbers are growing. Other than the potential for harm during and after the procedure, one of the concerns about the repair option is that data demonstrating that repair reduces subsequent risk of DCS are incomplete. There is one comparative study that followed divers with large PFOs discovered after DCS who self-selected into groups undergoing repair or not[4]. The study and its results are summarized in Figure 12.8.

In this study, divers who continued diving without repair had a markedly higher rate of DCS than those who had a repair, but caution is required in interpreting these data because the numbers of DCS cases arising after the repair decision were so small, and the divers were not randomized. Notwithstanding this concern, the study does provide some reassurance that there is a positive return on the risk exposure associated with having a repair. Many diving enthusiasts may well be prepared to take this risk for the apparent benefit of eliminating their anatomical right-to-left shunt. This may be particularly true of those conducting deep technical dives who may see little practical potential for improving the conservatism of their dives.

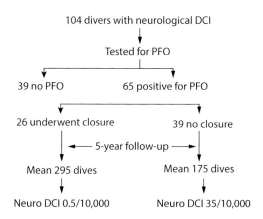

Figure 12.8 Key features and results of the study by Billinger and associates on the efficacy of repair of patent foramen ovale (PFO) in preventing serious neurological decompression sickness (DCS). The final results are based on very small numbers of cases (1 case of DCS in the closure group and 4 cases of DCS in the no closure group). DCI, decompression illness. (Data from Billinger M, Zbinden R, Mordasini R, et al. Patent foramen ovale closure in recreational divers: effect on decompression illness and ischaemic brain lesions during long-term follow-up. *Heart* 2011;**97**:1932–1937.)

Exercise

The relationship between DCS risk and exercise is a complex and evolving issue, and exercise needs to be considered in multiple contexts, specifically exercise before diving, exercise during diving and exercise after diving.

Until the early 2000s, little attention had been given to the issue of exercise before diving and its relationship with risk of DCS, other than general speculation that being physically fit was probably a good thing. Things changed with the publication of a remarkable series of experiments demonstrating that a single bout of heavy exercise approximately 20 hours before diving markedly reduced mortality in a rodent model of severe DCS. By 48 hours after exercise, the protective effect seemed to wear off. Translation of this finding into human research is incomplete, but there have been several studies demonstrating that heavy exercise between 2 and 20 hours before diving reduces VGE counts after diving. The mechanism for this protective effect is unclear. Early speculation that it was mediated by nitric oxide seemed disproved when protection persisted in the presence of a nitric oxide synthase inhibitor, although as a sidebar to this line of research it was discovered that exogenously administered nitric oxide also appeared to reduce post-dive VGE. It has been suggested that exercise produces some sort of endothelial conditioning effect that results in fewer suitable sites for micronuclei to grow when the surrounding tissue becomes supersaturated. Similarly, exercise may disturb stable micronuclei so that they subsequently involute, thus reducing the population transiently. Restoration of micronuclei numbers by whatever process is responsible for producing them would explain the decay in benefit over time following the exercise episode. There are no widely recommended practical strategies designed to take advantage of this phenomenon. Perhaps the best that can be said is that going for a run (or something similar) between 2 and 24 hours before diving may help reduce the risk of DCS.

The effect of exercise during diving may depend on its timing. The typical pattern is that activity during the bottom time sees the diver exercising moderately, and then ascent and decompression (if any) are largely done at rest. This is probably a disadvantageous pattern of exercise because it will result in increased perfusion and inert gas uptake (in some tissues at least) during the bottom phase of the dive and then decreased perfusion and inert gas elimination during the decompression. It is widely accepted that this explains the perception that dives involving hard work at the bottom are associated with greater risk of DCS. A reduction in risk may therefore be achieved by reducing work at depth and maintaining gentle levels of exercise during decompression. There is some evidence in support of these notions. Although a reduction in work at depth can be impractical in occupational diving, in recreational diving it is afforded by, for example, use of diver propulsion vehicles. Similarly, in a decompression diving situation, to maintain gentle exercise during decompression it is usually possible to fin gently against the resistance of the down line or decompression stage. In diving where hard work at the bottom cannot be avoided, the use of a longer safety stop (for a no decompression dive) or lengthening of the prescribed shallow stops in a decompression dive would be an appropriate precaution. There are no universally accepted guidelines for 'padding' decompression in this way.

Exercise after diving has generally been considered unwise, although the timing is unclear. Several concerns are noted, not the least of which is that there are many reports of symptoms of DCS arising during periods of work soon after diving. This, of course, may be coincidental, but there are plausible reasons to believe that exercise may have a causative role in such cases. First, exercise may promote the passage of VGE across pulmonary shunts into the arterial system, where they may be more harmful, as described in Chapter 10. Second (and similarly), exercise (particularly that involving lifting or straining) may promote right-to-left shunting of VGE across a PFO with the same result. Finally, it is speculated that where there are micronuclei in tissues supersaturated with inert gas, exercise may contribute to their excitation into growth, thus producing bubbles. This would be analogous to shaking an open bottle of carbonated drink, but the validity of this concern is unknown. At a practical level, mitigation of this risk involves refraining from exercise or lifting for a period after diving. This 'period' should definitely extend for at least several hours because this corresponds to the peak and duration of VGE formation after typical dives. Longer would be better, but how long is unknown.

Hydration

Hydration (or more correctly, dehydration) is one of the most widely recognized of the alleged risk factors for DCS among divers. For all the attention given to the matter, there is remarkably little proof that dehydration actually imputes increased risk.

There is one study in which pigs deprived of water and administered a diuretic during a saturation pressure exposure had more severe DCS than normally hydrated pigs after decompression. In addition, limited human data have shown that supplemental hydration just before diving reduces VGE numbers after diving, especially in subjects who appear prone to VGE formation. This finding is encouraging but falls short of proving that good hydration is protective in humans. Nevertheless, the proposition makes sense. There is evidence that divers are prone to dehydration through factors such as exposure to hot conditions, poor availability of water on boats, sea sickness and immersion diuresis. There is also evidence that realistic levels of 'dehydration' reduce regional tissue perfusion during exercise, and because perfusion is important for inert gas washout, it seems plausible that dehydration could impair this process. It is certainly true to say that no one has ever demonstrated dehydration to be beneficial.

It follows that maintenance of hydration can probably only be good. As a somewhat arbitrary guide, the supplementation of normal fluid intake with a litre of water over the hour before diving would make sense.

Temperature

It has long been observed that the risk of DCS seems higher when diving is conducted in cold conditions. The potentially dramatic effect of temperature on risk of DCS was demonstrated in a landmark study performed by the US NEDU[5]. It is a complicated study with multiple arms and profiles, but the most important observation was the comparison of outcomes when divers undertook a 120-foot for 30-minute dive with decompression as prescribed by a US Navy dive table under two different thermal conditions. In one set of dives (referred to as cold/warm), the divers were immersed in water at a temperature of 26°C for the bottom phase of the dive and 36°C for the decompression. In the second set of dives (referred to as warm/cold), the temperature conditions were reversed between the bottom and decompression phases. The divers wore no thermal protection. In the cold/warm series, there were no cases of DCS in 80 dives (0 per cent), whereas in the warm/cold series, there were 7 cases of DCS in 32 dives (22 per cent).

The water temperatures and the lack of exposure protection make the conditions difficult to interpret in real-world terms, but the dramatic change in DCS risk between the cold/warm and warm/cold conditions is highly relevant. It can be argued that the condition most analogous to real diving would be the markedly more hazardous warm/cold situation. Thus, divers tend to start a dive warm and become progressively colder during the dive. If there is a lesson to be learned from the NEDU temperature study it is that becoming cold during a dive should be avoided as much as possible.

Practical strategies to mitigate the risk of diving in cold water include optimizing exposure protection, which would include the use of drysuits with state of the art undergarments and possibly even active heating systems, which are now widely available. The ideal time to turn these heating systems on would be during decompression. Extreme divers in cold water caves have even established underwater habitats where the diver can remain under pressure, but not immersed, thus giving an opportunity to reduce conductive heat loss into the water and to take hot fluids orally. As previously, there is always the option of 'padding' or extending decompression for decompression dives conducted in cold water.

Some data suggest that remaining warm after diving (despite a cold environment) may reduce production of VGE and the incidence of DCS. It is therefore probably sensible to avoid becoming cold early after a dive, especially one that was provocative from a decompression point of view.

Almost paradoxically, however, there is a report of two cases of DCS arising in temporal relation to exposure to hot water in a shower early after diving. This single report has achieved considerable penetration into the diving community and is the cause of much anxiety about showers after diving. It is plausible that sudden warming of supersaturated superficial tissue could decrease gas solubility and precipitate symptomatic bubble formation. However, many divers take showers early in the post-diving period with no problems, and the risk of such events seems very low.

Obesity

It has long been believed that obesity is a risk factor for DCS, based largely on the 'first principle' belief that because nitrogen is highly soluble in fat, an obese person can absorb more nitrogen. Whether this is a practically relevant consideration is controversial. There is conflict in the literature with some studies (probably the majority of those that have addressed this issue) purporting to show an association between risk of DCS and obesity, whereas others have not. Whatever the truth of this matter, obesity is a condition that is often associated with reduced functional capacity and other health problems. Obese divers would benefit from losing weight for multiple reasons.

Age

There are some data suggesting that older divers are at higher risk of DCS and perhaps at higher risk of an incomplete recovery if they suffer serious event. However, once again, there is conflict in the literature on this subject. The fact that older divers are likely to have a lower functional capacity and a higher risk of cardiac events is probably of greater importance than concern about the risk of DCS.

Dive sequences

As alluded to earlier, multiple dives in a single day are common in recreational diving. Sequential dives conducted while dissolved inert gas in tissue remains after a previous dive are referred to as 'repetitive dives'. The definition of repetitive diving differs according to which table or decompression algorithm is used because there is variability in assumptions about total outgassing time. For example, the Professional Association of Diving Instructors, Inc. considers that complete outgassing occurs after 6 hours, whereas the Canadian Defence and Civil Institute of Environmental Medicine (DCIEM) table works on a much longer total outgassing time of 18 hours.

Irrespective of the definition, it is clear that if a second dive takes place in the presence of residual dissolved inert gas remaining after a previous one, then tissue gas loading during the second will compound on that remaining from the first. Perhaps for this reason it has frequently been taught that repetitive diving is a risk factor for DCS, although it is not clear why it should be, provided residual inert gas is adequately accounted for in calculation of no decompression limits or decompression protocols for subsequent dives. One argument that is sometimes advanced in this regard is that bubble formation after the first dive alters inert gas kinetics on the second dive, or those bubbles may undergo further growth after the second dive. There are no convincing data that clearly identify repetitive dives *per se* as being associated with increased risk. Indeed, the situation is made even less clear by the existence of an acclimatization phenomenon reported from occupational environments in which the incidence of DCS among a cohort of workers undertaking diving or compressed air work is reliably noted to fall over a multiday sequence of exposures. These exposures frequently differ (e.g. in being once daily) from the typical repetitive dives undertaken by recreational divers that may involve up to four or more short exposures per day. Nevertheless, the truth relating to risk in these situations is unclear. Part of the problem relates to the fact that so much of the diving undertaken by recreational divers is repetitive, so it is not surprising that many of the DCS cases arise in repetitive diving.

One particular form of repetitive diving that is associated with considerable controversy is so-called 'reverse profile' diving. This is the performance of a repetitive dive deeper than the previous dive (or than another dive in the repetitive sequence).

In this sense, the term 'reverse profile' is a misnomer because what is really being discussed is reverse depth diving. The origins of the edict that reverse profile diving is hazardous are unclear. Cursory manipulation of the repetitive function of common dive tables reveals that avoidance of reverse profiles results in more allowable bottom time over the sequence. That alone could be reason enough to avoid reverse profiles, but as in repetitive diving itself, it is not clear why reverse profile diving should be considered more hazardous provided residual inert gas from the previous shallower dive(s) is adequately accounted for in calculation of no decompression limits or decompression protocols for the subsequent deeper excursion.

REFERENCES

1. Tikuisis P, Gerth WA. Decompression theory. In: Brubakk AO, Neuman TS, eds. *Bennett and Elliott's Physiology and Medicine of Diving*. 5th ed. London: Harcourt Publishers; 2003:419–454.
2. Doolette DJ, Mitchell SJ. Hyperbaric conditions. *Comprehensive Physiology* 2011;**1**:163–201.
3. Doolette DJ, Gerth WA, Gault KA. *Redistribution of Decompression Stop Time From Shallow to Deep Stops Increases Incidence of Decompression Sickness in Air Decompression Dives*. Panama City, Florida: Navy Experimental Diving Unit; 2007: NEDU TR 11-06.
4. Billinger M, Zbinden R, Mordasini R, et al. Patent foramen ovale closure in recreational divers: effect on decompression illness and ischaemic brain lesions during long-term follow-up. *Heart* 2011;**97**:1932–1937.
5. Gerth WA, Ruterbusch VL, Long ET. *The Influence of Thermal Exposure on Diver Susceptibility to Decompression Sickness*. Panama City, Florida: Navy Experimental Diving Unit; 2007: NEDU TR 06-07.

This chapter was reviewed for this fifth edition by Simon Mitchell.

13

Decompression sickness: treatment

No-one who has seen the victim of compressed air illness, gravely ill or unconscious, put back into a chamber and brought back to life by the application of air pressure, will forget the extraordinary efficiency of recompression, or will be backward in applying it to a subsequent case of illness.

Robert Davis, 1935

INTRODUCTION

This chapter deals with the definitive management of decompression sickness (DCS). For information on the first aid management of the diving accident victim, see Chapter 48. DCS takes many forms, and although recompression is often the treatment of choice, the *optimal* treatment varies with circumstance. Consider the following cases:

- Saturation DCS as the diver very slowly approaches the surface.
- The same diver subjected to an extreme excursion from saturation.
- Inner ear DCS after helium breathing.
- A cerebrovascular incident after a short bounce to 50 metres.
- A joint bend developing hours after a long shallow dive.
- A dramatic crisis involving pulmonary, haematological and neurological systems after explosive decompression from saturation or from gross omitted decompression.
- Respiratory symptoms followed by the rapid development of paraplegia.
- Mild joint pain DCS after a shallow dive in a diver who has remained well within the established tables.

These cases cannot be managed optimally by a single regimen, yet the approach to their management is similar.

The guiding principle of treatment for DCS is recompression followed by a slow decompression back to atmospheric pressure, with the patient hopefully devoid of symptoms and signs. Oxygen breathing is used to increase the washout of inert gas and promote bubble resolution. Fluid replacement is recommended because divers are often dehydrated as a consequence of cold water diuresis, seasickness and bubble-induced fluid shifts out of the intravascular compartment. Many adjuvant therapies have been tried, most with little evidence of effect, including antiplatelet agents, corticosteroids, heparin and dextrans, whereas non-steroidal anti-inflammatory drugs (NSAIDs) and lidocaine have shown some promise.

If left untreated, the pain of joint DCS resolves spontaneously, usually within days or weeks. There have been reports of spontaneous resolution of cases of neurological DCS without recompression therapy; however, most patients require treatment or remain symptomatic. It is not known whether untreated DCS increases the likelihood of dysbaric osteonecrosis or subclinical neurological injury.

Care should be taken to avoid circumstances that will aggravate the 'bubbling' of DCS. These include excessive movement of the patient, exposure to altitude and the breathing of certain gases (e.g. nitrous oxide anesthesia).

RECOMPRESSION

The aim of recompression treatment is to produce the following[1]:

- An immediate reduction in bubble size, which will
  - Cause the surface tension acting on the bubble to increase and perhaps collapse the bubble.
  - Increase the surface area of the bubble relative to its volume, thus enhancing gas diffusion out of the bubble.
  - Reduce the length of any intravascular gas column and hence allow perfusion pressure to push bubbles out of the tissues into the venous circulation.
  - Reduce the compressive effect of bubbles on adjacent tissues.

- Reduce the bubble-tissue and bubble-blood interfaces and the secondary inflammatory reactions that follow.
- An increase in the diffusion gradient of gas out of the bubble (see Figure 10.3), which will
  - Relieve ischaemia and hypoxia.
  - Restore normal tissue function.

There are three factors to consider after deciding a diver needs recompression therapy:

1. The pressure (depth) required for therapy.
2. The gas mixture to be used.
3. The rate of decompression.

Depth of recompression

In deciding the depth of recompression, three different approaches are possible:

1. Recompress to a pressure (depth) dependent on the depth and duration of the original dive.
2. Recompress to a depth that produces clinical relief of symptoms and then tailor the gas mixtures for decompression from that depth.
3. Recompress to a predetermined fixed depth, i.e. according to standard tables of recompression therapy.

Only the third is in common practice these days, but each has some logic to it under certain circumstances.

RECOMPRESS TO A PRESSURE (DEPTH) DEPENDENT ON THE DEPTH AND DURATION OF THE ORIGINAL DIVE

This technique uses the principle that if a dive to 4 ATA produces DCS, then recompression to 4 ATA should relieve the symptoms. This approach was best typified by the now defunct concept of treating aviator DCS merely by descent to ground level.

This is not a particularly satisfactory technique because it is designed to cope with the total quantity of gas dissolved in the body during the original dive, irrespective of its distribution. Because DCS is the clinical manifestation of a gas bubble lodged in a vulnerable area, it is necessary to recompress to reduce the size of that particular bubble, irrespective of the total quantity of inert gas dissolved in the body. There is also evidence that once a bubble is formed, even compression to very high pressures may not completely eliminate that bubble, thus leaving bubble nuclei to re-expand on decompression.

The one advantage of this approach, apart from its simplicity, is evident when a diver develops DCS very soon after surfacing from a deep dive. Under these conditions, a prompt return to the original depth will ensure that there is no tissue-to-bubble pressure gradient that could cause bubble growth at a lesser depth.

RECOMPRESS TO A DEPTH OF RELIEF

This empirical approach was used first in underwater recompressions to reduce the depth exposure as far as possible. It is still applicable, both underwater and in chambers.

The freedom to be able to choose any depth to achieve an acceptable clinical result and then select an appropriate breathing gas is invaluable in serious cases (Figure 13.1).

As traditionally used for deep and saturation exposures, the patient is recompressed to the depth at which all major symptoms disappear, plus one additional atmosphere, based on the assumption that the additional pressure would result in a

reduction bubble size and allow increased surface tension to promote bubble resolution.

This approach is not without difficulty because it requires a sound knowledge of saturation decompression and the ability to mix and administer different gas mixtures. Nitrogen narcosis and central nervous system and pulmonary oxygen toxicity become important considerations. A recompression chamber (RCC) should have a mixed gas capability to support such operations.

RECOMPRESSION USING STANDARD RECOMPRESSION SCHEDULES

This approach uses standard recompression tables roughly divided into the following groups:

- Air tables.
- Oxygen tables.
- Oxygen tables with deep excursions.
- Helium-oxygen (heliox) tables.
- Saturation decompression.

Many such tables have been published by both commercial and military organizations around the world. Both air and heliox tables start at 30 and 50 metres, oxygen tables start at 9 to 18 metres,

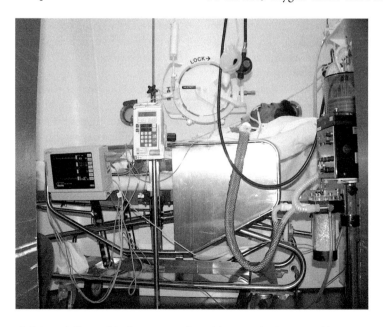

Figure 13.1 A severely injured diver with decompression sickness who is treated in a recompression chamber at 18 metres. Note the provision of both physiological monitoring and mechanical ventilation while under pressure. This is rarely required but available in many modern facilities. (Photograph by M. Bennett.)

deep excursions are commonly to 30 metres and saturation treatments depend on the depth of symptom relief.

These tables clearly state the gas mixture to be used (usually oxygen or heliox), the periods to be spent at each depth and the rate of decompression. Standard air, oxygen and gas mixture tables for recompression are presented in Appendix B and Appendix C.

Standard recompression tables

A prudent diving physician will advise non-experts to adhere to strict treatment guidelines, as depicted in the manuals, but retain his or her own flexibility to treat patients who did not respond or in facilities that may not be appropriate to apply the guidelines. For this reason, this text covers more than one set of treatment techniques. The standard tables are as follows.

AIR TABLES (US NAVY 1A, 2A, 3 AND 4 AND ROYAL NAVY 52, 53, 54, 55, 71, 72 AND 73)

These tables are used increasingly rarely. The US Navy (USN) first published their air recompression Tables 1 to 4 in 1945, and these were the standard treatment tables for more than 20 years. What is remarkable about these tables is that they were never tested on subjects with DCS. The test subjects made normal dives, which required decompression, but were then subjected to a treatment table instead. The treatment tables were deemed satisfactory if the subjects did not surface with DCS after one of the treatment tables!

During the 1960s, reported failure rates of up to 50 per cent on the air tables resulted in the development of the shallow oxygen tables.

Many experienced clinicians today are reluctant to use air tables because of the problems they bring and their variable benefits. The difficulties with air tables include logistical problems with prolonged decompression, aggravation of symptoms during ascent, nitrogen narcosis and DCS in the attendants and respiratory distress caused by the increased density of air under pressure (particularly if pulmonary involvement is already present). The results are often not adequate unless the symptoms are mild, recent and not the result of gross omitted decompression.

However, if oxygen is unavailable and the RCC can logistically support a treatment table lasting up to 40 hours, air tables may be considered.

OXYGEN TABLES (US NAVY 5 AND 6, ROYAL NAVY 61 AND 62 AND COMEX 12)

The introduction of standard oxygen tables using 100 per cent oxygen interspersed with short air breathing 'oxygen breaks' gives more flexibility and improved results (Figure 13.2). These tables are shorter, needing only 2 to 5 hours, require compression only to 18 metres (2.8 ATA) and are therefore logistically achievable. Divers Alert Network (DAN) reports that about 80 per cent of all DCS is treated with these tables. The physiological advantages are in the speed of bubble resolution and increased oxygenation of tissues.

Disadvantages include the less immediate reduction in bubble size (i.e. to less than half the volume reduction achieved with the 50-metre standard air tables), increased fire hazard, oxygen toxicity and the occasional intolerance of a distressed patient to a mask. Although the pressure gradient of nitrogen in the intravascular bubble-to-blood interface is increased with oxygen breathing, if the diver has previously dived in excess of 18 metres, there could well be a gas pressure gradient from tissue-to-extravascular bubble during the early phase of recompression.

With the foregoing qualifications, the use of oxygen tables has received worldwide acceptance as the starting point for all standard recompression therapy. Although some authors have reported significant failures with these tables, the success rate is higher than with the air tables that preceded them, and no better-performing alternative has been identified. Success rates for complete resolution of symptoms vary with both severity and the time to recompression, but they are often reported at 80 to 90 per cent.

Whenever oxygen is used, attention must be paid to oxygen toxicity. Unless one is following established safe protocols, it is suggested that the oxygen parameters should not exceed those likely to result in neurological or pulmonary toxicity (see Chapter 17). In cases of potential death or disability, exceeding these parameters may be acceptable.

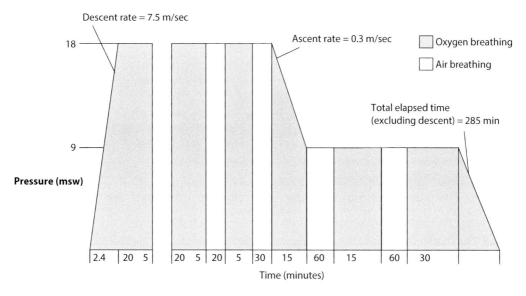

Figure 13.2 The US Navy Treatment Table 6 (or Royal Navy Table 62). Depths are expressed here as metres of sea water (msw). An initial period at 18 msw (60 feet) breathing 100 per cent oxygen with air breaks is followed by a slow ascent to 9 msw (30 feet).

OXYGEN TABLES WITH DEEP EXCURSIONS (US NAVY 6A) AND HELIOX TABLES (COMEX 30)

USN Table 6A involves the addition of an initial period of breathing air at 50 metres followed by a standard Table 6. This table was initially introduced as a treatment of cerebral arterial gas embolism (CAGE) in submarine escape trainees (with a low nitrogen load), although later studies have not shown any benefit from this deep excursion over the shallow 18-metre oxygen tables in divers.

Most centres now recommend starting with a standard USN Table 6 at 18 metres; however, in severe cases of DCS or cases not responding, the option exists to go on to a deeper table using a mixed gas such as a Comex 30 (Figure 13.3, Plate 3). Although based on little evidence, some centres advocate initial use of the Comex 30-metre table for severe neurological DCS. Heliox mixtures (50/50) are substituted for oxygen at depths greater than 18 metres. In refractory cases, there is then the opportunity to go to 50 metres using a modified USN Table 6A, Royal Navy (RN) Table 64 or Comex 50 breathing heliox mixtures.

A 2011 workshop reviewed the evidence for the use of 30-metre heliox recompression and made some recommendations concerning the appropriate use of these more challenging treatment schedules[2].

SATURATION TABLES (US NAVY 7)

Saturation treatments are used when divers have developed DCS during or just after decompression from saturation exposures. The customary treatment tables are inappropriate because of the extreme gas loads in 'slow' tissues and the often excessive oxygen exposures required. In general, increased pressure is applied, and the oxygen percentages are less. These tables may also be used after recompression to depth of relief in severe cases and when other tables have failed.

Gas mixture

Recompression results in a reduction of bubble size, but it may also be associated with a further uptake of gas into the bubble. Ideally, a breathing mixture would be selected that diffuses into the bubble at a slower rate than the inert gas diffuses out, resulting in bubble shrinkage. This is

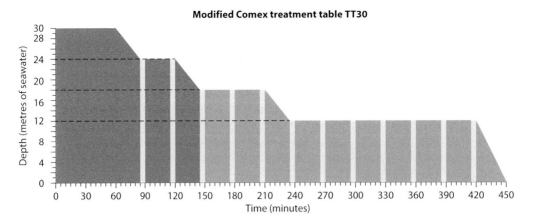

Modified Comex treatment table TT30

Figure 13.3 The Comex 30 treatment table. The maximum excursion is to 30 msw breathing 50 per cent oxygen in helium (heliox 50). This table is an adaptation by Dr Xavier Fructus of an older nitrox table developed by Dr Barthelemy at the French Navy diving facility (GERS) in the late 1950s. The final version of the Comex 30 heliox table appeared in the 1986 Comex medical book. Since then it has been modified by many users, so that multiple similar versions are in use around the world. The green areas on the graph represent the time spent by the patient breathing pure oxygen. The red areas on the Comex 30 table represent the patient breathing a 50/50 mix of oxygen and helium. Breaks in oxygen therapy are scheduled and are shown as the blue areas on the tables.

one reason that the oxygen tables are preferred to the air tables because no further inert gas can be absorbed.

There is anecdotal evidence that recompression using heliox has been beneficial in treating DCS after air dives. Hyldegaard and associates[3] demonstrated in a model of spinal DCS that, while breathing air, there is a steady increase in bubble size. When compression occurred while breathing oxygen, there was an initial increase and then decrease in bubble size, whereas with heliox there was a progressive shrinkage in bubble size.

The initial increase in bubble size with oxygen may be explained by the fact that at equal partial pressure differences the flux of oxygen in fat is twice that of nitrogen and four times that of helium[3]. This may explain the initial worsening of symptoms seen occasionally when patients with DCS are recompressed on oxygen.

There is little available evidence to suggest heliox tables are more effective than the oxygen tables, although many centres will move to a heliox table for the difficult or non-resolving acute case (Table 13.1). Heliox is also easier to breathe at depth than air – especially relevant to patients with respiratory 'chokes'.

In determining which therapeutic table should be selected, remember:

- The natural history of the disease:
  - The longer the surface interval before symptoms, the less likely they are to worsen over time.
  - Neurological symptoms have sequelae; many others do not.
- The value of pressure:
  - Recompression will prevent bubble growth and hasten resolution.
- The depth effect of recompression is less important the longer the symptoms have been present.

Delay to recompression

Once a manifestation of DCS has developed, the subsequent progress may be related more to the time elapsed before recompression than to the specific treatment table selected. With prompt treatment the destructive tissue distension effects of bubbles are lessened, as are the effects of ischaemia and the chemical and cytological reactions to the bubble.

Even using air tables, Rivera[4] demonstrated that if initial treatment was administered less than

Table 13.1 Comparison of the features of standard 18-metre oxygen tables and 30-metre heliox tables

Features	Oxygen tables (e.g. USN TT6, RN 62)	Heliox table (e.g. Comex 30)
Maximum depth (pressure)	18 msw (2.8 ATA)	30 msw (4.0 ATA)
Duration (not extended)	4 hr 45 min	7 hr 30 min (some versions vary)
Resources required	Relatively easily acquired, most recompression facilities can do these.	More complex, staff-intensive and requiring heliox supply. Many facilities not equipped for this.
Evidence base	Hundreds of thousands of applications with high success rates.	Some non-random comparisons with oxygen tables. Mixed results.
Common indications	All DCS.	Severe cases, particularly neurological, rapidly progressive forms of DCS. Cases not responsive to oxygen tables.
Gas switching	Air and oxygen only, with oxygen safe at maximum pressure.	Requires great care. Three breathing gases and oxygen not safe at maximum pressure.

DCS, decompression sickness; USN, US Navy.

30 minutes after symptoms developed, there was a 95 per cent probability of relief. This rate falls to 77 per cent if the delay exceeds 6 hours.

The delay among the dive, the development of symptoms and the presentation for treatment allows the clinician to assess the clinical importance and propose the most rational therapy.

To illustrate these principles, the approach to the patient who presents 30 minutes after a dive with an ascending paralysis is different from the patient who presents 48 hours after a dive with shoulder pain. The first patient's neurological injury is likely to progress with time, whereas the shoulder pain will not and may undergo spontaneous resolution.

The first patient should be treated aggressively, commencing with an 18-metre oxygen table or even a 30-metre heliox table. If using the former, consideration should be given to the options of going deeper and changing gas mixtures if early or full recovery is not evident.

Patients who delay seeking medical assistance may benefit from recompression even up to 14 days after injury; however, most diving physicians would not consider deep or saturation tables for patients with these late presentations. Consider two illustrative case histories (Case Report 13.1 and Case Report 13.2).

RECURRENCE OF SYMPTOMS

The fact that some authority has promulgated a therapeutic table does not make it effective, and there have been many modifications and deletions made to these tables during the professional lives of these authors.

As a good general rule, if symptoms recur *during* treatment, both the recompression schedule and the clinical management should be questioned. The physician should ensure that there has been adequate recompression and supportive therapy, including correct positioning, rehydration and so forth. The diagnosis should be reassessed, considering the following:

- Pulmonary barotrauma and each of its clinical manifestations (see Chapter 6).
- Complications of DCS, affecting target organs.
- Non-diving general medical diseases.

Nevertheless, patients with DCS do sometimes deteriorate during recompression therapy. The composition of the breathing mixture should be confirmed, as should the efficiency of the mask seal.

One air table (USN 4, RN 54) frequently caused DCS in attendants who did not even have

---

CASE REPORT 13.1

The patient made a dive to 18 metres for 60 minutes on scuba. There had been no dives for a month before this. The isolated symptom of left shoulder pain developed 5 hours after the dive and had been present for 24 hours before the diver presented for medical treatment.

Comment: This is not only a mild case of DCS, it is not going to get significantly worse as long as the patient avoids further exposure to hypobaric or hyperbaric conditions. By the time the medical assessment was made (29 hours after the dive), the tissues will have equilibrated fully with the atmospheric pressure, and thus there will be no significant pressure gradient pushing nitrogen into the bubble. On the contrary, there will be a mild gradient in the opposite direction. The administration of 100 per cent oxygen will enhance this gradient further.

The authors' approach to such a mild case would be to relieve the patient's symptoms and perhaps to reduce the possibility of subsequent bone damage (although there is no clear evidence that this latter is really possible) by recompression on an oxygen treatment table – probably at 18 metres. If recompression was not feasible, then surface oxygen would be appropriate.

CASE REPORT 13.2

This patient has symptoms identical to those of the patient in Case Report 13.1, but this time the left shoulder symptoms followed 10 minutes after a 30-metre dive for 30 minutes with a rapid ascent and omitted decompression. The diver has presented for assistance immediately after the symptom developed.

Comment: This is a very different situation from Case Report 13.1. Even assuming that the left shoulder pain is musculoskeletal and not referred neurological or cardiac, the likelihood of progression from the theoretical 'minor symptom' to a major case of DCS is much higher.

First, because the symptom developed soon after the dive, it is likely to become worse. Second, more symptoms are likely to develop (remembering that DCS manifestations may continue to arise over the next 24 hours). Third, the tissues surrounding the bubbles may well have nitrogen supersaturation pressures of almost 4 ATA. The bubble, existing on the surface, will have a nitrogen pressure of approximately 1 ATA, as the bubble is at the same ambient pressure as the body. Under these conditions, there will be a gradient between the tissues and the bubbles, increasing the size of the latter until the tissue gas tension becomes equated with the bubble gas tension.

The therapeutic approach to this diver is to recompress him to the maximum depth at which 100 per cent oxygen can be used therapeutically, i.e. USN Table 6 at 18 metres, and if a satisfactory response is obtained and maintained, to decompress him from that depth. Recompression treatment at 18 metres will not rapidly reverse the tissue-to-bubble nitrogen gradient and, if other more serious symptoms develop, it may be necessary to recompress him deeper on heliox (or an oxygen and nitrogen mixture). The authors of this text would select a 30-metre 50 per cent heliox treatment schedule (e.g. Comex 30). At this depth there would be no tissue-to-bubble nitrogen gradient.

---

a nitrogen load to start with. It is difficult to understand how it could then improve patients at the shallow stops. Oxygen is now used by both patient and attendant from 18 metres to prevent this problem. The short air embolism Table 5A, which many of us believed to be a contributor to deaths during treatment, has been removed from the *US Navy Manual*.

If similar and significant symptoms recur, they must be presumed to represent a re-expansion of a bubble, which was not completely removed, and treated accordingly.

Occasionally, there may be other explanations, such as:

- The inflammatory tissue reaction to the bubble.
- Lipid, platelet or fibrin deposits or emboli.
- Re-perfusion injury.
- Redistribution of gas emboli.

Although redistribution could be expected to respond to recompression therapy, it would be a great coincidence if it were to reproduce the same symptoms as the original lesion.

Recurrences of the original symptoms or the development of other serious symptoms should be seen as resulting from inadequate treatment or caused by aggravation of the problem by re-exposure to nitrogen at depth or on the surface. Recurrence of symptoms requires surface oxygen (if mild), hyperbaric oxygenation or a conventional therapy table.

Paraesthesia and other symptoms developing while undergoing recompression therapy may reflect the development of oxygen toxicity (see Chapter 17) and therefore are not necessarily an indication to extend the therapy.

It is not necessary to recompress repeatedly for minor and fluctuating symptoms, unless these symptoms have some ominous clinical significance. Minor residual musculoskeletal or peripheral nerve disease is very common, and chasing these symptoms to obtain a complete 'cure' becomes demoralizing and exhausting for both patient and attendants. It has become common practice to follow a formal recompression table with an 'oxygen soak' (typically a 9- to 14-metre oxygen table for 1 to 2 hours) on the following day, to reduce the incidence of minor persistent symptoms. It is probable that most of these symptoms are transient and more anxiety provoking than functionally important.

With spinal cord or cerebral damage, it is common practice to continue with intermittent hyperbaric oxygen therapy until all subjective and objective improvement has ceased. These authors use standard oxygen tables, as described earlier, on a daily schedule. Other regimens may be applied, but the use of repeated diving therapeutic tables,

such as extended Table 6 (USN) with its hyperbaric 'air breaks', is illogical and has increased complications to both attendant and patient. It is very unusual for even a patient with serious case to receive more than five or six treatment tables.

Both recompression and altitude exposure alter blood gases (oxygen, carbon dioxide and pH) and may affect these minor symptoms, presumably by affecting marginal ischaemia or nerve irritability from myelin sheath damage. Patients should be reassured that such minor symptoms – often persisting for weeks to months after DCS – are not uncommon and do not require intervention.

CEREBRAL ARTERIAL GAS EMBOLISM

Although recompression treatment of CAGE traditionally involved a deep excursion to 50 metres followed by a standard USN Table 6, diving physicians now use a standard 18-metre oxygen table such as USN Table 6.

If the CAGE is not caused by DCS and is a manifestation of pulmonary barotrauma, then the following other factors should be considered:

- The possibility of little or no inert gas loading in the tissues (thus making long saturation type treatments inappropriate and brief deep excursions more valuable).
- The presence of pulmonary tissue damage.
- The possibility of pneumothorax.
- Fitness for further diving and its investigations.

ADJUNCTIVE THERAPY

General medical treatment is required. This will vary according to the manifestations.

Position

Previously a head-down or Trendelenburg position was recommended for patients suspected of having CAGE to prevent re-embolization. The head-down position was originally used to divert emboli from the brain, given that the bubbles would preferentially rise to the higher vessels through the effect of buoyancy. This practice is no longer recommended because the increased venous pressure may cause increasing intracranial pressure and decreasing cerebral perfusion, thus aggravating the neurological disorder. In addition, increased venous return from the lower limbs may increase the possibility of paradoxical gas embolism through a patent foramen ovale. For the same reasons, the legs should not be raised. The patient should be supine or in the coma position and advised not to strain or perform Valsalva manoeuvres.

General care

The haematological effects of DCS may aggravate dehydration from immersion and cold-induced diuresis. This increases blood viscosity and reduces blood flow to the major organs. Rehydration is important, whether orally or intravenously, with a target of urinary output of 1 to 2 ml/kg per hour. Patients with serious cases should be intravenously hydrated with non–sugar-containing electrolyte fluids.

Hartman's solution, Ringer's lactate or physiological saline is preferable until the serum electrolytes and plasma osmolarity can be determined. Intravenous colloids are rarely used but may be of value, and low-molecular-weight dextran in saline has been used in the past to prevent rouleaux formation, expand the blood volume rapidly and reduce the likelihood of intravascular coagulation. Problems with using colloids include fluid overload, anaphylaxis, renal failure and bleeding – to date no advantage over crystalloids has been reported.

Glucose and other carbohydrate fluids must be avoided because cerebral injury may be exacerbated by hyperglycemia.

Urinary catheterization will be required for most patients with spinal DCS, as will careful skin and body maintenance.

During treatment, vital signs should be monitored, including an electrocardiogram (ECG), and this should not cause difficulties in most chambers.

Surface oxygen administration

One area that has been relatively overlooked recently is the administration of oxygen at normobaric pressure.

Albert R. Behnke
July 1990

The administration of 100 per cent oxygen will often relieve symptoms, if sometimes only temporarily, and it may reduce the likelihood that other symptoms will develop (a Divers Alert Network report suggests up to 50 per cent symptom resolution)[5]. This approach is particularly of value before subjecting the patient to altitude.

Oxygen has been demonstrated to:

- Enhance inert gas elimination.
- Prevent venous gas emboli, as detected by Doppler.
- Reduce the size of inert gas bubbles.
- Prevent development of DCS.
- Treat developed DCS.
- Prevent recurrences of DCS.
- Possibly improve oxygenation of damaged tissues.

In one series[6], surface oxygen was shown to be an effective treatment for DCS. Although this was a highly selected population, the series did demonstrate the value of surface oxygen, given early and for some hours, in remote areas where recompression facilities are not readily available. When it is used in transit, the DAN report of 1996 suggested that oxygen will result in some DCS cures and a reduction of DCS sequelae after recompression[5].

Although the value of administering 100 per cent oxygen with intermittent air breaks is unquestioned, problems do arise with inexperienced personnel. Commonly, an inadequate mask is used. Most available masks do not readily produce 40 per cent oxygen in the inspiratory gas even at very high flows. Other risks involve the inflammable nature of oxygen and the contribution to oxygen toxicity.

Some diving physicians prefer to use 100 per cent oxygen after recompression therapy to prevent the recurrence of DCS symptoms and avoid repeated treatments; however this practice is now unusual, and current practice tends toward repeated treatments for residual symptoms.

Drug therapy

Many classes of drugs have been tried to improve both symptoms and outcome from DCS. Few have stood the test of time. Drug use has often been based on the results of animal experimentation using extreme exposures and/or very rapid decompressions, and therefore of limited applicability. Some agents may be of value if they are administered before the actual decompression accident. There is some logic in the use of pharmacological agents to reduce, for example, platelet aggregation, microthrombi and neurological oedema. Other drugs proposed include those that increase tissue perfusion and/or expedite inert gas elimination. The clinical value of most drugs is less than remarkable.

LIDOCAINE

Lidocaine (formerly lignocaine in the United Kingdom) is recommended with caution, in the same dosage as used for cardiac dysrrhythmias, for severe cerebral and spinal DCS. There have been a couple of hopeful case reports and some experimental evidence to support this recommendation. A beneficial effect of lidocaine has been demonstrated in animal models of air embolism[7,8], and this benefit seemed confirmed when the drug was associated with a cerebral protective effect when it was used prophylactically in patients undergoing left-sided heart valve surgery[9]. Later studies did not confirm these findings, however, and many practitioners have abandoned this approach after unsuccessful use in their own practice.

ANTI-INFLAMMATORY AGENTS

NSAIDS have been advocated because of both their inhibitory effect on platelet aggregation and their wider anti-inflammatory and analgesic actions. On the one hand, the effect on platelet activation may modify the activation of the coagulation pathway by bubbles if given early enough after diving, and on the other, NSAIDS will temporarily relieve many of the symptoms of DCS and may hasten the resolution of those symptoms following recompression. The one double-blind randomized controlled study of these agents suggested that the results of recompression were similar with or without the NSAID tenoxicam, but on average one less recompression session was required[10]. Currently, many diving physicians recommend the adjunctive use of an NSAID for 5 to 7 days, beginning during or after the first recompression table.

ANTIPLATELET DRUGS

There is evidence that antiplatelet agents such as aspirin or dipyridamole, when given prophylactically, modify platelet action following decompression. However, there are no controlled studies to support the use of these drugs in the treatment of DCS. There are more arguments against the use of aspirin than for it, with the increased likelihood of aggravating inner ear or spinal cord haemorrhagic disease. Aspirin has a variety of other negative influences on susceptible individuals, such as bronchospasm, and there are reports in animal studies linking aspirin with an increased risk of dysbaric osteonecrosis.

AMINOPHYLLINE

Aminophylline, and probably other sympathomimetic drugs, may be contraindicated in dysbaric diving accidents. It results in the dilatation of the pulmonary vasculature and a profuse release of bubbles trapped in the pulmonary circulation into the systemic circulation.

ANTICOAGULANTS

Heparin and coumarin derivatives have been advocated because of their effect on the coagulation pathway. They were said to be indicated in cases of disseminated intravascular coagulation that had no evidence of systemic infarction and bleeding. These drugs are now rarely, if ever, used in DCS. Correction of specific coagulation defects seems a more logical approach to the rare complication of disseminated intravascular coagulation in DCS. It can be harmful following the haemorrhagic disorders of the spinal cord and inner ear and other DCS manifestations.

CORTICOSTEROIDS

The use of corticosteroids has previously been justified on the belief that this class of drugs may reduce cerebral oedema and modify the inflammatory process. This experience came not from treating DCS but from treating cerebral oedema associated with traumatic and vascular brain injury. Just as the use of corticosteroids has been discredited in brain injury, there are no definitive studies to support its use in DCS-related brain injury.

Although high-dose methylprednisolone initiated within 8 hours of traumatic spinal injury resulted in a significantly greater neurological recovery in a large randomized trial (the second National Acute Spinal Cord Injury Study [NASCIS 2][11]), there was no clinically significant improvement in function, and this practice has been abandoned because of serious side effects in some cases. In DCS there are no published trials supporting methylprednisolone use, and corticosteroids are no longer recommended. Some of the disadvantages of include severe sepsis, hemorrhage, hyperglycemia, anaphylaxis and an increased susceptibility to oxygen toxicity.

BENZODIAZEPINES

Diazepam (Valium) has been recommended for use in DCS. It may be of considerable value in reducing the incidence and degree of oxygen toxicity, especially in patients with serious cases who require extensive exposure to oxygen under pressure. It may also be useful in the occasional patient with a toxic-confusional state as a result of involvement of the neurological system from either DCS or CAGE. These patients can be very difficult to handle in the RCC, and they may not tolerate the oronasal mask without an anxiolytic. The dosage must be regulated according to the clinical state of the patient, but otherwise a 10-mg initial dose may be supplemented by 5 mg every few hours, without causing any significant drowsiness, respiratory depression or interference with the clinical picture.

Vestibular DCS may require suppressants, such as diazepam, to help control vertigo.

PERFLUOROCARBONS

These fascinating compounds have been developed in the efforts to produce an artificial blood substitute and to enable liquid respiration in patients with very poor lung function when they are acutely unwell in an intensive care setting. These compounds have the ability to absorb enormous volumes of oxygen and nitrogen and present several exciting possibilities for use in diving medicine. At this time, these agents are experimental only, and the authors of this text are not aware of any reported use in diving humans. This is likely to change, however, because several groups are interested in further investigation.

Potential uses include the treatment of DCS, in which the intravenous administration of a modest volume of perfluorocarbon may rapidly denitrogenate the tissues and eliminate any intravascular bubbles. Also of interest are the potential to increase the blood oxygen-carrying capacity with the administration of modest amounts of increased oxygen administration, the prevention of DCS by administration before diving and the extension of deep diving limits by the utilization of liquid breathing techniques (see the famous sequence in the movie *The Abyss*).

UNDERWATER TREATMENT

In-water air treatments

By far the most traditional of the non-chamber treatments of DCS is underwater recompression therapy. In this situation the water, instead of an RCC, exerts the pressure. Air supply is usually from compressors sited on the diving boat. Although this treatment is frequently disparaged, it has often been the only therapy available to severely injured divers, and it has had many successes, most of which have never been reported. This was certainly so in those remote localities such as Northern Australia, in the pearl fishing areas, where long periods were spent under water and standard diving equipment was used.

The failure of DCS to respond to recompression therapy is often related directly to the delay in treatment. Sometimes chambers are not readily available. For this reason, underwater air recompression was effectively used in Hawaii, with good results, within minutes of symptoms developing. This was also the experience of professional shell divers of Australia, at least until underwater oxygen therapy became available.

Despite the value of underwater air recompression therapy, many problems may be encountered, and this treatment should not be entered into without appropriate planning and resources.

Most amateurs or semi-professionals do not carry the compressed air supplies or compressor facilities necessary for the extra decompression. Most have only scuba cylinders or simple portable compressors that will not reliably supply divers (the patient and the attendant) for the depths and durations required. Environmental conditions are not usually conducive to underwater treatment. Often the depths required can be achieved only by returning to the open ocean. The advent of night, inclement weather, rising seas, tiredness and exhaustion and boat safety requirements make the return to the open ocean a very serious decision. Because of the considerable depth required, hypothermia becomes likely. Seasickness in the injured diver, the diving attendants and the boat tenders is a significant problem. Nitrogen narcosis produces added difficulties in the diver and the attendant.

The treatment often has to be aborted because of these difficult circumstances, thereby producing DCS in the attendants and aggravating it in the diver. Although in the absence of an RCC it may be the only treatment available to prevent death or severe disability, it should never be undertaken without careful consideration of the resources available and the environmental conditions.

Underwater oxygen therapy

The advantages of oxygen over air tables include increasing nitrogen elimination gradients, avoiding extra nitrogen loads, increasing oxygenation to tissues, decreasing the depths required for the reduced exposure time and improving overall therapeutic efficiency. The same caveats about organization, resources and sea conditions are applicable when comparing underwater air and underwater oxygen treatment (Table 13.2).

Beginning in 1970, this option has been applied to the underwater treatment of DCS. The procedures were developed in response to an urgent need for management of cases in remote localities – remote in both time and distance from hyperbaric facilities. As a result of the success of this treatment, and its ready availability, it is now practised even when experts are not available to supervise it.

The physiological principles on which this treatment is based are well known and not contentious,

Table 13.2 Minimum requirements for the safe conduct of in-water oxygen tables

Equipment
1. At least one G-sized (7000 litres) oxygen cylinder – medical grade.
2. Regulator and hoses (minimum 12 metres – marked in 1-metre intervals) rated as 'oxygen-safe' and maintained appropriately.
3. Full-face mask.
4. Suitable method for weighting diver and attendant to avoid unwanted changes in depth.
5. Hookah air supply for attendant diver.
6. Suitable diving platform (boat or wharf) above column of water to >9-metre depth.
7. Appropriate thermal protection for prolonged immersion.
8. A suitable communication system with divers.

Human resources
1. Appropriately trained individuals to oversee the procedures.
2. Attendant diver (breathing air).
3. Suitably trained attendant(s) to ensure appropriate decompression rate and gas supply.
4. Ability of the patient diver to be safely immersed for the duration of the table (e.g. not having seizures or unconscious).

Environmental factors
1. Protected site with calm water.
2. Freedom from unacceptable tidal fluctuation and current.
3. Water temperature compatible with thermal protection available.

although the indications for treatment have caused some confusion. As for conventional oxygen therapy tables, underwater oxygen was first applied mainly for minor cases of DCS, but it was subsequently found to be of considerable value in serious cases.

The techniques and equipment for underwater oxygen therapy are designed to make for safety, ease and ready availability, even in medically unsophisticated countries. Although accurate estimates are problematic, it is likely this approach is now in widespread use in the Pacific Islands and remote parts of Australia.

Hawaiians have included a deep air 'dip' before underwater oxygen treatment, in an attempt to force bubbles back into solution or to allow bubbles trapped in arteries to transfer to the venous system.

TECHNIQUE

Oxygen is supplied at maximum depth of 9 metres from a surface supply. Ascent is commenced after 30 minutes in mild cases, or 60 minutes in severe cases, if significant improvement has occurred. These times may be extended for another 30 minutes if there has been no improvement. The ascent is at the rate of 12 minutes/metre. After surfacing, the patient should be given periods of oxygen breathing, interspersed with air breathing, usually on a 1 hour on, 1 hour off basis, with respiratory volume measurements and chest x-ray examination if possible.

No equipment should be used with oxygen unless it is assessed 'oxygen safe' or if it is contaminated, dirty or lubricated with oil.

An air breathing diver attendant should always be present, and the ascent should be controlled by the surface tenders. The duration of the three tables is 2 hours 6 minutes, 2 hours 36 minutes and 3 hours 6 minutes. The treatment can be repeated twice daily, if needed.

The underwater oxygen treatment table is not meant to replace formal recompression therapy in chambers. It is an emergency procedure, able to be applied with equipment usually found in remote localities, and is designed to reduce the many hazards associated with conventional underwater air treatments. The customary supportive and pharmacological adjuncts to the treatment of recompression sickness should still be used, if available, and the superiority of experienced personnel and comprehensive hyperbaric facilities is not being challenged. Underwater oxygen treatment is considered as a first aid regimen, not superior to portable RCCs, but sometimes surprisingly effective and rarely, if ever, detrimental.

The relative value of proposed first aid regimens (underwater oxygen, underwater heliox, an additional deep descent and surface oxygen treatment) needs to be clarified.

USE OF UNDERWATER OXYGEN TREATMENT

Because this treatment is applied in remote localities, many cases are not well documented. Twenty-five cases were well supervised before this technique increased suddenly in popularity. Two such cases are described (Case Report 13.3 and Case Report 13.4).

There have now been many hundreds of cases of underwater air and underwater oxygen treatments recorded[12]. Apart from the relative paucity of complications, the major lesson learned was that prompt re-immersion of the diver allowed shorter duration of treatment and complete resolution of DCS manifestations. Many divers so treated resumed diving within days.

MEDICAL ATTENDANTS

General medical treatment is required during the recompression sessions. Patients should not be left unattended in RCCs, particularly while they are breathing increased oxygen concentrations.

First aid and resuscitation techniques are often required, as are accurate clinical assessments – and for these reasons it is desirable to have a trained medical attendant in the chamber. Most hospital-based hyperbaric facilities require their hyperbaric workers to have undergone a formal training program. It is necessary to consider the possibility that DCS may occur in the attendants, and hyperbaric attendants have an entire Australian Standard devoted to ensuring that facilities are aware of appropriate safety and training for these workers[13]. It is embarrassing to produce DCS in attendants during recompression therapy.

CASE REPORT 13.3

A 68-year-old male salvage diver performed two dives to 30 metres for 20 minutes each, with a surface interval of 1.5 hours, while searching for the wreck of *HMS Pandora* about 100 miles from Thursday Island in the Torres Strait.

No decompression staging was possible, allegedly because of the increasing attentions of a tiger shark. A few minutes after surfacing, the diver developed paraesthesiae, back pain, progressively increasing incoordination and paresis of the lower limbs.

Two attempts at underwater air recompression were unsuccessful when the diving boat returned to its base moorings. The National Marine Operations Centre was contacted for assistance.

It was about 36 hours after the dive before the patient was flown to the regional hospital on Thursday Island.

Both the Air Force and the Navy had been involved in the organization, but because of very hazardous air and sea conditions, and very primitive airstrip facilities, another 12 hours would be required before the patient could have reached an established recompression centre (distance, 3000 km [2000 miles]).

On examination at Thursday Island, the patient was unable to walk, with evidence of both cerebral and spinal involvement. He had marked ataxia, slow and slurred speech, intention tremor, severe back pain, generalized weakness, difficulty in micturition, severe weakness of lower limbs with impaired sensation, increased tendon reflexes and equivocal plantar responses.

An underwater oxygen unit was available on Thursday Island for use by the pearl divers, and the patient was immersed to 8 metres of depth (the maximum depth off the wharf). Two hours were allowed at that lesser depth, and the patient was then decompressed. There was total remission of all symptoms and signs, except for small areas of hypoaesthesia on both legs.

CASE REPORT 13.4

A 23-year-old female sports diver was diving with a 2000-litre (72 cubic feet) scuba cylinder in the Solomon Islands (nearest recompression chamber was 3500 km away and prompt air transport was not available); the dive depth was 34 metres and the duration approximately 20 minutes, with 8 minutes of decompression. Within 15 minutes of surfacing, she developed respiratory distress, then numbness and paraesthesiae, very severe headaches, involuntary extensor spasms, clouding of consciousness, muscular pains and weakness, pains in both knees and abdominal cramps. The involuntary extensor spasms recurred every 10 minutes or so.

The patient was transferred to the hospital, where neurological DCS was diagnosed, and she was given oxygen via a facemask for 3 hours without significant change. During that time an underwater oxygen unit was prepared, and the patient was accompanied to a depth of 9 metres (30 feet) off the wharf. Within 15 minutes she was much improved, and after 1 hour she was asymptomatic. Decompression at 12 minutes/meter was uneventful, and a commercial aircraft subsequently flew the patient to Australia.

RETURN TO DIVING AND FLYING

When considering a return to diving after an episode of DCS, it is important to consider the following:

- Has there been a good response to treatment?
- Are there any residual symptoms and signs attributable to DCS?
- Was the development of DCS consistent with the diving exposure?

- Does the individual have an increased susceptibility to DCS?
- Was there any evidence of associated pulmonary barotrauma?

Evidence supports the existence of bubbles for
some days or weeks after DCS and recompression
therapy – a function of the slower rate of gas elimination, especially in the presence of bubbles. For
this reason, the authors of this text recommend
a minimum period of 4 weeks before a return to
diving. Bubble micronuclei may exist indefinitely
within the tissues only to re-expand with an exposure to an inert gas load.

Patients with incomplete recovery after recompression should be followed up clinically with
appropriate investigations, e.g. brain imaging
techniques, electroencephalography (EEG), bone
scans and neuropsychological testing as indicated
by the clinical condition.

If there has been a less than complete recovery
following neurological DCS, the recommendation of the authors of this text is that the individual not dive again. Autopsy evidence suggests
that DCS may involve greater areas of the brain
and spinal cord than are detected clinically – a
characteristic of some degree of neurological
redundancy. A further insult may result in this
subclinical damage extending to become clinically evident. Therefore, the second episode of
neurological DCS may result in a significantly
worse outcome.

If the episode of DCS occurs after a relatively
trivial exposure, a cause for this increased susceptibility should be actively sought (e.g. pulmonary
barotrauma, patent foramen ovale). Evidence of
pulmonary barotrauma (see Chapter 6) usually
renders the individual permanently unfit to dive.

Many episodes of DCS result from a complete
disregard for decompression schedules or from
simply stretching accepted computer algorithms to
their limits. Rapid and frequent ascents and multiday repetitive diving are commonly reported.
Before a return to diving, the patient with DCS
should be counseled on safe diving practices.
Diving according to published dive tables (e.g. the
PADI tables) is now exceedingly rare, and almost all
diving is controlled by a personal diving computer.

Although greeted with some initial skepticism by
dive physicians, these computers do not seem to
have been associated with a higher incidence of
DCS – if anything, quite the reverse, with DCS
numbers falling across most jurisdictions.

Safe diving practices

- Use a decompression schedule that has been
tested and has a known and acceptable risk of
DCS (e.g. Canadian Defence and Civil Institute
of Environmental Medicine [DCIEM] tables;
see Appendix A) or a reputable personal diving
computer.
- Add a depth/time penalty for future diving;
i.e. for a dive to 16 metres for 35 minutes use
the decompression limits for a 40-minute,
18-metre dive. With a computer, stay well
within the no decompression limit rather than
dive to that limit.
- Restrict diving to two dives a day, with a long
surface interval.
- Have a rest day after each 3 days of diving.
- Perform slow ascent rates.
- Incorporate a 'safety stop' of 3 to 5 minutes at
3 to 5 metres on every dive.
- Ensure conservative flying after any diving
exposure.
- Consider substituting nitrox (oxygen
enriched air) for air, but dive according to
the air tables.

There is a lack of good scientific data on when it is
safe to fly or ascend to altitude following an episode
of DCS. Recommendations vary from 24 hours to
42 days. The bubble micronuclei discussed earlier
may expand with altitude exposure, with a resultant
return of symptoms. Because many diving destinations are in remote tropical areas, divers with DCS
are usually very reluctant and financially inconve-
nienced if they cannot return home for 4 to 6 weeks,
so this is a very real practical problem.

It is the policy of the authors of this text to recommend to these divers that they delay flying or
ascending to altitude for 2 weeks if possible, with a
preferred minimum of 1 week. These times should
be extended for divers with continuing symptoms
after recompression.

In rare situations one may attempt to remove asymptomatic bubbles and micronuclei by exposing the symptom-free diver to a few 2-hour sessions of breathing 100 per cent oxygen, before flying, and a further possibility is to charter an aircraft whose cabin pressures are kept at 1 ATA (not within many people's capability!).

REFERENCES

1. Moon RE, Gorman DF. Treatment of the decompression disorders. In: Brubakk AO, Neuman TS, eds. *Bennett and Elliott's Physiology and Medicine of Diving.* 5th ed. Edinburgh: Saunders; 2003:600–650.

2. Bennett MH, Mitchell SJ, Young D, King D. (2012) The use of deep tables in the treatment of decompression illness: the Hyperbaric Technicians and Nurses Association 2011 workshop. *Diving and Hyperbaric Medicine* 2012;**32**(3):171–180.

3. Hyldegaard O, Moller M, Madsen J. Effect of He-O$_2$, O$_2$, and N$_2$O-O$_2$ breathing on injected bubbles in spinal white matter. *Undersea Biomedical Research* 1991;**18**(5–6):361–371.

4. Rivera JC. *Decompression Sickness Among Divers: An Analysis of 935 Cases.* United States Navy Experimental Diving Unit research report 1-63. Panama City, Florida, Navy Experimental Diving Unit; 1963.

5. *DAN Report on Diving Accidents and Fatalities: 1996 Edition Based on 1994 Data.* Durham, North Carolina: Divers Alert Network; 1996.

6. How J, West D, Edmonds C. Decompression sickness in diving. *Singapore Medical Journal* 1976;**17**(2):92–97.

7. Evans DE, Catron PW, Mcdermott JJ, Thomas LB, Kobrine AI, Flynn ET. Effect of lidocaine after experimental cerebral ischaemia induced by air embolism. *Journal of Neurosurgery* 1989;**70**:97–102.

8. Dutka AJ, Mink R, Mcdermott J, Clark JB, Hallenbeck JM. Effect of lidocaine on somatosensory evoked response and cerebral blood flow after canine cerebral air embolism. *Stroke* 1992;**23**(10):1515–1521.

9. Mitchell SJ, Pellett O, Gorman DF. Cerebral protection by lidocaine during cardiac operations. *Annals of Thoracic Surgery* 1999;**67**:1117–1124.

10. Bennett MH, Mitchell S, Dominguez A. The adjunctive treatment of decompression illness with a non-steroidal anti-inflammatory drug (tenoxicam) reduces compression requirement. *Undersea and Hyperbaric Medicine* 2003;**30**(3):195–206.

11. Bracken MB, Shepherd MJ, Collins WF, *et al.* A randomized, controlled trial of methylprednisolone or naloxone in the treatment of acute spinal cord injury: results of the second National Acute Spinal Cord Injury Study. *New England Journal of Medicine* 1990;**322**:1405–1411.

12. Kay E, Spencer MP, eds. *In-Water Recompression.* UHMS workshop no. 48. Kensington, Maryland: Undersea Hyperbaric Medical Society; 1999.

13. Australian Standard (AS) 2299.2. Part 2. Hyperbaric oxygen facilities.

FURTHER READING

Bennett PB, Moon R, eds. *Diving Accident Management.* UHMS workshop no. 41. Durham, North Carolina: Undersea Hyperbaric Medical Society; 1990.

Bove AA. The basis for drug therapy in decompression sickness. *Undersea Biomedical Research* 1982;**9**(2):91–111.

Catron PW, Flynn ET Jr. Adjuvant drug therapy for decompression sickness: a review. *Undersea Biomedical Research* 1982;**9**(2):161–174.

Davis J, ed. *Treatment of Serious Decompression Sickness and Arterial Gas Embolism.* UHMS workshop no. 20. Durham, North Carolina: Duke University; 1979.

Moon RE. Adjuvant therapy for decompression illness. *South Pacific Underwater Medicine Society Journal* 1998;**28**(3):144–149.

Moon RE, Gorman DF. Treatment of the decompression disorders. In: Bennett PB, Elliott DH, eds. *The Physiology and Medicine of Diving*. London: Balliere Tindall; 1993.

Moon RE, Sheffield P, eds. *Treatment of Decompression Illness*. UHMS workshop no 45. Kensington, Maryland: Undersea Hyperbaric Medical Society; 1996.

Slark AG. *Treatment of 137 Cases of Decompression Sickness*. RNPL report 8/62. London: Medical Research Council; 1962.

US Navy Diving Manual, Volume 1: Air Diving. Flagstaff, Arizona: Best Publishing Company; 1996.

This chapter was reviewed for this fifth edition by Michael Bennett.

14

Dysbaric osteonecrosis

INTRODUCTION

Aseptic necrosis of bone has been described in diving lizards (mosasaurs) of the cretaceous period, although the association with human diving may not be entirely germane. In humans, infarction of areas of bone associated with exposure to pressure has been recognized since the turn of the twentieth century. The condition has been reviewed most recently in 2014[1]. Twynam first suggested a causal relationship between bone necrosis and pressure exposure in 1888 in a case report of a caisson worker constructing the Iron Cove Bridge in Sydney, although in retrospect the man appeared to have 'septic' necrosis.

In 1912, there were 500 cases of decompression sickness (DCS) reported among the caisson workers on the Elbe tunnel at Hamburg, and 9 had bone changes. Bassoe, in 1913, suggested a relationship between initial joint 'bends' and subsequent x-ray evidence of bone atrophy and sclerosis. Taylor, in 1943, noted that several months elapsed between the hyperbaric exposure and the joint symptoms and that shaft lesions are usually asymptomatic. Osteonecrosis has been observed following caisson work at a pressure of 117 kPa (less than 12 metres of sea water equivalent), and also for as short a time as 7 hours, divided into two shifts, at 242 kPa. This disease has gone by many names, but when there is a clear relationship between pressure exposure and the subsequent development of aseptic necrosis, we now use the term 'dysbaric osteonecrosis' (DON) (Table 14.1).

DON has been known to develop within 3 months of the presumed causative diving exposure and has occasionally resulted from 'once only' exposures. Three of five men who escaped from the submarine *Poseidon,* in 1931 in the China sea after being at a depth of 38 metres for 2 to 3 hours, subsequently developed osteonecrosis.

Table 14.1 Some synonyms for dysbaric osteonecrosis

Caisson arthrosis.

Caisson disease of bone.

Hyperbaric osteonecrosis.

Barotraumatic osteoarthropathy.

Avascular necrosis of bone[a].

Ischaemic necrosis of bone[a].

Aseptic necrosis of bone[a].

Diver's bone rot.

Diver's crumbling bone disease.

[a] To be distinguished from other causes of bone necrosis.

The first report of DON in a diver appears to have been by Grutsmacher in the German literature in 1941. The disease affected the shoulder joint. Osteonecrosis affecting hips and shoulders has frequently been reported in commercial diving fishers. It is rare in recreational sport scuba divers.

INCIDENCE

Detailed studies of the incidence of DON were not undertaken until the 1960s. Because the incidence of DON has fallen dramatically since that time, presumably following the advent of strict workplace health and safety rules based on sound decompression practices, most of the clinical and epidemiological work that informs the following discussion dates from the 1970s and 1980s. Figures should be considered cautiously because the radiologists or physicians in each survey may have used different radiological techniques and diagnostic criteria. Other factors influencing the results include the difficulty in obtaining adequate follow-up and the different decompression regimens used.

For example, at the Clyde Tunnel in Glasgow only 241 compressed air workers were surveyed of a total of 1362; 19 per cent of the workers surveyed had lesions, half of which were juxta-articular (next to a joint surface). By 1972, the UK Medical Research Council Decompression Sickness Council Panel had x-ray studies of 1674 workers, of whom 19.7 per cent had positive lesions. Also in 1972, a study by Jones and Behnke on the Bay Area Rapid Transit tunnelling project in San Francisco revealed no clinical or x-ray

evidence of necrosis. All prospective workers had pre-employment x-ray studies, and those workers with lesions were excluded. The pressure ranged from 9 to 36 lb/square inch (62 to 248 kPa) gauge, with only one decompression per day. However, the follow-up period was relatively short.

The reported incidence in divers is exceedingly variable, ranging from 2.5 per cent in the US Navy to a doubtful 80 per cent in Chinese commercial divers. Some representative surveys are listed in Table 14.2. The lower incidences are reported in military series and commercial diving operations where strict decompression schedules are adhered to, whereas the incidence is much higher in the self-employed diving fishers of Japan, Hawaii and Australia. The Australian diving fishers undertake relatively deep dives with long bottom times and often inadequate decompression. There is also a higher incidence among divers more than 30 years old, which may reflect increased exposure rather than age itself.

The Medical Research Council Decompression Sickness Central Registry has x-ray studies for nearly 7000 professional divers, and in 1989, Davidson reported there were only 12 cases of subchondral bone collapse, i.e. about 0.2 per cent[2]. Asymptomatic shaft lesions appeared in about 4 per cent. In 1989, Lowry reported that the prevalence of crippling osteoarthritis leading to total joint replacement had been conservatively estimated at more than 2 per cent in Australian abalone divers[1]. Most cases in most series involve shaft lesions, which have no long-term significance to health and well-being, except for the rare possibility of malignant change.

Earlier UK studies on professional divers indicated that lesions occurred significantly more commonly among the older men who had longer diving experience and also who had exposures to greater depths. Only 0.4 per cent of the compressed air divers who had never exceeded 50 metres had these lesions. The helium-breathing divers who did not exceed 150 metres had an incidence of 2.7 per cent, which rose to 7.6 per cent if they had been deeper. There was a definite increase in incidence among saturation divers and those with a history of DCS. Approximately one fourth of the lesions were potentially serious, closely associated with joints.

Another UK study of caisson workers, with 2200 subjects, showed an incidence of DON of

Table 14.2 Reported incidence of dysbaric osteonecrosis in divers

Investigators (year)	Type of diver	Total number	Percentage positive (%)
Ohta and Matsunaga (1974)[a]	Japanese shellfish	301	50.5
Fagan and Beckman (1976)	Gulf coast commercial	330	27
Elliot and Harrison (1976)	Royal Navy	350	4
Harvey and Sphar (1976)	US Navy	611	2.5
Wade et al. (1978)	Hawaiian fishing	20	65
Davidson (1981)	North Sea commercial	4422	4.4
Lowry et al.(1986)	Australian abalone	108	25
Kawashima and Tamura (1983)[a,1]	Japanese shellfish	747	56.4

[a] The Kawashima and Tamura survey is an extension of the Ohta and Matsunaga survey, and they have divers in common.

17 per cent. The lesions were more often in older men with more exposure to pressure and also correlated significantly with DCS. The incidence rose to 60 per cent for workers who had worked for 15 years in compressed air.

Although rare, several cases have been reported in aviators not exposed to hyperbaric conditions.

> Dysbaric osteonecrosis is rare in recreational scuba divers who breathe compressed air at depths of less than 50 metres and who follow the customary decompression tables.

Whether the incidence of bone lesions is related more to the cumulative effects of hyperbaric exposures than to the statistical chance of a single event increasing with multiple exposures is unknown.

The incidence of avascular necrosis of bone, within the general population not exposed to hyperbaric environments, is also not clearly defined.

The disease is rare in sport divers. A few cases (nearly all shoulder disease) have been reported, although it is likely that there are many other unreported sufferers. Gorman and Sandow[3] and Wilmhurst and Ross[4] published two typical case reports.

AETIOLOGY AND PATHOGENESIS

In terms of clinical pathology, DON is simply one in a long list of causes of aseptic necrosis, but perhaps one of the most fascinating. The most common cause of aseptic necrosis of the femoral head is fracture of the neck of the femur. The necrotic lesions of high-dose steroid therapy, even though multiple and bilateral, often involve the articular surface of the knee and ankle joints, virtually never seen with DON. This variation in distribution suggests that the pathogenesis may be different, even if the pathological features are identical. Osteonecrosis is also frequently reported in association with those diseases in which there is some disturbance of fat metabolism, e.g. diabetes mellitus, pancreatitis, alcoholism and cirrhosis, Gaucher's disease and hyperlipidaemia. Trauma and steroid administration are the most common associations. Aseptic osteonecrosis may occur without any known risk factors (idiopathic aseptic necrosis). Certain specific isolated-site bone necrosis disorders, such as Legg-Calvé-Perthes disease, may be associated with specific systemic or anatomical abnormalities (Table 14.3).

It has been postulated that many of these conditions may be associated with fat emboli and these emboli obstruct end arteries in rigid

Table 14.3 Some causes of aseptic necrosis

- Decompression sickness or dysbaric exposure.
- Trauma (e.g. fractured neck of femur, dislocated hip and unrelated fractures).
- Steroids (Cushing's syndrome and steroid therapy).
- Collagen diseases (e.g. lupus erythematosus, rheumatoid arthritis, polyarteritis nodosa).
- Occlusive vascular disease.
- Diabetes mellitus.
- Hyperlipidaemia.
- Liver disease (fatty liver, hepatitis, carbon tetrachloride poisoning).
- Alcoholism.
- Pancreatitis.
- Gaucher's disease.
- Gout.
- Haemophilia.
- Polycythaemia/marrow hyperplasia.
- Haemoglobinopathies (especially sickle cell).
- Sarcoidosis.
- Charcot joint.
- Specific bone necrosis disorders (Legg-Calvé-Perthes, Kienbock's, Freiberg's and Kohler's diseases).
- Radiotherapy.

haversian canals of bone, leading to avascular osteonecrosis. These fat emboli may arise from a fatty liver, coalescence of plasma lipoproteins, disruption of bone marrow or other fat tissue or a combination of the foregoing mechanisms. Enhanced coagulability may add to blood vessel obstruction.

The exact mechanism leading to bone necrosis in association with hyperbaric exposure has not been fully elucidated. The most widely held belief is that it results from the *decompression* phase and represents a delayed or long-term manifestation of DCS (see Chapter 12). There is a definite relationship between DON and exposure to inadequate decompression, experimental diving and clinical DCS.

There are, however, numerous variations on this basic concept. One theory is that the infarction is caused by *arterial gas emboli* produced during decompression. Certainly, 'silent' bubbles can be detected by Doppler techniques during clinically apparently safe decompression schedules. However, several series indicate a relationship with musculoskeletal DCS or total DCS, rather than specifically neurological or serious DCS, and it is

the latter that are more likely to be associated with intra-arterial bubbles.

Others propose that the fat in bone marrow takes up large amounts of nitrogen during longer pressure exposures. During or after decompression, gas is liberated from the fat, and expansion with decompression increases intramedullary pressure, thus compromising blood flow within non-compliant bone cavities[5]. Prompt recompression may prevent later deterioration because there is probably a critical period of bone ischaemia after which pathological changes become irreversible. Osteocytes are known to die after about 4 hours of anoxia. Some affected areas may spontaneously recover, whereas others progress to the typical necrotic lesions.

Bubbles have been found post mortem in the large venous sinusoids in animal experiments with DCS, and they may well have obstructed venous outflow from marrow, leading to areas of infarction. Bubble formation within bony lacunae and subsequent destruction of osteocytes are also possible following decompression.

Changes secondary to intravascular bubbles, whether arterial or venous, such as platelet

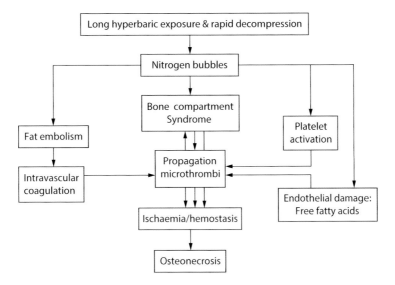

Figure 14.1 Suggested pathogenesis of dysbaric osteonecrosis. (From Kawashima M, Tamura H, Noro Y, et al. Pathogenesis and prevention of dysbaric osteonecrosis. In: *Proceedings of the 12th Meeting of the United States-Japan Cooperative Program in Natural Resources (UJNR) Panel on Diving Physiology, Washington DC, July 13–14.* Silver Spring, Maryland: National Undersea Research Program; 1993.)

aggregation and intravascular coagulation, may cause further vascular obstruction (Figure 14.1). Release of fat, thromboplastin and vaso-active substances could also trigger disseminated intra-vascular coagulation and exacerbate DON[2]. This model is supported by the post-dive observation of increased platelet adhesiveness and decreased platelet count in volunteers who display higher intravascular bubble counts on Doppler imaging[6].

It is possible that a number of factors may combine to produce necrosis in a given situation and that the aetiology is complex and multifactorial. Experimental evidence is available to suggest that both intravascular and extravascular aetiologies are consistent with the bone pathology, but a direct cause-and-effect relationship has not been proven. Asymptomatic or 'silent' bubbles during or after decompression are incriminated in those divers who have had neither DCS nor exposure to haz-ardous diving practices.

All embolism theories (gas, fat or other) do not adequately explain why other tissues do not appear to be embolized and why the femur and upper end of the humerus are particularly affected.

Oxygen toxicity is another possible cause of DON. Several mechanisms have been postulated.

One suggests that the local vasospastic reaction to high oxygen pressures leads to ischaemia. High oxygen pressures have been shown to cause swelling of fat cells, which may produce increased intramedullary pressure and ischaemia or, if insufficient to obstruct blood flow completely, could inhibit the clearance of gas from the marrow during decompression. Given the low rates of DON in those who practice oxygen decompression techniques, this seems an unlikely cause of DON.

An *osmotic* aetiology has also been suggested, incriminating the movement of water into or out of the bone. Rapid pressure changes during compression are associated with large gas gradients because the intravascular partial pressure of all inspired gases is transiently much higher than in the tissues. Thus, a gradient exists across the capillary wall, and water would then move into the vascular compartment. Expansion of the intravascular space within the rigid bone structure may to lead to local bone ischaemia. It has even been suggested that the absolute pressure within the medulla of bone may be transiently lower than that outside the cortex during a rapid compression, and that this alone could promote venous stasis and bone necrosis. It is unclear how this apparent violation of Pascal's Principle could occur, but such transient differences in pressure have been reported, with no clear explanation.

> Dysbaric osteonecrosis is thought to be a long-term effect of inadequate decompression.

Various animal models have been developed to study the aetiology of DON because of the obvious difficulties in early detection and monitoring of such a capricious and chronic disease. Much research thus involves the experimental induction of bone necrosis in animals such as guinea pigs and mice, but it is difficult to be convinced that these lesions are strictly comparable to those of divers and caisson workers. Studies in larger animals such as sheep that have a large fatty marrow compartment in long bones similar to humans have been more successful. These studies in sheep and human post-mortem studies tend to support raised intramedullary pressure combined with hypercoagulability mechanisms.

Any theory must account for the following observations:

- Dysbaric osteonecrosis may follow a single exposure to pressure.
- Although there appears to be a relationship between DCS and DON, not all divers with DON have a history of DCS.
- Not all divers who have DCS develop DON.
- Not all divers at high risk develop DON.

The development of effective strategies for prevention and treatment depends on further research elucidating the precise pathophysiological mechanisms involved.

PATHOLOGY

Histologically, the area of necrosis is usually much more widespread than is evident radiologically. Necrosis is first recognized by the absence of osteocytes in the bone lacunae. This probably starts within a few hours of infarction.

Revascularization then commences from areas of viable bone to form an area of vascular granulation tissue that extends into the infarcted area. Necrotic trabeculae are effectively thickened and strengthened by this new growth, and some lesions even disappear. The revascularization may be arrested before all areas of necrosis have been invaded. Continuing formation of new bone forms a zone of thickened trabeculae separated from necrotic bone by a line of dead collagen. This area of increased bone bulk is usually the first detectable radiological sign.

The necrotic trabeculae not strengthened by the revascularization process may eventually collapse under a load. It is at this stage that clinical symptoms, not necessarily temporally related to recent hyperbaric exposure, are noted. With lesions near articular cartilage, there is some flattening of the articular surface, and with further load, stress fractures appear in the subchondral bone. The underlying necrosis causes progressive detachment of the articular surface from its bed. This process resembles that of late segmental collapse, as seen in ischaemic necrosis following fractures of the neck of the femur. Secondary degenerative osteoarthritis often develops in affected joints.

Cases of malignant fibrous histiocytoma, superimposed on DON, may develop in conjunction with the prolonged reparative process set in train by the necrosis.

CLINICAL FEATURES

There may be a history of DCS or repeated inadequate decompression leading to investigation for possible disease. However, a definite connection between the site of DCS and the site of bone lesions has been notoriously difficult to establish. Early lesions are usually completely asymptomatic and may currently be detected only by bone scintigraphy (radioactive isotope scan), magnetic resonance imaging (MRI) or radiological examination. However, there are reports of persistent limb pain, in some cases quite severe, before the development of x-ray changes. Occasional patients have pain in the area of subsequent necrosis dating from the DCS incident. Persistent limb pain may be indicative of a bone compartment syndrome, which may progress to typical DON.

Symptoms of pain and restricted joint movement, usually affecting the hip or shoulder joint, may develop insidiously over months or years and are caused by secondary degenerative osteoarthritic changes.

An increase of 50 per cent in the total mineral content of the bone is necessary before it can be recognized as an area of increased density on the x-ray film, and these changes may take 3 to 6 months from the time of initial insult. MRI and, to a lesser extent, scintigraphy have emerging roles in earlier diagnosis, and reports have even suggested that causative bubbles may be visualized in the fatty marrow[7].

> X-ray lesions are usually found in the large long bones of the upper and lower limbs. These may be subdivided into juxta-articular (A) or head, neck and shaft (B) lesions.

There are two major sites for the radiological lesions, classified by their prognostic implications. These lesions may be present alone or in combination and are classified as juxta-articular lesions (A lesions) and head, neck and shaft lesions (B lesions).

Juxta-articular lesions

These are also referred to as joint lesions or A lesions and are potentially disabling. They may eventually result in collapse of the articular surface. The most common sites are the hips and shoulders. The lesions predominate in caisson workers and divers working in undisciplined or experimental conditions. Rare cases have been reported in other joints, e.g. the ankle. It is estimated that about one in five articular lesions will progress to articular surface collapse and up to one in five of these will be treated by arthroplasty or other surgical procedures.

Head, neck and shaft lesions

Lesions away from the articular surface are referred to as medullary or B lesions. They are usually asymptomatic and are seldom of orthopaedic significance. The most common sites are the shafts of the femur and humerus. These lesions do not extend beyond the metaphysis or involve the cortex of the bone. The shaft is not weakened, and pathological fracture is a rare complication.

New bone replacement has been observed in these lesions. Their importance lies in that they may demonstrate that people with the lesions are at greater risk of further DON, although this has not been proven statistically.

In assessing the radiological diagnosis of these lesions, it is important to realize that the X-ray will show only a fraction of the total lesion, and that some bone necrosis areas revealed by scintigraphy never become apparent on the x-ray studies.

Symptoms

Symptoms referable to juxta-articular lesions depend on the position and severity of the bone damage. Usually there is pain over the joint. This may be aggravated by movement and may radiate down the limb. There is often some restriction of movement, although a useful range of flexion may remain. In the shoulder, the signs are similar to those of a rotator cuff lesion, i.e. a painful arc from 60 to 180 degrees of abduction with difficulty in maintaining abduction against resistance. Lifting heavy weights may precipitate the onset of pain. Secondary degenerative osteoarthritis follows collapse of the articular cartilage and further reduces joint movement. The site of these lesions is approximately in the ratio of femur to the humerus, 1:2 to 1:3.

Neoplasia

Malignant tumours of bone (usually fibrous histiocytoma) have been reported in cases of aseptic necrosis, many of which were asymptomatic. The risk appears greatest with large medullary lesions.

RADIOLOGY AND DIFFERENTIAL DIAGNOSIS

Two main questions may arise in early or atypical lesions: Is the radiological lesion under examination either a variant of normal bone structure or perhaps a minor dysplasia of bone? Does the osteonecrosis have a cause other than the dysbaric environment?

Early diagnosis is based on minor alterations in the trabecular pattern of bone that result in abnormal densities or lucencies. Early detection of asymptomatic lesions may be verified only by serial radiological examinations, showing the progression of the lesion. Considerable skill is required in these assessments, and this work became the province of highly specialized panels of independent observers. Members compare their independent written reports before coming to a consensus position. In the United Kingdom a central registry for cases and x-ray studies was sponsored by a government body (the Medical Research Council). Lesions are classified as in Table 14.4 (Figures 14.2 through 14.9). This classification is useful to compare results among different studies. For a good review of this area see Williams and associates[8].

The first decision to make is whether the bone is normal[9]. Cysts and areas of sclerosis occur sporadically in otherwise normal persons but also in other diseases. Chance cortical bone defects must he eliminated, and the recognition of the normal bone island is essential.

These are dense areas of bone within the cancellous bone structure but that are sharply defined, round or oval, with the long axis running parallel to the long bone. Thought to develop early in life, they have a normal trabecular pattern around them and have no clinical significance.

Table 14.4 The United Kingdom Medical Research Council radiological classification of dysbaric osteonecrosis

A lesions (juxta-articular)
A1 Dense areas with intact articular cortex.
A2 Spherical opacities.
A3 Linear opacities.
A4 Structural failures.
    a Translucent subcortical band.
    b Collapse of articular cortex.
    c Sequestration of cortex.
A5 Secondary degenerative osteoarthritis.
B lesions (head, neck and shaft)
B1 Dense areas.
B2 Irregular calcified areas.
B3 Translucent and cystic areas.

In our enthusiasm to monitor divers at risk, we must also be aware of the dangers of irradiation – the promotion of malignancy being the most obvious. Even with good equipment and technique, a

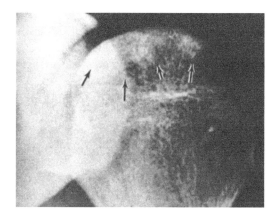

Figure 14.2 A1 lesions. Dense areas with intact articular cortex. At the top of the humerus are two areas where the trabecular pattern is blurred (arrows). The edge of the cortex looks 'woolly'.

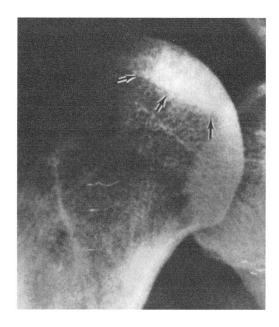

Figure 14.3 A2 lesion. Spherical segmental opacity (arrows). Originally called a 'snowcap lesion', this may remain symptomless.

diver receives one third of the annual maximum recommended dose of body irradiation for one long bone series. Unnecessary irradiation is to be avoided, and readers are advised to seek up-to-date recommendations on the frequency of long bone series in occupational divers. Currently, a common recommendation is a series at employment and then on leaving employment if more than 5 years have elapsed – with the former only required if the latter was not done on leaving the most recent employment. This practice protects both the diver and the employer from misinterpretation of bony changes.

Causes of radiological anomaly that may produce confusion in diagnosis include the following:

1. *Bone islands* (see earlier).
2. *Enchondroma* and other innocent tumours: These may calcify, causing an osteoclastic appearance in the shaft of the long bone. Medullary osteochondroma may show foci of calcification, which are more circular, whorled and in closer apposition than the foci of calcification of DON.

3. *Normal variants:* These include sesamoid bones, the shadow of the linea aspera and its endosteal crest.
4. *Osteoarthritis:* Osteoarthritis, not associated with juxta-articular DON, usually causes a reduction of the joint space, with sclerosis of the underlying bone on both sides of the joint. In DON, the cartilage space is not narrowed unless secondary osteoarthritis has occurred.

Other causes of osteonecrosis must be excluded (see Table 14.3). Both the radiological features and medical history are important in establishing

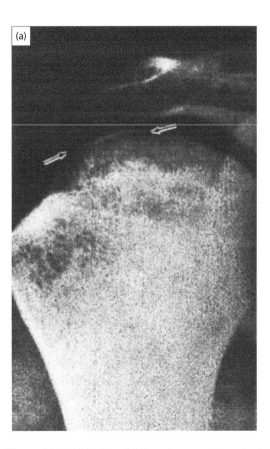

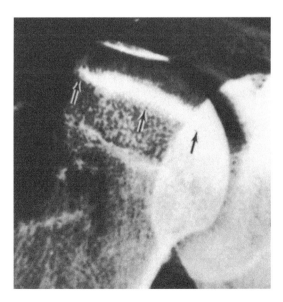

Figure 14.4 A3 lesion. Linear opacity. The dense line marked with arrows represents the lesion. The extremities of such linear opacities characteristically extend to the cortical margin.

Figure 14.5 A4 lesion. **(a)** Translucent subcortical band: this lesion (between arrows) is sometimes called a 'crescent sign'. Situated just under the articular cortical surface, the translucent line indicates that a sliver of the cortical surface is about to detach. *(Continued)*

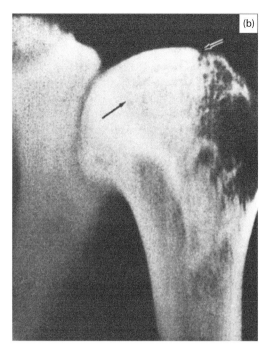

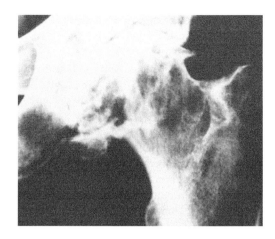

Figure 14.6 A5 lesion. Osteoarthritis. This condition can supervene on any lesion in which disruption of the articular surface has occurred. In osteonecrosis, the cartilage often remains viable so that a joint space of reasonable size continues to be radiologically visible despite severe osteoarthritis.

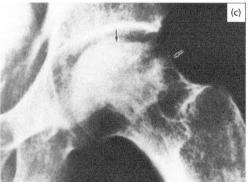

Figure 14.5 (Continued) A4 lesion. **(b)** Collapse of the articular cortex or subchondral depression: this tomogram shows a fracture line (arrows) developing between the sclerotic part of the bone above (which is being depressed into the femoral head) and the surrounding bone cortex. **(c)** Sequestration of the cortex: a loose piece of dead articular cortex has been pushed into the body of the femoral head, thus causing the latter to appear flattened (arrows).

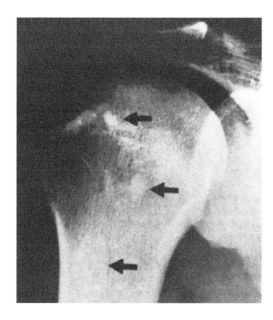

Figure 14.7 B1 lesion. Dense areas. These areas can be seen just at and below the junction of the humeral head and shaft (arrows). They are typical of the osteonecrotic lesions seen in such sites, and it is unlikely that they will ever cause disability.

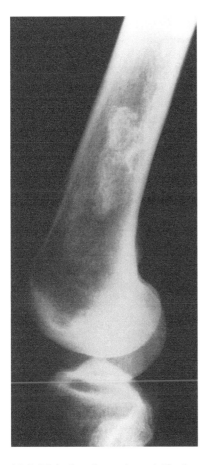

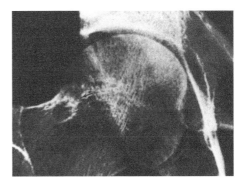

Figure 14.9 B3 lesions. Translucent areas and cysts. A single cyst (arrow) is usually seen in the femoral neck. Sometimes a line of small cysts appears at the point where the hip joint capsule attaches to the femoral neck. These irregularities may also be found at the junction of the shoulder joint capsule and humeral neck. Some experts believe these multiple lesions are not osteone-crotic, but rather relate to past damage at the point of a capsule's insertion into the neck of a bone.

Figure 14.8 B2 lesion. Irregular calcified areas. This condition is commonly seen in divers. Sometimes the appearance is that of rather foamy areas in the medulla at the lower end of the femur, often with a calcified margin. Sometimes femoral lesions have a hard, scal-loped edge around a translucent area. Endosteal thickening frequently accompanies these lesions.

the diagnosis. These causes should be rare in a fit, active diving population who have undergone medical assessment (see Chapters 53 and 54). Among the more important are the following:

1. *Trauma:* DON has been reported remote from the site of multiple fractures.
2. *Alcohol:* A history of heavy consumption or other organ damage may be obtained.
3. *Steroid therapy:* The likelihood of osteonecrosis increases with increased dose, the minimum being 10 mg prednisone or its equivalent per day for 30 days. Short courses of high-dose 'pulse' therapy have also been incriminated.
4. *Haemoglobinopathies:* Sickle-cell anaemia, thalassaemia and other variants may also be causative. Diagnosis is made by haematological investigations and by demonstrating lesions in the spine and skull.
5. *Specific bone necrosis syndromes* such as *Kienbock's disease* (spontaneous avascular necrosis of the carpal lunate) and Freiberg's disease (second metatarsal head): The osteo-chondroses of epiphyseal heads, such as *Legg-Calvé-Perthe's disease* (hip) *and Kohler's disease* (tarsal scaphoid), have specific age and clinical parameters.
6. *Collagen diseases:* Systemic lupus erythematosus and rheumatoid arthritis are associated with a very high incidence of osteonecrosis of the hip, both with and without steroid therapy.

The initial diagnosis of DON must be reason-ably certain because it has serious implications for the professional diver. Solitary lesions espe-cially require careful assessment, whereas multiple lesions make the diagnosis easier.

Symptoms and plain x-ray lesions are both relatively late manifestations, with MRI and scintigraphy (the latter now seldom used) both capable of identifying earlier lesions if sought (see later). The first radiological signs may be noted within 3 to 6 months of MRI changes, but they may take much longer – even years. The experienced radiologist looks for an increase in bone density as a result of the reactive changes to the presence of dead tissue, with new bone laid down on the surface of the dead bone.

The pathological lesion may never produce radiological changes. A 10-year radiological follow-up of 15 caisson workers revealed lesions in previously normal areas and worsening of known lesions despite cessation of further hyperbaric exposure[10]. Autopsy often reveals the pathological areas are far more extensive than the radiological demarcation. Diagnostic radiological parameters include the following:

Juxta-articular lesions (A lesions)

1. Dense areas with intact cortex (usually humeral head).
2. Spherical opacities (often segmental in humeral head).
3. Linear opacities (usually humeral head).
4. Structural failure showing as translucent subcortical bands (especially in heads of femur and humerus) and often collapse of articular cortex with sequestration.
5. Secondary degenerative arthritis with osteophyte formation.

There is usually no narrowing of the joint spaces until later stages. These lesions appear to be quite different from those of other causes of avascular necrosis.

Head, neck and shaft lesions (B lesions)

1. Dense areas, usually multiple and often bilateral, commonly in the neck and proximal shaft of the femur and humerus. These must be distinguished from normal 'bone islands'.
2. Irregular calcified areas in the medulla. These are commonly seen in the distal femur,

proximal tibia and the proximal humerus. They may be bilateral.
3. Translucent areas and cysts, best seen in tomograms of the head and neck of the humerus and femur.
4. Cortical thickening.

Emphasis is on minor variations of trabecular structure, and special radiographic techniques combined with skilled interpretation are required. Cylinder cone and tomography may be used. Computed tomography (CT) or bone scintigraphy may clarify a questionable area.

OTHER INVESTIGATIONS

The value of the plain x-ray examination in early diagnosis is being questioned, and other imaging techniques are being increasingly used.

Imaging techniques:

- Plain radiography.
- Scintigraphy.
- Computed tomography (including single photon emission computed tomography).
- Magnetic resonance imaging.

Bone scintigraphy (bone scans)

This investigation had an established role in the early detection of the bony reaction to osteonecrosis, before there are any changes on plain x-ray studies. Use has declined with the greater availability and lower cost of MRI (see later). Any lesion that stimulates bone formation is shown as a 'hot spot' by the radioactive bone-seeking tracer, on the scintigram (Figure 14.10). Technetium-99m–labelled methylene diphosphonate (MDP) is the most widely used tracer, but several newer diphosphonate compounds have been introduced that appear to have relatively higher skeletal affinity and may be more sensitive. These agents are injected intravenously, and images taken over time with a gamma camera. Scintigraphy-positive 'lesions' can be produced in animals as early as 2 to 3 weeks after decompression and have been shown to involve necrotic bone and osteogenesis at autopsy at 3 months, even though x-ray changes still had not developed in most cases.

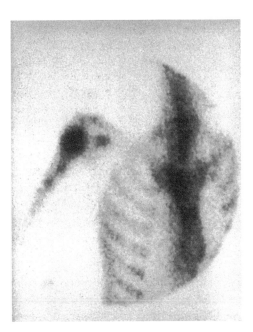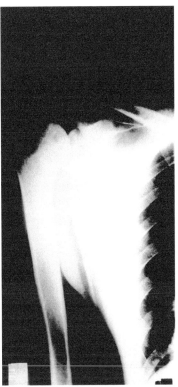

Figure 14.10 **(a)** Qualitative scintigram using technetium-99m–labelled methylene diphosphonate (MDP) that shows a 'hot spot', i.e. increased concentration of technetium with increased uptake of MDP, in the right shoulder of a 38-year-old diver who had performed many deep bounce dives on heliox. Most of these were experimental dives, although he never had treatment for decompression sickness and would admit only to the odd minor discomfort in a variety of joints after dives. Routine screening x-ray studies at the time showed a normal shoulder. **(b)** X-ray study of the right shoulder 4 months after the first scan. (Photographs courtesy of Dr Ramsay Pearson.)

Similar findings in humans with biopsy or radiological follow-up indicate that the 'hot spots' occur far earlier and are more numerous than the radiological changes. However, these 'hot spots' may resolve with no apparent longer-term changes and are therefore insufficient to establish a firm diagnosis. Overall, then, scintigraphy in early lesions is much more sensitive than radiology but has low specificity because any bone reparative reaction will be detected, no matter what the cause is.

Single position emission computed tomography

Single photon emission CT (SPECT) is said to improve specificity, and 'cold' areas occurring immediately after occlusion of blood supply may also be detected. Despite its promise, SPECT has not found a routine place in the diagnosis of DON, probably because of the high cost and poor availability of this technology.

Computed tomography

CT gives greater definition revealing both structural collapse and areas of new growth. CT scans may help in the diagnosis of early or doubtful changes on plain x-ray films. This imaging technique is essential if some of the surgical techniques, such as rotational osteotomy, are being contemplated.

Magnetic resonance imaging

MRI can detect necrosis of marrow fat within 2 to 4 days of the ischaemic episode and thus offers the best opportunity for early diagnosis. MRI studies may indicate far greater necrosis than conventional plain radiography and can also reveal bone lesions at other sites when a lesion has been detected on plain x-ray films. MRI of the shoulder joint has been suggested as the best surveillance technique for professional divers who are exposed deeper than 15 metres (Figure 14.11). At present, MRI is not routinely used as a screening tool because of the cost of examination.

Invasive investigations

Invasive investigations have been undertaken to aid in earlier diagnosis and therapeutic intervention. These techniques include arteriography, intraosseous phlebography, intramedullary pressure measurement and core biopsy. The latter three investigations are often combined in a technique described by Ficat in 1985[11] as functional exploration of bone, but this approach has not been widely adopted.

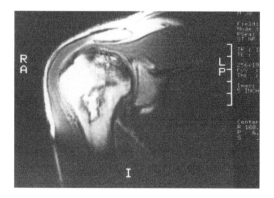

Figure 14.11 Magnetic resonance imaging of the right shoulder. On these slightly T1-weighted images there is evidence of marked distortion of the marrow signal with areas of necrosis indicated by the dark signal. There is also cortical irregularity. The process involves the articular surface of the glenohumeral joint.

PREVENTION

Early recompression of experimental limb bends in sheep prevents progression to DON, and this validates the clinical practice of recompression of all cases of DCS to reduce long-term damage.

Early recognition is imperative, and the following investigations are recommended for all professional divers exposed to frequent hyperbaric conditions at depths greater than 15 metres.

1. Baseline long bone x-ray studies.
2. MRI examination in doubtful plain x-ray findings or to define extent of lesions.
3. MRI 3 months after an episode of DCS involving the hips or shoulders.

Image-guided biopsy of suspicious lesions (or even surgical biopsy) may be appropriate in special circumstances.

The disease is rare in recreational scuba divers who follow decompression tables and use only compressed air to depths less than 50 metres. For these groups, unless there is a specific cause for concern, serial radiological investigation is certainly not warranted because of the unnecessary irradiation hazards and expense.

The problem of what to do when confronted with an asymptomatic B lesion is not yet clear. If the B lesion is thought to be provoked by nonadherence to established diving tables, these should clearly be followed in the future. Under these conditions, it is assumed that the B lesion is induced because of excessive provocation. If the diver has adhered to normal decompression tables, then it is presumed that he or she is particularly predisposed to DON, and consideration is given to restricting diving to reduce the risk of further lesions. It is generally accepted that the need for formal decompression staging should be avoided, as should experimental or helium diving. Doubtful cases should be treated as if positive until further radiological assessment clarifies the issue.

If a juxta-articular lesion is present, traditional teaching suggests that all exposure to compression should cease. There is, however, no evidence that this modifies the subsequent course of the problem. Today, a pragmatic approach is more common, with close attention given to the functional capacity of the individual diver along with counselling about avoiding further provocative diving if possible. Annual assessment of these divers will pay close attention to their continued functional capacity.

TREATMENT

Although healing is seen histologically, the possibility of resolution of radiologically positive asymptomatic lesions is less clear, although there are occasional reports in the literature. Nevertheless, the treatment of juxta-articular (A) lesions should be based on the finding that DON often progresses through the stages outlined later. One interesting study of the long-term outcome in affected divers who cease hyperbaric exposure after diagnosis suggests a high likelihood of further progression of lesions, and it has been suggested that progress may be unrelated to further diving exposure[10]. The asymptomatic head, neck and shaft lesions require no active therapy.

Hyperbaric oxygen therapy has been used successfully to treat the early stages of avascular necrosis (Ficat stages 1 and 2 – see the next section), but it is not clear whether DON is likely to respond in the same way.

Surgical treatment

Surgical treatment of disabling aseptic osteonecrosis must be based on the aetiology and may therefore have a rational basis in DON that is absent in idiopathic disease. Conversely, most surgical experience is with idiopathic osteonecrosis of the femoral head – the site at which osteonecrosis produces the most devastating disability. It is not yet clear whether the same approach will be more or less successful following DON. The type of treatment is determined by the staging of the disease process (as described by Ficat[11]), the age of the patient and the joints involved.

STAGING (FROM FICAT[11])

0 – Asymptomatic, pre-radiological (i.e. high index of suspicion confirmed by raised intramedullary pressure or positive scan).
1 – Symptomatic, pre-radiological.
2 – Symptomatic, radiological pre-destruction.

3 – Collapse of articular surface.
4 – Destruction of joint.

CURATIVE TREATMENT

Core decompression has its advocates, but the value of the procedure is still questionable. If accepted, it is indicated for stage 0 to 2. The results are, as expected, better for the earliest stages.

Vascularized fibular graft procedure has been used for stage 0 to 2 disease, mainly that affecting the hip. One comparative study suggests that results are better with this procedure than with core decompression[12].

RECONSTRUCTIVE TREATMENT

When gross damage to the articular surfaces exists, reconstructive techniques offer the best chance of rehabilitation.

1. Osteotomy of the femoral neck, either rotation or wedge, endeavours to move the weight-bearing axis away from a localized necrotic area.
2. Arthrodesis is possible for a young patient, with destruction of one hip only.
3. Arthroplasty is indicated for 'end-stage' joints especially if the patient is old or the disease is bilateral. Total joint replacement has proved useful in replacing severely affected hip and shoulder joints. The concern about this form of surgery is that the life of the prosthesis is unknown because it is used in a relatively young population with a long life expectancy.

RADIOLOGICAL TECHNIQUE

1. Good definition of the trabecular structure of the bone is important.
2. The gonads must be protected from ionizing radiation in young divers by the use of a lead shield, although this may hinder radiographical interpretation.
3. The following projections are required:
   (a) *Shoulder:* An anteroposterior projection of each shoulder joint. A 30 × 25 cm film is recommended. The patient is placed in a supine position with the trunk rotated at an angle of approximately 45 degrees to bring

the shoulder to be radiographed in contact with the table. This arm is partially abducted and the elbow is flexed. The radiologist should centre 2.5 cm below the coracoid process of the scapula and then cone to show as much humerus as possible, bringing in the lateral diaphragms to show only the head and shaft of the humerus. This view should show a clear joint space, and the acromion should not overlap the head of the humerus.

(b) *Hip:* An anteroposterior projection of each hip joint. A 30 × 25 cm film is recommended. The patient is placed in a supine position with the feet at 90 degrees to the tabletop. The edge of the gonad protector should be as near the femoral head as possible, but not in any way obscuring it. The radiologist should centre the cone over the head of the femur, i.e. 2.5 cm below the midpoint of a line joining the anterior, superior iliac spine and the upper border of the pubic symphysis.

(c) *Knee:* An anteroposterior and lateral projection of each knee. An 18 × 43 cm film is recommended. The radiologist should centre at the level of the upper border of the patella. The field should include the lower third of the femur and the upper third of the tibia and fibula.

REFERENCES

1. Uguen M, Pougnet R, Uguen A, Loddé B, Dewitte JD. Dysbaric osteonecrosis among professional divers: a literature review. *Undersea & Hyperbaric Medicine Society* 2014;**41**(6):579–587.
2. Davidson JK. Dysbaric disorders: aseptic bone necrosis in tunnel workers and divers. *Bailliere's Clinical Rheumatology* 1989;**3**:1–23.
3. Gorman DF, Sandow MJ. Posterior shoulder dislocation and humeral head necrosis in a recreational scuba diver. *Undersea Biomedical Research* 1992;**19**:457–461.
4. Wilmhurst P, Ross K. Dysbaric osteonecrosis of the shoulder in a sport scuba diver. *British Journal of Sports Medicine* 1998;**32**:344–345.
5. Lehner CE, Adams WM, Dubielzig RR, Palta M, Lanphier, EH. Dysbaric osteonecrosis in divers and caisson workers: an animal model. *Clinical Orthopedics and Related Research* 1997;**344**:320–322.
6. Pontier JD, Jiminez C, Blatteau JE. Blood platelet count and bubble formation after a dive to 30 msw for 30 min. *Aviation, Space and Environmental Medicine* 2008;**79**(12):1096–1099.
7. Stephant E, Gempp E, Blatteau J-E. Role of MRI in the detection of marrow bubbles after musculoskeletal decompression sickness predictive of subsequent dysbaric osteonecrosis. *Clinical Radiology* 2008;**63**:1380–1383.
8. Williams ES, Khreisat S, Ell PJ, King JD. Bone imaging and skeletal radiology in dysbaric osteonecrosis. *Clinical Radiology* 1987;**38**:589–592.
9. Hendry WT. The significance of bone islands, cystic areas and sclerotic areas in dysbaric osteonecrosis. *Clinical Radiology* 1997;**28**:381–393.
10. Van Blarcom ST, Czarnecki DJ, Fueredi, GA, Wenzel MS. Does dysbaric osteonecrosis progress in the absence of further hyperbaric exposure? A 10-year radiologic follow-up of 15 patients. *AJR American Journal of Radiology* 1990;**155**(1):95–97.
11. Ficat TP. Idiopathic bone necrosis of the femoral head: early diagnosis and treatment. *Journal of Bone and Joint Surgery British Volume* 1985;**67**(1):3–9.
12. Scully SP, Aaron RK, Urbaniak JR. Survival analysis of hips treated with core decompression or vascularized fibular grafting because of avascular necrosis *Journal of Bone Joint Surgery American Volume* 1998;**80**(9):1270–1275.

FURTHER READING

Jones JP, Ramirez S, Doty SB. The pathophysiologic role of fat in dysbaric osteonecrosis. *Clinical Orthopedics and Related Research* 1993;**296**:256–264.

Kawashima M, Tamura H. Osteonecrosis in divers – prevention and treatment. In: Shiraki K, Matsuoka S, eds. *Hyperbaric Medicine and Underwater Physiology*. Proceedings of the Third International Symposium of UOEH on Hyperbaric Medicine and Underwater Physiology. (III UOEH Symposium). University of Occupational and Environmental Health: Fukuoka; 1983.

Kawashima M, Tamura H, Noro Y, et al. Pathogenesis and prevention of dysbaric osteonecrosis. In: *Proceedings of the 12th Meeting of the United States-Japan Cooperative Program in Natural Resources (UJNR) Panel on Diving Physiology, Washington DC, July 13–14*. Silver Spring, Maryland: National Undersea Research Program; 1993.

Lowry CJ, Traugott FM, Jones MW. Dysbaric osteonecrosis – a survey of abalone divers. In: Edmonds C, ed. *The Abalone Diver*. Melbourne Diving Medical Centre/National Safety Council of Australia; 1986:50–62.

This chapter was reviewed for this fifth edition by Michael Bennett.

PART 4

Abnormal Gas Pressures

15

Inert gas narcosis

INTRODUCTION

Inert gas narcosis refers to a clinical syndrome characterized by impairment of intellectual and neuromuscular performance and changes in mood and behaviour. It is produced by an increased partial pressure of some inert gasses. In compressed air exposure, these changes, which have been observed for more than 100 years, are caused by nitrogen. The effects are progressive with increasing depth but not with increasing time at the same depth. The word 'inert' indicates that these gases exert their effect without undergoing metabolic change in the body, rather than inert gas in the biophysical sense.

Similar effects have been described with other metabolically inactive gases such as the rare gases (neon, argon, krypton, xenon), hydrogen and the anaesthetic gases, although at different partial pressures. Xenon is 'anaesthetic' at sea level and is used in some parts of the world as an anaesthetic agent. No narcotic effect of helium has been directly demonstrated at currently attainable pressures, although some narcotic properties have been postulated.

The 'inert' gas in compressed air is nitrogen, and its effects are also called nitrogen narcosis, depth intoxication, 'narks' and rapture of the deep

(*l'ivresse des grandes profondeurs*), the term coined by Cousteau. The narcosis, although highly variable, places a depth limit to safe diving with compressed air at approximately 40 to 50 metres. Effective work at greater depth requires the substitution of a less narcotic respiratory diluent such as helium or hydrogen.

Many 'unexplained' scuba deaths may have been associated with nitrogen narcosis.

HISTORY

Inert gas narcosis (IGN) was comprehensively reviewed in 2003, and interested readers are referred to that work for more detail[1]. The first recorded description of symptoms suggestive of air intoxication related to hyperbaric exposure was by Junod, who, in 1835, reported that 'thoughts have a peculiar charm and in some persons, symptoms of intoxication are present'. He was conducting research into the physiological effects of compression and rarefaction of air. J. B. Green in 1861 observed sleepiness, impaired judgement and hallucinations in divers breathing compressed air at 5.8 ATA, sufficient to warrant an immediate return to the surface. Paul Bert, in 1878, also noted that divers became intoxicated at great depth. In 1903, Hill and McLeod described impairment of intellectual functioning in caisson workers at 5.5 ATA. Damant, in 1930, likened the mental abnormalities and memory defects observed in men at 10 ATA to alcoholic intoxication and postulated that it was caused by the high partial pressure of oxygen.

Hill and Phillips suggested in 1932 that the effects could be psychological as a result of claustrophobia or perhaps caused by impurities in the air from the compressors (Case report 15.1). The Royal Navy appointed a committee to investigate the problems of deep diving and submarine escape, and their report in 1933 contained a section entitled 'semi-loss of consciousness'. Between 7 and 11.6 ATA, divers answered hand signals but in many cases failed to obey them. After return to surface, the divers could not remember the events of the dive. It was noted that all divers regained

---

CASE REPORT 15.1: DESCRIPTIONS OF DIVERS ABOUT THEIR EXPERIENCES AT BETWEEN 250 AND 300 FEET AS REPORTED BY HILL AND PHILLIPS

'You notice the dark more although it may not be darker; the light is a comfort and company. You notice things more if there is nothing to do; I get comfort from seeing the fish, it takes your mind off everything else'.

When asked for a description, an old hand at diving gave the following account: 'You have to be more careful in deep water; in deep water you know that you are concentrating... You think of each heave as you turn a spanner... If you go down with a set purpose it becomes an obsession; it will become the main thing and you will forget everything else'. He described how he thinks very deliberately; he says, 'I have finished my job, what shall I do next? – Of course, I have finished and now I must go up'. He described how he was aware of every action: 'If my hand goes out I think of my hand going out'. He gave the following as an analogy: 'if I saw a thing of value, say half-a-crown, in the street, I would pick it up. Down below I would look at it and think, "What is that, shall I pick it up? Yes, I will pick it up" and then I feel my hand go out'.

'I left the ladder determined to get to the bottom. At 250 feet I got a recurrence of the tingling and a feeling of lying on my back. I decided to rest a couple of minutes and then go on. I slid 10 feet and felt I was going unconscious. I made signals to be pulled up and kept repeating them. I lost the use of my limbs and let go everything. While hanging on to the rope I saw my own face in the front glass; it was outside the glass and looked all greenish; I was dressed in my shore-going suit. I heard the order, "Pull the diver up", again and again, as if someone in the suit was saying it'.

'Suddenly I came over rather "funny"; it was a distinct "different" feeling; I stood up, the tank wire in my right hand, and thinking it was a touch of CO_2, I began to breathe deep and hearty, thinking of course that in a couple of minutes I would be able to resume work. Then I seemed to go quite limp, a feeling of "no life or energy". This was new and strange to me, whether it was a part of CO_2, I didn't know, because I had never experienced a real dose of CO_2; anyhow, after stopping and doing the drill for CO_2, I thought I would be alright, but suddenly something definitely seemed to say – snap inside my head and I started to, what I thought, go mad at things'.

Description of interview of above diver after an aborted deep dive:

Practically no hypnoidal effort was required to produce the horrors of that morning's dive, and the picture of stark, mad terror....left an impression which is very difficult to describe. The impression was of sitting in the stalls and watching the acting of Grand Guignol. To such a pitch did he arouse his emotions that he clawed his face to remove the imaginary face-glass and tore his clothes which he mistook for his diving suit (Hill I, Phillips AE. Deep-sea diving. Journal of the Royal Navy Medical Service 1932;18:157–173).

full consciousness during the return to 1 ATA. The report also noted great individual variation in divers' reactions but was unable to elucidate the problem.

It was not until 1935 that Behnke, Thomson and Motley proposed the now generally held theory of the cause of this compressed air intoxication. They stated that the narcosis was the result of the raised partial pressure of the metabolically inactive gas, nitrogen. At a depth of 30 metres (4 ATA), compressed air produced a state of 'euphoria, retardation of the higher mental processes and impaired neuromuscular co-ordination'. This effect was progressive with increasing pressure so that at 10 ATA, stupefaction resulted. Unconsciousness developed between 10 and 15 ATA. They also invoked the Meyer-Overton hypothesis (see the later section on aetiology) to relate the narcotic effect to the high ratio of solubility of nitrogen in oil to water. It was not long after this major breakthrough that Behnke and Yarbrough reported that the substitution of helium for the nitrogen in compressed air eliminated narcosis.

The nitrogen partial pressure theory was not universally accepted. The 1933 Deep Diving Committee Report had raised the possibility that carbon dioxide retention was implicated. Case and Haldane, in 1941, reported that the addition of carbon dioxide to compressed air worsened the mental symptoms, although up to 6 per cent concentrations at 1 ATA had little mental effect. Bean, in 1947, demonstrated a reduction in arterial pH during compression and later also showed increased alveolar carbon dioxide concentrations. He explained these changes as being caused by reduced diffusion of carbon dioxide in the increased density of the air. He postulated that carbon dioxide was an alternative cause of depth narcosis. Seusing and Drube later supported Bean's views as recently as 1961. Also in 1961, Buhlmann believed that increased airway resistance led to hypoventilation and hypercapnia.

Rashbass in 1955 and Cabarrou in 1959 had already refuted the carbon dioxide theory, by observing signs of narcosis despite methods to ensure normal alveolar carbon dioxide levels. Later work (by Hesser, Adolfson and Fagraeus) showed that the effects of nitrogen and carbon dioxide are additive in impairing performance. Normal arterial carbon dioxide and oxygen levels, while the diver is breathing air and helium-oxygen at various depths, demonstrate the key role of nitrogen in the production of this disorder and the relative insignificance of carbon dioxide.

CLINICAL MANIFESTATIONS

Martini's law: Each 15-metre (50-foot) depth is equivalent to the intoxication of one martini.

Although there is marked individual variation in susceptibility to IGN, all divers breathing compressed air are significantly affected at a depth of 60 to 70 metres (Figure 15.1). The minimum pressure producing signs is difficult to define, but some divers are affected subjectively at less than 30 metres.

The higher functions, such as reasoning, judgement, recent memory, learning, concentration and attention are affected first. The diver may experience a feeling of well-being and stimulation similar to the overconfidence of mild alcoholic intoxication. Occasionally, the opposite reaction, terror, develops.

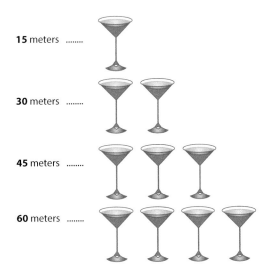

Figure 15.1 Martini's law illustrated. Diving on air at 60 metres is a dangerous challenge. (Illustration courtesy of http://p3respiratory6.wikispaces.com/)

This is more probable in the novice who is apprehensive in this new environment. Further elevation of the partial pressure of the inert gas results in impairment of manual dexterity and progressive deterioration in mental performance, automatisms, idea fixation, hallucinations and, finally, stupor and coma. Some divers complain of a restriction of peripheral visual field at depth (tunnel vision). They are less aware of potentially significant dangers outside their prescribed tasks (perceptual narrowing). More recently, abnormal emotional processing has been described, with a suggestion that the emotional responses to threat are muted with increasing IGN.

From a practical point of view, the diver may be able to focus attention on a particular task, but the memory of what was observed or performed while at depth may be lost when reporting at the surface. Alternatively, the diver may have to abort the dive because of failure to remember instructions. Repetition and drills can help overcome these problems through a 'practice effect'. Conversely, anxiety, cold, fatigue, sedatives, alcohol and other central nervous system depressant drugs aggravate narcosis.

Nitrogen narcosis has often been likened to alcoholic intoxication, especially the euphoria, lightheadedness and motor incoordination. There is some evidence that correlates subjective feelings of alcohol consumption and IGN, especially the variation in intensity experienced among individuals. In one elegant experiment reported in 2008, Hobbs[2] found evidence that heavier drinkers did not show a reduction in the effects of nitrogen narcosis at depth, but they did show tolerance for the combined effects of narcosis and alcohol. At much greater depths the parallel with general anaesthetic agents is probably closer.

Some of the reported observations at various depths breathing compressed air are shown in Table 15.1.

Table 15.1 Some observations on the effects of exposure to compressed air at increasing pressure/depth

Pressure (ATA)	Effects
2–4	Mild impairment of performance on unpractised tasks.
	Mild euphoria.
4	Reasoning and immediate memory affected more than motor coordination and choice reactions.
	Delayed response to visual and auditory stimuli.
4–6	Laughter and loquacity, which may be overcome by self-control.
	Idea fixation, perceptual narrowing and overconfidence.
	Calculation errors; memory impairment.
6	Sleepiness; illusions; impaired judgement.
6-8	Convivial group atmosphere: may be terror reaction in some; talkative; dizziness reported occasionally.
	Uncontrolled laughter approaching hysteria in some.
8	Severe impairment of intellectual performance.
	Manual dexterity less affected.
8–10	Gross delay in response to stimuli.
	Diminished concentration; mental confusion.
10	Stupefaction.
	Severe impairment of practical activity and judgement.
	Mental abnormalities and memory defects.
	Deterioration in handwriting; uncontrollable euphoria, hyperexcitability; almost total loss of intellectual and perceptive faculties.
>10	Hallucinogenic experiences.
	Unconsciousness.

The narcosis is rapidly evident on reaching the given depth (partial pressure) and is not progressive with time. It is said to be more pronounced initially with rapid compression (descent). The effect is rapidly reversible on reduction of the ambient pressure (ascent).

Other factors have been observed to affect the degree of narcosis. Cold, reduced sensory input, and both oxygen and carbon dioxide disturbances are interrelated in impairing the diver's underwater ability. In experimental conditions, with an attempt to control variables, alcohol and hard work have been shown to enhance narcosis. Moderate exercise and amphetamines may, in certain situations, reduce narcosis, but some studies have conversely suggested unpredictable or increased narcotic effects with amphetamines. Increased carbon dioxide and nitrogen tensions appear to be additive in reducing performance. Task learning and positive motivation can improve performance. Frequent or prolonged exposure produces some acclimatization, but this may reflect a reduction in psychological stress rather than representing true adaptation. For example, Hamilton and associates[3] have experimental evidence to suggest that the reported experience of adaption is more subjective than behavioural.

Direct pathological injury to the diver as a result of the high pressure of inert gas is unlikely. The danger is rather a result of how the diver may react in the environment while under the narcotic influence of nitrogen. Impaired judgement can lead to an 'out-of-air' drowning sequence, with no other apparent cause of death found. The diver affected by IGN may also be at increased risk of insidious hypothermia (see Chapter 28) because of decreased perception of cold and decreased shivering thermogenesis[4,5]. Jacques Cousteau[6] shared his experience of nitrogen narcosis (Case Report 15.2).

MEASUREMENT OF CENTRAL NERVOUS SYSTEM EFFECTS

Although suitable and reliable indices of IGN are not yet available, the search continues. Such tests would be useful in predicting individual susceptibility (diver selection), comparing the relative narcotic potencies of different respiratory diluents for oxygen, delineating the role of factors other than inert gas in producing depth intoxication and monitoring the degree of impairment during practical tasks.

Attempts to quantify the effects of IGN can be roughly divided into two methods. The first is a psychological behavioural approach measuring performance on tasks such as mental arithmetic, memory, reaction time and manual dexterity. The second relies on observing a change in some neurophysiological parameter. Some representative studies are discussed to illustrate points.

Behavioural approach

The aspects of behaviour usually studied may be divided into three categories: cognitive ability, reaction time and dexterity. The cognitive functions are the most affected and dexterity the least. One early study measured the performances of 46 men on simple arithmetic tests; reaction time and letter cancellation were measured at pressures from 3.7 to 10 ATA. This study demonstrated quantitatively the previously observed qualitative progressive deterioration with increasing pressure of compressed air. It also showed that individuals of high intelligence were less affected. The impairment noted on arrival at the target pressure was exacerbated by rapid compression.

Another study using simple arithmetic tests of manual skill showed that narcosis was maximal within 2 minutes of reaching depth, and continued exposure did not result in further deterioration, but rather there was a suggestion of acclimatization. Muscular skill was much less affected than intellectual performance. Other studies involving reaction time, conceptual reasoning, memory and psychometric tests all showed progressive deterioration with increasing pressure. Narcosis has also been measured by tests of intelligence and practical neuromuscular performance.

Some work on open water divers suggested a greater impairment of performance on manual tasks at depth when anxiety was present. Plasma cortisol and urinary adrenaline/noradrenaline (epinephrine/norepinephrine) excretion ratios were used to confirm the presence of anxiety noted subjectively. Divers were tested at 3 and 30 metres at a shore base and in the open sea. Intellectual functions, as assessed by memory test, sentence comprehension

CASE REPORT 15.2: A PERSONAL DESCRIPTION OF NITROGEN NARCOSIS BY JACQUES COUSTEAU

We continue to be puzzled with the rapture of the depths, and felt that we were challenged to go deeper. Didi's deep dive in 1943 of 210 feet had made us aware of the problem, and the Group had assembled detailed reports on its deep dives. But we had only a literary knowledge of the full effects of *l'ivresse des grandes profondeurs,* as it must strike lower down. In the summer of 1947 we set out to make a series of deeper penetrations.

…I was in good physical condition for the trial, trained fine by an active spring in the set, and responsive ears. I entered the water holding the scrap iron in my left hand. I went down with great rapidity, with my right arm crooked around the shotline. I was oppressively conscious of the diesel generator rumble of the idle *Elie Monnier* as I wedged my head into mounting pressure. It was high noon in July, but the light soon faded. I dropped through the twilight, alone with the white rope, which stretched before me in a monotonous perspective of blank white signposts.

At 200 feet I tasted the metallic flavour of compressed nitrogen, and was instantaneously and severely struck with rapture. I closed my hand on the rope and stopped. My mind was jammed with conceited thoughts and antic joy. I struggled to fix my brain on reality, to attempt to name the colour of the sea around me. A contest took place between navy blue, aquamarine and Prussian blue. The debate would not resolve. The sole fact I could grasp was that there was no roof and no floor in the blue room. The distant purr of the diesel invaded my mind – it swelled to a giant beat, the rhythm of the world's heart.

I took the pencil and wrote on a board, 'Nitrogen has a dirty taste'. I had little impression of holding the pencil, childhood nightmares overruled my mind. I was ill in bed, terrorised with the realisation that everything in the world was thick. My fingers were sausages. My tongue was a tennis ball. My lips swelled grotesquely on the mouth grip. The air was syrup. The water congealed around me as though I were smothered in aspic.

I hung stupidly on the rope. Standing aside was a smiling, jaunty man, my second self, perfectly self-contained, grinning sardonically at the wretched diver. As the seconds passed the jaunty man installed himself in my command and ordered that I unloose the rope and go on down.

I sank slowly through a period of intense visions.

Around the 264 foot board the water was suffused with an unearthly glow. I was passing from night to an imitation of dawn. What I saw as sunrise was light reflected from the floor, which had passed unimpeded through the dark transport strata above. I saw below me the weight at the end of the shotline, hanging twenty feet from the floor. I stopped at the penultimate board and looked down at the last board, five metres away, and marshalled all my resources to evaluate the situation without deluding myself. Then I went to the last board, 297 feet down.[*]

The floor was gloomy and barren, save for morbid shells and sea urchins. I was sufficiently in control to remember that in this pressure, ten times that of the surface, any untoward physical effort was extremely dangerous. I filled my lungs slowly and signed the board. I could not write what it felt like fifty fathoms down.

I was the deepest independent diver. In my bisected brain the satisfaction was balanced by satirical self-contempt.

I dropped the scrap iron and bounded like a coiled spring, clearing two boards in the first flight. There, at 264 feet, the rapture vanished suddenly, inexplicably and entirely. I was light and sharp, one man again, enjoying the lighter air expanding in my lungs. I rose through the twilight zone at high speed and saw the surface pattern in a blaze of platinum bubbles and dancing prisms. It was impossible not to think of flying to heaven (Cousteau JY. *The Silent World.* London: Reprint Society; 1954).

[*] 297 feet is 90.5 metres (don't try repeating this experiment!).

and simple arithmetic, showed evidence of narcosis in both 30-metre dives, but the decrement was greater in the ocean dives, possibly because of the greater psychological stress in the open sea. Unsurprisingly perhaps, these effects have not been reproduced in the laboratory.

Many experimental protocols have been criticized because the effects of motivation, experience and learning, for example, are difficult to control. Caisson workers participating in a card-sorting test showed some impairment at 2 to 3 ATA, especially those who had relatively little exposure to pressure. However, with repeated testing, i.e. practice, this difference disappeared, and no loss of performance was noted even deeper than 3 ATA. These experiments were repeated using 80 naval subjects at 2 and 4 ATA while breathing air and helium-oxygen mixtures. The only significant impairment was found at 4 ATA breathing air.

The effects of IGN on behaviour, as measured by the psychologist, were well reviewed by Fowler, Ackles and Porlier[7], and there has been relatively little work in this area since that time. More attention has been paid to the molecular mechanisms involved. Psychological studies suggest that the behavioural effects of all inert gases that produce narcosis are identical. Human performance under narcosis is explained using the 'slowed processing' model. Slowing is said to result from decreased activation or arousal in the central nervous system, manifested by an increase in reaction time, perhaps with a fall in accuracy. Increases in arousal, such as by exercise or amphetamines, may explain improved performance. Manual dexterity is less affected than cognitive functioning because dexterity requires fewer mental operations and there is less room for cumulative slowing of mental operations (processes). Although memory loss and impaired hearing are features of narcosis, these effects are more difficult to explain using the slowed processing model. A similar alteration in the processing of emotional experience has more recently been proposed by Löftdal and colleagues[8].

Studies of the subjective symptoms of narcosis have indicated that the diver can identify these symptoms and that they could relate the effect to the 'dose'. Euphoria, as described by terms such as 'carefree' and 'cheerful', is only one of these symptoms and may not always be present.

Other descriptive symptoms such as 'fuzzy', 'hazy' (state of consciousness) and 'less efficient' (work capability) and 'less cautious or self-controlled' (inhibitory state) may be more reliable indicators of effect on performance.

Behavioural studies have cast doubt on some traditional concepts of narcosis. True adaptation to narcosis has not been found in many performance tests. Where adaptation has been found, it is difficult to distinguish learned responses or an adaptation to the subjective symptoms from physiological tolerance. Carbon dioxide probably has additive and not synergistic effects in combination with nitrogen and probably acts by a different mechanism. Behavioural studies have not been able, so far, to demonstrate clearly the potentiating effects on IGN of anxiety, cold, fatigue, anti–motion sickness drugs and other sedatives (except alcohol).

Neurophysiological changes

Attempts have been made to confirm the subjective experiences and obtain objective evidence of performance decrement, with some neurophysiological parameter. The investigations included electroencephalographic records of subjects exposed to compressed air in chambers. Contrary to the expected findings of depression, features suggesting cortical neuronal hyperexcitability were noted at first. These included an increase in the voltage of the basal rhythm and the frequent appearance of low-voltage 'spikes' elicited by stimuli that do not have this effect at 1 ATA. Experiments in which the partial pressures of oxygen and nitrogen were controlled showed that in compressed air these changes are caused by the high oxygen partial pressure. If nitrogen-oxygen mixtures containing 0.2 ATA oxygen are breathed, these changes are absent. The depressant effects of nitrogen are then revealed. These consist of a decrease in the voltages of the basal rhythm and the appearance of low-voltage theta waves.

Blocking of electroencephalographic alpha rhythm by mental activity can be observed in half of the population. The observation that there is an abolition of this blocking on exposure to pressure introduced the concept of 'nitrogen threshold'. It was found that the time to abolition of blocking was inversely proportional to the square of the absolute pressure (T is proportional to $1/P^2$) for an individual, although there was marked variation among subjects. In some persons abolition of blocking was noted at depths as shallow as 2.5 ATA, where no subjective narcosis was evident.

Flicker fusion frequency was investigated in an attempt to obtain a measurement that could be applied to the whole population. Subjects were asked to indicate when the flickering of a neon light, at a steadily increasing rate, appeared continuous. This is termed a 'critical frequency' of flicker. After a certain time at pressure, the critical frequency dropped. The same relationship, T is proportional to $1/P^2$, resulted. Critical flicker fusion tests have been adapted for the in-water environment and continue to be used in the context of IGN assessment[8].

A more direct measure of central nervous system functioning may be obtained by observing the effect of inert gas exposure on cortical evoked potentials. Evoked potentials are the electroencephalographic response to sensory stimuli. A depression of auditory evoked responses on exposure to hyperbaric air has been shown to correlate with the decrement in mental arithmetic performance under the same conditions. The conclusion was that auditory evoked response depression was an experimental measure of nitrogen narcosis. However, other work was unable to support this hypothesis and concluded that there is a complex relationship among hyperbaric oxygen, nitrogen narcosis and evoked responses.

Auditory evoked responses as a measure of narcosis are problematic because of sound alteration with pressure and the ambient noise during hyperbaric exposure. Visual evoked responses (VERs) have been used in an attempt to produce more reliable information. VERs were studied in US Navy divers, and reliable and significant differences were reported while the divers were breathing compressed air *versus* helium-oxygen mixtures at pressure. A further study using VERs during a shallow 2-week saturation exposure with excursion dives suggested that some adaptation to narcosis occurred, but it was not complete. Reduction of frequency and amplitude of alpha activity when compared with pre-exposure and post-exposure surface levels were also noted. Nevertheless, the value of current methods of measurement of IGN, by the use of neurophysiological changes, is questionable.

AETIOLOGY

IGN is thought to be produced by the same mechanism as general anaesthesia with gases or volatile liquids. The inert gases and most volatile anaesthetic agents are simple molecules with no common structural feature, and they do not undergo chemical change in the body to exert their effect. This property suggests that a physical rather than chemical effect must be involved, and most research is based on the hypothesis that the mechanism is the same for all agents (the unitary hypothesis of narcosis). For this reason, the considerable efforts to understand the mechanism of action for anaesthetic agents are thought to have direct relevance for IGN.

At the turn of the twentieth century, Meyer and Overton noted a strong correlation between the lipid solubility of an anaesthetic agent and its narcotic potency, and this relationship has become known as the *Meyer-Overton Hypothesis*. Later, in 1923, Meyer and Hopf stated 'all gaseous and volatile substances induce narcosis if they penetrate cell lipids in a definite molar concentration which is characteristic for each type of cell and is approximately the same for all narcotics'. This means that the higher the oil-water partition coefficient (relative solubility) the more potent the inert gas. The hypothesis is that inert gas molecules are dissolved in the lipid membranes of neurons and somehow interfere with cell membrane function so that the higher the proportion of an agent dissolved in lipid, the more potent the agent as a narcotic (anaesthetic). In truth, it has long been realized there is more to anaesthetic action than this because there are some discrepancies in this relationship (Figure 15.2). For example, although both neon and hydrogen have been shown to be narcotic, neon appears to be more so despite a similar oil-water partition coefficient, and argon is about twice as narcotic as nitrogen but again has a similar oil-water solubility ratio. There are also anomalies among the volatile anaesthetics agents, but, in general, the relationship is much closer than with other physical properties. Intravenous general

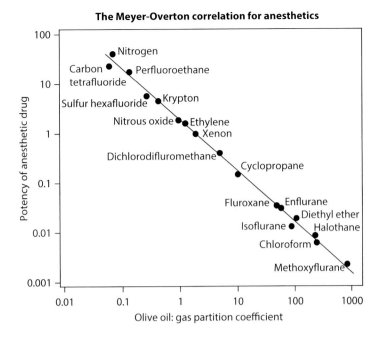

Figure 15.2 Graphical representation of the Meyer Overton hypothesis. Note the position of nitrogen as the least potent of the charted narcotic agents.

anaesthetic agents (e.g. thiopentone and propofol) do not fit this relationship and almost certainly produce narcosis through a different mechanism.

The *lipid solubility hypothesis* has been extended by the *critical volume* concept[10]. Here, the consequence of the narcotic agent dissolved in the lipid membrane is proposed to cause swelling of the membrane. At a critical volume, the swollen membrane somehow produces the clinical features of anaesthesia. Thus, there is a lipid volume change that differentiates the anaesthetized from the unanaesthetized state. Other factors, in particular pressure compressibility of the lipid, also affect volume. That some narcotic effects can be reversed by application of increased hydrostatic pressure lends weight to this hypothesis. (See also Chapter 20, on the high pressure neurological syndrome [HPNS]).

Exceptions in both animal and human studies have led to a further refinement – the *multi-site expansion model*[11]. This model postulates that expansion occurs variably at more than one molecular site and that pressure does not act equally at the same sites. Thus, hydrostatic pressure effects (see Chapter 20) or narcotic effects may predominate.

The *physical theories,* in general, support the concept that the site of action is a hydrophobic portion of the cell, the traditional view being that this is the cell membrane. Many studies show that membranes are resistant to the effects of anaesthetics, and other sites have been sought, such as the hydrophobic regions of proteins or lipoproteins. More recent studies have suggested that the site of action is a protein, rather than a lipid, and that narcotics act by competitive binding to specific receptors, thus affecting synaptic transmission. It has even been postulated that although impairment of cognitive function is a result of the inert gas narcotic effect, impaired motor ability is a consequence of raised hydrostatic pressure *per se*[12]. Not all experimental observations are easily reconciled, and the definitive description of the mechanism of action for volatile anaesthetic agents at the molecular level remains to be elucidated. For those interested in delving deeper into this area, see Pleuvry[13].

The site of action is most likely at a synaptic level, and many studies have looked at inhibitory and excitatory neurotransmitters and receptors in the central nervous system. Neurotransmitters studied include noradrenaline (norepinephrine), serotonin, dopamine, gamma-aminobutyric acid (GABA) and glycine. GABA is the most important inhibitory transmitter in the brain. Potentiation of inhibitory pathway synapse receptors (GABA receptors) is suspected to be a major component of IGN/anaesthesia, although action at a wide variety of neuronal sites is likely.

Exposure to narcosis raises extracellular dopamine in the area of the brain controlling the extrapyramidal system, at least in rats. This action may account for some of the neuromuscular disturbances of IGN. In contrast, dopamine is increased when HPNS is exhibited (see Chapter 20).

PREVENTION

In its simplest terms, prevention comes by avoiding exposure to partial pressures of inert gas known to produce intoxication. In practice, safe diving on compressed air requires an awareness of the condition and its effect on performance and judgement at depths greater than 30 metres. The maximum depth limit for an air dive should be between 30 and 50 metres, depending on the diver's experience and the task to be performed. Safe diving at a greater depth requires the substitution of a less narcotic agent to dilute the oxygen, such as helium, neon or hydrogen (one form of 'technical' diving).

There is a firm belief among divers that adaptation to IGN can develop over repeated daily exposures and that one can therefore 'work up' to deep dives. Several studies have shown that, although subjective adaptation can occur, measurement of standing steadiness or reaction time showed no improvement with repeated exposure[3]. As with alcohol, confidence is not matched by performance, thus possibly compromising safety.

Saturation at depths between 30 and 40 metres is said to allow the development of adaptation. Excursion dives to greater depths can then be made with more safety and improved work performance. A conventional working dive to 100 metres would be inconceivable using air as the breathing medium. However, operational dives may be performed to 100 metres if the excursion is from a saturated depth of 40 metres. At that depth, the diver becomes acclimatized to the nitrogen narcosis, with a progressive improvement of job performance, approaching 'surface' efficiency.

For most contemporary deep diving, the effect of IGN is avoided by substituting helium, or helium-nitrogen, as the diluent gases for oxygen. Oxygen cannot, of course, be used alone because of its toxicity at high pressure (see Chapter 17), but it can partially replace nitrogen in various nitrox mixtures. Hydrogen is also being used as a substitute for nitrogen and would be ideal except for the formation of an explosive mixture with oxygen.

Evidence that helium also has some narcotic effect arises from the observation that HPNS is not the same under hydrostatic pressure as it is under helium pressure. It has been postulated that both helium and oxygen need to be considered when calculating the narcotic effects of respired gases under great pressure[14].

Although amphetamines ameliorate narcotic slowing of reaction time, the use of drugs to reduce narcosis has, as yet, no place in diving. Conversely, divers should be warned of the risks of taking central nervous system depressant drugs, which, in the diver, may include alcohol, sedating antihistamines (in cold and sinus preparations) and anti–motion sickness drugs. These drugs may act synergistically with nitrogen in impairing performance and judgment, although this has been clearly shown only with alcohol[15].

REFERENCES

1. Bennett PB, Rostain JC. Inert gas narcosis. In: Brubakk AO, Neuman TS, eds. *Bennett and Elliott's Physiology and Medicine of Diving*. 5th ed. London: Saunders; 2003.
2. Hobbs M. Subjective and behavioural responses to nitrogen narcosis and alcohol. *Undersea and Hyperbaric Medicine* 2008;**35**(3):175–184.
3. Hamilton K, Laliberté MF, Fowler B. Dissociation of the behavioral and subjective components of nitrogen narcosis and diver adaptation. *Undersea and Hyperbaric Medicine* 1995;**22**(1):41–49.
4. Mekjavic IB, Passias T, Sundberg CJ, Ceiken O. Perception of thermal comfort during narcosis. *Undersea and Hyperbaric Medicine* 1994;**21**(1):9–19.

5. Mekjavic IB, Savic SA, Eiken O. Nitrogen narcosis attenuates shivering thermo-genesis. *Journal of Applied Physiology* 1995;**78**(6):2241–2244.

6. Cousteau JY. *The Silent World*. London: Reprint Society; 1954.

7. Fowler B, Ackles KN, Porlier G. Effects of inert gas narcosis on behavior: a critical review. *Undersea Biomedical Research* 1985;**12**:369–402.

8. Löftdahl P, Andersson D, Bennett M. Nitrogen narcosis and emotional processing during compressed air breathing. *Aviation Space and Environmental Medicine* 2012;**83**:1–5.

9. Balestra C, Lafère P, Germonpré P. Persistence of critical flicker fusion frequency impairment after a 33 msw SCUBA dive: evidence of prolonged nitrogen narcosis? *European Journal of Applied Physiology* 2012;**112**(12):4063–4068.

10. Miller KW, Paton WDM, Smith DA, Smith, EB. The pressure reversal of general anaesthesia and the critical volume hypothesis. *Molecular Pharmacology* 1973;**9**:131–143.

11. Halsey MJ, Wardley-Smith B, Green CJ. Pressure reversal of general anaesthesia: a multi-site expansion model. *British Journal of Anaesthesia* 1978;**50**:1091–1097.

12. Abraini JH. Inert gas and raised pressure: evidence that motor decrements are due to pressure per se and cognitive decrements due to narcotic action. *European Journal of Physiology* 1997;**433**:788–791.

13. Pleuvry BJ. Mechanism of action of general anaesthetic drugs. *Anaesthesia and Intensive Care Medicine* 2008;**5**(4):152–153.

14. Abraini JH. Some considerations regarding the narcotic potency of helium and oxygen in humans. In: Rostain JC, Marquis RE, eds. *Basic and Applied High Pressure Biology IV*. Medsubhyp Int 1995;**5**:77–82.

15. Fowler B, Hamilton K, Porlier G. Effects of ethanol and amphetamine on inert gas narcosis in humans. *Undersea Biomedical Research* 1986;**13**:345–354.

This chapter was reviewed for this fifth edition by Michael Bennett.

16

Hypoxia

INTRODUCTION

Hypoxia in the context of human physiology means an oxygen (O_2) deficiency, or a lower than normal partial pressure of O_2 (PO_2; also called the O_2 *tension*), in the tissue in question. The term strongly implies inadequate O_2 availability to bodily tissues. The brain, liver and kidney, which extract the greatest amount of O_2 from the blood to supply their energy requirements, are the first affected by falling O_2 levels in the body. Skin, muscle and bone are less vulnerable because of their lower energy requirements. O_2 does not directly supply the energy but is necessary to liberate the energy required for cellular metabolism from sugar (glucose).

Aerobic *('with O_2')* metabolism is much more efficient in the production of biological energy than anaerobic metabolism *('without O_2')* and is the key to complex life on Earth. For example, in the presence of O_2, 1 molecule of glucose can produce 38 molecules of the energy storage compound adenosine triphosphate (ATP), whereas in the absence of O_2, 1 molecule of glucose produces only 2 molecules of ATP (via the production of lactic acid). Thus, anaerobic conditions (hypoxia) drastically reduce the available energy.

Dry air, at a barometric pressure of 760 mm Hg, has a PO_2 of 159 mm Hg. When inspired, dry air becomes saturated with water vapour at body temperature. By this dilution the PO_2 drops to 149 mm Hg. Alveolar gas has a lower PO_2 than inspired air because it is further diluted by carbon dioxide (CO_2) and contact with de-oxygenated blood, to around 105 mm Hg. O_2 freely diffuses into the capillaries in the lung so that normal arterial blood levels are in the region of 100 mm Hg. As the blood moves through the tissue capillaries, O_2 moves by diffusion down partial pressure gradients to the cells, where it is consumed (Figure 16.1). After passage through the tissues the PO_2 falls to approximately 40 mm Hg in mixed venous blood coming back into the lungs.

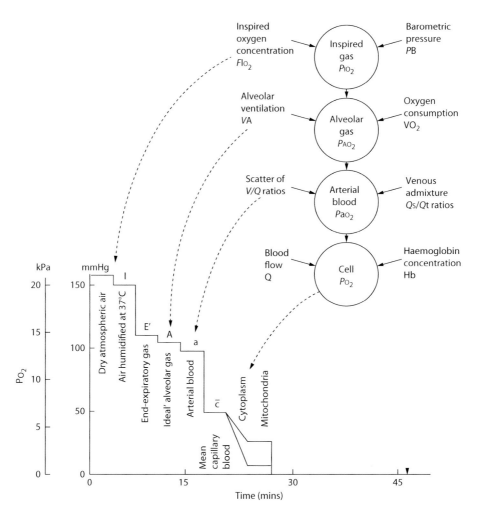

Figure 16.1 The oxygen cascade. On the left is shown the cascade with partial pressure of oxygen (PO_2) falling from the level in the ambient air down to the level in mitochondria, the site of utilization. On the right is shown a summary of factors influencing oxygenation at different levels in the cascade. (Redrawn from Nunn JF. *Applied Respiratory Physiology*. 3rd ed. London: Butterworth; 1987.)

The amount of O_2 stored in the body is limited, as are the high-energy phosphate bonds used to store energy. A person breathing air at sea level would hold approximately the following amounts of O_2, not all of which is available for use in vital organs such as the brain or heart:

In the lungs	450 ml
In the blood	850 ml
Dissolved in body fluids	50 ml
Bound to myoglobin in muscle	200 ml
	Total = 1550 ml

The result is that, unlike diving mammals, we do not have much reserve capacity and cannot stop breathing for long before severe hypoxia intervenes (Table 16.1). During a breath-hold, we are protected from hypoxia because our breakpoint is usually determined by the rising carbon dioxide tension. Hyperventilation prior to breath-holding reduces arterial carbon dioxide tension and extends our breakpoint, but at the risk of unconsciousness from hypoxia.

Basal O_2 consumption is of the order of 200 ml/minute, but in swimming and diving much higher

Table 16.1 Effects of hyperventilation on the breath-holding time and alveolar gas pressure at the breaking point in resting and exercising man

Effect	Without hyperventilation	With hyperventilation
Measurements while resting		
BH time (sec)	87	146
End-tidal PCO_2 (mm Hg)		
Before BH	40	21
Breaking point	51	46
End-tidal PO_2 (mm Hg)		
Before BH	103	131
Breaking point	73	58
Measurements while exercising		
BH time (sec)	62	85
End-tidal PCO_2 (mm Hg)		
Before BH	38	22
Breaking point	54	49
End-tidal PO_2 (mm Hg)		
Before BH	102	130
Breaking point	54	43

BH, breath-holding; PCO_2, partial pressure of carbon dioxide; PO_2, partial pressure of oxygen.
Source: From Craig AB. Causes of loss of consciousness during underwater swimming. *Journal of Applied Physiology* 1961;**16**:583–586.

consumption is possible (up to 3 litres/minute [lpm]). This explains why hypoxia develops so rapidly if respiration has stopped while exercise continues.

The delivery of O_2 at the cellular level requires an adequate inspired PO_2 (PIO_2), adequate lung function and adequate cardiac output. Further, because most O_2 in the blood is carried bound to haemoglobin, it also requires adequate functional haemoglobin levels. At arterial PO_2 (PaO_2) below 60 mm Hg, the amount of O_2 given up to the tissue is greatly reduced.

Although impairment of aerobic metabolism is probably the ultimate mechanism of death in most fatal diving accidents, hypoxia as a primary event is uncommon in conventional scuba diving (breathing air or nitrox). It is much more likely with mixed gas and rebreathing equipment.

The diving disorders mentioned here are discussed more fully in their specific chapters.

CLINICAL FEATURES

The physiological consequences of hypoxia in general medicine are well known and are not discussed here.

The symptoms and signs of hypoxia become obvious when the PaO_2 drops below about 50 mm Hg. This corresponds to an inspired concentration at sea level of 8 to 10 per cent. If the fall in PO_2 is rapid, then loss of consciousness may be unheralded. With slower falls, an observer may note lack of coordination or poor job performance. Euphoria, overconfidence and apathy are also been reported. Memory is defective and judgement impaired, leading to inappropriate or dangerous reactions to the emergency that may also endanger others. The diver may complain of fatigue, headache or blurred vision.

There are rarely any symptoms to warn the diver of impending unconsciousness from hypoxia.

Hyperventilation may develop in some cases, but it is usually minimal if the arterial CO_2 tension ($PaCO_2$) is normal or low.

There are marked individual differences in susceptibility to hypoxia. When combined with hypocapnia or hypercapnia, hypoxia will impair mental performance earlier than if the diver is normocapnic; mental performance may not be severely impaired until the alveolar-arterial PO_2 falls below 40 mm Hg. Hypoxia may precipitate or exacerbate other pathological conditions, such as coronary or cerebral ischaemia.

Cyanosis of the lips and nail beds may be difficult to determine in the peripherally vasoconstricted 'cold and blue' diver. Generalized convulsions or other neurological manifestations may be the first signs. Masseter spasm is common and may interfere with resuscitation. Eventually, respiratory failure, cardiac arrest and death supervene.

Diagnostic errors may arise because some of the foregoing manifestations are common to nitrogen narcosis, O_2 toxicity and CO_2 retention. The attending physician should also consider cerebral arterial gas embolism and decompression sickness (DCS), should the previously described features develop during or after ascent by a diver breathing compressed gases.

CLASSIFICATION

Hypoxia ('anoxia') has been classified into four types:

1. Hypoxic.
2. Stagnant.
3. Anaemic.
4. Histotoxic.

Hypoxic hypoxia

This designation covers all conditions leading to a reduction in arterial O_2 (Figure 16.2). A better term would be 'hypoxaemic hypoxia'. This is the common form of hypoxia seen in diving. Causes of hypoxaemia, with examples related to diving, are discussed in the following paragraphs.

INADEQUATE OXYGEN SUPPLY

This condition results from a decrease in O_2 pressure in the inspired gas, which may in turn be caused by an incorrect gas mixture or equipment failure. CO_2 retention is not a feature of this type of hypoxaemia.

ALVEOLAR HYPOVENTILATION

This condition occurs when the amount of gas flowing in and out of functioning alveoli per unit time is reduced. It may result from increased density of gases with depth or decreased compliance with the drowning syndromes, among other causes. The extreme example is breath-holding diving. There is associated CO_2 retention.

VENTILATION-PERFUSION INEQUALITY AND SHUNT

Perfusion of blood past alveoli that are not being ventilated causes non-oxygenated blood to move into the systemic circulation. This blood is referred to as a 'right-to-left shunt' because blood is shunted from the right side of the heart through the lungs but without picking up O_2 or releasing CO_2. The degree of arterial desaturation depends on the proportion of the cardiac output that is shunted (the shunt fraction). Lesser degrees of mismatching of perfusion and ventilation may be seen in near drowning, salt water aspiration syndrome, pulmonary O_2 toxicity and pneumothorax. Inequality of ventilation and perfusion may also occur in pulmonary DCS sickness and pulmonary barotrauma, as well as in deep divers using helium, in whom it is a consequence of lung cooling.

The arterial CO_2 response is variable with ventilation-perfusion disorders, with high levels in severe cases, but mild hypocapnia (low partial pressure of CO_2 [PCO_2]) is more usual if ventilation in the perfused lung is increased by hypoxic drive.

DIFFUSION DEFECT

This defect results from slowed diffusion of O_2 through a thickened alveolar-capillary barrier. This may occur after near drowning and as a result of pulmonary O_2 toxicity. CO_2 retention is not characteristic of this type of hypoxaemia because CO_2 diffuses through the barrier much more rapidly than O_2.

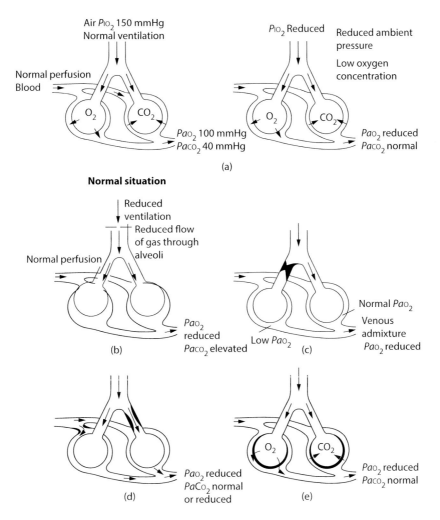

Figure 16.2 Mechanisms of hypoxaemia (hypoxic hypoxia). **(a)** Inadequate oxygen supply. **(b)** Alveolar hypoventilation. **(c)** Perfusion of non-ventilated alveoli causing venous admixture. **(d)** Ventilation-perfusion inequality. **(e)** Diffusion defect. $PaCO_2$, arterial partial pressure of carbon dioxide; PaO_2, arterial partial pressure of oxygen; PIO_2, inspired oxygen tension.

There is obviously great overlap among the different mechanisms by which the various conditions produce hypoxaemia.

Stagnant (ischaemic) hypoxia

Reduced tissue blood perfusion leads to hypoxia as a result of the continued metabolism of O_2 in the presence of a reduced supply, and it may be either regional or general. The extreme form is circulatory arrest. Syncope of ascent is a transitory manifestation resulting from inadequate cardiac output (see Chapters 6 and 47).

Reduced cardiac output may also be present in serious DCS when local ischaemia results from gas bubbles obstructing venous return. In addition, reduced cardiac output may be caused by gas emboli arising in both DCS and pulmonary barotrauma.

Many marine venoms induce stagnant hypoxia, and localized ischaemia is the cause of many of the symptoms and signs of these envenomations.

Anaemic hypoxia

This designation refers to any condition characterized by a reduction in haemoglobin concentration in the blood or alterations in the O_2-carrying capacity of haemoglobin. One cause is traumatic haemorrhage, with restoration of the blood volume with fluids.

Carbon monoxide poisoning (see Chapter 19), in which the formation of carboxyhaemoglobin reduces the O_2-carrying capacity of the blood, is most often a consequence of contamination of compressed air.

The capacity of haemoglobin to carry O_2 is also reduced in the presence of alkalaemia, e.g. low $PaCO_2$, and hypothermia.

Histotoxic hypoxia

This term refers to the situation in which adequate O_2 is delivered to the tissues, but there is a failure of utilization within the cell. Carbon monoxide poisons the enzyme cytochrome oxidase, which is a vital link in the use of O_2 to provide energy for normal cell function. Histotoxic hypoxia has also been postulated as a mechanism for inert gas narcosis (see Chapter 15) and O_2 toxicity (see Chapter 17).

HYPOXIA AND DIVING EQUIPMENT

Hypoxia secondary to inadequate inspired O_2 results from the failure or improper use of the diving equipment. Apart from running out of air on open-circuit scuba, this disorder occurs mainly with the use of closed-circuit or semi-closed-circuit rebreathing apparatus.

Of the following six causes only the first two mechanisms are possible with open-circuit scuba:

1. Exhaustion of gas supply.
2. Low O_2 concentration.
3. Inadequate flow rates.
4. Increased O_2 consumption.
5. Dilution hypoxia.
6. Hypoxia of ascent.

Exhaustion of gas supply

The 'out of air' situation remains a major cause of diving accidents, despite contents gauges, reserve supplies and training (Case Report 16.1).

Low oxygen concentration in the gas supply

Accidental filling of an air cylinder with another gas, such as nitrogen, may result in unconsciousness. Low-percentage O_2 mixtures (10 per cent O_2 or less), designed for use in deep or saturation diving, would lead to hypoxia if breathed near the surface.

Rusting (oxidization) of scuba cylinders can reduce the O_2 content, and It has led to at least one fatality and several 'near misses' (Case Report 16.2).

Inadequate flow rates

Many rebreathing diving sets have a constant flow of gas into the counterlung (see Chapters 4 and 62 for an explanation of this equipment). A set designed to use various gas mixtures has a means of adjusting these flow rates. The flow rate should be set to supply enough O_2 for the diver's maximum requirements, in addition to that lost through the exhaust valve. The higher the O_2 concentration of the gas, the lower the required flow rate will be, and *vice versa*.

If an inadequate flow rate is set for the O_2 mixture used, then the inert gas (e.g. nitrogen) will accumulate in the counterlung. Low concentrations of O_2 will then be inspired by the diver (Case Report 16.3). Other causes include blockage of the reducer by ice, particles among others.

Increased oxygen consumption

Most rebreathing sets are designed for maximum O_2 consumption between 1 and 2.5 lpm depending on the anticipated exertion. Commonly, the maximum O_2 uptake is assumed to be 1.5 lpm. Several studies have shown that divers can consume O_2 at higher rates than these. Values of more than 2.5 lpm for 30 minutes and more than 3 lpm for 10 to 15 minutes have been recorded without excessive fatigue underwater.

CASE REPORT 16.1

Two commercial divers were engaged in making a 110-metre mixed gas dive from a diving bell. The purpose of the dive was to tie in a 6-inch riser. While one diver was in the water at depth working on the riser, the diving bell operator excitedly informed topside that the bell was losing pressure and flooding. The surface operator, who was disconcerted by this information, opened valves to send gas to the bell. Communication with the bell operator was lost.

The diver who was in the water working on the riser was instructed to return to the bell, which he did. When the diver arrived at the bell, he found the bell operator unconscious and lying on the deck of the bell. The diver climbed out of the water into the bell, took off his Kirby-Morgan mask, and promptly collapsed. When topside personnel realized that they had completely lost communications with the bell, they made ready the standby divers. The first standby diver was dressed, put on his diving helmet and promptly collapsed unconscious on deck. At this point the bell with the diver and the bell operator was brought to the surface with the hatch open and without any decompression stops. The divers were extricated from the bell and recompressed in a deck decompression chamber. Both the diver and the bell operator died in the deck decompression chamber at 50 metres, of fulminating decompression sickness.

Examination of the rack (the collection of gas cylinders to be used during the dive) showed that the rack operator had mistakenly opened a cross-connect valve that should have been 'tagged out' (labeled to indicate that it should not be used). This valve permitted 100 per cent helium to be delivered to the diving bell and the standby divers, instead of the appropriate helium-oxygen breathing mixture.

Diagnosis: acute hypoxia and fulminant decompression sickness.

CASE REPORT 16.2

MB, a civilian diver, was asked to cut free a rope that was wrapped around the propeller of a diver's charter boat. Because of the very shallow nature of the dive (3 metres maximum), he used a small steel cylinder not often used by divers. After he entered the water, his diving partner noticed that he was acting in a strange manner and swam to him. At this point the diver was lying on the bottom and was unconscious but still breathing through his single hose regulator. The diving partner rescued the unconscious diver and got him on deck. His fellow divers prised the mouthpiece from him and gave him cardiopulmonary resuscitation, and the diver promptly regained consciousness.

On analysis, the gas in the cylinder was found to be 98 per cent nitrogen and 2 per cent oxygen. There was sea water present in the interior of the cylinder, together with a considerable amount of rust.

Diagnosis: acute hypoxia resulting from low inspired oxygen(see Chapters 6 and 47) concentration.

This increased exertion may be tolerated because of the cooling effect of the environment and/or greater tissue utilization with increased amount of O_2 physically dissolved in the plasma. This indicates that it is possible for a diver to consume O_2 at a greater than the often quoted rate under certain conditions. In rebreathing sets, a hypoxic mixture could then develop in the counterlung in response to accumulation of nitrogen (i.e. dilution hypoxia).

Dilution hypoxia

This term applies mainly to O_2 rebreathing sets. Dilution hypoxia is caused by dilution of the O_2 in the counterlung by inert gas, usually nitrogen.

CASE REPORT 16.3

AS was diving to 20 metres using a 60/40 oxygen-nitrogen mixture in a semi-closed-circuit rebreathing system. After 15 minutes he noted difficulty in obtaining enough gas. He stopped to try and adjust his relief valve and then suddenly lost consciousness. Another diver noticed him lying face down on the bottom. The second diver flushed the unconscious diver's counterlung with gas and took him to the surface, after which the set was turned to atmosphere, so that the diver was breathing air. The diver started to regain consciousness but was initially still cyanosed. He became aware of his surroundings and did not require further resuscitation. Equipment investigation revealed that carbon dioxide absorbent activity was normal, but reducer flow was set at 2 lpm instead of the required 6 lpm. This would supply inadequate oxygen for the diver's expected rate of utilization.

Diagnosis: hypoxia resulting from inadequate gas flow rate.

CASE REPORT 16.4

RAB was diving to 22 metres while using a semi-closed-circuit rebreathing set with a 40/60 oxygen-nitrogen mixture. After 36 minutes he was instructed to ascend slowly. At approximately 3 to 4 metres he noted some difficulty in breathing but continued to ascend and then started to climb on board, but he appeared to have some difficulty with this. When asked whether he was well he did not answer. He was cyanosed around the lips, and his teeth were firmly clenched on the mouthpiece. On removal of his set and administration of oxygen, he recovered rapidly but remained totally amnesic for 10 minutes. Examination of his diving equipment revealed that both main cylinders were empty and the emergency supply had not been used.

Diagnosis: hypoxia of ascent.

The unwanted nitrogen may enter the system by three methods:

1. From the gas supply.
2. From failure to clear the counterlung of air before use, thus leaving a litre or more nitrogen in it.
3. Failure to clear the lungs before using the equipment; e.g. if a diver breathes into the set after a full inhalation, he or she may add up to 3 litres of nitrogen to the counterlung. This may also occur if the diver surfaces and breathes from the atmosphere, to report activities or for some other reason.

Dilution hypoxia is more likely if O_2 is supplied only 'on demand' (i.e. when the counterlung is empty), rather than having a constant flow of gas into the bag. As the diver continues to use up the O_2, the nitrogen remains in the counterlung.

CO_2 will continue to be removed by the absorbent, thereby avoiding dyspnoea. Thus, the percentage of O_2 in the inspired gas falls as it is consumed. There is approximately 1 litre of nitrogen dissolved in the body, but the amount that would diffuse out into the counterlung to cause dilution hypoxia would be a small contribution.

Hypoxia of ascent

By one of the foregoing mechanisms, the percentage of O_2 being inspired may drop to well below 20 per cent. An inspired O_2 concentration of 10 per cent can be breathed quite safely at 10 metres because the partial pressure would still be adequate (approximately 140 mm Hg).

Hypoxia develops when the diver ascends sufficiently to reduce this PO_2 to a critical level (Case Report 16.4). The disorder is therefore most likely to develop at or near the surface.

HYPOXIA AND BREATH-HOLD DIVING

In a simple breath-hold, with no immersion or preceding hyperventilation, the breaking point (the irresistible urge to breathe) is initiated mainly by a rise in CO_2 level, and to a lesser extent by a fall in arterial O_2.

In breath-hold diving, hypoxic blackout is sometimes called breath-hold syncope or shallow water blackout. Because 'shallow water blackout' was first used in 1944 to describe loss of consciousness from the use of closed-circuit diving suits, it is best avoided in the breath-holding context. 'Hypoxic blackout' is a reasonable alternative.

There are two causes of this disorder – hyperventilation and ascent – and because they may occur concurrently, they are often confused. The hyperventilation effect is independent of depth and may be encountered in 1-meter-deep swimming pools, often by children trying to swim greater distances underwater.

Breath-hold divers who train to extend their breath-hold and also dive deep (e.g. free diving competitors, spear fishing) risk hypoxia of ascent, with loss of consciousness and subsequent drowning.

With hypoxia there is little or no warning of impending unconsciousness. With increased experience the breath-hold diver can delay the need to inhale by various techniques, without improving the O_2 status. Breath-hold time can be extended (but not with increased safety) by, for example, feet-first descent, training (adaptation), swallowing, inhaling against a closed glottis and diaphragmatic contractions.

One way of avoiding this hypoxia is to inhale 100 per cent O_2 before the breath-hold.

Hyperventilation

In 1961, Craig observed that swimmers who hyperventilated could stay longer underwater but then lose consciousness with little or no warning[1]. They were often competing, against others or themselves, and often exercising. The hyperventilation extended their breath-holding time because it washed out a large amount of CO_2 from the lungs, often to half the normal levels.

The build-up of CO_2 is the main stimulus forcing the swimmer to surface and breathe. After hyperventilating it takes much longer for this level (the 'breaking point') to be reached. Under these conditions, the diver may extend the breath-hold to the point that PaO_2 drops to a level inadequate to sustain consciousness. Increased exercise exacerbates this effect by increasing O_2 consumption.

The combination of these two effects (hyperventilation and exercise) can be deadly. One can demonstrate this dangerous combination in the following experiment: When the swimmer is concentrating on some purposeful goal, such as trying to spear a fish or retrieve a catch, he or she is more likely to ignore the physiological warning symptoms of an urge to breathe (resulting from the rise in CO_2 level in the blood) and delay the breaking point.

The dangers of hyperventilation and breath-hold diving are diagrammatically illustrated in Figure 16.3. It illustrates that, with earlier hyperventilation, the time to reach the irresistible urge to breathe (the breaking point) is prolonged. This extra time may allow the PaO_2 to fall to dangerous levels (hypoxic danger zone).

Ascent

Ascent hypoxia was first described in military divers losing consciousness as they surfaced with low O_2 levels in their rebreathing equipment.

In breath-hold divers, with descent the pressure rises proportionately in the alveolar gases, thus increasing the available O_2, CO_2 and nitrogen. Some O_2 can be absorbed and used, some CO_2 absorbed and buffered, and some nitrogen absorbed and deposited in tissues.

Thus, if a diver having 100 mm Hg O_2 and 40 mm Hg CO_2 in the alveolar gases was immediately transported to 2 ATA, the lungs would halve their volume; the O_2 would be 200 mm Hg, and the CO_2 80 mm Hg. Both would pass into the pulmonary capillary blood, the O_2 to be used and the CO_2 to be buffered. The alveolar PO_2 and PCO_2 therefore would decrease rapidly. By the time these values were both back to 'normal' levels, with O_2 at 100 mm Hg and CO_2 at 40 mm Hg, the diver would appear to be in a satisfactory respiratory status – until he or she ascended. With an expansion of the

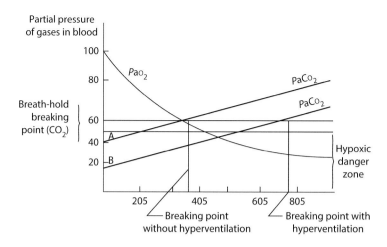

Figure 16.3 A diagrammatic representation of changes in arterial oxygen and carbon dioxide levels with breath-holding. Point A, without preceding hyperventilation; point B, with preceding hyperventilation. PaCO$_2$, arterial partial pressure of carbon dioxide; PaO$_2$, arterial partial pressure of oxygen.

lungs to twice their size at depth, the pressures in both gases would halve; i.e. the O$_2$ would drop to 50 mm Hg (approaching a potentially dangerous hypoxia level) and the CO$_2$ to 20 mm Hg – if the ascent was immediate.

Because ascents do take time, more O$_2$ will be consumed, extracted from the lungs during the ascent, and the CO$_2$ will increase toward normal as a result of the gradient between the pulmonary blood and alveoli.

The drop in O$_2$ is then able to produce the loss of consciousness, the 'syncope' or 'blackout', commonly noted among spear fishers. This condition is referred to as hypoxia of ascent. In deeper dives it becomes more likely, and with some very deep dives, the loss of consciousness may occur on the way to the surface in the top 10 metres (probably an explanation for the '7-metre syncope' described by French workers).

Other causes of hypoxia in breath-hold diving include salt water aspiration and the drowning syndromes (see Chapters 21, 22 and 24).

HYPOXIA AND DEEP DIVING

Animal experiments at great pressures are regularly undertaken to determine the limits of human exposure and thus ocean penetration. Ventilatory capacity is limited by restricted gas flow or increased work of breathing, both resulting from the effects of increased gas density or from pulmonary damage caused by the cooling effects on the lungs.

Hypoxia may be expected, as a result of such factors as an increased 'diffusion dead space' (caused by slowed diffusion of alveolar gases or incomplete mixing of fresh inspired gases and alveolar gases despite adequate inspired O$_2$ pressure and overall pulmonary ventilation).

The **Chouteau effect** (a disputed concept) is apparent clinical hypoxia despite normal inspired O$_2$ tension that, at least in goats, is rectified by a slight increase in the inspired O$_2$ tension (i.e. normoxic hypoxia). It has been explained by both an alveolar-arterial diffusion abnormality and a non-homogenous mixing of alveolar gas at very high pressures. Saltzman[2] has an alternative explanation, suggesting that at greater than 50 ATA there is decreased O$_2$ uptake, with decreased pH and increasing acidosis. Thus, there is a block in the utilization or transport of O$_2$.

MANAGEMENT

First aid management involves the basic principles of resuscitation, establishing an airway and ensuring that there is ventilation of the lungs and that the oxygenated blood is circulating; 100 per cent O$_2$ should be administered as soon as possible. Further management depends on the aetiology of the hypoxia.

In many cases there may be an overlap of different causes of tissue hypoxia, and all patients should receive a high inspired O_2 concentration.

Recompression or hyperbaric oxygenation may be indicated as a temporary measure to allow the foregoing regimens time to have an effect (see Chapters 6, 13 and 19).

Hypoxic hypoxia

These patients should be given supplemental inspired O_2 or ventilated with 100 per cent O_2 at whatever pressure is needed to ensure adequate arterial O_2 levels. Once these goals have been achieved, the pressure and percentage of O_2 can be progressively reduced while arterial gases or tissue O_2 is monitored by transcutaneous oximetry.

Stagnant hypoxia

The aim of therapy is to increase perfusion to the affected areas. This may require restoration of total circulatory volume, as well as vasodilator drugs, and hyperoxygenation as a temporary measure.

Anaemic hypoxia

Blood loss from trauma may require blood transfusion with packed red blood cells after crystalloid or colloid resuscitation. Synthetic blood substitutes show promise but have yet to be introduced to clinical practice.

In the case of carbon monoxide poisoning, hyperbaric oxygenation may be lifesaving during the early critical period.

Histotoxic hypoxia

This form of hypoxia can be treated only by removing the toxic substance and using hyperoxygenation as a temporary measure.

METHODS OF OXYGEN DELIVERY

There are various devices or apparatus for the therapeutic administration of O_2 (see also Chapter 49). Selection of the appropriate mode of administration depends on a number of factors:

1. Desired inspired O_2 concentration.
2. Need to avoid CO_2 accumulation.
3. Available O_2 (i.e. efficiency and economy).
4. Need to assist or control ventilation.
5. Acceptance of the method by the patient.

Various methods for the administration of O_2 are shown in Table 16.2 (see Chapter 49). Most plastic masks deliver less than 60 per cent of the

Table 16.2 Modes of oxygen therapy

Apparatus	Oxygen (lpm)	Concentration (%)
Nasal catheters	2–6	22–50
Semi-rigid masks (e.g. MC, Edinburgh, Hudson, Harris)	4–12	35–65
Venturi-type masks	4–8	24, 28, 35, 40, 50, 60
Soft plastic masks (e.g. Ventimask, Polymask)	4–8	40–80
Ventilators	Varying	21–100
Anaesthetic circuits	Varying	21–100
Demand valves	Varying	21–100
Hyperbaric oxygen	Varying	Varying

fraction of inspired O_2 unless a reservoir bag is incorporated, and this increases the risk of CO_2 retention.

REFERENCES

1. Craig AB. Causes of loss of consciousness during underwater swimming. *Journal of Applied Physiology* 1961;**16:**583–586.
2. Saltzman HA, Salzano JV, Blenkam GD, Kylstra JA. Effects of pressure on ventilation and gas exchange in man. *Journal of Applied Physiology* 1971;**30(4)**.

FURTHER READING

Andersson JPA, Liner MH, Runow E, Shagatay EKA. Diving response and arterial oxygen saturation during apnoea and exercise in breath-hold divers. *Journal of Applied Physiology* 2002;**93(3):**882–886.

Caine D, Watson DG. Neuropsychological and neuropathological sequelae of cerebral anoxia: a critical review. *Journal of the International Neuropsychological Society* 2000;**6:**86–99.

Dickinson P. Shallow water blackout. Drowning. Springer Berlin, Heidelberg 2014:571–575.

Lindholm P, Lundgren CEG. The physiology and pathophysiology of human breath-hold diving. *Journal of Applied Physiology* 2009;**106(1):**284–292.

Lumb A. Oxygen. In: Nunn's Applied Resipratory Physiology. 7th edition. Chapter 11. London: Churchill Livingstone; 2010.

Lundgren CEG, Ferrigno (eds). Physiology of breath-hold diving. 31st Undersea and Hyperbaric Medical Society Workshop. Undersea and Hyperbaric Medical Society: Kensington; 1985.

Schaefer KE. Circulatory adaptation to the requirements of life under more than one atmosphere of pressure. In: *Handbook of Physiology*. Section 2, *Circulation*. Volume 3. Washington, DC: American Physiology Society; 1965:1843–1873.

Sundal E, Irgens A, Troland K, Thorsen E, Gronning M. Prevalence and causes of loss of consciousness in former North Sea occupational divers. International Maritime Health 2013;**64(3):**142–7.

This chapter was reviewed for this fifth edition by Michael Bennett.

17

Oxygen toxicity

Oxygen toxicity is not encountered in routine scuba diving using compressed air. It is a consideration when higher partial pressures of oxygen are used in the inspired gas. Increased oxygen concentration and increased ambient pressure lead to higher partial pressures of oxygen. Divers may use high-oxygen gas compositions to reduce inert gas narcosis, reduce decompression obligations or prolong underwater time.

Central nervous system toxicity, manifested by convulsions, is potentially lethal in the diver.

Pulmonary toxicity is more likely in the longer exposures of saturation chamber diving or hyperbaric oxygen therapy.

Oxygen also has a major role in therapy of many diving disorders.

Toxicity can be avoided by controlling the inspired partial pressure of oxygen and/or the duration of exposure. It can be delayed by intermittent exposure.

INTRODUCTION

The normal partial pressure of oxygen (PO_2) in air is approximately 0.2 ATA. Although essential for survival, oxygen may become toxic at an elevated PO_2, and the complex systems we have for defending ourselves from oxygen toxicity are a testament to the evolutionary pressure to use this highly reactive molecule. A rise in the inspired oxygen fraction (FIO_2), an increase in the environmental pressure or a combination of both will elevate the inspired PO_2 (PIO_2).

High PIO_2 has several physiological effects on the body. Although increased PIO_2 has no direct effect on ventilation, there is a decrease in alveolar and arterial carbon dioxide (CO_2) buffering tension caused by the reduction in CO_2 carrying capacity of haemoglobin. Other physiological responses to high oxygen include vagally mediated bradycardia and vasoconstriction of intracranial and peripheral vessels. There is a small rate-dependent fall in cardiac output.

High PIO_2 is known to be associated with retinopathy of prematurity in pre-term infants and lung damage, convulsions, red blood cell suppression, visual defects, myopia and cataracts in adults. *In vitro*, toxic effects on cells of many other organs have also been demonstrated.

In diving, toxic effects on the central nervous system (CNS) and lungs are of prime importance, and only these are discussed in detail. The CNS threshold is above 1.5 ATA, and the pulmonary threshold is 0.55 ATA. At 1.6 ATA oxygen, pulmonary toxicity is the limiting factor regarding duration of exposure, whereas at higher pressures neurological toxicity is of prime concern.

In both the CNS and lungs there is a latent period before the onset of detectable toxicity. This delay enables high PO_2 to be used for increasingly short periods as the PIO_2 rises (Figure 17.1).

In diving and diving medicine, oxygen toxicity is possible in the following situations:

- Closed-circuit and semi-closed-circuit rebreathing equipment.
- Use of high FIO_2 mixtures.

- Saturation diving.
- Situations in which oxygen is used to shorten decompression times.
- Oxygen therapy for diving disorders (pulmonary only, and with prolonged use).
- Therapeutic recompression.
- Respiratory failure (e.g. near drowning).

HISTORY

Oxygen was 'discovered' in the latter half of the eighteenth century and immediately excited interest in its possible therapeutic effects. Following a series of experiments, in 1775 Priestley was among the first to suggest that there may be adverse effects of 'dephlogisticated air' – that is, air that was free from 'phlogiston', a substance thought to be released from a burning object[1]. Priestley had observed the rapid burning of a candle and speculated that 'the animal powers be too soon exhausted in this pure kind of air'. In fact, in 1772 Carl Scheele had already postulated the existence of a substance he called 'fire air' that supported combustion (later to be called 'oxygen' by Anton Lavoisier) following a similar experiment. Later, in 1789, Lavoisier and Sequin demonstrated that oxygen at 1 ATA does not alter oxidative metabolism but did note a damaging effect on the lungs.

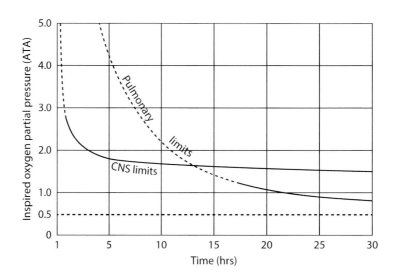

Figure 17.1 Predicted human pulmonary and central nervous system (CNS) tolerance to high-pressure oxygen.

In 1878, Paul Bert published his pioneer work *La pression barometrique,* in which he presented the results of years of study of the physiological effects of exposure to high and low pressures. He showed that although oxygen is essential to sustain life, it is lethal at high pressures. Larks exposed to air at 15 to 20 ATA developed convulsions. The same effect could be produced by oxygen at 5 ATA. Bert recorded similar convulsions in other species and clearly established the toxicity of oxygen on the CNS, also known as the *Paul Bert effect.* He did not report respiratory damage[1,2].

In 1899, the pathologist J. Lorrain Smith noted fatal pneumonia in a rat after exposure to 73 per cent oxygen at atmospheric pressure. He conducted further experiments on mice and gave the first detailed description of pulmonary changes resulting from moderately high oxygen tensions (approximately 1 ATA) for prolonged periods of time. Smith was aware of the limitations that this toxicity could place on the clinical use of oxygen. He also noted that early changes are reversible and that higher pressures shortened the time of onset. Pulmonary changes are also called the *Lorrain Smith effect.*

Although numerous animal studies were performed, evidence of the effect of high-pressure oxygen on humans was sparse until the 1930s. In 1933, two Royal Naval Officers, Damant and Philips, breathed oxygen at 4 ATA. Convulsive symptoms were reported at 16 and 13 minutes. Behnke then reported a series of exposures to hyperbaric oxygen. Exposure at 4 ATA terminated in acute syncope after 43 minutes in one subject and convulsions at 44 minutes in the other. At 3 ATA no effects were seen after 3 hours, but at 4 hours some subjects noted nausea and a sensation of impending collapse. At that time it was believed that 30 minutes of exposure at 4 ATA and 3 hours of exposure at 3 ATA were safe for men at rest. That the dose was important was confirmed in 1941 when Haldane reported a convulsion in less than 5 minutes at 7 ATA oxygen.

Meanwhile, at lower pressures, in 1939 Becker-Freyseng and Clamann found that 65 hours of exposure to 730 mm Hg oxygen at normal atmospheric pressure produced paraesthesiae, nausea and a decrease in vital capacity (VC).

At the beginning of World War II, some unexplained episodes of unconsciousness were noted in divers using closed-circuit rebreathing oxygen sets at what were considered safe depths. This prompted Donald, in 1942, to commence a series of experiments on oxygen poisoning (Figure 17.2)[3]. His observations in more than 2000 exposures form the basis of current oxygen diving limits. Unfortunately, many of his experiments were performed using rebreathing equipment, without CO_2 measurement. Among the more important findings were the marked variation of tolerance and the aggravating effects of exercise and underwater exposure. Donald suggested a maximum safe depth for oxygen diving of 8 metres.

Research since the 1980s has been primarily directed at elucidation of the mechanism of the toxicity. Workers have looked at such factors as the role of inert gas and CO_2, blockage of airways and atelectasis, changes in lung surfactant, changes in cellular metabolism, inhibition of enzyme system and the role of the endocrine system. Also, further efforts to delineate the pulmonary limits of exposure have been undertaken. This has become increasingly important with saturation diving

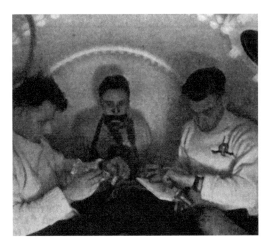

Figure 17.2 In 1942 and 1943, Donald carried out extensive testing for oxygen toxicity in divers. The chamber is pressurized with air to 3.7 bar. The subject in the centre is breathing 100 per cent oxygen from a mask. (From Donald KW. Oxygen poisoning in man: I, II. *British Medical Journal* 1947;**1**:667–672, 712–717.)

involving prolonged stays under increased ambient pressure and the use of oxygen mixtures to shorten decompression time.

AETIOLOGY

The precise mechanism of oxygen toxicity is unknown. Oxygen is a highly reactive element and has wide-ranging, dose-dependent effects in the body, including the regulation of blood flow, tissue oxygenation and energy metabolism in the brain. These effects are pressure dependent and are involved in the development of toxicity. There are a great many sites at which oxygen acts on metabolic pathways or on specific cellular functions. These sites may involve cell membranes, 'active transport', synaptic transmission, mitochondria or cell nuclei. Rather than causing an increase in metabolism, as suggested by early workers, hyperoxia has been demonstrated to depress cellular metabolism.

Many enzymes are inactivated by high PO_2, particularly those containing sulphydryl groups (-SH). It is postulated that adjacent -SH groups are oxidized to form disulphide bridges (-S-S-), thus inactivating the enzyme (this may be important in the development of cataracts). Enzymes containing -SH groups, and known to be susceptible, include glyceraldehyde phosphate dehydrogenase (a key enzyme in glycolysis), the flavoprotein enzymes of the respiratory chain and the enzymes involved in oxidative phosphorylation.

The *oxygen free radical theory of toxicity* is widely accepted as an explanation at the molecular level. The production of a range of free radicals is a normal consequence of aerobic metabolism, and for this reason, aerobic organisms (e.g. ourselves) have developed antioxidant mechanisms to cope with molecular oxygen exposure. In the presence of hyperoxia these mechanisms may be overwhelmed, leading to the formation of excess reactive oxygen forms and direct cellular toxicity through enzyme inactivation and structural damage (e.g. lipid peroxidation). These radicals are intermediates formed in many cellular biochemical enzyme catalyzed reactions and are the result of the reduction of the oxygen molecule by electrons. Superoxide anion (O_2^-) is formed when oxygen accepts a single electron and hydrogen peroxide (H_2O_2) two electrons. The final reaction is the acceptance by oxygen of four electrons to form water or a stable hydroxyl anion. Superoxide and peroxide can react to form the hydroxyl radical OH^-. All these species of oxygen, referred to as oxygen radicals, are highly oxidative.

Cells have a system of enzymes to scavenge these radicals called the tissue antioxidant system. Two of these enzymes, superoxide dismutase and catalase, are involved in maintaining adequate supplies of reduced glutathione (containing sulphydryl groups) to deal with the free radicals. Hyperoxia may cause this system to be swamped, and the excess free radicals may then produce cell damage. Examples of unwanted oxidation reactions are peroxidation of lipid in cell membranes and protein oxidation in cell membrane and cytoplasm. Both have been demonstrated in rat brain after hyperoxia[4]. Aerosolized (recombinant human manganese) superoxide dismutase preserves pulmonary gas exchange during hyperoxic lung injury in baboons[5]. Antioxidants such as glutathione have also been shown to offer some protection.

The characteristic feature of chronic pulmonary oxygen toxicity is pulmonary fibrosis (see later). In animal studies, paraquat, bleomycin and ozone have all been noted to produce pulmonary fibrosis. These agents are known to produce oxygen free radicals.

Gamma-aminobutyric acid (GABA) is a transmitter at CNS inhibitory nerve synapses. One of the demonstrated consequences of enzymatic changes induced by hyperoxia is a reduction in the endogenous output of GABA that results in the uncontrolled firing of excitatory nerves and the development of convulsions. Agents that raise brain levels of GABA appear to protect against convulsions. Lithium (useful in the treatment of bipolar disorder) has proved to be effective in inhibiting convulsions in rats. It was also shown to prevent the decrease in brain GABA that normally precedes the convulsions. In the rat lung lithium inhibits the development of oedema.

Exercise, hypoventilation and CO_2 inhalation predispose to convulsions, whereas hyperventilation may be protective. CO_2 may play a role in lowering seizure threshold at the cellular level, but more likely by influencing cerebral blood flow and hence the 'dose' of oxygen delivered to the brain.

At greater than 3 ATA PIO_2, oxyhaemoglobin is not reduced on passing through capillaries and so is not available for the carriage of CO_2 as carboxyhaemoglobin. Therefore, this route cannot eliminate CO_2. The resultant increase in brain CO_2 tension (PCO_2) has proved to be small (2.5 to 6 mm Hg). An equivalent rise is caused by breathing 6 per cent $FICO_2$ and does not cause convulsions in the presence of a normal PIO_2. It does, however, appear that the slight rise in PCO_2 reduces the cerebral vasoconstrictive effects of hyperoxia.

In contrast, CO_2 retention is unlikely to contribute to pulmonary toxicity, although related changes in acid-base balance may modify the syndrome via neurogenic and endocrine mechanisms. Very high levels of inspired CO_2 may actually protect against pulmonary damage.

Atelectasis (collapse of alveoli so they are no longer ventilated) results from absorption of oxygen during 100 per cent oxygen breathing and has been suggested as a contributory mechanism to oxygen toxicity in divers. Although atelectasis has been demonstrated, it is not an initiating factor, and toxicity also develops in the presence of inert gas. If the inert gas is at narcotic levels, it may actually enhance the onset of toxicity.

Human studies show no difference in the progression of pulmonary oxygen toxicity when comparing pure oxygen and diluted oxygen at the same PO_2. Rat studies indicate that the risk of CNS toxicity is enhanced by the presence of even small amounts of inert gas in the inspired mixture.

Endocrine studies show that hypophysectomy and adrenalectomy protect against hyperoxia. Adrenocorticotropic hormone (ACTH, corticotropin) and cortisone reverse this effect and, when given in normal animals, enhance toxicity. Adrenergic-blocking drugs, some anaesthetics, GABA, lithium, magnesium and superoxide dismutase have a protective effect. Adrenaline, atropine, aspirin, amphetamine and pentobarbital are among a host of agents that augment toxicity.

Light, noise and other stressful situations also affect CNS tolerance. Thus, the general stress reaction, and more specifically adrenal hormones, may have a role in enhancing CNS (and pulmonary) toxicity. Several observations suggest a role of the autonomic nervous system in modifying the degree of toxicity. Convulsions have been shown to hasten the onset of pulmonary oxygen toxicity in some animal studies. This may be related to an activation of the sympatho-adrenal system during convulsions.

Table 17.1 contains a list of factors that increase oxygen toxicity.

Table 17.1 Factors increasing oxygen toxicity

Physiological states	Gases
• Physical exercise	• Carbon dioxide
• Hyperthermia	• Nitrous oxide
• Immersion	• ? Inert gases
• Stress response	**Hormones and neurotransmitters**
Pathological states	• Insulin
• Fever	• Thyroxin
• Congenital spherocytosis	• ACTH
• Vitamin E deficiency	• Cortisol
Drugs	• Adrenaline, noradrenaline
• Amphetamine	• GABA
• Acetazolamide	**Chemicals**
• Aspirin	• Paraquat
• Atropine	• Ammonium chloride
• Disulfiram	**Trace metals**
• Guanethidine	• Iron
	• Copper

ACTH, adrenocorticotropic hormone; GABA; gamma-aminobutyric acid.

CENTRAL NERVOUS SYSTEM TOXICITY (THE 'PAUL BERT EFFECT')

In diving, CNS oxygen toxicity is more likely when closed-circuit or semi-closed-circuit rebreathing sets are used, and it is the factor limiting depth when oxygen supplementation is used. With compressed air, the effect of increased partial pressure of nitrogen (see Chapter 15) usually prevents the diver from reaching a depth and duration at which oxygen will become a problem (although occasional reports can be found). 'Technical' diving (see Chapter 62), in which a higher FIO_2 than air is commonly used, permits CNS toxicity (Case Report 17.1[6]). High oxygen pressures are used in therapeutic recompression for decompression sickness (DCS) and air embolism (see Chapters 6 and 13).

Clinical manifestations

A wide range of symptoms and signs has been described, the most dramatic of which is a grand mal–type convulsion. Consciousness is maintained up to the time of convulsion and there are apparently no changes in the electroencephalogram before convulsion.

In practice, there is no reliable warning of impending convulsions (but see Lambertsen's description later), and only about half of persons affected describe any premonitory symptoms. However, the list of such manifestations is long, and any unusual symptom should be suspect. The most commonly reported signs and symptoms are nausea, vomiting, light-headedness, dizziness, tinnitus, vertigo, incoordination, sensations of impending collapse or uneasiness (dysphoria), facial pallor, sweating, bradycardia, constriction of visual fields (tunnel vision), dazzle, lip twitching, dilatation of pupils, twitching of hand, muscular twitching elsewhere, hiccups, paraesthesiae (especially fingers), dyspnoea, disturbance of special senses, hallucinations and confusion.

Facial twitching is a common objective sign in chamber exposures to oxygen greater than 2 ATA, and it signifies an imminent convulsion.

CASE REPORT 17.1

A 47-year-old experienced underwater cave diver with no significant medical history was diving with two tanks – one containing compressed air, the other a 50 per cent mixture of oxygen and nitrogen (nitrox). Towards the end of the 47-metre, 19-minute dive, he was seen floating head down, unresponsive, with his mouthpiece out of his mouth and 'his fins [flippers] moving as if he was shivering' (as reported by another diver to the Coroner). The body was carried up to 15-metre depth and then allowed to ascend freely as the other divers decompressed. Cardiopulmonary resuscitation was attempted, but abandoned after 43 minutes, as there was no response.

Examination of the subject's diving equipment revealed that he had been breathing the 50 per cent oxygen/nitrogen mixture for most of the dive (at 47 metres, the PIO_2 would have been 5.7 ATA × 0.5, or 2.85 ATA). Each tank had a separate first stage connected in an unusual fashion by a two-way switch, which the diver had had made by a local engineering shop. This allowed the diver to switch from one tank to another rapidly. This switch supplied a single second-stage mouthpiece. The two tanks were different colours; the circuit from the black (compressed-air) tank was marked with yellow tape, while the circuit from the yellow (nitrox) tank was unmarked. The regulator had a small tear and a bite mark in the mouthpiece. The diver wore a face mask and separate mouthpiece rather than a full-face mask, which covers eyes, nose and mouth.

The *cause of death*, as determined by the Coroner, was drowning after oxygen toxicity.

(From Lawrence CH. A diving fatality due to oxygen toxicity during a 'technical' dive. *Medical Journal of Australia* 1996;**165**:262–263. ©Copyright 1996.*The Medical Journal of Australia*; reproduced with permission.)

Lip twitching may be seen if a mouthpiece is being used. Nausea, retching and vomiting are particularly noted after prolonged exposures between 1 and 2 ATA.

Central nervous system oxygen toxicity

- Twitching (especially lips).
- Nausea.
- Dizziness.
- Tinnitus.
- Tunnel vision.
- Dysphoria.
- Convulsions.

Many of these manifestations are associated with other potential causes. Facial pallor is thought to result from the intense peripheral vasoconstriction of hyperoxia and is not necessarily a sign of cerebral toxicity. Similarly, the paraesthesiae in fingers and toes do not necessarily indicate an impending convulsion. They may persist for hours after exposure and may represent an effect of local vasoconstriction on peripheral nerves or simply a tight-fitting wetsuit.

An important aspect of toxicity is the great variation in susceptibility. As well as the wide range of tolerance among individuals, there is marked variation in one person's tolerance from day to day[7]. Therefore, in any one diver, the time to onset of symptoms cannot be related to a predictable depth or time of exposure. Despite this variation, the greater the PO_2 and the longer the time of exposure, the more likely is the toxicity to develop.

Factors lowering threshold to central nervous system toxicity

- Severe exercise.
- Immersion in water rather than in air (e.g. a chamber).
- Hypothermia.
- Increased arterial carbon dioxide from any cause.

Exposure in water rather than in dry chambers markedly decreases the tolerance to oxygen. Many of the previously listed clinical features are much less apparent in the water, where convulsions are more often the first manifestation. A convulsion is much more dangerous under water because of the added complications of drowning and pulmonary barotrauma. Therefore, most authorities have set a maximum safe depth for pure oxygen diving at about 10 metres. Short dives may be safe at greater depths and prolonged ones at shallower depths (Table 17.2). Exposure in a compression chamber is considered to be less hazardous for an equivalent depth-time profile. Current decompression procedures, if performed in chambers, prescribe oxygen exposures at 18 metres (2.8 ATA), and seizure is rare.

Exercise has also been shown to hasten the onset of symptoms. Shallower maximum safe depths have been set for 'working' as opposed to 'resting' dives on oxygen. This observation is also of importance when oxygen is used to shorten decompression times in the water. Divers undergoing decompression should be at rest, e.g. supported on a stage – not battling swell, current and buoyancy to maintain constant depth. Hypothermia is likely to hasten the onset of symptoms.

Table 17.2 US Navy oxygen depth time limits in water

Normal operations			Exceptional operations		
Depth (ft)	Depth (m)	Time (min)	Depth (ft)	Depth (m)	Time (min)
10	3	240	30	9	45
15	4.6	150	35	10.7	25
20	6	110	40	12	10
25	7.6	75			

CO_2 build-up during exercise has been suggested as a potentiating factor in producing convulsions. Increased inspired PCO_2 may develop with inadequate absorbent systems and in poorly ventilated helmets and chambers, thus rendering the diver more susceptible to oxygen convulsions.

> The danger of convulsions prevents divers breathing 100 per cent oxygen deeper than 8 to 10 metres of sea water.

The role of inert gas in the exacerbation of oxygen toxicity needs to be more fully elucidated.

The frequency of presenting symptoms in 'wet' divers resting and working is shown in Table 17.3 from Donald's work[2,3]. In all cases exposure continued until the first symptoms developed ('end-point').

Convulsions, which may be the first manifestation of toxicity, are indistinguishable clinically from grand mal epilepsy (Case Reports 17.2, 17.3 and 17.4). A review of neurological toxicity in US Navy divers showed that convulsions were more likely to be the presenting feature in inexperienced divers breathing oxygen, compared with trained divers. It is inferred that some of the so-called premonitory symptoms may result from suggestion rather than oxygen. Of 63 divers, 25 had convulsions as the first clinical manifestation, 10 had focal twitching, and 13 more progressed to convulsions despite immediate reduction of PO_2. A more recent study revealed nausea as the most common manifestation, followed by muscle twitching and dizziness.

The following description of a typical convulsion has been given by Lambertsen[8], who performed much of the original work in the United States on this subject.

Localized muscular twitching, especially about the eyes, mouth and forehead usually but not always precedes the convulsion. Small muscles of the hands may also be involved, and incoordination of diaphragm activity in respiration may occur. After they begin, these phenomena increase in severity over a period, which may vary from a few minutes to nearly an hour, with essentially clear consciousness being retained. Eventually an abrupt spread of excitation occurs and the rigid tonic phase of the convulsion begins. Respiration ceases at this point and does not begin again until the intermittent muscular contractions return. The tonic phase usually lasts for about 30 seconds and is accompanied by an abrupt loss of consciousness. It is followed by vigorous clonic contractions of the muscle groups of head and neck, trunk and limbs, which become progressively less violent over about 1 minute. As the uncoordinated motor activity stops, respiration can proceed normally. Following the convulsion, hypercapnia is marked due to accumulation of carbon dioxide concurrent with breath holding. Respiration is complicated by obstruction from the tongue and by the extensive secretions, which result from the autonomic component of the central nervous system

Table 17.3 Incidence of symptoms resulting from exposure of divers to 'end-point' in water

Symptoms	388 resting divers (%)	120 working divers (%)
Convulsions	9.2	6.8
Lip twitching	60.6	50.0
Vertigo	8.8	20.8
Nausea	8.3	17.5
Respiratory disturbances	3.8	5.0
Twitching of parts other than lips	3.2	1.7
Sensation of abnormality (e.g. drowsiness, numbness, confusion)	3.2	
Visual disturbances	1.0	
Acoustic hallucinations	0.6	
Paraesthesiae	0.4	

CASE REPORT 17.2

BL, a 20-year-old trainee naval diver, was taking part in air diving training to a depth of 21 metres. He was using surface-supply breathing apparatus (SSBA), which consists of a demand valve and a hose to the surface connected to large cylinder via a pressure regulator adjusted according to the depth. After approximately 20 minutes, he was signalled with a tug on the hose to return to the surface because the cylinder was running low. He remained in the water at the surface while his hose was connected to another cylinder and then recommenced his dive. Some 12 minutes into the second dive, BL's surface attendant noted that there were no surface bubbles. The instructor told the attendant to signal BL via the hose tug system. There were no answering tugs on the line. The standby diver was then sent into the water to check BL. He found BL floating a metre off the bottom with his demand valve out of his mouth. He was brought rapidly back to the diving boat and cardio-pulmonary resuscitation was commenced using a portable oxygen resuscitator. After some time, probably about 15 minutes, the small oxygen cylinder of the resuscitator was noted to be low, so one of the group was instructed to connect the resuscitator to the emergency large oxygen cylinder. The oxygen cylinder was then found to have a line already attached to it – BL's SSBA! BL failed to respond to intense resuscitation carried on for more than 2 hours (inspired oxygen tension at 21 metres would have been 3.1 ATA).

Diagnosis: death resulting from central nervous system oxygen toxicity (presumably convulsions).

CASE REPORT 17.3

AM and his buddy, both military divers, were practising night-time underwater ship attack while using closed-circuit 100 per cent oxygen rebreathing sets. While approaching the ship, they exceeded the maximum safe depth to avoid being spotted by lights and had to ascend to the ship's hull (depth 9 metres). During their escape from the ship, AM had difficulty in freeing his depth gauge and, when he finally did examine it, discovered he was at 19 metres. He started to ascend and remembers 'two to three jerkings' of his body before losing consciousness. The buddy diver noted that AM 'stiffened' as he lost consciousness and then started convulsing, which continued while AM was being brought to the surface. Total time of dive was 28 minutes. At the surface, AM was pale with spasmodic respirations, and the lug on the mouthpiece had been chewed off. Artificial respiration was administered. AM was incoherent for 20 minutes and vomited once. A headache and unsteadiness in walking persisted for several hours after the incident. An electroencephalogram 3 days later was normal. (The buddy diver was exhausted on surfacing, felt nauseated and was unable to climb into the boat but recovered quickly.)

Diagnosis: near drowning secondary to central nervous system oxygen toxicity.

convulsive activity. Because the diver inspired a high pressure of oxygen prior to the convulsion, a high alveolar oxygen tension persists during the apnoea. The individual remains well oxygenated throughout the convulsion. Due to the increased arterial carbon dioxide tension, brain oxygenation could increase the breath-holding period. This is in contrast to the epileptic patient who convulses while breathing air at sea level.

The latent period before the onset of toxic symptoms is inversely proportional to the PIO_2. It may be prolonged by hyperventilation and interruption of exposure and shortened by exercise, immersion in water and the presence of CO_2.

CASE REPORT 17.4

TL was using a semi-closed-circuit rebreathing apparatus rigged for 60 per cent nitrogen. After 17 minutes at 22 metres, he suddenly noted a ringing noise in his head. He flushed through his set, thinking his symptoms were the result of carbon dioxide toxicity. He then noted that his surroundings were brighter than usual and decided to surface.

On surfacing he was noted to be conscious but pale and panting heavily. He moved his mouthpiece and while being brought on board 'went into a convulsion, where his whole face changed shape, his eyes rolled up into his head, his face turned a dark colour and his body began to cramp'. He recovered within 3 to 4 minutes, and 30 minutes later there was no abnormality on clinical examination.

Equipment examination revealed that the emergency oxygen cylinder was nearly empty, i.e. that he had used 64 litres of 100 per cent oxygen in addition to approximately the same amount of 60 per cent oxygen. The oxygen in his breathing bag would therefore have approximated 80 per cent and the inspired oxygen tension 2.4 ATA. The carbon dioxide absorbent was normal.

Diagnosis: central nervous system oxygen toxicity.

The 'oxygen off-effect' refers to the unexpected observation that the first signs of neurological toxicity may appear after a sudden reduction in PIO_2. Also, existing symptoms may be exacerbated. The fall in PIO_2 is usually the result of removing the mask from a subject breathing 100 per cent oxygen in a chamber. It may also occur when the chamber pressure is reduced or when the diver surfaces. It has been postulated that the sudden drop in cerebral arterial PO_2 in the presence of persisting hyperoxic-induced cerebral vasoconstriction results in cerebral hypoxia in a brain already impaired by oxygen poisoning.

The risk of oxygen toxicity in the presence of a diagnosis of epilepsy is unclear. The conservative assumption that such individuals are at increased risk is widely held, and epilepsy is one of the absolute contraindications to diving. Yet although there are some reports of seizures during and after hyperbaric therapy in these patients, no formal association has been described, and many patients with epilepsy are routinely treated in hyperbaric chambers without incident.

Some animal experiments have shown that older and male animals are more susceptible to oxygen toxicity, but this has not been conclusively demonstrated in humans.

The major differential diagnoses of neurological toxicity are cerebral arterial gas embolism (CAGE) and hypoglycaemia. The timing of symptoms and signs in relation to oxygen exposure, measurement of blood glucose and the subsequent recovery from oxygen toxicity are usually enough to distinguish among these entities.

Finally, there are anecdotal reports of a syndrome of fatigue, headache, dizziness and paraesthesiae in operational divers exposed to repeated oxygen at depth on a daily basis. This has not, however, been reported in patients having daily hyperbaric oxygen therapy at 2.4 ATA for 90 minutes daily.

Pathology

No pathological changes in the CNS directly attributable to oxygen toxicity have been observed in humans. Animal experiments with intermittent or continued exposure cause permanent neurological impairment with selective grey matter and neuronal necrosis (the *John Bean effect*)[9]. Changes have been reported on both light and electron microscopy in rats after exposure to 8 ATA oxygen. Lesions are found in specific areas, such as in the reticular substance of the medulla, the pericentral area of the cervical spinal grey matter, the ventral cochlear nuclei, the maxillary bodies and the inferior colliculi.

Pharmacological control of convulsions and pulmonary oedema does not alter the findings. Severe exposure eventually leads to haemorrhagic necrosis of the brain and spinal cord, but even single exposures (30 minutes at 4 ATA) produce ultrastructural changes in anterior horn grey matter.

Prevention

Predictable prevention of cellular changes by administration of drugs is not yet feasible. In animal experiments, many different pharmacological agents have been shown to have a protective effect against toxic effects of oxygen. The agents include disulfiram (also described in animals to potentiate toxicity), glutathione, lithium, iso-nicotinic acid, hydrazide, GABA and sympathetic blocking agents. None of these agents is in prophylactic clinical use at present. Prevention of convulsions by anaesthetics or anticonvulsant agents removes only this overt expression of toxicity, and damage at the cellular level will continue.

The only current safe approach is to place limits on exposure. These limits depend on the PO_2, the duration and the conditions of exposure (e.g. 'wet dive' or in a dry chamber, at exercise or rest, intermittent or continuous).

The Royal Navy and Royal Australian Navy place a limit for pure oxygen diving of 9 metres for a resting dive and 7 metres for a working dive. The US Navy relates the maximum duration of exposure to the depth (see Table 17.2).

The US Navy formerly required divers to undergo a test exposure of 30 minutes at 60 feet breathing 100 per cent oxygen to eliminate those divers who are unusually susceptible[10]. This does not take into account the marked variation in individuals from day to day or the marked influence of the exposure environment. Some individuals may be excessively oxygen sensitive, but the variability makes this uncertain and difficult to screen for. The oxygen tolerance test probably has no value in assessing normal dive candidates.

An awareness of levels at which toxicity is likely, and close observation for early signs such as lip twitching, should reduce the incidence of convulsions. If early signs are noted, the subject should signal his or her companion, stop excessive exertion and hyperventilate. However, premonitory symptoms or signs are unlikely in the working diver in the water.

In chamber therapy, most therapeutic tables do not prescribe 100 per cent oxygen deeper than 2.8 ATA. Periods of air breathing are used to interrupt the exposure to high levels of oxygen and thus reduce the likelihood of toxicity. Animal studies have demonstrated that interrupted exposure delays the onset of CNS toxicity by up to 100 per cent.

Electroencephalographic monitoring has not proved useful in predicting imminent convulsions.

When treating serious cases of DCS where the risks of oxygen toxicity are acceptable, drugs such as diazepam may be used to reduce the effects of toxicity. If available, most practitioners would prefer the option to use helium-oxygen mixtures to reduce the risk of toxicity.

Oxygen-breathing divers are advised to avoid the following:

- Exposure while febrile.
- Drugs that increase tissue CO_2, e.g. opiates, carbonic anhydrase inhibitors.
- Aspirin, steroids, sympathomimetic agents.
- Stimulants such as caffeine (e.g. coffee).
- Fluorescent lights.

Treatment

The initial aim of treatment is to avoid physical trauma associated with a grand mal convulsion. A padded tongue depressor to prevent tongue biting may be useful in a chamber. In contrast to epilepsy, hypoxia is not a concern, at least initially.

In the water, the traditional advice was that the diver should be brought to the surface only after the tonic phase of the convulsion ceased, but this practice has been challenged and is no longer the recommendation of the Diving Committee of the Undersea and Hyperbaric Medical Society[11]. The same action is often indicated in compression chambers, but with allowance made for decompression staging. If it is against the interests of the patient to ascend, it is usually a simple matter to reduce the oxygen in the breathing mixture[12].

Anticonvulsants may be used in exceptional circumstances. Phenytoin has been successfully used to stop convulsions in a patient with cerebral air embolism who was treated with hyperbaric oxygen. Diazepam is also very effective, as is the induction of anaesthesia with propofol.

Table 17.4 The management of oxygen toxicity in the recompression chamber

If oxygen intolerance occurs or is anticipated
- Halt ascent, remove mask at once and maintain depth constant.
- Protect a convulsing patient from injury caused by violent contact with fixtures, deckplates or hull, but do not forcefully oppose convulsive movements.
- With a padded mouthbit, protect the tongue of a convulsing patient.
- For non-convulsive reactions, have the patient hyperventilate with chamber air for several breaths.
- Administer sedative drugs on direction of a medical officer.
- Fifteen minutes after the reaction has entirely subsided, resume the schedule at the point of its interruption.
- If the reaction occurred at 18 metres, on the 135-minute schedule, on arrival at 9 metres switch to the 285-minute schedule (15 minutes air – 60 minutes oxygen, 15 minutes air – 60 minutes oxygen).

Source: From US Navy Diving Manual Revision 6. SS521-AG-PRO-010 (2008). Washington, DC: Naval Sea Systems Command; 2008.

PULMONARY TOXICITY (THE 'LORRAIN SMITH EFFECT')

Clinically obvious pulmonary oxygen toxicity does not manifest in short-duration oxygen diving. It assumes greater importance in saturation and long chamber dives and where a high PO_2 is inspired, such as in therapeutic recompression. Prolonged exposures to PO_2 as low as 0.55 ATA (e.g. in space flight) have been found to produce significant changes. A PIO_2 of 0.75 ATA has produced toxicity in 24 hours.

In animals, pulmonary oxygen poisoning causes progressive respiratory distress, leading to respiratory failure and finally death. The wide variation of tolerance among different species invalidates direct extrapolation of animal studies to humans, but early signs in humans are similar to those in animals. In patients receiving high concentrations of oxygen therapeutically, it is sometimes difficult to distinguish between the conditions for which the oxygen is given and the effects of oxygen itself (e.g. shock lung, respiratory distress syndrome).

Clinical manifestations

As in neurological toxicity, the factors affecting the degree of toxicity are the PIO_2, the duration of exposure and individual variation in susceptibility. Exposure to 2.0 ATA oxygen produces symptoms in some normal humans at 3 hours, but the occasional individual may remain symptom free for up to 8 hours.

The earliest symptom is usually a mild tracheal irritation similar to the tracheitis of an upper respiratory infection. This irritation is aggravated by deep inspiration, which may produce a cough. Smoking has a similar result. Chest tightness is often noted; then a substernal pain develops that is also aggravated by deep breathing and coughing. The cough becomes progressively worse until it is uncontrollable. Dyspnoea at rest develops and, if the exposure is prolonged, is rapidly progressive. The higher the inspired oxygen pressure, the more rapidly symptoms develop and the greater is the intensity.

Physical signs, such as rales, nasal mucous membrane hyperaemia and fever, have been produced only after prolonged exposure in normal subjects.

Pulmonary oxygen toxicity

- Chest tightness or discomfort.
- Cough.
- Shortness of breath.
- Chest pain.

The measurement of forced VC (FVC or VC) is one monitor of the onset and progression of toxicity, although it is less sensitive than the clinical symptoms. Reduction in VC is usually progressive throughout the oxygen exposure. The drop continues for several hours after cessation of exposure and many occasionally take several days to return to normal. Because measurement of VC requires the subject's full cooperation, usefulness may be limited in the therapeutic situation. Conversely, it is a useful tool in monitoring repeated exposures in hyperbaric workers. It has been used to delineate pulmonary oxygen tolerance limits in normal subjects – this is shown in Figure 17.3, which relates PO_2 to duration of exposure. The percentage fall in VC is plotted. The size of the fall in VC does not always indicate the degree of pulmonary toxicity as measured by other lung function tests, such as other lung volumes, static and dynamic compliance and diffusing capacity for carbon monoxide. Changes in diffusing capacity may be the most sensitive indicator.

Exposure at 3 ATA for 3.5 hours caused chest discomfort, cough and dyspnoea in most of 13 subjects. There was no significant change in post-exposure FVC. Maximum mid-expiratory flow rates were reduced, but airway resistance did not change[13].

Some studies in divers have indicated that the reduction in forced mid-expiratory flow rates may persist for at least 3 years after deep saturation dives and also after shallow saturation dives with the same hyperoxic exposure profile. Forced

expiratory volume in 1 second (FEV_1) and FVC were not significantly altered.

Some individuals, especially at higher PIO_2 (2.5 ATA), demonstrate a rapid fall in VC. The recovery after exposure is also more rapid than that after an equal VC decrement produced at a lower PO_2 for a longer time.

Although chest x-ray changes have been reported, there is no pathognomonic appearance of oxygen toxicity. Diffuse bilateral pulmonary densities have been reported. With continued exposure, irregularly shaped infiltrates extend and coalesce.

Pathology

The pathological changes in the lung as a result of oxygen toxicity have been divided into two types; acute and chronic[7], depending on the PIO_2.

Pressures of oxygen greater than 0.8 ATA cause a relatively acute toxicity that has been subdivided into exudative and proliferative phases. The exudative phase consists of a perivascular and interstitial inflammatory response and alveolar oedema, haemorrhage, hyaline membranes, swelling and destruction of capillary endothelial cells and destruction of type I alveolar lining cells. (This phase was the type described by Lorrain Smith.) Progression of the disease leads to the proliferative

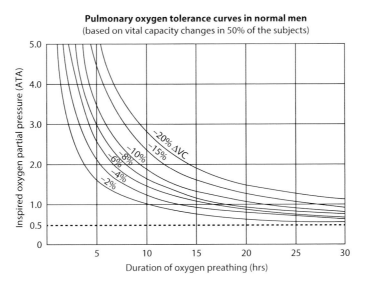

Pulmonary oxygen tolerance curves in normal men
(based on vital capacity changes in 50% of the subjects)

Figure 17.3 Relationship of partial pressure of oxygen breathed and duration of exposure with degree of pulmonary oxygen damage. ΔVC, vital capacity change.

phase, which, after resolution of the inflammatory exudate, is characterized by proliferation of fibroblasts and type II alveolar cells. There is an increase in the alveolar-capillary distance. Pulmonary capillaries are destroyed, and some arterioles become obstructed with thrombus.

A more chronic response usually follows PIO_2 between 0.5 and 0.8 ATA for longer periods. It is characterized by hyperplasia of type II cells, replacing type I cells and progressive pulmonary fibrosis, especially affecting alveolar ducts rather than alveolar septa. These features are also found in the adult respiratory distress syndrome (shock, drowning, trauma) for which high oxygen tensions are given. Whether oxygen actually causes the damage in these situations or exacerbates the condition by interacting with the initial pulmonary damage is not clear.

A consequence of these effects on pulmonary physiology is to increase ventilation-perfusion inequality. Obstruction of arterioles results in an increase in dead space.

Prevention

No specific therapy is available that can be used clinically to delay or modify the pulmonary damage caused by hyperoxia. Intermittent exposure may delay the onset of toxicity. Delay of pulmonary toxicity has been demonstrated in humans. It has been suggested that the rate of recovery is greater than the rate of development of cellular changes leading to toxicity.

When toxicity is evident, the PO_2 should be reduced. It is therefore important to be aware of the earliest signs of the syndrome.

Traditionally, the monitoring of VC has been employed as an indicator of toxicity. The maximum acceptable reduction in VC depends on the reasons for the exposure. Although a 20 per cent reduction may be acceptable in the treatment of severe DCS, a 10 per cent reduction would cause concern under operational diving conditions. One concept that has gained some popularity is that of the 'UPTD' or units of pulmonary toxic dose. UPTDs allow the expression of different exposures in time and PIO_2 related to a 'standard' exposure at 1.0 ATA expressed in minutes. Expected UPTDs can be calculated for any planned exposure and

that exposure can be modified to keep the decrement in VC within acceptable limits (see Clark and Thom[7] for a fuller explanation).

The degree of oxygen toxicity equivalent to a 2 per cent decrease in VC (approximately the decrement predicted for a standard US Navy Treatment Table 6 treatment for DCS) is completely reversible, asymptomatic and very difficult to measure under ordinary circumstances. With the elevated pressures of oxygen used in the treatment of serious diseases, such as severe DCS or gas gangrene, it may be reasonable to accept a greater degree of pulmonary toxicity to treat the patient. The primary requirement of any therapy is that the treatment should not be worse than the disease.

Pulmonary toxicity that produces a 10 per cent decrease in VC is associated with moderate symptoms of coughing and pain in the chest on deep inspiration. This degree of impairment of lung function has been shown to be reversible within a few days. It is suggested that a 10 per cent decrement in VC be chosen as the limit for most hyperbaric oxygen therapy procedures.

VC is a relatively crude measure of toxicity. Forced mid-expiratory flow measurements or the less practical diffusing capacity for carbon monoxide may prove to be more sensitive indicators for repeated or long-term exposures.

> Intermittent rather than continuous exposure to high oxygen pressure delays the onset of both neurological and pulmonary oxygen toxicity.

Adherence to proposed pressure-duration limits for pulmonary oxygen toxicity is difficult where extended durations and changing PO_2 are involved.

Methods for calculating cumulative pulmonary toxicity have therefore been devised (e.g. the UPTD), and they may have a role in prolonged decompression and hyperbaric oxygen therapy[7].

As discussed in the previous section on prevention of neurological toxicity, many drugs have been shown to be effective in animal experiments. They may have a role in the future in the prevention of pulmonary and other oxygen toxicity, at least for hyperbaric therapy exposure.

OTHER MANIFESTATIONS OF TOXICITY

It has been suggested that oxygen, although essential for survival of aerobic cells, should be regarded as a universal cellular poison. All organs and tissues of the body are susceptible to damage from oxygen free radical production. Nevertheless, in other organs receiving a high blood flow such as heart, kidney and liver, no toxicity has yet been detected in humans. It may be that CNS and pulmonary toxicity pre-empt its development in other organs.

Haematopoietic system

Oxygen, in space flight exposures, has been shown to have a deleterious effect on red blood cells that is manifested by abnormal cell morphology and/or a decrease in circulating red blood cell mass. This may be caused by depression of erythropoiesis, inactivation of essential glycolytic enzymes or damage to red blood cell membranes resulting from peroxidation of membrane lipid. Mice studies show irreversible damage to haematopoietic stem cells after 24 hours of exposure to 100 per cent oxygen.

There have also been occasional reports of haemolytic episodes following hyperbaric oxygen exposure, but these seem to be related to individual idiosyncrasies such as specific enzyme defects.

Eye

In 1935 Behnke reported a reversible decrease in peripheral vision after oxygen breathing at 3.0 ATA. Lambertsen and Clarke demonstrated a progressive reduction in peripheral vision after 2.5 hours of breathing oxygen at 3.0 ATA that reached about 50 per cent after 3.5 hours. Recovery was complete after 45 minutes of air breathing.

Progressive myopic changes have been well documented during hyperbaric therapy, and they have also been noted in divers. Reversal of this myopic shift usually occurs within a few weeks, but could take many months. Changes are probably related to an effect on the crystalline structure of the lens. Butler and colleagues demonstrated a myopic shift after 15 days of hyperbaric oxygen therapy and approximately 45 hours of diving exposure to 1.3 ATA oxygen[14].

Cataract formation has also been reported after extreme hyperbaric exposure (more than 100 treatment sessions), with lens opacities not completely reversible.

A reduction of the intraocular pressure may represent a toxic effect on the ciliary process. Retinal detachments, retinal micro-infarcts, changes in dark adaptation, photoreceptor damage and a decrease in the amplitude of the electroretinogram have all been recorded.

Other ocular effects of oxygen toxicity include retinopathy of prematurity in infants breathing supplemental oxygen. Initial retinal blanching resulting from vasoconstriction is followed by vessel obliteration and fibro-vascular proliferation, which may lead to retinal fibrosis and traction retinal detachments. Animal studies have demonstrated death of visual cells and retinal detachments on exposure to 0.9 to 3 ATA oxygen. Irreversible changes in the cornea and lens of guinea pigs develop after exposure to 3 ATA oxygen for between 4 and 16 hours.

Vasoconstriction

Other disorders that may be affected by the hyperoxic-induced vasoconstriction include Raynaud's phenomenon, Buerger's disease and migraine. Risk of closure of the ductus arteriosus has been proposed in the foetus exposed to increased oxygen.

Ear

Serous otitis media has been noted in aviators exposed to high concentrations of oxygen. It results from absorption of oxygen from the middle ear. A syndrome related to the middle ear was described in US Navy divers breathing 100 per cent oxygen from semi-closed-circuit and closed-circuit diving equipment. The symptoms were fullness, popping or crackling sensation in the ear and a mild conductive hearing loss. On examination the most common finding was fluid in the middle ear. The syndrome was first noted after rising from a night's sleep, not immediately after the dive itself, and it disappeared rapidly. There was no suggestion of barotrauma.

Cancer

Repeated or long-term exposure to high levels of oxygen free radicals could be expected to enhance tumour development. A literature review including human and animal studies failed to support a possible cancer-causing effect of hyperbaric oxygen[15].

> It is likely that, as more sensitive methods of detection are used, evidence of oxygen toxicity in many other cells and organs will be observed.

REFERENCES

1. Acott, C. Oxygen toxicity: a brief history of oxygen in diving. *South Pacific Underwater Medicine Society Journal* 1999;**29**(3):150–155.
2. Donald KW. *Oxygen and the Diver.* Harley Swan, UK: The Spa, Ltd.; 1992.
3. Donald KW. Oxygen poisoning in man: I, II. *British Medical Journal* 1947;**1**:667–672, 712–717.
4. Chavko M, Harabin AL. Regional lipid peroxidation and protein oxidation in rat brain after hyperbaric oxygen. *Free Radical Biology and Medicine* 1996;**20**(7):973–978.
5. Carraway MS, Crapo JD, Piantadosi CA. Aerolised manganese SOD decreases pulmonary injury in primates.1. Physiology and biochemistry. *Journal of Applied Physiology* 1997;**83**(2):550–558.
6. Lawrence CH. A diving fatality due to oxygen toxicity during a 'technical' dive. *Medical Journal of Australia* 1996;**165**:262–263.
7. Clark JM, Thom SR. Oxygen under pressure. In: Brubakk AP, Neuman TS, eds. *Bennett and Elliott's Physiology and Medicine of Diving.* 5th ed. London; Saunders; 2003:358–418.
8. Lambertsen. CJ. Effects of oxygen at high partial pressure. In: Fenn WO, Rahn H (Eds). Handbook of Physiology and Respiration. Bethesda, MD. *American Physiological Society* 1965;Section **3(2)**:1027-1046.
9. Bean JW. Effects of oxygen at increased pressure. *Physiology Reviews* 1945;**25**:1–147.
10. Butler FK, Knafel ME. Screening for oxygen intolerance in US Navy Divers. *Undersea Biomedical Research* 1986;**13**:193–223.
11. Mitchell SJ, Bennett MH, Bird N, *et al.* Recommendations for rescue of a submerged unresponsive compressed-gas diver. *Undersea and Hyperbaric Medicine* 2012;**39**(6):1099–1108.
12. *US Navy Diving Manual Revision 6. SS521-AG-PRO-010 (2008).* Washington, DC: Naval Sea Systems Command; 2008.
13. Clark JM, Lambertsen CJ, Gelfand R, Hiller WD, Unger M. Pulmonary function in men after oxygen breathing at 3.0 ATA for 3.5 h. *Journal of Applied Physiology* 1991;**71**(3):878–885.
14. Butler FK, Whit, E, Twa M. Hyperoxic myopia in a closed circuit mixed gas scuba diver. *Undersea and Hyperbaric Medicine* 1999;**26**(1):41–45.
15. Feldmeier JJ, Heimbach RD, Davolt DA, Brakora MJ, Sheffield PJ, Porter AT. Does hyperbaric oxygen have a cancer-causing or -promoting effect? *Undersea and Hyperbaric Medicine* 1994;**21**(4):467–475.

FURTHER READING

Bitterman N. Oxygen toxicity. *Undersea and Hyperbaric Medicine* 2004;31(1):63–72.

van Ooij PJ, Hollmann MW, van Hulst RA, Sterk PJ. Assessment of pulmonary oxygen toxicity: relevance to professional diving; a review. *Respiratory Physiology and Neurobiology* 2013;189(1):117–128.

Fock A, Harris R, Slade M. Oxygen exposure and toxicity in recreational technical divers. *Diving and Hyperbaric Medicine* 2013;43(2):67–71.

Sames C, Gorman DF, Mitchelll SJ, Gamble G. The long-term effects of compressed gas diving on lung function in New Zealand occupational divers: a retrospective analysis. *Diving and Hyperbaric Medicine.*

Beebe DC, Shui YB, Siegrfried CJ, Holekamp NM, Bai F. Preserve the (intraocular) environment: the importance of maintaining normal oxygen gradients in the eye. *Japanese Journal of Ophthalmology* 2014;58(1):225–231.

This chapter was reviewed for this fifth edition by Michael Bennett.

18

Carbon dioxide toxicity

RESPIRATORY PHYSIOLOGY

Carbon dioxide (CO_2) is normally present in the atmosphere in a concentration of 0.03 to 0.04 per cent by volume of dry air. This represents a partial pressure (PCO_2) of 0.23 to 0.30 mm Hg. It is one of the products of metabolism of protein, carbohydrates and fats produced in the mitochondria in roughly the same volume as oxygen is consumed. For example:

Glucose (a carbohydrate) + oxygen = carbon dioxide + water + energy

$$(C_6H_{12}O_6 + 6O_2 = 6CO_2 + 6H_2O + energy)$$

The resultant CO_2 has to be transported from the tissues by the circulation and eliminated by exhalation from the lungs.

The normal PCO_2 in arterial blood ($PaCO_2$) is about 40 mm Hg and for mixed venous blood is about 46 mm Hg. Some factors that determine arterial PCO_2 are summarised in Figure 18.1. PCO_2 in the alveolar gas ($PACO_2$) is in equilibrium with that of the pulmonary veins and is therefore also about 40 mm Hg. Being a product of metabolism, the amount of CO_2 produced is unchanged, so the $PACO_2$ is constant irrespective of depth (unlike oxygen and nitrogen, which reflect the pressures in the inspired gas).

CO_2 is the most potent stimulus to respiration. The central medullary chemoreceptors in the brain are stimulated by increases in arterial CO_2 and acidosis. In normal conditions, adjustments in ventilation keep the arterial and alveolar CO_2 partial pressure remarkably constant. The peripheral chemoreceptors (carotid and aortic bodies) are primarily responsive to hypoxaemia (increasing respiration) but also respond to increases in acidosis and CO_2 concentration.

The solubility of CO_2 is about 20 times that of oxygen so there is considerably more CO_2 than oxygen in simple solution (most of the oxygen is transported bound to haemoglobin). CO_2 is transported in the blood in both plasma and red cells. In each 100 ml of arterial blood, 3 ml are dissolved, 3 ml are in carbamino compounds (with haemoglobin and plasma proteins) and 44 ml are carried as bicarbonate (HCO_3^-).

At rest, approximately 5 ml of CO_2 per 100 ml blood are given up from the tissues and liberated in the lungs. About 200 ml of CO_2 are produced and excreted per minute. If this CO_2 is retained in the body (e.g. from rebreathing), the $PaCO_2$ will climb at the rate of 3 to 6 mm Hg per minute.

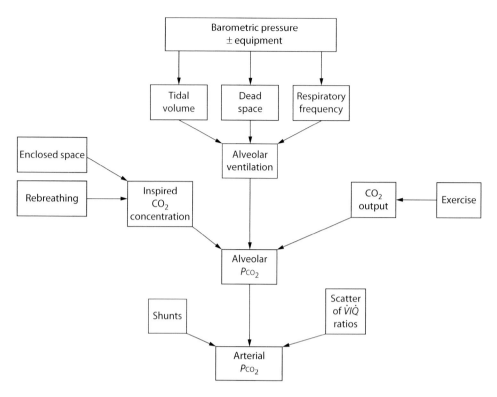

Figure 18.1 Some factors that influence the partial pressure of carbon dioxide (PCO_2). V/Q, ventilation-perfusion. (Adapted from Nunn JF. Applied Respiratory Physiology. 3rd ed. London: Butterworth; 1987.)

With exercise, much larger amounts of CO_2 are produced. The working diver can produce more than 3 litres of CO_2 per minute for short periods, and 2 litres per minute for more than half an hour, usually without serious alteration in $PaCO_2$ – as a result of a concomitant increase in respiration.

Because ventilation matches any increased CO_2 production, while diving, the arterial and hence alveolar CO_2 tensions should be maintained at approximately 40 mm Hg despite increasing environmental pressure. Therefore, the alveolar CO_2 percentage decreases with increased depths. In contrast, because the source is from the inspired gas, the alveolar partial pressure of oxygen (PO_2) and the partial pressure of nitrogen (PN_2) increase with depth, but the percentages show little change.

$PaCO_2$ is the primary drive to respiration, as discussed earlier, and it is intimately related to alveolar ventilation. As every breath-hold diver knows, deliberate hyperventilation can drive the $PaCO_2$ down and extend breath-hold time

(see Chapters 16 and 61). The exact relationship between $PaCO_2$ and alveolar ventilation is shown in the following equation:

$$P_ACO_2 \rightarrow kVCO_2/Va + P_ICO_2$$

Where k is a conversion factor to convert conditions at STPD (standard temperature and pressure, dry) to BTPS (body temperature and pressure, saturated); VCO_2 is the CO_2 production in litres per millimetre STPD; Va is the alveolar ventilation in litres per minute BTPS; and $PICO_2$ is the inspired carbon dioxide partial pressure.

Alterations in $PaCO_2$ have widespread effects on the body, especially on the respiratory, circulatory and nervous systems. Apart from the hypocapnia produced by hyperventilation, the more frequent derangement in diving is hypercapnia, an elevation of CO_2 in blood and tissues. This may be an acute effect or chronic. Where hypercapnia produces pathophysiological changes dangerous to the diver, the term 'CO$_2$ toxicity' (or CO_2 poisoning) is used.

ACUTE HYPERCAPNIA

Causes

Excluding asphyxia and drowning, there are five main mechanisms of CO_2 toxicity in diving:

1. Failure of an absorbent system, e.g. in closed-circuit or semi-closed-circuit rebreathing apparatus, submarines, saturation complexes.
2. Inadequate ventilation of an enclosed environment, e.g. in standard dress or other helmet diving and compression chamber diving where flushing is required to remove CO_2.
3. Inadequate pulmonary ventilation, e.g. in deep diving where the work of breathing dense gases is greater, or with increased resistance from the equipment.
4. Physiological adaptations to diving ('CO_2 retainers').
5. Contamination of breathing gases by CO_2.

Whatever the cause, CO_2 toxicity is much more rapid when the diver is exercising and producing large amounts of CO_2.

> Serious carbon dioxide toxicity is most commonly encountered in divers using closed-circuit or semi-closed-circuit rebreathing equipment. It is also seen where there is inadequate ventilation of an enclosed space such as a helmet, recompression chamber or submarine.

In diving operations that rely on recycling of respiratory gases, the most common method of CO_2 removal uses the reaction between alkali metal (sodium, lithium) hydroxide reagents (e.g. Protosorb, Sodasorb, Baralyme, Dragersorb) and carbonic acid:

$$H_2O + CO_2 = H_2CO_3$$

$$H_2CO_3 + 2NaOH = Na_2CO_3 + 2H_2O$$

$$Na_2CO_3 + Ca(OH)_2 = 2NaOH + CaCO_3$$

Other techniques, some still being developed, include cryogenic freeze-out of CO_2 with liquid air or oxygen, molecular sieves, electrolytic decomposition into carbon and water and the use of peroxides and superoxides that generate oxygen while removing CO_2.

FAILURE OF THE ABSORBENT SYSTEM

This failure in rebreathing sets may have the following causes:

Inefficiency of absorbent material

This may be caused by large granule size, poor packing (resulting in poor contact between absorbent and gas because of 'channeling' of gases), low environmental temperature, low alkali content, low water content or sea water contamination.

Equipment design faults

The canister should be of adequate size and adequate length compared with its cross-sectional area. It should be insulated against extreme temperature changes. In circuit rebreathing equipment, the gas space between the absorbent granules ideally should exceed the maximum tidal volume, so that there is time for absorption during the next part of the respiratory cycle. In pendulum rebreathing equipment, excessive functional dead space between the diver's mouth and the canister causes inhalation of expired CO_2.

Operator error

CO_2 build-up may result if the diver fails to pack the canister properly with active absorbent, undertakes excessive exertion or exceeds the safe working life of the set (Case Report 18.1).

INADEQUATE VENTILATION OF THE ENVIRONMENT

In helmet and recompression chamber dives, there must be a sufficient volume of gas supplied to flush the enclosed system of CO_2. In the same way that $PaCO_2$ is dependent on alveolar ventilation, the level of CO_2 in the enclosed space is inversely proportional to the ventilation of that space. When corrected to surface volumes, this means progressively greater amounts of gas must be supplied as the diver or chamber goes deeper.

INADEQUATE PULMONARY VENTILATION

At depth, this situation is primarily the result of the increased density of the respired gases. This causes an increased resistance to gas flow,

---

CASE REPORT 18.1

AB, an experienced open-circuit diver and recent *aficionado* of deep, closed-circuit rebreather diving using mixed gases, was diving to 85 metres on a wreck. Shortly after reaching the bottom, he became agitated and was acting irrationally. His diving companion tried to assist but was unable to calm him down. The diving companion indicated that AB should begin his ascent but was not able to make his intention understood. After approximately 1 minute of struggling, AB became unconscious with his mouthpiece still *in situ*. His companion held him and began an ascent to his first decompression stop.

At approximately the 70-metre depth, they encountered the next pair of divers descending, and AB was transferred to their care and assisted to 35 metres, where the second pair of divers was obliged to stop for decompression. They inflated AB's buoyancy vest and he ascended unconscious and unaccompanied rapidly to the surface.

AB surfaced near the boat and was rapidly retrieved from the water and oxygen administered – initially by bag and mask ventilation, although he rapidly resumed breathing. He was transferred to a hyperbaric facility and recompressed after formally being intubated and ventilated because of his depressed state of consciousness. He had omitted significant decompression obligations and had experienced a rapid ascent, so he was presumed to be highly likely to have significant decompression illness on top of the primary cause of this event. His condition improved rapidly and he was extubated the following morning, with normal neurological function. He had no recall of beginning to feel breathless toward the end of the descent.

An examination of his equipment revealed a misassembled absorbent system whereby circuit gas was able to by-pass the absorbent canister and flow freely from the expiratory limb of the circuit to the inspiratory limb. On arrival at the recompression facility, an arterial blood gas had returned a $PaCO_2$ value of 78 mm Hg.

On reflection, AB admitted to making the same error on a previous occasion, but he had been able to exit the water before any serious consequences had ensued.

Diagnosis: CO_2 intoxication secondary to absorbent system failure resulting from misassembly. Closed-circuit rebreather diving is complex and requires meticulous attention to detail. Perhaps it is best suited to obsessive-compulsive personality types (see Chapter 62).

---

both in the breathing apparatus and in the diver's own airways. Using the less dense helium as the diluent gas instead of nitrogen avoids this problem. Tight wetsuits, harnesses and buoyancy compensators further restrict thoracic movement and place an increased workload on the diver's respiratory muscles. The extent to which this load is overcome varies greatly among divers, but there is often some elevation of the alveolar PCO_2.

PHYSIOLOGICAL ADAPTATIONS TO DIVING ('CO₂ RETAINERS')

In the diving literature, CO_2 is often incriminated as a major factor producing loss of consciousness, with rebreathing equipment and while employing high oxygen pressures in gas mixtures. There have been many adequately investigated cases to verify this.

There are also divers who tolerate high PCO_2 levels – 'CO₂ retainers' (see later). These divers are more likely to experience neurological oxygen toxicity at lower oxygen pressures or durations. The explanation given is that the higher $PaCO_2$ causes cerebral vasodilation and thus a larger oxygen load to the brain. These problems are more likely with oxygen or gas mixture diving equipment and with rebreathing sets (see Chapters 4 and 63).

High oxygen levels in the inspiratory gas have been thought since the 1950s (e.g. several reports from Lanphier from 1950 to 1958) to reduce the respiratory response to CO_2. Most later reports suggest that at an aerobic work rate, ventilation is not altered whether the subject breathes 100 per cent oxygen or air.

Kerem and his co-workers[1] demonstrated that while breathing high oxygen pressures, established divers had significantly lower sensitivity to high CO_2 levels. These Investigators concluded that the divers had an impaired CO_2 response that was either inherent or acquired. Kerem and colleagues also demonstrated that the mean end-tidal PCO_2 was significantly higher than that in non-divers and diving trainees, when breathing nitrox with 40 per cent O_2 at both 1 and 4 ATA.

In relation to open-circuit equipment using air (scuba), the relevance of CO_2 as a contributor to significant diving problems is more dubious. Many divers do, however, reduce their ventilation voluntarily to conserve air and allow mild elevations of their $PaCO_2$. This practice of long inspiratory and expiratory pauses that reduce minute ventilation is called 'skip breathing' and often results in headache at the end of a dive that clears rapidly after surfacing. This practice is not generally advised, but it is common among relatively inexperienced divers trying to extend their dive time. A link with serious diving injury has not been established.

The general physiology literature assumes that $PaCO_2$ is held remarkably constant during both rest and exercise, within a very narrow range of a few millimitres of mercury. Dempsey and Pack[2], in a text on the regulation of breathing, stated that 'significant, sustained CO_2 retention is extremely rare in health, even under the most extreme conditions of exercise intensity and flow limitation'.

Yet, significant exercise (O_2 uptake >60 per cent of maximal) under water and using scuba, produces an elevation of $PaCO_2$ and is sometimes marked ($PaCO_2$ >60 mm Hg). With increasing depth, a progressively greater amount of energy is required to breathe and rid the body of CO_2. At extreme depth, the work of breathing may produce enough CO_2 to exceed the ability to expire CO_2, and this has been postulated as a mode of death in some deep divers.

Different regulators produce varying degrees of resistance to ventilation, with the potential for CO_2 retention. Resistance also rises with inadequate maintenance of the regulator or the deposition of foreign bodies and salt particles. Maintaining regulator performance to an acceptable level can be difficult. The CO_2 retention is usually minor and does not lead to CO_2 toxicity. It does, however,

increase with exposure to depth and with low scuba cylinder pressure driving the gas through the regulator.

Perhaps more important than the consistent but mild CO_2 build-up with normal scuba diving is the occasional atypical subject who responds inadequately, either at depth or on the surface, to raised CO_2 levels. It may be that these divers progressively elevate their CO_2, as an alternative to increasing their ventilation, when the resistance to breathing increases. Under these conditions, it is theoretically possible that toxic levels may eventuate.

In diving parlance these divers are referred to as 'CO_2 retainers', a concept based heavily on the work of Lanphier. This concept has received widespread acceptance in the diving medical fraternity, but is not widely accepted among more conventional physiologists.

If, indeed, there are such divers who are CO_2 retainers, then the explanation for this is conjectural. Some investigators have suggested that the ability to tolerate higher than normal CO_2 levels will permit the subject to achieve greater diving success. These divers may succeed with deep breath-hold diving, tolerate the high CO_2 levels in helmet diving or tolerate increased breathing resistance from equipment or increased gas density with depth. In this situation the CO_2 retainer would be self-selecting – being more successful during diver training and therefore over-represented in the established diver population – where they have been observed by physiologists such as Lanphier.

A more plausible explanation for high $PaCO_2$ levels in divers, for the various reasons referred to previously, is that divers develop an adaptation allowing them to tolerate the higher levels of CO_2 encountered while diving. Similarly, as 'skip breathers' continue to dive, this breathing pattern becomes habitual, and a tolerance to CO_2 would develop.

'Skip' or 'controlled' breathing may not only put divers at risk of problems from CO_2 toxicity, oxygen toxicity, nitrogen narcosis and pulmonary barotrauma, but it also induces bewilderment among diving respiratory investigators.

There have been cases reported of divers who had otherwise unexplained episodes of unconsciousness and who were later shown to have a markedly reduced ventilatory response to elevated $PaCO_2$. It is suggested that a combination of CO_2 toxicity and nitrogen narcosis may have induced unconsciousness in some of these divers, but in others the depth is too shallow to incriminate significant nitrogen narcosis.

Some of the divers who have lost consciousness with scuba at depths around 30 metres have not only been very experienced divers, but also have had asthma. The traditional CO_2 retention in these subjects may be a contributing factor.

Equating the respiratory response to CO_2 among divers with that of patients with chronic obstructive pulmonary disease or those with sleep apnoea has little clinical or research merit.

In 1992, Donald[4] reviewed many of the studies frequently referenced both here and by others and not only cast considerable doubt on their methodology and conclusions, but also argued against any continuing support for the concept of CO_2 retainers as a separate group of divers.

CONTAMINATION

Some buoyancy vests are fitted with a CO_2 cartridge to inflate the vest in an emergency. A diver who, in a panic situation, inflated the vest and then breathed this gas would rapidly develop CO_2 toxicity.

In limestone cave diving, gas pockets may form under the roof. A diver may be tempted to remove the regulator and breathe in this gas, which, not being replenished, will gradually accumulate CO_2. Such a diver may then develop CO_2 toxicity.

In practice, 'contamination' is much more likely the result of the failure of absorbent systems, as described earlier.

Clinical features

These features depend on the rate of development and degree of CO_2 retention. They vary from mild compensated respiratory acidosis, detected only by blood gas and electrolyte estimations, to rapid unconsciousness with exposure to high $PICO_2$ (Case Report 18.2). Although CO_2 is a respiratory stimulant, most of its effects result from the acidosis it produces and are neurologically depressant.

At 1 ATA, a typical subject breathing air to which 3 per cent CO_2 has been added doubles the respiratory minute volume. There is no disturbance of central nervous system function. A 5 to 6 per cent CO_2 supplement may cause distress and dyspnoea accompanied by an increase, mainly in tidal volume but also in respiratory rate. There is a concomitant rise in blood pressure and pulse rate. Mental confusion and lack of coordination may become apparent. A 10 per cent inspired CO_2 eventually causes a drop in pulse rate and blood pressure and severe mental impairment. A 12 to 14 per cent level will cause loss of consciousness and eventually death by central respiratory and cardiac depression if continued for a sufficient time ($PaCO_2$ greater than 150 mm Hg); 20 to 40 per cent inspired CO_2 rapidly causes midbrain convulsions – extensor spasms – and death.

These effects occur at progressively lower inspired concentrations with increasing depth because toxicity depends on partial pressure, not inspired concentration.

If the inspired CO_2 is allowed to increase gradually (as may occur with a rebreathing set with failing absorbent), the following sequence is observed on land. The subject notices dizziness, unsteadiness, disorientation and restlessness. There is sweating of the forehead and hands, and the face feels flushed, bloated and warm. Respiration increases in both depth and rate (Case Report 18.3). Muscular fasciculation, incoordination and ataxia are demonstrable. Jerking movements may occur in the limbs. The subject becomes confused, ignores instructions and pursues tasks doggedly. Gross tremor and clonic convulsions may appear. Depression of the central nervous system may lead to respiratory paralysis and eventually death if the high $PICO_2$ is not discontinued.

Underwater, the diver may not notice sweating and hot feelings, given the cool environment. Incoordination and ataxia are much less obvious because movements are slowed through the dense medium and the effect of gravity is almost eliminated. Hyperpnoea may not be noted by the diver performing hard work or engrossed in a task. With the rapid development of hypercapnia, there may be no warning symptoms preceding unconsciousness. During the recovery period, the diver may remember an episode of lightheadedness or transitory amblyopia, but these occupy only a few seconds and there is therefore insufficient time to take appropriate action.

CASE REPORT 18.2

WS, a very fit dive instructor, experienced two episodes of unconsciousness under similar conditions, about 1 year apart. They both were associated with diving between 30 to 50 metres depth, non-stressful and requiring little exertion. They both occurred 10 or more minutes after reaching the sea bed, and there were no problems during descent, and specifically no difficulty with middle ear autoinflation.

Other divers on the same dives used similar scuba equipment and gases from the same compressor (his own dive shop) and experienced no difficulty.

The first episode resulted in a sensation of imminent loss of consciousness, to a severe degree, and caused him to ditch his weight belt and ascend, with help. With the ascent he regained his normal state of awareness. On his second episode he totally lost consciousness and was brought to the surface by one of the companion divers. He was fully conscious and alert within a few minutes of surfacing. Following this dive he was aware of a dull headache.

The only contributory factors that could be ascertained were as follows:

He was renowned for consuming extremely small quantities of air, and he did admit to employing 'skip breathing' in the earlier part of his diving career – although such a voluntary decision was not made in recent years. He had asthma of moderate degree. He had not taken any anti-asthmatic medication before the dives. He then sold his diving practice and refrained from diving activities.

Provisional diagnosis: combined carbon dioxide/nitrogen narcosis effect with possible asthma contribution.

Whatever the explanation, remember the maxim that any diving accident not explained and not prevented will recur under similar conditions.

CASE REPORT 18.3

JF was doing a compass swim using a closed-circuit 100 per cent oxygen rebreathing set at a maximum depth of 5 metres. He had difficulty keeping up with his companion and noticed that his breathing was deep and the gas seemed hot. He ventilated his counterlung with fresh oxygen but still had breathing difficulty. Just before being called up after 33 minutes in the water, his companion noted that JF 'got a new burst of speed, but kept adding more gas to his counterlung'.

On reaching the tailboard of the boat, JF complained that he was nearly out of gas. His eyes were wide, his face flushed and his respirations panting and spasmodic. He then collapsed and stopped breathing. His face mask was removed, and he was given mouth-to-mouth respiration, then 100 per cent oxygen as breathing returned. He was unconscious for 5 minutes, and headache and amnesia extended for several hours after the dive.

Oxygen percentage in the counterlung was 80 per cent and the activity time of the unused absorbent was reduced to 32 minutes (specification 61 minutes). The canister (plus absorbent) from JF's set was placed in another set, and a fresh diver exercised in a swimming pool using this. He was unable to continue for more than 5 minutes because of a classic CO_2 build-up.

Diagnosis: CO_2 toxicity.

A throbbing frontal or bitemporal headache may develop during a slow CO_2 build-up (while still conscious) or after a rapid build-up (during recuperation).

> An exercising diver in the water may have little warning of carbon dioxide toxicity prior to becoming unconscious.

If the diver is removed from the toxic environment before the onset of apnoea, recovery from an episode of acute CO_2 toxicity is rapid, and the diver appears normal within a few minutes. He or she may complain of nausea, malaise or severe headache for several hours. The headache does not respond to the usual analgesics or ergotamine preparations.

Early workers in this field observed the 'CO_2 off effect', i.e. a brief deterioration in the clinical state when a significant CO_2 exposure is abruptly suspended and the diver breaths normal air. This observation has been less often reported more recently.

CO_2 retention enhances nitrogen narcosis (see Chapter 15), and it renders the diver more susceptible to oxygen toxicity (see Chapter 17). Conversely, there is evidence that nitrogen narcosis does not exacerbate CO_2 retention by depressing ventilatory response. The hyperoxia of depth may slightly reduce ventilatory drive. It is also believed that CO_2 increases the possibility of decompression sickness by increasing tissue perfusion and by increasing red blood cell agglutination (see Chapter 11).

Prevention and treatment

Although it is often the practice to familiarize divers who use rebreathing sets with the syndrome of CO_2 toxicity under safe control conditions, so that appropriate action can be taken at the first indication, this may not assist divers while underwater. In the water there may be few warning symptoms before the problem results in incapacitation. Familiarization will at least alert divers to the problem. Divers should be encouraged to report any unusual symptoms to their companions.

The ideal prevention is by CO_2 monitoring and using an alarm system to warn of rising levels. CO_2 has been referred to as 'the dark matter of diving' because a workable system of real-time monitoring while immersed has proven elusive. At present, and despite concerted efforts from a number of manufacturers, this monitoring is practical for recompression chambers, habitats and submarines, for example, but not yet for self-contained rebreathing apparatus.

If CO_2 levels are not monitored, then attention must be paid to adequate ventilation of chambers, avoidance of hard physical work, keeping within the safe limits of the CO_2 absorbent system and other factors. Even with these precautions, accidents will still happen.

It critical to appreciate that the percentage of CO_2 in the inspired gas becomes increasingly important as the pressure increases. Although 3 per cent CO_2 in the inspired air at the surface produces little effect, at 30 metres (4 ATA) it is equivalent to breathing 12 per cent on the surface and would be incapacitating. At very great depth, minimal percentages of CO_2 are dangerous.

The diver using underwater rebreathing apparatus should be well trained in what to do when CO_2 toxicity is suspected. The diver should stop and rest, thus reducing muscular activity and CO_2 production. At the same time he or she should signal the diving partner because assistance may be required and unconsciousness may be imminent. Either the diver or the companion should flush the counterlung with fresh gas, ditch the affected diver's weights and reach the surface by using positive buoyancy. In deep diving, it may be necessary to return slowly to a submersible chamber. On arrival at the surface or submersible chamber, the diver should immediately breathe from the atmosphere.

Attempts to identify and therefore isolate the CO_2 retainers have been unsuccessful. Personnel selection is therefore not feasible at this stage. Prevention includes advising against any skip breathing or other gas conservation techniques, but it is difficult to enforce. Equipment should not impose a significant breathing resistance, even at maximal workloads. The replacement of helium for nitrogen in mixed gas diving is often effective.

First aid treatment simply requires removal from the toxic environment. Maintenance of respiration and circulation may be necessary for a short period. PCO_2 and pH return to normal when adequate alveolar ventilation and circulation are established.

CHRONIC HYPERCAPNIA

The need for defining tolerance limits to CO_2 for long exposures is becoming increasingly important with the development of saturation diving, the use of submersibles and extended submarine patrols (see Chapter 67).

Marked adaptation to inspired CO_2 levels between 0.5 per cent and 4 per cent has been demonstrated. This adaptation is characterized by an increased tidal volume, a lower respiratory rate and a reduction in the ventilatory response to hypercapnia produced by exercise.

Biochemically, there is a reversal of the initial increase in hydrogen ion concentration, a rise in the plasma bicarbonate and a fall in the plasma chloride, i.e. mild compensated respiratory acidosis. There is a slight rise in $PaCO_2$. These latter changes are almost complete in 3 to 5 days' exposure, although there is a significant reduction in the ventilatory response in the first 24 hours. There is also a rise in serum calcium and other mineral changes.

While at rest, the average diver can tolerate a surface equivalent of up to 4 per cent inspired CO_2 (a $PICO_2$ of 30 mm Hg), without incapacitating physiological changes. During exercise, alveolar ventilation does not increase sufficiently to prevent a significant degree of CO_2 retention as shown by an elevation of $PaCO_2$. This loss of the ventilatory response to CO_2 (of the order of 20 per cent in submariners) may also be of great significance in the saturation diver, particularly during exercise.

REFERENCES

1. Kerem D, Melamed Y, Moran A. Alveolar PCO_2 at rest and exercise in divers and non-divers breathing O_2 at 1ATA. Undersea and Biomedical Research 1980;7(1):17–26.
2. Dempsey J, Pack A, eds. *Regulation of Breathing*. 2nd ed. New York: Deckker, Inc.; 1995.
3. Donald K. Are divers really different? In: *Oxygen and the Diver*. Hanley Swan, UK: The Spa, Ltd.; 1992.

FURTHER READING

Camporesi EM, Bosco G. Ventilation, gas exchange and exercise under pressure. In: Brubakk AO, Neuman TS, eds. *Bennett and Elliott's Physiology and Medicine of Diving*. 5th ed. London: Saunders; 2003:77–114.

Clark, JM, Sinclair RD, Lenox JB. Chemical and non-chemical components of ventilation during hypercapniac exercise in man. *Journal of Applied Physiology* 1980;**48**:1065–1076.

Dempsey J, Pack A, eds. *Regulation of Breathing*. 2nd ed. New York: Deckker, Inc.; 1995.

Donald K. Are divers really different? In: *Oxygen and the Diver*. Hanley Swan, UK: The Spa, Ltd.; 1992.

Donald K. Carbon dioxide and hyperbaric oxygen. In: *Oxygen and the Diver*. Hanley Swan, UK: The Spa, Ltd.; 1992.

Florio J. Studies in rescued divers. In: Lanphier EH, ed. *The Unconscious Diver: Respiratory Control and Other Contributing Factors*. 25th Undersea Medical Society Workshop, Madison, Wisconsin 18–20 September 1980. Bethesda, Maryland: Undersea Medical Society; 1980.

Gelfand K, Lambertsen CJ, Peterson RE. Human respiratory control at high ambient pressures and inspired gas densities. *Journal of Applied Physiology* 1980;**48**:528–539.

Kerem D, Daskalovic YI, Arieli R, Shupak A. CO_2 retention during hyperbaric exercise while breathing 40/60 nitrox. *Undersea and Hyperbaric Medicine* 1995;**22**(4):339–346.

Lanphier EH. Carbon dioxide poisoning. In: Waite CL, ed. *Case Histories of Diving and Hyperbaric Accidents*. Bethesda, Maryland: Undersea and Hyperbaric Medical Society; 1988.

Lumb A. Carbon Dioxide. Chapter 7. In: *Nunn's Applied Respiratory Physiology*, 7th edition, Churchill Davidosn, London 2010.

Lumb A. Control of breathing, Chapter 5, *Nunn's Applied Respiratory Physiology*, 7th Edition, Churchill Livingstone, London: 2012.

MacDonald JW, Pilmanis AA. Carbon dioxide retention with underwater work in the open ocean. In Lanphier EH, ed. *The Unconscious Diver: Respiratory Control and Other Contributing Factors.* 25th Undersea Medical Society Workshop, Madison, Wisconsin 18–20 September 1980. Bethesda, Maryland: Undersea Medical Society; 1980.

Morrison JB, Florio JT, Butt WS. Effects of CO_2 insensitivity and respiratory pattern on respiration in divers. *Undersea Biomedical Research* 1981;**8**:209–217.

Parkes MJ. Evaluating the importance of the carotid chemoreceptors in controlling breathing during exercise in man. *Biomedical Research International* 2013:2013:893506.

Schagatay E. Human breath-hold ability and its underlying physiology. *Human Evolution* 2014;29(1-3):125–140.

Wasserman K. Testing regulation of ventilation with exercise. *Chest* 1976;**70**:173S–178S.

This chapter was reviewed for this fifth edition by Michael Bennett.

19

Breathing gas preparation and contamination

INTRODUCTION

Contamination of a diver's breathing gas can cause a variety of effects. These range from relatively mild discomfort resulting from an oily taste or odour to a mild headache, respiratory changes or respiratory distress, impaired cognition and consciousness, cardiac arrhythmias and death through toxicity or drowning. In earlier editions of this text, this chapter began by stating that the death of a diver as a result of breathing a contaminated gas mixture is an uncommon event. Unfortunately, this statement has become less true with the increased use of various forms of mixture diving and rebreathers. Readers need be aware of the causes of contamination and the methods of prevention and treatment.

AIR COMPRESSORS

Suitable technologies to compress breathing gas are essential to the conduct of underwater diving. Early 'standard dress' divers used simple hand pumps to provide a constant flow of compressed air to their helmets. Modern demand regulators used in both scuba diving and commercial surface-supply breathing apparatus (SSBA) require a supply of compressed gas at around 5 to 10 bar pressure that can be delivered either from the first-stage regulator on a dive cylinder or from the surface via a diving umbilical hose. Compressors are therefore necessary either to supply breathing gas directly to the diver or to fill the dive cylinders.

High-pressure air compressors

Compressors used to fill scuba cylinders take in air at atmospheric pressure and compress it to 200 to 300 bar. The high-pressure air is then filtered, dried and often stored in storage cylinders until it is decanted into scuba cylinders. Alternatively, small compressor units may be used to fill the diver's cylinder directly

If the air was compressed to high pressure in one step, there would be two major problems. First, the gas would become very hot, and subsequently a large volume of condensation would form when the gas cooled. Second, it would be difficult to design seals to prevent air leakage around the large pistons required. Because of these problems, most systems compress the air in three or four stages.

The basic design of a three-stage system is shown in Figure 19.1. At each stage the gas is compressed by a piston that moves up and down in a cylinder with inlet and outlet valves controlling the airflow. These compressors are oil lubricated, and small amounts of oil mist mix with the air as it is compressed. This must be removed, along with the water vapour in the air.

In the first stage, the air is compressed to about 8 bar. It then passes through cooling coils, and the resultant drop in temperatures causes some reduction in the pressure. Some compressors have an interstage filter between the first and second stages, although this is not standard in the diving industry. The second stage of compression raises the pressure further before the air is again cooled. In conjunction with an interstage filter, water and oil are condensed and filtered out. The final stage compresses the air to the pressure required for the storage tanks or scuba cylinders. A final filter system should be incorporated, which may include a fine filter (to remove further moisture), activated carbon (for odour) and molecular sieve material (to remove moisture and oil particles). In an environment where there is likely to be high levels of carbon dioxide, it may advisable to add an extra filter with carbon dioxide absorbent (e.g. soda lime). If carbon monoxide is of particular concern a catalytic converter element such as Hopcalite medium may also be added. A four-stage compressor differs from the three-stage device shown only in that there are smaller pressure increase steps over each stage.

The cylinder, piston and valves in each stage of the compressor are smaller than the preceding because the volume of gas decreases in accordance with Boyle's Law. In the previous example, if the volume of the first stage cylinder was 1000 ml, to match the pressures given, the second stage would need to be less than 200 ml and the third stage about 25 ml.

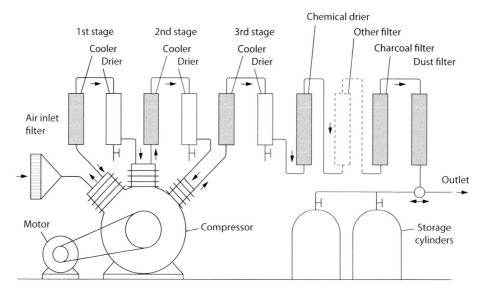

Figure 19.1 Diagramme of a three-stage compressor.

The moisture that condenses is the water vapour in the air that was compressed. If the relative humidity of the air entering the compressor was 50 per cent, condensation would occur when the air pressure is increased to more than 2 bar (if the temperature remains constant). It is difficult and expensive to remove water from compressed air by chemical means only, so this is achieved throughout the process primarily by means of condensation as the air passes through pipes cooled by either fans (air) or water. Interstage separators, fitted with drains, then remove this excess (condensed) water. The process is optimized at the final filter stage by the fitting of a pressure maintaining valve (PMV). The PMV maintains pressure within the final filter (to around 160 to 190 bar, depending on the final pressure) and so increases the efficiency of (chemical) filtration.

A refrigeration system is sometimes used to increase condensation (Figure 19.2). This is fitted

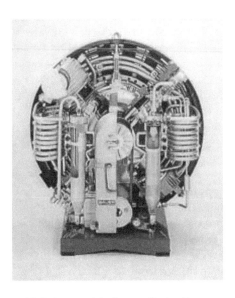

Figure 19.2 A portable four-cylinder Bauer compressor (Bauer AG, Schrobenhausen, Germany) in which some of the components have been cut away to show the internal design. To reduce the size of the compressor, the cylinders are arranged in a radial pattern. The spiral coils are to cool the air between stages of compression; cooling is aided by a fan attached to the far side of the unit. Contaminants are removed from the compressed air by chemicals in prepared packs that fit into two cut-away vertical cylinders in front of the compressor.

after the final (after) cooler and is usually sold separately from the compressor. Both a high outlet valve pressure and refrigeration will also increase the removal of any contaminants that condense with, or in, the water.

There is a divergence of opinion on how best to lubricate compressors. Some advocate synthetic oils, and others recommend mineral oils. The manufacturers' instructions are the best guide to selecting the lubricant. Standard motor oils should not be used because they may break down under high pressures and heat.

Attempts have been made to design compressors that do not need lubrication. Another option is to use water as coolant and lubricant. Neither approach has won general acceptance. The reality is that all high-pressure compressors require oil, at least in the crank case.

Compressors range in size from small units that can be carried by one person to large units that weigh several tonnes. In output terms, these range from as little as 28 to 1500 litres per minute and even larger.

Low-pressure air compressors

SSBA involves much more complex equipment than scuba to provide safety for deeper occupational diving operations. Compressed air may be supplied from large cylinders filled before the dive or from a low-pressure compressor that runs throughout the dive. The air passes through a diver's control panel and then via an umbilical hose to the diver's helmet or demand mask. When a low-pressure compressor is used, a large-volume storage vessel and/or high-pressure cylinders may be incorporated into the system as a back-up. 'Hookah' is a colloquial term sometimes used to refer to minimalist versions of SSBA in which a simple low-pressure compressor supplies a mouth-held regulator via a floating hose. Hookah is commonly used in the seafood harvesting sector and by some recreational divers.

There is a larger variety of compressor types in use for SSBA and hookah diving, with currently used options including reciprocating piston and rotary screw-type compressors. Low pressure air compressors are either lubricated and sealed with oil, or of an oil-free "dry" design and there are advantages and disadvantages to each of the multiple available configurations. Because the compressor is running at the dive site and is usually powered by a diesel or petrol internal combustion engine, there is probably a greater risk of unexpected intake of contaminants compared with a properly installed high-pressure compressor at a fixed location. The quality of compressors used in practice varies dramatically, from well-filtered and well-monitored systems to inexpensive compressors designed for workshop compressed air and sometimes equipped with only makeshift filtration.

GASES FOR MIXED GAS AND TECHNICAL DIVING

Commercial mixed gas diving usually involves helium-oxygen gas mixtures prepared by commercial gas supply companies or mixed on the dive site by highly qualified life support technicians and dive supervisors. The large supply cylinders used are generally prepared by mixing gases from a high-purity supply, and the final mix is analyzed multiple times to check that the composition is correct. This process is costly in time and equipment.

The gas that fills the cylinders used in military and recreational technical mixed gas diving is generally sourced from large cylinders and then transferred into the smaller cylinders used by the diver. The mixture is often blended on site as each cylinder is filled.

In the recreational diving industry where nitrox is commonly used, oxygen is generally sourced in large cylinders from a commercial supplier. The oxygen is decanted into the cylinders, where the pressure is measured, and the cylinder is 'topped-up' with air to a pre-determined pressure to produce the mixture required. The mixture is then analyzed for its oxygen content. This procedure is known as 'partial pressure blending'. If the gases supplied were of sufficient purity, significant contamination should be prevented. (Purity of supplied gas can vary, especially in some countries with lower standards of oversight). It is essential that the oxygen content is measured using two analyzers to verify the final mixture. The diver should also analyze the gas to ensure there has been no error. Failure to do so has sometimes been associated with serious consequences.

Another method of mixing (known as 'continuous flow blending') involves the air being first passed through a membrane system that removes some nitrogen and so creates a higher-oxygen mixture. This is then compressed. To reduce the risk of fire or explosion, the mixture must have an oxygen concentration of 40 per cent or lower. An alternative method of continuous flow blending for nitrox is carried out by introducing metered amounts of oxygen into the intake airflow stream of the compressor via mixing coils. It is important that the gas is mixed thoroughly before entering the compression stage to ensure that the oxygen concentration is lower than 40 per cent. The output is sampled and adjusted until the desired mixtures are obtained. This process can be used only on suitable compressors and to a maximum of 40 per cent oxygen concentration.

Trimix can be produced by combining helium with oxygen and air or a suitable nitrox mixture. Accurate measuring equipment is required, as are suitable valves to control the flow of gases. Once the trimix is produced, it is rolled or agitated for an hour or so to allow the gases to homogenize. To confirm the final mixture the oxygen content needs to be measured, although, ideally, the helium content should also be analyzed.

In any of these systems where air is one of the source gases used, or where a mixture is blended and then compressed by a high- or low-pressure compressor, the same potential sources of contamination exist as for air. Potential problems are multiplied by the complexity of the system and the fact that lubrication oil life can be much reduced through oxidation by oxygen-rich mixtures.

As an alternative to compressors, oil-free reciprocating 'booster pumps' are sometimes used to avoid these risks and to avoid the risk of oxygen fire and explosion when filling cylinders with oxygen-rich mixtures.

SOURCES OF CONTAMINANTS

A contaminant in compressed gas may have been in the air before compression, added during compression because of some fault in the compressor system or have been present or generated within the storage system.

There are many potential contaminants in the atmospheric air taken in by compressors, particularly if the compressors are located in an industrial area or near any running internal combustion engines (e.g. near a boat jetty). Carbon monoxide and nitrogen oxides are components of polluted city air in levels that may be toxic, particularly when the inspired partial pressure is raised by breathing at depth. They may also enter the compressed air if the compressor is driven by, or operated near, an internal combustion engine that produces these compounds. Volatile hydrocarbons and organic compounds, such as methane, may also be present in environmental air.

Compressor lubricating oil may also contaminate the air if excessive oil vapour or even liquid oil passes around the piston rings to enter the supply and overload filters. This is most likely when the rings are damaged or if the air intake is restricted. In reality, some oil is present in the air delivered by even the best-maintained oil-lubricated compressor, and this may increase at higher temperatures. Hence, the drainage from the interstage and final aftercooler separators will always be oily. A well-maintained, modern compressor will have lower levels present in the compressed air produced, but an older, less well-maintained compressor will have higher levels.

More complex forms of contamination can also arise from within the compressor. High temperatures ('hot spots') and high pressures within the compressor produce an ideal environment for contaminants to form. Both these factors promote chemical reactions and hence the production of contaminants. If an unsuitable lubricating oil is used in the compressor, it may produce oil vapour, which may contaminate the air as oil, break down to produce volatile hydrocarbons or burn and form carbon monoxide. The same trouble can also result if the compressor overheats, causing 'cracking' (oil breakdown) or 'flashing' (oil combustion). The air becomes contaminated with volatile hydrocarbons or combustion products such as carbon monoxide and nitrogen oxides. Many low molecular weight volatile contaminants can cause some level of anaesthesia, and the effect is magnified by increased pressure and inert gas narcosis. This may lead to impaired cognition, a reduced seizure threshold and a greater potential for cardiac

arrhythmias while diving. It has been suggested that these contaminants could be contributory to some morbidity and mortality in divers.

Overheating may also be caused by poor design or maintenance of the compressor – a restriction in the compressor intake, a dirty filter, excessive length of intake or a kinked intake hose can all cause problems such as overheating and reduced output.

Therefore, a compressor that may produce satisfactory air when tested running under normal circumstances may deliver contaminated air if it temporarily overheats. This may lead to part of a batch of cylinders being filled with contaminated gas, whereas others are not.

Other problems include leaks between the compressor stages, via piping, loose fittings or head gaskets or around the pistons.

Overall, the most common dangerous contaminant remains carbon monoxide, whether from excessive intake levels or from within the compressor. In some ways this is most dangerous when the air is otherwise clean because carbon monoxide is odourless and tasteless and will not be detected by the diver. Conversely, many potential contaminants have readily noticeable and generally unpleasant smell and taste and are obvious from the first breath.

> Contaminants in compressed gas may have been present in the gas before compression, added during compression or resident in the storage system.

Some divers believe that using an electric compressor prevents carbon monoxide contamination. It removes one common cause of carbon monoxide – that of the driving motor exhaust. However, it does not reduce the other external and internal sources of carbon monoxide described earlier.

With more and more divers visiting dive destinations in developing countries, especially in the tropics, gas contamination is becoming an increasing problem. Problems are most likely when small, low-cost, compressors designed for filling a few cylinders are overused to fill cylinders for hours at a time in hot and humid environments, thus leading to overheating and ineffective filtration through water-saturated filters. These risks are compounded where there is lack of knowledge of appropriate purity standards, poor regulatory oversight or just lack of a proper air quality testing program.

Contamination from other sources

Air contamination from residues within the storage cylinder is not common. Residues of cleaning and scouring materials and scale formed by rusting can contribute vapours or dust if the cleaning operation is not conducted properly or if the cylinder or storage vessel is allowed to deteriorate. Water may be introduced into storage cylinders if there has been a failure of the drying system. There have been problems with paint systems that have been used to protect the interior of steel storage cylinders, where pressure cycling can cause the release of solvent vapour.

Lubricants used on regulators and reducers can sometimes cause fears of contamination. A diver may taste the lubricant in the regulator and think that the air is contaminated, and, if the wrong lubricants have been used, these fears may be justified. With enriched oxygen mixtures, only lubricants approved for use with oxygen should be used, to reduce the risk of fire.

The most difficult source of contamination to isolate is intermittent inlet contamination. For example, one report details a company that had an air compressor inlet on the roof (a not uncommon position). On rare occasions, its air was contaminated with organic chemicals. Only after much work and customer dissatisfaction was the source identified. A nearby factory sometimes used spray painting equipment with an exhaust fan. With a particular wind direction, these fumes would blow across to the compressor inlet.

There is a low risk of contamination in mixture diving when the source gases are produced by liquefaction. This reduces the risk of contamination because most of the potential impurities are separated by their higher boiling points. For mixtures prepared by mixing compressed air with other components, there are potential problems with the air and in the mixing process.

There is a possibility of increasing the concentration of trace contaminants when using recycled and reclaimed gases for deep diving operations and gases compressed in submarines. The compounds that are not removed in any purification process can accumulate with recycling until they are at level that causes a problem. For this reason, a thorough risk analysis should be done to determine likely contaminants, including those that could be infrequent (e.g. methane from animals or from sewerage). A suitable screening gas analysis program for the identified contaminants is highly desirable.

In rebreather diving, contamination with expired carbon dioxide as a result of failure of the 'scrubber' is a potential problem that periodically leads to fatalities.

> With an increase in depth, and hence partial pressure of contaminants, toxicity will increase.

GAS PURITY STANDARDS

Standards specify the composition and the maximum allowed concentration of contaminants in breathing air and for gases used in deep diving. Greater purity is demanded for gases used in deep diving because of the effect of higher inspired partial pressures for all gases in a mixture. Standards vary among organizations with respect to the acceptable level of contaminants, how these are to be detected and for which contaminants the gas should be tested.

Table 19.1 shows some of the available standards. Readers who may rely on these data should review the source documents for verification and more specific information. The standards are updated periodically, so it is important for users to monitor any changes and act accordingly.

Detailed consideration of the standards could lead to the opinion that most limits are rather conservative. Safety margins are incorporated for two reasons. First, the standards are generally based on extrapolation of the effects of the contaminants in isolation at 1 ATA (i.e. the surface equivalent value [SEV]). This may not be entirely valid for contaminants in combination at high pressures. Second, a safety margin will help to allow for any deterioration in the air quality among tests.

Standards are only lists of the maximum allowed concentration of some common impurities. Air may

Table 19.1 Air purity standards (summarized)

Substance	Standards US Navy (2008)	AS/NZ 2299.1-2015	HSE DVIS9[a] (2008)	CGA g-7.1-2011
Oxygen (% by volume)	20–22	21 ± 1	21 ± 1	20–22
Carbon dioxide (ppm$_v$)	1000	600	500	1000
Carbon monoxide (ppm$_v$)	20	5	3	10
Oil (mg/m^3)	5	0.5	0.5	5
Water (mg/m^3)	—	50	25[b]	[c]
Odour and taste	Not objectionable	Not objectionable	None	None
Volatile hydrocarbons (ppm$_v$)	25	—	—	25

AS/NZ, Australia/New Zealand; CGA, Compressed Gas Association; HSE, Health and Safety Executive.

[a] Based on European Standard EN12021 Compressed Air for Breathing Apparatus.

[b] Applies to air leaving compressor.

[c] Varies with environment but approximately 24 ppm.

meet these specifications and still contain toxic substances. A greater variety of contamination problems occurs in caisson work where industrial equipment is being operated. Mineral dust from excavation and blasting is a common problem. Unusual contamination has also occurred in recompression chamber operations, especially if therapeutic or research equipment is used in the chamber. Because exposure times are generally greater in chambers, the toxic contamination has more time to exert its effect, particularly during saturation dives. Toxic substances that may be present include mercury from manometers, ammonia or Freon from leaking air conditioning plants, anaesthetic residues and other vapours from pharmaceutical preparations used during hyperbaric treatments. Potential hazards can be minimized by conducting an appropriate risk assessment.

In using gas mixtures prepared for deep diving, problems can result from the great pressure at which the mixtures are used. This will increase the risk of toxicity because of the higher partial pressures of contaminants. For example, and ignoring the dilution by water vapour in the lungs, at 1 ATA a carbon dioxide concentration of 2 per cent in inspired air means an inspired partial pressure (FICO$_2$) of 15.2 mm Hg, and this is well-tolerated. At 5 ATA (40 msw), however, the same concentration means an FICO$_2$ of 60.8 mm Hg – which will cause dyspnoea, increased work of breathing, distress and ultimately unconsciousness. The same

problems will result from a concentration of only 0.2 per cent at 50 ATA. Therefore, standards need adjustment if they are used for depths and times greater than those assumed by their designers.

In the hyperbaric chamber environment (and elsewhere), toxicological problems can be introduced by the use of cleaning agents, among other sources. This is a growing problem with the rise in the prevalence of multi-resistant organisms that require extensive decontamination of therapeutic chambers between uses. The basic rule must be 'if in doubt, leave it out'. Useful guidelines are available from reference to experience with long-term exposures in spacecraft and nuclear submarines. However, with the increase in hyperbaric treatment centres and greater reporting and communication among these centres, information on potentially problematic substances in a hyperbaric environment is more readily available.

The reasons for listing the components and the concentrations commonly specified are outlined in the following subsections:

Nitrogen and oxygen

The concentration of oxygen in compressed air standards is close to the level in clean, dry air. Any significant deviation is most unusual. If the nitrogen concentration was elevated, it could increase the risk of decompression sickness, narcosis or hypoxia. If the oxygen concentration was increased, the risk of oxygen toxicity, and fire hazards in hyperbaric chambers, would rise. The oxygen may be elevated by connecting to a bulk oxygen supply. This may be accidental, but it has been deliberate in the misguided belief that increasing oxygen concentration will increase the endurance available from a cylinder.

Carbon dioxide

A typical specified carbon dioxide level of 0.05 per cent (500 parts per million [ppm]) means that at 10 ATA the partial pressure of carbon dioxide would still be well below that required to cause any physiological effect. It has been argued that the British and Australian/New Zealand standards may be too strict because some other standards set a maximum limit of 0.1 per cent. This would not be toxic to the depth limits of compressed air diving and would be easier for compressor operators to meet.

The carbon dioxide level, even if it is within the specification used, should be considered in relation to the level in the ambient air. Global increases in carbon dioxide levels, further increased in cities and industrial areas, can cause compressor intake air to have carbon dioxide levels in excess of standards, even though they are physiologically safe. Some compressors use intake scrubbing of carbon dioxide from ambient air with absorbent canisters.

Carbon monoxide

This toxic gas binds tightly to the oxygen binding sites of haemoglobin to form carboxyhaemoglobin – preventing the carriage of oxygen. If sufficient haemoglobin binds with carbon monoxide, the diver will become hypoxic. The formation of carboxyhaemoglobin will also interfere with the transport of carbon dioxide away from the tissues by preventing its combination with haemoglobin. Carbon monoxide also causes oxidative stress and direct cellular toxicity.

The sometimes described cherry red colour of these victims is an unreliable clinical sign, especially in patients with cardiorespiratory impairment. Exertion and increased ventilation will hasten the development of symptoms. Subjects

with a low haemoglobin level are more susceptible to carbon monoxide poisoning.

The concentrations required for poisoning are considerably greater than the maximum carbon monoxide level of 3 to 10 ppm specified in most standards. Exposure to ambient air with carbon monoxide levels higher that 100 ppm is considered dangerous to human health. A limit of 25 to 50 ppm is a suggested maximum level for occupational workers exposed for up to 8 hours a day.

For divers breathing air, the higher partial pressure of oxygen tends to protect against the effects of increased carbon monoxide partial pressure while at depth. The toxic limits of carbon monoxide at depth and how they are modified by varying ambient and oxygen partial pressures have not been established. Divers are probably at greatest risk of unconsciousness as they surface and lose the protection offered by the increased transport of oxygen in plasma that occurs at depth when the partial pressure of oxygen in inspired air is elevated.

A lower maximum carbon monoxide concentration is needed for deep and saturation divers. This is because the exposure times are longer. In addition, the oxygen partial pressure is usually limited to about 0.4 ATA, so the protection from an elevated oxygen pressure is reduced.

Oil

Oil occurring as a mist or vapour can cause compressed air to have an unpleasant odour and taste. Its direct, toxic effects in normal people are not known except that in high concentrations oil vapour can cause lipoid pneumonia. In some people, low concentrations of oil vapour can trigger asthma. Condensed oil, especially if combined with solid residues, can cause malfunctions of equipment. The other problem with oil is that it can decompose if overheating occurs and can generate hydrocarbons and toxic compounds of carbon, nitrogen and sulphur, depending on the oil composition.

Some compressed air standards distinguish oil from other hydrocarbons and specify maximum limits for each. Most hydrocarbons in high-pressure systems can be serious fire hazards. Some have other undesirable effects, such as being carcinogenic.

CASE REPORT 19.1

An experienced diver was diving in an area subject to tidal currents. He planned to dive at 'slack water' and anchored his boat a short time before the low tide. The hookah compressor was correctly arranged with the inlet upwind of the exhaust and the dive commenced. After an hour at 10 metres, the diver felt dizzy and lost consciousness but was fortunately pulled aboard by his attendant and revived.

Diagnosis: carbon monoxide poisoning, confirmed by blood analysis.

Explanation: As the tide turned, so did the boat. This put the compressor inlet downwind of the motor exhaust. The carbon monoxide from the exhaust was drawn into the compressor inlet and was breathed under pressure by the diver.

CASE REPORT 19.2

A 35-year-old man, with 20 years of diving experience and no relevant medical history, undertook a solo crayfish dive. He told the boat operator that he would be 15 minutes, but he failed to surface. A search by police divers found him the following day at a depth of 9 msw. The autopsy was limited because of destruction of the body by sea lice. The police investigation suggested that he was diving over-weighted with 17.5 kg on the weight belt, which was not released. All his equipment was intact and working correctly and the cylinder pressure was 194 bar, so he died very early in the dive.

Analysis of the cylinder contents revealed an extremely high carbon monoxide level, 13,600 ± 300 ppm (NZ standard <10 ppm), as well as increased levels of carbon dioxide and methane. A second cylinder owned by the diver returned similar analysis. Both cylinders were filled at the same time at the same dive shop.

The coroner's finding was that 'death [was] due to asphyxia due to his cylinder gas being contaminated with carbon monoxide, brought about by an idiosyncratic malfunction of the air compressing equipment'. There was no evidence of any other cylinders filled on that day reported as contaminated, so this was an isolated finding, the cause of which was unknown. (This case is from the New Zealand diving fatality data and was reported in Millar IL, Mouldey PG. Compressed breathing air: the potential for evil from within. *Diving and Hyperbaric Medicine* 2008;**38**(3):151.)

Water

Control of water vapour is needed to reduce corrosion and oxidation damage to equipment. A low water concentration may also prevent ice formation and supply blockage or a free-flowing regulator when diving in cold water as a result of adiabatic cooling during pressure reduction. Some investigators think that this problem has been overstated because the areas susceptible to blockage are at lower pressure than the cylinder. In these areas, the air will not be saturated because the gas has expanded. Water condensation can also impair the efficiency of the filters used to remove other contaminants. This is more common with some of the molecular sieve filter systems.

Deaths have been reported from diving with steel cylinders containing water. Rusting occurs if these cylinders are left unused for long periods. Rusting consumes oxygen and leaves a mixture that caused death from hypoxia. The other problem is that the rusting process weakens the cylinder and may cause it to become an 'unguided missile' if the gas rapidly discharges. Severe injuries and deaths have been caused by exploding cylinders.

Solid particles

These particles must be controlled by filters to protect the diver and the equipment. The effect of the particles depends on their size and composition. Particles such as pollens can cause hay fever and asthma in susceptible divers. Pollens have been found inside scuba cylinders. Other particles have various undesirable physiological effects depending on their size and composition. Any dust that causes coughing could be particularly hazardous, especially for a novice diver.

In diving equipment, abrasive particles such as mineral dust would accelerate wear on the equipment by abrasive erosion. Soluble particles such as salt crystals can accelerate corrosion by promoting electrolysis. Organic dust can also contribute to a fire hazard. There have been cases of filters breaking down, letting material through and contributing particles of filter material to the air supply. Large concentrations of particulates can become a fire hazard.

Nitrogen dioxide and nitrous oxide

Some of the oxides of nitrogen, and nitrogen dioxide in particular, are intensely irritating, especially to the lungs, eyes and throat. These symptoms can occur when an individual is exposed to gas with a concentration of nitrogen dioxide greater than 10 ppm. At lower concentrations, the initial symptoms are slight and may not be noticed, or they may disappear. After a latent period of 2 to 20 hours, further signs that may be precipitated by exertion appear. Coughing, difficulty in breathing, cyanosis and haemoptysis accompany the development of pulmonary oedema. Unconsciousness usually follows.

The typical maximum level of no higher than 2 ppm is also the maximum allowed level for 24-hour exposure in some standards. If the effect is increased with pressure, then 0.2 ppm may be a more appropriate limit. In industrial cities, 2 ppm is often exceeded.

Nitrous oxide is an anaesthetic agent, but only at high concentrations. A low concentration of it is specified because, if nitrous oxide is generated within the compressor a precursor, nitric oxide must have been formed. Nitric oxide can also be converted to nitrogen dioxide at higher pressures and temperatures. Therefore, a compressor that adds nitrous oxide to the air being compressed can also form nitrogen dioxide.

Odour and taste

Odour and taste are controlled to avoid air that is unpleasant to breathe. They also provide a back-up for the other standards because if the air has an odour, it contains an impurity.

Volatile hydrocarbons

Volatile hydrocarbons such as benzene, toluene, xylene and ethane, among others, exist as gases at temperatures usual to diving situations and, as such, can be absorbed and distributed throughout the body in a similar manner to volatile anaesthetic agents. However, their side effects, such as impaired consciousness and increased cardiac irritability, present additional dangers to the diver. These gases may also be carcinogenic and present a fire hazard, so they need to be limited to a maximum of 5 ppm.

Most air purity standards do not require testing for these hydrocarbons, with the exception of the Canadian CSA 275.2 2004 standard (5 ppm of volatile non-methane hydrocarbons and 5 ppm of halogenated hydrocarbons); and the US CGA G-7.1-2011 standard (25 ppm of volatile hydrocarbons).

PREVENTION

Contamination should not occur if clean, dry air is pumped by a suitable, well-maintained compressor into clean, corrosion-free cylinders. Any deviation from this procedure will lead to the risk of contamination.

> Prevention of contamination involves the use of suitable, well-maintained compressors, adequate filters, clean cylinders and regular analysis of the gas.

Filtering will be necessary to remove any contaminants introduced by compression. It will also be needed if the air compressed comes from a polluted area. Water removal will be needed in most situations. The choice of filtering agents and the frequency of replacement are the purview of a specialized field of engineering, and these issues should be considered with experts in the field. The following methods and agents are commonly used.

1. Silica gel, to remove water vapour.
2. Activated alumina, to remove water vapour.
3. Activated charcoal, to remove oil mist and volatile hydrocarbons.
4. Activated zeolites and molecular sieves, to remove oil and water.
5. Reverse flow or centrifugal filters, to remove solids and large liquid drops.
6. Hopcalite (a combination of manganese and copper oxide) acts as a catalyst to converts carbon monoxide to carbon dioxide.
7. Soda lime, to remove carbon dioxide.
8. Cryogenic cooling, to remove impurities with a higher boiling point (normally water and carbon dioxide).
9. Refrigerant dryer, to reduce final outlet temperature to a pressure dew point low enough to facilitate the condensation of most of the moisture (water and oil) and thus extend the life of the chemical reagents.

Some companies incorporate several filtering agents into a cartridge, thereby simplifying the servicing of the compressor.

The lifespan of some filters can be reduced by certain conditions. For example, activated charcoal is exhausted faster when it is used with nitrox rather than air.

TREATMENT

For most of the conditions caused by contaminated air, the first step is to replace the contaminated air supply with an appropriate uncontaminated breathing gas. Underwater, this will mean reverting to an alternative source. On the surface, breathing fresh air may suffice in mild cases. However, rest, breathing high concentration oxygen and general first aid measures may be required. In more severe cases, resuscitation may be needed.

It is generally believed that patients with serious cases of carbon monoxide toxicity benefit from hyperbaric oxygen therapy, and this is widely used.

Treatment of nitrogen dioxide poisoning requires rest in all cases. This may prevent the condition from progressing. If the exposure was thought to be to a toxic concentration or if the patient develops further symptoms, then 100 per cent oxygen is indicated. If pulmonary oedema develops, it should be appropriately managed.

DETECTION OF CONTAMINATION

The accurate assessment of the concentration of contaminants is best left to specialists, such as air pollution analysts. The tests outlined give the user a reasonable assessment of air quality. Some tests should not be used for samples where a death or legal action may be involved because they require large amounts of air for an imprecise answer. In some countries, there is a requirement that air testing be conducted by an independent tester rather than by the supplier.

For most compressor operators, the purchase of an indicating tube gas analyzer system is a sound investment. These are made by Mine Safety Apparatus (Pittsburgh, USA), Auer (Berlin, Germany) and Dräger (Lubeck, Germany), among other companies. The devices operate by passing a metered volume of air through a glass tube filled with chemicals. These chemicals react with the contaminant and cause a colour change. A scale on the tube indicates the amount of contaminant present in the sample. Tubes from different manufacturers cannot be mixed because the tube systems use different flows and volumes of gas.

The oxygen concentration may be checked using an oxygen electrode, analyzer or indicator tube. This is particularly important for diving with gases other than air.

Carbon dioxide can be measured using an indicating tube or a variety of chemical and physical techniques. Infrared absorption is commonly used.

Oil and dust can be determined by filtering and weighing, with the increase in the dry weight indicating the weight of oil and dust. A solvent such as hexane may be used to dissolve the oil; the remaining weight is particulate matter.

This procedure requires an accurate balance and is not commonly used in the diving industry. An indication of the presence of oil can be obtained by directing a jet of air on to a clean sheet of white paper and then examining the paper under ultraviolet light. Some oils will fluoresce, although, despite some exceptions, synthetics generally do not. Indicating tubes can be used, as well as a newer dedicated device for detection of oil aerosols in compressed air.

Nitrogen oxides may be detected using indicating tubes. These tubes may also be used for detection of water vapour, but a method involving a measurement of the dew point is more suitable.

Combinations of gas chromatography and mass spectrometer systems have, until recently, been needed to obtain an accurate identification of trace contaminants in divers' air. These expensive laboratory-based systems need a competent operator and a large stock of reference samples to give satisfactory service. Laboratories involved with air pollution measurement may be able to provide these facilities. Gas analysis technology is advancing rapidly, however, and there are now handheld photo-ionization detectors (PIDs) and modestly priced flame ionization detectors (FIDs) that can detect and/or quantify contamination at levels relevant to diving. Work is continuing on 'gas detectors on a chip' that promise to enable real-time monitoring of gases in the future, potentially at both the compressor output and within the breathing circuit, especially of rebreather equipment.

FURTHER READING

Burman F. Compressed gas (air) supply system. Presented at the Ninth European Committee for Hyperbaric Medicine (ECHM) Consensus Conference, Belgrade, Serbia, 2012.

Compressed Gas Association. *CGA G-7.1-2011. Commodity Specification for Air.* 6th ed. Chantilly, Virginia: Compressed Gas Association; 2011.

Health and Safety Executive. *Diver's Breathing Air Standard and the Frequency of Examination and Tests.* DVis9(Rev1). Suffolk: HSE Books; 2008.

Millar IL, Mouldey PG. Compressed breathing air: the potential for evil from within. *Diving and Hyperbaric Medicine* 2008;3(3):145–151.

Standards Association of Australia. *AS/NZS 2299.1:2015 Occupational Diving Operations. Part 1. Standard Operational Practice.* Sydney: Standards Australia/Standards New Zealand; in press.

US Navy Diving Manual Revision 6. SS521-AG-PRO-010 (2008). Washington, DC: Naval Sea Systems Command; 2008.

This chapter was reviewed for this fifth edition by John Lippmann.

High-pressure neurological syndrome

> The high-pressure neurological syndrome (HPNS), also called the high-pressure nervous syndrome, is a condition noted in deep diving. With divers breathing helium mixtures, it is noticeable from about 150 to 200 metres. The first effects are tremors, but the condition progresses to lapses of consciousness at depths in excess of 300 metres. In animals compressed to greater depths, convulsions and death occur. HPNS should not be confused with nitrogen narcosis, neurological decompression illness or central nervous system oxygen toxicity.
>
> HPNS is a complex phenomenon described by neurological, psychological and electroencephalographic changes. The gas composition, the rate of compression and the absolute pressure affect these parameters. HPNS appears to be ameliorated by gases having an anaesthetic or narcotic effect and by slowing the rate of compression.
>
> Increased hydrostatic pressure appears to be the most important contributor to the development of HPNS, which remains a major limitation to deep diving. It is not a concern within the depth range of compressed air diving.

HISTORY

Alternative respiratory gases to compressed air have been sought because of the restriction to effective diving at depths greater than 40 to 60 metres of sea water (msw) as a result of nitrogen narcosis and the high density of air (see Chapter 15). Projection of knowledge concerning inert gas narcosis, especially lipid solubilities, suggested that substituting helium for nitrogen would prevent severe narcosis until pressures were greater than 40 ATA. However, in the 1960s, difficulties were encountered beyond a depth of 200 metres (pressure of 20 ATA) when using a helium-oxygen breathing mixture. This syndrome, which is also characterized by a disturbance of the nervous system, is quite different from the effects of nitrogen (i.e. inert gas narcosis). Because the most prominent feature noted was tremors, the condition was initially referred to as helium tremors[1], although it is now realized that the use of helium is merely an association and that helium itself is not the cause[2].

In retrospect, a series of experiments in the 1880s recorded abnormal excitement, disturbed locomotion and paralysis in marine animals exposed to a high-pressure environment. During the 1920s, a series of publications dealt with the effects of high hydrostatic pressures. Halsey[3] cited a paper published in 1936 in which manifestations that may have been the high-pressure neurological syndrome (HPNS) were reported in vertebrate animals.

In the 1960s, British, US, Russian, and French investigators noted tremors and performance impairment in divers compressed to depths of 200 to 400 msw (20 to 40 ATA)[4]. Coarse tremors were often associated with other symptoms such as nausea, vomiting, dizziness and vertigo. Decreased ability to carry out fine movements was observed. In animals, similar changes were noted that, under further pressure, progressed to generalized convulsions.

This complex of features has become known as the 'high-pressure neurological syndrome' or the 'high-pressure nervous syndrome', abbreviated HPNS in either case. HPNS should not be confused with inert gas narcosis (see Chapter 15), neurological decompression sickness (see Chapter 11), central nervous system oxygen toxicity (see Chapter 17) or other gas toxicities.

AETIOLOGY

HPNS has been observed in all animals studied that have a central nervous system at least as complex as that of a flatworm[5]. Studies in non–air-breathing aquatic animals demonstrate that the effect is not dependent on elevated gas pressure and is at least partly the result of increased hydrostatic pressure[3]. In air-breathing animals, including humans, HPNS develops while breathing helium and oxygen under high ambient pressure. The inspired gases may modify the manifestations of HPNS[6] (see later), thus complicating comparative studies, but breathing gases under pressure *per se* is not the primary cause.

Animals breathing a helium-oxygen mixture under increasing pressure develop fine and then coarse tremors. These tremors proceed to localized myoclonic episodes and then to generalized clonic seizures. If compression is stopped, the animal will continue to show this seizure activity for as long as 12 hours. Reduction in pressure relieves the symptoms. If compression is continued, tonic-clonic seizures may continue and lead to death. HPNS is reversible up to a certain stage. Using a slower rate of compression can increase the depths at which convulsions occur.

The addition of nitrogen, hydrogen or nitrous oxide to oxygen-helium mixtures significantly delays the onset of both convulsions and tremor. The anti-tremor effect is only about one half that of the anticonvulsant effect. The potency of these gases in alleviating some features of HPNS is proportional to their narcotic potency.

Increased hydrostatic pressure appears to increase excitability of the central nervous system[7], and this may be counteracted to some degree by the use of narcotic drugs[8]. These agents appear to act at different locations, and therefore a different clinical pattern develops if HPNS is modified by nitrogen, barbiturates or ketamine. Barbiturates and anticonvulsants significantly elevate the tremor and convulsion threshold pressures, and they may be synergistic with narcotic and anaesthetic gases. Studies in rats indicate that some of the adverse symptoms of HPNS can be reduced by intravenous alcohol; however, at higher doses, a characteristic pattern of unsteady locomotion was observed[9].

The exact mechanism of production of HPNS is not understood. Some aetiological factors that have been proposed in the past include a temperature effect, gas-induced osmosis, a modified form of inert gas narcosis and hypoxia or hypercapnia caused by the respiratory limitations imposed by increased gas density. Halsey presented evidence that tends to discount these theories[3].

At a simplistic level, one explanation may be a subtle pressure effect on the architecture of excitable membranes in the nervous system. Thus, if an excitable membrane is 'crushed' even subtly, in a way that alters geometry and function of transmembrane proteins, membrane surface receptors and ion channels, then derangement of normal function could result. Such a mechanism offers a convenient segue into explaining the ameliorating effect of narcotic gases whose 'space-occupying dissolution' into the membrane may restore the membrane's original architecture, virtually the reciprocal explanation for pressure reversal of general anaesthesia by anaesthetic vapours.

In reality (and as is the case for explaining the mechanism of anaesthesia by anaesthetic vapours), the explanation is not likely to be as simple as that. There is considerable evidence for the role of neurotransmitters in pathogenesis. These include gamma-aminobutyric acid (GABA), dopamine, serotonin, acetylcholine and N-methyl-D-aspartate (NMDA). The monoamine-depleting drug reserpine lowers the pressure required to produce convulsions. Drugs such as sodium valproate, which enhance the activity of GABA, prevent or reduce some of the changes associated with the syndrome.

Focal injection of NMDA antagonists in rats has been shown to be protective against convulsions. At 81 ATA, primates pre-treated with an NMDA receptor antagonist showed a delayed onset of face tremor and myoclonus with abolished severe whole body tremor and seizure activity. The electroencephalographic (EEG) increase in alpha activity was also abolished, thereby indicating that NMDA transmission plays a significant part in the manifestations of HPNS[10].

The serotonin syndrome has features similar to those of HPNS. At least in rats, a modified form of the syndrome appears at increased pressure – consistent with the hypothesis that elevation of 5-hydroxytryptamine (5-HT) or activation of receptors has occurred. Elevation of striatal dopamine in rats exposed to pressure can be blocked by 5-HT receptor antagonists and, concurrently, observable motor features of HPNS can be reduced[11].

Changes in neuronal calcium ions induced by high-pressure helium have been postulated as a mechanism for the excitatory phenomena of HPNS[12].

CLINICAL FEATURES

The components of the breathing gas mixture, the rate of compression and the time for adaptation influence the presentation. Breathing helium-oxygen, mild effects are seen at pressures of 100 metres, and these effects progress to become debilitating at depths greater than 300 metres. Adding 5 to 10 per cent nitrogen (or hydrogen) to the helium-oxygen respiratory gas mixture reduces symptoms and may permit useful work to be performed after more rapid compression

and/or deeper exposure (see later). There is a marked individual variation in susceptibility.

Symptoms

Many different symptoms have been reported from various studies, but most symptoms seem to involve a disturbance of central nervous system function. Effects reported include tremor of the hands and arms that may extend to the whole body, occasional muscle jerks, light-headedness or dizziness, headache, euphoria, drowsiness and loss of consciousness. There is a tendency to fall asleep if not stimulated. Dysphoria and even paranoia are possible. Gastro-intestinal symptoms such as nausea sometimes progressing to vomiting, epigastric sensations, diarrhoea, loss of appetite and aversion to food (leading to weight loss in prolonged exposures) and abdominal cramps may result from a disturbance of the vestibulo-ocular reflex.

Dyspnoea at depths in excess of 300 metres may be a manifestation of HPNS, but this can be difficult to separate from the effects of dense gas and increases in the work of breathing. It can develop or intensify suddenly and may be precipitated by exercise. The distress is greater during inspiration, but surprisingly it is ameliorated by using nitrogen in the breathing mixture, which paradoxically increases gas density and thus the work of breathing.

Signs

Tremor may appear in depths as shallow as 150 metres (16 ATA), and it progressively intensifies with increasing depth and pressure. This sign is increasingly reported on deep technical dives where the compressions are extremely fast. The tremor is seen both at rest and on movement. The tremor frequency is 8 to 12 Hz, which differs from that caused by Parkinson's disease and cerebellar disease, which have a frequency of 3 to 8 Hz. It may be thought of as an extension or exaggeration of the normal physiological resting tremor. The amplitude but not the frequency of the tremor increases with faster rates of compression or increasing absolute pressure. There is a gradual return toward normal following cessation of compression, but it may not be complete until the diver is decompressed. Divers learn to adapt to the tremor, thus leading to an apparent improvement after a day or two.

Opsoclonus is an involuntary, constant, random jittering of the eyes. It is said to be one of the earliest signs of HPNS, and it develops at a depth of 160 metres (17 ATA)[8].

Disturbances of long-term memory and decreases in psychomotor performance have been reported following exposures that produced HPNS. The performance impairment abates somewhat during a stay at constant pressure, but at depths greater than 300 metres, full recovery has not been recorded. Other neuropsychological changes have been reported in some divers. The question remains as to what degree of cognitive performance decrement is acceptable from an occupational and safety standpoint.

Psychomotor tests involving manual dexterity reveal a considerable performance decrement, correlated with the tremor, and averaging 1 per cent, for each 20 metres of depth. Manual dexterity gradually starts returning toward normal levels after 1½ hours at a constant pressure.

Electrophysiological changes

The EEG records during exposure of divers reveal an increase in theta activity and a decrease in alpha waves. Increased theta activity may be seen from depths of 60 metres while breathing air or from 150 metres while breathing helium-oxygen mixtures.

Sleep disruptions such as an increase of awake periods and a decrease in sleep stages 3 and 4 and rapid eye movement sleep has been reported at depths of 450 metres.

Somatosensory evoked potentials increase in amplitude, but they are accompanied by an increase in threshold for sensory stimulation. Shortened latency of peaks following the initial cortical P1 is consistent with a state of hyperexcitability in the brain.

The evoked cortical responses may also be altered during deep dives. A progressive decline in the auditory evoked response, by as much as 50 per cent at 457 metres, has been observed. This may be the result of increased sound conduction in high-density gas. Visual evoked responses have not shown any consistent changes.

PREVENTION AND CONTROL

It is unlikely that HPNS will be able to be entirely prevented. Nevertheless, several approaches are possible either to delay onset or to modify its clinical effects.

Reduction in the rate of compression reduces the incidence and severity of HPNS. This can be achieved by a slower overall rate or by inserting stops to allow for acclimatization as greater depths are reached. Very slow rates of compression do improve or even prevent symptoms of HPNS in some subjects. Indeed, nausea can be virtually eliminated. Nevertheless, at depths exceeding 300 metres, even with 6 days of compression, some signs of HPNS are still present. With increasing depth, symptoms become more serious and severely limit the ability to perform useful work[13]. Performance decrements induced by compression improve during a stop at constant pressure, but total recovery has not been recorded at pressures greater than 300 msw[14]. Very slow compression rates are economically disadvantageous in occupational (saturation diving) settings, and they simply cannot be considered in technical 'bounce' diving applications. Thus, at a practical level, slowing compression rates is frequently not particularly useful.

Modification of the breathing gas mixture has been used to delay or modify HPNS. Interestingly, the narcotic effect of nitrogen has been used to counter some of the symptoms. Small amounts of nitrogen (5 to 10 per cent) introduced into the helium-oxygen mixture have been shown to markedly reduce tremor but not EEG abnormalities.

Hydrogen has also been studied in breathing gas mixtures[14,15]. Hydrogen is less dense than helium and thus would be even better for respiratory mechanics. Being more lipid soluble than helium, hydrogen has a greater narcotic potency, and this can be used to reduce some of the symptoms of HPNS. It appears that the narcotic potency of hydrogen is too great for it to be used alone with oxygen in very deep applications, but hydrogen-helium-oxygen mixtures with about 50 per cent hydrogen have allowed working dives to 500 metres to be achieved without significant symptoms of HPNS and with minimal performance decrement[15]. Electrophysiological changes and sleep disruptions were still present.

The advantages of added nitrogen include decreased cost, increased thermal comfort, a reduced distortion of speech and a reduction in the HPNS. In adding nitrogen to a deep diving mixture to reduce HPNS, the user must be careful not to increase the narcotic potency of the gas to a higher level than desired at the intended depth of use (see Chapter 62). The advantages of helium and hydrogen include a reduction in the narcotic effect and a reduction in the work of breathing.

Drugs such as alcohol, anaesthetics and anticonvulsants have been suggested to control HPNS. Ketamine is effective in preventing HPNS in rats. Barbiturates have an anticonvulsive effect over a wide range of pressures. Valproate is effective in baboon experiments in reducing HPNS at pressures greater than 40 ATA[16]. Other anticonvulsants have only a limited effect. Common anticonvulsant drugs such as phenytoin and carbamazepine had no effect on prevention of tremor, myoclonus and seizures in rats. This finding suggests that HPNS-induced seizures are of an unusual type, and that conventional anticonvulsant treatment would be of limited value for HPNS in humans[17]. Currently, the use of drugs to modify HPNS has no place in human exposure.

Brauer raised two possible problems in trying to control HPNS. First, the efforts to ameliorate HPNS may be effective only on the early manifestations. In so doing, a situation may be created where the first sign may be more serious HPNS, which, in animals, has been fatal. The second problem is that, in baboons, delaying the development of HPNS can induce a new set of symptoms that may involve brain damage[5]. This is all speculative, and it is clear that more work is required in this area.

HPNS is a major limiting factor in deep diving[14]. The extremely long duration of deep dives that involve very slow rates of compression to mitigate HPNS followed by slow decompression to avoid decompression sickness have curbed commercial interest in such diving. Thus, research into HPNS has progressed little since the 1990s. Extrapolation from lower primates to humans suggests that human divers are approaching depths at which seizures may be anticipated.

REFERENCES

1. Bachrach HJ, Bennett PB. The high pressure nervous syndrome during human deep saturation and excursion diving. *Forsvarsmedicin* 1973;**9**:490–495.

2. Bennett PB, Mcleod M. Probing the limits of human deep diving. *Philosophical Transactions of the Royal Society of London; Series B, Biological Sciences* 1984;**304**:105–117.

3. Halsey MJ. Effects of high pressure on the central nervous system. *Physiological Reviews* 1982;**62**:1341–1377.

4. Bennett PB, Rostain JC. The high pressure nervous syndrome. In: Bennett PB, Elliott DH, editors. *The Physiology of Diving and Medicine of Diving.* 4th ed. Philadelphia: Saunders; 1993.

5. Brauer RW. Hydrostatic pressure effects on the central nervous system: perspectives and outlook. *Philosophical Transactions of the Royal Society of London: Series B, Biological Sciences* 1984;**304**:17–30.

6. Abraini JH. Some considerations regarding the narcotic potency of helium and oxygen in humans. In: Rostain JC, Macdonald AG, Marquis RE, editors. *Basic and Applied High Pressure Biology.* IV. *Medsubhyp International* 1995;**5**:77–82.

7. Miller KW, Paton WDM, Smith RA, Smith EB. The pressure reversal of general anaesthesia and the critical volume hypothesis. *Molecular Pharmacology* 1973;**9**(2):131–143.

8. Jain KK. High-pressure neurological syndrome (HPNS). *Acta Neurologica Scandinavica* 1994;**90**:45–50.

9. Garcia-Cabrere I, Berge OG. Interaction of ethanol and the high pressure nervous syndrome in rats. *Undersea Biomedical Research* 1990;**17**(5):375–382.

10. Pearce PC, Halsey MJ, MacLean CJ, *et al.* The effects of the competitive NMDA receptor antagonist CPP on the high pressure neurological syndrome in a primate model. *Neuropharmacology* 1991;**30**(7):787–796.

11. Kriem B, Abraini JH, Rostain JC. Role of 5-HT 1b receptor in the pressure-induced behavioral and neurochemical disorders in rats. *Pharmacology, Biochemistry and Behavior* 1996;**53**(2):257–264.

12. Philp RB, Kalogeros G, McIver DJ, Dixon SJ. Effects of elevated pressures of inert gases on cytosolic free Ca^{2+} of cultured neuroblastoma cells stimulated with carbachol: relevance to high pressure neurological syndrome. *Cell Calcium* 1994;**15**(2):117–121.

13. Bennett PB. Physiological limitations to underwater exploration and work. *Comparative Biochemistry and Physiology: A, Comparative Physiology* 1989;**93**:295–300.

14. Rostain JC. The high pressure nervous syndrome: neurological and cognitive studies. In: *Long-term Health Effects of Diving: An International Consensus Conference.* Bergen, Norway: Norwegian Underwater Technology Centre and University of Bergen, Norway; 1994.

15. Abraini JH, Gardett-Chauffour MC, Martinez E, *et al.* Psychological reactions in humans during an open sea dive to 500 m with a hydrogen-helium-oxygen mixture. *Journal of Applied Physiology* 1994;**76**(3):1113–1118.

16. Pearce PC, Clarke D, Dore CJ, *et al.* Sodium valproate interactions with the HPNS: EEG and behavioral observations. *Undersea Biomedical Research* 1989;**16**(2):99–113.

17. Wardley-Smith B, Dore C, Hudson S, Wann K. Effects of four common anticonvulsants on the high pressure nervous syndrome in the rat. *Undersea Biomedical Research* 1992;**19**(1):13–20.

This chapter was reviewed for this fifth edition by Simon Mitchell.

PART 5

Aquatic Disorders: The drowning syndromes

21

Drowning

Drowning is defined as the death of an air-breathing animal as a result of submersion in fluid. When patients lose consciousness because of aspiration causing hypoxia, but subsequently recover, the term 'near drowning' is used. When symptoms are not severe enough to classify as near drowning, another term, the 'aspiration syndrome', is employed.

In divers, and others who submerge after losing consciousness, the pathology of drowning is complicated by the effects of barotrauma in air spaces (e.g. middle ear, sinus, face mask) and decompression artefact.

When I use a word it means just what I choose it to mean – neither more nor less.

Humpty Dumpty, from Lewis Carroll

General reviews indicating the importance of this topic to diving medicine have been presented by diving clinicians such as Sir Stanley Miles, Kenneth Donald, Carl Edmonds, Barbara Tabeling, Christopher Dueker, Tom Neuman and others (see the Further Reading list at the end of this chapter and also Chapters 24 and 25).

Other specialists such as forensic pathologists, epidemiologists, animal researchers and respiratory and emergency clinicians have an equal involvement, but they approach the topic from different aspects. This diversity of interests has had implications not only on terminology, but also on conventional beliefs and prejudices.

TERMINOLOGY

The drowning syndromes have been researched extensively for centuries, yet we cannot even agree on the definition.

Drowning, until the nomenclature was changed by the World Congress on Drowning in 2002, meant the death of an air-breathing animal as a result of submersion in a liquid. There were a number of related clinical diagnoses:

Near-drowning referred to a serious clinical syndrome with the loss of consciousness from the submersion, but not resulting in death. It was therefore a lesser condition, but one that could lead to drowning.

Delayed drowning or *secondary drowning* occurred when the victim appeared to recover from the near drowning incident, but then proceeded to die. This had important management implications.

The *aspiration syndrome* referred to the lesser effects of aspiration of fluid into the lungs, without death or loss of consciousness.

There was an escalating range in the severity of symptoms and signs among aspiration, near drowning and drowning. They were incorporated together as *the drowning syndromes* because they needed to be seen as a continuum, for a comprehensive understanding of this disorder.

Post-immersion syndromes referred to the complications that develop after immersion and subsequent rescue. These included pulmonary (infections and inflammations), brain, haematological, renal and multi-system disorders. They also had clinical and management implications.

Other nomenclatures have been proposed over the centuries, based on the type (sea water and fresh water drowning) and amount of fluid inhaled (wet and dry drowning). Modell's classification of 1971[1], which was based on survival and on whether aspiration occurred, failed because although death was a clear differentiator, aspiration was not.

These classifications were less clinically valuable and may even be artefactual or misleading. They probably did add to the confusion and deserved the approbation of the World Congress on Drowning.

Thus, by 2002, when the World Congress on Drowning convened, it confronted the problem of a complicated nomenclature, some of which was not very informative. To promote an international statistical conformity for surveillance and comparison of research and epidemiological data, it was decided to use just one all-embracing term – *drowning* – to cover all such clinical eventualities and not imply an outcome. The World Congress thus succeeded in demographic standardization, but in doing so managed to oversimplify a genuinely complex subject. The Congress then relented with one demarcation qualification – based on outcome, whether the drowning was fatal or non-fatal. In doing so, the Congress managed to re-define a previously well-defined term ('drowning') and add an oxymoron ('non-fatal drowning'). Other subsequent classifications included warm water or cold water drowning. The International Liaison Committee on Resuscitation's (ILCOR) complex definition in 2010 similarly combined all forms of aspiration, from the most innocuous to the drowning deaths, into the one category (see Chapter 22). This all-embracing approach was not a problem for statisticians, but it resulted in a loss of information and direction for clinicians, most of whom revert to the more useful older definitions.

For clinicians, who need to make management decisions based on the client's presentation, it is still preferable to distinguish among the following:

- Those who died (drowning).
- Those who lost consciousness and were at risk of dying (near drowning).
- Those who had minor inhalation and transitory symptoms (aspiration).
- Those who had later complications of the aspiration. These include the various forms of organ damage, such as lung, brain and kidney disease.

DEMOGRAPHY

Drowning causes half a million deaths per year, worldwide. In many countries, drowning is one of the most common causes of all deaths for children less than 12 years old. In the United States and Australia, it is the second leading cause of death, after motor vehicle accidents, in children less than 12 years old.

The worldwide death rate from drowning is 6.8 per 100 000 person years. The rate of drowning in different populations varies widely according to their access to water, the climate and the national swimming culture. The incidence in most developed countries has now dropped to less than 2 per 100 000. In Africa and in Central America, the incidence is 10 to 20 times higher than this. Island nations with dense populations, such as Japan and Indonesia, are more vulnerable than are large continental nations.

Key risk factors for drowning are male sex, age less than 14 years, alcohol use, low income, poor education, rural residency, aquatic exposure, risky behavior and lack of supervision. Epilepsy increases the risk of drowning by 15 times. The exposure-adjusted, person-time risk of drowning is 200 times higher than that from traffic accidents. For every person who dies of drowning, at least another 4 persons receive care in the emergency department for 'non-fatal drowning'.

There is a predictable age distribution for specific types of drowning. Most swimming pool deaths occur in children, surf deaths occur mostly in teenagers and young adults, ocean deaths occur in sailors and fishers throughout the whole adult range and bathtub drowning occurs in either young babies or older infirm persons. Homicides occur in all ages.

Alcohol consumption is involved in more than half the adult male drowning cases. This may result from the following:

- Increased risk-taking activities.
- Reduced capacity to respond to a threatening situation.
- Loss of heat secondary to peripheral vasodilatation.
- Interference with the laryngeal reflex.
- Increased vagal response.
- Increased tendency to vomit.
- Suicidal intentions.

> 'Bacchus hath drowned more men than Neptune'. Old English Adage.

The demographic features of general drowning accidents are not reflected in the drowning of divers (see Chapter 25). Although it should be the simplest and most informed topic in diving medicine, drowning is plagued with paradoxes. It is responsible for most diving fatalities, but unless other explanations are added, it is a totally inadequate explanation. Divers, unlike other aquatic adventurers, carry their own breathable gas supply (their life support system) with them, and unless this is interrupted in some way, drowning per se is inexplicable. It is a grossly oversimplified diagnosis without determining what has compromised this respirable gas supply or what complications have ensued.

BEHAVIOUR DURING DROWNING

Over the range of animals tested and observed, consciousness is usually lost within 3 minutes of submersion and death between 4 and 8 minutes, as a result of cerebral hypoxia.

Observations of *human* drowning parallel those of the animal experiments, involving a panic reaction with violent struggling followed by automatic swimming movements. There may be a period of voluntary breath-holding or involuntary laryngospasm as fluid strikes the nasopharynx or larynx. During this period of apnoea, hypoxia, hypercapnoea and acidosis develop, and respiratory attempts may result in much swallowing of water and even vomiting. With increasing hypoxia, unconsciousness supervenes, and any laryngospasm abates. Inhalation of water into the lungs may then have many respiratory, cerebral, haematological and biochemical consequences. These are documented later.

Some misunderstandings need to be addressed.

- The lungs do not usually 'flood' with water. Once death has occurred, and respirations have stopped, aspiration ceases. Hypoxaemia becomes evident from minimal aspirations (1 to 3 ml/kg body weight). Volumes greater than 11 ml/kg are needed before blood volumes are altered, volumes greater than 22 ml/kg are needed to produce obvious biochemical alterations and volumes greater than 44 ml/kg are needed to induce ventricular fibrillation. In humans, volumes exceeding 22 ml/kg are uncommon and they are usually much less, as inferred from the lung weights at autopsy.
- Laryngospasm does not typically persist until death. It is a possible but temporary response.
- There is no such clinical entity as 'dry drowning'. This is a pathological finding in some cases of drowning and in which the aspirated fluid has subsequently been absorbed.
- For many years, drowning was characteristically associated with a 'fight for survival', but this is not inevitable, and it is uncommon in divers underwater. It is more common in swimmers on the surface.

From observations in children exposed to drownproofing, as it is euphemistically called, there is usually a failure of the infant to struggle. Breath-holding and automatic but ineffectual paddling-type movements are evident as the infant sinks to the bottom.

In many diving-related circumstances drowning may proceed in a quiet and apparently unemotional manner. Examples of these *quiet* or *silent drownings* include the following:

1. Hyperventilation before breath-hold diving (see Chapters 3, 16 and 61) is a common cause of drowning in otherwise fit individuals who are good swimmers, often in a swimming pool in which they could have stood up. Hyperventilation followed by breath-hold diving can result in loss of consciousness secondary to hypoxia. This occurs before the blood carbon dioxide levels rise sufficiently to force the diver to surface and/or breathe. In these cases, loss of consciousness can occur without any obvious warning, and the underwater swimmer then aspirates and drowns quietly.

2. Hypothermia and/or cardiac arrhythmias, leading to loss of function and drowning, have been well described by Keatinge and others[2].

3. Drugs and alcohol increase the likelihood of drowning by impairing judgement, reducing the struggle to survive and possibly reducing laryngospasm. It is likely that nitrogen narcosis may have a similar effect in divers.

4. Diving problems may produce hypoxia. These include the dilution hypoxic effects with mixed gas breathing and ascent hypoxia (see Chapter 16) and carbon monoxide toxicity resulting from the interference with oxygen metabolism. These effects are likely to cause loss of consciousness without excess carbon dioxide accumulation, dyspnoea or distress.

5. Water aspiration causing hypoxia (see Chapter 24). In animals, 2.2 ml of fresh water inhaled per kg body weight drops the arterial partial pressure of oxygen (PaO_2) to approximately 60 mm Hg within 3 minutes, or to 40 mm Hg with sea water. A similar situation was observed clinically in the salt water aspiration syndrome of divers.

6. Other causes of unconsciousness leading to drowning have been described, e.g. diving-induced cardiac arrhythmias, cerebral arterial gas embolism, some marine animal envenomations and coincidental medical illnesses such as epilepsy or cerebral haemorrhage.

Sudden death induced by vagal inhibition can follow a sudden immersion (this is not drowning, although it can be confused with it, and the drowning syndromes may be precipitated by sudden cold water impact with the pharynx or larynx).

ANIMAL EXPERIMENTS

In the early 1900s many animal experiments conducted both in Europe and North America demonstrated that if an animal was immersed and drowned in water containing chemical traces or dyes, these would spread through the tracheobronchial tree to the alveolar surfaces. In the case of fresh water, this was also absorbed into the bloodstream.

A consistent fall in arterial oxygen content was observed, followed by a rise in arterial carbon dioxide and sometimes cardiac arrhythmias.

Swann and his colleagues from Texas[3,4], in a series of accurate but misleading experiments, flooded animals' lungs with fresh or salt water and demonstrated the significant differences between the two, attributable to osmotic pressures. In both cases, flooding of the lungs produced a reduction in PaO_2 and pH, with a rise in the arterial partial pressure of carbon dioxide ($PaCO_2$).

Because *fresh water* was osmotically much weaker than blood, it moved into the bloodstream and produced haemodilution – reducing blood concentrations of proteins, sodium, chloride and so forth. The subsequent reduction in the osmotic pressure of the blood caused haemolysis and a liberation of both haemoglobin and potassium, with resultant metabolic and renal complications, aggravated by hypoxia. Deaths were often cardiac and resulted from ventricular fibrillation.

When, however, the animals' lungs were flooded with *sea water* – which has a higher osmotic concentration than blood – water was drawn from the bloodstream into the lungs, thereby producing pulmonary oedema and haemoconcentration. This caused an increase in the haematocrit, blood proteins and electrolytes.

For many years physicians attempted to correct these presumed electrolyte, metabolic and cardiac abnormalities in human drownings, but their cases did not replicate the animal model (Figure 21.1).

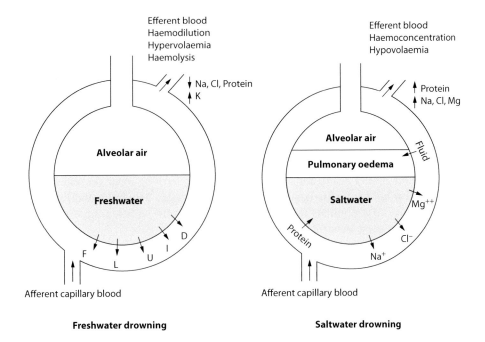

Figure 21.1 Biochemical and circulatory changes after flooding animals' lungs with fresh water and sea water. Cl, chloride; K, potassium; Mg, magnesium; Na, sodium.

Earlier workers had shown that in dogs that drowned, there were still large volumes of air in the lungs, as there are in humans.

Colebatch and Halmagyi[5], working in Australia in 1961, produced an animal model more relevant to the clinical management of patients, by aspiration of only 1 to 3 ml/kg body weight. By using these smaller volumes, these researchers demonstrated the sudden arterial hypoxia, not directly proportional to the amount of fluid inhaled. Pulmonary hypertension, vagal inhibition and reduced compliance were also observed. These investigators demonstrated that the weight of the lungs increased threefold the weight of the instilled sea water. Sea water aspiration usually caused significant pulmonary oedema, but aspirated fresh water was often absorbed from the lungs within 2 to 3 minutes.

Subsequent animal experiments by Modell[6] and others, using intermediate volumes of aspirant, demonstrated that shunting of blood was the predominant cause of persistent arterial hypoxaemia, as a result of perfusion of blood through non-ventilated areas of lung. Destruction of lung surfactant in fresh water installation also resulted in alveolar wall damage and pulmonary oedema.

'DRY' DROWNING

This misnomer continues to be reported, despite the absence of experimental and clinical support for drowning without aspiration. The proponents originally quoted the observations of Charles Cot[7], a Belgian doctor who reported in the French literature in 1931. He observed the 'dry' lungs of dogs fished from the Seine. Because there was no reason to believe that the dogs had drowned, as opposed to being disposed of in the water after death, this support was dubious.

The colourful terminology ensured the popularity of 'dry drowning', and many clinicians observed that persons who drowned may not have had obvious water in the lungs at autopsy. This was attributed to laryngospasm caused by asphyxia, continuing until death. Virtually every review of drowning over the rest of that century acknowledged this concept, without question, although the incidence was often increased to 20 to 40 per cent. It did conflict with the findings of earlier animal experiments.

Clinicians who dealt with sea water drownings, such as in scuba divers, never witnessed this paradox – indeed, they marveled at the degree of foam in the lungs and airways, whereas clinicians who dealt with fresh water drownings were much more enthusiastic about the 'dry drowning' pathological observation. Now the incidence of presumed 'dry' drownings has sunk to less than 2 per cent, even among the earlier proponents of this concept. It is a pathological entity, not a clinical one.

As it has been stated, fresh water is absorbed very rapidly from the lungs after death, and therefore autopsy findings cannot be used to imply (let alone prove) the absence of a previous aspirant. This is especially so when these investigations are performed sometime after the event or after cardiopulmonary resuscitation. 'Dry drowning' is probably an artefact of fluid absorption from the lungs, or it may indicate death from other causes. The deleterious effects of the aspiration can proceed even after the absorption of the fluid.

In the absence of more information, it would be prudent to presume that all victims of near drowning or drowning have aspirated and base one's first aid and management on this presumption. This is supported by the knowledge that laryngospasm does not usually continue until death, and thus even if it does occur during the drowning process, it will not prevent aspiration as hypoxic death is approached.

RADIOLOGY AND PATHOLOGY

Death may occur during immersion, soon after or from delayed complications.

> In recreational scuba deaths, drowning is the most common cause – but it is usually a secondary effect, with the primary cause leading to loss of consciousness. Drowning reflects the fact that unconsciousness occurred in a watery environment.

Accidents (e.g. hypoxia, gas toxicities, immersion pulmonary oedema, dysbarism, medical illnesses, trauma) that occur while someone is immersed or submerged may result in the secondary complication of drowning, with all its pathological sequelae. Drowning then complicates

the interpretation of the diving accident and contributes to a combined disorder.

Certain external characteristics of drowned victims are common, although these are more specific for immersion than for drowning (see Chapter 51). These include the following: pale, wrinkled, 'washerwoman's' skin; post-mortem decomposition; lacerations and abrasions from impact with rocks, coral, shells, motor boats and their propellers; post-mortem injuries from aquatic animals, varying from the nibbling of protuberances (fingers, ears, nose and lips) by crustaceans and fish to the large tearing wounds of sharks and crocodiles.

Radiology, and especially *computed tomography scans,* may be of value in drowning cases. These studies are likely to detect pulmonary interstitial oedema, sub-glottic fluid in the trachea and main bronchi, frothy airway fluid, hyper-expanded lungs, high-attenuation particles (indicating sand or other sediment), pleural effusion, haemorrhage or effusion in the middle ear and para-nasal or mastoid sinuses, gas and fluid in the stomach and other contributory causes of death.

The theory and the procedures for *autopsies* of drowning victims are surprisingly contentious for such a common disorder. An autopsy can imply, but not reliably prove, that death is the result of drowning. There is no pathological feature that is pathognomonic for drowning.

Respiratory system

At autopsy, the main macromorphological changes associated with drowning are caused by the penetration of the liquid into the airways. These are external foam from the mouth and nose, frothy fluid in the airways and overexpansion of the lung. They are not specific to drowning and can be found, usually to a lesser degree, in other cardiorespiratory disorders.

The mushroom-like foam or 'plume' from the mouth and nostrils, often exacerbated by resuscitation efforts, is composed of the drowning aspirant (usually sea water), pulmonary oedema, mucus and pulmonary surfactant, together with fine air bubbles. It extends into the lower airways, is relatively resistant to collapse and may last some days. It is particularly common with salt water drowning. It is thought to develop only if there is some inspiratory action (i.e. it is not a passive, post-mortem event). Respiratory epithelial cells and CD68+ alveolar macrophages have been detected in the foam.

The lungs are water-logged, often heavier than normal, and overdistended *(emphysema aquosum)*. The lung weights reduce over the subsequent few days, as fluid is redistributed, and sometimes fluid accumulates in the pleural cavity. This is another reason for performing early autopsies. The overdistension may cause the ribs to be imprinted on the pleural surfaces, and the lungs may extend over the mediastinal midline. The lung surfaces may be pale and mottled, and areas of distended alveoli or bullae may be evident, as may subpleural haemorrhages (Paltauf's spots). The lungs retain their shape and size on sectioning.

Pleural effusions are common and increase with the duration between death and autopsy.

When non-breathing bodies are immersed, significant quantities of fluid usually do not enter the lower respiratory system, but some may enter with the descent of the body as a result of replacement of the contracting gas space (Boyles' Law). This is unlike the foam referred to earlier.

Histological evidence of focal alveolar damage and emphysema is frequent. Microscopic changes may demonstrate toxic effects both of chemicals and of the specific aspirant. The surfactant changes, including denaturation, can progress even after apparent clinical improvement. Epithelial and endothelial changes, with detachment of the basilar membrane and cellular disruption, have been described. Sand, marine organisms, algae and diatoms may be observed in the lungs.

The finding of water, effusion or blood in the middle ears, mastoid or para-nasal sinuses is not evidence of drowning *per se*, but it may indicate descent of the body while still alive (see Chapter 51). Other explanations include the inflow of water after death and the effects of venous congestion during the agonal struggle.

Usually the death results from hypoxia from the *acute pulmonary damage* and the shunting of blood through non-aerated tissue. Sometimes there is progressive or irreversible lung damage, for various reasons. They include progressive surfactant damage, pneumonitis from the aspirant,

vomitus and foreign bodies. Even victims who appear normal on arrival at hospital can deteriorate over the next 6 to 12 hours. Respiratory infections and abscesses are not infrequent if death is delayed. Pulmonary oxygen toxicity, associated with prolonged resuscitation attempts, may also be present (see Chapter 17).

Other organs

The *stomach* often contains free fluid, water inhaled during the incident, together with debris and organisms. Wydler's sign is a three-layer separation of foam, fluid and solids in the stomach.

Local haemorrhages in the upper torso musculature are sometimes claimed to be drowning induced, but this finding is controversial and non-specific.

The major effects on the *neurological* system are those of hypoxic brain damage with petechial haemorrhages and subsequent cerebral oedema and raised intracranial pressure.

Autopsies on drowning victims who submerged while still alive, although unconscious, may also show other cranial haemorrhages, which are sometimes misinterpreted as a cause of the accident. Meningeal haemorrhages, both dural and arachnoid, may be observed. These are usually not extensive and are quite different from the brain haemorrhages of arterial gas embolism or decompression sickness or from the petechial haemorrhages of asphyxia. They are probably derived from the bleeding of descent sinus barotrauma, which ruptures into the cranial cavity when the enclosed gas spaces expand during ascent.

There is often considerable venous congestion of the viscera, especially the brain, kidneys and other abdominal organs. Hypoxic cerebral necrosis and acute renal tubular necrosis with blood pigment casts are both described.

Because of the relatively small amount of fluid usually aspirated in drowning, it is considered unlikely that victims die acutely of *electrolyte imbalance* and/or associated *ventricular fibrillation*.

Cardiac arrhythmias may be initiated by hypoxia, but this is not demonstrable at autopsy. Cases of prolonged QT interval causing death from immersion have been postulated, but support for this as a common cause of death is lacking in drowning surveys.

The possibility of vagally induced death immediately following immersion has also been proposed when dealing with water colder than 15°C.

In the event of delayed drowning deaths, the lungs, brain or kidneys may all be involved.

Laboratory findings

A series of biochemical tests has been designed to verify drowning as the cause of death. The rationale is that the inhaled fluid, because it has different osmotic pressures, electrolytes and particulates compared with the pulmonary blood flowing past it, will change the latter and alter the character of the blood in the pulmonary veins, the left side of the heart and the systemic arterial system.

Thus, one can compare the left-sided heart blood with the right-sided heart blood and deduce the nature of the aspirate. In fresh water drowning, the left-sided heart blood should have a lower osmotic pressure and a dilution of most electrolytes. The hypo-osmolarity could result in haemolysis with a raised serum haemoglobin and potassium levels. Sea water aspirate should draw fluid from the circulating blood, thereby causing a rise in specific gravity and most blood constituents in the arterial blood. Such changes can be verified in animal experiments when the lungs are flooded with large volumes of fluid and the parameters are measured immediately post mortem.

Neither situation is likely in human drowning, in which the volume of aspirate is relatively small. There are usually many hours between death and autopsy, thus allowing blood constituents and electrolytes to equilibrate. Effective resuscitation is also likely to diminish any variations in venous and arterial blood.

For the foregoing reasons, the Gettler test (chloride variation) and sodium, magnesium, calcium, strontium, haematocrit, haemoglobin, pulmonary surfactant protein and specific gravity levels are unlikely to contribute to the autopsy diagnosis of drowning, although all have had their proponents. Some pathologists use the measurement of vitreous electrolytes to support the diagnosis. Atrial natriuretic peptide levels may increase in drowning, but also in immersion *per se,* in cardiac disease and in any hypervolaemic state. They also only persist for short periods.

Identification and comparison of environmental and systemic diatoms and algae in the lungs, blood, kidneys and vertebrae have been recommended. The single-celled diatoms, usually 10 to 80 micrometres long, are ubiquitous with about 15 000 different species – some inhabiting most waterways. They do not enter the tissues from the lungs unless there is an active circulation. Their presence in both the water environment and the body tissues does not prove drowning, merely the aspiration of that water while the body's circulation is still functional. The silica shell makes diatoms stable and thus detectable by complex autopsy procedures. Despite its potential, the detection of diatoms is not often employed in pathological laboratories because of its complexity and the possibility of contamination. In addition, pollution of waterways reduces the presence of diatoms.

Further discussion relevant to drowning is found in Chapters 22 to 25.

REFERENCES

1. Modell JH. *Pathophysiology and Treatment of Drowning and Near-drowning.* Springfield, Illinois: Charles C Thomas; 1971:8–9, 13.
2. Keatinge WR, Prys-Roberts C, Cooper KE, Honour AJ, Haight J. *Survival in Cold Water.* Oxford: Blackwell Scientific Publications; 1969.
3. Swann HG, Brucer M, Moore C, Vezien BL. Fresh water and sea water drowning: a study of the terminal cardiac and biochemical events. *Texas Reports on Biology and Medicine* 1947;**5**:423–437.
4. Swann HG, Spofford NR. Body salt and water changes during fresh and sea water drowning. *Texas Reports on Biology and Medicine* 1951;9:356–382.
5. Colebatch HJH, Halmagyi DFJ. Lung mechanics and resuscitation after fluid aspiration. *Journal of Applied Physiology* 1961;**16**:684–696.
6. Modell JH. Drowning. *New England Journal of Medicine* 1993;328(4):253–256.
7. Cot C. *Les asphyxies accidentelles.* Paris: N. Maloine; 1931.

FURTHER READING

Brown SD, Gaitanaru D. Drowning and near-drowning. In: Brubakk AO, Neuman TS, editors. *Bennett and Elliott's Physiology and Medicine of Diving.* 5th ed. Philadelphia: Saunders; 2003.

DiMaio D, DiMaio VJ. Death by drowning. In: *Forensic Pathology.* 2nd ed. Boca Raton, Florida: CRC Press; 2001.

Drowning and near-drowning workshop. *South Pacific Underwater Medical Society Journal* 2002;**32**(4):189–206.

Dueker C, Brown S. *Near Drowning.* 47th Workshop. Undersea and Hyperbaric Medicine Society. Kensington, Maryland: Undersea and Hyperbaric Medicine Society; 1999.

Edmonds C. Drowning syndromes: the mechanism. *South Pacific Underwater Medicine Society Journal* 1998;**28**(1):2–9.

Edmonds C, Walker D, Scott B. Drowning syndromes with scuba. *South Pacific Underwater Medicine Society Journal* 1997;**27**(4):182–190.

Idris AH, Berg R, Bierens J, Bossaert L, Branche C, Gabrielli A, *et al.* Recommended guidelines for uniform reporting of data from drowning: the "Utstein style." *Circulation* 2003;**108**:2565–2574.

Layon AJ, Modell JH. Drowning: update 2009. *Anesthesiology* 2009;**110**:1390–1401.

Levy AD, Harcke HT, Getz JM, Mallak CT, Caruso JL, Pearse L, Frazier AA, Galvin JR. Virtual autopsy: two- and three-dimensional multidetector CT findings in drowning with autopsy comparison. *Radiology* 2007;**243**:862–868.

Piette MHA, DeLetter EA. Drowning: still a difficult autopsy diagnosis. *Forensic Science International* 2006;**163**:1–9.

Pounder DJ. *Bodies from Water.* 1992. University of Dundee, Forensic Medical Lecture notes.

Rao D. Drowning. *Forensic Pathology Online.* 2013. www.forensicpathologyonline.com/E-Book/asphyxia/drowning

Szpilman D, Joost JLM, Bierens MD, Handley AJ, Orlowski JP. Drowning: current concepts. *New England Journal of Medicine* 2012;**366**:2102–2110.

Van Beeck EF, Branche CM, Szpilman D *et al.* A new definition of drowning. *Bulletin of the World Health Organization* 2005;**83**(11):801–880.

Zhu BL, Quan L, Li DR, *et al.* Postmortem lung weight in drownings: a comparison with acute asphyxiation and cardiac death. *Leg Med (Tokyo).* 2003;**5**(1):20–26.

HISTORICAL REFERENCES

Bajanowski J, Brinkmann B, Stefanec AM. *et al.* Detection and analysis of tracers in experimental drowning. *International Journal of Legal Medicine* 1998;**111**(2):57–61.

Banting FG, Hall GE, James JM, *et al.* Physiological studies in experimental drowning. *Canadian Medical Association Journal* 1938;**39**:226.

Cantwell GP, Verive MJ, Shoff WH, *et al.* Drowning. *Medscape.* 2011. http://emedicine.medscape.com/article/772753-overview#showall

Colebatch HJH, Halmagyi DFJ. Lung mechanics and resuscitation after fluid aspiration. *Journal of Applied Physiology* 1961;**16**:684–696.

Colebatch HJH, Halmagyi DFJ. Reflex airway reaction to fluid aspiration. *Journal of Applied Physiology* 1962;**17**:787–794.

Colebatch HJH, Halmagyi DFJ. Reflex pulmonary hypertension of fresh water aspiration. *Journal of Applied Physiology* 1963;**18**:179–185.

Conn AW, Barker GA, Edmonds JF, Bohn MB. Submersion hypothermia and near-drowning. In: *The Nature and Treatment of Hypothermia,* vol 2. Pozos RS, Wittmers LE Jr, editors. Minneapolis, Minnesota: University of Minnesota Press; 1979.

Cot C. *Les asphyxies accidentelles.* Paris: N. Maloine; 1931.

Craig AB Jr. Underwater swimming and loss of consciousness. *JAMA* 1961;**176**:255–258.

Davis JH. Autopsy findings in victims of drowning. In: Modell JH, editor. *Pathophysiology and Treatment of Drowning and Near Drowning.* Springfield, Illinois: Charles C Thomas; 1971.

Donald KW. Drowning. *British Medical Journal* 1955;**2:**155–160.

Edmonds C. A salt water aspiration syndrome. *Military Medicine* 1970;**135**(9):779–785.

Giammon ST, Modell JH. Drowning by total immersion: effects on pulmonary surfactant of distilled water, isotonic saline, and sea water. *American Journal of Diseases of Children* 1967;**114:**612–616.

Golden FSC, Tipton MJ, Scott RC. Immersion, near drowning and drowning. *British Journal of Anaesthesia* 1997;**79:**214–225.

Halmagyi DFJ. Lung changes and incidence of respiratory arrest in rates after aspiration of sea and fresh water. *Journal of Applied Physiology* 1961;**16:**41–44.

Halmagyi DFJ, Colebatch HJH. The drowned lung: a physiological approach to its mechanism and management. *Australasian Annals of Medicine* 1961;**10:**68–77.

Halmagyi DFJ, Colebatch HJH. Ventilation and circulation after fluid aspiration. *Journal of Applied Physiology* 1961;**16:**35–40.

Karpovich PV. Water in lungs of drowned animals. *Archives of Pathology* 1933;**15:**828.

Keatinge WR. *Survival in Cold Water.* Oxford: Blackwell Scientific Publications; 1969.

Keatinge WR, Prys-Roberts C, Cooper KE, Honour AJ, Haight J. Sudden failure of swimming in cold water. *British Medical Journal* 1969;**1:**480–483.

Kringsholm B, Filskov A. Kock K. Autopsied cases of drowning in Denmark, 1987-89. *Forensic Science International* 1991;**52:**95–92.

Lougheed DW, James JM, Hall GE. Physiological studies in experimental asphyxia and drowning. *Canadian Medical Association Journal* 1939;**40:**423.

Lowson JA. Sensations in drowning. *Edinburgh Medical Journal* 1903;**13:**31–45.

Martin E. Hepatic lesions in death from drowning. *Annales de médecine légale* 1932;**12:**372.

Miller R. *Anaesthesia.* 3rd ed. Edinburgh: Churchill-Livingstone; 1990.

Modell JH. *Pathophysiology and Treatment of Drowning and Near-drowning.* Springfield, Illinois: Charles C Thomas; 1971:8–9, 13.

Modell JH. Drowning. *New England Journal of Medicine* 1993;**328**(4):253–256.

Modell JH, Davis JH. Electrolyte changes in human drowning victims. *Anesthesiology* 1969;**30:**414–420.

Modell JH, Graves SA, Ketover A. Clinical course of 91 consecutive near-drowning victims. *Chest* 1976;**70:**231–238.

Modell JH, Moya F. Effects of volume of aspirated fluid during chlorinated fresh water drowning. *Anaesthesia* 1966;**27:**662–672.

Modell JH, Moya F, Newby EJ, Ruiz BC, Showers AV. The effects of fluid volume in sea water drowning. *Annals of Internal Medicine* 1967;**67:**68–80.

Moritz AR. Chemical methods for the determination of death by drowning. *Physiological Reviews* 1944;**24:**70.

Mueller WF. Pathology of temporal bone haemorrhage in drowning. *Journal of Forensic Sciences* 1969;**14**(3):327–336.

Neuman TS. Near drowning. In: Bove A, Davis J, editors. *Bove and Davis' Diving Medicine.* 3rd ed. Philadelphia: Saunders; 1997.

Noble CS, Sharpe N. Drowning; its mechanisms and treatment. *Canadian Medical Association Journal* 1963;**89:**402–405.

Pearn J. Pathophysiology of drowning. *Medical Journal of Australia* 1985;**142:**586–588.

Plueckhahn VD. Alcohol and accidental drowning. *Medical Journal of Australia* 1984;**141:**22–26.

Swann HG, Brucer M, Moore C, Vezien BL. Fresh water and sea water drowning: a study of the terminal cardiac and biochemical events. *Texas Reports on Biology and Medicine* 1947;**5:**423–437.

Swann HG, Spofford NR. Body salt and water changes during fresh and sea water drowning. *Texas Reports on Biology and Medicine* 1951;**9:**356–382.

Tabeling BB. Near drowning. In: *The Physician's Guide to Diving Medicine.* New York: Plenum Press; 1984.

This chapter was reviewed for this fifth edition by Carl Edmonds.

22

Pathophysiological and clinical features of drowning

> Human series of near drowning cases do not show the electrolyte, haematological and cardiac changes seen in animals whose lungs are flooded.
>
> Aspiration causes lung changes and hypoxaemia, which in turn may result in acute respiratory distress syndrome, hypoxic brain damage or cardiac, multisystem or renal disease.
>
> Many patients have survived without brain damage despite total immersion for durations of 15 to 45 minutes. Thus, resuscitation has to be implemented energetically.
>
> Many patients deteriorate or die hours or days after rescue and resuscitation, and therefore observation in hospital is required over this time.
>
> Most patients recover without sequelae, but those with hypoxic encephalopathy may have residual neurological and neuropsychiatric problems.

INTRODUCTION

The pathophysiological process of drowning has been the focus of many attempts to classify and sub-classify, with terms such as 'drowning' *versus* 'near drowning', 'wet drowning' *versus* 'dry drowning' and 'secondary drowning' enjoying periods of popularity. However, a 2010 international consensus determined that these terms contribute little to understanding of the problem and discouraged their use[1]. A unifying definition of drowning published by the International Liaison Committee on Resuscitation (ILCOR) is as follows: 'a process resulting in primary respiratory impairment from submersion/immersion in a liquid medium. Implicit in this definition is that a liquid/air interface is present at the entrance of the victim's airway, preventing the victim from breathing air. The victim may live or die after this process, but whatever the outcome, he or she has been involved in a drowning incident'.

PATHOPHYSIOLOGY

The effects of drowning are multiple, but the initial and primary insult is to the respiratory system, with hypoxaemia being the inevitable result (Case Report 22.1).

The sequence of events that occur with drowning includes the following:

1. Initial submersion in water preventing air breathing. This is usually followed by voluntary breath-holding. Duration of the breath-holding

---

CASE REPORT 22.1

Ernie Hazard, age 35: 'I was thinking "This is it. Just take a mouthful of water and it's over." It was very matter of fact. I was at a fork in the road and there was work to do – swim or die. It didn't scare me. I didn't think about my family or anything. It was more businesslike. People think you always have to go for life, but you don't. You can quit....'

The instinct to breathe underwater is so strong that it overcomes the agony of running out of air. No matter how desperate the drowning person is, he or she does not inhale until on the verge of losing consciousness. That is called the 'break point'.

The process is filled with desperation and awkwardness: 'So this is drowning...so this is how my life finally ends.... I can't die, I have tickets for next week's game'.... The drowning person may even feel embarrassed, as if he or she has squandered a great fortune. He or she has an image of people shaking their heads over this dying so senselessly. The drowning may feel as if it is the last, greatest act of stupidity in his or her life. The thought shrieks through the mind during a minute or so that it takes the panicky person to run out of air.

Occasionally, someone makes it back from this dark world. In 1892, a Scottish doctor, James Lowson, was on a steamship bound for Colombo. Most of the 180 people on board sank with the ship, but Lowson managed to fight his way out of the hold and over the side:

'I struck out to reach the surface, only to go further down. Exertion was a serious waste of breath and after 10 or 15 seconds the effort of inspiration could no longer be restrained. It seems as if I was in a vice which was gradually being screwed up tight until it felt as if the sternum of the spinal column must break. Many years ago my old teacher used to describe how painless and easy death by drowning was – "like falling about a green field in early summer" – and this flashed across my brain at the time. The "gulping" efforts became less frequent and the pressure seemed unbearable, but gradually the pain seemed to ease up. I appeared to be in a pleasant dream, although I had enough willpower to think of friends at home and the site of the Grampians, familiar to me as a boy, that was brought into my view. Before losing consciousness the chest pain had completely disappeared and the sensation was actually pleasant.

'When consciousness returned I found myself on the surface. I managed to get a dozen good inspirations. Land was 400 yards distant and I used a veil of silk and then a long wooden plank to assist me to shore. On landing and getting on a sheltered rock, no effort was required to produce copious emesis. After the excitement, sound sleep set in and this lasted three hours, when a profuse diarrhoea came on, evidently brought on by the sea water ingested. Until morning break, all my muscles were in a constant tremor which could not be controlled'.

From Junger S. *The Perfect Storm*. London: Fourth Estate; 1997, with quotes from James Lowson in *The Edinburgh Medical Journal*.

---

depends on several factors, which include general physical condition, exercise, prior hyperventilation and psychological factors (see Chapter 61). This is frequently a period when the victim swallows substantial amounts of water.

2. Fluid aspiration into the airway at the point of breaking the breath-hold. Eventually, the rising arterial carbon dioxide tension ($PaCO_2$) compels inspiration, and fluid is aspirated.

Laryngeal spasm may follow the first contact of the glottis with water. While laryngospasm is maintained, the lungs may remain dry; however, the inevitable result of the associated hypoxaemia is that the spasm will eventually also break, and if the victim remains immersed, then aspiration of water into the lungs will follow. Vomiting of swallowed liquid may occur, and this may also be aspirated into the lungs.

3. Progressive hypoxaemia. This may initially result from oxygen use during voluntary breath-holding and any subsequent laryngospasm, but ultimately it is aspiration of water or regurgitated stomach contents into the gas-exchanging segments of the lungs that provokes persistent and progressive hypoxaemia. The inhalation of water can occur through involuntary diaphragmatic contractions even if the victim is not breathing *per se*. The presence of water instead of air and the dilution of surfactant function with consequent alveolar atelectasis result in a ventilation-perfusion (V/Q) mismatch with a preponderance of low V/Q units and extensive venous admixture. The resulting hypoxaemia leads to unconsciousness, bradycardia and ultimately asystolic cardiac arrest. Hypoxic brain damage follows within a very short space of time.

CLINICAL FEATURES

The *respiratory* manifestations of drowning include the following:

- Dyspnoea.
- Retrosternal chest pain.
- Blood-stained, frothy sputum.
- Tachypnoea.
- Cyanosis.
- Pulmonary crepitations and rhonchi.
- Hypoxaemia.

Pulse oximetry typically reveals low oxygen saturations, but a pulse oximeter may not read at all on a cold, peripherally shut-down victim. An arterial blood gas determination reveals hypoxaemia (lower limit of the 'normal' range for arterial oxygen tension [PO_2] is 80 mm Hg [10.5 kPa]). There is often acidaemia that usually has a metabolic component, but that may be mixed and very severe in a respiratory peri-arrest situation. Carbon dioxide levels are frequently elevated in a peri-arrest condition, but they may be normal or even low during spontaneous breathing or manual ventilation.

Initial chest x-ray studies may be normal, or they may show patchy opacities or pulmonary oedema. Significant hypoxia may be present even when chest x-ray changes are subtle or even absent.

Complications may include pneumonitis, pulmonary oedema, bronchopneumonia, pulmonary abscess and empyema. Severe pulmonary infections with unusual organisms leading to long-term morbidity have been reported. Progression to the acute respiratory distress syndrome (ARDS) is not uncommon in drowning situations.

Central nervous system effects of hypoxia include variable impairment of consciousness, ranging from awake to comatose, with decorticate or decerebrate responses. If hypoxia is prolonged, a global hypoxic brain injury can result with cerebral oedema, raised intracranial pressure and sustained coma. Seizure activity is common in this setting.

Cardiovascular manifestations are largely the result of the effects of hypoxaemia on the heart. Progressive bradycardia leading to asystolic cardiac arrest is not uncommon. After rescue and resuscitation, supraventricular tachycardias are frequent, but various other dysrhythmias may occur. When the hypoxic acidotic insult has been severe, hypotension and shock may persist despite re-establishment of a perfusing rhythm. The central venous pressure may be elevated as a result of right-sided heart failure exacerbated by elevated pulmonary vascular resistance, rather than by volume overload. Mixed venous oxygen tension may also be low, indicating tissue hypoperfusion.

Multi-system organ failure may develop secondary to the hypoxaemia, acidosis and resultant hypoperfusion. Decreased urinary output occurs initially and occasionally progresses to acute tubular necrosis and renal failure. Haemoglobinaemia, coagulation disorders and even disseminated intravascular coagulation may complicate the clinical picture.

Laboratory findings include decreased arterial oxygen with variable $PaCO_2$ values, metabolic and respiratory acidosis, haemoconcentration, leucocytosis, increased lactic dehydrogenase, occasional elevated creatinine levels and haemolysis as indicated by elevated free haemoglobin. Serum electrolytes are usually within the normal range.

> The arterial oxygen tension is always low, but the carbon dioxide tension may be low, normal or elevated.

Recovery from drowning is often complete in survivors. However, residual neurological deficiencies may persist in the form of either cognitive impairment or extrapyramidal disorders.

SURVIVAL FROM DROWNING

Treatment at the scene of an accident is sometimes of little ultimate consequence with many disorders, but in drowning it often determines whether the victim lives or dies. The standard of first aid and resuscitation training of the rescuers therefore influences outcome.

In human drowning, deterioration after initial resuscitation is frequently recorded, and this influences management (see Chapter 23).

The temperature of the water and thus the degree of hypothermia may also be factors. Poorer results are achieved in warm water drowning.

In what was previously referred to as 'dry' drowning (in which the distal airway remains relatively dry because of early laryngospasm), the patient is hypoxic and, if rescued in time, may– make a rapid recovery. However, when laryngospasm relaxes and fluid aspiration occurs as it eventually does if the victim remains immersed, the result is drowning.

Other factors that influence outcome include the following: the presence of chlorine, other chemicals and foreign bodies; the aspiration of stomach contents; and the subsequent development of pneumonitis, respiratory infection and multi-organ failure.

One likely cause for delayed death is progressive lung injury[2]. ARDS develops in a significant proportion of drowning cases; usually hours or days after the aspiration. Other causes of death in the days after the event include cerebral hypoxia, secondary infections (usually of the lungs), renal failure and iatrogenic events.

Factors that negatively influence survival have been well documented by Modell[3]:

- Prolonged immersion.
- Delay in effective cardiopulmonary resuscitation.
- Severe metabolic acidosis (pH <7.1).
- Asystole on admission to hospital.
- Fixed dilated pupils.
- Low Glasgow Coma Scale score (<5).

Nevertheless, none of these predictors is infallible, and survival with normal cerebral function has been reported with all the foregoing factors.

Claims of survival after extended duration underwater without ventilation of the lungs have been used to encourage rescuers to persevere with resuscitation efforts. There have been cases reported in victims who have been submerged for between 15 and 45 minutes[4-7] and who have survived without neurological sequelae. The explanations given for such prolonged durations of survival are as follows:

1. Hypothermia is protective and develops very rapidly with aspiration of water. In swimmers and divers, hypothermia may be present before the incident.
2. The 'diving reflex' is a possible, but contentious, explanation. Within seconds of submersion, the diving reflex may be triggered by sensory stimulation of the trigeminal nerve and by reflex or voluntary inhibition of the respiratory centre in the medulla. This produces bradycardia and shunting of the blood to the areas more sensitive to hypoxia – the brain and coronary circulations. It is independent of baroreceptor or chemoreceptor inputs. The diving reflex is more intense in the frightened or startled animal, compared with animals which dive or submerge voluntarily, but it is not known whether this finding is applicable to humans. Water temperatures higher than 20°C do not inhibit the diving reflex, but progressively lower temperatures augment it.
3. Gas exchange in the lungs can continue after submersion. With or without the effects of laryngospasm, there may be several litres of air remaining within the lungs, thus allowing for continued exchange of respiratory gases. Increased pressure (depth) transiently enhances oxygen uptake by increasing the PO_2 in compressed lungs. In an unconscious state, with low oxygen use and the effects of hypothermia, a retained respiratory gas volume could add considerably to the survival time, although it is not often considered in the literature on drowning.

Whether fluid enters the lungs in an unconscious victim depends on many factors, including the spatial orientation of the body. For example, a dependent position of the nose and mouth, facing downward, is not conducive to fluid replacement of the air in the lungs.

Even though spectacular and successful rescue can be achieved after prolonged submersion, it is more frequent that this is not so. Many victims lose consciousness and die after only a few minutes of submersion.

REFERENCES

1. Soar J, Perkins GC, Abbas G, *et al.* European Resuscitation Council guidelines for resuscitation 2010, section 8. Cardiac arrest in special circumstances: electrolyte abnormalities, poisoning, drowning, accidental hypothermia, hyperthermia, asthma, anaphylaxis, cardiac surgery, trauma, pregnancy, electrocution. *Resuscitation* 2010;**81**:1400–1433.
2. Oakes DD, Sherck JP, Maloney JR, *et al.* Prognosis and management of victims of near drowning. *Journal of Trauma* 1982;**22**:544.
3. Modell JH. Drowning. *New England Journal of Medicine* 1993;**328**(4):253–256.
4. Siebke J, Breivik H, Rod T, Lind B. Survival after 40 minutes' submersion without cerebral sequelae. *Lancet* 1975;**1**(7919):1275–1277.
5. Young RSK, Zaincraitis ED, Dooling EO. Neurologic outcome in cold water drowning. *JAMA* 1980;**244**:1233–1235.
6. Sekar TS, Mcdonnell KF, Namsirikul P, *et al.* Survival after prolonged immersion in cold water without neurological sequelae. *Archives of Internal Medicine* 1980;**140**:775–779.
7. Nemiroff MJ, Saltz GR, Weg JC. Survival after cold-water near-drowning: the protective effect of the diving reflex. *American Review of Respiratory Disease* 1977;**115**(4):145.

This chapter was reviewed for this fifth edition by Simon Mitchell.

23

The management of drowning

> Initial resuscitation attempts may be vital in determining the outcome. All divers should be adept at basic resuscitation. Dive leaders and boat operators should have a more advanced training, including the use of oxygen.
>
> Ventilatory support is the mainstay of treatment of hypoxaemia. To be effective, endotracheal intubation may be required.
>
> Causes of drowning that require special management should be considered. Rescuers should be aware of the possibility of cranial or cervical spine injury.
>
> Resuscitation should continue until the return of acceptable physiological parameters, especially core temperature.
>
> Continuing intensive care management for respiratory failure may be necessary.
>
> Central nervous system preservation remains the main therapeutic challenge.

AT THE SITE

Rescue and initial resuscitation

In the diving setting, the management of a drowning situation often begins with witnessing a diver become unconscious underwater. Before resuscitation efforts can begin, the victim must be retrieved to the surface. Related considerations were reviewed by the Undersea and Hyperbaric Medical Society (UHMS) Diving Committee[1], and their findings are outlined here.

The overarching goal of this initial phase of the rescue is to retrieve the diver to the surface as quickly as possible, even if the victim has a mouthpiece in place and appears to be breathing (which would be a most unusual circumstance). More typically, the victim is found unconscious with the mouthpiece out. No attempt should be made to replace it; however, if the mouthpiece is retained in the mouth, then the rescuer should make an attempt to hold it in place during the ascent. An ascent should be initiated immediately. If there is significant risk to the rescuer in ascending (if the rescuer has a significant decompression obligation), then making the victim buoyant and sending him or her to the surface may be the only option, depending on the degree to which the rescuer wishes to avoid endangering himself or herself.

The committee flagged one exception to the advice to surface immediately. In the situation where a diver is in the clonic phase of a seizure with the mouthpiece retained, then the mouthpiece should be held in place and ascent delayed until the seizure abates. To be clear, however, this does not apply to the more common situation of the seizing diver whose mouthpiece is out. In the latter situation, the ascent should be initiated while the diver is still seizing. This dichotomy arises because of the committee's perception of the shifting balance of risk between pulmonary barotrauma and drowning in situations where the airway is at least partially protected or not. Thus, where the airway is completely unprotected (mouthpiece not retained), the risk of drowning outweighs the risk of barotrauma imposed by seizure-induced apposition of the glottis tissues. Where the airway is partly protected (mouthpiece retained and held in place), the opposite holds true. This matter is discussed in more detail in the committee report[1].

At the surface, the victim should be made positively buoyant face-up, and a trained rescuer should attempt to give two mouth-to-mouth rescue breaths. Experience has shown that this is often all that is required to stimulate the victim to breathe. Pausing to give rescue breaths will slightly delay removal from the water for definitive cardiopulmonary resuscitation (CPR) and is therefore a gamble that the victim has not yet having suffered cardiac arrest. However, given the extremely poor outcome expected if a drowning victim suffers a hypoxic cardiac arrest and the time it usually takes to remove a diver from the water, the committee determined that this was a gamble worth taking. The best chance of survival lies in preventing hypoxic cardiac arrest, and establishing oxygenation is the means of such prevention. If the diver has already had a cardiac arrest, then a small extra delay in initiating CPR imposed by performing in-water rescue breaths is not likely to alter the outcome. There is some human evidence suggesting a survival advantage for in-water rescue breathing in non-diving drowning situations[2].

Once at the surface and in a situation where the surface support is not immediately to hand, a choice must be made whether to wait for rescue or initiate a tow to shore or nearest surface support. The committee determined that if surface support is less than a 5-minute tow away, then a tow should be commenced with intermittent rescue breaths administered if possible. If surface support or the shore is more than a 5-minute tow away, then the rescuer should remain in place, continuing to administer rescue breaths for 1 minute. If there is no response in this time, then a tow toward the nearest surface support should be initiated without ongoing rescue breaths. These guidelines are summarized in Figure 23.1.

It is notable that these guidelines contain no reference to in-water chest compressions. Although techniques for in-water chest compressions have been described[3,4], the committee did not consider there was adequate evidence of efficacy to justify the extra difficulty and stress to the rescuer for their inclusion in the rescue protocol.

The victim should be kept horizontal as much as possible during and after removal from the water. The patient should be moved with the head in the neutral position if cervical spine injury is suspected. Scuba divers are most unlikely to have suffered cervical spine trauma. A basic life support algorithm should be initiated immediately, beginning with assessment of the airway (Figure 23.2).

AIRWAY

Vomiting and regurgitation frequently follow a submersion incident. Foreign particulate matter causing upper airway obstruction should be removed manually or later by suction. Obstruction of the upper airway by the tongue is common in the unconscious patient.

Two methods are used to overcome the obstruction:

Head-tilt/chin-lift is accomplished by pushing firmly back on the patient's forehead and lifting the chin forward by using two fingers under the jaw at the chin. The soft tissues under the chin should not be compressed, and unless mouth-to-nose breathing is to be employed, the mouth should not be completely closed. This technique should be avoided if cervical spine injury is suspected.

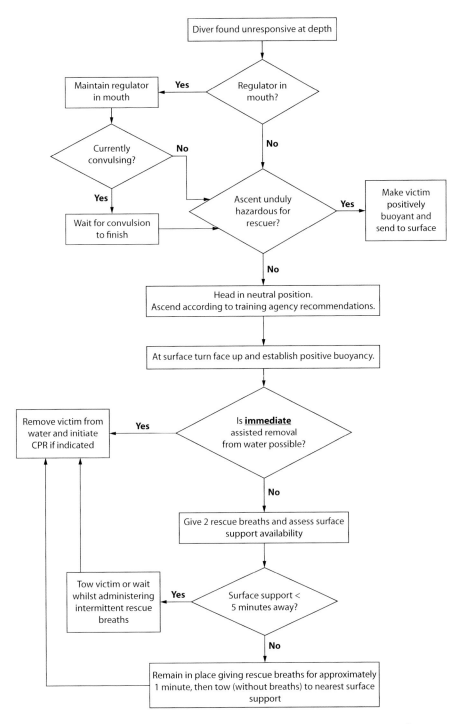

Figure 23.1 Undersea and Hyperbaric Medical Society Diving Committee guidelines for rescue of an unresponsive diver from depth. It is recommended that the interested diver read the original paper which contextualizes these recommendations more thoroughly. CPR, cardiopulmonary resuscitation. (From Mitchell SJ, Bennett MH, Bird N, Doolette DJ, *et al.* Recommendations for rescue of a submerged unconscious compressed gas diver. *Undersea and Hyperbaric Medicine* 2012;**39**:1099–1108.)

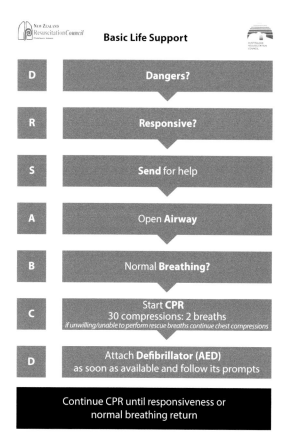

Figure 23.2 Basic life support algorithm. AED, automatic external defibrillator; CPR, cardio-pulmonary resuscitation. (From the Australian Resuscitation Council.)

Jaw-thrust describes the technique of forward displacement of the lower jaw by lifting it with one hand on either side of the angle of the mandible. Unless cervical spine injury is suspected, this technique is often combined with head-tilt.

Time should not be wasted in trying to clear water from the lower airways. If airway obstruction is encountered and has not responded to normal airway management, the *Heimlich manoeuvre* (sub-diaphragmatic thrust) has been suggested[5]. This manoeuvre, which was proposed as a routine step to clear water from the airway, has not received the widespread endorsement of resuscitation councils around the world. It should be used with caution and only as a last resort because of the risks of regurgitation of gastric contents, rupture of the stomach and causing delay in initiating effective ventilation. Persistent airway obstruction may result from a foreign body, but other causes include laryngeal oedema or trauma, bronchospasm and pulmonary oedema.

BREATHING

Respiration can be assessed by placing one's ear over the victim's mouth while looking for chest movement, listening for air sounds and feeling for the flow of expired air. If breathing is detected, oxygen should be administered and the victim maintained in the 'recovery' position to avoid aspiration of fluid or vomitus.

If breathing is absent, mouth-to-mouth or mouth-to-nose breathing is instituted. Initially, two full breaths of air, with an inspiratory time (for the victim) of 1 to 1.5 seconds, are recommended. For adults, an adequate volume to observe chest movement is about 800 ml. If no chest movement is seen and no air is detected in the exhalation phase, then head-tilt or jaw-thrust manoeuvres should be revised. Failing that, further attempts at clearing the airway with the fingers (only if the victim is unconscious!) should be undertaken. With mouth-to-mouth respiration, the rescuer pinches the victim's nose and closes it gently between finger and thumb. Mouth-to-nose rescue breathing may be more suitable in certain situations, such as when marked trismus is present or when it is difficult to obtain an effective seal (e.g. injury to mouth, dentures).

Paramedics or other practitioners with advanced skills are likely to use a bag-mask-reservoir device connected to an oxygen source for manual positive pressure ventilation in the field. Useful adjuncts in resolving upper airway obstruction may include a nasopharyngeal airway, oropharyngeal airway or supraglottic airway device such as a laryngeal mask. Endotracheal intubation in the field should be undertaken only by highly trained and experienced practitioners.

The rate of chest inflation should be about 12 per minute (one every 5 seconds) with increased rate and decreased volume in young children.

It must be made clear that the recent advocacy for 'compression-only CPR' in which rescue breathing is omitted and first responders provide only chest compressions to victims of community cardiac arrest is not relevant to CPR in the context of drowning. The cause of cardiac arrest in the community is usually some sort of cardiac disease, whereas it is hypoxia in drowning. Compression-only CPR works in community cardiac arrest because the victim is not hypoxic at the onset of cardiac standstill, and the lungs are filled with air to functional residual capacity. In contrast, hypoxia is usually the cause of cardiac arrest in drowning, and the lungs are frequently compromised by aspirated fluid and alveolar collapse. Failing to ventilate the lungs during resuscitation of a drowning victim is likely to bias against a good outcome[1].

CIRCULATION

The presence of a carotid or femoral pulse should be sought in the unconscious non-breathing victim. This is often difficult because the patient is usually cold and peripherally vasoconstricted. Although it is possible that external cardiac compression (ECC) could precipitate ventricular fibrillation in a hypothermic patient, if in doubt it is safer to commence ECC than not.

If no carotid pulse is detected, ECC should be commenced after two initial breaths. Higher rates of compression are now recommended, with greater outputs achieved at 100/minute compared with the traditional 60/minute standard. Controversy still exists over the mechanism of flow in external compression, with the evidence for the older 'direct compression' model being challenged by the 'thoracic pump' theory.

Cardiac compression should be performed with the patient supine on a firm surface. The legs may be elevated to improved venous return. The rescuer kneels to the side of the patient. The heel of the rescuer's hand should be placed in line with the patient's sternum. The lower edge of the hand should be about two fingers above the xiphisternum (i.e. compression is of the lower half of the sternum). The second hand should be placed over the first, and the compression of the sternum should be about 4 to 5 centimetres in adults in the vertical plane. To achieve this, the rescuer's elbow should be straight, with the shoulders directly over the sternum. A single rescuer may be able to achieve rates of only 80/minute because of fatigue, but if several rescuers are present, it may be possible to maintain high rates.

Further help should be sought immediately, by a third person, if possible, without compromising resuscitation efforts.

Advanced life support and transport

A regional organized emergency medical service (e.g. paramedics) that carries specialized apparatus such as oxygen, endotracheal tubes, suction and intravenous equipment should be activated, if available. In any case, the patient should be transferred to hospital as soon as possible. The early administration of oxygen by suitable positive pressure apparatus, by personnel trained in its use, may be the critical factor in saving lives. For this reason, oxygen administration equipment should be carried on all dive boats. Patients who regain consciousness or who remain conscious after drowning events may have significant pulmonary venous admixture with resultant hypoxaemia. All such patients should receive supplementary oxygen and be further assessed in hospital. Respiratory and cardiac arrests have occurred after apparently successful rescue[6].

Although endotracheal intubation remains the best method for securing an airway and achieving adequate ventilation, the necessary expertise may not be available until the victim is transferred to hospital. In such cases, the use of airway devices such as the laryngeal mask airway may improve ventilation while the patient is being transported to hospital. Other airways such as the pharyngotracheal lumen airway and the Combitube tube are alternatives, but they require more training and have their own problems. One potential problem with all supraglottic devices, and with mouth-to-mouth and bag-mask ventilation techniques for that matter, is that the airway pressures required to inflate a 'wet', non-compliant lung may be very high and not easily achieved with these devices or methods. Endotracheal intubation may the only way to achieve adequate tidal volumes in such patients.

Properly trained and equipped personnel attending a case in the field may be able to invoke advanced resuscitation techniques such as the airway interventions mentioned earlier and the monitoring methods, drug administration strategies and arrhythmia treatments specified in Figure 23.3.

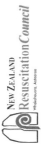

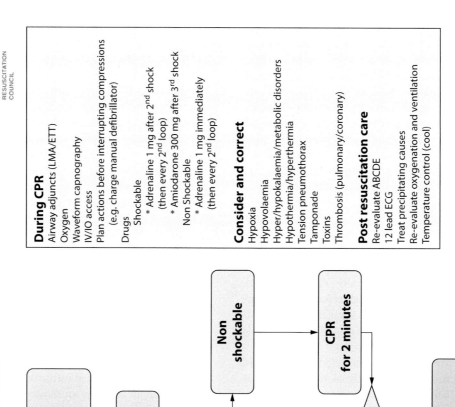

Figure 23.3 Advanced life support algorithm. CPR, cardiopulmonary resuscitation; ECG, electrocardiogram; ETT, endotracheal tube; IV, intravenous; IO, intra-osseous; LMA, laryngeal mask airway. (From the Australian Resuscitation Council.)

HOSPITAL

Hospital management is subdivided into initial emergency department management and continuing therapy in the intensive care unit. All patients should receive oxygen (see Chapter 49) while undergoing evaluation.

Emergency department

On arrival, the emphasis is on evaluation and resuscitation of respiratory failure. Preliminary assessment includes airway, circulation and level of consciousness re-evaluation. Continuous monitoring of pulse, blood pressure, pulse oximetry and electrocardiography are commenced.

The severity of the case determines the appropriate care. If submersion victims show no signs of aspiration on arrival in the emergency department, there may be no need for hospital admission. Patients who are asymptomatic and have normal chest auscultation, chest x-ray findings and arterial blood gases will not subsequently deteriorate[7-9]. They may safely be discharged after 6 hours. In contrast, patients with mild hypoxaemia, auscultatory rales or rhonchi or chest x-ray changes should be admitted for observation because they may deteriorate.

In moderately hypoxaemic patients who have not lost consciousness and who are breathing spontaneously, the use of non-invasive ventilatory support with face mask or nasal continuous positive airway pressure (CPAP) may be an alternative to sedation and endotracheal intubation, provided adequate gas exchange is achieved[10].

Seriously affected patients should be admitted to an intensive care unit or a high-dependency unit. Patients with symptomatic hypoxaemia or disturbed consciousness may rapidly deteriorate further as a result of progressive hypoxaemia. Patients who have had a cardiac arrest or are unconscious and/or severely hypoxaemic require ventilatory support and should be intubated using a rapid sequence induction technique. A nasogastric tube should be inserted and the stomach emptied before induction, if possible.

Concurrent with resuscitation measures, a careful search for any other injuries, such as cranial or spinal trauma, internal injuries and long bone fractures, should be undertaken. Initial x-ray studies should include the chest and cervical spine. Cerebrovascular accident, myocardial infarction, seizure or drug abuse should be suspected if the cause of the incident is not readily apparent. One study revealed that 27 per cent of recreational diving deaths appeared to have a cardiac event as the disabling injury[11], so a high index of suspicion for myocardial ischaemia should be maintained. A 12-lead electrocardiogram would be advisable early in the evaluation.

Similarly, in the scuba diver, other disorders such as pulmonary barotrauma and cerebral arterial gas embolism may have initiated or complicated the drowning. These conditions may require specific treatment such as recompression, hyperbaric oxygen or drainage of a pneumothorax. Nevertheless, it should never simply be assumed that a diver 'must have' suffered pulmonary barotrauma and arterial gas embolism just because the diver was brought to the surface rapidly or unconscious. There have been many unconscious ascents from significant depths in which it appears that pulmonary barotrauma did not occur. Moreover, such an assumption would indicate hyperbaric therapy. Although recompression should not be withheld from a patient who clearly warrants it, it is logistically difficult and more hazardous for an intensive care patient, and recompression should not be used speculatively.

The main goal of therapy is to overcome major derangement of hypoxaemia with its subsequent acidosis. The benchmark should be an arterial oxygen tension (PaO_2) of at least 60 mm Hg. This may be achieved by administration of oxygen by mask in milder cases, possibly with CPAP, but some patients will require more aggressive therapy, employing intermittent positive pressure ventilation (IPPV) with a high fractional inspired oxygen concentration (FIO_2).

High ventilatory pressures may be required to obtain adequate tidal volumes. Progress should be monitored by serial arterial blood gas determinations and continuous pulse oximetry.

The institution of continuous positive end-expiratory pressure (PEEP) with either IPPV or spontaneous ventilation, (i.e. CPAP) will decrease the pulmonary shunting and ventilation-perfusion inequality and increase the functional residual capacity, thus resulting in a higher PaO_2. Nebulized bronchodilator aerosols may be used to control bronchospasm. In sedated patients, fiberoptic bronchoscopy can be used to remove suspected particulate matter, and repeated gentle endotracheal suction will assist in the removal of fluid from the airway.

Early on in the resuscitation sequence, large-bore *intravenous access* should be established and warmed crystalloid fluids commenced. Moderate volumes may be required initially because of tissue losses, immersion diuresis and dehydration, but care should be taken not to overhydrate. Simultaneously, blood for haematology and biochemistry laboratory work can be drawn for baseline assessment. Testing should include cardiac enzymes. Intra-arterial pressure monitoring is useful and allows frequent arterial blood gas determinations to guide ventilation and acid-base management.

If *cardiac arrest* is diagnosed, the rhythm should be rapidly determined, and defibrillation and/or intravenous adrenaline (epinephrine) should be administered according to advanced life support protocols (see Figure 23.3). Other arrhythmias should also be appropriately treated if they have not responded to correction of hypoxaemia and restoration of adequate tissue perfusion.

In the past, it was common to attempt to correct *metabolic acidosis* by giving bicarbonate. The use of bicarbonate in this setting is controversial, and some clinicians may prefer to hyperventilate a patient to create a respiratory compensation for the metabolic acidosis. A more modern alternative intravenous alkalinizing agent is tromethamine acetate (tris-hydroxymethyl aminomethane [THAM]). THAM has the apparent advantage that its action does not result in the generation of carbon dioxide (as occurs with sodium bicarbonate), and as such it may be a better choice in hypercapnic patients who have mixed acidaemia or in patients who are difficult to ventilate. These descriptors may apply to drowning victims.

Some drowning victims have been noted to be markedly hypoglycaemic, and an association with alcohol intoxication, physical exhaustion and hypothermia is relevant. Blood glucose concentrations should be rapidly determined along with blood gases on arrival at hospital, and intravenous glucose therapy should be instituted if appropriate. Untreated hypoglycaemia may aggravate hypoxic brain lesions. However, intravenous glucose must be used with care because hyperglycaemia is also potentially harmful to injured neurons. Hyperglycaemia resulting from massive catecholamine release or other causes may require insulin infusion.

Hypothermia may complicate drowning and pose difficulties with resuscitation end points in the event of cardiac arrest (see Chapter 28). The emergency department management of hypothermia depends on severity, and low-reading thermometers are required because severe hypothermia may otherwise be overlooked. Warmed intravenous fluids and inspired gases, insulation, forced-air warming blankets and radiant heat may be sufficient, but in severe cases, gastric lavage, peritoneal lavage or even cardiopulmonary bypass has been employed. Resuscitation should continue at least until core temperature approaches normal. Care should be taken to avoid hyperthermia because even mild degrees of cerebral hyperthermia can be profoundly disadvantageous to the injured brain.

Hypovolaemia may result from the combined effects of immersion diuresis and pulmonary and tissue oedema. Circulatory support maybe required to provide adequate perfusion of vital tissues. The maintenance of effective cardiac output may require the correction of hypovolaemia, which may be unmasked by the instigation of body rewarming. PPV also decreases venous return to the heart and thus lowers cardiac output. This can usually be overcome by volume restoration or even augmentation. If after volume replacement the patient does not rapidly regain adequate cardiac output, then inotropic support will be required.

Although not studied specifically in the context of drowning, there is compelling evidence from large randomized studies suggesting that resuscitation of intensive care patients with crystalloid fluids results in better outcome (and less requirement for renal replacement therapy) than does resuscitation using colloids. If colloids are used, small volumes of concentrated albumin may be optimal. Care must be taken not to overhydrate drowning patients.

Once intravascular volume is normalized and adequate cardiac output is established, fluid administration should be parsimonious. Diuretics (e.g. frusemide) have also been employed where overhydration is suspected. A urinary catheter with hourly output measurements is essential to determine renal perfusion and function and is a good indication of adequate volume. *Electrolyte disturbances* are usually not a significant problem in the initial phases, but any abnormality should be corrected.

Antibiotics given prophylactically are of dubious benefit. Antibiotics should be employed only where clearly clinically indicated, guided by sputum and blood cultures. Routine use may encourage colonization by resistant organisms.

Intensive care

The general principles of intensive therapy are followed, but with special emphasis on respiratory function because near drowning is a common cause of the acute respiratory distress syndrome (ARDS).

The following clinical parameters, established on arrival in the emergency department, should be regularly monitored:

- Routine clinical observations such as pulse, blood pressure, temperature, respiratory rate, minute volume, inspiratory and PEEP pressures, electrocardiography, pulse oximetry and urine output.
- Where indicated, invasive monitoring such as central venous pressure, pulmonary artery wedge pressure and cardiac output by a pulmonary artery catheter.
- Blood tests such as arterial blood gas and acid-base status, haemoglobin, packed cell volume, white cell count, serum and urinary electrolytes, serum and urinary haemoglobin and myoglobin levels, serum creatinine, urea, glucose, protein and coagulation status.
- Regular chest x-ray examination to detect atelectasis, infection, pneumothorax, pulmonary oedema, pleural effusions and other disorders.
- Serial measurement of pulmonary mechanics, by measurement of airway pressures and compliance, which are also useful in monitoring progress. In the less severely ill patient, simple spirometry is a useful guide to recovery.

The optimal method of *ventilation* aims to produce an adequate oxygen tension at the lowest FIO_2 (preferably FIO_2 of 0.6 or less to avoid pulmonary oxygen toxicity; see Chapter 17) with the least haemodynamic disturbance and the least harm to the lung. CPAP can be dramatic in improving oxygenation by reducing intrapulmonary shunting. Pressures of 5 to 10 centimetres of water are usual, but greater pressures may be required. Patients receiving PPV tend to retain salt and water, so fluid intake should be reduced to about 1500 ml/day with low sodium content. Fluid overload may have a deleterious effect on pulmonary function.

Various modes of ventilation have been employed. These include spontaneous respiration with CPAP, IPPV with and without PEEP, synchronous intermittent mandatory ventilation, pressure support and high-frequency ventilation. Increasing experience in the management of ARDS has led to the development of so-called 'lung protective ventilator strategies' characterized by relatively long inspiratory times, high end-expiratory pressures and relatively small tidal volumes. This may require acceptance of both a degree of 'permissive hypercapnia' and mild respiratory acidosis that in the short term may be treated with bicarbonate or THAM, before medium-term compensation through renal retention of bicarbonate. Postural changes (e.g. prone ventilation) are sometimes experimented with in individual patients. There is no universally applicable formula for ventilating these patients, and much individualization of regimens occurs in high-level intensive care units. These types of strategy may be necessary in severely affected drowning victims.

Femoro-femoral or full *cardiopulmonary bypass* has been employed both for rewarming hypothermic patients and for establishing adequate oxygenation in severe cases[12]. Severe ARDS has been successfully managed with variable periods (up to weeks) of extracorporeal membrane oxygenation (ECMO).

Because of improvements in cardiorespiratory support, preservation of the *central nervous system* is now the major therapeutic challenge[13]. The application of various brain protection techniques including deliberate hypothermia, hyperventilation, barbiturate coma and corticosteroids has not altered cerebral salvage rates in the specific context of drowning[14,15]. Studies in community cardiac arrest do provide circumstantial support for the use of hypothermia after prolonged resuscitation. Although some intensive care units may try this in drowning victims, it is certainly not considered a standard of care. It is notable that corticosteroids have not been shown to reduce cerebral oedema or intracranial pressure (ICP) and are not recommended.

Central nervous system function is assessed clinically and potentially by electroencephalography. ICP monitoring has been advocated where intracranial hypertension is suspected, with prompt therapy for any sudden elevation.

Serial creatinine estimations often reveal mild *renal impairment* in patients requiring intensive care. Severe acute renal failure[16] requiring dialysis is less common, but it may develop in patients who presented with severe metabolic acidosis and elevated initial serum creatinine levels. Occasional cases of rhabdomyolysis have also been reported[17].

Hyperpyrexia commonly follows drowning, and its effect may be deleterious, especially to the injured brain. External cooling and antipyretic drugs to prevent shivering and to keep the temperature lower than 37°C may be indicated.

Continuing hyperexcitability and rigidity may require the use of sedative and relaxant drugs.

PROGNOSIS

It is difficult to prognosticate in individual cases because data from the literature, much of it in the paediatric age group, arise from widely different situations. These situations range from childhood bath and pool incidents in fresh water to boating, swimming and diving activities in the open sea. Nevertheless, several reasonably consistent observations emerge.

Factors that negatively affect outcome include submersion time, time to initiation of effective CPR, severe metabolic acidosis, Glasgow Coma Scale (GCS <5), cardiac arrest and the presence of fixed dilated pupils. However, complete recoveries have been reported despite the presence of one or more of these adverse predictors.

Poor prognostic factors

Prolonged submersion.
Prolonged time to effective cardiopulmonary resuscitation.
Cardiac arrest.
Absence of spontaneous respiration.
Prolonged coma.

Several pooled series indicate that 90 per cent of patients who arrive at least arousable with spontaneous respiration and purposeful response to pain will survive neurologically intact. In contrast, of the patients in this series who arrived comatose, 34 per cent died, and 20 per cent of the survivors had neurological damage[18].

Unresponsive coma, decorticate and decerebrate rigidity, areflexia and fixed dilated pupils are not in themselves diagnostic signs of death, although they are, of course, signs of a poor prognosis. Patients who arrive in hospital in asystole usually have a poor prognosis, and one series reported a 93 per cent mortality rate after cardiac arrest. Current treatment regimens do not alter the outcome.

The rapid development of severe hypothermia, either before or during the final submersion, is probably protective and helps to explain some spectacular recoveries after prolonged periods of submersion. The role of the diving reflex remains controversial.

REFERENCES

1. Mitchell SJ, Bennett MH, Bird N, Doolette DJ, et al. Recommendations for rescue of a submerged unconscious compressed gas diver. *Undersea and Hyperbaric Medicine* 2012;**39**:1099–1108.
2. Szpilman D, Soares M. In-water resuscitation: is it worthwhile. *Resuscitation* 2004;**63**:25–31.
3. March NF, Mathews RC. New techniques in external cardiac compression: aquatic cardiopulmonary resuscitation. *JAMA* 1980;**244**(11):1229–1232.
4. Kizer KW. Aquatic rescue and in-water CPR. *Annals of Emergency Medicine* 1982;**11**:166.

5. Heimlich HJ, Patrick EA. Using the Heimlich manoeuvre to save near drowning victims. *Postgraduate Medicine* 1988;**84**(2):62–67, 71–73.

6. Maniolos N, Mackie I. Drowning and near drowning on Australian beaches patrolled by lifesavers: a 10-year study, 1973–1983. *Medical Journal of Australia* 1988;**148**(4):165–171.

7. Causey AL, Tilleli JA, Swanson ME. Predicting discharge in uncomplicated near-drowning. *American Journal of Emergency Medicine* 2000;**18**(1):9–11.

8. Pratt FD, Haynes BE. Incidence of secondary drowning after saltwater submersion. *Annals of Emergency Medicine* 1986;**115**:1084–1087.

9. Szpilman D. Near drowning and drowning classification: a proposal to stratify mortality based on the analysis of 1,831 cases. *Chest* 1997;**112**(3):660–665.

10. Dottorini M, Eslami A, Baglioni S, Fiorenzano G, Todisco T. Nasal-continuous positive airway pressure in the treatment of near-drowning in freshwater. *Chest* 1966;**110**(4):1122–1124.

11. Denoble PJ, Caruso JL, Dear G de L, Pieper CF, Vann RD. Common causes of open-circuit recreational diving fatalities. *Undersea and Hyperbaric Medicine* 2008;**35**:393–406.

12. Bolle RG, Black PG, Bowers RS, *et al.* The use of extracorporeal rewarming in a child submerged for 66 minutes. *JAMA* 1988;**260**:377–379.

13. Modell JH. Current concepts: drowning. *New England Journal of Medicine* 1993;**328**(4):253–256.

14. Gonzalez-Rothi RJ. Near drowning: consensus and controversies in pulmonary and cerebral resuscitation. *Heart Lung* 1987;**16**(5):474–482.

15. Modell JH. Treatment of near drowning: is there a role for H.Y.P.E.R. therapy? *Critical Care Medicine* 1986;**14**:593–594.

16. Spicer ST, Quinn D, Nyi Nyi NN, Nankivell BJ, Hayes JM, Savdie E. Acute renal impairment after immersion and near-drowning. *Journal of the American Society of Nephrology* 1999;**10**(2):382–386.

17. Simcock AD. The resuscitation of immersion victims. *Applied Cardiopulmonary Pathophysiology* 1989;**2**:293–298.

18. Modell JH, Graves SA, Ketover A. Clinical course of 91 consecutive near-drowning victims. *Chest* 1976;**70**(2):231–238.

This chapter was reviewed for this fifth edition by Simon Mitchell.

24

Salt water aspiration syndrome

Divers who aspirate small quantities of sea water may develop a respiratory disorder with generalized symptoms mimicking those of an acute viral infection. Severe cases merge into near drowning.

The symptoms develop soon after the dive and usually persist for some hours, and they are aggravated by activity and cold exposure.

Superficially, there are similarities between the salt water aspiration syndrome and other diving disorders, but the characteristics and natural history differentiate it from pulmonary barotrauma, decompression sickness, Key West scuba divers' disease, immersion pulmonary oedema, hypothermia, infections and asthma.

Treatment includes rest and oxygen inhalation.

HISTORY

A common diving illness in the Royal Australian Navy (RAN) in the 1960s was the salt water aspiration syndrome (SWAS)[1]. Its frequency may have been the result of the strenuous training imposed on novice divers, the absence of purge valves in second stage regulators or the extreme buddy breathing trials in which increasing numbers of trainees shared the one mouthpiece until finally one diver broke for the surface. In the RAN series, most patients with SWAS presented after night diving, when the influence of a cool environment may have aggravated the clinical situation.

In another entirely different diving environment, the professional abalone divers were almost routinely suffering from a brief, overnight affliction that they called 'salt water fever', which they correctly attributed to excessive water intake through the mouthpiece. The mouthpiece was connected to the surface-supplied air compressor, via an upstream or tilt valve. This simple piece of equipment was not very efficient in maintaining a water-free air supply and was recognized as a 'wet' breathing system. The air intake was sited below the exhaust valves, thus ensuring a nebulized water inhalation. It was replaced by the current first and second stage regulators in the 1980s by most professional divers.

The divers aspirated small quantities of sea water and developed a respiratory disorder, but with generalized symptoms mimicking those of an acute viral infection. More severe cases merged into near drowning.

A prospective survey was carried out on 30 consecutive patients who presented for treatment[1]. In none of these dives was the depth or duration exposure sufficient to implicate decompression sickness. The symptoms were documented and investigations were performed. To validate the cause, a simple experiment was performed on 'volunteers', who were both medical practitioners and divers, in which 'doctored' demand valves (second stage regulators) were used with the face immersed in sea water and the line pressure progressively reduced. Various respiratory measurements were monitored that replicated those in the survey. Unfortunately, more formal investigations were not pursued, and this experiment still awaits a more disciplined and sophisticated approach to define the degree and type of aspirate required.

The degree to which the same findings can be applied to fresh water aspirations and quantification of the influence of environmental factors on symptoms, also await clarification.

The frequency of SWAS has diminished somewhat with improved equipment and more lenient demands placed on novice divers, but it is still frequent enough among trainees to cause problems and diagnostic difficulties. Other seafarers to present with a similar disorder, but possibly not as frequently, are snorkellers, surfers and helicopter water rescuees.

The importance of SWAS lies in the understanding of near drowning cases and in its confusion with other diving or infectious diseases.

AETIOLOGY

Salt water aspiration (SWA) is a ubiquitous consequence of diving in the ocean, as well as among surfers, snorkellers, helicopter rescuees and ocean swimmers, who now recognize SWAS.

With divers, a watertight seal of the demand valve should ensure that water does not enter the spaces that carry the inspiratory and expiratory air.

This depends on the integrity of the mouthpiece, inspiratory valve or diaphragm (rubber or silicone) and the expiratory or exhaust valves. Any damage, wear, perforation, displacement or foreign body can disrupt these seals. This is more likely with increasing pressure gradients across the seals, such as with increasing respiration.

Whether the diver is aware of the 'leaking' probably depends on many factors, such as the volume, the site of entry (the proximity of the leak to the air inlet) and the attention paid to other activities. Sometimes the diver will recollect a specific incident leading to the aspiration (often inducing a cough), or he or she may notice a 'bubbling' or 'wet' sensation in the regulator. Other times, the diver may not notice anything, as occurs with the inhalation of many nebulized particles.

SWA in divers may occur in certain circumstances, namely:

1. In inexperienced divers because they commonly overbreathe the regulator.
2. Excessive respiratory flow and volumes, as with exercise and anxiety.
3. Increasing depth and thus density of the inspired gas.
4. During buddy breathing or re-inserting the regulator underwater.
5. From a faulty, corroded or damaged regulator.
6. Foreign body (salt crystals, weed, sand) interference with the diaphragm or exhaust valve seating.
7. Failure of the mouthpiece seal, as from tears.
8. Being towed at speed.
9. With upstream regulator valves, as in some surface supply units.
10. Whenever the air intake is below the exhaust outlet – a positional effect.
11. Removing the regulator on the surface.

As we know from respiratory medicine, larger volumes of fluid in the upper respiratory tract stimulate a laryngeal response varying from coughing to laryngospasm. Nebulized droplets with diameters of 1 to 10 micrometres are distributed to the terminal bronchi, with less deposition in the upper respiratory tract. The aspiration volumes in diving probably depend on the previously listed 10 circumstances.

CLINICAL FEATURES

The following observations were made on clinical cases of SWAS[1,2]:

Immediate symptoms

On specific interrogation, a history of aspiration was given in 90 per cent. Often, the novice diver did not realize the significance of the aspiration as the causal event of the syndrome.

Most divers noted an immediate post-dive cough, with or without sputum. It was usually suppressed during the dive. Only in the more serious cases was the sputum bloodstained, frothy and copious (as seen routinely in near drowning cases).

Subsequent symptoms

The following symptoms were observed:

- Rigors, tremors or shivering – 87 per cent
- Anorexia, nausea or vomiting – 80 per cent
- Hot or cold (feverish) sensations – 77 per cent
- Dyspnoea – 73 per cent
- Cough – 67 per cent
- Sputum – 67 per cent
- Headaches – 67 per cent
- Malaise – 53 per cent
- Generalized aches – 33 per cent

The signs and symptoms usually reverted to normal within a few hours and rarely persisted beyond 24 hours, unless the case was of greater severity.

RESPIRATORY SYMPTOMS

There was often a delay of up to 2 hours before dyspnoea, cough, sputum and retrosternal discomfort on inspiration were noted. In the mild cases, respiratory symptoms persisted for only an hour or so, whereas in the more severe cases, they commenced immediately following aspiration and continued for days. The respiratory rate roughly paralleled the degree of dyspnoea. Physical activity and respiratory stimulants appeared to aggravate the dyspnoea and tachypnoea, as did movement and exercise.

Auscultation of the chest revealed crepitations or occasional rhonchi, either generalized or local, in about half the cases. Rarely, they were high pitched and similar to those observed in obstructive airways disease.

Administration of 100 per cent oxygen was effective in relieving respiratory symptoms and removing any cyanosis.

X-ray study of the chest revealed areas of patchy consolidation, or a definite increase in respiratory markings, in about half the cases. These usually cleared within 24 hours, but they remained longer in severely affected patients. X-ray studies taken after the incident and repeated within a few hours sometimes showed a variation of the site of the radiological abnormality.

Expiratory spirometry performed repeatedly over the first 6 hours showed an average drop of 0.7 litres from the baseline in both forced expiratory volume in 1 second and vital capacity measurements. Even those patients who had no respiratory symptoms had a reduction in lung volumes. Arterial blood gases revealed oxygen tensions of 40 to 75 mm Hg with low or normal carbon dioxide tensions, indicative of shunting (perfusion) defects.

GENERALIZED SYMPTOMS

Patients often complained of being feverish. Malaise was the next most prominent feature. Headaches and generalized aches through the limbs, abdomen, back and chest were important in some cases, but usually not dominant. Anorexia was transitory.

The feverish symptoms were interesting – and are also seen in near drowning cases. Shivering, similar in some cases to a rigor and in other cases to generalized fasciculations, was more common in the colder months. It was precipitated or aggravated by exposure to cold, exercise or breathing 10 per cent oxygen (a research procedure, not recommended clinically). It was relieved by administration of 100 per cent oxygen. It occurred especially in patients exposed to cold because of duration and depth of dive, inadequate thermal clothing and environmental conditions during and after the dive.

The association of shivering with hypoxia and cold had been described previously[3]. The shivering occurs concurrently with the pyrexia, which also takes an hour or two to develop.

Pyrexia was verified in half the cases, up to 40°C (mean, 38.1°C; standard deviation [SD] = 0.6), and the pulse rate was elevated (mean, 102 per minute; SD = 21), over the first 6 hours.

Some patients obtained relief from these symptoms by either hot water baths or showers or by lying still in a warm bed.

In some patients, there was an impairment of consciousness, including transitory mild confusion or syncope with loss of consciousness on standing. These were clinically approaching the near drowning cases described (see Chapter 22), and they were treated accordingly.

INVESTIGATIONS

Haemoglobin, haematocrit, erythrocyte sedimentation rate and electrolytes remained normal. The white blood cell count was usually normal, although mild leucocytosis (not in excess of 20 000 per cubic millimetre) was observed in a few cases, with moderate polymorphonuclear leucocytosis and a shift to the left.

Lactic dehydrogenase estimations revealed a mild rise in some cases. X-ray and lung volume changes were as described earlier.

Examination of the diving equipment may reveal the cause of the aspiration. Inspection of the second stage regulator, breathing against the regulator with the air supply restricted and having another diver use the equipment under similar conditions all may identify the problem. See the section on re-enactment of a diving incident in Chapter 51.

DISCUSSION

A detailed investigation into the causes of *recreational scuba diving deaths*[4,5] revealed that SWA was part of the sequence leading to death in 37 per cent of the cases – often a consequence of equipment problems or diving technique. In these cases, 'leaking regulators' were either observed and commented on by the victim beforehand or were demonstrated during the subsequent diving investigation.

The degree of aspiration increases with the volume of air required (e.g. with exertion, swimming against currents, panic) and/or with a diminished line pressure to the second stage.

SWA often formed a vicious circle with panic and exhaustion.

Hypoxia from SWA aggravated the problems of fatigue and exhaustion and was a precursor to loss of consciousness (with or without dyspnoea) in both near drowning and drowning cases.

In *recreational scuba,* the diver may attribute SWA-induced post-dive lethargic symptoms to sub-clinical decompression sickness or the unusual physical demands of the dive activity. If the diver is exposed to cold and develops the generalized symptoms characteristic of a feverish reaction, he or she will be unlikely to relate this to an unnoticed aspiration some hours earlier.

Whether the clinical manifestations are entirely caused by the hyper-osmotic sea water or whether there is a contribution to the pulmonary inflammatory response from the various organisms, vegetation and particulate matter in sea water is not known. Extrapolating from the animal experiments on aspiration, it would seem that the required inhaled volume of hyper-osmotic sea water would be more than 100 ml in humans. Small particle nebulization is not essential, but it is possibly relevant in those divers who were not aware of aspiration.

There is no distinct division in the initial presentations among SWAS, near drowning and drowning cases. Aspiration syndromes merge with near drowning – the intensity of the symptoms and the degree of consciousness often depending on environmental circumstances, the activity of the victim and the administration of oxygen.

DIFFERENTIAL DIAGNOSIS

In the differential diagnosis of SWAS, the possibility of other occupational diseases of divers must be considered:

1. *Acute infection* – The aspiration syndrome may mimic an acute respiratory infection that develops soon after a dive. It is often claimed that a mild upper respiratory infection is likely to be aggravated by diving. This is questionable with the number of divers who continue to dive, uneventfully, despite such infections. Differentiation between SWAS and an acute infection can be made from the

history of aspiration, serial chest x-ray studies, spirometry and a knowledge of the natural history of the infectious diseases. In the first few hours of this syndrome, the possibility of both influenza and early pneumonia are often considered – to be dismissed as the symptoms clear within hours.

2. *Decompression sickness* with cardiorespiratory or musculoskeletal manifestations – If there is a likelihood of cardiorespiratory symptoms of decompression sickness ('chokes'), recompression therapy is indicated. Decompression sickness should be considered in patients who conduct deeper, prolonged or repetitive diving. The specific joint pains and abnormal posturing characteristic of the 'bends' are quite unlike the vague generalized muscular aches, involving the limbs and lumbar region bilaterally, seen with SWAS. The immediate beneficial response to the inhalation of 100 per cent oxygen in SWAS is of diagnostic value. With decompression sickness, any relief is more delayed. Chest x-ray studies, lung function tests and blood gas analyses may be used to confirm the diagnosis. Decompression sickness responds rapidly to recompression therapy (as does SWAS to hyperbaric oxygenation). Otherwise, except for the occurrence of a latent period, the clinical history of the two disorders is dissimilar.

3. *Pulmonary barotrauma* – Serious cases of pulmonary barotrauma result in pneumothorax, air emboli and mediastinal emphysema occurring suddenly after a dive. In minor cases of pulmonary barotrauma, confusion with the SWAS may arise. In these patients, the diagnosis and treatment of the former must take precedence until such time as the natural history, chest x-ray findings, spirometry and blood gas analysis demonstrate otherwise. Oxygen is appropriate first aid treatment for both disorders. Hyperbaric oxygen is also an effective (but unnecessary) treatment for SWAS.

4. *Hypothermia* – The effects of cold and immersion are usually maximal at, or very soon after, the time of rescue. The clinical features are likely to be confused with SWAS only when both conditions exist. The body temperature is higher than normal in SWAS and lower than normal in hypothermia.

5. *Key West scuba divers' disease*[6] – This and other infective disorders resulting from contaminated equipment may cause some confusion. Fortunately, these illnesses usually take longer to develop (24 to 48 hours) and to respond to therapy. There is thus little clinical similarity in the sequence and duration of the clinical manifestations.

6. *Asthma* – Some patients have hyperreactive airways to hypertonic saline (sea water), analogous to an asthma provocation test (see Chapter 55). Such patients have the clinical signs of asthma (expiratory rhonchi, especially with hyperventilation, typical expiratory spirometry findings and positive asthma provocation tests). They respond to salbutamol or other beta agonists.

7. *Immersion pulmonary oedema* – This disorder may be either a complication or an initiator of SWAS.

TREATMENT

Most of the clinical manifestations of SWAS respond rapidly to rest and the administration of oxygen. Warming the patient is of symptomatic benefit. In general, no other treatment is required.

There is a possibility that some of the clinical manifestations may not entirely be caused by to the aspiration of water, but by the body's (and specifically the respiratory tract's) response to aspirated organisms, foreign bodies or irritants carried to the lungs with the sea water aspiration.

REFERENCES

1. Edmonds C. A salt water aspiration syndrome. *Military Medicine* 1970;**135**(9):779–785.
2. Mitchell S. Salt water aspiration syndrome. *South Pacific Underwater Medicine Society Journal* 2002;**32**(4):205–206.
3. Bullard R. Effects of hypoxia or shivering on man. *Aerospace Medicine* 1961;**32**:1143–1147.

4. Edmonds C, Walker D. Scuba diving fatalities in Australia and New Zealand. *South
Pacific Underwater Medicine Society Journal*
1989;**19**(3):94–104.

5. Edmonds C, Walker D. Scuba diving
fatalities in Australia and New Zealand.
*South Pacific Underwater Medicine Society
Journal* 1991;**21**(1):2–4.

6. Kavanagh AJ, Halverson CW, Jordan CJ,
et al. A scuba syndrome. *Connecticut
Medicine* 1963;**27**(6):315.

*This chapter was reviewed for this fifth edition by
Carl Edmonds.*

25

Why divers drown

Historically, drowning has been incriminated as the cause of death in 74 to 82 per cent of recreational diving deaths, compared with the more high-profile diseases of decompression sickness (<1 per cent) and contaminated air supply (<1 per cent).

Comparisons of divers who drown with those who survive from near drowning reveal the importance of the following:

- Personal factors, including both medical and physical fitness.
- Diving experience.
- Faulty equipment and misuse of equipment.
- Hazardous environments.
- Neutral buoyancy being maintained during the dive and not being dependent upon the buoyancy compensator.

Other factors that increase the likelihood that diving problems will have an unsuccessful outcome include the following:

- An inadequate air supply.
- The failure to employ correct buddy diving practices.
- Inadequate buddy communication.
- Failure to achieve positive buoyancy after a diving incident.
- Inappropriate or delayed rescue and resuscitation.

SNORKELLERS

Diving includes snorkelling. Snorkellers who rarely leave the surface still expose themselves to many hazards, including drowning (see Chapter 61). There are few well-documented series of these incidents. Walker described 90 snorkelling deaths between 1972 and 1987, although many had no forensic assessment[1]. Edmonds and Walker described 60 such deaths between 1987 and 1996, all of which had coroners' inquiries and/or autopsy investigations[2]. Lippmann and Pearn described a further 130 cases, up until 2006[3].

Surface drownings caused about 25 to 45 per cent of the snorkellers' deaths. Drowning followed hypoxia from breath-hold diving, usually after hyperventilation, in 15 to 20 per cent (see Chapters 16 and 61 for these conditions).

Surface drownings tended to occur in an older but wider range age group than the hypoxic drownings, but at a younger age than those who die of the other major cause, cardiac disease. These snorkellers were often aquatically inexperienced, less fit tourists who engaged in commercial reef-snorkelling trips or solo swimming. Frequently, they had medical disorders that made them more vulnerable, such as epilepsy, respiratory diseases such as asthma, salt water aspiration and vomiting. Adverse environmental factors, such as currents and choppy surface conditions, were contributors in 15 per cent. The absence of fins in 40 per cent made coping with aquatic conditions more difficult. Overall, the physical unfitness and aquatic inexperience that led to panic and aspiration dominated the situation.

DIVERS

Drowning among divers is very different in both aetiology and responses from drowning in the general population. Divers do not fear immersion, as do many of the customary drowning victims. The usual drowning victims, falling from a boat or deck, are often unprepared for the withdrawal of a respirable atmosphere, surprised by the sudden cold exposure, choking from a gasp and aspiration of water, illogical and unreasoning in survival attempts. Even swimmers presume that air will be constantly available. The scuba diver is fully prepared, enjoying this leisure activity and protected from the environment, carrying his or her own air supply. The diver has also planned for accidents that could cause drowning by employing buoyancy apparatus and an emergency air supply and with companions trained for rescue. The situation of drowning in divers is thus different from most of those described in Chapter 21.

In a prelude to the 1997 Undersea and Hyperbaric Medical Society (UHMS) Workshop on Near Drowning, the Chairman made the following statement in the pre-workshop correspondence: 'As you know, the drowning literature ignores diving, whilst the diving literature ignores drowning'[4].

It is paradoxical that drowning, which causes more than 80 times the number of deaths in recreational divers than either decompression

sickness or contaminated air, does not rate more than a paragraph or two in some diving medical texts.

In reviewing the literature on drowning, before the 1997 Workshop[4], the only papers that could be found that specifically related any of the drowning syndromes to scuba diving were one on the salt water aspiration syndrome[5] and one with an anecdotal review followed by a case report[6]. Nevertheless, of the major seminal reviews presented on this subject, many have been by diving physicians[7–10].

A normally functioning diver, with adequate equipment in a congenial ocean environment, is protected from drowning by carrying his or her own personal life support – the scuba equipment. Drowning would occur only in the presence of the following:

- Diver fault (pathology, psychology or technique).
- Failure of the equipment to supply air.
- Hazardous environmental influences.

Nevertheless, the most common ultimate cause of death in recreational scuba divers is drowning. Factual information that clarifies the causes and management is of value in preventing further fatal outcomes.

Previous surveys illustrated the importance of drowning as the ultimate cause in 74 to 82 per cent of recreational scuba diving fatalities[11–15]. Of note in the more detailed surveys[13–18] was the high frequency of multiple contributing factors to each death. Drowning tended to obscure those preceding factors. The drowning sequelae and drowning pathology were results of the environment in which the accident occurred, not the initiating or primary causes of the accident.

For example, any loss of consciousness or capability when engaging in terrestrial activities is unlikely to cause death. It would do so more frequently if the victim was diving underwater.

Survey results

The aspiration of sea water that causes clinical features in scuba divers who retain consciousness is discussed in Chapter 24. Sometimes, this progresses to the other manifestations of near drowning and drowning, and these conditions were compared in one survey of fatalities (drownings) and survivors (near drownings)[16] in recreational diving. The observations were as follows.

PERSONAL CONTRIBUTIONS

Population

Of the 100 fatalities, 89 per cent occurred in male divers and 11 per cent occurred in female divers. Of the 48 survivors, 52 per cent were male and 48 per cent female. Compared with the diving population at the time (30 per cent female, 70 per cent male), male divers were overrepresented in the scuba drowning cases, as they are in almost all other forms of drowning[9]. The surprise was that female divers appeared to be overrepresented in the 'survivor' series.

Whether female divers had more accidents or whether they only reported them more frequently could not be deduced. However, it does appear as if accidents in female divers result in fewer deaths.

Training

In the fatalities, 38 per cent of these divers had no known formal qualification. This group was approximately equally divided among:

- Those in whom documentation was inadequate.
- Those without training, but who were experimenting with scuba under their own or their friends' cognizance.
- Those who were engaged in introductory dives, brief resort courses or 'dive experiences' with a recognized commercial organization.

Of the survivors, 81 per cent had completed basic training, and only 4 per cent had no training.

Surprising numbers in both groups were under formal training at the time – 8 per cent of the fatalities and 15 per cent of the survivors.

Experience

Experience did not directly correlate with training. In both the fatality and survivor series, the divers were equally represented among inexperienced divers (<5 dives), novice divers (5 to 20 dives) and experienced divers – one third each.

Of the fatalities, more than half these divers were experiencing diving situations to which they had not been previously exposed, whereas one third had previous experience of the conditions in which they died. The others were unable to be assessed.

The buddy or dive leader appeared to be considerably more experienced than the diver in most of these cases, thereby possibly explaining why the diver died and the buddy lived.

Victim's behaviour

In 100 diving fatalities, more than a third were observed to have either a panic response or rapid or abnormal movements (Table 25.1). The survivors reported these sensations in more than one half of cases. The increased incidence in the surviving group could be attributed to this being a reported sensation, whereas the fatality figure represented only the observed behaviour.

More than half the divers who died showed no change in their behavior before drowning, with loss of consciousness being the first objective warning in one third. It was the first manifestation noted in one fourth of the survivors.

Of interest was the absence of panic in many of the cases, even though it is a frequent cause of other diving deaths[11–13,17]. Drowning scuba divers frequently drown quietly – possibly because of the effects of previous aspiration (hypoxia), depth (narcosis) or training ('don't panic').

A request for a supplementary air supply was made by twice as many divers who died (21 per cent) as survivors. This may bring into

Table 25.1 Behaviour among fatalities and survivors of drowning in divers

Victim's behaviour	Fatalities (observed)	Survivors (reported)
Panic	21%	27%
Rapid or abnormal movements	16%	31%
Nothing unusual	63%	42%
Loss of consciousness	33%	25%
Air requested	21%	10%

question the value of relying on a buddy to respond to such a request. Alternatively, with the survivors, more frequently buddies offered the emergency air supply – a preferred sequence. Occasionally, there was the apocryphal underwater tussle for a single regulator. When the low-on-air diver went for an air supply, he or she more frequently sought the companion's primary regulator than the octopus.

Medical conditions (history)

This is a contentious area, not only regarding the incidence of medical disorders but also their significance. Authors differ in their assessments of this, and none are free of selection bias.

Medical history data from fatality records are inevitably underestimates. In one analysis[13], when a purposeful attempt was made to acquire the medical history, in less than half of the cases could this be obtained.

In this survey no attempt was made to draw statistical differences regarding the correlation between past illnesses and drowning; however, there was no doubt as to the contribution in the survivor group (Table 25.2). Some of both groups should not have been classed as medically fit for diving (see Chapters 53 to 59).

ENVIRONMENTAL FACTORS
Water conditions

The adverse influences of water conditions were expected (see Chapter 5). Probably the only surprise was the frequency with which drowning occurred in calm waters – in more than half the cases. Strong tidal currents were slightly more frequent in the fatality group.

Table 25.2 Medical disorders among fatalities and survivors of drowning in divers

Medical disorders	Fatalities[a]	Survivors
Asthma	10%	19%
Cardiovascular disease	6%	2%
Drug intake	10%	8%
Very unfit	5%	4%
Panic	7%	8%

[a]History often not sought.

Fresh water or sea water

Most of the accidents occurred in the ocean, without obvious differences between the fatality (93 per cent) and survivor groups (98 per cent). The extra difficulty of performing rescues in cave diving (2 per cent) was expected.

Depth of incident

The depth of the aspiration or drowning incident was not necessarily the depth of the original problem. Thus, a diver who used most of the air supply and then panicked and ascended may not have exhibited any evidence of aspiration until reaching the surface.

As in previous surveys[11,13], many problems developed on the surface. Approximately half the fatalities occurred on the surface or on the way to the surface. Frequently, the diver no longer had adequate air to remain underwater. Another 20 per cent occurred in the top 9 metres, and the rest were distributed over the remaining depths. This finding implies that just reaching the surface is not enough. Successful rescue then requires the victim to remain there.

The survivors more accurately reported the depth at which the incident developed, as opposed to the depth at which the incident was noted by others. Nevertheless, almost two thirds of these incidents occurred in the top 10 metres.

In the fatality and the survivor groups, the dive was the deepest of their diving career in 26 per cent and in 33 per cent, respectively. In almost half the 'inexperienced' and 'novice' divers, the depth was beyond that which had previously been undertaken. This finding suggests that these groups are especially susceptible to the various problems associated with depth (panic, air consumption, visibility, narcosis and logistical difficulty with rescue).

This suggests that it is not so much the environment that is the problem, but the diver's limited experience of that environment. The risk of 'diving deeper' without extra prudence and supervision is apparent. Any dive deeper than that previously experienced should be classified and treated as a 'deep dive', irrespective of the actual depth.

Visibility

Visibility was usually acceptable, but it seemed to be more frequently adverse in the fatalities (38 per cent) compared with the survivors (18 per cent).

Conclusions

The cases, in general, demonstrated the adverse effects of various environments, especially with tidal currents, white (rough) water, poor visibility and deeper diving than previously experienced. There was not a great deal of difference between the two groups, except in the higher incidence of strong tidal currents, night diving and cave diving in the fatalities. The figures, however, were small. Such adverse environments may affect the victim directly or may negatively influence rescue and resuscitation.

EQUIPMENT

In most fatalities, the equipment showed no structural abnormality, and only in 20 per cent were there significant or serious *faults* contributing to the fatality. This finding corresponded with the reported incidence by the survivors (18 per cent).

Equipment faults were most frequently found with buoyancy compensators and regulators (both first and second stages).

The incidence of equipment *misuse* was more frequent but more difficult to ascertain in the fatality series – and it depends on one's definition (fatalities 43 per cent, survivors 38 per cent). Misuse of equipment included the use of excessive weights (fatalities 25 per cent, survivors 27 per cent). It also included the failure to carry equipment that could have been instrumental in survival (e.g. buoyancy compensator, contents gauge, snorkel) – in 12 per cent and in 8 per cent, respectively. Difficulties in using buoyancy compensators were also frequent.

DIVING TECHNIQUE

Various diving techniques contributed to the drowning incidents or influenced rescue and survival. They included a compromised air supply, buoyancy factors, buddy rescue and resuscitation attempts.

Air supply

In 60 per cent of the fatalities, either an out-of-air (OOA) or a low-on-air (LOA) situation had developed. There was insufficient air in the tank for either continuing the planned dive or returning to safety underwater. In the survivors, there was a lower incidence (35 per cent) of compromised air supply, but it was still very high. The survivors were more likely to have air in their tanks to cope with the emergency.

The failure to use the available contents gauge, in both groups, was a source of concern, which could sometimes be attributed to the conditions placing other stress on the diver (e.g. depth, anxiety, tidal current, deepest dive ever). In many more cases, there was a voluntary decision to dive until the tank was near reserve or 'ran out'.

One surprising feature was the failure in both groups (8 per cent and 13 per cent) to reopen the valve of the scuba tank after initially testing the tank pressure before the dive. Thus, even though there was plenty of air in the tank, it was unavailable other than to sometimes allow a rapid descent to a few metres. Only then was the diver aware that further air was not available. In none of these cases was there a buddy check of equipment – breathing near the water surface and checking the equipment before descent.

In a smaller number of cases there was a failure to ensure that the cylinder tap was adequately turned on. Reducing tank pressure resulted in a restriction of air supply – sometimes obvious only at depth.

Buoyancy factors

Buoyancy was frequently a vital factor in reaching the surface and in remaining there as an unconscious diver and being found, rescued and resuscitated in time. The three major influences on this are buoyancy compensators, weights and the companion (buddy) diver practice.

Buoyancy compensators

In the survivor group. the buoyancy compensator was inflated by the victim or rescuer (35 per cent and 25 per cent) in twice as many cases as in the fatality group (15 per cent and 16 per cent). This figure is even more relevant when the delay in producing buoyancy in the fatality group is considered (see later).

Weights

These weights were as shown in Table 25.3.

Although in 30 per cent of the fatality cases the weights were ditched, in practice this was not as valuable as it sounds. In most of the instances in which the rescuer ditched the weights, the victim was probably no longer salvageable because of the delay (see later).

The survivor group not only ditched the weights more frequently, but often this was done by the victim. When it was done by the rescuer, it was usually performed early in the incident.

Buoyancy action by survivors

The fatality and survivor groups differed in that the survivors more often performed an action (ditching weights, inflating buoyancy compensator) that resulted in their achieving positive buoyancy during and following the incident.

An interesting observation was made when the victim and buddy were both in difficulty, usually based on an LOA/OOA situation. In the ensuing situation, irrespective of whose problem developed first, the overweight diver tended to be the one who died, and the buoyant diver was the one that survived. In the 14 instances, the ratio was 6:1.

All this gives support to the current instructor agencies' emphasis on buoyancy training, although one could argue for its inclusion in introductory courses more than in advanced courses.

Table 25.3 Use of weights among fatalities and survivors of drowning in divers

Weights	Fatalities (observed)	Survivors (reported)
Not worn	1%	6%
Not ditched	66%	48%
Entangled	3%	2%
Victim ditched	10%	19%
Rescuer ditched	20%	25%

COMPANION DIVER PRACTICE, RESCUE AND RESUSCITATION

In most cases of significant aspiration of water, rescue depends on rapid action undertaken by either the victim or the companion (buddy) diver. Once a diver gets into difficulty and is unable to carry out safety actions by himself or herself, the diver is heavily reliant on the buddy or dive leader. The fatality and survivor populations were very different in this respect.

Fatalities

In the fatality group, less than half the victims had an experienced buddy available to assist them. In 21 per cent of the fatalities, the dive was a solo one. In 38 per cent, the diver had separated from his or her buddy, and in 12 per cent the diver had separated from the group, before the serious incident. Thus, a voluntary separation happened in 50 per cent of the cases before the fatality. The separation was initiated in most cases because the victim could not continue (usually because of an LOA situation). The victim then attempted to return alone, essentially making it a solo dive.

The diver was separated from the buddy or the group during the actual incident, and often by the incident, in 21 per cent of cases. However, in almost half of these cases, the separation was produced because the diver was following the buddy or the group. The others occurred during the 'rescue'.

Thus, separation made early rescue and resuscitation improbable. In 9 per cent, the victim was swimming behind his or her companion or companions, and thus the victim was not visible to the 'buddy' at the time of the incident.

In summary, 80 per cent of the victims did not have a genuine buddy, by virtue of their elected diving practice. In fewer than 1 in 10 deaths was there continued contact with the buddy or group during and following the incident.

The victims seemed flagrantly to disregard the 'buddy' system – as did their companions, the organization that conducted the dive or the 'dive leader'. Group diving conferred little value because the 'leader' often had insufficient contact with individual divers to be classified as a buddy, and the responsibility of others was not clear – especially toward the last of the 'followers'.

In only 20 per cent was the diver reached within 5 minutes of the probable incident time, and thereby have a real chance of successful resuscitation. In another 12 per cent, the diver was recovered within 6 to 15 minutes, and theoretically there was a slight chance of recovery with these divers, had the rescue facilities been ideal and had fortune smiled brightly.

Resuscitation was not a feasible option for most of the eventual fatalities, who were obviously dead or showed no response to the rescuers' attempts, in 9 out of 10 cases. This is explained by the excessive delay in the rescue in most cases.

Survivors

In the surviving group, most were rescued by their companion. Some form of artificial respiration or cardiopulmonary resuscitation was required in 29 per cent of the cases. Oxygen was available and used, usually in a free-flow system, in 52 per cent of cases.

No specific data were available on the buddy divers assisting the survivors, other than the subjective assessment of whether the survivor believed the buddy to be of much value, as follows:

- The buddy was immediately available to the survivor in 71 per cent of cases.
- The buddy was considered to be of assistance in 58 per cent of cases.
- The buddy supplied an independent air source in 15 per cent of cases.
- The buddy inflated the buoyancy compensator in 25 per cent of cases.
- The buddy ditched the weight belt in 25 per cent of cases.
- The buddy attempted buddy breathing in 4 per cent of cases.

In 52 per cent of cases, the diver surfaced under control of the buddy.

The attitude toward buddy diving practice in the survival group appeared to be very different from that in the fatality group.

The frequency of oxygen use probably represented a more sophisticated and organized diving activity, which may also be related to more conscientious buddy behaviour.

The axiom is that to rescue an incapacitated diver successfully, one must know where he or she is and reach the diver quickly. This implies some form of buddy responsibility. Once reached, the buddy divers seemed to be of considerable value – implying good training or initiative in this aspect of diver safety.

In recent years there has been a promotion of solo diving and reliance on oneself, as compared with buddy diving practices. The foregoing data indicate that the traditional buddy concept, correctly practised, is of more value.

CONCLUSIONS

There are many lessons for recreational divers to learn from the data now available, as well as from the diving medical experience and the regulatory requirements of commercial diving, to reduce the incidence of drowning with scuba. They can be summarized as follows:

1. Diver fitness. Ensure both medical and physical fitness, so that there is no increased likelihood of physical impairment or loss of consciousness or difficulty in handling unexpected environmental stresses.
2. Experience. Ensure adequate experience of the likely dive conditions (dive under the supervision of a more experience diver when extending your dive profile).
3. Equipment. Failure to possess appropriate equipment is a risk, but not as much as equipment failure and misuse. Misuse includes the practice of overweighting the diver, as well as an overreliance on the buoyancy compensator.
4. Environment. Hazardous diving conditions should be avoided, and one should use extreme caution with tidal currents, rough water, poor visibility, enclosed areas and excessive depths.
5. Neutral buoyancy (dive). Ensure neutral buoyancy while diving. This implies not being overweighted and not being dependent on the buoyancy compensator.
6. Air supply. An inadequate supply of air for unexpected demands and emergencies may convert a problematical situation into a dangerous one. It also forces the diver to experience surface situations that are worrying and conducive to anxiety, fatigue, unpleasant decision making and salt water aspiration.

Equipment failure is not as common a cause of LOA/OOA as is failure to use the contents gauge and/or a decision to breathe the tank down to near reserve pressure.

7. Buddy diving. Use traditional buddy diving practice – two divers swimming together. Solo diving, for the whole or part of the dive, is much more likely to result in an unsatisfactory outcome in the event of diving problems. It is the divers who are committed to the traditional buddy diving practices who are likely to survive the more serious of the drowning syndromes.

8. Positive buoyancy (after the incident). Positive buoyancy is frequently required if problems develop. Failure to remove the weight belt during a diving incident continues to be a major omission, and it must reflect on training standards. In most situations, unbuckling and then ditching (if necessary) the weight belt is the most reliable course of action once a problem becomes evident. Buoyancy compensators cause problems in some emergency situations, and not infrequently they fail to provide the buoyancy required expeditiously, especially at depth. They are of great value in many cases – but they are not to be relied on.

9. Buddy communication. If feasible, inform the buddy before ascent. If correct buddy diving practice is being carried out, the buddy will automatically accompany the injured or vulnerable diver back to safety.

10. Rescue. Employ the rescue, water retrievals, first aid facilities (including oxygen) and medical evacuation systems that were planned before the dive.

These factors differentiate a drowning fatality from a successful rescue.

REFERENCES

1. Walker DG. The investigation of critical factors in diving related fatalities. Published annually in the *South Pacific Underwater Medical Society Journal* 1972–1989.
2. Edmonds C, Walker D. Snorkelling deaths in Australia. *Medical Journal of Australia* 1999;**171**:591–594.
3. Lippmann JM, Pearn JH. Snorkeling-related deaths in Australia, 1994–2006. *Medical Journal of Australia* 2012;**197**(4):230–232.
4. Dueker C. Dueker CW Drowning Syndrome-The Mechanism. Chapter 1. In: Dueker C, Brown S, editors. *Near Drowning.* 47th Workshop. Undersea and Hyperbaric Medicine Society. Kensington, Maryland: Undersea and Hyperbaric Medical Society; 1999.
5. Edmonds C. A salt water aspiration syndrome. *Military Medicine* 1970;**135**(9):779–785.
6. Zwingelberg KM, Green JW, Powers EK. Primary causes of drowning and near drowning in scuba diving. *The Physician and Sportsmedicine* 1986;**14**:145–151.
7. Donald KW. Drowning. *British Medical Journal* 1955;**2**:155–160.
8. Tabeling BB. Near drowning. In: Carlston CB, Mathias RA, Shilling CW, editors. *The Physician's Guide to Diving Medicine.* New York: Plenum Press; 1984.
9. Neuman TS. Near drowning. In Bove A, Davis J, editors. *Diving Medicine.* Philadelphia:. Saunders; 1990.
10. Edmonds C. Drowning syndromes: the mechanism. *South Pacific Underwater Medicine Society Journal* 1998;**28**(1):2–12.
11. Mcaniff JJ. *United States Underwater Diving Fatality Statistics/1970–79.* Washington, DC: US Department of Commerce, NOAA, Undersea Research Program; 1981.
12. Mcaniff JJ. *United States Underwater Diving Fatality Statistics/1986–87.* Report number URI-SSR-89-20. Kingston, Rhode Island: University of Rhode Island, National Underwater Accident Data Centre; 1988.
13. Edmonds C, Walker D. Scuba diving fatalities in Australia and New Zealand: the human factor. *South Pacific Underwater Medicine Society Journal* 1989;**19**(3):104.
14. Edmonds C, Walker D. Scuba diving fatalities in Australia and New Zealand: the environmental factor. *South Pacific Underwater Medicine Society Journal* 1990;**20**(1):2–4.

15. Edmonds C, Walker D. Scuba Diving Fatalities in Australia & New Zealand. The Equipment Factor. *South Pacific Underwater Medicine Society J.* 1991;**21**(1):2–4.

16. Edmonds C, Walker D, Scott B. Drowning syndromes with scuba. *South Pacific Underwater Medicine Journal* 1997;**27**(4):182–190.

17. Divers Alert Network. *Report on Diving Accidents and Fatalities.* Durham, North Carolina: Divers Alert Network; 1996.

18. Lippmann J, Baddeley A, Vann R, Walker D. An analysis of the causes of compressed-gas diving fatalities in Australia from 1972–2005. *Undersea and Hyperbaric Medicine* 2013;**40**(1):49–61.

This chapter was reviewed for this fifth edition by Carl Edmonds.

PART 6

Other Aquatic Disorders

26

Seasickness (motion sickness)

INTRODUCTION

Almost everybody is susceptible to motion sickness[1]. In general, the population can be divided roughly into one third who are highly susceptible, one third who react only under rough conditions and one third who become sick only under extreme conditions. Although anyone with a normally functioning vestibular system is susceptible, people who are totally deaf and have unresponsive vestibular systems are very resistant.

In diving, two situations predispose to seasickness. The first is on the boat going to the dive site, and the second is while the diver is in the water, particularly if attached to the boat, for example, on a shot line during decompression. Most divers are less susceptible to seasickness while swimming underwater than when they are on the boat. For this reason, many divers hurry to enter the water after exposure to adverse sea conditions en route to the dive site. Problems develop because divers are inadequately prepared and equipped as a result of haste or from the debilitating and demoralizing effects of seasickness.

SYMPTOMS

Usually, the first sign of seasickness is pallor, although this occasionally may be preceded by a flushed appearance[1]. This may be followed by yawning, restlessness and a cold sweat, often noticeable on the forehead and upper lip. Malaise, nausea and vomiting may progress to prostration, dehydration and electrolyte and acid-base imbalance, although these latter and more serious manifestations usually appear only in intractable seasickness during long periods at sea. During this progression, there is often a waxing and waning of symptoms, especially before the actual development of vomiting, and vomiting itself often brings temporary relief.

Tolerance develops to a particular motion, and a person may become acclimatized to specific conditions. If there is a change in the intensity or nature of the motion, the individual may again be susceptible. Continuous exposure to constant conditions usually produces tolerance within 2 to 3 days. Tolerance can also develop to repeated shorter exposures. There is a central nervous system habituation to such a degree that after the person disembarks and the motion is stopped, the person feels that he or she is rocking at the frequency of the original ship exposure.

There is considerable variation in susceptibility to seasickness. With increasing age individuals tend to become more resistant, and at least one study suggests that girls and women are more susceptible[2]. This susceptibility is said to result from a lack of experience with the situations that produce seasickness. Overindulgence in food and alcohol before exposure, and especially the night before, predisposes to motion sickness. Both the number of meals and their energy content correlate with susceptibility to airsickness[2]. The position on board the vessel can also be important, with least stimuli if the victim is amidships and using the horizon as a visual reference. Any attempt to read aggravates motion sickness. Psychological factors play a part, especially with seasickness that develops before boarding the vessel. Once one person becomes seasick, there is often a rapid spreading among others present.

AETIOLOGY

Motion sickness is caused by a mismatch or conflict of sensorineural information[3]. Normally, the vestibular stimuli are consistent with the visual and proprioceptive stimuli, all informing the brain of the position of the body – even when it is in motion. When the environment starts moving as well, the information becomes conflicting. The motion sickness occurs at the onset and cessation of sensory rearrangements; when input of vision, vestibular and proprioception is at variance with the stored patterns of recent stimuli information.

PREVENTION

For boat passengers and sailors, acclimatization will develop if progressively increasing periods are spent at sea. Otherwise, it usually takes 2 to 3 days of continuous exposure to adapt to new conditions. The sources of vestibular and proprioceptive stimulation should be reduced to a minimum. This usually means either lying down or being as still as possible. Unnecessary head movements should be avoided. In small craft, staying along the centre line of the craft, toward the stern, incurs the least complex motion. Conflicting visual stimulation is reduced by keeping the eyes closed or by focusing on the horizon. Vulnerable individuals should definitely avoid reading, and noxious stimuli such as smells should be avoided.

Drugs for general use

Most drugs for preventing and treating seasickness are either antihistamines or anticholinergics. This reflects the importance of histaminergic and cholinergic transmission of neural inputs to the vestibular apparatus, the solitary tract nucleus and the vomiting centre itself. Drugs that target the chemoreceptor trigger zone, such as the 5-hydroxytryptamine antagonist ondansetron and the dopamine antagonist droperidol, are not considered particularly effective in motion sickness.

Commonly used antihistamines include cyclizine, dimenhydrinate, promethazine and cinnarizine; and the most commonly used anticholinergic is hyoscine or scopolamine (whose most widely available preparation is a transdermal patch). Various attempts have been made to compare the efficacy of these agents, both within and between the two classes. Graybeil and colleagues[4] compared drugs alone and in combinations. They found that the best combination was promethazine hydrochloride 25 mg in combination with 25 mg ephedrine sulphate. Scopolamine was the most effective single drug, but it was more effective also when combined with ephedrine sulphate or d-amphetamine sulphate than as a single drug. In a trial reported by Pyykko and associates[5], dimenhydrinate was more effective than one scopolamine patch and about equal to two and had the advantage of needing a shorter period to become effective. Other studies place cyclizine and dimenhydrinate as equal in performance but suggest that cyclizine reduced gastric symptoms and drowsiness[6]. Use of combined preparations (e.g. hyoscine and dimenhydrinate[7]) may be more effective than a single compound.

Drugs for divers

The main problem for divers is that all these drugs have some side effects, and none are truly proven safe for diving. Antihistamines may cause dry mouth and drowsiness, whereas anticholinergics also cause dry mouth, variable levels of sedation and occasionally blurred vision. The effects on arousal leave open the possibility of an interaction between motion sickness drugs and nitrogen narcosis. Another frequently cited concern is the question of whether there is any interaction between the drugs and risk of oxygen toxicity. There has been limited investigation of these issues. In hyperbaric chamber dives to 36 metres, transdermal scopolamine was not found to cause decrements in cognitive performance or manual dexterity[8]. Both scopolamine[9] and cinnarizine[10] were found not to increase risk of central nervous system oxygen toxicity in rats. Although not a trial in divers or diving, it is perhaps notable that dimenhydrinate was found to induce significant neurocognitive impairment in volunteer subjects, whereas cinnarizine and transdermal scopolamine were not[11].

In electing to use anti–motion sickness agents, divers must accept that the safety case for use in diving has not been comprehensively made for any drug. However, on balance (which includes consideration of the debilitating effects of seasickness on divers who nevertheless enter the water), the risk *versus* benefit equation probably favours use of a preventive agent in susceptible divers. At the present time, the evidence suggests that use of a non-sedating antihistamine such as cinnarizine or an anticholinergic in the transdermal form (scopolamine) is acceptable. Unfortunately, both these agents can be difficult to source in Australia and New Zealand. Use of the sedating antihistamines (e.g. cyclizine) or those shown to affect performance significantly (e.g. dimenhydrate) should be avoided. Any drug used for this purpose must be tried previously to ensure that no untoward reactions occur.

TREATMENT

If a sufferer is seriously ill or if vomiting has commenced, the pylorus will be constricted, and oral drugs may not reach their site of absorption. The drugs must be administered parenterally. Some agents are suitable for intramuscular injection if an intravenous line is not available. Sufferers severely affected by seasickness should not dive, and they should lie down and try to sleep. A mild degree of sedation is sometimes very helpful if the patient is being supervised by someone suitably qualified. This can often be achieved by use of an antihistamine that is not only antiemetic but also sedating (e.g. cyclizine). Under these circumstances, a drug such as droperidol in very small doses may also be helpful, but there should be no diving if sedating strategies are used. If there is a prolonged period of interrupted oral intake, intravenous fluid and electrolyte replacement may be required; seagoing medical officers have observed that the fluid may be more important than the drug.

REFERENCES

1. Money KE. Motion sickness. *Physiological Reviews* 1970;**50**:1–50.
2. Lindseth G, Lindseth PD. The relation of diet to airsickness. *Aviation, Space, and Environmental Medicine* 1995;**66**:537–541.
3. Gordon CR, Spitzer O, Doweck I, Shupak A, Gadolth N. The vestibulo-ocular reflex and seasickness susceptibility. *Journal of Vestibular Research* 1996;**6**:229–233.
4. Graybiel A, Wood CD, Knepton J, Hoche JP, Perkins GF. Human assay of antimotion sickness drugs. *Aviation, Space, and Environmental Medicine* 1975;**46**:1107–1118.
5. Pyykko I, Schalen L, Jantti V. Transdermally administered scopolamine vs. dimenhydrate. *Acta Otolaryngologica (Stockholm)* 1985;**99**:588–596.
6. Weinstein SE, Stern RM. Comparison of Marzine and Dramamine in preventing symptoms of motion sickness. *Aviation, Space, and Environmental Medicine* 1997;**68**:890–894.
7. Cooper C. Motion sickness a guide to prevention and treatment. *Medicine Today* 2000;**1**:50–56.
8. Williams TH, Wilkinson AR, Davis FM, Frampton CM. Effects of transcutaneous scopolamine and depth on diver performance. *Undersea Biomedical Research* 1988;**15**:89–98.
9. Bitterman N, Eilender E, Melamed Y. Hyperbaric oxygen and scopolamine. *Undersea Biomedical Research* 1991;**18**:167–174.
10. Arieli R, Shupak A, Shachal B, Shenedrey A, Ertracht OD, Rashkovean G. Effect of the anti-motion sickness medication cinnarizine on central nervous system oxygen toxicity. *Undersea and Hyperbaric Medicine* 1999;**26**:105–109.
11. Gordon CR, Gonen A, Nachum Z, Doweck I, Spitzer O, Shupak A. The effects of dimenhydrate, cinnarizine, and transdermal scopolamine on performance. *Journal of Psychopharmacology* 2001;**15**:167–172.

This chapter was reviewed for this fifth edition by Simon Mitchell.

27

Thermal problems and solutions

BASIC TEMPERATURE PHYSIOLOGY

For a diver in the water or a pressure chamber, the heat transfers are often greater than normally experienced on land. Most readers will not need a more detailed discussion of basic temperature physiology. Any who do are advised to read any of the basic or, if preferred, more advanced texts on the subject.

With the exception of the animals that hibernate, mammals require a relatively stable body temperature to operate. For a person to be comfortable, the deep body temperature must remain at about $37 \pm 1°C$. Temperatures above this initially cause sweating, and higher temperatures may lead to heat exhaustion, heat stroke and the potential for subsequent death from hyperthermia. Below the comfort range, shivering can progress to the various stages of hypothermia, potentially leading to coma and death. Hypothermia is covered in Chapter 28.

Humans maintain their body temperature by balancing heat production and loss. Heat is produced by the biochemical processes that convert food to energy and waste products. Heat can also be gained from the external surroundings. This occurs in a hot climate or by touching, or being exposed to, something that is warmer than the person; including the ingestion of food and drink.

Most heat is lost from a warm body by transfer to a cooler environment. The other avenue of losing heat is in warming material that enters the body. Warming and humidifying air before it reaches the lungs are continuous heat drains. Ingestion of cool food and drinks plays only a small part.

A constant temperature is maintained if the production and loss of heat remain equal. The body can achieve this in a variety of ways. In a warm environment, the amount of heat produced is set by the activity of the metabolic processes and the exercise undertaken. So, the production side of the equation is fixed. Heat loss to the environment can be adjusted. It is influenced by skin temperature, which is monitored by, and to some extent under the control of, the nervous system. If more heat needs to be lost, nervous stimuli will initiate peripheral vasodilatation, causing increased blood flow to the skin and more heat to be transferred. If still greater heat loss is needed, the body can sweat. The consequent evaporation cools the skin and enables more heat to be lost.

In a cold environment, if peripheral vasoconstriction and the subsequent reduction of blood flow to the skin are insufficient to conserve heat, more heat can be produced by muscular activity, such as shivering. The main other methods of maintaining body temperature are behavioural and include, for example, putting on or taking off clothes and moving to a warmer or cooler place.

DIVER IN SHALLOW WATER

The temperature of the oceans range from –2°C (28.4°F), which is the freezing point of sea water of normal salinity, to a surface temperature in some places of almost 38°C (100°F). In most regions, the annual range of temperature in open ocean is less than 10°C. This narrow range is caused by the high heat capacity of water that dampens the seasonal change in temperature. The thermal environment is usually predictable enough to allow precautions to be taken when diving.

In most circumstances, the diver's problem is to maintain body heat. Cooling occurs because water is a good conductor and has a high specific heat.

For most dives in shallow water, an increase in insulation reduces heat loss to an acceptable level. Increased insulation is also required for survival during prolonged exposure to cold water. The temperature at which extra insulation is required depends on the duration of the dive, the heat production the diver can maintain and the diver's internal insulation. This internal insulation is related to the amount of body fat carried and to the

previous exposure to cold, which generates a degree of tolerance.

Wetsuits are the most common protective clothing used in temperate water. They are made from sheets of rubber that has gas bubbles injected into it as it solidifies. A surface layer of fabric gives the rubber strength and protection. The fabric adds little to the insulation, which mainly comes from the trapped gas bubbles. Some heat is also conserved, especially with a well-fitting wetsuit, because the layer of water between the wetsuit and the skin is trapped and warms up, thus helping to reduce heat loss. Because the bubbles in the rubber obey Boyle's Law, their volume decreases with depth, so the insulation diminishes as depth increases (Figure 27.1).

Drysuits are made from a fabric-rubber composite sheet. They derive their name from the intention that the wearer of the suit should remain dry under the watertight barrier of the fabric. Because of this, a warm layer of clothing can be worn, and a layer of air is trapped in the suit. As a gas space, the undersuit layer follows Boyle's Law, so gas must be added to the suit during descent

(a)
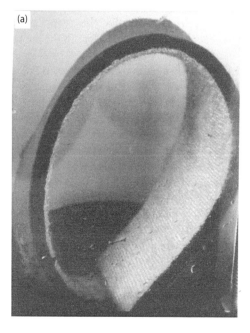

(b)
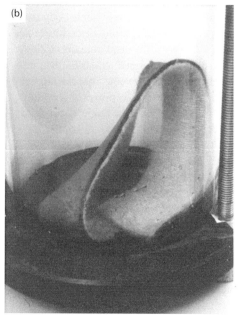

Figure 27.1 Compression of a wetsuit under pressure. A piece of 7-mm (1/4-inch) Neoprene, initially at 1 ATA **(a)** and then at 4 ATA (30 metres/100 feet) **(b)**. Note how much the Neoprene has compressed.

and vented during ascent to preserve the insulating layer and control buoyancy.

A wetsuit or drysuit provides adequate thermal comfort in relatively shallow water. The drysuit is the preferred option for colder, deeper and longer dives. A common problem with both suits is the loss of dexterity caused by cooling of the hands in cold water.

The insulating efficiency of these suits is demonstrated by a comparison of the likelihood of survival of subjects immersed in water at 5°C. Without protection, most would die within 3 hours. However, a thin man in a thick wetsuit would be expected to survive for up to 20 hours (see Figure 28.1 in Chapter 28).

Heat loss during immersion is much greater from some body surfaces than from others. Areas of high heat loss include skin over-active muscles and areas of the body with little subcutaneous fat. In cold water, a diver in a wetsuit will lose a substantial amount of heat from the head unless it is appropriately insulated. The effective insulation of hands presents a problem for long dives in cold water, which cause loss of dexterity. Despite the use of commonly available gloves, this can be a factor limiting performance unless active warming is provided.

DEEP DIVER

A diver at substantial depth is generally breathing an oxygen-helium mixture from a supply of dry gas. Because of the higher specific heat of the helium, extra heat is required to warm the gas. This can cool the diver to an extent that requires the use of external heat to warm the gas. Norwegian commercial diving guidelines recommend that, for dives deeper than 150 metres, the breathing gas must be warmed. Failure to warm the gas can cause dyspnoea (see later).

Various techniques of diver warming have been investigated and/or used. They include the use of electrical and chemical energy and even nuclear energy. Heat from the decomposition of concentrated hydrogen peroxide or from other hydrogen catalytic reactions has been tested. Drysuits with inner garments using aerogel materials have been shown to extend dive duration greatly. However, hot water supplied from a boiler on the surface remains the most common commercial diving system. This water is pumped down to the diver and circulates through the space between diver and wetsuit.

If the breathing gas is not heated, a deep diver can suffer from dyspnoea induced by the cold gas. This can manifest as substernal discomfort and chest tightness that may spread to cover the whole substernal area. The more important response for its effect on safety is the production of large amounts of thick mucus that can plug the airways and equipment. With high heat loss, shivering may be uncontrollable, and the diver may be unable to hold the mouthpiece. Rest and breathing warm gas cure the condition. Warming the inhaled gas prevents it.

Dehydration is a hazard of diving with a heated suit. One study showed that the level of dehydration could be as high as 4 to 5 per cent of the body weight of the diver. This is a level that can cause decreased mental and physical performance.

DIVING IN HOT ENVIRONMENTS

Hot water is a less common problem than cold, but cases of divers overheating have occurred. This may happen when diving in water that is artificially heated, as in a power station. It can also occur if a diver needs the protection of a drysuit when diving in warm water because of a risk of disease. Some divers, including police and maintenance or repair contractors, occasionally have to dive in sewerage processing plants and other places with a high risk of infection. These divers can be at risk of overheating caused by the thermal protection of the drysuit.

In some circumstances, a wetsuit with cooler water pumped down to it provides a satisfactory method of maintaining body temperature. If a drysuit is needed for protection, a cooling vest containing ice pouches can be used to help prevent the diver from overheating. It may also be feasible to circulate cold water through the vest to provide a longer period of tolerance.

There is also a risk of **hyperthermia** on the surface while waiting to dive, particularly if the diver is in the sun, or if the diver exerts himself or herself. In this situation, a bucket of cold water poured over the diver, or a quick immersion to cool off, is generally an adequate method of cooling the diver. Deaths from heat stroke have occasionally occurred during military training when divers, wearing an insulating suit, were required to exercise. This is an entirely preventable condition if the supervisors are aware of the problem.

DIVER IN A RECOMPRESSION CHAMBER

Problems with the heat balance of divers in recompression chambers (RCCs) have caused deaths from hyperthermia and difficulties from hypothermia.

In any RCC with a carbon dioxide absorbing system, overheating may be a problem in a warm climate, and a method of cooling and dehumidification is needed. If the carbon dioxide is removed by reaction with soda lime, water is produced, and this is added to the water produced by the diver as sweat, thereby humidifying the air in the RCC. The atmosphere becomes saturated with water vapour, and the diver can no longer rely on sweating as a method of cooling the body. This situation leads to an increase in body temperature. The problem is compounded because, as temperature rises above normal, the body produces more heat as the chemical reactions in the body accelerate.

Because helium is a good conductor of heat, a diver in a helium atmosphere heats or cools more rapidly than in an air-filled space. In an air-filled RCC, a person in light clothes is comfortable in a temperature range from about 20°C to 30°C. For a diver in an oxygen-helium atmosphere, the thermal comfort range is narrower and warmer than for a diver in air. The acceptable temperature increases with depth because there is more helium in the atmosphere as the pressure is increased. A diver is comfortable at about 29°C at shallow depths, and this increases to about 34°C as the pressure is increased. There is an associated narrowing of the temperature range in which a diver is comfortable, to less than 1°C.

With this narrowing of the comfort range, there is also an increase in the rate at which cooling and overheating occur if the temperature goes beyond the comfort zone. Therefore, it is necessary to monitor temperature control with a helium-rich atmosphere in the RCC closely. In any RCC, dehumidification is required if the RCC temperature is warm.

The problems of humidity and overheating are least with an RCC in which carbon dioxide is removed by flushing the chamber with compressed air. This also removes water vapour, and the diver can keep cool by sweating.

FURTHER READING

Crawshore LI, Wallace HL, Dasgupta S. Thermoregulation. In: Auerbach PS, editor. *Wilderness Medicine.* 5th ed. Philadelphia: Mosby Elsevier; 2007.

Flynn ET. Temperature effects. In: Lundgren CEG, Miller JN, editors. *The Lung at Depth.* New York: Marcel Dekker; 1999.

Larsson A, Gennder M, Ornhagen H. *Evaluation of a Heater for Surface Independent Divers.* FOA Report C50094-5. Stockholm: National Defense Research Establishment; 1992.

Mekjavic IB, Tipton MJ, Eiken O. Thermal considerations in diving. In: Brubakk AO, Neuman TS, editors. *Bennett and Elliot's Physiology and Medicine of Diving.* 5th ed. Philadelphia: Saunders; 2004:115-152.

Nuckols ML. Analytical modeling of a diver dry suit with enhanced micro-encapsulated phase change materials. *Ocean Engineering* 1999;**26**:547-564.

United States Navy. *Report TA 04-16, NEDU TR 05-02.* Panama City, Florida: Navy Experimental Diving Unit; 2005.

United States Navy. *Report TA 04-04, NEDU TR 05-08.* Panama City, Florida: Navy Experimental Diving Unit; 2005.

US Navy Diving Manual Revision 6 SS521-AG-PRO-010 (2008). Washington, DC: Naval Sea Systems Command; 2008.

This chapter was reviewed for this fifth edition by John Lippmann.

28

Cold and hypothermia

INTRODUCTION

Immersion in cold water may result in a variety of adverse events. In some cases, the exposure may be rapidly fatal as a result of cold shock. Victims who survive this period may not be able to rescue themselves because of a loss of motor power. Prolonged exposure raises the possibility of progressive hypothermia, which can be exacerbated during time spent above water in exposed environments.

If heat loss from the body is greater than heat production, then body temperature falls and hypothermia is likely. In all except the warmest seas, divers must wear some form of thermal protection to maintain a favourable balance between heat production and heat loss to the water. As discussed in Chapter 27, a wetsuit generally provides adequate insulation for short exposures in tropical and temperate water. In colder climates (and especially for long exposures), a drysuit, which provides more insulation, may be required. In prolonged exposures in extreme conditions, active heating of

the drysuit and possibly the breathing gas may be necessary.

Failure to maintain heat balance results in a fall in body temperature. If this is mild (1°C to 2°C), the diver feels cold and may shiver. This shivering, and a loss of dexterity, may affect delicate manual tasks. A continued loss of heat may cause the body temperature to fall to a level where the diver is incapable of self-care and is liable to drown. At still lower body temperatures, death occurs even if drowning is prevented.

Hypothermia is a common cause of death in marine disasters. None of the 1498 passengers who entered the water after the sinking of the *Titanic* survived. Although many could swim and had life jackets, few lived longer than 40 minutes. Almost all passengers in the life boats were saved. Figure 28.1 shows the relationship of expected survival time with water temperatures. Curves of this type should be used with caution. For example, most would predict that people could not swim the English Channel, but the swimmers do not take much notice.

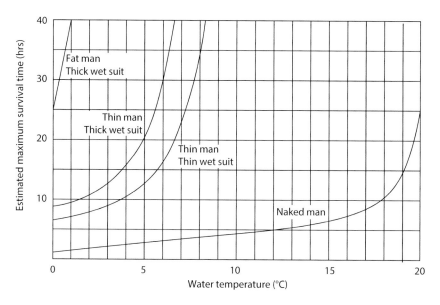

Figure 28.1 Survival expectancy related to water temperature.

The realization that hypothermia was one of the most common causes of death of sailors during the Second World War led to the development of covered inflatable life rafts and exposure suits that give better protection in cold water. Information on all aspects of hypothermia, including some not considered in this discussion, is available in several reviews. Keatinge's text is famous[1]. Other reviews should be consulted by readers likely to deal with hypothermia in a clinical setting[2–4].

In this chapter the emphasis is on the clinical features, prevention and treatment of hypothermia as encountered by the diving physician.

INITIAL REACTIONS TO IMMERSION IN COLD WATER

In many cases, good swimmers have died within a few metres of safety after short periods of cold immersion. Some workers postulated that these deaths were caused by inhaling water, whereas others suggested a cardiac aetiology. The Royal Navy studies in this area were reviewed by Tipton[5]. He provided a range of rational potential explanations for these fatalities based around a complex series of early physiological responses. Tipton divided them into several groups, which are summarized here.

Cardiovascular responses

There is an immediate increase in heart rate of about 20 beats/minute and an increase in cardiac output. There is a fall in peripheral perfusion as a consequence of vasoconstriction. Not surprisingly, these changes are accompanied by an increase in blood pressure.

These responses may explain some of the sudden deaths. Swimmers with coronary disease are at risk because of the simultaneous increase in cardiac work (tachycardia, increased preload and afterload secondary to peripheral vasoconstriction) and decrease in coronary perfusion (because of the tachycardia). The second group at risk comprises those with cerebrovascular disease. The sudden hypertension may trigger a cerebrovascular incident.

Respiratory responses

The initial gasp on entering cold water may be followed by uncontrollable hyperventilation. There may be a 10-fold increase in ventilation; three- to fourfold increases are common. This response can lead to water inhalation and drowning, which is more likely to occur in rough water or where there is a period when the head is immersed. The victim simply cannot hold his or her breath, so even a good swimmer may aspirate water.

A less obvious problem is that the hyperventilation causes hypocapnia. Tipton[5] cited a study in which the arterial carbon dioxide fell 12 mm Hg after an iced water shower for 1 minute. He suggested that this fall could cause enough reduction in cerebral blood flow to explain the disorientation and clouding of consciousness that has been noted.

Cold and hyperventilation can trigger bronchoconstriction in persons with asthma. In addition, in physiologically normal subjects there is a shift in end-expiratory volume so that the subject is breathing close to total lung capacity. This is an inefficient form of respiration because the lung volume is on an unfavourable part of its compliance curve, and this will rapidly induce fatigue.

Figure 28.2 presents a more complete version of possible cold shock responses.

Musculoskeletal responses

Another crucial response to immersion in cold water is a decrease in swimming performance. Tipton and colleagues[6] had subjects swim at a range of temperatures. Only half could complete a 90-minute swim in 10°C water. A decrease in stroke length and a reduction in distance travelled for a given energy expenditure were observed in the subjects who did not complete the cold water swim. People with more fat over the arms fared better, a finding suggesting that part of the decrease in performance may have been caused by local cooling rather than generalized hypothermia. In sudden immersion in even colder water, a rapid deterioration of physical performance (before the onset of significant hypothermia) has emerged as a crucial contributor to death by drowning because there is a very limited time beyond which the victim is physically unable to effect self-rescue.

Immersion in cold water usually causes

- Tachycardia.
- Hypertension.
- Hyperventilation.
- Rapidly decreasing muscle performance.

SIGNS AND SYMPTOMS OF HYPOTHERMIA

The degree of hypothermia that ensues after immersion depends on environmental and physiological factors.[2,3,7] Environmental factors include the water temperature and flow, the duration of exposure, the insulating materials (e.g. fabrics, fat, grease) and the gas mixture employed. Physiological factors include somatotype, activity during exposure, the degree of cold adaptation and the use of drugs that induce vasodilation or prevent heat-saving vasoconstriction.

With rare exceptions, the lethal lower limit for humans has been 23°C and 25°C (rectal). The effects of hypothermia are set out in the following paragraphs.

Mild hypothermia

The core temperature is in the range of 33°C to 35°C. The victim is handicapped by the cold but is breathing and fully conscious. The victim is probably shivering and experiencing local reactions including the sensation of coldness in the extremities. Numbness occurs as the peripheral sensory nerves are affected. Vasoconstriction, particularly in combination with immersion, leads to a centralization of blood volume and a diuresis that can cause dehydration.

Difficulty in performing co-ordinated fine movements, in response to motor nerve involvement, may result in a dangerous situation in which a diver cannot effectively manage a task or the equipment. This loss of control because of cold hands may also be a problem even in divers with normal body temperature. Indeed, maintenance of hand function despite adequate 'whole body' thermal protection is one of the most challenging aspects of prolonged dives in very cold water. In water near freezing, it is possible to encounter situations where, despite the use of dry gloves with insulating 'under-gloves', the diver is warm but the hands are useless.

A major danger with mild hypothermia is that lethargy and sluggish reactions may lead to an accident or drowning. Other local reactions, such as immersion foot and frostbite, are more applicable to general and military medicine than to diving medicine.

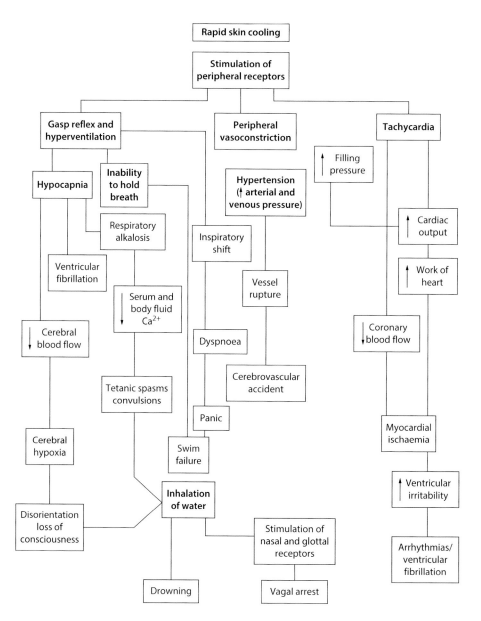

Figure 28.2 A more complete version of possible cold shock responses. ↑ increase, ↓ decrease. (Adapted from Tipton MJ. The initial responses to cold-water immersion in man. *Clinical Science* 1989;77:581–588.)

Moderate hypothermia

With a core temperature between 30°C and 33°C, a diver is slow to respond or unconscious. Shivering is a variable response; if present, it often ceases in this temperature range and is replaced by muscle rigidity. Heart rate and cardiac output fall.

The electrocardiogram (ECG) may show prolonged Q-T intervals, and a J wave may be present. Nodal rhythm, atrio-ventricular block, atrial fibrillation and ventricular fibrillation can develop. Respiratory frequency falls with the reduction in tissue oxygen needs. Many of the victims of maritime accident cases of hypothermia succumb at this stage because they are no longer able to contribute to their rescue, to keep swimming or even keep to their head above water.

Severe hypothermia

The victim has a core temperature below 30°C. He or she is unconscious or semi-conscious, and muscle rigidity can be confused with rigor mortis. Respiration and pulse may be depressed or not detectable; indeed, respiration may be reduced to one to two gasps per minute. There is a high risk of ventricular fibrillation. Any electrical activity on the ECG or electroencephalogram (EEG) is evidence of continued life. Bizarre ECGs should not be considered artefacts. In a field situation, the pupillary light reflexes may be helpful, but their absence is not evidence of death.

Recognition that severe hypothermia can 'imitate death' has given rise to 'The Alaskan dictum', which states: 'do not assume a patient is dead until he is warm and dead'. This may lead to unsuccessful attempts at revival, but this is preferable to unnecessary deaths. The chilled brain has a greatly increased tolerance to hypoperfusion, and remarkable recoveries have been recorded. For example, the paper by Gilbert and colleagues[8] provided dramatic anecdotal support for the Alaskan dictum. These workers reported the resuscitation of a victim with a core temperature of 13.7°C. A skier became trapped in an ice gully and was continuously flooded by freezing water. She struggled for about 40 minutes and was trapped for a further 40 minutes before she was extracted and basic first aid was started. This was replaced by cardiopulmonary resuscitation (CPR) and positive pressure ventilation with oxygen during a 1-hour flight to hospital. Given advanced hospital care, she has made a good recovery. Similarly, in her review, Larach[9] mentioned cases where survivors were neurologically intact after more than 4 hours of cardiac arrest associated with hypothermia.

Clinical phases of progressive hypothermia:

1. Mild – 35°C to 33°C
2. Moderate – 33°C to 30°C
3. Severe – less than 30°C

SYSTEM REVIEW

A review of systems is performed[3,7].

Cardiovascular system

The initial stimulatory response to immersion in cold water is discussed earlier. Later, as temperature falls, both chronotropy and inotropy are reduced, leading to a reduction in cardiac output and blood pressure. Ultimately, cardiac arrest may occur at about 20°C (rectal) or earlier. Various arrhythmias are common: atrial fibrillation occurs at about 30°C, and ventricular fibrillation usually occurs below 25°C. The blood becomes more viscous, and because hypothermia reduces the effective release of oxygen from haemoglobin, tissue hypoxia may develop.

In the past, it was emphasized that movement of the throat, limbs or chest during rescue or resuscitation could trigger ventricular fibrillation in a hypothermic heart. However, Larach[9] presented data showing this to be a rare complication.

Effects of hypothermia on inert gas exchange in divers are sometimes raised as an issue, but it is not clear that 'hypothermia' *per se* is required for water temperature to influence gas exchange. This is largely a semantic argument, however. There is convincing evidence that becoming 'cooler' during decompression is disadvantageous from a decompression sickness risk perspective when compared with remaining 'warm' during decompression (see Chapter 12). This is probably because being cooler results in reduced perfusion of peripheral tissues, with correspondingly impaired washout of inert gas. Temperature may also influence the solubility of inert gas in tissue, and a reduction in gas solubility in peripheral tissues during a hot post-dive shower has been invoked as an explanation for contemporaneous onset of decompression sickness symptoms in a small number of cases (see Chapter 12). It is not certain whether these symptoms were coincidental with the shower or whether the temperature effect was 'causative'.

Central nervous system

With a core temperature below 35°C, impairment of speech, fixation of ideas, sluggish reactions and mental impairment occur. Depersonalization, amnesia, confusion and delirium are possible. Unconsciousness may develop at about 30°C, and by 27°C most reflexes are lost. Exposure to cold initially causes reflex hyperventilation, but with increasing hypothermia the respiratory centre is depressed, and this contributes to hypoxia and acidosis.

As alluded to previously, hypothermia is neuroprotective and may be beneficial in cold water drowning (assuming it did not cause the drowning in the first place!). Indeed, an extensive experimental literature demonstrates hypothermia to be neuroprotective in most carefully conducted *in vitro* and *in vivo* experiments. Harnessing this protective effect for clinical benefit in humans has been more problematic, although there are conspicuous examples in which it is usually successful. One is the use of deep hypothermic circulatory arrest for certain thoracic vascular procedures where simple cardiopulmonary bypass with or without selective cerebral perfusion is not possible. The mechanism of this protection is not certain. Although it is widely assumed that it accrues from a reduction in the cerebral metabolic rate for oxygen, hypothermia confers extra protection in experiments where cerebral electrical activity is already ablated by pharmacological means. Other mechanisms have been proposed to explain such observations. For example, it is thought that hypothermia may independently suppress the release of harmful excitotoxins by hypoxic neurons.

Gastrointestinal system

Some slowing of intestinal activity and retardation of the rate of destruction of bacteria occur. Paralytic ileus may develop in cases of severe hypothermia.

Renal system

Cold and immersion initially cause an increase in central blood volume and a diuresis. Hyponatraemia and hypovolaemia may follow. As the temperature falls further, cardiac output and hence glomerular filtration are reduced, resulting in decreased urinary output.

Liver

There is a decrease in liver function that is probably a direct temperature effect on enzyme activity. As a consequence, metabolites such as lactate may accumulate. Drugs accumulate because their clearance is slowed or stopped.

Locomotor system

Shivering is a heat-producing response to cold. It mainly affects the large proximal muscles, but it also causes a loss of co-ordination and difficulty in the performance of fine tasks. There is a loss of muscle power. Swimming ability is decreased, with increasing discomfort and fatigue. Apathy and euphoria may combine with fatigue to stop the diver from taking appropriate action for rescue. As previously mentioned, the cooling of peripheral muscles in very cold water can impair the ability to self-rescue before the onset of significant core hypothermia, which may lead to drowning.

Cutaneous reactions

Any prolonged immersion results in softening and swelling of the skin, rendering it susceptible to injury and infection. This 'washerwoman's skin' is characterized by soft ridges, especially over the tips of fingers and toes.

In cold water, there may be a sudden release of histamine in susceptible persons that causes cold or allergic urticaria. In some cases the skin rapidly becomes hot, red and oedematous. Symptoms may occur during or after exposure. Occasional deaths have been reported (see Chapter 42).

PREVENTION OF HYPOTHERMIA

The most important and effective means of preventing hypothermia during diving is wearing exposure protection that is appropriate to the expected water temperature and duration of the dive. Broadly speaking, exposure protection can be divided into three categories: stinger suits, wetsuits and drysuits.

Stinger suits are usually made of Lycra or a similar material and are intended mainly to prevent skin contact with marine stingers. Although some of the heavier materials have some insulating properties, stinger suits provide minimal thermal protection, and their use is best restricted to warmer tropical waters.

Wetsuits come in a variety of styles and thicknesses. They work on the principle that water enters the suit but then is trapped and warmed, and heat loss to the environment is subsequently prevented by the insulating properties of the Neoprene foam of which the suits are made. This action relies substantially on a snug fit, which prevents circulation of water through the suit. The insulating properties of the suit are determined by fit, thickness and degree of body coverage; and various designs are made to be suited to conditions. Thin suits (e.g. 3-mm Neoprene) with short legs and arms are designed for tropical use. Thick suits (e.g. 7-mm thick, often with overlapping layers) that cover the entire body, including head, feet and hands, can be used in cold temperate water, especially for short-duration dives.

Long-duration dives in temperate waters usually require a drysuit. These also come in various styles. Some of these suits effectively provide a waterproof 'shell' with little inherent heat insulation capability, whereas others are constructed of material that provides some insulation. Nevertheless, in both cases, it is the 'undergarments' chosen that largely determine the insulating properties of the combination. Heavier insulating undergarments that trap more still air between the diver and the drysuit shell are generally warmer. Some divers use argon to inflate their drysuits (gas must be added during descent) because of its low thermal capacity. However, several studies of this strategy have failed to show a clear advantage over air.

In non-diving immersions (e.g. after maritime accidents), hypothermia can be delayed or prevented by use of a variety of strategies:

- Wear a wetsuit or a survival suit to reduce heat loss.
- If wearing a life jacket, try to adopt a spheroidal position (foetal position), with the head out of the water and the legs pulled up to the chest and the arms wrapped around the legs. This has been referred to as the Heat Escape Lessing Posture (HELP). It may increase the survival time by 50 per cent. 'Drown-proofing', where the victim rests with head under water

between breaths, is not advocated because of the increased heat loss from the head.

- Do not swim unless very close to safety; groups of survivors should remain huddled tightly together to conserve heat (and to give the rescuers a larger target to find). For completeness, it should be mentioned that the literature is not unanimous on this point, and the question of whether or not exercise causes an improvement in the balance between heat production and heat loss is highly nuanced. It is probably true to say that for an exposure where the eventual duration is uncertain (but potentially long), the safest option is to avoid exercise.
- Wear clothing to reduce heat loss. In particular, a hood or some other head protection is important in conserving heat.
- Avoid or delay immersion if any other options are feasible.

TREATMENT OF HYPOTHERMIA

It is desirable to obtain a measurement of the victim's temperature if this is possible. A rectal temperature should be obtained, and a low-reading thermometer may be required. This is the best measurement of those commonly used. Where it is not possible to obtain a rectal temperature, the tympanic membrane temperature is a useful measure that can be obtained with minimal disturbance to the patient or protective insulation, but it requires a special digital thermometer. Others choose oesophageal temperature as their preferred measure of deep body temperature[2], but this is unlikely to be available in the field.

In mild cases of hypothermia, removal from the cold environment, protection from wind, the use of blankets and the use of hot water bottles in a sleeping bag are all remedies that have worked and may be all that is required.

Shivering slowly restores body heat if further heat loss is prevented. Heat loss from the head should be minimized, as should evaporative heat loss from wet clothing. In an exposed situation, two large plastic bags, one over the victim's body and one over an insulating layer such as a sleeping bag, have been recommended. This prevents evaporative cooling as well as avoiding the need to strip the wet clothes from the survivor. In an unexposed environment, wet clothes should be replaced with dry clothes or an alternative (e.g. a blanket or sleeping bag), and the victim should be protected from air movement as much as possible. When removing the clothes in patients with moderate to severe cases of hypothermia, the garments should be cut to avoid excessive movement of these patients.

The specific treatment of serious hypothermia includes measures discussed in the following sub-sections.

First aid

It is important to keep the patient horizontal during and following removal from the water, especially after prolonged immersions. A rescue basket, a stretcher or a double-strop system, with one loop lifting the patient under the arms and another under the knees, can be used. This prevents a sudden fall in blood pressure that can occur with the loss of hydrostatic pressure on the legs[10]. There have been cases where the patient was alive and responsive in the water but apparently dead by the time he or she reached a rescue helicopter after being lifted in a vertical position. This shock reaction is thought to be caused by blood pooling in the legs.

> The pulse may be difficult to detect in a hypothermia casualty, and blood pressure may be unrecordable despite the presence of tissue perfusion.

If drowning has occurred, then CPR takes precedence over the management of hypothermia, although any practicable steps should be taken to try to prevent further heat loss. Remember that signs of life can be very difficult to detect in a hypothermic victim. A normal life support algorithm and resuscitation algorithm should be followed, but with some modification. Concern is sometimes expressed over the potential for airway manipulation to precipitate ventricular fibrillation in a cold patient, but maintaining an airway and ensuring ventilation take precedence over such concerns[11].

Correction of ventricular fibrillation by electrical defibrillation may not be effective when the core temperature is below 30°C (or even until higher temperatures), but expert consensus holds that defibrillation should be tried up to three times no matter what the temperature, after which (if unsuccessful) CPR should be maintained while rewarming continues[11]. When 30°C is reached, further attempts at defibrillation should be made.

Although there are few relevant human data, it is usually recommended that resuscitation drugs are not administered until the victim is warmer than 30°C. This is because these drugs are not thought to be particularly effective in a very cold patient, and the drugs may accumulate with repeat dosing (from delayed distribution and metabolism), resulting in a toxic picture once the patient is rewarmed[11].

Hospital care

The victim with severe hypothermia needs hospital care during and after rewarming. Most patients should be kept immobile, handled gently and given supplemental oxygen. Intravenous fluids should be warmed to at least body temperature. Although one animal study suggested that centrally administered intravenous fluid can be as hot as 65°C[12], expert consensus suggests that 42°C is a sensible maximum[11]. Intravenous fluid infusion is not an effective means of rewarming (the required volumes would be too high), but the goal of warmed fluids is to avoid further cooling with cold fluid. A balanced electrolyte solution (not normal saline), with supplemental glucose if the patient is hypoglycaemic, is suggested. Administration of 500 ml at once then 100 ml/hour is a simple guide to overcome haemoconcentration and possible shock as the peripheral vessels expand, but experienced clinicians will tailor fluid administration to the needs of individual patients.

Methods of rewarming

Rewarming should begin as soon as possible. A review of therapy stressed the shortage of trials comparing methods of rewarming patients with moderate or severe hypothermia[13]. The choice of rewarming method often depends on the skills and equipment available rather than on best evidence. Some of the options are outlined here.

Most victims of mild hypothermia will recover if they are allowed to rewarm passively with good thermal protection including blankets and caps. To speed the process, they can lie under a forced air warmer and be disturbed as little as possible. This seems to be the best rewarming treatment in a small hospital. It is non-invasive, safe, easy to use and readily available[14]. There has been previous advocacy for the use of graded temperature baths[15]. An initial water temperature of 36°C, to reduce the pain response and risk of atrial fibrillation, and then an increase over 5 to 10 minutes to 40°C to 42°C, until the rectal temperature is above 33°C, has been recommended, but this approach has been omitted from more recent definitive reviews[11]. It is logistically difficult, and it is probably unnecessary with the present wide availability of forced air warmers in hospitals.

A forced air warmer is also a valid option for active rewarming in patients with more serious cases who are spontaneously breathing and have a perfusing rhythm. For patients requiring resuscitation (circulatory and/or ventilator support), the gold standard for active rewarming is cardiopulmonary bypass or extracorporeal membrane oxygenation. These have the advantage of supporting circulation and ensuring adequate oxygenation in addition to rewarming. However, they are extremely invasive procedures that require large teams of expert staff, and they are available only at some large centres. Other relevant techniques include warming and humidification of inspired gases and peritoneal and gastric lavage with warmed fluid.

PROLONGED IMMERSION

The problems of a diver who has been immersed for a long period have not been investigated in a systematic manner. It is known from rescues of divers with adequate insulation that survival for at least 24 hours can be expected. About one third of the crew of the USS *Indianapolis* survived for about 4 days in life jackets after being sunk near the Philippines. The main problems for the survivors were dehydration and mental issues. It is not clear whether these mental problems stemmed from lack of sleep, anxiety related to the delayed rescue or severe dehydration[16].

Beckman and Reeves[17] stressed that, in such patients, hypoglycemia, dehydration, haemoconcentration and adrenocortical stress response are factors to be considered along with hypothermia. This would suggest that fluids with glucose may be needed, as well as heating, but how the warming should be administered in these patients is open to question. Probably the best advice is to be prepared for complications.

REFERENCES

1. Keatinge WR. *Survival in Cold Water*. Edinburgh: Blackwell Scientific Publications; 1977.
2. Giesbrecht GG. Cold stress, near drowning and accidental hypothermia: a review. *Aviation, Space, and Environmental Medicine* 2000;**71**:733–753.
3. Short BH. Cold induced thermoregulatory failure. 1. Physiology and clinical features. *Australian Military Medicine* 2000;**9**:29–33.
4. Short BH. Cold induced thermoregulatory failure. 1. Management and outcomes. *Australian Military Medicine* 2000;**9**:88–90.
5. Tipton MJ. The initial responses to cold-water immersion in man. *Clinical Science* 1989;**77**:581–588.
6. Tipton M, Eglin C, Gennser M, Golden F. Immersion deaths and deterioration in swimming performance in cold water. *The Lancet* 1999;**354**:626–629.
7. Serba JA. Thermal problems: prevention and treatment. In Bennett P, Elliott D, editors. *The Physiology and Medicine of Diving*. 4th ed. London: Saunders; 1993.
8. Gilbert M, Busund R, Nilson PA, Solbø JP. Resuscitation from accidental hypothermia of 13.7°C with circulatory arrest. *The Lancet* 2000;**355**:375–376.
9. Larach MG. Accidental hypothermia. *The Lancet* 1995;**345**:493–498.
10. Golden FS, Hervey GR, Tipton MJ. Circum-rescue collapse. *Journal of the Royal Naval Medical Service* 1991;**77**:139–149.

11. Soar J, Perkins GC, Abbas G, *et al.*
    European Resuscitation Council guidelines
    for resuscitation 2010 section 8. Cardiac
    arrest in special circumstances: electrolyte
    abnormalities, poisoning, drowning, acci-
    dental hypothermia, hyperthermia, asthma,
    anaphylaxis, cardiac surgery, trauma,
    pregnancy, electrocution. *Resuscitation*
    2010;**81**:1400–1433.
12. Sheaff CM, Fildes JJ, Keogh P, Smith RF,
    Barrett JA. Safety of 65°C intravenous
    fluid for the treatment of hypother-
    mia. *American Journal of Surgery*
    1996;**172**:52–55.
13. Rogers I. Which rewarming therapy
    in hypothermia? A review of the ran-
    domised trials. *Emergency Medicine*
    1997;**9**:213–220.
14. Koller R, Schnider TW, Niedhart P. Deep
    accidental hypothermia and cardiac
    arrest- rewarming with forced air.
    Acta Anaesthesiologica Scandinavica
    1997;**41**:1359–1364.
15. Hoskin RW, Melinyshyn MJ, Romert TT,
    Goode RC. Bath rewarming from immersion
    hypothermia. *Journal of Applied Physiology*
    1986;**61**:1518–1522.
16. Herman JK. Survivor of the Indianapolis.
    US Navy Medicine 1995;**86**:13–17.
17. Beckman EL, Reeves E. Physiological impli-
    cations as to survival during immersion in
    water at 75°F. *Aerospace Medicine*
    1966;**37**:1136–1142.

*This chapter was reviewed for this fifth edition by
Simon Mitchell.*

29

Infections

LOCAL INFECTIONS

Introduction

A variety of pathogenic organisms may be encountered through contact with water. These include bacteria, viruses, protozoa and parasites. Infection associated with swimming or diving may be acquired in a number of ways. Waterborne pathogens may enter the body through intact or damaged skin or through mucous membranes. Common portals of entry include eyes, ears, nose, throat, lungs and gastrointestinal or genitourinary tracts. The infection may remain localized to the site of entry or progress to severe, systemic disease.

The microscopic flora of water is determined by such factors as its proximity to human habitation, the content of organic matter, pH, temperature, light, salinity, oxygenation and rainfall. Some microorganisms are found naturally in water, others are periodically washed into water from soil and others favour the artificially created environments of swimming spas, baths and aquaria.

The exact mode of penetration of the organism into a body site depends on the interplay of several factors involving water, pathogen and host. For example, divers may lose the bacteriostatic benefits of cerumen, normal flora and acidic pH in the external ear with repeated immersion, thus predisposing to external ear infections. Factors affecting host defences to permit infection by aquatic microorganisms include trauma, aspiration and immunosuppression.

Marine bacteria were, until relatively recently, thought to cause few infections in humans. Since the 1970s, however, these organisms have been isolated from a variety of human infections. Such pathogens may obtain entry by trauma from coral, rock or marine animal spines, teeth or shell or from ingestion or aspiration of water.

The morbidity resulting from diving with certain pre-existing infections is perhaps more important and certainly more common than infections directly caused by swimming or diving. These infections are mainly those affecting the respiratory system and may cause or complicate barotrauma.

Upper respiratory infections render the sufferer liable to barotrauma of sinuses and/or middle ear as a result of blockage of equalizing air passages (see Chapters 7 and 8). Lower respiratory infections, in which there may be bronchospasm, mucus plugs and obstruction of smaller airways, may predispose to gas trapping and pulmonary barotrauma (see Chapter 6).

It has been suggested that the spread of respiratory infections is enhanced by diving, and this does appear to be clinically so in some cases. Sharing of regulators, or of drinking vessels on dive boats, may be a cause of cross-infection. Special problems of infection control arise in the closed environments of dive boats, saturation chambers, undersea habitats, submarines and hyperbaric facilities.

Aetiology

Infections associated with the marine environment and aquatic activities are common. The reasons are the increasing use of water for recreational activities and, unfortunately, increased sewage pollution of oceans and inland waterways.

Infecting organisms are usually bacteria, but protozoa, viruses, fungi and helminths may also be involved. Sea water contains many bacteria known to be potentially pathogenic for humans (Table 29.1).

The outcome of exposure to water-borne organisms depends on a number of factors. Factors relating to the organisms themselves include the causal organism, inoculum size and virulence. Host factors include the site of inoculation, gastric acidity (for gastrointestinal infection) and host immunity. Interaction between the organism and host factors determines the outcome of exposure, i.e. whether infection occurs and, if it does, whether mild or severe disease results.

Many water-borne organisms that were previously considered non-pathogenic or of doubtful pathogenicity have been implicated as definite pathogens, with some causing severe, even fatal, disease. Certain species may be associated with disease more often. For example, *Aeromonas sobria* and *Aeromonas hydrophilia* cause most clinically significant *Aeromonas* infections. Severe invasive disease caused by non-cholera *Vibrio* species is most commonly associated with *Vibrio vulnificus*[1]. This organism can cause overwhelming septicaemia with rapid progression to death within 48 hours. Production of virulence factors by bacteria (e.g. cytolysins, proteolytic enzymes) may be seen with some organisms and correlates with invasiveness and pathogenicity.

Table 29.1 Some potentially pathogenic bacteria found in water environments

Acinetobacter lwoffi	Mycobacterium marinum
Actinomyces species	Mycoplasma phocacerebrale[a]
Aeromonas hydrophilia	Plesiomonas shigelloides
Aeromonas sobria	Proteus mirabilis
Alcaligenes faecalis	Pseudomonas aeruginosa
Bacillus subtilis	Pseudomonas species
Clostridium botulinum	Salmonella enteritidis
Edwardsiella tarda	Serratia species
Enterobacter species	Staphylococcus aureus
Enterococcus species	Staphylococcus epidermidis
Enterococcus faecalis	Vibrio alginolyticus[a]
Erysipelothrix species[a]	Vibrio cholera
Escherichia coli	Vibrio parahaemolyticus[a]
Flavobacterium species	Vibrio vulnificus[a]
Klebsiella pneumoniae	

[a] More likely to be involved in marine acquired infection.

Host factors may potentiate the development of infection. Severe or even fatal infections caused by *V. vulnificus* predominantly occur in immunosuppressed persons, e.g. those with chronic renal disease or liver disease (particularly alcoholic liver disease) or those receiving immunosuppressive therapy. A strong relationship is seen with haemochromatosis, and fulminant infection also predominantly occurs in male patients; female hormones are thought to be protective against the *Vibrio* endotoxin[1]. Severe infections in otherwise healthy individuals are not common, but they do occur frequently enough to cause concern.

In the external ear and elsewhere in the body, environmental factors such as prolonged immersion resulting in skin maceration or high humidity aid bacterial proliferation and penetration even through intact skin. Bacteria have been shown to survive longer in moist skin and may then gain entry following relatively minimal integumentary damage. The softened, macerated skin of immersion is, of course, more prone to damage from minor trauma.

Sites of infection

As with most infective diseases, aquatically derived infections are generally categorized according to the apparent site of entry of the organism.

WOUND INFECTIONS

Integumentary trauma is a common association of aquatic activities, be they recreational or occupational. Skin abrasions or cuts caused by contact with coral, rocks, jagged metal on wrecks and fish spines or teeth are common. Organisms subsequently isolated may be found in sea water or are normal human skin flora. They include *Staphylococcus aureus*, pyogenic streptococci, *Vibrio* organisms, *Enterobacter*, *Pseudomonas*, and *Bacillus*. Although potential pathogens may be present either in the water or in the skin, many marine infections arise because the pathogen is part of the normal flora of the agent producing the trauma, such as coral (see later), fish spines or seashells. In this context, various species

of halophilic or marine *Vibrio* organisms are frequently involved.

A vivid illustration of the potential for introduction of infection is a study of the teeth of a great white shark, which were found to harbour potentially pathogenic species of *Vibrio*, *Staphylococcus* and *Citrobacter*. Swabs of shark bite injuries have grown *Vibrio parahaemolyticus*, *Aeromonas caviae*, *Vibrio alginolyticus*, *Vibrio carcharia* and *A. hydrophila*, among others. *A. hydrophila* and *A. sobria* wound infections have followed diving in polluted waters. *Aeromonas* species can cause severe progressive wound infections with cellulitis leading to osteomyelitis.

Marine-acquired wound infections range from mild local inflammation, cellulitis, lymphadenitis and abscess formation to severe spreading infection with systemic effects and even septicaemia. The more severe infections are often associated with *V. vulnificus* or *Aeromonas*.

Treatment

Wounds should be thoroughly cleaned and débrided of devitalized tissue and foreign material. This may require local or general anaesthesia.

Significant local manifestations such as cellulitis and lymphangitis indicate the need for a broad-spectrum systemic antibiotic (e.g. doxycycline, co-trimoxazole) after a swab is taken for culture and sensitivity. In such cases, bed rest, elevation of the affected limb and other general supportive measures are also required. The potential for infection in relatively minor wounds to progress to catastrophic sepsis relatively quickly should always be borne in mind by those caring for patients wounded in aquatic environments. Signs of systemic infection should prompt early institution of intravenous antibiotic therapy and referral for definitive care.

Wounds sustained in or out of the water, including ulcerations resulting from poorly fitting fins, are notoriously slow to heal in divers who spend considerable time in the water. Secondary infection is common and is aided by softening and maceration of the skin from immersion, as well as by swimming in contaminated water. A prolonged period of time out of the water with frequent dressings with antiseptic powder or ointments may be required to achieve healing. Prompt drying after immersion and taping or other protection of vulnerable chafing areas may be of prophylactic value.

CORAL CUTS

This specific wound infection deserves separate mention because it is so common and potentially troublesome. Corals frequently cause lacerations and abrasions to inexperienced divers. These injuries may initially appear minor, but because of foreign material such as pieces of coral, nematocysts and infected coral secretions, they often become inflamed and infected.

Clinical features

The laceration, usually on the hand or foot, causes little trouble at the time of the injury. Some hours later there may be a 'smarting' sensation and a mild inflammatory reaction around the cut. This may result from the presence of discharging nematocysts. In the ensuing 1 to 2 days, local swelling, erythema and tenderness develop around the site. Usually this abates in 3 to 7 days.

Occasionally, an abscess or ulcer forms and discharges pus. This can become chronic, and osteomyelitis of the underlying bone has been reported. Cellulitis may also occur. Fever, chills, arthralgia, malaise and prostration occur in some cases, suggesting a severe bacterial infection. Healing may take months to years if complications ensue.

First aid

The wound should be thoroughly cleaned using a soft brush and a mild antiseptic solution. All foreign material should be removed. These measures incur some discomfort to the patient and may necessitate the prior use of topical or injected local anaesthetic.

Treatment

After cleaning, the wound should be dressed with a soft absorbent dressing. Antibiotic ointment several times daily (e.g. mupirocin [Bactroban]) is effective if applied early. Systemic antibiotics are indicated if there are signs of local or systemic spread of infection. Tetanus prophylaxis is advisable.

Prevention

Coral cuts can be avoided by the use of protective clothing, gloves and swim fins with heel covers and prompt treatment of minor abrasions. Good training in buoyancy control for divers also prevents damage to the coral.

OTITIS EXTERNA

Although otitis externa occurs without indulging in aquatic activities, swimming increases the risk about three to five times. In divers, external ear infection is one of the most common and troublesome disorders encountered, particularly in tropical environments.

Aetiology

Hot, humid conditions such as in tropical climates or recompression chambers provide ideal conditions for relevant organisms. Retention of fluid within the external auditory canal following immersion, particularly in contaminated water, adds to the risk. Exostoses, which are common in swimmers and divers, predispose to retention of cerumen, epithelial debris and water. Local trauma, such as attempts to remove cerumen by cotton swabs or syringing, are often associated with subsequent infection. Swimmers with dermatological conditions, such as seborrhoea, neurodermatitis and eczema, have an increased incidence.

The bacterial flora is usually mixed, with *Pseudomonas aeruginosa*, *S. aureus* and *Proteus* species predominating. Less commonly, diphtheroids, *Escherichia coli*, *Streptococcus faecalis*, *Aspergillus niger* and *Candida albicans* are involved.

> *Pseudomonas aeruginosa* is the most common organism found in otitis externa in divers.

Prolonged exposure to water (especially warm water) changes the healthy ear flora from gram-positive cocci and diphtheroids to gram-negative bacilli, and this change often precedes the acute symptoms of otitis externa. In divers, *P. aeruginosa* is probably the most frequently associated organism in otitis externa. The external ear canal provides an environment particularly conducive the growth of this organism. The organism can also be found in fresh water lakes, some of which are associated with a high risk of infection to swimmers.

Pseudomonas, Escherichia species and fungi are the most common pathogenic organisms in saturation diving environments, where there is commonly a high ambient temperature and relative humidity. Other marine bacteria causing otitis externa include *Achromobacter xylosoxidans, E. coli and Enterobacter, Klebsiella, Proteus* and *Vibrio* species.

Clinical features

The infection may be either circumscribed (furuncle) or diffuse. Symptoms include itching or pain in the ear made worse by jaw movements and traction on the tragus. Examination reveals localized tenderness, moist debris in an oedematous and erythematous external canal and possible conductive hearing loss. The eardrum may not be visualized. Regional lymphadenopathy and, rarely, a purulent discharge may be present. Divers may complain of vertigo resulting from obstruction of one ear canal and the consequent unequal ingress of cool water on one side compared with the other. This effectively elicits a transient 'caloric' response.

Treatment

Management consists of analgesia with topical and/or oral analgesics and gentle cleaning of the canal. This should be followed by antibiotic steroid ointments, which should completely fill the ear canal or be impregnated in a wick, or regularly applied antibiotic drops. Ciprofloxacin-hydrocortisone ear drops may be useful for *Pseudomonas* otitis externa. Antifungal agents are often included in these preparations. Systemic antibiotics may be required. Patients with severe or unresponsive cases should have culture and sensitivity tests to aid antibiotic therapy. Diving should cease until the condition has cleared.

Prevention

The ears should be rinsed with fresh water to remove salt water or contaminants. Salt crystallizes on drying in the ear canal and, being hygroscopic, retains moisture. Alcohol-based drops routinely instilled in the canal following every dive to ensure adequate drying are strongly recommended in high-risk settings (e.g. multiple dives over multiple days in a tropical environment). Acetic acid–based preparations are also useful for this purpose and have been shown to reduce the incidence of otitis externa during saturation dives, an incidence that otherwise approaches 95 per cent. Glacial acetic acid 5 per cent in propylene glycol is very effective, as is 5 per cent acetic acid in 85 per cent isopropyl alcohol (Aqua Ear).

Otitis externa can be a major problem in saturation diving and on long-duration diving expeditions, but active prophylaxis can significantly reduce the incidence. Diligent adherence to a prophylactic regimen of drying and appropriate drops applied after every dive is the key to avoiding this problem.

OTITIS MEDIA

This infection is not nearly as common as otitis externa, but it may occasionally complicate middle ear barotrauma (see Chapter 7), especially when the barotrauma follows an acute upper respiratory infection (Case Report 29.1). The most commonly involved organisms are haemolytic streptococci, pneumococci or staphylococci. A severe case of suppurative otitis media in a diver that was caused by *V. alginolyticus* has been reported. This patient had a long history of upper respiratory infections and otitis media since childhood but continued to dive in warm sea water. These or other mixed flora gain entry to the middle ear via the Eustachian tube or less commonly through a perforation of the tympanic membranes as a result of the middle ear barotrauma. The presence of water, fluid or blood provides a culture medium. Clinical features and management are similar to those of other causes of otitis media, except that the condition is typically noted 4 to 24 hours after diving. Otitis media is usually treated with systemic antibiotics.

SINUSITIS

Acute sinusitis is also a recognized infection in divers. The aetiology, clinical course and bacteriological findings are similar to those of otitis media. It sometimes follows sinus barotrauma (see Chapter 8).

Chronic sinusitis is a possible long-term occupational disease of divers. The potential contribution of dental disease to maxillary sinusitis should not be overlooked. Orbital cellulitis, with the

---

CASE REPORT 29.1

AM had been diving intermittently for some years. He had mild symptoms of a 'cold' but was able to equalize his ears satisfactorily and so went ahead with the planned dive. He was unable to descend beyond 5 metres because of pain in both ears and inability to autoinflate. After surfacing, the pain subsided, but otoscopic examination revealed grade 3 aural barotrauma in the right ear and grade 2 in the left. A few hours after the dive, he developed increasingly severe pain in the right ear, which was accompanied by tinnitus and later pyrexia. On examination, his temperature was 38.2°C, and the tympanic membrane appeared lustreless and erythematous with an outward bulge. Audiometry revealed mild conductive hearing loss in the right ear. The administration of antibiotics and decongestants resulted in symptomatic improvement in 24 hours. Seven days later, the appearance of both tympanic membranes was normal, as was the audiogram.

Diagnosis: otitis media complicating middle ear barotrauma.

---

infection extending from the sinus, has also been observed. This is a medical emergency requiring intensive antibiotic therapy.

EYE

Keratitis caused by *P. aeruginosa* has been reported following exposures similar to those resulting in pseudomonas folliculitis (see later). *P. aeruginosa* has also been associated with corneal ulcer and endophthalmitis.

V. alginolyticus has also been reported to cause conjunctivitis[1], as has *Chlamydia* following swimming in certain lakes.

Keratitis caused by *Acanthamoeba* has been associated with exposure of the eye to contaminated water (e.g. hot tubs), especially in wearers of contact lenses. This organism is ubiquitous in aquatic environments, and more cases may be expected. Treatment is with oral ketoconazole and topical miconazole or neomycin or propamidine isethionate. Surgery such as keratoplasty or even enucleation may be required in complicated cases.

GASTROENTERITIS

Gastrointestinal infection may result from ingestion of water containing pathogenic organisms while swimming. It is also a common complication of drinking untreated water during travel to remote locations on diving trips.

For such infections, the size of inoculum is important. For example, an inoculum of less than 100 bacteria is unlikely to cause significant infection or disease in normal hosts. An exception to this is infections with *Shigella* species, which may occur with ingestion of as few as 10 to 100 organisms. Gastric acidity is an important host defence. In people taking antacids or with achlorhydria, the infective dose of organisms is considerably lower.

The most severe form, with profuse watery diarrhoea and dehydration and prostration, is caused by *Vibrio cholerae*. Non-cholera *Vibrio* species, found in sea water, can also cause gastroenteritis with nausea, vomiting, diarrhoea, fever and abdominal pain.

Other bacteria also found in water, and associated with gastroenteritis, include *Bacillus cereus, E. coli, Salmonella* species and *Campylobacter jejuni*.

Severe infections have occurred following consumption of shellfish, oysters and fish contaminated with marine organisms, especially *V.vulnificus* (see later).

Swimmers in fresh water are also at risk of protozoan parasites such as *Giardia lamblia, Naegleria fowleri* and *Cryptosporidium parvum*.

GENITOURINARY INFECTIONS

The increase in diving in cold environments and in prolonged technical dives has almost certainly resulted in the increased use of drysuits. These are inconvenient if the user needs to urinate during the dive unless the diver is fitted with a so-called 'pee valve', in which case the male user wears a 'uritip'-type condom connected to a drain tube and valve that can be opened to the water. There are also adaptors that allow female divers to use a pee valve. This allows urination during diving.

There have been several case reports of divers developing urinary tract infections and early signs of urosepsis resulting from *Pseudomonas* infections that probably arose from growth of the organism in inadequately washed drain tubes and consequent introduction of the organism to the urethra[2]. Divers using these devices need to pay careful attention to cleaning them with an antiseptic after use and to flushing them again with antiseptic solution immediately before use.

Specific pathogens

VIBRIO

The genus *Vibrio* (gram-negative bacillus) are so-called 'halophilic' organisms that tend to live in marine or brackish water but have also been reported from inland waterways[1]. *Vibrio* species are well known human pathogens, with the most famous (*V. cholerae*) being the causative agent for cholera. Several other species of *Vibrio* cause infection in humans. All are indigenous to marine environments and are natural flora of shellfish (Table 29.2). They thrive in warmer temperatures.

V. vulnificus is the most virulent and is capable of causing severe rapidly progressive wound infections, gastroenteritis and severe systemic illness in swimmers and divers.

Other vibrio organisms, such as *V. alginolyticus,* have also been seen in marine wound infections (Case Report 29.2), but they do not seem to be as invasive as *V. vulnificus.* Nevertheless, a case of epidural abscess caused by this organism has been reported, manifesting 3 months after an open head injury incurred diving in sea water. *Vibrio damsela* wound infection has followed injury from a stingray barb.

Clinical presentations

These include wound infection, gastroenteritis, cellulitis, fasciitis, septic thrombophlebitis, vasculitis, conjunctivitis, otitis externa, otitis media and septicaemia.

A case of endometritis following sexual intercourse while swimming in sea water known to harbour *V. vulnificus* has been reported (Case Report 29.3), again indicating the virulent nature of this organism.

Diagnosis

There must be a high index of suspicion in the presence of signs of sepsis early after wounding in the marine environment. Microscopy and culture of wounds and blood should be undertaken, using appropriate media for marine organisms.

Treatment

In severe infections, surgical débridement and broad-spectrum antibiotic administration before confirmation of the organism may be necessary. Tetracyclines in combination with gentamicin or one of the third-generation cephalosporins such as ceftriaxone, or a fluoroquinolone such as ciprofloxacin, may be appropriate. It is generally recommended that empirical therapy be commenced in suspected systemic infections while awaiting the results of antibiotic sensitivity testing. Early and aggressive treatment reduces the risk of progression to life-threatening complications.

ERYSIPELOTHRIX

Infections (erysipeloid) with the gram-positive bacillus *Erysipelothrix rhusiopathiae* or *Erysipelothrix insidiosa* are found worldwide. Abrasions resulting from contact with fish, shellfish, meat or poultry may lead to the infection, which is usually limited to the skin. In the marine context, this organism

Table 29.2 Pathogenic marine Vibrio organisms causing wound and other infections

Vibrio vulnificus	Wound infection, cellulitis, septicaemia, pneumonia, meningitis, endometritis, peritonitis, gastroenteritis
Vibrio parahaemolyticus	Otitis, conjunctivitis, osteomyelitis, gastroenteritis
Vibrio alginolyticus	Cellulitis, Epidural Abscess, Otitis, Pneumonia
Vibrio damsela	Septicaemia, otitis
(Non-01) *Vibrio cholerae*	Gastroenteritis, wound infection

CASE REPORT 29.2

A 20-year-old man struck his forehead on a submerged object while diving off a platform along the coast of Guam. He sustained an 8-cm laceration and lost consciousness for 2 minutes after the incident. The laceration was repaired, and x-ray studies were taken that revealed a comminuted fracture of the frontal bone extending through the frontal sinus, with minimal depression of the fragments. A computed tomography scan showed the fracture site but no other evidence of intracranial disease.

The patient underwent frontal craniotomy with exenteration of the frontal sinus and realignment of the frontal bone fragments 3 days after the accident. Results of bacterial cultures of the subdural and epidural spaces were negative. The patient did well post-operatively, but he did experience cerebrospinal fluid rhinorrhea.

The patient remained asymptomatic for 3 months until intermittent fever and headache developed. A repeat computed tomography scan revealed a displaced frontal fracture site, as well as a large epidural fluid collection. Physical examination was completely normal other than the bony defect. Laboratory studies showed only that spinal fluid cultures were negative.

In the operating room, osteomyelitis of the frontal bone was noted. The entire frontal plate of involved bone was excised. A 25-ml collection of purulent material was recovered from the epidural space. Gram stain of this material revealed pleomorphic, curved, gram-negative rods.

The aerobic culture of the epidural space and frontal bone tissue revealed heavy growth of *Vibrio alginolyticus* in a pure culture.

The patient was treated with a 4-week course of intravenous chloramphenicol at a dosage of 50 mg/kg per day without complication. The patient recovered without neurological sequelae and was discharged without medication other than phenytoin for seizure prophylaxis. The patient was seen in follow-up 6 months later and was completely asymptomatic (From Opal SM, Saxon JR. Intracranial infection by Vibrio alginolyticus following injury in salt water. *J Clin Microbiol* 1986;23:373–374.).

CASE REPORT 29.3

A 32-year-old woman presented with a 24-hour history of severe pelvic pain described by the patient as 'worse than having a baby'. She also complained of right lower quadrant pain, low back pain and frequent urination with burning and constant cramping. On physical examination, the patient appeared to be 'toxic' with a temperature of 38.4°C. Her lungs were clear, and her abdomen was non-tender. On pelvic examination, there were no external lesions, but a non-bloody, purulent vaginal discharge was noted. The uterus was also very tender. An intrauterine device, which had been in place for 1 year, was removed through the cervix and sent to the microbiology laboratory for aerobic culture.

The patient initially received 4.8×10^6 units of benzyl penicillin (penicillin G) in divided doses intramuscularly. She also received oral doxycycline, 100 mg per day for 14 days. Two days later, she was much improved with little discomfort.

After isolation of *Vibrio vulnificus* from this unusual site (endocervix), the patient was interviewed as to possible sources of exposure to this marine bacterium. The patient had not eaten any seafood in the 2 weeks before the onset of symptoms. However, about 18 hours before the onset of pelvic pain she had been swimming in Galveston Bay and had engaged in sexual intercourse while in the water.

V. vulnificus has repeatedly been isolated from Galveston Bay, with a peak incidence during periods of warm temperatures and moderate salinities (From Tison DL, Kelly MT. Vibrio vulnificus endometritis. *J Clin Microbiol* 1984;20:185–186).

may be involved in skin infections after contact and wounding with crustaceans, coral, marine mammals and fish.

Clinical features

There is a history of skin injury, which may appear to heal during a 1- to 7-day latent period. Then a sharply defined purplish-red area spreads outward from the injury site, which becomes indurated. There is an associated itch, pain or burning sensation. Oedema develops, and adjacent joints become stiff and painful. Regional lymphadenitis or systemic manifestations such as endocarditis have been reported but are rare. Secondary infection may result in abscess formation.

Prevention and treatment

All small marine cuts and injuries should be thoroughly cleaned and treated actively with antiseptic solutions. Definite lesions are best treated with local antibiotic powder or ointment and systemic penicillin or tetracycline.

PSEUDOMONAS

P. aeruginosa has been previously mentioned as a common cause of otitis media. Although it is not known to survive in salt water, this organism may persist for a long time in fresh water. It thrives in a warm, moist environment.

Pseudomonas folliculitis

This condition, also known as 'splash rash', is usually seen after exposure to whirlpools, spas and hot tubs, but it has also been described after swimming pool exposure.

A papulo-pustular eruption develops some 8 to 48 hours after exposure to a recirculating water environment. The lesions may be pruritic or even tender and usually occur on the axillae, groin, trunk and buttocks. Fever, malaise, dizziness, headache, sore eyes and throat and regional lymphadenopathy may develop.

Pseudomonas urethritis and *keratoconjunctivitis* have also been reported following immersion in whirlpools or spas, as well as in drysuit divers (see earlier).

Diving suit dermatitis

Several similar cases have been reported in divers. The distribution of the rash coincided with the area covered by the suit. The wetsuit, which provides optimal conditions for *P. aeruginosa,* was shown to be the source of the organism in at least one diver.

These conditions are usually self-limiting in 1 to 2 weeks, but pustules or abscesses may recur for several months. Cultures of skin lesions and environmental source reveal the same serotype of *P. aeruginosa.*

Prevention requires improved disinfection and drying of diving suits.

Treatment is usually symptomatic, but in severe cases, systemic antibiotics may be required. This infection can be troublesome because *Pseudomonas* is resistant to many antibiotics. Fluoroquinolones such as ciprofloxacin and aminoglycosides such as gentamicin are usually effective.

TRICHOPHYTON

Tinea pedis dermatophytosis, caused by a *Trichophyton* species or *Epidermophyton floccosum,* is common in swimmers and divers because of such factors as moist environment, bare feet on wet decks and floors of communal showers. It is usually of nuisance value only, but secondary infection may lead to lymphangitis and lymphadenitis.

Treatment with a topical imidazole agent or terbinafine is effective. Occasionally, systemic griseofulvin or terbinafine is required.

MALASSEZIA FURFUR

Pityriasis versicolor caused by *Malassezia furfur* becomes obvious in swimmers and divers because of their exposure to sunlight when the small, patchy areas fail to tan evenly.

Treatment is usually sought for cosmetic reasons only, and it includes topical fungicides, imidazole creams and lotions. Rarely, systemic terbinafine may be required. Although this treatment eradicates the infection, the areas of discoloration may persist for many months.

MYCOBACTERIUM MARINUM

This acid-fast atypical tuberculous bacillus *Mycobacterium marinum* (previously also called *Mycobacterium balnei*) is the cause of cutaneous granulomata that have been called 'swimming pool granuloma' or 'swimmer's elbow'. *M. marinum* is also known to occur in sea water. This organism may gain entry to the skin via an abrasion from a swimming pool wall or ship's hull. Granulomata usually develop on fingers, hands, elbows or knees. There is one report of the infection following the bite of a dolphin, and the infection has also been noted in tropical fish tank enthusiasts (fish-fancier's finger). Immunosuppressed individuals appear to be particularly susceptible.

Clinical features

The granulomata usually develop over bony prominences (i.e. sites of abrasion). The onset is noted 3 to 4 weeks after the predisposing injury (8 weeks in the case of dolphin bite). The granulomata may develop as discrete red papules covered with fine scales and may be large enough to be fluctuant. Aspiration may then reveal thick pus. The papules or cysts may become indurated or even ulcerate. Spontaneous resolution can occur in 1 to 2 years, but cases have persisted for 45 years. There is no evidence of systemic involvement. Synovitis was a common presenting feature in one series.

Diagnosis

This infection is identified by punch skin biopsy of the ulcer and demonstration of the organism either by direct staining (acid-fast) or culture on Lowenstein-Jensen media at 30°C to 33°C. Growth takes up to 3 weeks. Results of skin testing with tuberculin are positive in 85 per cent of cases.

Treatment

Drug therapy should be guided by response to *in vitro* sensitivity tests. Infections have responded to treatment with trimethoprim-sulphamethoxazole, tetracyclines (especially minocycline) and the tuberculosis drugs rifampicin and ethambutol. The drugs have to be continued for at least 4 weeks, with some authorities suggesting much longer regimens. The use of local warmth may be beneficial, and it has been suggested that the infection is confined to the skin because of the inability to grow at body core temperature. Surgery, either alone or in combination with antibiotics, has also been reported to be useful. Antibiotics are essential if the infection has extended to deep tissues such as tendon sheaths, joints or muscle.

Prevention

These measures include adequate chlorination of swimming pools, smooth tiles and, in the case of divers, protective gloves and clothing.

SCHISTOSOME DERMATITIS

This condition, also known as 'swimmer's itch', bathers' itch and marine dermatitis, is likely to be contracted near the surface of the water. It is caused by penetration of the skin by cercariae of non-human schistosomes. The cercaria is the larval developmental stage in the life cycle of the fluke. The organism is found in certain fresh or brackish lakes and swamps where a suitable ecological niche exists.

The life cycle of the organism involves shore-loving birds and various gastropod molluscs such as snails of the seashore. The adult fluke is a parasite and lives in the mesenteric vessels of vertebrates, including water birds. The fluke lays its eggs, which pass into the bird's gut, and faeces, and are deposited in the lakes that the birds inhabit. The eggs hatch in the water and become young miracidia, which spend most of their lives in the body of the water snails. In the water snails, the miracidia develop into free-swimming larvae, termed cercariae, which are capable of penetrating the skin of wading birds – or humans. If the cercariae enter the birds, then the life cycle starts anew. If they penetrate the skin of humans, they die because of an active foreign body reaction they induce in human tissue. The condition may then become manifest.

Clinical features

Humans become involved accidentally in this cycle. The cercariae are able to penetrate human skin but not blood vessels. This penetration causes a prickling sensation while in the water or soon after leaving it and is thought to be a mechanical irritation.

The pruritus subsides, to return a day later with increasing intensity in association with an erythematous papular eruption. There may be some associated inflammatory swelling. The rash is present for about 1 week and then fades, leaving a brown pigmentation that persists for some time. The degree of reaction varies greatly, and previous exposure causes hypersensitivity to develop in many persons. The foreign protein of the dead cercariae causes antibody production. This antigen-antibody reaction occurs at the site of each dead larva and is responsible for the itchy papules. Lesions occur only on parts of the body that have been exposed to water.

Prevention and treatment

For prevention, persons at risk should wear protective clothing and vigorously rub any exposed areas immediately after leaving the water. Dimethylphthalate is of value as a repellent.

Treatment is symptomatic (e.g. calamine lotion).

MYCOPLASMA PHOCACEREBRALE

For many years, the identity of the organism causing so-called 'seal finger' was unknown. Seal finger is named for an association with seal bites, the manual handling of dead seals or other interactions involving contact with seals by aquarium workers, divers and veterinarians. It is characterized by pain and cellulitic swelling of the hand, and if untreated or if treatment is unduly delayed, it can result in loss of digits and joint ankylosis with permanent reductions in manual function. The causative agent was identified when *Mycoplasma phocacerebrale* was isolated from both affected tissues and the mouth of a seal that delivered the bite[3]. There should always be a high index of suspicion for seal finger if cellulitis (particularly of the hand) develops in someone who has been in contact with seals, even if this person has not been bitten. The antibiotic treatment of choice is tetracycline.

GENERAL INFECTIONS

Swimming and diving in polluted waters

Ingestion of polluted drinking water has long been known to pose a risk of hepatitis, typhoid, cholera, dysentery and other gastrointestinal diseases[4]. With the greater worldwide awareness of increasing environmental pollution has come awareness that the swimmer or diver may also be exposed to the risk of these and other infections. Where monitoring is in place, beaches worldwide are periodically closed because of sewage pollution. The safety of many unmonitored locations is uncertain[5].

In coastal waterways close to large population centres, the water may be heavily contaminated with a wide range of organisms, but especially faecal coliforms and streptococci, *Salmonella* species, enteroviruses and rotaviruses[6-8]. Bodies of water that do not 'flush' well such as enclosed bays and harbours are more likely to contain significant numbers of pathogens.

Bacterial counts are often used to indicate water quality. Although such testing has been suggested for common faecal bacteria such as total coliforms, faecal coliforms, *E. coli*, faecal streptococci and enterococci, water is usually tested directly for coliforms and faecal streptococci only, to achieve timely and relatively inexpensive results. Sources of faecal contamination to surface waters include wastewater treatment plants, on-site septic systems, domestic and wild animal manure and storm runoff[9]. High coliform counts correlate with the presence of pathogens such as *Salmonella*, *Shigella* and *Aeromonas*, but not so well with pathogenic viruses.

High faecal streptococcal counts in marine recreational water have been associated with various illnesses, and the US Environmental Protection Agency sets a limit of 35 colony-forming units/100 ml for safe exposure[9].

Viruses (especially enteric) can enter the marine environment in massive quantities in urban sewage disposal and are not all destroyed by normal sewage treatment processes. Some viruses can survive for long periods of time in sea water and may be associated with enteric disease among swimmers (especially children). Enteric and respiratory viruses that are shed directly into water from bathers may be a source of infection. One report suggested an association between water quality and gastroenteritis in swimmers at several US beaches. Polio vaccine viruses, adenoviruses and Coxsackievirus have been recovered from sewage-affected coastal water.

Professional divers may have to work in severely polluted water. Wetsuits and normal masks provide little protection to the skin or gastrointestinal tract. Vaccination against hepatitis A should be considered. Special procedures and equipment

Table 29.3 Potentially pathogenic microorganisms isolated from polluted waters[a]

Gram-negative bacteria	Gram-positive bacteria
Coliforms	*Staphylococcus*
Escherichia coli	*Streptococcus*
Klebsiella	*Bacillus*
Enterobacter	**Viruses**
Citrobacter	*Enteroviruses*
Edwardsiella	*Reovirus*
Legionella pneumophila	*Adenovirus*
Campylobacter	*Hepatitis A virus*
Serratia	**Protozoa**
Proteus	*Entamoeba*
Oxidase-positive groups	*Giardia*
Aeromonas	*Acanthamoeba*
Plesiomonas	*Naegleria*
Pseudomonas	*Hartmanella*
Chromobacterium	
Yersinia	
Vibrio cholerae	
Vibrio parahaemolyticus	
Vibrio alginolyticus	
Group F 'Vibrio-like' organisms	
Lactose-positive 'Vibrio-like' organisms	
Anaerobes	
Bacteroides	
Clostridium	
Fusobacterium	
Eubacterium	

[a] This list does not imply that all of these microorganisms are present in any given body of water.

such as full hoods and occlusive drysuits may be required in such situations (see Chapter 66).

Table 29.3 lists pathogenic organisms isolated from polluted waters. The role of these organisms in the production of disease in swimmers and divers requires further epidemiological studies.

Vibrio vulnificus

V. vulnificus (see earlier) thrives in warm coastal sea water. It is a particularly virulent organism, and severe infections that may proceed to septicaemia have resulted from marine trauma[10], especially from shellfish or crabs, but also from aspiration of sea water, gastroenteritis and aquatic sexual intercourse.

CLINICAL MANIFESTATIONS

The patient may present with fever, chills, headache and myalgia. Bullous skin lesions may develop, as may necrotizing fasciitis and myositis. Septicaemia with hypotension and shock has a high mortality rate. Disseminated intravascular coagulation and respiratory distress syndrome have also been described with *V. vulnificus* infection. Patients succumbing to this infection may have underlying

General infections 351

disease, such as diabetes, liver disease (especially haemochromatosis) or renal failure, or they may be immunosuppressed.

TREATMENT

Wounds should be thoroughly cleaned as soon as possible, and penetrating or more serious injuries should be surgically explored and débrided under antibiotic cover[11]. Appropriate antibiotics to commence while awaiting the results of sensitivity testing include tetracycline and gentamicin or an extended-spectrum cephalosporin such as cefotaxime. Intensive care support is often required for multi-system failure. The infection is not contagious.

> *Vibrio* infections should be suspected in any patient presenting with fever and shock in association with wound infections, pneumonia or gastroenteritis when there is a recent history of immersion in salt water.

Schistosomiasis

Schistosomiasis (bilharzia), a disease caused by trematodes (flukes), is one of the most important causes of morbidity in the tropics. Humans are the definitive host of pathogenic schistosomes. The life cycle is similar to that described earlier under schistosome dermatitis, with humans replacing birds. *Schistosoma japonica* infection was described in the Philippines in World War II in US servicemen. It is also endemic in the Yangtze River area of China. *Schistosoma haematobium* and *Schistosoma mansoni* occur in Africa, the Middle East and South America. The infection is derived from contact (bathing or swimming) with infected water. Several weeks following skin penetration, an allergic reaction develops (Katayama syndrome), which may be severe with fever, cough, headache, abdominal pain, splenomegaly and patchy pneumonia. These symptoms then subside for several months. The parasite can damage liver gut, lung (multiple small abscesses) and bladder. Severe central nervous system involvement may develop with *S. japonicum* infection.

If immersion occurs in potentially infected water, showering and vigorous towelling may prevent penetration of the skin by cercariae.

Schistosomiasis was reported in three scuba divers from a dam in the Transvaal. Schistosome infestations are not contracted from salt water or properly chlorinated swimming pools.

Leptospirosis

Human infections with leptospirae usually follow ingestion of water or food contaminated with these spirochaetes. Less often the organism gains entry via a break in the skin or mucous membrane. Fishery workers and recreational water users are at risk. Several epidemics from swimming in fresh water have been reported. Rats, swine, dogs and cattle are the principal sources of infection. Certain species (e.g. *Leptospira icterohaemorrhagiae*, *Leptospira canicola*, *Leptospira pomona* or *Leptospira australis*) may predominate in a given geographical area.

CLINICAL FEATURES

The incubation period is usually 1 to 2 weeks and is followed by a sudden onset of fever, malaise, nausea, myalgia, conjunctival injection and headache. This period, during which the spirochaetes are present in the blood, may be followed by organ involvement, particularly of the liver (jaundice), kidney (renal failure) or lungs. There may also be meningism (benign aseptic meningitis), nausea and vomiting. The disease may persist for up to 3 weeks. Severe leptospirosis with profound jaundice (Weil's disease) develops in up to 10 per cent of cases.

TREATMENT

The role of antibiotics in mild febrile forms of the disease is controversial, but doxycycline and ampicillin have been advocated[12]. More severe cases respond to penicillin G, ampicillin and amoxicillin intravenously, as well as erythromycin. Complete resolution of the disease process is usual.

PREVENTION

This disorder is prevented by avoidance of exposure to potentially contaminated water, rodent and other host control and possible vaccination of dogs to reduce contamination. Doxycycline (200 mg weekly) may be indicated for short-term protection where risk of exposure is high.

Pharyngoconjunctival fever

This is an acute illness caused by several types of adenovirus[13]. It has an incubation period of 5 to 9 days and is characterized by fever, malaise, pharyngitis, cervical lymphadenopathy, cough, conjunctivitis and sometimes diarrhoea. Outbreaks of pharyngoconjunctival fever have been reported in swimmers. Similar viruses are probably often involved in swimming pool conjunctivitis epidemics, and sporadic outbreaks are reported. No serious morbidity and no deaths have been reported.

Primary amoebic meningoencephalitis

The free-living amoeba of the species *N. fowleri* causes this severe, often fatal, illness. This protozoan organism is found in fresh water and prefers warmer temperatures; it is found more frequently in lakes, hot springs, swimming pools or industrial thermal waters. The organism cannot survive long in a marine environment.

Naegleria species gain entry to the central nervous system via the mucosa of the nasopharynx and the cribriform plate. The amoeba then multiplies in the meninges and olfactory bulbs and eventually elsewhere in the brain. Cases have been reported from Australia, Belgium, the Czech Republic, the United Kingdom, New Zealand and the United States. It is likely that many others have been diagnosed as having acute pyogenic meningitis, with failure to demonstrate the infecting organism[14].

CLINICAL FEATURES

The incubation period is about 3 days to 2 weeks. The presentation is similar to that of acute pyogenic meningitis, with the patient in good health before the sudden onset of frontal headache, mild fever and lethargy, sometimes associated with sore throat and rhinitis. The headache and pyrexia progress over 3 days with vomiting, neck rigidity, disorientation and coma. The cerebrospinal fluid changes are those of bacterial meningitis, usually under increased pressure. The coma deepens, and death in cardiorespiratory failure supervenes on the fifth or sixth day of the illness. A high index of suspicion and an absence of the expected pathogenic bacteria in the purulent cerebrospinal fluid raise the diagnosis[14]. This is confirmed by observing the motile amoebae in a plain wet mount of fresh cerebrospinal fluid.

Pathological findings at post-mortem examination reveal a slightly softened, moderately swollen brain, covered by hyperaemic meninges. There is a purulent exudate over the sulci and in the basal subarachnoid cisterns. Small, local haemorrhages are seen in the superficial cortex, but the olfactory bulbs are markedly reddened and in some cases haemorrhagic and necrotic. On microscopic examination, there is a mild fibrinopurulent meningeal reaction, and amoebae may be seen in the exudate. The degree of encephalitis varies from slight amoebic invasion and inflammation to complete purulent, haemorrhagic destruction. The nasal mucosa is severely ulcerated, and the olfactory nerves are inflamed and necrotic. There is no evidence of amoebic invasion elsewhere in the body.

TREATMENT

There is a very high mortality. Of the approximately 200 cases reported to early 2012, only 12 patients survived. Amphotericin B is the drug of choice, in high dosage intravenously and small doses intraventricularly or intrathecally. Concurrent miconazole and rifampicin have also been used.

PREVENTION

Pollution of waterways by sewage and domestic wastewater must be controlled if this disease is to be prevented. Swimming and diving should be avoided in potentially contaminated water, especially if the water or environmental temperature is high.

Key West scuba divers' disease

This syndrome was described in classes at the US Navy's scuba training establishment at Key West, Florida. It was reported to occur 36 hours after first use of one particular type of scuba regulator, and it was noted in several students at each new course.

CLINICAL FEATURES

The disease is characterized by the onset of malaise, anorexia, myalgia, fever often greater than 38°C, headache and substernal tightness. One death has been attributed to this condition. Apart from these features, physical examination, chest x-ray features, urine examination and throat and blood culture results for bacteria are negative. Viral studies are also non-contributory. The illness subsides spontaneously in 72 hours. Continued use of the same regulator does not result in recurrence of the illness unless there is an intervening period without diving.

A multitude of organisms, including mainly *Pseudomonas* and *Fusarium,* has been found on the low-pressure diaphragm and interior of the corrugated air hoses of the twin-hose regulators. Decontamination of these parts appears to prevent the illness.

Salt water aspiration syndrome is caused by aspiration of small amounts of salt water during diving, and it mimics an acute respiratory infection (see Chapter 24). It bears some resemblance to Key West scuba divers' disease. It is not thought to be a contagious disease but is included because of its importance in the differential diagnosis of infectious illness. It usually resolves without antibiotic therapy.

Near drowning and pulmonary infection

During recovery from aspiration of both fresh and salt water, some patients develop severe infections of the lungs. This is one of the many possible reasons for the delayed hypoxia seen in such patients. Post-mortem examinations performed on those who die more than 12 hours after near drowning frequently show evidence of bronchopneumonia or multiple abscesses. However, the changes are often those of irritant pneumonitis rather than infection (see also Chapters 21 and 22).

Although in many cases it may be difficult to determine whether the infection was acquired in hospital, there have been numerous reports of cases in which organisms causing pneumonia have also been isolated from the drowning site. Organisms isolated in near drowning victims include *Aeromonas, P. aeruginosa, Pseudomonas putrefaciens, Klebsiella pneumoniae, Burkholderia pseudomallei* (melioidosis), *Chromobacterium violaceum, V. vulnificus, Streptococcus pneumoniae, Legionella* and the fungal organisms *Aspergillus* and *Pseudallescheria boydii*[15,16]. Patients with some

of these primarily pulmonary infections have also developed septicaemia and metastatic abscesses.

Rapid development of *Aeromonas* pneumonia and sepsis with highly positive blood cultures has been reported after immersion in healthy young men[17].

Prophylactic antibiotics have not proved useful and may in fact encourage infection with resistant organisms. Microscopy and culture of sputum or tracheal aspirate should be performed regularly, and appropriate antibiotic therapy should be instituted.

Special environments

ENCLOSED ENVIRONMENTS

The human-microbe-environment relationship is both subtle and complex. A change in any one of the elements may have substantial effects on the others.

An increasing problem in the closed environments in undersea habitats, submarines and hyperbaric facilities is contamination by microorganisms, and the flora in such situations can be very rich (see also Chapters 64 and 67 to 69). Cross-infection of divers through the use of common equipment, diving practices such as buddy breathing and habitation in small enclosures aggravate these problems. The concentration of pathogenic organisms may lead to an increased rate of skin, respiratory and systemic infections.

The most common organism isolated from skin infection in saturation divers is *P. aeruginosa,* an organism that is seldom found in routine skin infections elsewhere. The factors encouraging infection are not entirely clear, but the hyperbaric atmosphere may play a role apart from the humidity and temperature. Evidence has been presented to suggest that the organism is not necessarily introduced into the system by the infected diver, and it may persist in the fresh water system for several months[18].

Whenever a group of people live together in close proximity for days or weeks, they undergo an initial period of illnesses. After recovering from these infections, they are then immune to subsequent infections, as long as they live in isolation with their antigenic peers. They are, however, extremely susceptible to infections from exogenous sources or when the period of isolation ends and they re-establish contact with outside personnel. Such examples are seen with the *Polaris* submarine crews and people living in Antarctica, among others. This is readily explained by the limited sources of infection.

Other interesting changes in saturation complexes may be found because of the effects of pressure, temperature, gas changes and relative humidity on the survival, selectivity and transport mechanisms of microorganisms. It was found that humidities in the region of 50 per cent were the most detrimental to air-borne bacteria; however, this may not be applicable to marine organisms transported mechanically from the marine environment, which may assume a predominant role in the air flora of submersible habitats. In less-controlled saturation systems, with high humidity, there may be a greatly increased propensity to infection.

HYPERBARIC EFFECTS

Oxygen under high pressure is of value in treating certain infections and may be lifesaving or limb saving in cases of clostridial gas gangrene and necrotizing fasciitis. It has also been of value in the treatment of chronic osteomyelitis and other infections.

Oxygen under pressure may have a multitude of effects on the human-microbe-environment interaction. Pulmonary oxygen toxicity is thought to impair bacterial defence mechanisms and thus cause increased susceptibility to infections, particularly of the respiratory tract, whereas oxygen and *Pseudomonas* infection appear to be additive in damaging the lung to produce the acute respiratory distress syndrome.

Enhancement of viral infection by hyperbaric oxygen has been demonstrated in cell cultures, by an acceleration of virus maturation and by production of abnormally high yields or faster host cell destruction. These effects do not depend on continual exposure during the infectious cycle and therefore may be applicable to all types of hyperbaric exposures. The change appears to be produced by changes in the membrane of the cell and lysosomes.

Experimental studies on rats exposed to 100 per cent oxygen at 3 ATA for 15 minutes before they were infected with Coxsackievirus demonstrated

an inhibition of interferon activity, greater viral proliferation and less leakage of lysosome enzymes, together with increased host mortality.

Hyperbaric changes in physiology of the host have been inferred from tissue cultures. There appear to be alterations in cell permeability and in metabolism of amino acids and ribonucleic acid precursors. The divers' steroid levels are increased, both in saturation and brief diving excursions, this increasing susceptibility to bacterial and viral infections.

In some cases, there does seem to be a tendency to impede the host's reaction, together with increased susceptibility to infection. Organisms may change, both in incidence and activity, when they are associated with a hyperbaric environment. Deep diving or a hyperbaric helium environment can increase the resistance to penicillin of *S. aureus* and to gentamicin and rifampicin by *E. coli* and *Salmonella typhimurium*[19]. Hyperbaria also seems to increase the effects of some antibiotics (e.g. in increasing permeability of tetracyclines in cerebrospinal fluid).

The foregoing information remains patchy, selective and incomplete. In the practice of hyperbaric oxygen therapy, opportunistic infections do not seem to be a practical problem. In relation to saturation diving environments, this area remains a productive field for future developments – but little research activity has been reported to date.

REFERENCES

1. Oliver JD. Wound infections caused by *Vibrio vulnificus* and other marine bacteria. *Epidemiology and Infection* 2005;**133**:383–391.
2. Harris R. Genitourinary infection and barotrauma as complications of 'p-valve' use in drysuit divers. *Diving and Hyperbaric Medicine* 2009;**39**:210–212.
3. White CP, Jewer DD. Seal finger: a case report and review of the literature. *Canadian Journal of Plastic Surgery* 2009;**17**:133–135.
4. Cabelli VJ, Dufour AP, McCabe LJ, Levin MA. Swimming-associated gastroenteritis and water quality. *American Journal of Epidemiology* 1982;**115**:606–616.

5. Prieto MD, Lopez B, Juanes JA, Revilla JA, Llorca J, Delgado-Rodriguez M. Recreation in coastal waters: health risks associated with bathing in sea water. *Journal of Epidemiology and Community Health* 2001;**55**:442–447.

6. Pruss A. Review of epidemiological studies on health effects from exposure to recreational water. *International Journal of Epidemiology* 1998;**27**:1–9.

7. Birch C, Gust I. Sewage pollution of marine waters: the risks of viral infection. *Medical Journal of Australia* 1989;**4**(18):609–610.

8. Keuh CSW, Grohmann GS. Recovery of viruses and bacteria in waters off Bondi beach: a pilot study. *Medical Journal of Australia* 1989;**4**(18):632–638.

9. United States Environmental Protection Agency. *Water: Monitoring and Assessment 5.11. Fecal Bacteria.* http://water.epa.gov/type/rsl/monitoring/vms511.cfm

10. Hill MK, Sanders CV. Localized and systemic infection due to *Vibrio* species. New Challenges from Infectious Diseases. *Infectious Disease Clinics of North America* 1988;**2**(3):687–707.

11. Wiliamson JA, Burnett PJ, Rivken JW, Jacqueline F. *Venomous and Poisonous Marine Animals: Medical and Biological Handbook.* Sydney: University of New South Wales Press; 1996.

12. Pappas G, Cascio A. Optimal treatment of leptospirosis: queries and projections. *International Journal of Antimicrobial Agents* 2006;**28**:491–496.

13. Bell JA, Rowe WP, Engler JI, Parrott RH, Huebner RJ. Pharyngoconjunctival fever: epidemiology of a recently recognized disease entity. *Journal of the American Medical Association* 1955;**157**:1083–1092.

14. Myint T, Ribes JA, Stadler LP. Primary amebic meningoencephalitis. *Clinical Infectious Diseases* 2012;**55**:1737–1738.

15. Ender PT, Dolan MJ. Pneumonia associated with near-drowning. *Clinical Infectious Diseases* 1997;**25**:896–907.

16. Dworzack DL, Clark RB, Padjitt PJ. New causes of pneumonia, meningitis, and disseminated infections associated with immersion. New Challenges from Infectious Diseases. *Infectious Disease Clinics of North America* 1988;**3**:615–633.

17. Ender PT, Dolan MJ, Dolan D, Farmer JC, Melcher GP. Near-drowning–associated *Aeromonas* pneumonia. *Journal of Emergency Medicine* 1996;**14**(6):737–741.

18. Ahlen C, Mandal MH, Iverson JI. Identification of infectious *Pseudomonas aeruginosa* strains in an occupational saturation diving environment. *Occupational and Environmental Medicine* 1998;**55**:480–484.

19. Hind J, Atwell RW. The effect of antibiotics on bacteria under hyperbaric conditions. *Journal of Antimicrobial Chemotherapy* 1996;**37**:253–263.

FURTHER READING

Buck JD, Spotte S, Gadbaw JJ. Bacteriology of the teeth from a great white shark: potential medical implications for shark bite victims. *Journal of Clinical Microbiology* 1984;**20**:849–851.

Gregory DW, Schaffner W. *Pseudomonas* infections associated with hot tubs and other environments. *Infectious Diseases Clinic of North America* 1987;**1**:635–648.

Iredell J, Whitby M, Blacklock Z. *Mycobacterium marinum* infection: epidemiology and presentation in Queensland 1971–1990. *Medical Journal of Australia* 1992;**157**:596–598.

Johnston JM, Izumi AK. Cutaneous *Mycobacterium marinum* infection ('swimming pool granuloma'). Clinics in Dermatology 1987;**5**(3):68–75.

Joseph SW, Daily OP, Hunt RJ, Seidler DA, Colwell RR. *Aeromonas* primary wound infection of a diver in polluted waters. *Journal of Clinical Microbiology* 1979;**10**:46–49.

Royle JA, Isaacs D, Eagles G, *et al.* Infections after shark attacks in Australia. *Medical Journal of Australia* 1997;**16**(5):531–532.

Saltzer KR, Schutzer PJ, Weinberg JM, Tangoren IA, Spiers EM. Diving suit dermatitis: a manifestation of *Pseudomonas* folliculitis. *Cutis* 1997;**59**:245–246.

Sausker WF. *Pseudomonas aeruginosa* folliculitis ('splash rash'). *Clinical Dermatology* 1987;**5**:62–67.

Tsakris A, Psifidis A, Douboyas J. Complicated suppurative otitis media in a Greek diver due to a marine halophilic *Vibrio* species. *Journal of Laryngology and Otology* 1995;**109**:1082–1084.

Van Asperen IA, de Rover CM, Schijven JF, *et al.* Risk of otitis externa after swimming in recreational fresh water lakes containing *Pseudomonas aeruginosa. British Medical Journal* 1995;**311**(7017):1407–1410.

This chapter was reviewed for this fifth edition by Simon Mitchell and Michael Bennett.

30

Scuba divers' pulmonary oedema

INTRODUCTION

Pulmonary oedema occurs when fluid passes from the pulmonary capillaries to accumulate in the pulmonary alveoli and causes effects similar to those of the drowning syndromes (see Chapters 21 to 24).

There are three forms of immersion pulmonary oedema (IPE), induced while swimming, free diving or scuba diving. They have some similar features, but there are significant differences in their demographics, causation and therapeutic implications. The swimming-induced cases tend to occur in persons who are young and very fit, but exposed to extreme exertion. The free divers experience breath-holding and barotraumatic influences that are described elsewhere (see Chapters 3, 6 and 61).

In the colourful parlance of scuba divers, IPE is referred to as 'drowning from within'. Scuba divers' pulmonary oedema (SDPE) can occur in apparently healthy individuals, most frequently in middle-aged women. In a survey of scuba divers, about 1 per cent described it. An individual predisposition is a likely factor because recurrences are common with diving, snorkeling and swimming.

There are many other causes of pulmonary oedema in diving medicine.

PULMONARY OEDEMA

Pulmonary oedema is the accumulation of fluid in the lungs. It may be a transudate (from high pulmonary capillary-to-alveolar pressure gradients) or an inflammatory exudate with protein, red cells or other components (capillary damage), or it may represent lymph accumulation[1].

Pulmonary oedema is well described in a variety of disorders in the general medical literature and results from failure of the heart to remove fluid from the lung circulation ('cardiogenic pulmonary oedema'), a direct injury to the lung parenchyma ('non-cardiogenic pulmonary oedema') or, more rarely, neurogenic factors.

Cardiogenic pulmonary oedema can develop from congestive cardiac failure, infarction, cardiomyopathies, myocarditis, arrhythmias, hypertension, tamponade, fluid overload and other conditions.

Non-cardiogenic pulmonary oedema can develop from pulmonary obstruction, thoracic surgical procedures, infections, allergies, toxic inhalants, trauma, aspiration and other conditions. In the respiratory and anaesthetic medical literature, non-cardiogenic pulmonary oedema can result from a restriction of inspiration causing negative pressure pulmonary oedema (NPPE)[1,2].

The development of pulmonary edema during swimming and diving is well established. The question whether pulmonary edema develops during exercise on land may be more controversial[3]. There are some terrestrial environmental provocations, such as in exertional pulmonary oedema, both in athletes (long-distance running and rugby footballers) and race horses, and in the high-altitude pulmonary oedema of climbers[4,5].

Exercise-induced pulmonary edema could occur by the following mechanisms[3]: an increase in capillary hydrostatic pressure, an increase in capillary permeability or an inability of the lymphatic system to clear fluid extruded from the vessels.

IMMERSION PULMONARY OEDEMA

Although the first aid treatment for all three groups of IPE may be similar, subsequent investigations and preventive measures differ.

As a group, these disorders were well reviewed by Koehle and associates in 2005[6]. These investigators reviewed 60 cases from the literature. There were 34 scuba divers, 18 swimmers and 8 free divers. There was a history of prior or subsequent pulmonary oedema in at least 13 cases. The symptoms included cough in 82 per cent, dyspnoea in 80 per cent and haemoptysis in 62 per cent. Less common were weakness and confusion. Chest pain was not a feature. Although physical examination was not well described, chest crackles (rales) and wheezing were noted in 25 per cent and 10 per cent, respectively. Most IPEs were verified radiologically. The mean oxygen partial pressure was 66.2 mm Hg (± 17.4) with an arterial oxygen saturation of 88.8 per cent (± 7.3). In the majority, symptoms resolved in 5 minutes to 24 hours, and 2 cases were fatal.

Swimming-induced pulmonary oedema

Healthy swimmers performing under extreme exertion, such as in Israeli and US combat forces, can develop swimming-induced pulmonary oedema (SIPE)[6-11]. Pathophysiological explanations for SIPE include increased cardiac output from physical exertion, pulmonary vascular blood pooling secondary to immersion, increase in pulmonary vascular resistance in response to cold exposure and increased perfusion in dependent parts of the lung as a result of hydrostatic pressure gradients – the lower lung with side-stroke swimming.

Overhydration may have contributed in some cases, and others occurred in relatively warm waters, up to 23°C.

In triathletes, IPE seemed to occur mostly in women and soon after the commencement of the swimming sector. There was no such observation in the triathlons' cycling or running sectors, a finding indicating that immersion probably is the provoking stress. Some of the athletes had repeated episodes, and in a survey, 1.4 per cent of female triathletes had a history of this disorder[8].

Clinical features included dyspnoea, cough, sputum, haemoptysis, 'inspiratory crackles', wheezing, low arterial oxygen (corrected with oxygen inhalation) and temporary restrictive lung function on spirometry. The chest radiographs became normal after 12 to 18 hours. Pulmonary investigations, including broncho-alveolar lavage, indicated that the pathological feature was capillary stress failure with no evidence of inflammation.

Free diving and pulmonary barotrauma of descent

This is a well-recognized and understood cause of pulmonary oedema. It results from the excessive pressure gradient that develops between the pulmonary capillary and the alveoli, after the residual lung volume has been reached during descent (Boyles' Law effect; see Chapters 3 and 6).

SCUBA DIVERS' PULMONARY OEDEMA

SDPE was first recorded in 1981[12]. It is usually described as an uncommon disorder[6,13,14], often in apparently healthy individuals[6,13,15,17], with only a hundred or so cases being well documented. Comprehensive reviews were prepared by Lundgren and Miller in 1999[17], Slade and associates in 2001[18], Koehle and colleagues in 2005[6], Edmonds in 2009[7] and Coulange and colleagues in 2010[16].

Pons and associates[13] conducted a survey on divers, and of the 460 responders, 5 (1.1 per cent) had a history suggestive of pulmonary oedema. The actual incidence is unknown, but possibly this disorder is underdiagnosed[7,14,18,19]. Divers Alert Network (DAN), the international emergency diving service, has reported a few calls each month from divers with symptoms suggestive of this disorder[20]. Some of the divers with SDPE had also noted similar problems during surface swimming, especially with exertion[6,13,21].

Six deaths have been documented; one in a diver with hypertension, dyslipidaemia and arteriopathy and the other five in divers with no previous cardiopulmonary problems[14,22,23]. Three had at least one previous well-documented episode. However, other deaths, like so many deaths in the underwater environment, could have been attributed to drowning. Because the pathology of drowning is similar to that of SDPE, and the latter diagnosis is frequently not considered at autopsy, there is a strong possibility that some deaths from SDPE are incorrectly identified as drowning deaths – especially if this was the first such incident encountered by the diver. Other deaths from SDPE are known but await reporting.

SDPE is significantly more frequent in female divers and older divers, and it tends to recur[16,22–24]. Exertion is not a requirement in SDPE and is sometimes specifically denied[15,19,23,25]. Others have recorded a history of exertion in about half the cases[16].

Clinical features

SDPE manifests clinically with fast shallow respirations, dyspnoea, fatigue, cough and sometimes bloodstained expectoration, hypoxia and auscultatory signs of pulmonary oedema. Commonly, the first reported respiratory symptoms occur after reaching shallow depths or during the ascent, although a sensation of feeling cold may precede the symptoms. Some divers have observed sea water aspiration, anxiety and/or exertion before the respiratory distress[7,16,22,23].

Investigations reveal temporary restrictive spirometry and reduced compliance, hypoxaemia and characteristic radiological (plain x-ray study or computed tomography [CT] scan) abnormalities.

ECG and echocardiographic anomalies have been described. Increased troponin and natriuretic peptide levels have been reported[16].

Symptoms usually resolve rapidly (minutes or hours) after the immersion is terminated, although death has occasionally supervened – usually while still immersed. The hypoxaemia, respiratory function, radiology (chest X-ray or CT scan) and cardiac investigations also resolve within hours or days in most cases, after rescue from the water[13–15,26].

Predisposition

An individual predisposition for pulmonary oedema is a likely factor because a diver[6,12–14,18,19,21] or swimmer[13,21] with pulmonary oedema is more likely to experience other episodes of SDPE, previously or subsequently. Yet when diving under similar conditions, the diver may have been spared. Whether the variation in presentation relates to the individual diver, the dive profile, environmental conditions or the dive equipment, is conjectural.

Most of the surveys have shown an average age of between 35 and 60 years, significantly older than the diving population from which they came, and these are frequently experienced divers[6,14,19,21,26]. The detrimental effects of age could be enhanced by its correlation with hypertension, ischaemic or other heart diseases and reduced respiratory function.

Causes

The aetiology of SDPE is unknown, but because no single cause has been demonstrated, various possible complementary causes have been incriminated, based on the clinical histories and known physiological stressors, both cardiogenic and noncardiogenic. They include cold-induced pulmonary oedema, immersion and hydrostatic pressures, NPPE, exertion, pre-existing cardiac disease, stress and aspiration.

COLD-INDUCED HYPERTENSIVE PULMONARY OEDEMA

Wilmshurst and colleagues[12] first described SDPE and attributed it mainly to the effects of cold, which induced hypertensive pulmonary oedema. In their series, those who developed this condition on one or more occasions were abnormal, compared with divers who never had pulmonary oedema. It was proposed that 'labile hypertensives', with an exaggerated vaso-constrictor response to cold, would be particularly prone to develop pulmonary oedema because of an increase in after-load cardiac stress from hypertension and a pre-load stress from the pulmonary vascular blood volume increase that occurs with immersion.

This report was followed by further work by Wilmshurst and associates in 1989[21], comparing divers and swimmers who had pulmonary oedema with controls. These investigators hypothesized that a pathological hypertensive response to cold and/or raised oxygen pressure induced cardiac decompensation that resulted in pulmonary oedema during immersion. The divers in the pulmonary oedema group were followed up for an average of 8 years, at which time seven divers had become hypertensive. All the cases occurred in waters colder than 12°C. Thus, the hypotheses proposed by Wilmshurst and colleagues incriminated a vascular hyperreactivity to a cold stimulus.

This explanation has been supported by some reports[12,14,21], but not others, which observed SDPE in relatively warm waters[13,15,18,19,23–25]. Cold exposure may not have been an important factor even in the cold water cases because most divers were protected by insulating wetsuits or drysuits, although they were still presumably exposed to cold air inhalation irrespective of the water temperature.

Pons and colleagues[13] reported results that did not support the observations of Wilmshurst and associates, by finding no cardiovascular difference between these subjects and healthy controls. Forearm vascular resistance, vaso-active hormone levels and left ventricular function were the same in subjects with aquatically induced pulmonary oedema as in controls. Hypertension and the vascular hyperreactivity to cold exposure may contribute to SDPE – but the extent of this awaits clarification.

IMMERSION AND HYDROSTATIC PRESSURES

Intrathoracic blood pooling can be induced when the body is submerged[17,18,21,27,28]. It causes the following changes: an increase of about 500 ml of pulmonary blood; reduced compliance; an increase in pulmonary arteriole transmural pressures;

a reduction of the vital capacity; increased cardiac output, stroke volume and atrial pressure; and an increase in the work of breathing[27–29].

The thoracic blood pooling and the raised pulmonary artery pressure are postulated to cause increased capillary permeability leading to pulmonary oedema[6,21]. Other investigators believe that this is not a likely explanation for the development of this form of oedema[13,15]. Many case histories include expectoration of bloody froth, which does indicate some pulmonary capillary damage[13,14,18].

Because the weight of water increases with depth, there is variable hydrostatic pressure on sections of the lungs at different levels (depths). When the pressure at the air intake level is shallower than the thorax, there is increased negative pressure required for inspiration. The pressure at the air intake is 1 ATA with head-out immersion, but it is at the same depth as the regulator when using scuba underwater. The negative inspiratory pressure from immersion *per se* thus varies with the spatial positioning of the body. It is increased when the free or snorkel diver is immersed but breathing surface air or when the scuba diver assumes a head-up vertical position. With rebreathing equipment, there is an inspiratory resistance if the diver's thorax is below the counterlung bag.

'Simulated diving' in the dry hyperbaric chamber, where none of the hydrostatic pressures of the water environment can be incriminated, still induces raised pulmonary artery pressure. The increased inspiratory resistance could be a factor.

NEGATIVE PRESSURE PULMONARY OEDEMA

The effects of inspiratory and expiratory pressures were first demonstrated in 1927[30]. Negative inspiratory pressure has been postulated as a cause of NPPE and SDPE by most reviewers[13–18,20]. It is a feasible possibility in scuba divers, more so than in swimmers. In the scuba diving environment, negative pressure during inspiration can arise from the following:

- Immersion *per se*, especially with a head-up/vertical or head-out position.
- Inspiratory breathing resistance from diving equipment (regulator, snorkel).
- Reduced gas supply or pressure.
- Increased gas density with depth.

- Increased ventilation, as occurs with exertion, anxiety and hyperventilation.
- In rebreathing equipment, when the counter-lung is positioned above the lung.
- Equipment impositions such as tight wetsuits, buoyancy compensators and so forth, which may impose greater inspiratory effort.

Thorsen and colleagues[31] demonstrated that increasing the inspiratory restrictive load in divers with head-out immersion reduced the diffusing capacity of the lung. This finding may indicate subclinical pulmonary oedema. No changes occurred in pulmonary function with either of the conditions, separately. In another study, this disorder was not provoked when divers were subjected to considerable negative pressure inspiration, even when these pressures were extreme (50 cm H_2O) and close to being intolerable over a 1-hour period[32].

The maximum negative inspiratory pressures likely to be encountered from the breathing apparatus are 25 to 32 cm H_2O[17]. In the diving literature, 15 to 20 cm H_2O inspiratory resistance is considered moderate, and 20 to 25 cm H_2O inspiratory resistance is considered high[33].

EXERTION

This is more characteristic of SIPE than SDPE, which often involves little exertion. Pulmonary oedema is reported in the general medical literature, in rugby players, cyclists, marathon runners, racehorses and swimmers. West[5] stated: 'Pulmonary capillaries have a dilemma. Their walls must be extremely thin for efficient gas exchange, but be immensely strong to resist the mechanical stresses that develop during heavy exercise. Elite human athletes at maximal exercise develop changes in the structure of the capillary wall as evidenced by red blood cells (and protein) in their alveoli. Racehorses routinely break their pulmonary capillaries while galloping'.

Wagner and associates[34,35] claimed that the high cardiac output associated with high-intensity exercise elevates the pulmonary vascular pressure to such a degree that fluid leaks across the capillary endothelium into the interstitial tissue.

Zavorsky in 2007[36] reviewed the general medical literature and supported the observation that exercise provoked pulmonary oedema. His experiments

supported a dose-response relationship of strenuous exercise and pulmonary oedema.

Most patients with SIPE have exercised excessively. Some, especially the older subjects, may have had a cardiac basis, as with some cases of SDPE. In these patients, troponin level determinations and other cardiac investigations may be warranted[26].

CARDIAC PATHOLOGY

Magdar and his co-workers[37] at the Karolinska Institute in Sweden compared the different clinical manifestations of myocardial ischaemia induced by exercise in the terrestrial and aquatic environment. In those experiments, subjects with cardiac ischaemia (middle-aged men) were exercised in both environments, with electrocardiographic monitoring to ST depression. Clinically, the cardiac ischaemia manifested with dyspnoea in the water (both 18°C and 25.5°C) and with the more traditional pain of angina pectoris on land. This may well have been the first description of mild pulmonary oedema when swimming, and with rigorous scientific observation.

The recognition of dyspnoea as a manifestation of ischaemic heart disease while immersed is thus understandable, as is the alleviation of this symptom following successful coronary artery surgery[24,36,38].

Cochard and associates[14] described six episodes of pulmonary oedema among five experienced divers, 37 to 56 years old. Three of these divers had hypertension, one had cardiac ischaemia with ventricular dysfunction and one died after a cardiac arrest.

Garcia and colleagues[38] described 10 cases in divers 46 to 74 years old who developed pulmonary oedema, all of whom had cardiovascular disease. The disorder developed in five divers before surfacing. Eight divers were taking beta-blockers, and this association has been noted in other case histories as has the relationship with hypertension[18,26,38]. It is possible that drugs that produce pulmonary vascular hypertension could be detrimental in contributing to SDPE and that drugs such as sildenafil may reduce it.

Kenealy and Whyte[19] observed repeated SDPE in a 69-year-old woman in a shallow pool heated to 28°C. Chest x-ray studies verified the diagnosis, and

subsequent investigation revealed mild cardiomyopathy and an ejection fraction of 37 per cent (see
Chapter 39).

It is presumed that impairment of cardiovascular function makes divers less able to tolerate the various physiological changes imposed by
diving[21]. Most of the SDPE cases that have cardiopulmonary studies undertaken have shown no significant functional abnormalities, possibly because
these investigations have been delayed for some
days after the incident.

In 2013 Gempp et al described 54 consecutive
survivors of SDPE, 15 of whom had a reversible
myocardial dysfunction[42]. These had early elevated
cardiac troponin T and natriuretic peptides, ECG
changes and/or wall motion abnormalities with
reduced ejection fraction on the echocardiogram.
Symptoms and laboratory findings usually resolve
within 72 hours and replicate Takotsubo cardiomyopathy. This disorder has been identified in
cases of apparent SDPE, and may be much more
frequent than is currently recognized.

Many reported cases of SDPE do not specify
when their cardiac assessment was made. Then,
the assumption of "no cardiac abnormality" is not
supportable. SDPE could be an immersion induced
Takotsubo. Cardiac investigations in cases of
SDPE must take place promptly and, if abnormal,
should be repeated.

The demographics of aged females in the
SDPE cases may reflect the same distribution in
Takotsubo. The medical and cardiac "clearance to
resume diving", based on investigations many days
after the event, can be misleading – and explain the
unfortunate subsequent incidents and deaths.

ASPIRATION

Some patients with SDPE observed the intake of
sea water associated with rough seas, exertion and
overbreathing the regulator.

Salt water aspiration and near drowning are recognized as common causes of pulmonary oedema.
The salt water aspiration syndrome was first
described in 1971[39]. The clinical manifestations
were verified by inducing salt water aspiration in
healthy volunteers and recording the physiological results. The clinical case histories and clinical
examinations indicated pulmonary oedema of a
non-cardiogenic, pulmonary origin, with typical

hypoxaemic and spirometric impairments similar to those of SDPE. More gross clinical findings
are observed in near fatal drowning cases, and the
autopsy findings of fatal SDPE and drowning cases
are similar (see Chapter 21).

STRESS

The stress, which is present in so much recreational
diving and endurance swimming, may explain
why immersion induces pulmonary oedema.
See Chapter 45. The "stress cardiomyopathy" of
Takotsubo and other reversible cardiomyopathies
is believed to be precipitated by sympathomimetic
stimulation with catecholamine excess.

GENERAL DISCUSSION

Observations from the general medical literature
enhance our understanding of the possible aetiologies of SDPE. There are many causes of pulmonary oedema unrelated to diving, but aquatically
induced pulmonary oedema has specific stressors.
Extrapolating from the terrestrial to the diving
situation may not be appropriate. The three types
of aquatically induced pulmonary oedema appear
to share provoking causes, but to varying degrees.

The reasons for SIPE have been reasonably well
established, and they include severe exertion and
immersion, including thoracic blood pooling and
the hydrostatic effects on the pulmonary circulation. We also understand the major reason for pulmonary oedema with breath-hold diving, namely
pulmonary barotrauma of descent. We can avoid
the occurrence of these two causes of IPE. We do
not know the relative importance of the possible
causes of SDPE and prevention is less predictable.

The varying severity of SDPE, both clinically
and pathologically, bears a strong resemblance to
the drowning syndromes – salt water aspiration,
near drowning and fatal drowning. Minor degrees
of aspiration may be sub-clinical and unnoticed
by some divers, but they may still damage the
capillary-alveolar wall. This may be evidenced by
the temporary impairments in spirometry and
arterial oxygen levels that seem to accompany 'normal' scuba diving. There may well be a causal relationship between aspiration of sea water damaging
pulmonary capillaries and the other physiological
aberrations associated with immersion and scuba

diving, inducing SDPE. It may be compounded by the abnormal hydrostatic pressures with immersion, the cardiopulmonary effects of cold and immersion and the production of negative inspiratory pressures induced with scuba diving.

These physiological changes that accompany immersion and the negative inspiratory pressures that are associated with scuba diving increase the likelihood of pulmonary capillary stress. These aggravating stressors are described earlier, but we have no understanding of the degree that they may be relevant to SDPE.

Most would agree with Cochard and associates[14] that the explanation for SDPE is probably multi-factorial, a combination of factors imposed on the cardiovascular and respiratory systems. However, explaining SDPE by the known physiological stressors from the diving environment is based on presumptions that need validation. For example, a deleterious influence of tight wetsuits was not confirmed in one experiment[40]. Most of the other hypotheses have never been tested.

Negative inspiratory pressure has been postulated in SDPE by most observers[13–18,20,21]. Nevertheless, pulmonary oedema is not usually reported in the numerous 'head-out' immersion experiments. There were some effects on lung function from head-out immersion in young men, when this was combined with a mild negative inspiratory pressure of 9 cm H_2O/second/litre[31]. In the absence of clinical symptoms, and with the failure to reduce either forced vital capacity or maximal expiratory flows, this contribution to pulmonary oedema remains unconvincing. More recent experiments with excessive negative inspiratory pressures also cast doubt on this as a sole cause[32].

To date, there is no known association demonstrated between SDPE and decompression illness, although many cases seemed to occur during or after ascent. Pulmonary filtration of bubbles during decompression in scuba divers may increase pulmonary hypertension and damage capillary integrity, thereby increasing the likelihood of pulmonary oedema.

The observed association of SDPE symptoms with ascent could equally be explained by the hydrostatic positional effects on negative inspiratory pressures, described earlier, by the reduction of inspiratory oxygen pressures during ascent or by the redistribution of pulmonary oedema fluids from the expansion of thoracic gas according to Boyle's Law.

The association of pulmonary oedema with hypertension and/or cardiac failure is confused by their individual correlations with age, beta-blockers and ischaemic heart disease, thus complicating the relative significance of each of these factors[18,19,26,38,41,42]. Reversible myocardial dysfunction has been demonstrated in patients with SDPE[41,42]. The similarity to Takotsubo disease is striking, in some cases, with transient echocardiographic, ECG and cardiac enzyme anomalies, but normal coronary angiograms.

Older divers experience greater pre-load and after-load on cardiac function than younger divers, when exposed to cold conditions[43]. This exposure is common both from the diving environment and from the inhalation of cold, dense gases (Charles' Law).

Some convincing contributing factors are idiosyncratic to the affected diver and implied by the association with increased age, increased individual susceptibility, tendency to recurrences and the detection of relevant cardiac disease. Some researchers have incriminated genetic factors similar to those evident in altitude sickness[20].

Thus, SDPE, especially in older divers, should be an indication for prompt and comprehensive cardiac investigation. Unless the cause can be identified, verified and corrected, divers with SDPE should be advised of the possible risks of continuing with the activity that provoked it and should be advised against further diving or energetic swimming.

DIFFERENTIAL DIAGNOSIS

Diving-related diseases that can produce pulmonary oedema in their own right, and cause diagnostic confusion, are the salt water aspiration syndrome, drowning, respiratory oxygen toxicity, gas contaminations, cold urticaria, the Irukandji syndrome (jellyfish envenomation) and diving-induced asthma[7,41]. Pulmonary decompression sickness, pulmonary barotrauma and the so-called 'deep diving dyspnoea' are diving disorders that may cause diagnostic confusion. Cardiac diseases, including Takotsubo, need to be considered.

Anxiety-produced hyperventilation may also cause some diagnostic confusion, but this has none of the other respiratory manifestations of SDPE.

INVESTIGATIONS

The major problem in management of SDPE is hypoxaemia. Thus, blood gases are extremely important, interpreted with an appreciation of the inspiratory oxygen percentage and the degree of positive pressure employed in the resuscitation. Indeed, the arterial oxygen correction should guide this therapy.

Radiology from chest x-ray studies to CT scans will indicate the degree of oedema, as will the performance of lung function tests as soon as possible.

Because a cardiovascular cause of SDPE occurs in an appreciable number of these cases, especially in older patients, this needs to be assessed in the acute phase. Elevated cardiac troponin T levels and naturaemic peptides may indicate this condition, as may other cardiac enzymes and electrocardiographic and echocardiographic abnormalities. These abnormalities, together with evidence of hypertension, hyperlipidaemia, respiratory disease or diabetes, may need follow-up[42].

Usually, the cardiac and respiratory laboratory anomalies correct within days or weeks.

TREATMENT

Assuming the supine horizontal position on the surface of the water, and ditching weights, may reduce the immersion effects, whilst awaiting rescue. Over-inflating the buoyancy compensator could impair respiration, and so is not advised. Switching to high-oxygen gases would be advised for technical divers. These recommendations have not been validated.

The diver should immediately be rescued from the water and rested. Oxygen 100 per cent should be administered while waiting for medical evacuation to the nearest intensive care unit. Positive pressure respiration may be needed in severe cases, and positive end-expiratory pressure may be of value[44]. The remarkable success of this treatment usually makes other pharmacological interventions, such as diuretics, unnecessary – although these drugs are advocated by some physicians[20,41].

Although improvement is relatively rapid after leaving the water, some patients have required intensive resuscitation. Cases of unconsciousness have been well recorded, as have deaths. In most patients, there is complete resolution of clinical features within a day or two.

Medical assessment is required to verify SDPE and exclude any predisposing features. Although SDPE may develop in apparently healthy divers, sometimes it is based on transitory cardiac or respiratory disorders. Investigations to exclude predisposing factors need to be undertaken promptly to detect transitory pathology, such as Takotsubo, diabetes or asthma. SDPE, should be an indication for comprehensive assessment, not only for possible therapy but also to avoid further SDPE episodes.

For the patients who have reversible myocardial dysfunction, a more conservative approach to the recommendations regarding fitness to resume diving may be warranted. Some physicians believe that all individuals with SDPE should be advised to forgo scuba diving. It seems reasonable that unless the cause can be identified, verified and prevented, divers with SDPE should be advised of the possible risks of continuing with the activity that provoked it and should be advised against further diving, snorkeling or energetic swimming. Those who continue to dive should be advised of the risks and ensure they are thermally well protected, not overhydrated, have minimal regulator resistance, avoid excessive exertion, avoid drugs such as beta-blockers, use companion divers and always have emergency oxygen available at the dive site[15,22,23,41]. However, these opinions are contentious and do not necessarily apply to all cases of IPE from other causes[20].

IPE from other causes are dealt with elsewhere. Free diving and pulmonary barotrauma of descent, with its treatment, are discussed in Chapters 3 and 6. An occasional case of pulmonary oedema has been reported in relatively short breath-hold dives to shallow depths (6 metres), but whether the causal relationship is with IPE or pulmonary barotrauma of descent is contentious[45]. There have been at least four reported cases of pulmonary oedema occurring during hyperbaric oxygen therapy in patients with cardiac disease. These may be related to the direct cardiac effects, increased peripheral vasoconstriction and pulmonary capillary permeability associated with this environment[46].

There have been serious cases of IPE that have not responded as rapidly as would be desired or that continued to deteriorate to a fatal or near fatal outcome even though the diver reached the surface or the shore[22–24].

REFERENCES

1. Lang SA, Duncan PG, Shephard DA, Ha HC. Pulmonary oedema associated with airway obstruction. *Canadian Journal of Anaesthesia* 1990;**37**:210–218.
2. Buda AI, Ingels B, Daughters GT, Stinson EB, Alderman EL. Effect of intrathoracic pressure on left ventricular performance. *New England Journal of Medicine* 1979;**301**:453–459.
3. Bates ML, Farrell ET, Eldridge MW. The curious question of exercise-induced pulmonary edema. *Pulmonary Medicine* 2011;**2011**:361931.
4. West JB, Tsukimoto K, Mathieu-Costello O, Prediletto R. Stress failure in pulmonary capillaries. *Journal of Applied Physiology* 1991;**70**:1731–1742.
5. West JB. Vulnerability of pulmonary capillaries during exercise. *Exercise and Sport Sciences Reviews* 2004;**32**(1):24–30.
6. Koehle MS, Lepawsky M, McKenzie DC. Pulmonary oedema of immersion. *Sports Medicine* 2005;**35**(3):183–190.
7. Edmonds C. Scuba divers' pulmonary oedema: a review. *Diving and Hyperbaric Medicine* 2009;**39**(4):226–231.
8. Miller CC, Calder-Becker K, Moldave F. Swimming induced pulmonary edema in triathletes. *American Journal of Emergency Medicine* 2010;**28**(8):941–946.
9. Adir Y, Shupak A, Gil A. Swimming induced pulmonary edema. *Chest* 2004;**126**:394–399.
10. Weiler-Ravell O, Shupak A, Goldenberg I, Halpern P, Shoshani O. Pulmonary oedema and haemoptysis induced by strenuous swimming. *BMJ* 1995;**311**:361–362.
11. Shupak A, Weiler-Ravell O, Adir Y. Pulmonary oedema induced by strenuous swimming. *Respiratory Physiology* 2000;**121**(1):25–31.
12. Wilmshurst P, Nuri M, Crowther A, Betts I, Webb-Peploe MM. Forearm vascular response in subjects who develop recurrent pulmonary oedema when scuba diving: a new syndrome. *British Heart Journal* 1981;**45**:349.
13. Pons M, Blickenstorfer D, Oechslin E, Hold G, Greminger P. Pulmonary oedema in healthy persons during scuba diving and swimming. *European Respiratory Journal* 1995;**8**:762–767.
14. Cochard G, Arvieux J, Lacour J-M, Madouas G, Mongredien H, Arvieux CC. Pulmonary edema in scuba divers. *Undersea and Hyperbaric Medicine* 2005;**32**(1):39–44.
15. Hampson NB, Dunford RG. Pulmonary oedema of scuba divers. *Undersea and Hyperbaric Medicine* 1997;**24**:29–33.
16. Coulange M, Rossi P, Gargne O. Pulmonary oedema in healthy scuba divers: new physiological pathways. *Clinical Physiology and Functional Imaging* 2010;**30**:181–186.
17. Lundgren CE, Miller JN. *The Lung at Depth: Lung Biology in Health and Disease.* Vol 132. New York: Marcel Dekker; 1999.
18. Slade JB, Hattori T, Ray CS, Bove AA, Cianci P. Pulmonary oedema associated with scuba diving. *Chest* 2001;**120**:1686–1694.
19. Kenealy H, Whyte K. Diving related pulmonary oedema as an unusual presentation of alcoholic cardiomyopathy. *Diving and Hyperbaric Medicine* 2008;**38**:152–154.
20. Harper B. Immersion pulmonary oedema. *Alert Diver* 2011;**Fall.** p46–49, Fall edition. 2011. www.alertdiver.com/IPE.
21. Wilmshurst PT, Nuri M, Crowther A, Webb-Peploe MM. Cold-induced pulmonary oedema in scuba divers and swimmers and subsequent development of hypertension. *Lancet* 1989;**1**:62–65.
22. Edmonds C, Lippmann J, Lockley S, Wolfers D. Scuba divers' pulmonary oedema: recurrences and fatalities. *Diving and Hyperbaric Medicine* 2012;**42**(1):40–44.
23. Smart DR, Sage M, Davis FM. Two fatal cases of immersion pulmonary oedema. *Diving and Hyperbaric Medicine* 2014;**44**(2):97–100.

24. Allen J. A cardiac near-catastrophe. *Alert Diver (SEAP edition)* 2000;**Oct–Dec:**17–18.

25. Edmonds C. Scuba divers pulmonary oedema: a case report. *Diving and Hyperbaric Medicine* 2009;**39**(4):232–233.

26. Edmonds C. Pulmonary oedema, dyspnoea and diving. *South Pacific Underwater Medical Society Journal* 2001;**31**(2):75–78.

27. Lundgren CE, Pasche AJ. Physiology of diving: immersion effects. In: Shilling CW, Carlston CB, Mathias RA editors. *The Physicians' Guide to Diving Medicine.* New York: Plenum Press; 1984:86–98.

28. Hong SK. Breath-hold diving. In: Bove AA, editor. *Bove and Davis' Diving Medicine.* 3rd ed. Philadelphia: Saunders; 1997.

29. Hong SK, Cerretelli P, Cruz, JC, Rahn H. Mechanics of respiration during submersion in water. *Journal of Applied Physiology* 1969;**27**(4):535–538.

30. Moore RL, Binger CA. The response to respiratory resistance: a comparison of the effects produced by partial obstruction in the inspiratory and expiratory phases of respiration. *Journal of Experimental Medicine* 1927;**45**(6):1065–1080.

31. Thorsen E, Skogstad M, Reed JW. Subacute effects of inspiratory resistive loading and head-out water immersion on pulmonary function. *Undersea and Hyperbaric Medicine* 1999;**26**:137–141.

32. Sheilds S. Submarine and Underwater Medicine Unit, Royal Australian Navy, personal communication.

33. Warkander DE, Nagasawa GK, Lundgren CEG. Effects of separate inspiratory and expiratory resistance on ventilation at depth. *Undersea Biomedical Research* 1990;**17**(Suppl):44.

34. Wagner PD, Gale GE, Moon RE. Pulmonary gas exchange in humans exercising at sea level and simulated altitude. *Journal of Applied Physiology* 1986;**61**:260–270.

35. Wagner PD. Exercise, extra-vascular lung water and gas exchange. *Journal of Applied Physiology* 2002;**92**:2224–2225.

36. Zavorsky GS. Evidence of pulmonary oedema triggered by exercise in healthy humans and detected with various imaging techniques. *Acta Physiologica* 2008;**189**(4):305–317.

37. Magder S, Linnarsson D, Gullstrand L. The effect of swimming on patients with ischemic heart disease. *Circulation* 1981;**63**(5):979–986.

38. Garcia E, Padilla W, Morales VJ. Pulmonary oedema in recreational scuba divers with cardiovascular diseases. *Undersea and Hyperbaric Medicine* 2005;**32**(4):260–261.

39. Edmonds C. A salt water aspiration syndrome. *Military Medicine* 1970;**135**:779–785.

40. Mahon RT, Norton D, Krizek S. Effects of wet suits on pulmonary function studies in basic underwater demolition/seal trainees in the United States Navy [abstract]. *Undersea and Hyperbaric Medicine* 2002;**29**(2):134.

41. Mitchell S. Immersion pulmonary oedema. *Diving and Hyperbaric Medicine* 2002;**32**(4):200–202.

42. Gempp E, Louge P, Henkes A, *et al.* Reversible myocardial dysfunction and clinical outcome in scuba divers with immersion pulmonary edema. *American Journal of Cardiology* 2013;**111**(11):1655–1659.

43. Wilson T, Gao Z, Hess KL, *et al.* Effect of aging on cardiac function during cold stress in humans. *American Journal of Physiology Regulatory, Integrative and Comparative Physiology* 2010;**298**:R1627–R1633.

44. Bersten AD, Holt AW, Vedig AE, Skowronski GA, Baggoley C. Treatment of severe cardiogenic pulmonary oedema with continuous positive airway pressure delivered by face mask. *New England Journal of Medicine* 1991;**325**:1825–1830.

45. Gempp E, Shardella F, Cardinale M, Louge P. Pulmonary oedema in breath-hold diving. *Diving and Hyperbaric Medicine* 2013;**43**:162–163.

46. Dassan M, Paul V, Chadha S, *et al.* Acute pulmonary edema due to hyperbaric oxygen therapy. *Chest* 2014;**145**(3 Suppl):74A.

This chapter was prepared for this fifth edition by Carl Edmonds.

31

Trauma from marine creatures

INTRODUCTION

For animals not equipped with venoms and poison, defence against predators relies on either camouflage or aggression. Traumatic damage by the predator may be achieved from biting, bumping, spearing, electrical charges or corrosive materials.

Many marine animals avoid humans, but this attitude can be altered by familiarity with divers, who do not confront the animals aggressively. Increased proximity promotes the possibility of injury to both species.

Feeding activity is also related to aggression. Many divers make the error of feeding these animals. This results in conditioning them into associating humans with food. Often the animal will then attack other divers to acquire this food. In this manner divers have evoked feeding attacks from animals that would normally not have behaved in this manner. Examples include reef sharks, eels, groupers, dolphins and many fish.

SHARKS

General information

Most of the 470 species of sharks are marine inhabitants, but many enter estuaries, and some travel far up rivers, whereas a few, such as the bull shark, can thrive in fresh water environments. Most sharks live in the relatively shallow waters off the continents or around islands and inhabit the temperate or tropical zones, but some are deep dwelling, to more than 2000 metres (Figure 31.1).

Some, such as the great white shark, are pelagic, and although poikilothermic, they have adapted to colder ocean temperatures. In other species, the activity and food requirements may be more related to the environmental temperature. Shark attacks tend to be more frequent when the water temperature reaches 20°C or more because of these reasons and because of the increased frequency of humans bathing in warm water.

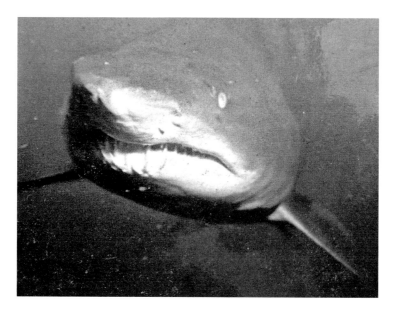

Figure 31.1 Grey nurse shark.

Even though Australia is renowned as one of the most dangerous areas in the world for shark attacks, there is an average of only one fatality per year, among millions of bathers at risk. The fatality rate from shark attacks in the open ocean is about 30 per cent. Rescue and first aid groups sometimes exaggerate the risk for ulterior reasons.

Shark attack remains a genuine but unlikely danger to seafaring people. Although rare, the attack is often terrifying in intensity, and the degree of mutilation has a strong emotive effect.

Data on shark attacks

There has been little factual research on shark attacks, perhaps because of the understandable difficulty of experimenting with these animals. Basically, our statistical information comes from two sources – detailed data collection from specific case histories, as exemplified by the work of Coppleson and data collection agencies such as from the US-based International Shark Attack File. Neither source is comprehensive, and neither is adequate by itself. The detailed case histories demonstrate the range of possibilities, whereas the attack file information indicates probable behaviour. The difficulty in obtaining accurate

details of any specific shark attack is understandable when one considers the suddenness of the accident and the emotional reactions of the participants.

The problem in assessing the statistical information is that many of the data are insufficient and unreliable. Application of the statistics to an open-water situation is not warranted. Nevertheless, much interesting information is available.

Shark attacks, comprising about 100 per year, are more frequent when there are more people at risk (i.e. during warm weather, on weekends and holidays). Attacks are more likely at the sharks' natural feeding times, at dusk, near deep channels, in turbid waters, in estuaries and near abattoirs and fishing grounds – where animal products are dumped.

Anatomy and physiology

Of the more than 400 species of sharks, only 30 have been implicated in attacks on humans, and only 4 species are frequently involved – the great white, oceanic whitetip, bull and tiger sharks. They allegedly have low intelligence, but this has not interfered with their ability to survive far longer than humans in the evolutionary time scale.

They are well equipped to locate prey and others of their own species, conduct seasonal migrations and identify specific localities. They react to multiple stimuli, with the sense of smell being a principal means of locating prey. They can detect some substances in minute quantities (e.g. blood in less than one part per million). Although their visual acuity for differentiating form or colour may not be selective, their ability to discriminate movements and minor contrast variations in low-light conditions is extremely efficient.

Sharks have an ability to detect low-frequency vibrations (e.g. the flapping of an injured fish). Their hearing is especially sensitive to low-frequency sounds, and they have an extraordinary faculty for directional localization of this sound. Their taste is not well developed, but preferences for some foods have been suggested (no – not humans). The lateral line is a multi-sensory system commencing at the head and passing along the shark's body. This system receives a variety of information, including vibrations of low frequency, temperature, salinity, pressure and minute electrical fields such as those produced by other fish or humans in the vicinity.

The feeding response is related more to the presence of specific stimuli than to the nutritional requirements of the animal. The presence of chemical stimuli, such as those released from freshly killed animals, can attract sharks and may result in the so-called 'feeding frenzy'. Sharks may swim together in an orderly and smooth manner, but when abnormal vibrations are set up (e.g. by one of the animals being shot or hooked), then the abnormal activity of that animal may trigger feeding responses in the others, and this may intensify into the feeding frenzy.

Attack patterns

There are several different types of attack. These may be identified by the behaviour of the animals and the subsequent nature of the injury. Four types represent different degrees of a feeding attack, and the others represent a territorial intrusion.

1. Sharks in a feeding pattern tend to circle the victim and gradually increase their swimming speed. As the circles begin to tighten, the sharks may commence a crisscross pattern (i.e. going across the circle). At this stage, they may produce injury by *contact,* when they bump or brush the prey. The shark's abrasive skin can cause extensive injuries, and it is thought that the information obtained by the animal at this time may influence the progression of the feeding pattern.

2. The *shark bite* is usually performed with the animal swimming in a horizontal or slightly upward direction, with the head swung backward and the upper teeth projecting forward. This results in a great increase in the mouth size and a display of the razor-sharp teeth. The force of the attack is often enough to eject the victim well clear of the water. The bite force may be up to 1000 kilograms per square centimetre. Once the animal has a grip on the prey, if the feeding pattern continues, the mouthful will usually be torn out sideways or the area totally severed.

3. A variant, often used by the great white shark when attacking a larger animal that could possibly inflict damage, is the *'bite and spit'* behaviour. This is seen not only against seals and sea lions, but also against other prey that may have a similar silhouette on the surface – such as surfboard riders, surface swimmers and so forth. The shark may make one sudden dash, take one bite and then release the prey, which then bleeds to death. Once the prey has stopped moving, the shark can then continue the feeding pattern in relative safety.

4. If other sharks are in the vicinity, they may reflexly respond to the stimuli created by the attack and commence a feeding pattern behaviour called a *feeding frenzy.* In this instance the sharks are likely to attack both the original prey and the predator or any other moving object. During this feeding frenzy, cannibalism has been observed, and the subsequent carnage can be extensive.

5. The fifth type of attack is termed *agonistic* and is that of an animal having its territorial rights infringed by an intruder – either a swimmer or a diver. This is quite unlike the feeding pattern. The shark tends to swim in a far more awkward manner, exaggerating a lateral motion with his head, arching the spine and angling its pectoral fins downward. In this position, it appears to be more rigid and awkward in its movements than the feeding animal. It has been compared, both

in appearance and motivation, to a cornered animal, adopting a defensive and snapping position. If the intruder diver vacates the area, confrontation will be avoided and an attack aborted.

6. When a diver jumps from a boat onto a shark (who may be following and scavenging refuse from the craft), the animal may reflexly snap at the intruder, in *defence*.

Clinical features

The lesions produced by shark bites are readily identifiable. The rim of the bite has a crescent shape, delineating the animal's jaw line (see Plate 5). There will be separate incisions from each tooth along the line, with occasional fragments of the teeth in the wound (the teeth were embedded in the shark's gums, more than fixed in the jaw). Identification of the shark species is possible from these teeth. There may be crushing injuries to the tissues, and variable amounts of the victim may be torn away. Haemorrhage is usually severe, in excess of that noted in motor vehicle accidents – probably because of ragged laceration of vessels, preventing vaso-constriction.

A great variety of damage is noted in different attacks. In some cases, merely the brushing and abrasive lesions of the skin may be present. In others, the teeth marks may be evident, encircling either the victim's body or even the neck – when the shark has had an appreciable amount of the victim within its mouth but has still not completed the attack. In most cases, there is a single bite, but occasionally several attacks and bites are made on the one victim. Amputations and extensive body wounds are common. In victims not killed immediately, the major problems are massive haemorrhage and shock. Adjacent people are rarely attacked.

Treatment

The most valuable first aid measures are to protect the patient from further attack and to reduce or stop haemorrhage. The rescuer is rarely injured because the shark tends to concentrate on the original victim. Once the patient is removed from the shark and prevented from drowning, attention should be paid to the prevention of further blood loss. This is achieved by any means available (e.g. pressure on the site of bleeding or proximal to this site, tourniquets or pressure bandages, clamping of blood vessels). One should use any material available. The mortality rate is such that there need be no apprehension regarding either the use of tourniquets or contamination of wounds.

The patient should be lying down with legs elevated. He or she should be covered lightly with clothing or a towel and reassured as much as possible. Medical treatment is best commenced before transfer of the patient to the hospital. Infusion of blood, plasma or other intravenous replacement fluid should be given top priority until shock has been adequately controlled. This can be ascertained by the clinical state of the patient, the pulse rate, blood pressure, central venous pressure and so forth. The use of morphine intravenously is likely to give considerable benefit, despite its mild respiratory depressant effect. Assessing and recording vital signs become integral parts of the management; these signs should be monitored throughout the transfer of the patient to the hospital.

At all stages, first aid resuscitation takes priority over the need for hospitalization. Transport to hospital should be performed in a gentle and orderly manner. Excess activity aggravates the bleeding and the shock state in these patients. Case reports abound with statements that the victims died in transit. They could more accurately state that the victims died because they were in transit – before clinical stabilization.

After the clinical state is stabilized, the patient is transferred by the least traumatic means available. The surgical procedures are not significantly different from those used for a motor vehicle accident case. With the patient under anaesthesia, the areas are swabbed, and bacteriological culture and sensitivity tests are obtained. X-ray studies or screening should be performed, both to detect bone damage and to identify foreign bodies. Surgical excisions of obviously necrotic material and removal of foreign bodies are required. The surgical techniques should otherwise be of a conservative type, especially if the blood supply is intact. Tendon suture should not be attempted unless the wound is very clean. Skin grafting is performed early, to preserve nerves, tendons, vessels, joints and muscles.

A severed limb should be wrapped, moistened, placed in a plastic bag and kept cold (not frozen) as advised by the hospital and transferred with the patient.

Broad-spectrum antibiotics are required, and bacteriological contamination is sometimes extensive, both with marine and terrestrial organisms. *Clostridium tetanus* and *Clostridium welchii* have both been isolated from shark wounds, although the contamination almost certainly occurred after the injury.

Consideration should be given to other medical problems that may exist, such as near drowning, decompression sickness or pulmonary barotrauma, and that may be a consequence of the dive profile disrupted by the shark attack.

Prevention

Prevention of shark attack depends on the marine locality. The following procedures are relevant in different situations.

HEAVILY POPULATED BEACHES

The most effective method to prevent shark attack is by the use of enclosures or meshing. Total bay enclosures are effective in sheltered areas, if consistent surveillance is carried out to ensure the integrity of the net. Areas exposed to adverse weather or surf are best protected by meshing.

Meshing involves the intermittent use of a heavy-gauge net, which is submerged from buoys on the seaward side of the breaking waves for 24 hours and then retrieved. Sharks tend to swim into it. The net wraps around the animal and interferes with its gill function. Because most sharks are unable to reverse, they will struggle and attempt to push themselves forward through the mesh. This causes the shark to be further immobilized and thus produces death by suffocation. Most of the sharks are dead by the time the mesh is retrieved, and the others are killed at the time of the retrieval.

Using this technique, the shark population becomes decimated. The experience on the relatively heavily shark-populated beaches of Australia and South Africa is similar. Shark attacks could still occur despite meshing. Nevertheless, the results are dramatic. Not only does the shark population decrease, shark sightings also decrease, and the shark attacks are almost eliminated. The population develops more confidence in the safety of their surfing area, and increased tourism often compensates for the cost of the shark meshing.

ALTERNATIVE TECHNIQUES

Bubble curtains, sound and ultrasonic waves and electric repellents, for example, do not have the same success as enclosure or meshing techniques. Many methods of repelling sharks will, given different conditions and different-sized animals, result in an alerting or an attraction response in the very animals they are meant to deter. Such is certainly the case with some electrical and explosive devices. The observation that some of these techniques work, initially should not engender confidence for a longer-term deterrent or for the deterrence of larger animals.

SURVIVAL SITUATION

The crashing of an airplane or the noise associated with a ship sinking often attracts sharks. Thus, the survivors of such accidents are then susceptible to shark attack. The most effective way to prevent this is to use life rafts and have the survivors move into them as quickly as possible. As an alternative, the Johnson Shark Screen is very effective. The Shark Screen is a bag of thin, tough plastic with a collar consisting of three inflatable rings. The survivor partially inflates one of the rings, by mouth, and then climbs into the bag. He or she fills it with water by dipping the edge so that it becomes full, thus appearing to any shark as a large, solid-looking black object. The other rings can be inflated at leisure. The bag retains fluids and excreta that could have stimulated a shark attack. It also attenuates the bioelectric and galvanic fields produced by the survivors.

"Shark Chaser" was of value only to the manufacturer. It consists of a dye and copper acetate. The black dye was meant to confuse the shark's visual localization, whereas the copper acetate was thought to be a deterrent chemical, mimicking decaying shark tissue. It does not work. Another chemical, produced by the peacock or Moses sole, has been investigated, but it has not been effectively marketed.

SWIMMERS

Swimmers are advised not to urinate in the water or swim with abrasions or bleeding wounds. They are also advised to move gently and not thrash around on the surface. They should stay with a group, or at least with a buddy. This is cynically claimed to reduce the chance of shark attack by

50 per cent but, in fact, it probably reduces it far more. Swimmers are also advised not to swim in water with low visibility, near drop-offs or deep channels or during late afternoon or night, when sharks tend to be involved in feeding.

DIVERS

The incidence of shark attacks on scuba divers appears to be increasing and now comprises one third of all shark attacks. Conventional wetsuits offer no protection despite popular hopes to the contrary. Specially designed wetsuits that either camouflage the diver or disrupt the sharks' visual input have been advocated repeatedly, and they are currently coming back into fashion. Divers are advised in the same way as swimmers, but with added precautions.

Underwater explosives tend to attract sharks. Shark attacks are more likely at increased depth and can be provoked by feeding, playing with or killing sharks. If one is diving in shark-infested waters, the use of a shark billy (a stout rod with a metal spike) can be effective in pushing the animals away. Powerheads, carbon dioxide darts and the drogue dart (this has a small parachute attached with disrupts the shark's orientation and swimming efficiency) are all specialized pieces of equipment that may be appropriate in certain situations.

Portable electric devices are enjoying a recurrence of popularity, having been discarded after a series of experiments in the mid-twentieth century. They are currently employed by divers and surfers, a successful result of astute marketing more than research. Shark attacks on divers who wore these devices have not dented the enthusiasm of the diving technophiles, but they should be aware that the electrical current that dissuades small sharks may attract larger ones.

Divers are advised not to catch fish or shellfish or tether them near their body because this may attract sharks. If sharks are encountered, it is advised to descend to the sea bed or to the protection of rocks, a cliff face or some other obstacle to interfere with the normal feeding attack pattern described earlier. If the diver recognizes an agonistic attack pattern from the shark, he or she should vacate the area, swimming backward.

Chain mail (stainless steel) suits discourage sharks from continuing an attack, but they incur buoyancy problems for divers and swimmers that outweigh the risks of shark attack. Experiments are being conducted on the use of Kevlar incorporated into wetsuits as a shark bite–resistant material.

It is sometimes claimed that women should not dive or swim while menstruating. There is no evidence to support the belief that decomposing blood will attract sharks; in fact, the experimental and statistical evidence suggests the opposite.

CROCODILES, ALLIGATORS AND CAIMAN

Crocodiles cause as many human fatalities as do sharks, in the areas where both are found. This was not always so, but although there may be a diminishing number of shark attacks as a result of meshing, there is an increased crocodile attack frequency because they have been protected and grow larger (Figure 31.2). There is also an increase of tourism into remote crocodile territories.

These animals become more aggressive during breeding times. The young are hatched from eggs and are protected by both parents.

They range in size from 1 to 10 metres long, and the larger specimens (more than 2 metres) are the ones potentially dangerous to humans. The largest animals weigh up to a ton. The species considered to be human eaters are the Australian salt water crocodile and the Nile crocodile, which grow to 8 metres; and the American crocodile and alligator, which grow to 3.5 metres. South American caimans are of the same family as alligators and grow up to 5.5 metres, but they are usually shorter.

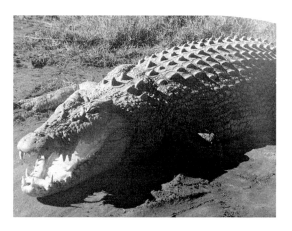

Figure 31.2 Crocodile.

Even the Indian mugger crocodile may attack humans if it is provoked while nesting. All crocodilians are carnivorous, and deaths have been recorded in snorkel and scuba divers.

These animals are often believed to compete with fishers by damaging nets, and they may prey on both domestic animals and humans.

Alligators are slower moving and generally less dangerous to humans. Crocodiles have narrower snouts than alligators, and the fourth tooth in each side of the lower jaw is usually visible when the mouth is closed.

Salt water crocodiles may also be found in fresh water. They may have swum inland from an estuary or traveled many kilometres overland. Fresh water crocodiles are also found in lakes and rivers that have no connection with the sea, and in some countries they may be both large and dangerous.

If humans or other animals intrude into the territory, the crocodile sometimes gives a warning by exhaling loudly or even growling at the intruder.

For reptiles, they have very complex brains and are intelligent enough to stalk a human, strong enough to destroy a water buffalo, and gentle enough to release their own young from the eggs – with their teeth. They even carry the newly hatched babies in their massive jaws.

Crocodiles tear their food from the carcass, by twisting and turning in the water to achieve this. They then swallow it whole. Once an attack pattern has begun, the crocodile attacks repeatedly until the prey is captured, and it may follow the victim from the water if necessary. If the animal captures large prey, it may hide the carcass underwater, entangled in submerged trees or under ledges, until it is ready to resume feeding.

The animal often lies along the banks of rivers, with only the nostrils protruding above water to breathe. The prey, especially land animals such as horse, cattle, giraffe, rhinoceros, kangaroo and wallaby, come to the river bank to drink and may be grabbed in the jaws of the crocodile and twisted off its feet. This movement sometimes breaks the neck of the victim. Once the prey is in the water, it is more vulnerable to panic and drowning. Although this 'death roll' is the classical attack pattern, crocodiles can move fast on land and in water, and recent attacks in Australia have included attacks with the victim free swimming in deep water, on dry land and in boats. When crocodiles attack small motor boats, they focus on the outboard motor – presumably because of the vibrations emanating from it.

On land, the attacks are more common at night when the animals stalk for food. They can move surprisingly fast – faster than most humans, issue a hissing sound and sometimes attack by sweeping the victim with their powerful tail.

The first aid, medical treatment and investigations are the same as for shark attack. Occasionally, a tooth fragment is found by x-ray examination of the wound.

OTHER BITING MARINE ANIMALS

Little space has been allocated to the other marine animals that are said to bite because it is difficult to find more than a few cases of a verified fatal bite on a human.

Barracuda

These fish inhabit tropical and subtropical waters, grow up to 3 metres long and swim fast (Figure 31.3). Barracuda have occasionally been known to attack, and they cause straight or V-shaped wounds. They are sometimes attracted by brightly coloured objects and lights, such as from diving at night.

Grouper

There have been reported cases of a grouper attacking a human, with death resulting. As a general rule, these heavyweight bulldogs of the sea have built up a reputation for friendliness more than forcefulness (Figure 31.4). They are, however, feared in some areas (e.g. the pearl-diving beds between New Guinea and Australia). These fish can act aggressively if speared.

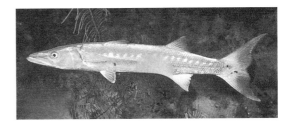

Figure 31.3 Barracuda.

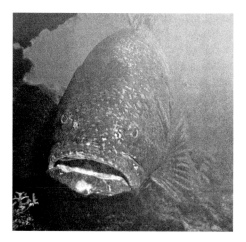

Figure 31.4 Grouper.

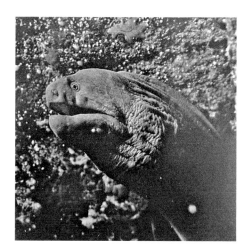

Figure 31.6 Moray eel.

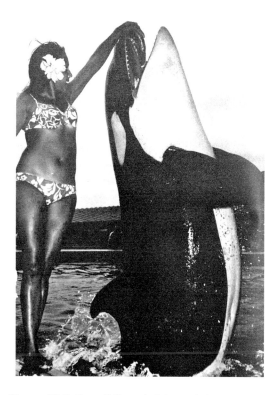

Figure 31.5 Orca (killer whale), on right.

Killer whale (orca)

This animal is the largest of the dolphin family and inhabits all oceans (Figure 31.5). It acquired its name from its tendency to travel in packs, feeding on other marine creatures such as seals, larger whales and so forth. Orcas shepherd prey into deep water and cause death by battering and drowning. Human injuries and fatalities have resulted from this mechanism, and this is no longer a relatively innocuous human predator.

Eel

Many eel attacks have been reported. Moray eels can grow up to 3 metres long and up to 30 centimetres in diameter (Figure 31.6). They occasionally attack without provocation, but an attack is usually precipitated by an intrusion into their domain, or after they have been injured or caught on lines or spear guns. Divers who feed the eels inadvertently encourage them to be more adventurous and less fearful, thus increasing the attack potential – for food. Certainly, once they do attack, they are likely to be difficult to dislodge and may even resume the attack after being dislodged. The wound is likely to be badly lacerated and heavily infected. The medical and surgical treatments conform to those normally used with other damaged and infected tissues.

Pinnipeds

Even the usually placid walrus, if sufficiently provoked by hunters, can retaliate with ferocity. The California sea lion and its Australian cousins have inflicted minor attacks on humans, usually after human intrusion into the breeding harems.

The more infamous *leopard seal* is a solitary animal in the Antarctic and cooler southern waters (Figure 31.7). It stalks penguins, seals and other warm-blooded prey, even humans. It swims above them until finally the prey has to surface to breathe. Then the leopard seal strikes. If a leopard seal is sighted, diving should be suspended. If underwater at the time of sighting, divers should not surface in mid-water, but follow the sea bed to the shore, before departing.

Biting fish

The piranha (*Serrasalmus* spp) have probably the worst reputation of all small fish, and although they are carnivorous and can be very ferocious and vicious, they do not deserve their very bad press. They are abundant in the rivers of South America, and most of the 20 or more species are harmless. They may grow to 45 centimetres, but some are only a couple of centimetres long. The black piranha and its relatives do cause concern. In sufficient numbers, they are believed to be able to remove the flesh from large animals within minutes. Although attacks on humans are rare, there are some well-documented cases from the Amazon.

Taylor fish or bluefish (*Pomatomus saltatrix*) also work in large schools and occasionally have caused injury to bathers. They commonly travel in large numbers along the East Coast of the United States and have been known to drive swimmers from the water in Miami, Florida. Fingers and toes can be badly injured and occasionally even amputated.

Spanish mackerel (*Scomberomorus maculatus*) in shoals have also occasionally attacked and injured swimmers. Other fish that are not commonly known to bite humans may do so under certain circumstances. The very beautiful and famous batfish (*Platax* spp) around Heron Island in the Great Barrier Reef, among many other diving destinations, are unfortunately fed by divers and, because of this, unpleasant nips may be inflicted on divers' exposed skin.

Most puffer fish (tetrodotoxic fish) are also able to inflict injury because their jaws are designed to crunch crustaceans. They are slow-swimming fish and therefore can be approached by divers, with occasional unfortunate results. One such fish, called Thomas the Terrible Toadfish, inflicted multiple injuries to waders, at Shute Harbour on the Great Barrier Reef. He attacked so many bathers' feet that he also became known as Thomas the Terrible Toe Fish.

ELECTRIC RAYS

These rays are slow and very ineffective swimmers, usually lying submerged in the mud or sand at shallow depths, in temperate climates (Figure 31.8). They can produce an electric discharge between 8 and 220 volts, and this is passed between the electrically negative underside of the ray and the positive topside. These animals are easily identified by thick electric organs on each side of the spine. The discharge is

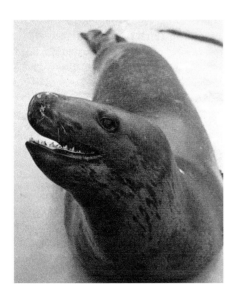

Figure 31.7 Leopard seal.

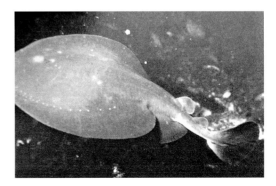

Figure 31.8 Electric ray.

automatic when the fish is touched, or even during an approach. There is then a latent period before the fish regains its full electrical potential. The electric discharge may well cause much amusement to other divers, but it can sometimes be disabling.

OCTOPUS AND SQUID

Octopoda, of the class Cephalopoda, have been the source of much folklore (Figure 31.9). Although most of these animals avoid human contact as much as possible, many of them are able to inflict significant bites, puncture wounds from the beak (mouth) or the modified claws on the tips of the tentacles of the giant squid. Other injuries have been produced by the sepia or ink, from the venom associated with salivary glands of the octopus and the animal's ability to adhere to and hold a swimmer or diver underwater, with the suction pads from the tentacles.

Although there has been a great deal of fantasy in some of the descriptions of octopus attacks, there have nevertheless been a dozen or so well-recorded episodes in which injury has occurred to humans. Attacks are known to this author, including one that resulted in the death of a diver. Most injuries follow the intrusion of the diver wielding a spear gun.

SWORDFISH AND SAWFISH

This group includes the swordfish, sailfish, marlin, garfish and sawfish.

There are documented cases of both death and injury from these fish. The trauma is caused by the saw or sword, which is an extension of the jaw. Even the smaller species, which can skim above the surface of the water, have caused many injuries to fishers. The garfish can sometimes ascend 2 metres above the sea level and are possibly attracted by lights used by fishers at night. The penetrating injuries from the relatively small spear-shaped jaws have resulted in both penetration of body cavities and injuries to the face and head.

Both sawfish and the swordfish achieve their damage by the use of their large appendage, in either an attacking or a defensive role. Occasional attacks have occurred underwater, in which case death is usually caused by blood loss. Other attacks have occurred after the fish has been caught and

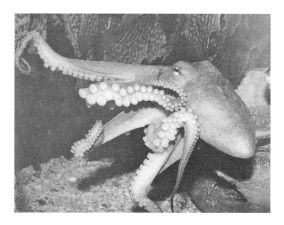

Figure 31.9 Octopus.

brought on board. This is commonly recorded by fishers trawling for marlin and swordfish.

FURTHER READING

Australian Shark Attack File. http://taronga. org.au/animals-conservation/conservation-science/australian-shark-attack-file/australian-shark-attack-file 2013.

Baldridge D. *Shark Attack*. USA: Berkley Pub Group, Penguin Books; 1975. Available from author: Box 1521б, Sarasota, FL 33579.

Coppleson V. *Shark Attack*. Sydney: Angus and Robertson; 1958.

Edmonds C. *Dangerous Marine Creatures*. Flagstaff, Arizona: Best Publishing; 1995.

Edwards H. *Crocodile Attack*. Adelaide, South Australia: J.B. Books; 1998.

International Shark Attack File. 2013. http://www. flmnh.ufl.edu/fish/sharks/isaf/isaf.htm

KwaZulu-Natal Sharks Board. 2013. www.shark. co.za

Myers RF, Bergbauer M, Kirschner M. *Dangerous Marine Animals*. London: Sea and Seashore Life Book Publishers; 2009.

Sutherland SK. *Australian Animal Toxins*. Melbourne: Oxford University Press; 1983.

US Navy Diving Manual. Appendix 5C. Hazardous Marine Creatures. Flagstaff, Arizona: Best Publishing; 2008.

This chapter was reviewed for this fifth edition by Carl Edmonds.

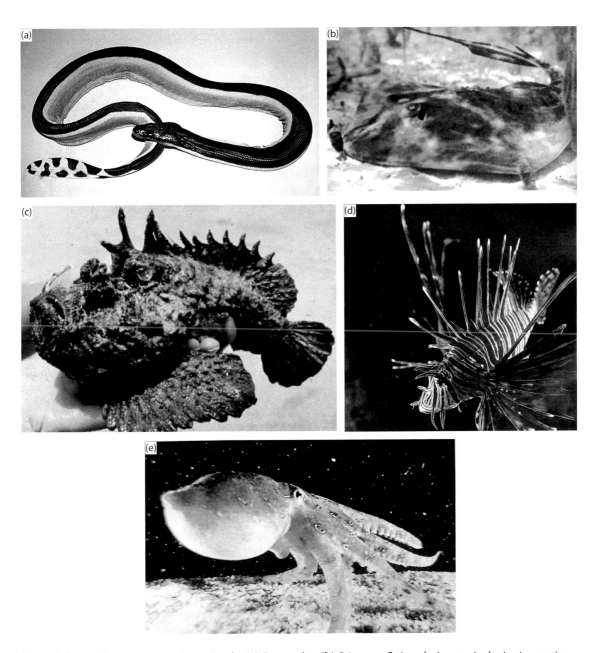

Plate 4, front. Dangerous marine animals. **(a)** Sea snake. **(b)** Stingray. Spine during typical stinging action. (Courtesy of Dr R. Thomas.) **(c)** Stonefish. (Courtesy of R. Taylor.) **(d)** Lion fish. (Courtesy of K. Gillett.) **(e)** Blue-ringed octopus. (Courtesy of K. Gillett.)

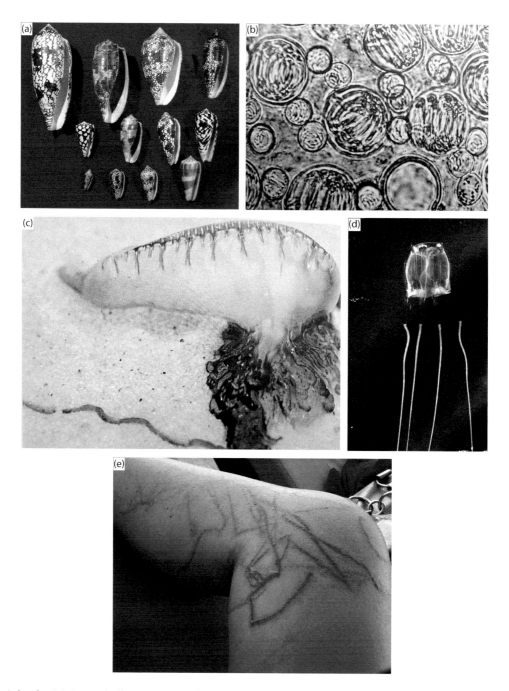

Plate 4, back. **(a)** Cone shells. (Courtesy of Dr R. Chesher.) **(b)** Nematocysts. The stinging cells of *Cnidaria* (jellyfish) with one discharged and empty (lower, right corner). (Courtesy of K. Gillett.) **(c)** Portuguese man-o'war (*Physalia* species). (Courtesy of K. Gillett.) **(d)** Irukandji. (Courtesy of K. Gillett.) **(e)** Large box jellyfish (chirodropid) stings, e.g. *Chironex*, Morbakka, showing lines delineating the tentacle contact. Erythema with nodules and vesicles produce a ladder pattern and later scarring.

32

Venomous marine animals*

PRESSURE BANDAGE IMMOBILIZATION

This important first aid method was developed in Australia in 1978. It was designed for envenomations that are not characteristically associated with a local inflammatory reaction (swelling, pain, erythema).

Some venoms, especially those with a higher molecular weight, are absorbed from the wound site by the lymphatic vessels before entering the circulation. The aim of this first aid treatment is to retard venom transport via the lymphatic system. This is achieved with a dual approach.

First, the lymphatic vessels at the bite site are compressed by firm but comfortable bandaging,

---

* Note: In this chapter, reference is made to traditional pharmaceuticals because these were the ones originally employed and assessed with these injuries. For example, diazepam may be mentioned in a situation in which current clinicians may prefer more modern anxiolytics. Whether the currently fashionable drugs are more appropriate, effective or safer may be contentious. Adhering to the original medications at least has the virtue that they will be still recognizable in a few years' time.

preferably with elastic or crepe bandage – but any cloth will do. This bandaging is then extended up then down to as much of the rest of the bitten limb as possible, preferably leaving the digits exposed to monitor circulation, and with the injury site marked on the bandage. Bandaging can be applied over clothing or over other bandaging. Second, proximal movement of lymph in the vessels is slowed or stopped by splinting and immobilizing the limb, and other body movement, thus reducing the 'muscle pump' effect of muscle contraction and lymph flow. Enclosing the affected upper limb in a sling, or strapping the affected lower limb to the opposite leg, may also reduce mobility. If the envenomation wound is not on a limb, a pressure pad and immobilization need to be instituted as far as possible.

Correctly applied, this technique can retard venom movement into the circulation until the bandage is removed, hours later. There is little threat to limb tissue oxygenation, which is just one of the major problems in using tourniquets with a similar intent.

There are two serious limitations to this technique. First, to prevent a tourniquet-like result, it should not be used if the venom is causing inflammation (swelling) under the bandage. Most of these inflammatory venoms (e.g. from fish stings and some land snake bites) localize themselves by inducing vaso-constriction, and the circulation should not be further compromised. Second, the technique merely delays the effect of the venom. It is not a definitive treatment in itself. It allows for the orderly transfer of the victim to hospital, where all the preparations for treatment, acquisition of antivenom, resuscitation and anti-allergy preparations are employed – before removal of the bandage.

In summary, the pressure bandage immobilization method of first aid is as follows:

- Apply a firm, broad elastic bandage or similar wrapping (even clothing or strips or pantyhose will do in an emergency) over the bite site, at the same pressure as employed for a muscle sprain. Do not occlude the circulation.
- Apply more bandage over as much of the rest of the bitten limb as practical. Ensure that fingers or toes are not covered. It is often prudent to

bandage over the top of clothing, such as jeans, rather than move the limb to remove clothing.
- Immobilize the limb and the patient. Ensure that the bitten limb is kept motionless by applying a splint and instructing the patient to cease all use of the limb, local muscle contracture and any general activity. Transport should come to the patient, not *vice versa*.

In marine envenomation, the pressure bandage immobilization technique is applicable to sea snake bites, and probably to blue-ringed octopus and cone shell envenomations, and it is not indicated for cnidarian injuries, fish stings, injuries from urchins or sponges or any minor injuries.

SEA SNAKE BITES

General information

The sea snake (family Hydrophiidae) is found in warmer waters of the Indo-Pacific and Red Sea. The subfamily Hydrophiinae, typified by the yellow-bellied sea snake, spends its life at sea. It has recently been observed in the Caribbean and so may be spreading from its Indo-Pacific habitat. It is a fish eater and thus needs a venom for capture of its prey. These snakes are efficient swimmers and are equipped with paddle-shaped tails for this reason. They can submerge for 2 hours. They are inquisitive, and sometimes aggressive, especially if handled or trodden on. They are attracted by fast-moving objects (e.g. divers being towed by a boat), and under these circumstances they can congregate and become troublesome. They are also caught in trawling nets, especially in the tropics. The other subfamily, Laticaudinae, comprises the banded sea snakes and spend their time between sea and land. Land snakes may also be found in the water, sometimes causing difficulty with identification. No land snake has the flattened tail.

Sea snake venom is 2 to 10 times as toxic as cobra venom, but sea snakes tend to deliver less of it, and only about one fourth of those bitten by sea snakes ever show signs of envenomation. There is sometimes reluctance to inject venom even when they do bite. Nevertheless, the venom able to be injected by one fresh adult sea snake of certain species is enough to kill three men. In most species the apparatus for delivering the venom is poorly developed even though the mouth can open widely, whereas in a few others the mouth is small and the snake has difficulty in obtaining a wide enough bite to pierce the clothing or any other protective layer. The bite causes little inflammatory response, and the current venom detection kit is not of value.

Sea snake venom appears to block neuromuscular transmission by acting on the post-synaptic membrane and may affect the motor nerve terminals. It blocks the effects of acetylcholine. Autopsy findings include patchy and selective necrosis of skeletal muscles, as well as tubular damage in the kidneys if the illness lasts longer than 48 hours.

Clinical features

An initial puncture at the time of biting is usually observed. Fang and teeth marks may vary from 1 to 20, but usually there are 4, and teeth may remain in the wound. After a latent period without symptoms, lasting from 10 minutes to several hours, generalized features develop in approximately one fourth of the cases. Pain and swelling are minor.

Mild symptoms include a psychological reaction such as euphoria, anxiety or restlessness. The major symptoms are paralysis or myolysis and are evident usually within the first 6 hours.

The tongue may feel thick. Thirst, dry throat, nausea and vomiting occasionally develop. Generalized stiffness and muscle aching may then supervene. If weakness does progress to paralysis, it is often the ascending Guillain-Barré type, with the legs involved an hour or so before the trunk, followed by the arms and neck. The other manifestation of paralysis is one that extends centrally from the area of the bite (e.g. from a bite on the hand to the forearm, arm, other arm, body and legs). Usually, the proximal muscle groups are the most affected, and trismus and ptosis are characteristic. Muscular twitching, writhing and spasms may be seen, and the patient may develop difficulty with speech and swallowing as the paralysis extends to the bulbar areas. Facial and ocular palsies then develop. Respiratory distress, from involvement of the diaphragm, may result in dyspnoea, cyanosis and finally death in a small number of the cases affected. Cardiac failure, convulsions and coma may be seen terminally.

Myoglobinuria may develop. When this is seen, one must consider the other possible effects of myonecrosis, namely acute renal failure with electrolyte and potassium changes, uraemia and aggravation of the muscular paralysis and weakness. This myonecrotic syndrome with renal failure usually supervenes on the other muscular paralysis and may thus prolong and aggravate this state. Coagulopathies are not characteristic of sea snake envenomation.

When recovery occurs, it is usually rapid and complete.

First aid

Current treatment is the use of the pressure bandage immobilization technique (see earlier).

Reassurance is needed, and exertion is to be avoided. The limb is immobilized, as is the patient. If possible, the snake (dead, to avoid further envenomations) should be retained for identification because although it may be harmless, the treatment certainly is not.

In the event of respiratory paralysis, artificial or mouth-to-mouth respiration may be required. Full cardiorespiratory resuscitation may be required in some cases.

Medical treatment

Once the patient is transported to adequate medical facilities, and the clinicians have reviewed and prepared the therapy indicated, the pressure bandage may be removed. Once this happens, the envenomation will have its effect on the patient, and then the treatment, including the antivenom regimen, can be instituted.

Apart from the foregoing first aid procedures, full cardiopulmonary resuscitation may be required. Fluid and electrolyte balance must be corrected, and acute renal failure is usually obvious from the oliguria, raised serum creatinine level and electrolyte changes. A high serum potassium level is particularly dangerous, and treatment by haemodialysis is then required. This may result in improvement in the muscular paralysis and the general clinical condition. The acute renal tubular necrosis and the myonecrosis are considered temporary, if life can be maintained.

Treatment may be necessary for the cardiovascular shock and convulsions.

Sea snake antivenom from the Australian Commonwealth Serum Laboratories (CSL) can be used cautiously in serious cases, with evidence of paralysis or myolysis. It contains 1000 units per ampoule. Care must be taken to administer it strictly in accordance with the directions in the current package. The antivenom can be dangerous to patients who are allergic to it. Emergency preparations for anaphylactic shock are required. Some authorities advise anti-allergy pre-treatment, although this is questionable unless special predispositions exist. The sea snake antivenom is composed of two antivenoms, and each has a very specific action. Unfortunately, although it does counter the most common sea snake venoms, there are others that are not covered. If sea snake antivenom is unavailable, tiger snake antivenom or polyvalent land snake antivenom could be used, although their value is not certain. Any antivenom can cause serum sickness for up to a fortnight later, and staff and patients need to be aware and prepared for this possibility.

Patients with sea snake bite should be hospitalized for 24 hours because of the delay in developing symptoms. Sedatives may be required, and it is reasonable to administer diazepam as required. This will assist in sedating the patient, without interfering significantly with respiration. Preparation for treatment of anaphylaxis should remain available.

Prevention

This is usually achieved by not handling sea snakes. It is suggested that the feet be shuffled when walking along a muddy sea bed, and that protective clothing be worn when underwater. The wetsuit is usually sufficient, and if a diver is collecting sea snakes, it is wise to use specialized sea snake tongs.

FISH STINGS

General information

Many fish have spines and a venom apparatus, usually for protection but occasionally for incapacitating their prey. Spines may be concealed, only becoming obvious when in use (e.g. stonefish or *Synanceia* species), or they may be highlighted as an apparent warning to predators (e.g. butterfly cod or firefish).

Some fish envenomations have resulted in death, especially by the stonefish and stingray. These are described separately. Others, such as the infamous scorpion fish and firefish (family Scorpaenidae), catfish (family Plotosidae and Ariidae) and stargazers (family Uranoscopidae), have also been responsible for occasional deaths in humans. As a general rule, fish that have been damaged (e.g. those from fishing nets) cause fewer problems clinically, probably because some of the envenomation system may have been previously triggered. However, even dead fish can be venomous when handled. Those wounds that bleed profusely are also less likely to cause intense symptoms. Some spines are inexplicably not associated with venom sacs.

Other fish may produce injury by their knife-like spines, which may or may not be venomous. Examples include old wife (family Enoplosidae), surgeonfish and unicorn fish (family Acanthuridae) and ratfish (family Chimaeridae).

Identification of the species of fish responsible is not always possible. Fortunately, there is not a great variety in the symptoms.

Clinical features

If venom is injected, the first symptom is usually local pain that increases in intensity over the next few minutes. It may become excruciating, but it usually lessens after a few hours ('with the change of the tide' – an old mariner's attempt at reassurance). The puncture wound is anaesthetized, but the surrounding area is hypersensitive. Pain and tenderness in the regional lymph glands may extend even more centrally to the abdomen or chest.

Locally, the appearance is that of one or more puncture wounds, with an inflamed and sometimes cyanotic zone around this wound. The surrounding area becomes pale and swollen, with pitting oedema.

Generalized symptoms are sometimes severe. The patient is often very distressed by the degree of pain, which is disproportionate to the clinical signs. This distress can merge into a delirious state. Malaise, nausea, vomiting and sweating may be associated with mild temperature elevation and leucocytosis. Respiratory distress may develop in severe cases. Occasionally, a cardiovascular shock state may supervene and cause death.

First aid

The patient should be laid down and reassured.

The affected area should be rested in an elevated position. Arrangements can then be made to immerse the wound in hot water (ideally up to 45°C, but no hotter than the patient can comfortably tolerate) for 30 to 90 minutes – or until the pain no longer recurs. As well as the wound, some normal skin, from victim and rescuer, must also be tested in the hot water to ensure that scalding is not induced. The injured skin may well be hypoaesthetic, or the pain relief from the hot solution may seem preferable to the pain from the scalding – and thus not give adequate warning of this danger. The wound should be washed and cleaned.

Fishers often make a small incision across the wound and parallel to the long axis of the limb, to encourage mild bleeding and relieve pain if other methods are not available.

First aid treatment of fish stings (venom injected by spine):

- Lay the patient down with the affected limb elevated.
- Wash the surface venom away and gently remove the spine or integument if present.
- Immersion in hot water (up to 45°C) will reduce the pain. The rescuer should test the temperature on himself or herself first and also include normal skin of the victim, to avoid scalding.
- Inject local anaesthetic (without adrenaline) into and around the wound.
- Clean the wound. Apply local antiseptic or local antibiotic.

Medical treatment

This treatment includes first aid, as described earlier. Local anaesthetic, e.g. 5 ml of 1% lidocaine without adrenaline (epinephrine), if injected through the puncture wound, will give considerable relief. It may

need to be repeated every 30 to 60 minutes. Local or regional anaesthetic blocks may also be of value.

Symptomatic treatment may be needed for generalized symptoms of cardiogenic shock or respiratory depression. Systemic analgesics or narcotics are rarely needed; however, they may be of value in severe cases. Symptomatic treatment is given for the other clinical features present.

Exploration, débridement and cleansing of the wound, with removal of any broken spines or their integument, are best followed by the application of local antibiotic such as neomycin or bacitracin. Tetanus prophylaxis may be indicated. Broad-spectrum antibiotics (e.g. doxycycline) may be needed if the infection spreads, as may occur with delayed cleansing.

Stonefish antivenom (see later) is approved only for *Synanceia* species, but it is currently also being applied for difficult cases of other Scorpaenidae species.

The basic physiological signs (e.g. temperature, pulse and respiration; blood pressure [BP]; central venous pressure [CVP]; urine output), serum electrolytes, blood gases, electroencephalogram and electrocardiogram are monitored if indicated. For serious or extensive lesions, a soft tissue x-ray study, ultrasound examination or magnetic resonance imaging scan may be needed to demonstrate foreign body or bone injury.

A recurrence of symptoms 1 to 2 weeks after the injury usually indicates a foreign body reaction (treated by excision of the irritant) or an infection (treated by antibiotics).

Stonefish

GENERAL INFORMATION

This fish grows to about 30 cm in length and is usually in warm tropical and subtropical waters. It lies dormant in the shallows, buried in sand, mud, coral or rocks, and is practically indistinguishable from the surroundings. The 13 erectile dorsal spines, capable of piercing a sandshoe, are covered by loose skin or integument. When pressure is applied over them, they become erect, and two venom glands discharge along ducts on each spine, into the penetrating wound. The fish may live for many hours out of the water.

The venom is an unstable protein, with a pH of 6.0 and a molecular weight of 150 000. It produces an intense vaso-constriction, and therefore it tends to localize itself. It is destroyed by heat, alkalis and acids. The toxin is multi-component with neurotoxic, myotoxic, cardiotoxic and cytotoxic properties. It causes muscular paralysis, respiratory depression, peripheral vasodilation, shock and cardiac arrest. It is also capable of producing cardiac dysrhythmias.

Each spine has 5 to 10 mg of venom associated with it, and this venom is said to be neutralized by 1 ml antivenom from the Australian CSL. Occasionally, a stonefish spine may have no venom associated with it. It is thought that the venom is regenerated very slowly, if at all.

CLINICAL FEATURES

Whether the local or generalized symptoms predominate seems to depend on many factors, such as the geographical locality, number of spines involved, protective covering, previous stings, and first aid treatment, among other factors.

Local

Immediate pain is noted. This increases in severity over the ensuing 10 minutes or more. The pain, which is excruciating in severity, may be sufficient in some patients to cause unconsciousness and thus drowning. Ischaemia of the area is followed by cyanosis, which is probably caused by local circulatory stasis. The area becomes swollen and oedematous, often hot, with numbness in the centre and extreme tenderness around the periphery. The oedema and swelling may become quite gross, extending up the limb. Paralysis of the adjacent muscles is said to immobilize the limb, as may pain.

The pain is likely to spread proximally to the regional lymph glands (e.g. axilla or groin). Both the pain and the other signs of inflammation may last for many days. Necrosis and ulceration can persist for many months.

General

Signs of mild cardiovascular collapse are not uncommon. Pallor, sweating, hypotension and syncope on standing may be present. Respiratory failure may result from haemorrhagic pulmonary oedema, depression of the respiratory centre,

cardiac failure and/or paralysis of the respiratory musculature. Bradycardia, cardiac dysrhythmias and cardiac arrest are also possible.

Malaise, exhaustion, fever and shivering may progress to delirium, lack of co-ordination, generalized paralysis, convulsions and death. Convalescence may take many months, and it may be characterized by periods of malaise and nausea.

TREATMENT

See the previous discussion of first aid and medical treatment for fish stings. Stonefish antivenom is approved only for *Synanceia* species, but is currently also being applied for difficult cases of other Scorpaenidae species.

Stonefish antivenom may be administered with 1 ml neutralizing 10 mg of venom (i.e. the venom from one spine). Follow the directions in the CSL product statement inclusion. Anti-allergy preparations should be taken. Further doses can be given if required, but this antivenom should never be given to people with horse serum allergy. It should be protected from light and stored between 0°C and 5°C, but not frozen. It should be used immediately on opening.

Systemic analgesics and narcotics are seldom indicated or useful, although intravenous narcotics are sometimes used. Tetanus prophylaxis is recommended. Systemic antibiotics may be used because secondary infection is likely. Débridement should be considered if significant tissue damage and necrosis are present, or if foreign material could be left in the wound.

Appropriate resuscitation techniques may have to be applied. These include endotracheal intubation with controlled respiration, chest compressions and defibrillation. Monitoring procedures may need to include records of clinical state (pulse, respiration), BP, CVP, pulse oximetry, electrocardiogram, lung function tests, arterial gases and pH. Clinical complications of bulbar paralysis should be treated as they arise.

PREVENTION

One should wear thick-soled shoes when in dangerous areas and be particularly careful on coral reefs and while entering or leaving boats. A stonefish sting is said to confer some degree of immunity for future episodes.

Stingrays

GENERAL INFORMATION

This vertebrate lies in the sand, and the unwary victim may tread on its dorsal surface or dive over it. As a response to this pressure, the stingray swings its tail upward and forward, driving the spine into the limb (usually the ankle) or body of the victim. An integument over the serrated spine is ruptured. Venom escapes and passes along grooves into the perforated wound. Extraction of the spine results in a laceration caused by the serrations and retro-pointed barbs, and it may leave fragments of spine or sheath within the wound.

The venom is a protein (molecular weight greater than 100 000) heat labile, water soluble and with an intravenous median lethal dose (LD_{50}) of 28.0 mg/kg body weight. Low concentrations cause electrocardiographic effects of increased PR intervals associated with bradycardia. A first-degree atrio-ventricular block may occur with mild hypotension. Larger doses produce vaso-constriction, second- and third-degree atrio-ventricular block and signs of cardiac ischaemia. Most cardiac changes are reversible within 24 hours. Some degree of respiratory depression is noted with greater amounts of venom. This is probably secondary to the neurotoxic effect of the venom on the medullary centres. Convulsions may also occur.

Fishers who handle these fish in nets are less seriously affected because the integumentary sheath is probably already damaged.

CLINICAL FEATURES

Local

Wounds may be lacerations with haemorrhage or punctures with pain, or a mixture. Pain is usually immediate and is the predominant symptom, increasing over 1 to 2 hours and easing after 6 to 10 hours, but it may persist for some days. The pain may be constant, pulsating or stabbing. Bleeding may be profuse and may relieve the pain. A mucoid secretion may follow. Integument from the spine may be visible in the puncture wound, which may gape and extend for a few centimetres in length. The area is swollen and pale, with a bluish rim, centimetres in width, spreading around the wound after an hour or two. Local necrosis, ulceration and secondary infection are common and if unchecked may cause incapacity for many months. Osteomyelitis in the underlying bone is a possible complication.

Aggravation of pain and inflammation within days may be caused by secondary infection, whereas aggravation after a week is usually the result of a retained foreign body.

General

The following manifestations have been noted: anorexia, nausea, vomiting, diarrhoea, frequent micturition and salivation. There is extension of pain to the area of lymphatic drainage. Muscular cramp, tremor and tonic paralysis may occur in the affected limb or may be more generalized. Syncope, palpitations, hypotension, cardiac irregularities (conduction abnormalities, blocks) and ischaemia are possible. Respiratory depression may occur, with difficulty in breathing, cough and pain on inspiration. Other features include nocturnal pyrexia with copious sweating, nervousness, confusion or delirium.

The symptoms may last from hours (the venom effect) to many months (a foreign body and/or infection).

Fatalities have occurred, especially if the spine perforates the pericardial, peritoneal or pleural cavities. Death may result from the envenomation (cardiac arrhythmias), trauma, haemorrhage or delayed tissue necrosis and infection.

TREATMENT

See the earlier discussion of first aid and medical treatment for fish stings.

The special problems of penetration of body cavities and immediate and delayed haemorrhage must be monitored with stingray injuries. Delayed problems are frequent.

PREVENTION

Divers are advised to shuffle the feet when walking in the water. This gives the ray time to remove itself – which it cannot do with a foot on its dorsum. Although wearing rubber boots decreases the severity of the sting, the spine penetrates most protective material. Care is needed when handling fishing nets and when diving under ledges.

CNIDARIAN INJURIES

General information, including Portuguese man o' war

Cnidaria is a phylum of 9000 species containing jellyfish, sea anemones, fire coral, stinging hydroids among others. It constitutes one of the lowest orders of the animal kingdom and has members that are dissimilar in general appearance and mobility.

The common factor among the cnidarians (also called coelenterates) is the development of many nematocysts or stinging capsules. These capsules are of two types – one that adheres to the animal's prey, either by sticky mucus or by a coiled spring; and the other that acts as a needle, penetrating the prey and discharging venom into it. This may be as long as 0.5 mm. The triggering mechanism that is responsible for the discharge of the nematocyst is thought to be initiated by many factors – such as trauma or the absorption of fresh water into the nematocyst capsule, thus causing it to swell.

The functions of the nematocysts are to incapacitate and retain prey, which is food for the Cnidaria. The nematocysts of different types of Cnidaria may be identifiable and therefore of value in the differential diagnosis of marine stings. In some centres, serological and immunological tests may also be available to identify different species. Nematocysts may be removed from the skin by the use of transparent adhesive tape, for later identification.

There may be a characteristic pattern of nematocyst stings, depending on their aggregation on the tentacle of the Cnidaria and on the morphology of the tentacles. Thus, the *Portuguese man o' war* (often called the *bluebottle*) usually produces a single, long strap with small blisters along it. The *mauve stinger* has two to four short red lines. The *Chironex* has multiple long, red lines, often with the tentacle adherent because of a thick, sticky substance, when the patient is first seen. *Stinging hydroids* and *fire coral,* being non-mobile, sting only when touched by the diver.

Clinical factors may vary from a mild itch locally, to severe systemic reactions, to allergic responses and to death. The local symptoms vary from a prickly or stinging sensation developing immediately on contact to a burning or throbbing pain. The intensity increases over 10 minutes or so, and the erythema may develop papules, vesicles or even pustules, with necrotic ulcers in severe cases. The pain may spread centrally, with lymphadenopathy, and may be associated with abdominal and chest pain.

Generalized symptoms include fever, increased secretions, gastrointestinal disorders, cardiovascular failure, respiratory distress and signs of a toxic-confusional state.

The intensity of both local and generalized manifestations of Cnidaria stinging may vary according to the following: the species involved (*Chironex* is often lethal, whereas the blubber jellyfish can often be handled with impunity); the extent of the area involved; the body weight of the victim, with injury more severe in children than in adults; thickness of the skin in contact; and individual idiosyncrasies such as allergic reactions, pre-existing cardiorespiratory disease and other conditions. Because the most dangerous Cnidaria is the *Chironex,* this genus is dealt with in detail. The *Portuguese man o' war* or bluebottle *(Physalia)* sting is one of the most common problems encountered by bathers.

First aid treatments have been based on the use of empirical and fashionable treatments, such as vinegar, dehydrating agents (alcohols) or denaturing agents (acetic acid, ammonia, papaine in meat tenderizers) to reduce the discharge of further nematocysts. Some of these treatments have triggered nematocyst discharge and aggravated the symptoms.

Current treatments include the gentle removal of tentacles, washing with sea water and possibly hot water soaks (up to 45°C, as described for fish stings – see earlier). The use of anti-burn preparations and cold packs and the application of local anaesthetic ointments and steroids to reduce symptoms of pain or itch, respectively, have all been employed. A 50 per cent water, 50 per cent baking soda combination has been proposed. The heat treatment (up to 45°C) is the currently fashionable first aid, although it has not been demonstrated for all Cnidaria, and it is applied for as long as necessary to reduce pain (usually about 20 minutes).

Prevention of Cnidaria stings is achieved by not swimming in areas they inhabit, by using some water-repellent sunscreens and by wearing a protective suit, such as the Lycra suits or 'stinger suits'. The reason most cnidarians do not injure humans is that the nematocyst is incapable of penetrating the depth of skin necessary to cause symptoms. Variations of this mode of injury occur in four instances:

1. *Direct entry.* Coral cuts are often experienced in the tropics, and in these cases there is a laceration of the skin that allows nematocysts to discharge directly into the wound tissues. This is supplemented by a foreign body reaction to the nematocysts, coral pieces and organisms. Pacific Islanders once spread cnidarians over their spears for greater effect.
2. *Nudibranchs,* especially the *Glaucus,* ingest certain cnidarians and use their nematocysts for their own purposes. This means that humans who come in contact with these nudibranchs may then sustain an injury having a distribution that corresponds to the area of contact with the nudibranch.
3. *Ingestion and inhalation.* Allergy and anaphylaxis may develop from contact, inhalation or ingestion. Some cnidarians are poisonous to eat.
4. *Irukandji.* Some jellyfish produce a minimal sting but inject a toxin that causes severe generalized muscular spasms, especially affecting the large muscle masses of the spine and abdomen, up to 2 hours later (discussed later in this chapter).

Chironex (box jellyfish, sea wasp)

GENERAL INFORMATION

These large cnidarians, called Cubomedusae, *Chironex fleckeri,* are restricted to the warm waters of the Indo-Pacific region. Fatalities are more numerous in the waters off Northern Australia. Related species of chirodropids may be found in other tropical areas, such as the Indo-Pacific equatorial waters and the Middle East.

Chironex is said to be the most venomous marine animal known. It is especially dangerous to children and patients with cardiorespiratory disorders (patients with asthma and coronary artery disease). Its box-shaped body can measure 20 cm along each side, and it has up to 15 tentacles measuring up to 3 metres in length on each of its 4 pedalia. The animal is usually small at the beginning of the monsoon or hot season, and it increases in size and toxicity as it matures during this season. It is especially found after bad weather and on cloudy days, when it moves into more shallow water. It is almost invisible in its natural habitat, being pale blue and transparent. It tends to avoid noise, such as in harbours with motor boats and near the turbulence of surf – but this should not be relied upon. It is actively mobile, but it often drifts with the wind and tide when near the surface.

The severity of the sting increases with the size of the animal, the extent of contact with the victim and the delicacy of the victim's skin. Deaths have occurred with as little contact as 6 to 7 metres of tentacle, in adults – and much less in children. Adjacent swimmers may also be affected to a variable degree. The tentacles tend to adhere with a sticky, jelly-like substance. They can usually be removed by bystanders because of the protection afforded by the thick skin on the palmar aspect of their hands. This protection is not always complete, and stinging can occur even through surgical gloves.

TOXIN

The venom is made up of lethal, dermatonecrotic and haemolytic fractions with specific antigens, and cross-immunity probably does not develop to other species. The effects on the cardiovascular system include an initial rise in arterial pressure that is followed by hypotensive-hypertensive oscillations. The hypotensive states are associated with bradycardia, cardiac irregularities (especially delay in atrio-ventricular conduction), apnoea and these oscillating arterial pressures. The cardiovascular effects are caused by cardiotoxicity, brainstem depression and/or baroreceptor stimulation (a vasomotor reflex feedback system). Ventricular fibrillation or asystole precedes cerebral death. Only a few stinging incidents, about 2 per cent, result in death.

Clinical features

The patient usually screams as a result of the excruciating pain, occurring immediately on contact, and increasing in intensity, often coming in waves. The patient then claws at the adherent tentacles (whitish strings surrounded by a transparent jelly). He or she may become confused, act irrationally or lose consciousness and may drown because of this.

> *Chironex* stings are excruciatingly painful and potentially fatal.

Local

Multiple interlacing whiplash lines – red, purple or brown – 0.5 cm wide, develop within seconds. The markings are in a 'beaded' or 'ladder' pattern and are quite characteristic. These acute changes last for some hours. They are also described as transverse wheals. If death occurs, the skin markings fade. If the patient survives, the red, swollen skin may develop large wheals, and, after 7 to 10 days, necrosis and ulceration develop over the area of contact. The skin lesions may take many months to heal if deep ulceration occurs. Itching may also be troublesome and recurrent. Pigmentation and scarring at the site of these lesions may be permanent.

General

Excruciating pain dominates the clinical picture, whereas impairment of consciousness may lead to coma and death. The pain diminishes in 4 to 12 hours. Amnesia occurs for most of the incident following the sting. If death occurs, it usually does so within the first 10 minutes; survival is likely after the first hour.

Cardiovascular effects dominate the generalized manifestations. The patient may develop cardiac shock, appearing cold and clammy with a rapid pulse, disturbance of consciousness, hypotension, tachycardia and raised venous pressure. The cardiac state may oscillate within minutes from episodes of hypertension, tachycardia, rapid respirations and normal venous pressure to hypotension, bradycardia, apnoea and elevated venous pressure. The oscillation may give a false impression of improvement just before the patient's death.

Respiratory distress, cyanosis, pulmonary congestion and oedema may be caused by the cardiac effects or by direct midbrain depression. Paralysis and abdominal pains may occur. Malaise and restlessness may persist, with physical convalescence requiring up to a week. Irritability and difficulty with psychological adjustment may take weeks or months to disappear. Immunity to the sting is said to occur following repeated and recent contacts, although it is likely that the cross-immunity among the species is incomplete or absent.

TREATMENT

First aid

Prevent drowning. Apply copious quantities of vinegar to reduce the likelihood of discharge of previously undischarged nematocysts. This should be done for at least 30 seconds. This may be repeated. Remove the tentacles with their undischarged nematocysts. Do this gently but quickly, pulling in one direction only. Rough handling or rubbing will cause further nematocysts discharge. Some researchers are concerned that even vinegar could increase venom discharge from partly triggered nematocysts; however, vinegar is one of the few substances that can inactivate nematocysts.

If vinegar is not available, other materials may be of value, but there is much conflict over which substances may aggravate the condition. Local remedies, such as lemon or lime juice, have yet to be evaluated, but it is possible that stale wine or even Coca-Cola, applied locally, may reduce the nematocyst discharge. Water warmer than 43°C is being considered for this purpose, as is topical lidocaine, but validation of the effectiveness of these approaches are still awaited.

Pressure bandage immobilization was proposed by some authorities as a way of reducing venom absorption, but most experts have been more circumspect – observing that it could result in pressure trauma inducing extra nematocyst discharge and increased concentration of the venom. It is not recommended.

Cardiopulmonary resuscitation may be required. It should be continued and reapplied whenever there is any deterioration in the patient's cardiorespiratory status. Do not assume because there is initial improvement that the patient will not have a relapse.

Treatment of *Chironex* sting:

- Rescue the patient from the water.
- Apply vinegar in copious quantities, before gently removing the tentacles.
- Perform artificial respiration and external chest compressions as required.
- Administer box jellyfish antivenom, if available.
- Apply local anaesthetic ointment.
- Administer intravenous narcotics or general anaesthesia.
- Use steroids.

Medical treatment

Intermittent positive pressure respiration, possibly with oxygen, replaces mouth-to-mouth artificial respiration, if needed. This will require constant attention because of the varying degree of respiratory depression. General anaesthesia with endotracheal intubation and controlled respiration is needed if analgesia cannot otherwise be obtained.

Local applications include lidocaine or other local anaesthetic ointment. This may assist even after the first few minutes, during which time the traditional vinegar is believed to be of prophylactic value. Analgesics include morphine 15 mg or pethidine (Demerol) 100 mg, intravenously in divided doses. This may also protect against shock.

Hydrocortisone 100 mg is administered intravenously every 2 hours if needed. Local steroid preparations are valuable for treating dermal manifestations such as swelling, pain and itching.

Chlorpromazine 100 mg intramuscularly, or diazepam 10 mg intravenously, or their more contemporary equivalents, may be of value after the immediate resuscitation because they assist in sedating and tranquilizing the patient without causing significant respiratory depression. Other drugs may be used but are unproven in this clinical disorder. These include noradrenaline (Levophed) or isoprenaline (Isuprel) drips for hypotension, respiratory or cardiac stimulants, verapamil and others. Continuous electrocardiographic monitoring is indicated, as are pulse rate, BP, CVP, respiratory rate, arterial gases, pulse oximetry and pH levels. External cardiac massage and defibrillation are performed if required.

Chironex (box jellyfish) antivenom has been developed by the Australian CSL and is derived from the serum of hyper-immunized sheep. It is of value against both the local and general manifestations, but it is specifically of value for life-threatening cardiac or respiratory manifestations. One to three vials, possibly with magnesium sulphate, are injected intravenously over 5 to 15 minutes, or as varied and directed by the CSL product literature enclosed with the antivenom.

PREVENTION

Prevention includes the wearing of adequate protective clothing (e.g. overalls, wetsuits, Lycra or body stockings). One should restrict swimming or wading to the safe months of the year. Care is especially needed on cloudy days toward the end of the hot season. Dragging a section of a beach with 2.5-cm mesh has been used, not very successfully, to clear an area for bathing. Information should be sought about the prevalence of dangerous cubozoans in the area. In some places, this important information is withheld by tour operators, and even some government bodies, to facilitate tourism,

Irukandji syndrome

Some jellyfish produce a minimal or negligible sting, but they inject a toxin that causes a catecholamine storm, with cardiovascular manifestations and severe generalized muscular spasms, especially affecting the large muscle masses of the spine and abdomen, up to 1 to 2 hours after the sting. Because of the latent period, the relationship may not be realized, and diagnostic problems arise. Although the Irukandji syndrome has mainly been reported from the tropical and subtropical parts of the Indo-Pacific, especially Northern Australia, Malaysia and Thailand, it occurs in other areas (e.g. other Indo-Pacific Islands, Florida, Hawaii, West Indies, Caribbean [Bonaire]) and from other jellyfish or marine animals.

The name Irukandji was given by Dr Flecker, from a local aboriginal tribe living near Cairns, Australia, where the injury was first described. Similar clinical syndromes have now been reported from many other warm water areas throughout the world. In 1964, another Cairns physician identified the common cause of the syndrome in that area, and it was a small box jellyfish, now known as *Carukia barnesi*.

This animal is rarely observed by the victim, although the stinging may occur near the surface and in either deep or shallow waters. It is traditionally a small box jellyfish with a transparent body about 1 to 2 cm long and with four tentacles varying from a few centimetres up to 1 metre in length, depending on the degree of contraction. Nematocysts, appearing as clumps of minute red dots, are distributed over the body and tentacles. The delayed injury is proportional to the duration, extent and location of the sting.

Similar clinical symptoms may accompany stings from many other cnidarians, especially other carybdeids such as the *Morbakka* – commonly found in Thailand and that also cause substantial pain and morbidity. Similar symptoms have been associated with other cnidarians, and the Irukandji syndrome has even been confused with decompression sickness in divers.

Stinging incidents occur in clusters in the same locality, often in late summer, where clear warm ocean waters approach the land. Others occur well out to sea, in depths of 10 to 20 metres, and so they are a frequent concern to pearl divers.

CLINICAL FEATURES
Local

A few seconds after contact, a stinging sensation may be felt. This sensation increases in intensity for a few minutes and diminishes during the next half hour. It is usually sufficient to cause children to cry and adults to leave the water, but it may be much less noticeable. It may recur at the commencement of the generalized symptoms but is overshadowed by them.

In the Australian context, where *Carukia barnesi* and *Malo kingi* are commonly incriminated, a red reaction 5 to 7 cm in diameter surrounds the area of contact within 5 minutes. Small papules appear and reach their maximum in 20 minutes, before subsiding. 'Kissing' lesions occur, where the original skin lesion comes into contact with other skin, for example, near joints. The red colouration can occasionally last up to 3 hours, and there is a dyshidrotic reaction (skin dry at first, with excessive sweating later) over

the area. Occasionally, in severe cases the area may remain swollen for many hours. Other variations in local reactions can result from different Irukandji-inducing cnidarians.

There is usually a latent period of 5 to 120 minutes between contact and the development of generalized symptoms. The patient may not relate these symptoms to the local reaction unless specifically questioned about this.

General

Pain usually dominates the clinical presentation. Abdominal pains, sometimes severe and associated with spasm and board-like rigidity of the abdominal wall, often come in waves. Muscular aches such as cramps and dull boring pains occur, with increased tone and muscle tenderness on examination. This especially involves the spine, but it also involves hips, shoulders, limbs and chest. Headache may also be severe.

Profuse sweating, anxiety, a sensation of doom and restlessness may develop, as may retching, nausea and vomiting.

Respiratory distress with coughing may be associated with grunts preceding exhalations. Pulmonary oedema has been described, usually many hours after the stinging, and it may be indicated by radiology or screening, blood gases and troponin estimations. There may be increased BP and pulse rate, with possible arrhythmias and even cerebral haemorrhage from the venom-induced catecholamine release.

Later symptoms include numbness and tingling, itching, smarting eyes, sneezing, joint and nerve pains, weakness, rigors, dry mouth and headache. Temperature usually remains normal.

Symptoms diminish or cease within 4 to 12 hours. Occasionally, malaise and distress may persist, and convalescence may take up to a week.

PREVENTION

One should wear protective clothing (e.g. wetsuits, Lycra). Once stinging incidents have been reported in an area, immersion should be avoided.

FIRST AID

It is commonly recommended that the copious use of local applied vinegar for at least a minute may reduce subsequent discharge of nematocysts.

Others disagree and use hot water (45°C, as described earlier) to denature the venom protein. The delay between stinging and development of symptoms may make either approach problematic but probably will cause no harm.

The use of compression bandages has been recommended by some people, but this is contentious. The concern is that these bandages may themselves traumatize the nematocysts and increase their discharge rate. Immobilization seems prudent.

MEDICAL TREATMENT

1. During the severe phase with abdominal pains, spasms and coughing, opioids in increasing doses may be required. Fentanyl, pethidine and morphine have been effective.
2. Promethazine, with an intravenous dose of 0.5 mg/kg, to a maximum of 25 mg, not only reduces the symptoms of nausea and vomiting, but also reduces the subsequent amount of narcotic required.
3. Alpha blockers have been recommended for the control of hypertension, as a result of catecholamine release. Phentolamine may be given as a bolus dose and subsequent infusion (1 to 5 mg initially and 5 to 10 mg/hour). Hydralazine has also been used. Deaths have occurred from cerebral haemorrhage following the venom-induced catecholamine storm.
4. Other medications that have been used include diazepam and antihistamines. Magnesium sulphate infusions have been employed by some physicians and denigrated by others. General anaesthesia with assisted respiration could be used if the conventional techniques prove insufficient.
5. Monitoring of fluid and electrolyte status, together with cardiorespiratory parameters, would seem indicated. Pulmonary oedema has been treated with intubation and controlled ventilation, high inspiratory oxygen and positive end expiratory pressure.
6. Attention must be paid to the possibility of pulmonary oedema development. Any patient who has required narcotics or has other indications of significant envenomation should be investigated with chest radiology or scanning, electrocardiography and echocardiography, blood gases and troponin estimations because of this risk.
7. During the latter part of the illness, when only fleeting neuralgic and arthralgic symptoms predominate, simple analgesics may be effective.

The following recommendations, devised by Little and Mulcahy, appear reasonable:

If there are only local symptoms, treat symptomatically and observe for 2 hours. Observe until the victim is asymptomatic, and if no medication is needed for 6 hours, then discharge the patient with the advice to return to the emergency department if symptoms recur.

If systemic symptoms develop at any time, then admit the victim to hospital, give intravenous promethazine 0.5 mg/kg (maximum, 25 mg). Add intravenous pethidine (0.25 to 0.5 mg/kg) every 5 minutes if required. If more than 2 mg/kg pethidine is required, then check the creatine kinase, urea and electrolyte levels, and perform a full blood count.

If further analgesia is required, give fentanyl 0.5 mcg/kg and observe closely. This may be repeated. A chest x-ray study or computed tomography scan should be performed with electrocardiography and echocardiography considered. If signs or symptoms of pulmonary oedema develop (which may occur after 10 to 12 hours), then repeat the creatine kinase determination and admit the patient to a coronary care or intensive care unit.

CONE SHELL STINGS

General information

These attractive univalve molluscs are highly favoured by shell collectors of the tropics and warm temperate regions. They have a proboscis extendible from the narrow end, which is able to reach most of the shell. Holding the shell even by the 'big end' may not be safe and may court a sting with a resultant 25 per cent mortality rate. The cone shell inhabits shallow waters, reefs, ponds and rubble. Its length is usually up to 10 cm. It has a siphon, sometimes ringed with orange, that detects its prey and may be the only part visible if the cone burrows under the sand. The proboscis, which delivers the *coup de grace,* carries 1 to 10 radular teeth that penetrate and inject venom into its prey and thus immobilize the victim.

Probably only the fish-eating cones are dangerous to humans, but because these are difficult to distinguish at first sight, discretion is recommended. The venom is composed of two or more substances. One interferes with the neuromuscular activity and elicits a sustained painful muscular contracture; the other causes paralysis by abolishing the excitability of muscle fibres and summates with tubocurare, but it is uninfluenced by eserine. The major effect appears to be directly on skeletal muscular activity. Children are particularly vulnerable.

> Cone shell venom causes skeletal muscle paresis or paralysis, with or without myalgia.

Clinical features

LOCAL

The initial puncture effects may vary from painless to excruciating pain and may be aggravated by salt water. The wound may become inflamed and swollen, sometimes pale and ischaemic, with a cyanotic area surrounding it, and it may be numb to touch.

GENERAL

Numbness and tingling may ascend from the bite to involve the whole body, and especially the mouth and lips. This may take 5 to 10 minutes to develop. Skeletal muscular paralysis may spread from the site of injury and may result in anything from mild weariness to complete flaccid paralysis. Difficulty with swallowing and speech may precede total paralysis. Visual disturbances may include double and blurred vision (paralysis of voluntary muscles and pupillary reactions). These changes may take place within 10 to 30 minutes of the bite. Respiratory paralysis may dominate the clinical picture. This results in shallow, rapid breathing and a cyanotic appearance, proceeding to apnoea, unconsciousness and death. Other cases are said to

result in cardiac failure, although this is probably secondary to the respiratory paralysis. The extent of neurotoxic damage is variable. If the patient survives, he or she will be active and mobile within 24 hours. Neurological sequelae and the local reaction may last many weeks.

Treatment

FIRST AID

The following recommendations are made, depending on the presence of paralysis.

Without paralysis

The limb can be immobilized and a pressure bandage applied rapidly to reduce the speed of venom absorption. The patient should be rested and reassured until he or she is transported to an intensive care unit and the pressure bandage is removed.

With paralysis

Mouth-to-mouth respiration, or other supportive ventilation, may be needed. This may have to be continued for hours or until medical facilities are reached. This artificial respiration is the major contributor to saving the patient's life.

Cardiopulmonary resuscitation is needed if the patient has neither pulse nor respiration. The patient may be able to hear but not communicate and thus requires reassurance. If the patient is in shock, ensure that he or she is lying down with the feet elevated.

MEDICAL TREATMENT

With respiratory paralysis, administer artificial respiration with intermittent positive pressure adequate to maintain normal arterial gases and pH. Endotracheal intubation or insertion of a laryngeal mask prevents aspiration of vomitus and facilitates tracheo-bronchial toilet, when indicated. Routine care and management of the unconscious patient are required. Chest compression, defibrillation, vasopressors and so forth may be indicated by the clinical state and electrocardiogram. Local anaesthetic can be injected into the wound, to relieve local pain. Respiratory stimulants and drugs used against neuromuscular blockade are not indicated.

Prevention

The people at risk (e.g. shell collectors, visitors to the reefs in tropical and sub-tropical areas, school children) need to be educated about this danger. They should avoid contact with the cone shell. Probably no part of it can be touched with impunity, unless the animal is dead. Despite advice to the contrary, touching the 'big end' is not always safe. If these shells must be collected, it is advisable to use forceps and a tough receptacle.

BLUE-RINGED OCTOPUS BITES

General information

This animal usually weighs 10 to 100 g and is currently recognized mainly in the Australasian and Indo-Pacific region. Its span, with tentacles extended, is from 2 to 20 cm, but it is usually less than 10 cm. The blue-ringed octopus is found in rock pools, clumps of cunjevoi and shells, from the tidal zone to a depth of 10 metres. The colour is yellowish brown with ringed marking on the tentacles and striations on the body. These markings change to a vivid iridescent blue when the animal is feeding or becomes angry, excited, disturbed or hypoxic. The heavier specimens are more dangerous, and handling these attractive creatures has resulted in death within minutes. Many such incidents have probably escaped detection by the coroner. Autopsy features are non-specific, and the bite fades after death.

The toxin ('maculotoxin') is more potent than that of any land animal. Analysis of posterior salivary extracts demonstrates a toxin of low molecular weight, identical to tetrodotoxin. The effects are that of a neurotoxin and a neuromuscular blocking agent. It is not curare-like, and it is not influenced by neostigmine and atropine, at least during the acute phase. Hypotension may develop.

> The maculotoxin of the blue-ringed octopus is identical to tetrodotoxin from the puffer fish. It is a neurotoxin and a neuromuscular blocker, resulting in painless skeletal muscle paralysis.

Clinical features

LOCAL

Initially, the bite is usually painless and may thus go unnoticed. The 1-cm circle of blanching becomes oedematous and swollen in 15 minutes. It then becomes haemorrhagic and resembles a small blood blister. If the patient survives the next hour, he or she notices a local stinging sensation for about 6 hours. A serous or bloody discharge may occur. Local muscular twitching may persist for some weeks.

GENERAL

A few minutes after the bite, a rapid, painless paralysis dominates the clinical picture, which progresses in this order: abnormal sensations around mouth, neck and head; possible nausea and/or vomiting; dyspnoea with rapid, shallow and stertorous respirations leading to apnoea, asphyxia and cyanosis; visual disturbances, with involvement of the extraocular eye muscles resulting in double vision, blurred vision and ptosis, whereas intraocular paralysis results in a fixed dilated pupil; difficulty in speech and swallowing; general weakness and lack of co-ordination progressing to complete paralysis.

The duration of paralysis is usually between 4 and 12 hours, but it can be longer, and the weakness and lack of co-ordination may persist for another day. The patient's conscious state is initially normal, even though he or she may not be able to open the eyes or respond to the environment. The respiratory paralysis (causing hypoxia and hypercapnia) finally results in unconsciousness and then death, often within minutes of the commencement of symptoms, unless resuscitation is continued. Cardiovascular effects of hypotension and bradycardia are noted in severe cases.

There may be a cessation at any stage of the previously described clinical sequence (i.e. the effects may cease with the local reaction, may lead to partial paralysis or proceed to complete paralysis and death). Less severe bites may result in generalized and local muscular contractions, which may continue intermittently for 6 hours or more. This occurs with a sub-paralytic dose. Other symptoms noted in mild cases include a lightheaded feeling, depersonalization, paraesthesia, weakness and exhaustion.

Treatment

FIRST AID

Before paralysis

Immobilization of the limb and application of a pressure bandage (see earlier) reduce the absorption of venom. Rest the patient, preferably lying on the side in case of vomiting, and do not leave the patient unattended. Only after hospitalization, where preparations have been made for respiratory support, should the pressure bandage be removed.

With respiratory paralysis

Apply assisted respiration to ensure that the patient does not become hypoxic. Attention must be paid to the clearing of the patient's airway of vomitus, tongue obstruction, dentures and other obstructions. If an airway is available, this should be inserted – but it is not essential. Artificial respiration may have to be continued for hours, until the patient reaches hospital. If delay has occurred, then chest compression may also be required. Reassure the patient, who may hear but not communicate, that you understand the condition. Enlist medical aid, but never leave the patient unattended to obtain this help.

The general first aid protocols recommend that cardiopulmonary resuscitation is commenced on any victim who is unconscious and is not breathing.

MEDICAL TREATMENT

For respiratory paralysis, artificial respiration with intermittent positive pressure respiration is necessary to maintain normal arterial blood gases. Endotracheal intubation or laryngeal mask airway insertion also prevents aspiration of vomitus and facilitates tracheo-bronchial toilet, when indicated. Usual management of the unconscious patient is required.

Edrophonium (Tensilon) and neostigmine are of no value during the deeply paralyzed state. Other central respiratory stimulants may be of use in borderline cases or during the recovery period. Local anaesthesia infiltration to the painful area relieves local pain. For delayed allergic reactions, intravenous hydrocortisone for systemic effects, subcutaneous adrenaline for bronchospasm or an oral antihistamine for skin lesions is indicated.

Prevention

Contact with the octopus should be avoided, and empty shells should be treated with suspicion. Requests by scientific groups for collection of these specimens should be tempered with caution. A public program on the dangers of this animal should be directed especially to children, who are attracted by the bright colouration.

OTHER MARINE ANIMAL INJURIES

Only a few of these injuries are mentioned in this text. Injuries from the sea urchin, electric rays and corals are selected for inclusion because of their interest and frequency in tropical and temperate regions.

Sea urchins

Of the 6000 species of sea urchins, approximately 80 are thought to be venomous or poisonous to humans. They belong to the phylum Echinodermata, named after the hedgehog *(Echinos)* because of the many-spined appearance. In some sea urchin injuries, such as from the ubiquitous *Diadema setosum,* (the *long-spined* or *black sea urchin*), the damage is mainly done by the breaking off of the sharp brittle spines after they have penetrated the diver's skin. Sometimes, the spines have disappeared within a few days, but in other cases they become encrusted and may remain for many months, to emerge at sites distant from the original wound. They are commonly covered by a black pigment, which can be mistaken for the actual spine during attempted removal.

Other sea urchins, such as the *crown of thorns, Acanthaster planci,* can also cause damage when the spines pierce the skin, but they seem to have a far more inflammatory action, indicative of a venom. Vomiting is a frequent accompaniment. Injuries from the crown of thorns have been more commonly reported since divers attempted to eradicate them from reefs.

The most toxic sea urchins are the Toxopneustidae, which have short, thick spines poking through an array of flower-like pedicellariae. Deaths have been reported from these sea urchins. The venom is thought to be a dialyzable acetylcholine-like substance.

TREATMENT

The long spines tend to break easily and therefore need to be extracted without any bending. A local anaesthetic may be required if surgical extraction is attempted. Drawing pastes such as magnesium sulphate have been used. Some find relief with the use of heat, and others have removed the spines by the use of a snake-bite suction cup.

Various interesting treatments have been developed. In Nauru, it is claimed that urinating on the wound immediately after the injury produces excellent results. This presumably relieves the bladder, if not the pain. The use of meat tenderizer owes more to good advertising than to therapeutic efficiency.

One technique, which would be described as barbaric if not for the fact that it seems to work, is to apply extra trauma and movement to the area – to break up the spines within the tissue. It does seem as if, in this case, activity is more beneficial than rest and immobilization. With the latter, the limb tends to swell and become more painful.

Antiseptics and local antibiotics are sometimes employed to reduce infections, but most of the unpleasant sequelae result from the foreign bodies remaining in the wound.

Occasionally, patients present after eating sea urchins. In Tonga, sea urchins are used as an aphrodisiac; however, the ovaries may be poisonous and produce both gastrointestinal and migraine-like symptoms.

Sponges

These sedentary animals require some defence from mobile predators, and they have developed a skeleton of calcareous and silicaceous spicules. They also have a form of toxin that is not well understood. About a dozen sponges are toxic, among the 5000 or so species, and they are mainly found in the temperate or tropical zones. Skin lesions have developed from sponges that have been deep frozen or dried for many years.

CLINICAL FEATURES

One group of symptoms relates to the contact dermatitis associated with the areas of sponge contact. After a variable time, between 5 minutes and 2 hours, dermal irritation is felt. It may be precipitated by wetting or rubbing the area. It may progress over the next day or so and feel as if ground glass has been abraded into the skin. Hyperaesthesia and paraesthesia may be noted. The symptoms can persist for a week or more, with inflammatory and painful reactions around the area. The degree of severity is not related to the clinical signs, and some patients may be incapacitated by the symptoms without any objective manifestations.

The dermal reaction may appear as an erythema, with or without papule and vesicle development. There is sometimes desquamation of the skin in the second or third week, but in other cases skin lesions have recurred over many months.

TREATMENT

The only adequate treatment is prevention, by using gloves when handling sponges and not touching anything that has been in contact with them.

The use of alcohol, lotions or hot water usually aggravates the condition. Local application of cooling lotion such as calamine may be of some value, but treatment with conventional dermatological preparations has limited success.

Coral cuts

GENERAL INFORMATION

Corals, because of their sharp edges combined with human awkwardness underwater, often cause lacerations. The sequelae of this injury may well equal the intensity of the more impressive marine animal injuries. Not only is the coral covered by infected slime, but also pieces of coral or other foreign bodies often remain in the laceration. It is possible that some of the manifestations, especially initially, result from the presence of discharging nematocysts. There have also been occasional patients who have been infected by the marine organism *Erysipelothrix*. Certain *Vibrio* organisms are also present in the marine environment (see Chapter 29) and can cause serious infection. These may need to be cultured in a saline medium if identification is to be made.

CLINICAL FEATURES

A small, often clean-looking laceration is usually seen on the hand or foot. It causes little inconvenience at the time of injury and may go unnoticed. A few hours later, there may be a 'smarting' sensation, especially during washing. At that stage, there is a mild inflammatory reaction around the cut. Within the next day or two, the inflammation becomes more widespread with local swelling, discolouration and tenderness. In severe cases, there may be cellulitis, abscess formation with chronic ulceration or even osteomyelitis.

After healing, there may be a small numb area of skin with a fibrous nodule beneath it, a keloid reaction to the foreign body (coral).

TREATMENT

This involves thorough cleansing of the area, removal of the foreign material and the application of an antiseptic solution. Diluted bleach is often employed by the yachting community. If available, antibody powder or ointment (e.g. neomycin or bacitracin) is effective.

One sequela of coral cuts is sometimes a very unpleasant pruritus that can be troublesome for many weeks. It responds to the use of a local steroid ointment.

FURTHER READING

Atkinson PR, Boyle A, Hartin D, Mcauley D. Is hot water immersion an effective treatment for marine envenomation? *Emergency Medical Journal* 2006;**23**:503–508.

Auerbach PS. *A Medical Guide to Hazardous Marine Life.* Chicago: Mosby–Year Book; 1991.

Australian Resuscitation Council. *Guideline 9.4.5. Envenomation – Jellyfish Stings.* 2010. www.resus.org.au

Barnes JH. Cause and effect of Irukandji stingings. *Medical Journal of Australia* 1997;**167**:649–650.

Burnett JW. Taking the sting out of jellyfish envenomation. *Alert Diver SEAP* 2000;**April–June:** 14–15.

CSL Antivenom Handbook. 2nd ed. Melbourne: Commonwealth Serum Laboratories; 2001. http://www.toxinology.com/generic_static_files/cslavh_contents.html (But see also White, later in this list.)

Edmonds C. *Dangerous Marine Creatures.* Flagstaff, Arizona: Best Publishing; 1995.

Fenner PJ. Venomous marine animals. *South Pacific Underwater Medical Society Journal* 2004;**34**:196–202.

Fenner PJ, Lippmann JM, Gershwin LA. Fatal and severe box jellyfish stings in Thai waters. *J Travel Medicine* 2010;**17**(2):133–138.

Gershwin L, Richardson AJ, Winkel KD, *et al.* Biology and ecology of Irukandji jellyfish (Cnidaria: Cubozoa). *Advances in Marine Biology* 2013;**66**:1–85.

Hadok JC. 'Irukandji' syndrome: a risk for divers in tropical waters. *Medical Journal of Australia* 1997;**167**:649–650.

Halstead B. *Poisonous and Venomous Marine Animals of the World.* Vols. 1–3. Washington, DC: US Government Printing Office; 1965.

Halstead BW, Auerbach PS, Campbell DR. *A Colour Atlas of Dangerous Marine Animals.* London: Wolfe Medical Publications; 1990.

Lippmann JM, Fenner PJ, Winkel K, Gershwin LA. Fatal and severe box jellyfish stings, Including Irukandji stings, in Malaysia, 2000–2010. *Journal of Travel Medicine* 2011;**18**(4):275–281.

Little M, Mulcahy RF. A years experience of Irukandji envenomation in far north queensland. *Med J Aust.* 1998;**169**:638–41.

Loten C, Stokes B, Worsley D, *et al.* A randomised controlled trial of hot water (45°C) immersion versus ice packs for pain relief in bluebottle stings. *Medical Journal of Australia* 2006;**184**:329–333.

Sutherland SK. *Australian Animal Toxins.* Melbourne: Oxford University Press; 1990.

Taylor G. Are some jellyfish stings heat labile? *South Pacific Underwater Medical Society Journal* 2000;**30**(2):74–75.

Tibballs J. Australian venomous jellyfish, envenomation syndrome, toxins and therapy. *Toxicon* 2006;**48**:830–859.

US Navy Diving Manual. Appendix 5C. Hazardous Marine Creatures. Flagstaff, Arizona: Best Publishing; 2008.

Welfare P, Little M, Pereira P, Seymore J. An in-vitro examination of the effect of vinegar on discharged nematocysts of *Chironex fleckeri. Diving and Hyperbaric Medicine* 2014;**44**(1):30–34.

White J. *A Clinician's Guide to Australian Venomous Bites and Stings: Incorporating the Updated CSL Antivenom Handbook.* Melbourne: Commonwealth Serum Laboratories; 2013.

Williamson JA, Fenner PJ, Burnett JW, Rifkin JF. *Venomous and Poisonous Marine Animals.* Sydney: University of New South Wales Press; 1996.

This chapter was reviewed for this fifth edition by Carl Edmonds.

33

Fish poisoning

INTRODUCTION

Food poisoning from ingested marine animals is a serious hazard to many populations. Three fourths of the world's population lives within 15 km of a coastline. This poisoning is important in tropical or temperate climates, where the outbreaks tend to be sporadic and unpredictable. Commercially valuable industries have been curtailed or prohibited because of the serious threat from this high-protein, readily available food. In cold climates, poisoning from marine and polar animals is also of serious import, but it is more predictable and can be avoided.

Diseases that can destroy whole communities, change the fate of military operations, devastate fishing industries, yet still arise sporadically in a previously safe marine environment, are worthy of considerable investigation and research. Such has not been the case. This subject is sadly neglected, both in medical research and in medical training.

For those physicians associated with marine medicine, yachting, diving or travel, and those who practise near coastlines, a knowledge of seafood poisoning is essential. It is also important to those involved in public health, industrial medicine and the general health of island communities.

Space allows the description of only a few of the more significant fish poisonings. Ciguatera, tetrodotoxin and scombroid poisoning are discussed because of their commercial implications. Shellfish and crustacean poisoning is summarized. No reference is made to barracuda poisoning, hallucinatory fish poisoning, mercury poisoning, other pollutants, seal liver poisoning, shark and ray poisoning, turtle poisoning and many others. One complicating factor is that there may be more than one type of marine poison responsible for the clinical manifestations in the patient.

Viral and bacterial contamination of fish and shellfish is also common, and it is dealt with in general medical texts.

Perhaps the least-understood effects are the **subacute and chronic marine toxicology effects.** The original description of mercury poisonings from marine foods concentrated on 111 cases, including 43 deaths, from the contaminated Minamata Bay in Japan. Another outbreak in Sweden was followed by the observation of hazardous levels in the United States and Canada. Only after the acute effects were countered did the long-term toxicity of this toxin receive attention. Shark meat with high concentrations of mercury is still sold as 'flake' in large supermarkets and fish shops. The metal has a propensity to cause neural degeneration and is thought to be especially dangerous to children and pregnant women.

Since that time, many other chronic marine toxins have been proposed, often as a result of human ingestion of top marine predators that concentrate the toxins as they move up the food chain. Thus, shark, tuna, eel and the large crustaceans become harbingers of this toxicity. Beta-methylamino-l-alanine (BMAA) is produced by cyanobacteria microorganisms and is concentrated up the marine food chain until the food (e.g. shark fin soup, cartilage pills) is consumed by humans. It has been incriminated as a contributor to Alzheimer's and Parkinson's diseases and motor neurone disease. Much investigation is required, and this field is still in its infancy.

CIGUATERA POISONING

On a worldwide basis, ciguatera poisoning is the most common and most serious of the marine toxins, affecting some 10 000 to 50 000 people per year. It is mainly a disorder of the tropics and, to a lesser degree, the semitropical and temperate zones. It is mostly found between 35 degrees of latitude north and south. International transport of fish cuisine has greatly extended the geographical sites of ciguatera outbreaks into temperate climates and more sophisticated cultures. The fish cannot be identified as poisonous by their external appearance.

The fish implicated in this poisoning are usually reef fish. These fish may ingest *Gambierdiscus toxicus* (the originator of ciguatoxin), which lives on coral and sea weed, or they may acquire it from the eating other contaminated fish. Ciguatoxin is harmless to the fish, but it tends to concentrate as it travels up the food chain to the more active carnivorous predators. It is for this reason that the larger predator fish tend to be more toxic.

Local knowledge indicates areas in which the fish are poisonous. This knowledge is not entirely reliable, however, because the areas change. Poisoning is more likely when reefs have been disturbed by natural damage, such as hurricanes, or by human-made damage, such as constructions, atomic explosions or disruptions of the ecology with agricultural run-offs, thus permitting proliferation of *G. toxicus*.

Various techniques have been promulgated in folklore to predict which fish will be safe to eat. Observations that are totally irrelevant, despite parochial beliefs, include:

- The presence of worms in the fish.
- Whether ants or flies refuse it.
- Whether a silver coin will turn black if inserted.
- Whether grated coconut will turn green if cooked with the fish.

Traditional measures of feeding potentially dangerous fish first to either the cat (sometimes carried on boats for this purpose) or the older members of primitive tribes, have been recorded. The senior author of this text, who is a cat-lover, and the publishers, deplore this attitude.

In a survival situation, the advice is do not eat the viscera of the fish (e.g. liver, gonads, intestines) and avoid the exceptionally large reef predators and those species often implicated in ciguatera poisoning. These include barracuda, grouper, mackerel, snapper, sea bass, mahi-mahi, surgeon fish, parrot fish, wrasses, jacks and many others. Moray eels are particularly toxic. Boiling the fish many times and discarding the water after each boiling may be helpful. As an alternative to this last technique, the fish may be sliced and continually soaked in water, which should be changed every 30 minutes or so. Eat only small quantities.

Symptoms may vary, and they may be modified by the presence of other marine poisons such as maitotoxin, scaritoxin and okadaic acid, among others. Ciguatoxins increase sodium channel permeability, release norepinephrine and may increase calcium uptake in cells.

Clinical features

Symptoms usually develop 2 to 12 hours after ingestion of the food. More severe cases tend to occur earlier. Gastrointestinal symptoms develop in 6 to 24 hours and last 1 to 4 days. Cardiac symptoms occur early in this phase, and neurological symptoms appear a little later.

Generalized nonspecific symptoms may develop, including weakness and dull aches in the limbs and head. These muscle pains may progress to more severe weakness, with or without cramps. The myalgia differentiates this disorder from tetrodotoxin poisoning. Paraesthesiae and numbness are noted around the mouth and sometimes peripherally. Gastrointestinal problems include anorexia, nausea, vomiting and diarrhea. Severe neurological disturbances may develop in 12 to 36 hours and include delirium, cranial nerve involvement, lack of co-ordination and ataxia, with occasional extrapyramidal disorders, convulsions, coma and even death. Death is likely to be caused by respiratory failure, although in severe cases there is evidence of hypotension, cardiac dysrhythmias and other cardiovascular problems.

Skin lesions are characteristic and include erythema, pruritus, or a burning sensation – sometimes with vesicular formation. They may be very severe for a few days but then usually subside. Hair and nail loss may supervene. In severely affected patients, these skin lesions may be troublesome for many weeks. In female patients, the vagina may be affected, sometimes severely, causing symptoms of cystitis or dyspareunia. Less commonly, male patients may notice pain during ejaculations, and the toxin may be transmitted in semen, thus causing local symptoms in women.

The death rate in different series varies from 0.1 to 10 per cent. In severe outbreaks, the presentation of the disease can be acute and widespread. In most Indo-Pacific regions, the disease tends to be sporadic and mild. In these cases, the main symptoms can clear within 1 or 2 days, although residual weakness and paraesthesiae, together with a reversal or distortion (dysaesthesia) of temperature perception, may persist for long periods. This last symptom is characteristic of ciguatera, but it may also be found in neurotoxic shellfish poisoning.

Severe cases may take many months or up to a year for full recovery. Exacerbations can be precipitated by alcohol, nicotinic acid, caffeine and other vaso-active drugs. The production of an erythematous area associated with a burning sensation following intake of alcohol is typical of this disorder and may persist for some months. The illness can also recur following stress or the ingestion of certain fish or of animals fed fish meal (e.g. pork, poultry). Immunity does not develop, and subsequent poisonings may be even more severe.

Although ciguatoxin analysis is not yet adequate for human cases, it can be demonstrated in uneaten fish remains. The time delay makes this problematic in the diagnosis of clinical cases in the acute stage.

Treatment

Treatment includes the removal of unabsorbed material by induction of vomiting or gastric lavage in patients who do not have respiratory depression. Activated charcoal may be taken orally. Rest and observation in a hospital are required until the patient has recovered. Respiratory support may be required.

The medical treatment is basically symptomatic; however, there have been many different pharmacological remedies proposed. None are consistently effective. Intravenous mannitol has been recommended, if it is given within the first few days – but may still be of value for up to 2 weeks. A dose of 20 per cent intravenous mannitol of 250 ml slowly to a maximum of 1 g/kg, piggy backed to a 5 per cent dextrose infusion, is recommended. Some studies have questioned its value, but what works in one area may not work in others because the ciguatoxin has diverse regional variations.

Drugs that have been suggested include lidocaine, steroids or calcium gluconate 10 per cent intravenously to relieve the neuromuscular or neurological features and perhaps increase muscle tone. Calcium channel blockers may help in patients with residual symptoms.

As a general rule, pharmacological treatment does not have nearly the effectiveness of general medical care. Symptomatic treatment, while avoiding vaso-active drugs and substances, seems most valuable. Diazepam can be given safely, and patients with severe cases may require the assistance of a neurologist or an organically oriented psychiatrist for pharmacological advice. A tricyclic antidepressant may be of benefit if given in small doses (e.g. amitriptyline 25 to 50 mg at night).

TETRODOTOXIN POISONING

Of all that are in the waters you may eat these: whatever has fins and scales you may eat. And whatever does not have fins and scales you shall not eat; it is unclean for you.

Deuteronomy. 14:9,10.

Tetrodotoxin poisoning follows the ingestion of puffer fish, ocean sunfish or porcupine fish. The name 'puffer' derives from the ability of the fish to inflate itself by taking in large quantities of air or water. The scales have been modified to form protective plates or spikes. These fish are recognized as poisonous throughout the world, although they are more common in tropical and temperate regions. The toxin is concentrated mainly in the ovaries, liver and intestines. Lesser amounts occur in the skin, but the body musculature is usually free of poison. The toxicity is related to its reproductive cycle.

With two exceptions, these fish are usually considered inedible. The first exception is the uninformed consumer. Captain James Cook on September 7, 1774, sampled this fish in New Caledonia, with near fatal results. The other exception is the Asiatic gourmet consuming 'Fugu'. After a prolonged apprenticeship, specially licensed chefs in Japan are allowed to prepare this fish and receive considerable kudos by retaining enough of the toxin to produce a numbing effect in the mouth – but not enough to cause death. Nevertheless, accidents do happen, and poisoning from Fugu affects about 50 cases per year. The fatality rate is about 7 per cent.

The toxin interferes with neuromuscular transmission in motor and sensory nerves and in the sympathetic nervous system, by interfering with sodium transfer. It also has a direct depressant effect on medullary centres, skeletal muscles (reducing excitability), intracardiac conduction and myocardial contractility. Hypotension result from the effects on the preganglionic cholinergic fibres or from the direct effect on the heart. Respiratory depression precedes cardiovascular depression.

Clinical features

The onset and severity of symptoms vary greatly according to the amount of toxin ingested. Usually, within the first 1 to 2 hours, the patient notices muscular weakness and other effects of blockage of the motor and sensory systems.

Paraesthesia around the mouth may also extend to the extremities, or it may become generalized. Autonomic effects include salivation, sweating, chest pain, and headache, Gastrointestinal symptoms of nausea, vomiting and diarrhoea may develop, and there is sometimes a decrease in temperature, pulse rate and blood pressure.

A coagulation disturbance, which is an occasional complication, may lead to systemic bleeding or desquamation from haemorrhagic bullae.

Neurological involvement may commence as muscular twitching and lack of co-ordination and may proceed to complete skeletal muscular paralysis, including respiratory paralysis.

Bulbar paralysis may produce interference with speech and swallowing. The pupils, after initially being constricted, may become fixed and dilated. The clinical picture is therefore one of generalized paralysis with the patient maintaining a fully conscious state while oxygenation is maintained. This is important in the management because the patient is able to hear and understand the statements made by people around him or her.

The high death rate from this disorder results from respiratory paralysis, and if death occurs, it does within 24 hours of ingestion. It is a reflection of incorrect diagnosis or inadequate resuscitation techniques in most cases. Death has occurred within 17 minutes of ingestion, but it is more likely in the following 4 to 6 hours, from respiratory failure.

The onset of symptoms may be delayed for up to 20 hours, and so observation and hospitalization are required.

Treatment

Before the patient shows signs of paralysis or weakness, the use of an emetic or gastric lavage may be of value in removing poisonous material. Activated charcoal may be taken orally. Lavage may also be employed if controlled respiration has required the insertion of an endotracheal tube, which prevents aspiration of stomach contents.

After weakness has become apparent, the treatment is entirely symptomatic and consists of maintenance of an adequate respiratory state, monitoring of vital signs and measurement of arterial blood gas and biochemical profile. The patient may require a mechanical ventilator for up to 24 hours before regaining muscular control. Because consciousness is retained in the absence of skeletal or respiratory movement, the periodic administration of a minor tranquilizer such as diazepam seems prudent. Continuous explanation and reassurance should be given, even though the patient cannot respond physically to these communications.

Various pharmacological treatments have been proposed, including intravenous calcium gluconate 10 per cent, anticholinesterases, respiratory stimulants, steroids and others. There is no firm evidence that these drugs are of value. Monoclonal antibodies to tetrodotoxin are currently being developed.

General nursing care, with special attention to pressure areas and to eye and mouth toilets, is axiomatic in these paralyzed and debilitated patients.

Prevention

'Scaleless' fish should not be eaten unless they are known to be harmless. If one chooses to eat Fugu in Japan, it should be purchased from a first-class restaurant with a licensed cook. All the viscera and skin must be removed.

In a survival situation, these fish should be eviscerated, and only the musculature should be consumed. The meat should be cut or torn into small bits and soaked in water for at least 4 hours. The fish should be kneaded during this time and the water changed at frequent intervals. The toxin is partly water soluble; therefore this soaking may help to remove it. One should not eat more than is required to maintain life. Feeding of the fish to test animals has been suggested.

SCOMBROID POISONING

This disorder is possible wherever mackerel-like fish, tuna, bonito, mahi-mahi, albacore, sardines and anchovies are caught and eaten without adequate care or preparation. It has also occurred in epidemics related to contaminated canned tuna and other large fish.

The fish, which are normally safe to eat, become poisonous when handled incorrectly. If these fish are left for several hours at room temperature or in the sun, the histidine in their muscular tissues is changed by bacterial action into saurine, a histamine-like substance. The bacteria implicated include *Proteus morganii*, *Clostridium*, *Salmonella* and *Escherichia*, among others. Laboratory verification of contaminated fish is obtained by demonstrating a histamine content in excess of 100 mg/100 g of fish muscle.

Clinical features

The fish may have a characteristic 'peppery' taste. After half an hour to 1 hour, other symptoms characteristic of histamine toxicity develop in severe cases. Gastrointestinal symptoms associated with headache, palpitations and tachycardia with hypotension are followed by a typical 'allergic-type' syndrome. The allergic may involve the skin with a urticarial reaction, the respiratory system with bronchospasm or the cardiovascular system in the form of anaphylactic shock. Usually, the symptoms abate within 24 hours.

Treatment

First aid treatment includes the removal of unabsorbed material by vomiting or gastric lavage if the patient is not too severely distressed. Treatment involves the customary techniques for handling dermatological, respiratory or cardiovascular manifestations of allergy and anaphylaxis. These include antihistamines (including histamine-2 blockers such as cimetidine), adrenaline (or other sympathomimetic drugs) and steroids.

Prevention

Prevention is possible by correct care, storage and preparation of the fish. Prompt refrigeration and not leaving the fish exposed to the sun or room temperature have reduced the incidence of this disease. It is believed that pallor of the gills, or an odour or staleness, may indicate that saurine is present in the fish.

SHELLFISH AND CRUSTACEAN POISONING

Shellfish include oysters, clams, mussels and cockles, among others. Crustaceans include lobsters, crayfish yabbies, prawns, crabs and others. Five different types of poisoning may develop from ingestion of these animals.

Gastrointestinal type

This is the most common type of shellfish poisoning, and it develops some hours after ingestion of contaminated shellfish. Viruses, marine *Vibrio* organisms, *Escherichia coli* and other bacteria and organisms have been implicated. Usually, manifestations last about 36 hours, but they vary according to the organism and are treated along general medical guidelines.

Allergic type

The allergic reaction appears to be a typical hypersensitivity reaction to a protein in the shellfish. It is likely that the victim was previously exposed to the same or similar protein to which he or she developed an antibody reaction. Symptoms appear after the second and subsequent exposures and are aggravated by exercise, heat and emotion. There may be a history of allergy to other foreign proteins (e.g. hay fever, antitoxins, horse serum). The clinical features are dermatological, respiratory and/or cardiovascular and may therefore mimic scombroid poisoning (see earlier). Antihistamines, adrenaline (or sympathomimetic drugs) and steroids tend to be used in patients with these three manifestations.

Hepatic disease

There appears to be a hepatotoxin especially concentrated in molluscs and perhaps related to the presence of a toxic dinoflagellate. This toxin may result in severe hepatocellular disease with the clinical picture of acute yellow atrophy. Viral infection, causing infectious hepatitis, has also been reported.

Paralytic shellfish poisoning

> The waters that were in the rivers were turned into blood, and the fish that were in the rivers died; and the river stank.
>
> *Exodus 7:20-21*

Paralytic shellfish poisoning is caused by the ingestion of a neurotoxin, called saxitoxin, which is concentrated in shellfish and produced by a marine protozoon, a dinoflagellate. Many species of these dinoflagellates may be involved, but the most common is *Alexandrium catenella*. Other species have also been incriminated, as have other toxins, thus explaining the variability of clinical manifestations with this disease. A dose of 1.0 to 1.5 mg of saxitoxin can be fatal in humans. Saxitoxin acts by blocking sodium channels in nerve and muscle cells. It is derived from the dinoflagellates, which are filtered by mussels, clams, oysters and scallops, and it makes consumption of these shellfish hazardous when the sea water dinoflagellate count is as low as 200/ml. Neither steaming nor cooking affects the potency of the toxin, and commercial processing does not eliminate it.

Paralytic shellfish poisoning is associated with 'red tide' or other 'water bloom' – a discolouration of the sea resulting from masses of dinoflagellates. The Red Sea was so named because of the occasional appearance of this colouration during these red tides. Native North Americans avoided shellfish for this reason. The first clinical description of this disorder dates back to 1689, but there have been many outbreaks since, with 54 such occurrences in Alaska, affecting 117 individuals, between 1973 and 1992.

The symptoms usually appear within 0.5 to 3 hours, never more than 12 hours after ingestion. The prognosis is good for people surviving an additional 12 hours, although weakness and disability can occur for weeks afterward.

The clinical symptoms are mainly those related to developing neuropathy, affecting peripheral nerves, the central nervous system, the autonomic nervous system and skeletal muscle.

The clinical effects and treatment are similar in many ways to those of tetrodotoxin and ciguatera poisoning.

Amnesic shellfish poisoning

This disorder is, more accurately, domoic acid poisoning. It was first described in 1958. There have been a couple of severe outbreaks from ingestion of shellfish contaminated with various marine organisms including a pennate diatom *(Nitzschia)*, and some phytoplankton outbreaks have occurred in Japan, Prince Edward Island in Canada and the West Coast of the United States.

Domoic acid is an excitatory neurotransmitter that specially affects the hippocampus, thalamus and frontal lobes of the brain – with temporary or permanent damage.

Initially, there are gastrointestinal symptoms, 1 to 24 hours after ingestion, with neurological manifestations and memory loss developing within 48 hours and possibly progressing to seizures, multiple central nervous system effects and cardiac disorders. Bronchial secretions may be profuse and require individuals to be treated with endotracheal intubation.

Survivors often have neurological improvement for up to 12 weeks after ingestion.

The treatment is symptomatic because no antidote exists.

FURTHER READING

Clark RF, Williams SR, Nordt SP, Manoguerra AS. A review of selected seafood poisoning. *Undersea and Hyperbaric Medicine* 1999;**26**(3):175–185.

Edmonds C. *Dangerous Marine Creatures.* Flagstaff, Arizona: Best Publishing; 1995.

Friedman MA, Fleming LE, Fernandez M, *et al.* Ciguatera fish poisoning: treatment, prevention and management. *Marine Drugs* 2008;**6**(3):456–479.

Halstead B. *Poisonous and Venomous Marine Animals of the World.* Vols. 1–3. Washington, DC: US Government Printing Office; 1965.

Medline Plus, US National Library of Medicine. *Poisoning: Fish and Shellfish.* http://www.nlm.nih.gov/medlineplus/ency/article/002851.htm

Palafox NA, Jain LG, Pinano AZ, *et al.* Successful treatment of ciguatera fish poisoning with intravenous mannitol. *JAMA* 1988;**259**:2740–2742.

Ragelis EP. *Seafood Toxins*, American Chemical Society. Symposium Series, Washington DC. Chapter 3. Volume 262; 2009.

Sutherland SK, Tibballs J. *Australian Animal Toxins.* 2nd ed. Melbourne: Oxford University Press; 2001.

Williamson JA, Fenner PJ, Burnett JW, Rifkin JF. *Venomous and Poisonous Marine Animals.* Sydney: University of New South Wales Press; 1996.

This chapter was reviewed for this fifth edition by Carl Edmonds.

34

Underwater explosions

INTRODUCTION

Although most information on this topic has been acquired from naval research work, it is relevant to some civilian divers. Explosives are used in salvage, mining and dredging operations, as well as in war-like activities that involve divers and shipwreck survivors. During World War II, there were many deaths among immersed divers and swimmers following air, surface ship or submarine attack.

For an explosion with the same energy and at the same distance, an underwater blast is more dangerous than an air blast. This is because in air the blast energy dissipates more rapidly and tends to be reflected at the body surface, whereas in water the blast wave travels through the body and causes internal injuries.

PHYSICS OF BLAST WAVES

Some knowledge of underwater explosions is of assistance in understanding their clinical manifestations.

An explosion is a very fast chemical reaction. The process propagates through the explosive at 2 to 9 km/second. The products of the reaction are heat and combustion products such as carbon dioxide. A bubble of gas is produced in the water. The gas

in the bubble may be at a pressure of 50 000 atmospheres and a temperature of 30 000°C. The bubble rapidly expands in a spherical form, thus displacing water. This rapid expansion generates the first pressure wave as the pressure in the gas bubble produces a pressure pulse that is transmitted through the water. It is sometimes called the short pulse or primary pulse. The initial pressure change of the pulse is steep, increasing to a peak pressure within a few microseconds. The pressure in the bubble falls as it expands and the gas cools. The fall of pressure at the end of the explosion reflects the end of the expansion of the gases and takes milliseconds.

The outward momentum of the water that has been displaced by the bubble enlarges the bubble past its equilibrium volume, and a series of volume swings can be initiated. These volume oscillations of the bubble cause a series of pressure waves.

Near the point of detonation, the velocity of the first pressure wave is great, and it is related to the speed at which the explosive detonates. Some explosives produce high pressures for a short period. Other types, with a slower reaction rate, produce less intense pressure waves that have a longer duration. At a point some distance from the detonation, the velocity of the pressure waves slows to that of sound in water, about 1.5 km/second. From then on, the pressure waves follow the laws of sound in water. The energy of the waves decreases with distance, and the waves are reflected and absorbed in a similar fashion to sound waves.

In water, the pressure pulse is not absorbed as rapidly as in air. In air, the gas surrounding the explosion is compressed and so absorbs energy from the explosion. In water, which is far less compressible, there is little absorption. So the pressure pulse is transmitted with greater intensity over a longer range. Thus, the lethal range of an explosion is normally far greater than the same mass of explosive in air.

A pressure wave is transmitted over a greater range in water than in air.

The energy in a typical blast is distributed in the following proportions: the initial pressure wave has approximately one fourth the energy, subsequent waves total one fourth and the other manifestations, such as heat and turbulence, comprise the remaining half. In an explosion, most of the damage is caused by the initial pressure wave.

Other waves may result from an explosion. If the initial waves reach the sea bottom, they may be reflected or absorbed. The proportions depend on the nature of the sea bed. If it is hard and smooth, there is little absorption and much reflection; conversely, a soft sea bottom absorbs more. The angle of incidence (i.e. the angle at which the waves strike the sea bed) is equal to the angle of reflection. The reflected wave coming from the sea bed may combine with the other waves to cause increased damage. If the sea bed is distant from the point of detonation, this effect is negligible.

At the water surface, the reflected wave is a negative pressure pulse rather than a positive pulse. As a result of this, a diver may experience a less intense pressure wave if he or she is close to the surface. The negative reflected pulse tends to cancel the positive direct path pulse.

At the surface, a series of events may modify the pressure waves. Above a certain intensity, the surface of the water is broken or shredded and thrown up into a dome, termed the *dome effect*. This dissipates a small part of the pressure wave, and the remainder is reflected back into the water. Other disturbances that may be observed on the surface following the

dome phenomenon include the slick and plume. The *slick* is a rapidly expanding ring of darkened water resulting from the advancing of the pressure waves. The *plume* is the last manifestation of the explosion and is the result of gas reaching and breaking the surface of the water. Although the plume may be spectacular, it does little damage.

The surface phenomenon varies with the size and depth of the explosion. With a deep or small explosion, the dome may not form because there may be insufficient energy to shred the water. The slick tends to be retained to a greater depth because it is dependent only on the presence of the pulse wave. Shallow explosions tend to create a large plume (Figure 34.1).

Thermal layers may also reflect the pressure waves from the explosion, as may other objects such as large ships. The size of the charge, depth of detonation and distance from target have an influence on the potential damage by the initial and subsequent pressure waves.

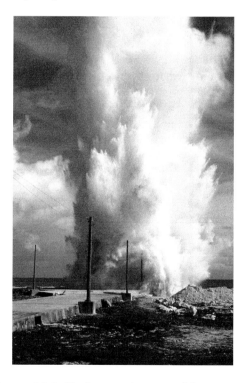

Figure 34.1 Shallow underwater blast undertaken for reef passage clearance using a slowly detonating explosive (ammonium nitrate – fuel oil mixture). Note the large plume.

Charge size, distance and risk of injury

The risk of injury or death depends on several variables: the size of the charge, the victim's distance from it and the nature of the sea bottom. US sources give the relationship shown in the following equation for estimating the effect of a TNT charge[1]. Other explosives behave differently; the longer pulse from a more slowly detonating explosion can cause more damage than the same pressure from a more rapidly detonating explosive.

$$P\left(lb/\text{square Inch}\right) = \frac{\sqrt[3]{13000 \times \text{charge size}\,(lb)}}{\text{Distance from charge}\,(\text{feet})}$$

where P = pressure.

Pressures greater than 2000 lb/square inch cause death, and pressures greater than 500 lb/square inch are likely to cause death or serious injury. Pressures in the range 50 to 500 lb/square inch are likely to cause injury, but those less than 50 lb/square inch are unlikely to cause any harm.

MECHANISM OF INJURY

In air explosions, the main causes of damage are fragments from the charge container and shrapnel and foreign bodies drawn into the explosive wave, as well as the pressure wave[2-4]. In the water, particles are retarded by the medium. Also, with air explosions much of the pressure wave is reflected at the body surface because this is an interface between media of different densities. Intestinal injury as a result of blast damage rarely occurs from explosions in air.

In water, the blast wave passes through the body because it has a consistency similar to that of water. The individual molecules are displaced very little, except in areas capable of compression (i.e. in gas spaces). Damage is mainly at the air-tissue interfaces within the body. The gas in the gas-filled cavities is almost instantaneously compressed as the pressure wave passes, and the walls of these spaces are traumatized as a result.

Damage can be expected in the lung, air-filled viscera in the abdomen, sinus cavities and ear.

In the lungs, the damage is not caused by pressure transmitted via the upper airways, but it is the result of transmission of the wave directly through the thoracic wall. The pressure wave reaches the gas-tissue interface at the respiratory mucosa, and it is there that the tissues are 'shredded' or torn apart.

> Injury from an underwater blast occurs mainly at gas-tissue interfaces.

Animal experiments

The effects of underwater blast on animals have been studied extensively. As would be predicted, the respiratory and gastrointestinal tracts were the most significantly affected. Pathological examinations revealed injury to the lungs and gas-filled abdominal viscera. Central nervous system lesions were also observed.

The respiratory damage included alveolar haemorrhage, mucosal injury to the bronchi and trachea, acute interstitial emphysema, pneumothorax and haemothorax. Intestinal injury consisted mainly of subserous and submucosal haemorrhage and perforation of the gas-filled viscera. Renal and hepatic systems were not affected, with no evidence of gallbladder or urinary bladder damage. When both the thorax and abdomen were immersed, the lungs were consistently more affected than the intestines. When only the abdomen was immersed, then it was most affected, with bleeding via the rectum.

These and other observations demonstrate the importance of the air-tissue interface in damage from an underwater blast. Wolf[5] cited experiments to confirm this phenomenon. When three loops of bowel were prepared and occluded, with one collapsed, another filled with saline and a third filled with air, only the air-containing loop sustained injury.

There is some contention regarding the cause of death in animals exposed to underwater explosions. In most cases, early deaths are probably because of pulmonary lesions. These animals usually exhibit low arterial oxygen saturation, sometimes correctable by 100 per cent oxygen inhalation, with respiratory acidosis and carbon dioxide retention. Some early deaths may be caused by central nervous system involvement. Petechial haemorrhage and oedema have been noted in the brain. These may be caused by a rapid increase in the venous pressure, following compression of the chest and abdominal venous reservoirs by the pressure wave. With this transmission of pressure into the cerebral venous system, small blood vessels may rupture. Another postulate is that pressurizing the air in the alveoli, or rupture of alveoli, may result in the production of air emboli. Air has been demonstrated in the cerebrovascular system of animals that were in the upright position during the blast.

> Brain damage is thought to be caused by a rapid rise in venous pressure following compression of the chest and abdomen by the pressure wave.

Late deaths result from the complications of respiratory, abdominal and neurological injuries. These include bronchopneumonia, peritonitis and coma and its sequelae.

CLINICAL FEATURES

Information on the clinical features of underwater explosions in humans is mainly derived from case reports[2–4]. Most of the physical parameters such as distance from the blast and intensity are not known, and thus clinical correlation with the physical parameters is not possible. Autopsies are usually complicated by the effects of drowning and immersion.

Huller and Bazini[6] reported on 32 casualties from an Israeli destroyer. While the victims were in the water, they were exposed to blast from an exploding missile. Nineteen had both pulmonary and abdominal injuries. Five had only abdominal injuries, and 8 had only pulmonary injuries. It is not possible to determine whether there was any physical reason for this distribution of symptoms.

Of the 24 laparotomies performed, 22 had tears of the bowel and 11 had subserosal bleeding in other parts of the bowel. In 1 case the perforations were found only at a second operation, and

Table 34.1 Pulmonary symptoms and radiological findings

Pulmonary symptoms (27 patients)	Percentage
Haemoptysis	56
Dyspnoea	41
Abnormal auscultatory findings	41
Chest pain	22
Cyanosis	19
Radiological findings	**Percentage**
Mild to severe infiltrates	100
Pneumomediastinum	22
Haemothorax	19
Interstitial emphysema	11
Pneumatocele	11
Pneumothorax	4

Source: From Huller and Bazini (1970).

in 1 case there was also a lacerated liver. One had an isolated rupture of the spleen, but this may have been caused by an incident before the patient entered the water. An unexpected finding was that 4 patients had electrocardiographic changes consistent with myocardial injury. Three patients died of cardiorespiratory failure within 8 hours of surgery. One survived 48 hours before dying of peritonitis and sepsis.

In other reports, neurological involvement has been described. Middle ear damage with hearing loss is common. Abnormalities of consciousness, varying from mild delirium to coma, have been reported. Patients may suffer severe headaches, and there may be interference with the spinal cord and the autonomic nervous system. It is possible that the paralytic ileus that is quite common in this disorder is at least partly caused by a neuronal reflex phenomenon. Subdural haematomas have been reported. Pain has been reported in the testes and legs, as well as in the abdomen and chest (Table 34.1).

MANAGEMENT

Blast injuries cause severe body trauma, and affected patients should be evaluated in much the same way as any other trauma patient while remaining mindful that an absence of obvious external injury does not rule out internal injury. It follows that the patient should be admitted to hospital for observation, even though he or she may not appear seriously affected in the early stages. Exposure to altitude may aggravate or precipitate respiratory difficulties. Pneumothoraces and gastrointestinal perforations should also be considered before the patient is evacuated by air.

> The patient may not appear to be seriously injured in the early stages, and there may be no external signs of injury.

The patient should have no oral intake and be maintained on intravenous fluids with gastric suction until the full extent of the damage has been assessed. It is easy to suggest that the appropriate studies to ascertain the degree of lung or abdominal injury should be performed, but for abdominal injury there is no clear recent opinion on what these should be. A previous review[3] suggested that computed tomography (CT), if available, may provide evidence of large collections of fluids and haematomas that require operation. Smaller lesions that may require operation can be missed with CT. Intraperitoneal air suggests injury, but it is a non-specific sign because it may not indicate perforation. The review also considered other options. Peritoneal lavage provides evidence of perforation and bleeding but does not identify haematomas. Even laparoscopic and endoscopic assessments were not considered reliable diagnostic tools.

When there are signs of peritonitis, such as rebound tenderness, rigidity or decreased bowel sounds, a decision has to be made on surgical intervention. These signs may be caused by haemorrhagic lesions throughout the bowel that produce peritonism without perforation. Before surgical exploration, there should be a reasonable presumption of gastrointestinal perforation, which is a clear indication for surgical management. Bleeding from the rectum is common and is not itself an indication for surgery.

> Management is similar to that of severe body trauma from other causes.

Treatment of the respiratory damage is based on general medical principles. Care must be taken in the use of positive pressure ventilation. The administration of high fractions of inspired oxygen may be needed if there is significant hypoxaemia. Pure oxygen for a period may be considered in patients with signs of cerebral or cardiac air embolism.

Antibiotics may be indicated, and supportive care should be tailored to the individual case. Intubation, ventilation and intensive care are necessary in some cases. Intravenous fluids and transfusions may be required.

Hyperbaric oxygen therapy has been proposed to reduce cerebral oedema, eliminate cerebral bubbles and improve tissue oxygenation. However, hyperbaric oxygen treatment is likely to delay and complicate cardiopulmonary support and surgery, and its risks *versus* benefits must be carefully considered, even in sophisticated hyperbaric units. However, if cerebral arterial gas embolism is the dominant feature hyperbaric oxygen is essential.

PREVENTION

The obvious preventive measure is to avoid diving in areas where explosions are possible. If this is unavoidable, the diver should wear protective clothing. This may be a drysuit, which gives the most protection. An air-containing vest gives some protection because it reflects much of the pressure pulse at the first water-air interface and absorbs some of the remainder. If it is possible for the diver to reach the surface and float face-up, the effect of the pressure wave will be decreased. If the diver is near the surface, the pressure wave may be attenuated by reflected waves.

> Elevation of the chest and abdomen out of the water reduces the severity of blast injury.

Lifting the chest and abdomen out of the water lessens the effect of the blast. This is especially so if the swimmer can lie on some piece of debris or solid support. Facing away from the explosion is said to give some protection.

REFERENCES

1. Physics. In: *US Navy Diving Manual Volume 1. NAVSEA 0994-LP-001-9010.* Washington, DC: Naval Sea Systems Command; 1996.

2. Guy RJ, Glover MA, Cripps NPJ. The pathophysiology of primary blast injury and its implications for treatment. Part I. The thorax. *Journal of the Royal Naval Medical Service* 1998;**84**:79–86.

3. Guy RJ, Glover MA, Cripps NPJ. The pathophysiology of primary blast injury and its implications for treatment. Part II. Injury and implications for treatment. *Journal of the Royal Naval Medical Service* 1999;**85**:13–24.

4. Guy RJ, Glover MA, Cripps NPJ. Primary blast injury: pathophysiology and implications for treatment. Part III. Injury to the central nervous system and limbs. *Journal of the Royal Naval Medical Service* 2000;**86**:27–31.

5. Wolf NM. *Underwater Blast Injury: A Review of the Literature.* US Navy Submarine Medical Research Laboratory report number 646. Groton, CT: US Navy; 1970.

6. Huller T, Bazini Y. Blast injuries of the chest and abdomen. *Archives of Surgery* 1970;**100**:2–30.

This chapter was reviewed for this fifth edition by Simon Mitchell.

PART 7

Specific Diving Diseases

35

The ear and diving: anatomy and physiology

INTRODUCTION

This section on the ear and diving (Chapters 35 to 38) is included because ear problems comprise the most common occupational diseases of diving, and the diving physician needs a working knowledge of otology. It is not always possible to obtain specialist assistance at an early stage in the assessment of a diving accident (i.e. when effective therapeutic decisions are made).

The ideal combination is a diving physician and an otologist, both of whom have an appreciation of the other's specialty. It is for the diving physician that this section is included.

EXTERNAL EAR

The *external ear* comprises the pinna and the external ear canal, which captures sound waves and directs them to the middle ear – separated from the external ear by the ear drum or tympanic membrane (Figure 35.1)

The external ear canal is approximately 3 cm long; the outer third is surrounded by cartilage and soft tissue, and the inner two thirds are surrounded by bone. It is lined by stratified squamous epithelium that tends to migrate outward, carrying casts of dead epithelial cells, foreign bodies (e.g. dust) and cerumen.

Cerumen or wax forms in the outer one third of the canal. At body temperature, the wax has bacteriostatic fatty acids and produces a hydrophobic lining that prevents the epithelium from becoming wet. This keeps the external ear canal from becoming soggy and creating a culture medium for infections of the external canal – *otitis externa* (see Chapter 29). The pH of the external canal lining is usually slightly acidic, which also acts as a bacteriostatic factor.

Interference with the function of the external canal can be produced by removal of the cerumen, whether by *syringing of the ear,* long periods of *immersion* or *traumatic gouging* of the canal with cotton buds, fingernails, hair pins and other objects. The mere presence of cerumen or wax should not be an indication for external ear toilet or syringing. On the contrary, syringing is likely to aggravate the subsequent otitis externa if it is performed before immersion (Case Report 35.1).

With immersion, divers can lose most of the cerumen from their ears, and it is rare to see a diver in frequent practice who has a significant amount of cerumen blockage unless he or she wears a hood that limits the entry of water.

In hyperbaric environments, as encountered by saturation and commercial divers, the

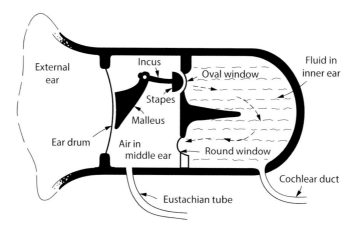

Figure 35.1 Ear anatomy.

CASE REPORT 35.1

During a diving medical seminar in Tahiti, a heated discussion ensued on the value of ear syringing to remove cerumen. Of the 44 divers present, only 3 were required by a Club Méditerranée physician to have cerumen removed from their ears, even though in none of these cases was the external ear obstructed. Otitis externa developed in 4 ears during the subsequent week – 1 bilateral and 2 unilateral cases – in the 3 divers who had their ears syringed. It demonstrated statistically what most of us knew clinically.

---

temperature and humidity encourage the growth of *Pseudomonas aeruginosa,* which causes the most common problem among these divers – otitis externa.

Patients with seborrhoeic dermatitis, often manifesting as dandruff, may have episodes of external ear itchiness. If they respond to this by scratching the ear, they will gouge out furrows of wax and excoriate the skin – thus breaking the two protective linings. Otitis externa may develop within hours. If they refrain from inflicting this trauma, and especially if they treat the inflammation and itch with the use of a non–water-based antiseptic or steroid ointment, then this unpleasant sequence of events will not occur.

Patients with an occluding cerumen plug or otitis externa should not dive, but they sometimes do. The obstruction of one external auditory canal may greatly restrict water entry, resulting in asymmetrical caloric stimuli and vertigo while diving and/or conductive hearing loss on the surface.

A long-term reaction to cold water in the external ear canal is the development of *exostoses* – usually from three sites around the ear canal. Being osteomata, exostoses are very hard white masses and are tightly covered by epithelium. Sometimes they grow to such a size that they occlude the external ear canal and cause conductive deafness. They take many years to grow and are also seen in surfers and swimmers. They may require removal by an otological surgeon, but sometimes complications ensue. Less extensive lesions can still produce problems by interfering with the drainage of cerumen, debris and water – thereby predisposing to otitis externa. Otitis externa may complete the partial occlusion of the canal that was initiated by the exostoses.

MIDDLE EAR

The *tympanic membrane,* separating the external and middle ears, is a thin but tough and flexible conical membrane. It mirrors the pathological features in both the external ear and the middle ear.

The *middle ear* is a gas-containing cavity separated from the external ear by the tympanic membrane and from the inner ear by the round and oval windows (Figure 35.2). Between the tympanic membrane and the oval window, three small bones are linked together – the ossicular chain, comprising the malleus, incus and stapes. These bones transmit the sound wave pressures on the ear drum across the middle ear and into the fluid-filled inner ear.

During otoscopy, the promontory and handle of the malleus can be seen impinging on the tympanic membrane. The stapes is attached by a strong, fibrous band to the oval window. An inward movement of the oval window is transmitted through the inner ear hydraulic system (peri-lymph) and is reflected by a similar but opposite movement of the round window, outward into the middle ear.

The *middle ear cleft* extends from the middle ear cavity into the air cells of the mastoid, petrous and zygomatic portion of the temporal bone postero-laterally, as well as into the Eustachian tube infero-medially. The middle ear is lined with mucosa that constantly absorbs oxygen from the enclosed space, thereby giving the middle ear a negative pressure (0 to –20 mm H_2O) relative to the environment. This is intermittently equalized by environmental pressure through the Eustachian tube. This tube is 3.5 to 4.0 cm long and is directed downward, forward and medially from the middle ear to the nasopharynx. It is usually closed, but it opens briefly and frequently. It is lined by respiratory epithelium and is subject to all the allergies, irritants and infections of this tissue.

The purposes of the Eustachian tube are to aerate the middle ear and maintain equal pressures across the tympanic membrane – between the middle ear and the environment. At the nasopharyngeal opening, the pressure is at environmental or ambient levels, whereas the middle ear opening of the Eustachian tube is at middle ear pressure. If there is a blockage of the Eustachian tube,

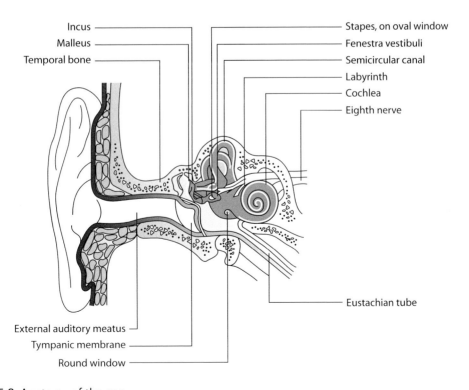

Figure 35.2 Anatomy of the ear.

the middle ear cannot be aerated regularly, and therefore a significant negative pressure develops at a rate of 50 mm H_2O per hour as oxygen is absorbed from this cavity by the mucous membrane. This results in a retracted tympanic membrane and an effusion, both of which partly reduce the negative pressure.

The Eustachian tube usually opens once a minute while one is awake and every 5 minutes during sleep. Swallowing and yawning commonly open this tube and allow replenishment of the gas to the middle ear from the nasopharynx, without any active or artificial overpressurization.

In divers, the Eustachian tube may be opened voluntarily by increasing the pressure in the nasopharynx by 50 to 250 mm H_2O in excess of the pressure in the middle ear (see Chapter 7). Then gas passes from the nasopharynx into the middle ear, thus alleviating the middle ear negative pressure produced as the diver descends. If equalization of the pressures is not achieved during descent, by the time a gradient of 400 to 1200 mm H_2O is reached, this pressure may produce a 'locking effect' on the valve-like cushions of the Eustachian tube that prevents further active or passive opening.

If the pressure in the middle ear exceeds that in the nasopharynx by 50 to 200 mm H_2O, then the Eustachian tube usually opens passively, and gas passes from the middle ear into the nasopharynx. This occurs when the diver ascends toward the surface.

The foregoing pressures are pressure differences between the spaces mentioned. They should not be directly extrapolated to water depths because of the considerable tissue movement and distortion that reduce some of the pressure gradients during ascent and descent. Thus, a diver with a very mobile tympanic membrane and a small-volume middle ear cleft would be able to tolerate a much greater descent without experiencing any change in middle ear pressures. In practice, it is found that if the Eustachian tubes are not open, the diver may experience some subjective sensation at a depth of 0.3 m H_2O. Discomfort or pain may be felt at a depth as shallow as 2 metres – this is also the depth at which the locking effect can develop, and the tympanic membrane may rupture from a dive to 2 to 10 metres.

Abnormalities of Eustachian tube function in divers or other groups exposed to variations in ambient pressure result in middle ear barotrauma and indirectly in inner ear barotrauma, with mucosal and membrane haemorrhage and ruptures. These clinical entities are dealt with in the discussion of barotrauma in Chapter 7 and in the differential diagnosis of deafness and disorientation (see Chapters 37 and 38).

INNER EAR

The inner ear is composed of the cochlea, a snail-like structure responsible for hearing, and the vestibular system, which is responsible for the orientation in space (i.e. appreciation of acceleration, equilibrium, balance and positioning) (Figure 35.3).

Sound and hearing

The hearing part of the inner ear, the cochlea, is composed of three adjoining tubes or scalae:

- The scala vestibuli (or inner tube) is connected to the middle ear by the oval window membrane and the foot plate of the stapes. It contains perilymph, which is similar in composition to extracellular fluid.
- The scala tympani (or outer tube) is connected to the middle ear via the thin and fragile but flexible, round window membrane. This also contains perilymph, which is continuous with that of the vestibuli. The vestibuli and the tympani communicate at the apex.
- The scala media (or middle) tube lies between the other two channels, demarcated from the scala vestibuli by a fragile Reissner's or vestibular membrane. This separates the fluid of the two tubes but is so thin that it does not impede the pressure waves (sound) passing between them. Between the scala media and the scala tympani, there is the much thicker basilar membrane, which does impede sound waves and supports the 25 000 reed-like basilar fibres, which are connected to the sound receptors, called hair cells. Each sound frequency causes a vibration at a different sector of the basilar membrane. Near the

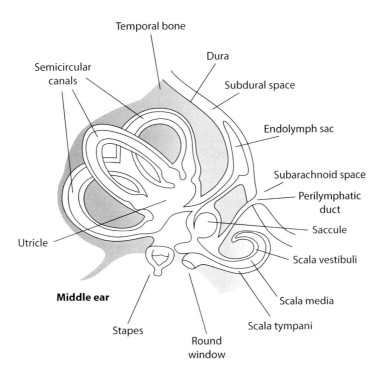

Figure 35.3 Inner ear anatomy.

oval and round windows, the basilar fibres are short and rigid, and they are sensitive to high-frequency sounds, whereas further up the cochlea, they become longer and more flexible and respond to low-frequency sounds. Damage to specific areas produces specific hearing loss. The fluid within the media is endolymph, similar in composition to intracellular fluid.

The integrity of the foregoing membranes, together with the different composition and electrical potential of the inner ear fluids, is required for normal hearing.

Sound is caused by the vibrations or pressure waves at frequencies between 20 and 20 000 cycles per second (20 to 20 000 Hertz), transmitted to the ear in air or water.

The external ear directs the lower-frequency sound to the tympanic membrane. This vibrates and transmits these vibrations through the ossicular chain of the middle ear to the oval window and thence to the cochlea fluid of the inner ear, thereby distorting the basilar membrane and triggering off

the nerve impulses from the hair cells (transducers). Thus, pressure waves are converted into electrical impulses that are passed to the brain via the eighth (auditory) nerve, where they are identified and interpreted as sound. The pressure wave disperses by distending the round window into the middle ear. Once the sound stops, these structures resume their normal position.

The hair cells of the cochlea may also be stimulated by vibration of the bones of the skull. Sounds that cause this vibration and are heard in this manner are transmitted by bone conduction. This method of hearing is less sensitive than the air conduction pathway, but it is important for hearing underwater. It is the pathway by which people with external and middle ear damage can still hear.

Perilymphatic aqueducts of variable size may connect the perilymph fluid of the cochlea and vestibular system to the cerebrospinal fluid in the brain's subarachnoid space. This also allows transmission of pressure between the two hydraulic systems and explains why Valsalva manoeuvres, coughing and so forth can cause a pressure wave in the perilymph that is transmitted from intrathoracic pressure to the venous system and the cerebrospinal fluid.

Symptoms of cochlea impairment include tinnitus, dysacusis and hearing loss.

Balance and spatial orientation

The balance organ of the inner ear is called the vestibular apparatus, and it includes three semicircular canals, positioned at right angles to each other. They measure movement of the enclosed fluid in any plane, by end organs (transducers). The semicircular canals detect change of movement of the head and supply this information by nerve impulses to the central nervous system.

These canals connect with the utricle and the saccule, which are ballooned, fluid-filled cavities, also at right angles to each other. They contain otoliths (ear stones) – sensory end organs (also transducers) able to detect movement of fluid and influenced by gravity. They supply gravitational information of the position of the head in space.

The vestibular system is very dynamic, with constant input from all areas at all times. The end organs fire electrical discharges even in the resting state. If there is a stimulus in one area, then there should be a corresponding stimulus in a complementary area on the other side; otherwise, conflicting messages are received by the brain. These impulses, giving information regarding position and movement in space, are transmitted to the brain by the vestibular part of the eighth cranial nerve to the brainstem and finally the cerebellum, where balance is monitored, co-ordinated and interpreted.

The membranous labyrinth is somewhat like an inflated inner tube of an automobile tire, and it contains endolymph, which also fills the scala media. Around the membranous labyrinth there is perilymph, which fills the scala vestibuli and tympani and is also connected to the cerebrospinal fluid by the perilymphatic duct.

Vestibular damage may lead to symptoms of disorientation and imbalance, vertigo and associated vagal complaints such as nausea, vomiting and syncope. Nystagmus, the clinical sign that corresponds to symptomatic vertigo, is a typical flickering eye movement with a slow component moving the eyes to one side and a fast or 'correcting' component bringing the eyes back to their original position. With an irritating lesion in one vestibular system, the nystagmus (fast component) is to that side. A destructive lesion causes it to go to the opposite side. Nystagmus, like vertigo, can be suppressed by other sensory input, cortical inhibition, some drugs and other factors.

If the vestibular system is damaged irreparably, the clinical features may diminish over the subsequent weeks or months as the brain accommodates to the inequality by suppressing responses from the undamaged side (cerebral inhibition). Nevertheless, the damage can still be demonstrated by provocative tests (e.g. caloric electronystagmograms) or movements (sudden head turning) (see Chapter 36). If the damage is more central, such as in the cerebellum, then nystagmus may persist even though the vertigo can be partly inhibited.

Under normal circumstances, balance control is characterized by much redundancy, and so one area of the visual-proprioceptive-vestibular complex may be damaged without inevitable imbalance or ataxia.

CLINICAL OTOSCOPY

Visual inspection of the external ear canal and tympanic membrane is one of the more valuable clinical examinations to be made on diving candidates. Otological disorders such as cholesteatoma may be diagnosed, or there may be a condition such as otitis externa, which is aggravated by diving, or a perforated tympanic membrane making the diver susceptible to vertigo and otitis media. An external ear blockage predisposes to vertigo and external ear barotrauma. As well as allowing identification of both external and middle ear barotraumas, a major value of otoscopy is the verification of a successful middle ear autoinflation under voluntary control (see Chapter 7).

The tympanic membrane is viewed while the candidate attempts to inflate the middle ear by active manoeuvres. Commonly, one ear is easier to autoinflate than the other, and so when diving the main attention is focused on the slower ear. Physicians experienced in diving medicine spend considerable time ensuring that diving candidates understand the techniques and sensations experienced during middle ear autoinflation. Inadequate middle ear autoinflation is responsible for the most common and preventable diving illness – middle ear barotrauma of descent.

In one Australian series, the tympanic membrane was viewed initially in 87 per cent of diving candidates, with 84 per cent being mobile during the autoinflation. In the remaining 13 per cent of diving candidates, 12 per cent claimed subjective autoinflation. The otoscopic view was obstructed by cerumen in 9 per cent, by an unusual canal alignment or structure in 3 per cent and by exostoses in 1 per cent.

Pneumatic otoscopy can demonstrate the mobility of the ear drum, but it is of no value in verifying the voluntary control of autoinflation, required by divers.

FURTHER READING

Edmonds C, Freeman P, Thomas R, Tonkin J, Blackwood FA. *Otological Aspects of Diving.* Sydney: Australasian Medical Publishing; 1973.

Farmer JC. Otological and paranasal problems in diving. In: Bennett PB, Elliott H, eds. *The Physiology and Medicine of Diving.* 4th ed. London: Saunders; 1993.

Hunter ES, Farmer JC. Ear and sinus problems in diving. In: Bove A, Davis J, eds. *Bove and Davis' Diving Medicine.* 4th ed. Philadelphia: Saunders; 2004.

Molvaer OI. Otorhinological aspects of diving. In: Brubakk AO, Neuman TS, eds. *Bennett and Elliott's Physiology and Medicine of Diving.* 5th ed. London: Saunders; 2003.

This chapter was reviewed for this fifth edition by Carl Edmonds.

36

The ear and diving: investigations

INTRODUCTION

Otological investigations vary among different clinics depending on their sophistication, skills and clinical orientation. This discussion is confined to investigations that have been found of value in clinical diving medicine.

Simple tests of hearing are mentioned in Chapter 37, and tests of balance in Chapter 38, and these investigations are applicable in remote areas. A specialized diving medical unit employs pure tone audiometry, impedance audiometry and the electronystagmogram (ENG). Otological clinics have far more specialized procedures.

PURE TONE AUDIOMETRY

This technique measures the ability to hear pure tones in octaves between 125 and 8000 Hz (cycles per second) (Figure 36.1). The hearing loss in each frequency is measured in decibels – a logarithmic scale, which means that a loss of 10 dB represents a 10-fold change in intensity of the noise, 20 dB a 100-fold change, 30 dB a 1000-fold change and so forth. Testing is done initially for air conduction, but if this is significantly impaired, then bone conduction should be measured. With sensorineural deafness, the loss is the same for both air and bone conduction.

If bone conduction is adequate and normal, then it infers that the cochlea is picking up sound waves transmitted via the bone, and therefore the sensorineural component of the hearing is normal. If there is a considerable discrepancy, with poor air conduction but normal bone conduction, then this suggests 'conductive' deafness (i.e. involving the external or middle ear; see Figure 36.1).

A very quiet area, usually a soundproof audiogram booth, is necessary for reliable testing. In patient with severe unilateral deafness, sound levels of 40 to 60 dB can be heard by cross-hearing, and therefore masking is needed in the good ear while the damaged one is being tested above this level.

As a general rule, conductive deafness tends to be first noted in the lower frequencies, 250 to 3000 Hz, and the sensorineural damage is first noted somewhere between 4000 and 8000 Hz. If there is serious and significant nerve damage, then all frequencies may be involved.

More elaborate audiology procedures, using such devices and techniques as recruitment, brainstem and Bekesy audiometry, short-increment sensitivity index (SISI) and pure tone decay, are used

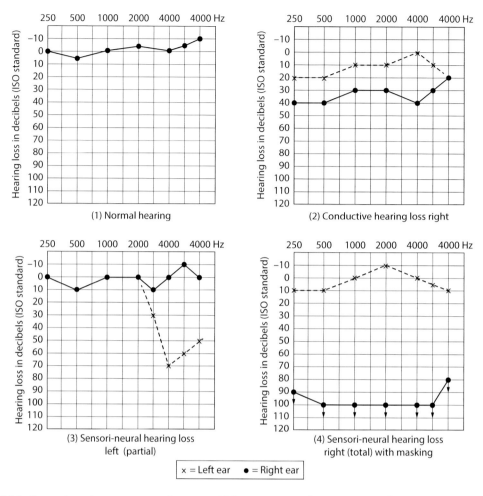

Figure 36.1 Examples of pure tone audiograms. ISO, International Organization for Standardization.

by otologists – but they are of little interest to the diving physician. Speech discrimination testing is of value if there is distortion of hearing.

The most valuable of all ear function tests is the comparison of repeated pure tone audiograms. If these measurements are made before the diver commences his or her hyperbaric experiences, and routinely during the diving career, then cumulative damage can be readily identified.

Pure tone audiometry should also be performed immediately if there is any subjective complaint of hearing loss or evidence of an inner ear disorder such as tinnitus or vestibular symptoms. Once evidence of sensorineural impairment is found, then serial audiometry should be performed to ensure that therapeutic measures are having their desired effect.

TYMPANOMETRY

Indirect assessments of the function of the middle ear cavity and the Eustachian tube are obtained from most of the otological investigations. Techniques to measure the middle ear pressures and movements directly are now available to clinicians.

The tympanometer (impedance audiometer) is designed to facilitate the quick, objective testing of middle ear function by measuring the mobility of the middle ear system (usually called compliance), the pressure within the middle ear cavity and the variation in middle ear mobility reacting to variations of pressure from −300 to +300 mm H_2O applied in the external ear. It can also react to voluntary autoinflation of the middle ear through the Eustachian tube – and herein lies its specific value to the diving clinician.

A graph is produced on an XY plotter and is termed a tympanogram, with the peak height on the Y axis showing the compliance and its position on the X axis showing the middle ear pressure (Figure 36.2). The middle ear pressure can be changed with successful middle ear autoinflation manoeuvres.

The middle ear pressures, recorded as the position of the tympanogram peak on the X axis, change with different diving environments and accidents. There may be a decrease of middle ear pressure when 100 per cent oxygen is breathed or an increase in middle ear pressure when a helium-oxygen mixture (heliox) is breathed. In the first case, nitrogen is lost and oxygen is absorbed from the middle ear, and this is one of the causes of serous otitis media with oxygen-breathing divers. The reason for the increase in middle ear pressure while breathing heliox is that the helium moves into the middle ear faster than the nitrogen moves out.

Pathological conditions that may cause a **positive pressure peak** are as follows: acute otitis media in the very early stages; middle ear barotrauma of descent (after subsequent ascent) after haemorrhage and exudation in the middle ear; and overpressure from middle ear barotrauma of ascent (see Figure 36.2).

A **negative pressure peak** may develop with middle ear barotrauma of descent, while the diver is still at depth. Negative pressure peaks are related to inadequate Eustachian tube patency and are associated with absorption of gas from the middle ear cavity. Eustachian tube blockage, insufficient autoinflation and oxygen inhalation are typical causes. The negative middle ear pressure may result in effusion, and if the middle ear accumulates a significant amount of fluid, the pressure peak may disappear and the tympanogram becomes flat.

Middle ear barotrauma of descent, producing congestion and swelling within the middle ear, results in a decreased amplitude of the peak of the tympanogram, thus demonstrating reduced **compliance**. These rise as the structures and lining of the middle ear return to normal.

With **perforation of the tympanic membrane,** no pressure gradient can exist across the membrane, and therefore there is no peak. This information is used clinically to show the patency of grommets inserted into the tympanic membrane, but it is also of value in demonstrating a perforated tympanic membrane that cannot be seen otoscopically.

Tympanograms with increased amplitude or notches may be caused by an ear drum abnormality or ossicular discontinuity. Increased amplitude or notching occurs with healed perforations, and a W-shaped pattern can be produced. Ossicular chain discontinuity may cause a high peak or deep or multiple notches.

The presence of a respiratory wave in the tympanogram implies a continuously open (patent) Eustachian tube – an occasional sequela of middle ear barotrauma, especially with overly forceful Valsalva manoeuvres.

A way of verifying inner ear fistula that is currently under investigation integrates an impedance audiometer and an ENG, with both horizontal and vertical leads. The induction of nystagmus during the external ear pressure change may give some support to the diagnosis, but this procedure should be performed only if facilities exist for immediate inner ear surgery – if the procedure enlarges the fistula.

Diving tympanogram

In 1973, Edmonds and colleagues verified voluntary autoinflation attempts by divers, by using a manually controlled tympanogram. The pressure in the external ear was changed from −300 to +300 mm H_2O, and this tympanogram was used as the control. The pressure in the external ear was then moved to zero, and a Valsalva manoeuvre was performed by the subject. A tympanogram was then repeated, moving from −100 to +300 mm H_2O. If the Valsalva was successful, this demonstrated a significant movement of the peak, thus validating the increase in the middle ear pressure (because the Valsalva manoeuvre forced more air into this cavity). At the completion of this second tympanogram, at +300 mm H_2O, the

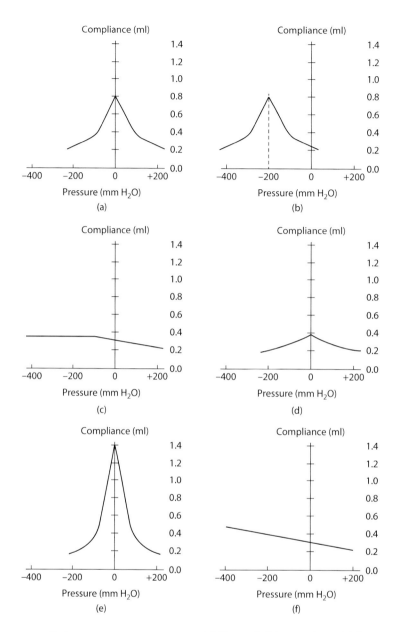

Figure 36.2 Diagrammatic tympanogram responses. **(a)** Normal; **(b)** negative middle ear pressure (e.g. Eustachian tube obstruction); **(c)** fluid-filled middle ear cavity (e.g. haemorrhage from severe middle ear barotrauma); **(d)** reduced compliance (e.g. otosclerosis or mucosal congestion in the middle ear from barotrauma); **(e)** increased compliance seen with disarticulation of the ossicles, scarred or very mobile tympanic membranes; **(f)** perforated tympanic membrane.

subject was then asked to perform the Toynbee manoeuvre, and the third tympanogram was recorded, passing from +300 to −300 mm H$_2$O. If the Toynbee manoeuvre was successful, the peak of the tympanogram returned toward the control, or even beyond it, to indicate a reduction of middle ear pressure (Figure 36.3).

This method is an objective way of measuring the effects of voluntary autoinflation and deflation on the middle ear. This technique included

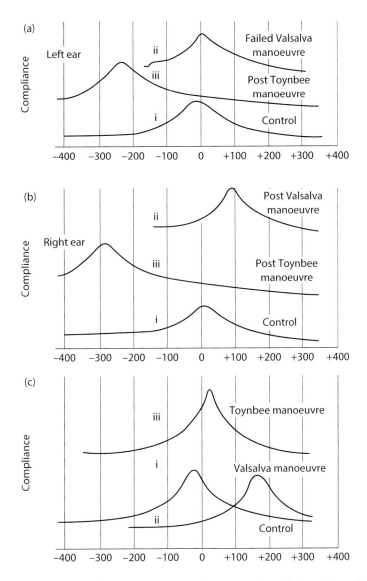

Figure 36.3 Diving tympanogram: the tympanometry demonstration of the effect of Valsalva and Toynbee manoeuvres on middle ear pressures. **(a)** Left ear: (i) normal control tympanogram, passing from 400 mm H_2O on the left to +300 mm H_2O on the right (note: opposite to the conventional technique); (ii) Valsalva manoeuvre attempted at the neutral position (peak of control tympanogram) and a repeat tympanogram from 100 mm H_2O to +300 mm H_2O shows no substantial movement of the peak (i.e. middle ear pressures were not induced by the procedure). The Valsalva manoeuvre failed; (iii) Toynbee manoeuvre performed at +300 mm H_2O with the subsequent tympanogram showing a 225 mm H_2O negative pressure being produced in the middle ear. The Toynbee manoeuvre was successful. **(b)** Right ear: (i) normal control tympanogram; (ii) Valsalva manoeuvre produced an 80 mm H_2O positive pressure in the middle ear; (iii) Toynbee manoeuvre at +300 mm H_2O produced a 280 mm H_2O negative pressure to the middle ear. The Valsalva and Toynbee manoeuvres were successful. Note: For patients' tolerance, the technique has been modified to extend between 300 and +300 mm H_2O. **(c)** Diving tympanogram demonstrates an increase in middle ear pressure from 25 mm H_2O (normal) to +175 mm H_2O with Valsalva manoeuvre and then a partially successful Toynbee manoeuvre, reducing the middle ear pressure to +25 mm H_2O.

modifications of the conventional tympanogram, to avoid inadvertent opening of the Eustachian tube (and consequent release of post-Valsalva pressure), induced by positive pressures encountered during the traditional procedure.

Modified diving tympanogram

A modification of the foregoing procedure was promoted by Lehm and Bennett to employ the simplified portable automatic tympanometer (e.g. MicroTymp, Welch Allyn, Skaneateles Falls, New York), which has fixed pressure gradients and a digital readout.

Three tympanograms were performed on each ear. The first tympanogram was performed before any attempt to ventilate the middle ear actively (the 'static tymp' test). The subjects were then asked to perform a Valsalva manoeuvre and requested not to talk or swallow until a second tympanogram was completed on both ears. Subjects were then asked to swallow three times, and a third tympanogram was performed. The presence of normal Eustachian tube function and correct performance of the manoeuvre were recorded if the peak pressure became more positive following the Valsalva manoeuvre and returned to baseline or more negative after swallowing. A failure to move the peak pressure wave indicates a likely problem with autoinflation.

The tympanometer is a valuable instrument for use in both the clinical and research aspects of diving medicine.

VESTIBULAR FUNCTION TESTING

When there is an imbalance in the neural activity from the vestibular systems, involuntary eye movements develop and are termed *nystagmus*. This is the physical sign that corresponds to the sensation of vertigo.

Spontaneous nystagmus is an important sign of vestibular disorder. **Positional vestibular testing** refers to the effects of certain head, neck and eye positions in producing abnormal vestibular responses in some patients.

The Hallpike caloric tests were the traditional tests used to demonstrate the activity of the vestibular system stimulated by water at temperatures of 30°C and 44°C (i.e. 7°C above and below body temperature), with the subject lying supine and the head elevated to 30 degrees. The temperature change causes convection currents in the horizontal or lateral semicircular canal, and this stimulates the vestibular system. The response to hot and cold water on both sides is compared, and conclusions are drawn on whether there is unequal function of the two vestibular systems to identical stimuli and whether there is preponderance of responses to one side. The first suggests a peripheral lesion and the second a more central one.

In the event of no response from one side, greater stimuli may be given, such as iced water calorics (more practical than the standard calorics under most operational hyperbaric conditions) or even drug provocation.

If nystagmus is estimated clinically (i.e. by unaided observation or by the use of Frenzel's glasses), it is a crude sign and is associated with many misinterpretations. With peripheral vestibular lesions, the eye movements are sometimes best observed by having the subject close the eyes and perform distracting exercises such as mental arithmetic. The eyes can then be seen rolling with fast and slow components beneath the closed lids. These primitive techniques of assessing vestibular function in the field are rarely needed currently. Vestibular function assessment has been revolutionized by the addition of the ENG to detect spontaneous nystagmus and the effects of both positional and caloric provocation.

Electronystagmogram

ENG assessment of nystagmus is an objective and quantitative measure of the ocular movement, and it is a sensitive measurement of vestibular dysfunction. The ENG is far more sensitive than the clinical sensation of vertigo, and therefore it depicts subclinical levels of vestibular disease. It may demonstrate abnormality long after the symptoms have disappeared.

The recordings are measurements of movement of the eye that causes a deflection on its electrical field. This is possible because the retina has a negative charge compared with the cornea, and as the eyes move so does the electrical field, detected by electrodes adjacent to the eyes. In some units, infrared tracking devices in a dark room have now replaced electrical leads to measure eye movement.

In clinical practice, the conventional ENG is a graphic record of vestibular function made during various positions and during caloric stimulation – the Hallpike tests described earlier. Thus, the horizontal electrodes are commonly used. In diving research, it is recommended that the tracings embrace both horizontal and vertical movements.

By the use of this very valuable and objective test, vestibular dysfunction can be demonstrated. The duration of the nystagmus can be observed, reviewed and measured, and the degree of nystagmus can be quantified by different parameters (rate, height and deflection of the slow and fast components). The vestibular responses can be stimulated in a provocative but selective manner by the use of the Hallpike caloric test, positional tests and even changing pressures – locally in the external ear or by altering the subject's ambient pressure in compression chambers.

Stress may be used to increase the sensitivity of the ENG to demonstrate perilymph fistulae. In these cases, either pressure (tympanometry) may be applied to the external canal (Hennebert's sign) or a loud noise of 95 dB at 500 Hz (Tullio phenomenon) may be used. Alternately, body sway–type tests can be used. The frequencies of the stimuli can be reduced to those more likely to have vestibular effects, such as 50 or 25 Hz, and the intensity can be increased to 130 dB, with the patient standing on a platform to measure postural stability during low-frequency stimulation.

The ENG has revolutionized the approach to vertigo and its relationship with diving, and it has allowed physicians to clarify and verify clinical impressions, often by demonstrating significant pathophysiological features in cases that may otherwise have been classified as functional. ENG has an occasional application as an electrodiagnostic procedure in recompression chambers, with the electrode leads under pressure and the measuring equipment outside the chamber, to assist in diagnosis and to monitor the effects of therapeutic intervention such as recompression and gas mixture alterations.

ENGs may be used to differentiate end-organ (vestibular) disease from central (brain) causes of vertigo and dizziness. The ENG in peripheral vestibular end-organ disease produces spontaneous nystagmus greater than 7 degrees/second, as a result of a reduction in the tonic discharge from the affected vestibule. The nystagmus (fast phase) is thus toward the side of increased vestibular activity. It is strongest when the subject looks to the same side as the fast phase. It is suppressed by visual fixation (more than 40 per cent) and is augmented by eye closing and mental concentration (e.g. mathematical calculations).

Sophisticated computerized balance and movement tests are used in many balance disorder clinics.

RADIOLOGY AND SCREENING TECHNIQUES

The value of plain x-ray studies of the otological area is limited to demonstration of middle ear, mastoid and para-nasal cavities. They are of value in assessing the safety of deaf divers to undergo compression.

More recently, the use of computed tomography, magnetic resonance imaging and other scanning techniques has allowed identification of more anatomical and pathological structures. These methods have been used to demonstrate the degree of barotraumas, integrity of the round window membrane, gas and haemorrhagic lesions in the inner ear, among other conditions.

Brain scans and arterial Doppler measurements are applicable in some differential diagnoses.

Future developments in this field are expected, but in practice the value of the sophisticated scanning techniques is limited at this stage.

FURTHER READING

Black FO, Lilly DJ, Peterka RJ, Hemenway WG, Pesznec SC. The dynamic posturographic pressure test for the presumptive diagnosis of perilymph fistulas. *Neurologic Clinics* 1990;**8**:361–374.

Edmonds C, Freeman P, Tonkin J, Thomas R, Blackwood F. *Otological Aspects of Diving*. Sydney: Australasian Medical Publishing; 1973.

Elner A, Ingelstedt S, Ivarsson A. A method for studies of the middle ear mechanics. *Acta Otolaryngologica* 1971;**72**:191.

Farmer JC. Otological and paranasal problems in diving. In: Bennett PB, Elliott H, eds. *The Physiology and Medicine of Diving*. 4th ed. London: Saunders; 1993.

Flood M, Fraser G, Hazell JWP, Rothera MP. Perilymph fistulae. *Journal of Laryngology and Otology* 1985;**99**:671–676.

Gersdorff MC. Tubal-impedance-manometry. *Archives of Oto Rhino-Laryngology* 1977;**217**:319–407.

Ingelstedt S, Invarsson A, Jonson B. Mechanics of the human middle ear. *Acta Otolaryngologica* 1967;**228**(Suppl):1–58.

Kohut RI. Perilymph fistulas: clinical criteria. *Archives of Otolaryngology Head and Neck Surgery* 1992;**118**:687–692.

Lehm JP, Bennett MH. Predictors of middle ear barotrauma associated with hyperbaric oxygen therapy. *South Pacific Underwater Medicine Society Journal* 2003;**33**:127–133.

Mcneill C. Testing for Perilymphatic Fistula: A Subjective Procedure for Audiologists. M.A. thesis (audiology). Sydney: Macquarie University; 1992.

Pyykko I, Ishizaki H, Aalto H, Starck J. Relevance of the Tullio phenomenon in assessing perilymphatic leak in vertiginous patients. *American Journal of Otology* 1991/92;**13**(4):339–342.

Riu R, Hottes L, Giullerma R, Badres R, LeDen R. La trompe d'eustache dans la plongée. *Revue de Physiologie Subaquatique et Médecine Hyperbare*, 1969:194–198.

This chapter was reviewed for this fifth edition by Carl Edmonds.

37

The ear and diving: hearing loss

CLINICAL FEATURES

Deafness is one of the most common symptoms encountered in diving medicine. For accurate diagnosis, an objective measurement of the hearing loss is required, using pure tone audiograms (PTAs). Figure 37.1 illustrates the mechanisms of sound transmission.

In some cases, the complaint is not supported by conventional audiometric testing. The diver may refer to a feeling of 'fullness' or 'blockage' within the middle ear. This is a sensation associated with congestion and swelling of the tympanic membrane and mucosal lining of the middle ear cavity. It is commonly caused by middle ear barotrauma of descent, and it frequently resolves within a week or so. Hearing loss is usually identified and clarified by a combination of clinical history, otoscopy, tympanometry and PTAs.

Hearing loss can be associated with tinnitus, dysacusis or, if the associated vestibular system is involved, vertigo (see Chapter 38).

Objective hearing loss in divers may be of four types (see Chapter 36):

- Conductive – caused by problems of the conductive apparatus (external ear, tympanic membrane, ossicles, middle ear). This is common.

- Sensorineural – in which the problem lies in the cochlea or the auditory nerve. This is less common, but very important.
- Central – resulting from lesions of the auditory pathways in the brain, central to the cochlear nuclei. This is rare because the hearing centres are bilaterally represented.
- Mixed – various combinations of the foregoing three types.

The type of hearing loss can be inferred from the *patient's speech*. Soft but articulate speech associated with a moderately severe hearing loss is suggestive of conductive deafness. Loud, clear speech suggests an acquired bilateral sensorineural hearing loss. Slurred, hesitant, inarticulate and inaccurate speech is more likely with central lesions. Impaired speech discrimination may be obvious during the interview.

The otological examination may include the *tuning fork tests*. The Rinne test becomes abnormal when the tuning fork is heard louder by bone conduction (fork base held on the mastoid bone) than by air conduction (tines of fork placed over the auditory meatus). This result indicates 'conductive' deafness. A Barany noise box may 'mask' the other ear during the tests, which may extend between 64- and 4096-Hz tuning forks.

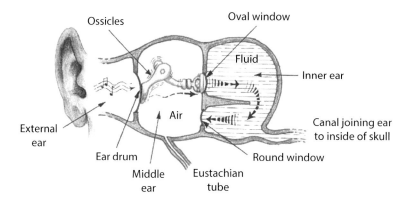

Figure 37.1 Sound transmission, conducted through the external and middle ears, into the sensorineural inner ear.

The Weber test is performed with a 256- or 512 Hz-tuning fork. It is placed on the vertex of the skull, and the subject indicates in which ear he or she hears the tuning fork. The patient hears it in the affected ear with conductive deafness, the unaffected ear with sensorineural deafness or both ears in mixed or bilateral deafness (or in normal hearing).

The Schwabach test is performed by comparing the patient's and the examiner's ability to hear the tuning fork tests by bone conduction.

Operational hearing tests

In remote environments, use can be made of even more primitive techniques. The ticking or alarm from a wrist watch or digital gaming device has a reliable sound intensity and frequency. The frequency is commonly about 4000 to 6000 Hz, and this is the area that is less noticeable to the diver than the usual voice frequencies of 250 to 2000 Hz. Comparison is made between the diver's two ears and the examiner's. The finding that the watch can be heard only in one ear, or that the hearing acuity for the watch ticking is less than that of the examiner's, suggests that a PTA is required. For divers who have subjective sensations of 'dullness', these basic hearing tests give some reassurance to the examiner that a gross sensorineural hearing loss is less likely.

As a rough general indicator, for use in remote or isolated areas, an approximation of the diving accident victim's hearing can thus be made by:

Speech.
Associated symptoms (e.g. tinnitus, vertigo).
Hearing tests with watch, electronic devices and whispered speech.
'Tuning fork' tests – Rinne, Weber and Schwabach.

The type and existence of hearing loss are confirmed by audiometric testing (see Chapter 36). Most value is obtained by comparison of the diver's post-incident audiograms with those performed before diving training, or previous annual audiograms if he or she is a frequent or professional diver. If hearing loss is demonstrated, bone conduction testing should be performed. A classification of the types of hearing loss can be made, based on whether it is predominantly conductive or sensorineural.

CLASSIFICATION OF HEARING LOSS IN DIVING

Conductive hearing loss.
  a. External ear obstruction.
    i. Cerumen.
    ii. Otitis externa.
    iii. Exostoses.

b. Tympanic membrane perforation.
  i. Middle ear barotrauma of descent.
  ii. Forceful autoinflation.
  iii. Shock wave.
c. Middle ear cleft disorder.
  i. Middle ear barotrauma of descent.
  ii. Otitis media.
  iii. Forceful autoinflation.
  iv. Increased gas density in middle ear.
  v. Ossicular disruption.
Sensorineural hearing loss.
  a. Noise-induced hearing loss.
  b. Decompression sickness.
  c. Inner ear barotrauma.
Other forms of hearing loss.
Dysacusis.

CONDUCTIVE DEAFNESS

External ear obstruction

Obstruction of the external ear is not uncommon in divers. It is easily diagnosed both by history and by otoscopic examination. It may also induce vertigo under certain circumstances (see Chapter 38). The causes are as follows:

1. *Cerumen plug.* Conductive deafness may result from the movement of cerumen in the external ear as a result of gas space alterations with diving. Water may cause swelling of the desquamated tissue and cerumen, possibly obstructing an external canal that was already partly blocked.
2. *Otitis externa.* Infection is aggravated by immersion of the ear in water (see Chapters 29 and 35).
3. *Exostoses.* Exostoses may be single or multiple (see Chapter 35). Although complete obstruction of the external canal is infrequently caused by these alone, it may develop in the presence of cerumen or otitis externa.

Tympanic membrane perforation

Perforation of the tympanic membrane is a not uncommon complication of diving. There is usually a well-defined reason. The patient may complain of a sensation of air hissing through the tympanic membrane, especially during autoinflation of the middle ear.

Caloric stimulation may produce transient vertigo underwater (see Chapters 7 and 38). The hearing loss is conductive, but usually only 5 to 15 dB on a PTA. The lower frequencies are most affected. Hearing loss is rectified when the tympanic membrane is almost closed. This may take hours to a few days with small perforations or weeks with larger ones.

Clinical management includes keeping the ear dry. Divers are advised not to aggravate the problem by further pressure changes (e.g. flying, diving, nose-blowing or middle ear autoinflation [which divers with ear symptoms tend to do]). Prophylactic oral antibiotics are rarely indicated. In some cases, the diver may become aware of the perforation only at a later date (e.g. when returning from a diving expedition or after performing a Valsalva manoeuvre).

The causes of perforation of the tympanic membrane during diving include the following:

1. *Middle ear barotrauma of descent* (see Chapter 7).
2. *Forceful autoinflation.* The Valsalva manoeuvre may cause perforation of the tympanic membrane, especially if the membrane has been damaged previously (e.g. by middle ear barotrauma, otitis externa, scarring, old perforations).
3. *Shock wave.* This may result from an underwater explosion or the pressure wave from another diver's fin. These patients often develop vertigo, and there are often no signs of middle ear barotrauma of descent on otoscopy.

Middle ear disease

Dullness of hearing, dampening of sound, deafness and 'fullness' or 'blockage' within the ear are common symptoms reported by divers. The most common cause is middle ear barotrauma of descent.

Middle ear diseases associated with diving are as follows:

1. *Middle ear barotrauma of descent.* This is also known as 'ear squeeze' (see Chapter 7).
2. *Otitis media.* The hearing loss is of the conductive type. Infection may follow contamination

of the middle ear with nasopharyngeal organisms, introduced with autoinflation. It may progress because of the culture media of blood and effusion, caused by middle ear barotrauma of descent. The patient usually presents with pain that has developed within 6 to 24 hours of a dive. Prognosis and treatment are based on general medical principles (see Chapter 29).

3. *Forceful autoinflation of the middle ear.* This is associated with middle ear barotrauma of descent, and it may be an indirect cause of some of the damage noted with this disorder. Damage may affect the tympanic membrane, ossicles, oval window, cochlea or round window. Damage of the last three structures may result in a sensorineural deafness. Dysacusis may also develop (see later).

4. *Increased gas density.* With exposure to increased pressure and increased depth, more gas molecules pass into the middle ear to maintain its volume. The gas is denser – causing a depth-related, reversible hearing loss resulting from increased impedance of the middle ear transformer. This explains some of the hearing loss noted in recompression chamber experiments and helmet diving. The use of helium, which reverses this increased gas density, unfortunately changes the middle ear resonant frequency, thereby also interfering with normal hearing. Underwater, bone conduction is the major sound pathway for hearing.

5. *Ossicular disruption.* This disorder may follow middle ear barotrauma and may also cause a mixed hearing loss. It is identified on the tympanogram (see Chapter 36).

> Hearing loss in diving may be either conductive or sensorineural; the latter is more serious, and the former is more common.

SENSORINEURAL DEAFNESS

Noise-induced deafness

Extreme noise exposure may result in temporary or permanent threshold shifts that manifest as sensorineural deafness. The sensorineural deafness is usually bilateral and partial. This may be experienced in compression chambers or with diving helmets or compressors, for example.

The hearing loss is confined almost entirely to frequencies higher than the frequency of the offending noise, with the greatest shift for tones about half an octave above the exposure tone, but all the higher frequencies may be more or less affected. Hearing for lower tones remains almost unaffected.

Exposure to a 1000-Hz signal at 120 dB (the threshold of discomfort) for half an hour usually causes a temporary threshold shift of about 35 dB over the upper half of the speech range. These changes are normally reversible, but the frequencies that are most vulnerable and least likely to recover are those between 3000 and 6000 Hz. Paradoxically, the threshold shift may be a protective mechanism that protects against even greater damage.

> Frequencies between 3000 and 6000 Hz are particularly susceptible to noise-induced deafness.

Repeated exposure to loud noise may cause a permanent threshold shift in which the multiple threshold shifts summate, especially if there is little time between the exposures. Prolonged and repeated exposure to noise is also likely to occur in attendants who work with compressors and compression chambers. Under these conditions, it would be expected that the noise-induced deafness would be bilateral.

Divers in the armed services are often trained in gunnery and explosives – both predispose to sensorineural deafness.

Pre-existing sensorineural deafness seems to sensitize the ears to further damage from other causes.

Decompression sickness

The clinical manifestations of decompression sickness are discussed in Chapter 12.

Inner ear barotrauma

Ear barotrauma is discussed in Chapter 7.

Pure tone audiograms should be performed on all divers, recreational and commercial, before exposing them to hyperbaric conditions. Without these pre-incident audiograms, an assessment of hearing damage is more difficult, especially because it predominantly involves the asymptomatic high frequencies in mild or early cases. In mild sensorineural deafness, unlike the conductive deafness that interferes with speech frequencies, the diver may not be aware of the deafness.

DYSACUSIS

This term, which has been used to denote 'faulty' hearing, does not encompass hearing loss, but the terms are not mutually exclusive - both may exist from the same cause. In diving medicine the most common types of dysacusis are painful hearing and echo hearing.

Dysacusis, manifesting as *painful hearing*, may follow injury to the inner ear from noise damage, secondary to middle ear barotrauma or from successful but excessive Valsalva manoeuvres. There may be an associated hearing loss, either temporary or permanent. The pain, which is usually associated with loud noises, may persist for a variable time.

Any excessive noise may produce pain, especially the sound levels of 120 dB or greater. This is possible in either helmet diving or in compression chambers. It has been known to damage the vestibular part of the inner ear and produce the *Tullio phenomenon* (vertigo and nystagmus associated with excessive noise stimulation).

A dysacusis effect from a *patulous Eustachian tube* may manifest as an echo, excessive awareness of the patient's respiration or speech (causing the patient to speak softly) or the reverberation of sounds as from footsteps. The Eustachian tube may be overstretched and made 'patulous' by the excessive pressure employed during the Valsalva manoeuvre. Other medical causes should be excluded.

The clinical otoscopic sign of tympanic membrane movement during respiration is considered pathognomonic of a patulous Eustachian tube in the general population. This is not necessarily so among divers, many of whom are quite capable of opening the Eustachian tube at will and during normal breathing.

The symptoms may be relieved or abolished by reclining or lowering the head between the legs – thus increasing venous and lymphatic congestion in the soft tissue of the Eustachian tube. The symptoms are also temporarily relieved by sniffing, or by the nasal congestion associated with upper respiratory tract infections.

The disorder may be transitory, or it may last for many months. Treatment is not usually indicated, and those procedures that have been employed in otological practice (e.g. paraffin or Teflon paste injections around the Eustachian cushions) may not be appreciated by divers, who need patent Eustachian tubes for their diving activities.

FURTHER READING

Antonellip J, Parnell GJ, Becker GD, Paparella MM. Temporal bone pathology in scuba diving deaths. *Otolaryngology Head and Neck Surgery* 1993;**109**:514–521.

Demard F. Les accidents labyrinthiques aigus au cours de la plongée sous-marine. *Forsvarsmedicin* 1973;**9**(3):416–422.

Edmonds C, Freeman P, Tonkin J, Thomas R, Blackwood F. *Otological Aspects of Diving.* Sydney: Australasian Medical Publishing; 1973.

Edmonds C. Diving and inner ear damage. *Diving and Hyperbaric Medicine* 2004;**34**:2–4.

Edmonds C. Round window rupture in diving. *Forsvarsmedicin* 1973;**9**(3):404–405.

Elliott E, Smart DR. A literature review of the assessment and management of inner ear barotrauma in divers and recommendations for returning to diving. *Diving and Hyperbaric Medicine Journal* 2014;**44**(4):243–5.

Farmer JC. Otological and paranasal problems in diving. In: Bennett PB, Elliott H, eds. *The Physiology and Medicine of Diving.* 4th ed. London: Saunders; 1993.

Farmer JC, Thomas WG, Youngblood DG, Bennett PB. Inner ear decompression sickness. *Laryngoscope* 1976;**86**:1315–1327.

Freeman P, Edmonds C. Inner ear barotrauma. *Archives of Otolaryngology* 1972;**95**:556–563.

Gempp E, Louge P. Inner ear decompression sickness in scuba divers: a review of 115 cases. *European Archives of Otor-hino-laryngology* 2013;**270**:1831–1837.

Hunter ES, Farmer JC. Ear and sinus problems in diving. In: Bove AA, Davis J, eds. *Bove and Davis' Diving Medicine*. 4th ed. Philadelphia: Saunders; 2004.

McCormick JG, Holland W, Holleman I, Brauer R. Consideration of the pathophysiology and histopathology of deafness associated with decompression sickness and absence of middle ear barotrauma. Proceedings of UMS annual scientific meeting. *Undersea Biomedical Research* 1974;**1**(1).

Nishioka I, Yanagihara N. Role of air bubbles in the perilymph as a cause of sudden deafness. *American Journal of Otology* 1986;**3**(6):430–438.

Pulec JG, Hahn FW. The abnormally patulous Eustachian tube. *Otolaryngologic Clinics of North America* 1970;**3**(1):131–140.

Pullen FW. Perilymphatic fistula induced by barotrauma. *American Journal of Otology* 1992;**13**(3):270–272.

Smerz RW. A descriptive epidemiological analysis of isolated inner ear decompression illness in recreational divers in Hawaii. *Diving and Hyperbaric Medicine* 2007;**37**(1):2–9.

Yanagita N, Miyake H, Sakakibara K, Sakakibara B, Takahashi H. Sudden deafness and hyperbaric oxygen therapy: clinical reports of 25 patients. In: *Fifth International Hyperbaric Conference*. ICHM publ, Amsterdam. 1973:389–401.

This chapter was reviewed for this fifth edition by Carl Edmonds.

38

The ear and diving: vertigo and disorientation

DISORIENTATION

The diver needs an accurate appreciation of his or her spacial orientation, depth and distance from boat or shore, to enable safe return. With the advent of free diving and scuba diving – without an attachment to the surface – the importance of *spatial orientation* underwater has increased.

Under terrestrial conditions, spatial orientation (the position of one's body in space) depends mainly on information from three inputs – vision, proprioception and the vestibular system. Vision usually dominates the other two, unless there is abnormal sensory input, damage or stimulation of the other systems.

> Awareness of body position in space involves integration of visual, proprioceptive and vestibular input information.

The most likely cause of disorientation under water is the *reduction of sensory input*. With greatly impaired vision and reduced proprioception in an unfamiliar environment, disorientation is more likely. Also, in contrast to the situation on land, there is an added dimension of vertical movement. This becomes important when the diver has lost sight of the sea bed and is distant from the surface. Other sensory inputs are also modified (e.g. the speed of sound is increased, making localization and discrimination more difficult).

This lack of orientation may be independent of any vestibular problem and occurs in predictable environment conditions, such as the following:

- Night diving.
- Diving in murky or white water (water with bubbles).
- Diving without a companion, buddy line, surface line, float or boat contact.
- Diving far from the surface, sea bed or other marine objects.

Under these conditions, the novice diver especially may become disorientated and also develop symptoms of an agoraphobic reaction (see Chapter 41), a sensation of depersonalization, derealization or isolation, associated with anxiety that may extend to panic.

Clues to spatial orientation are employed by the experienced diver underwater. Exhaust bubbles can be felt on the skin, moving toward the surface. In certain positions, inhalation or exhalation may be expedited, especially with the use of twin hose regulators and rebreathing equipment. Inhalation is easier if the breathing bag is below the diver in the water. If the breathing bag or the relief valve is above the diver, then it is easier to exhale. Heavy objects with negative buoyancy (e.g. weight belts, pressure gauge, knife) still obey gravity and press or fall downward. Buoyancy compensators pull upward. Gas spaces within the body can be felt to expand during ascent and contract during descent. This may be noted in the diver's lungs, middle ear, drysuit or face mask. When the diver is immobile, the legs tend to sink and the chest to rise – negatively buoyant fins increase this tendency. These clues are of value to the alert, experienced and composed diver, but they are ignored by the trainee or during a panic situation.

> Diving reduces visual and proprioceptive input, thus placing greater reliance on the vestibular system.

Psychological factors are believed to influence disorientation. Neuroticism, and its associated anxiety state, may result in neglect of many of the orientation clues that have been learned and may interfere with an appreciation of their significance.

Disorientation may be an early manifestation of a toxic-confusional state caused by *abnormal gas pressures* (e.g. carbon dioxide toxicity, hypocapnia, oxygen toxicity, hypoxia, nitrogen narcosis, high-pressure neurological syndrome, carbon monoxide toxicity). These toxicities are mentioned in other chapters and are evident by appraising the diving profile and analysis of the breathing gases. Disorientation in these states, although possibly of extreme importance as an early symptom, may be overshadowed by subsequent events – unconsciousness or drowning.

> Despite the multitude of causes of disorientation under water, the most common is inadequate sensory input experienced by the novice diver.

In other diving accidents, there may also be a prodromal sensation of disorientation, but this becomes obliterated with the impairment of cerebral function. Such instances are seen with cerebral arterial gas embolism, decompression sickness and syncope of ascent, among others.

There are many other coincidental disorders that may contribute to disorientation. Examples include cardiovascular disease, cerebrovascular disease and drugs (sometimes related to the diving, e.g. anti-seasickness medications, decongestants).

VESTIBULAR DISORDER

The anatomy and physiology of the bilateral and integrated vestibular system are described in Chapters 35 and 36.

The most dramatic and demonstrable cause of disorientation underwater is vertigo. The diving-induced causes are detailed later in this chapter. The perennial problem of differentiating vertigo from other disturbances of equilibrium such as dizziness, giddiness, unsteadiness, faintness, lightheadedness, swaying and other conditions is nowhere more prominent than in the early diving literature.

In this chapter, the term 'vertigo' is reserved for conditions in which there is a hallucination of movement, resulting in the impression that objects are moving in a certain direction (objective vertigo) or the patient is moving in a certain direction (subjective vertigo).

Because vertigo is associated with nystagmus and this can be demonstrated objectively, differentiation is made between the specific causes of vertigo from those of disorientation in general.

Even under good diving conditions, there is interference of visual cues and weightlessness causing loss of proprioceptive input. Extraordinary significance is then placed on vestibular responses – greatly in excess of that customary on land. Vertigo is aggravated if the vestibular stimulation is increased, as is likely in the aquatic and dysbaric environments.

If vertigo occurs to such a degree that the diver cannot compensate, or if it is associated with vomiting, visual disturbances or unconsciousness, then safety will be seriously impaired.

When the disorientation of the diver results from a disorder of the vestibular system, it is more commonly a transient and mild effect of the unequal stimulation of the two labyrinths (from pressure changes and/or caloric stimuli). The disorder may persist for as long as the unequal stimuli remain and perhaps for a few minutes longer. During this period, however, accidents may occur either directly from the effects of vertigo and disorientation or indirectly by influencing the dive profile.

Sometimes, peripheral vestibular disorders may be more severe and longer lasting (e.g. for many weeks) – until the pathological features are repaired or until central compensatory mechanisms inhibit the unequal vestibular responses. This condition may be seen in decompressions sickness, especially with deep and mixed gas diving, or the more frequent inner ear barotrauma. In these cases, the clinical effects may be catastrophic and endanger even the habitat or saturation diver – let alone the free swimming recreational scuba diver.

Central vestibular disease interfering with vestibular and cerebellar relationships may produce very long-lasting signs, but in divers these central signs are less common than the peripheral manifestation of vestibular disease.

Once a vestibular disorder has developed, a full otological investigation is indicated – of middle ear and inner ear function, both auditory and vestibular.

Investigations of cases of vertigo in diving should include the following:

- Physical and otological examination.
- Pure tone audiometry.
- Electronystagmography (ENG) – with positional, sometimes caloric or even dysbaric provocation.

In vestibular disease, there is a nystagmus demonstrable at the time of the abnormal sensation and for a variable time thereafter.

Vertigo is likely to be even more serious in breath-hold diving. Aspiration or vomiting is more significant. Orientation cues, such as the direction of bubbles, are less appreciated by free divers. With scuba, there is an adequate air supply to permit the diver to wait and settle – to see whether the vertigo is transitory.

Apart from the diving-induced causes of vertigo, many other causes may have to be considered – causes unrelated or only peripherally related to the diving. These include the following:

- Ear infections.
- Benign paroxysmal positional vertigo (cupulolithiasis).
- Vestibular neuronitis.
- Ménière's disease.
- Coincidental neurological disease (e.g. multiple sclerosis).
- Cerebrovascular disease.
- Acoustic neuroma.
- Drugs (e.g. some anti-malarial agents).

CLASSIFICATION OF VERTIGO IN DIVERS

Vertigo caused by unequal vestibular stimulation.

1. Caloric stimulation.
   a. Unilateral external auditory canal obstruction.
      i. Cerumen.
      ii. Otitis externa.
      iii. Miscellaneous.
   b. Tympanic membrane perforation.
      i. Shock wave.
      ii. Middle ear barotrauma of descent.
      iii. Forceful autoinflation.
2. Barotrauma.
   a. External ear barotrauma.
   b. Middle ear barotrauma of descent.
   c. Middle ear barotrauma of ascent.
   d. Forceful middle ear autoinflation.
   e. Inner ear barotrauma.
      i. Perilymph fistulae.
      ii. Other pathological features.
3. Decompression sickness.
4. Miscellaneous (e.g. Tullio phenomenon).

Vertigo caused by unequal vestibular responses.

1. Caloric responses.
2. Barotrauma.
3. Gas toxicity.
4. Motion sickness.
5. Sensory deprivation.

Non-diving aetiologies of vertigo.

UNEQUAL VESTIBULAR STIMULATION

Exposure to both hyperbaric and aquatic environments results in stimuli to both vestibular apparatuses. Under most diving conditions, the stimuli on each side are equal, but in certain situations this is not so, especially when there is a pathological process involving one external or middle ear. Under these conditions, a dominant stimulus effect on one side may produce vertigo.

Caloric stimulation

When the diver immerses himself or herself, there is normally an equal flow of cold water into both external auditory canals. This stimulation is symmetrical, and no vertigo is expected – nor does it occur in most dives. If the stimulus is greater on one side, vertigo would be expected – with an intensity and duration related to this inequality.

In the production of caloric vertigo, the spatial position of the diver is pertinent. In an experimental situation, caloric stimulus produces the most intense vertigo and nystagmus when the subject is either lying supine with the head elevated at 30 degrees or lying prone with his head depressed at an angle of 30 degrees. In both these positions, the horizontal semicircular canal becomes vertical. This has been demonstrated in the supine position during the traditional Hallpike caloric tests (see Chapter 36).

This 'Hallpike' head position is adopted by divers occasionally (e.g. when cleaning the hulls of ships). The diver assumes the most vestibularly sensitive 'prone with head-down' position when descending obliquely, swimming horizontally when underweighted or with positively buoyant fins. Resumption of an upright posture abolishes the vertigo (Figure 38.1).

In these positions, vertigo may result when there is unilateral obstruction to water flow into one external canal, when a tympanic membrane perforates or where there is bilateral and equal caloric stimulus but with unequal vestibular responses (see later).

UNILATERAL EXTERNAL AUDITORY CANAL OBSTRUCTION

Unilateral obstruction of the external ear canal does not cause permanent vestibular damage, and the only effect on audiometry is that from the canal obstruction (i.e. remedial conduction deafness). Two common causes observed are cerumen and otitis externa (Case Report 38.1), although others include exostosis, foreign body, ear plug, air bubble in the external canal and an asymmetrical hood such as with a hole over one ear only that may allow water to flow into one ear only and produce this effect.

TYMPANIC MEMBRANE PERFORATION

Perforation of the tympanic membrane is a dramatic cause of transient but often disabling vertigo. Initially, there may be a 'pop' or loud noise or pain associated with a sensation of cold water rushing into the middle ear. Vertigo follows almost immediately and usually lasts for less than a minute, although it feels longer. This small amount of cold water rapidly warms to body temperature, thereby removing the caloric stimulus.

Vertigo is especially likely if the diver is descending, encouraging more water flow into the middle ear.

On surfacing, the diver may have bloodstained fluid running from the external ear that is expelled when the gases that have remained in the middle ear expand during ascent and force blood out through the perforation.

There may be no vertiginous symptoms when there is no entry of water into the middle ear cavity because this space is occupied by blood, or if the perforation occurs during ascent. These patients usually notice the hissing of gas through the perforation with ascent or autoinflation. Occasionally, vertigo first develops while they are driving after the dive. Whether this is caused by head movements aggravating positional vertigo, air currents replacing water in producing caloric stimulation or eddy current movements of the tympanic membrane and ossicles is unknown.

There are three major predisposing causes of tympanic membrane perforation leading to vertigo while diving: a shock wave, middle ear barotrauma of descent and forceful autoinflation of the middle ear.

1. *Shock wave.* This is a disorder easily diagnosed by history, and it was common when Navy divers were subjected to underwater explosions, especially when they were faced at right angles

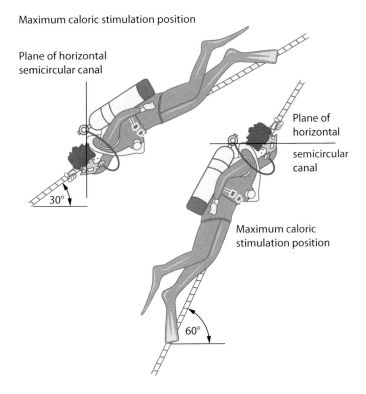

Maximum caloric stimulation position

Plane of horizontal
semicircular canal

30°

Plane of
horizontal

semicircular
canal

Maximum caloric
stimulation position

60°

Figure 38.1 Caloric stimulation related to spatial orientation.

CASE REPORT 38.1

This diver had no difficulty in autoinflating his ears during a descent to 10 metres. While swimming along a horizontal underwater line, he felt as if he were rotating to one side around the line. Because the line was on the sea bed, he knew that his sensation was incorrect, and he decided to surface. The vertigo, which lasted for some 10 to 20 seconds, did not trouble him during the ascent, and he had no further difficulty.

On clinical examination, there was no abnormality other than the presence of a large plug of hard cerumen in the left ear. Before removal of the plug, it was decided to carry out electronystagmography (ENG) with caloric testing, to ascertain whether sufficient water passed this obstruction. The positional ENG result was normal, but the caloric demonstrated a false picture of a total left canal paresis. The cerumen was removed, and no evidence of external or middle ear barotrauma was observed. The cerumen plug was large enough to obstruct the free flow of water, but not enough to prevent some water from equalizing the changing pressures within the external ear. The caloric stimulus was therefore much greater in the unobstructed ear, thus producing transient vertigo. No further incidents occurred after the plug was removed.

Diagnosis: vertigo from a unilateral caloric stimulus secondary to unilateral auditory canal obstruction by a cerumen plug.

to the source (see Chapter 34). In recreational diving, the most common underwater shock wave that produces perforation of the tympanic membrane and vertigo is caused by being 'finned'. When a diver swims past another diver, considerable pressure waves are felt from the fin (or flipper) movements. Perforation of the tympanic membrane is possible, especially if the middle ear is not adequately autoinflated. The shock wave, which is a water pressure wave, is probably also responsible for the entry of water into the middle ear following the perforation. Most patients have no permanent vestibular or hearing sequelae, although these sequelae could occur in patients with more severe cases with inner ear barotrauma.

2. *Middle ear barotrauma of descent* (see Chapter 7).
3. *Forceful autoinflation of the middle ear.*

Barotrauma

As a cause of vertigo, there are five clinically important types of barotrauma (see Chapter 7):

1. External ear barotrauma of descent ('reversed ear').
2. Middle ear barotrauma of descent ('ear squeeze').
3. Middle ear barotrauma of ascent ('alternobaric vertigo').
4. Forceful autoinflation of middle ear.
5. Inner ear barotrauma.

Vertigo secondary to barotrauma is more likely when the diver is upright (vertical) than when he or she is horizontal or in the traditional 'caloric' position. It is possible, but ethically questionable, to reproduce this barotrauma-induced vertigo in a compression chamber with ENG monitoring to verify this clinical observation.

This spatial orientation may infer involvement of the utricular or saccular divisions. The unequal pressure gradients may themselves produce vestibular disorder or they may, especially when associated with forceful autoinflation, result in inner ear barotrauma, producing a much more permanent effect.

EXTERNAL EAR BAROTRAUMA OF DESCENT ('REVERSED EAR')

This disorder is discussed in Chapter 7.

MIDDLE EAR BAROTRAUMA OF DESCENT ('EAR SQUEEZE')

This disorder is also discussed in Chapter 7.

Case 38.2 demonstrates in an objective manner that vertigo and nystagmus can be precipitated with the middle ear pressure changes during descent.

Case 38.3 demonstrates that middle ear barotrauma of descent can initiate vertigo and nystagmus, that this manifestation may continue and that the condition need not be merely transitory.

Because there is no evidence of abnormal cochlear or vestibular function before the dives referred to in Case Reports 38.2 and 38.3, there is no reason to believe that the vestibular response is the result of an underlying vestibular inequality. In both cases, an inability to equalize the middle ear space, and presumed inequality of middle ear pressure, is the cause of the abnormal vestibular response.

These descriptions are thus similar in concept, although opposite in direction, to the alternobaric vertigo described by Lundgren and confirmed independently with ENG by Edmonds (divers) and Tjernstrom (aviators). The nystagmus responses described in this and previous reports are inhibited by eye opening, thereby indicating the peripheral nature of the disorder. Persistent nystagmus implies more persistent barotraumatic disease in the vestibule.

Dysbaric ENG studies may supplement formal vestibular function tests in aviators and divers and may be needed to demonstrate vestibular disease. It is related to Hennebert's sign.

MIDDLE EAR BAROTRAUMA OF ASCENT ('ALTERNOBARIC VERTIGO')

An unequal release of gas from the middle ear cavities, especially during the initial stages of ascent, results in a pressure difference between the two middle ears and unequal stimuli to the vestibular systems (see Chapter 7). The nystagmus is toward the side of the block, with the diver's spinning sensation toward that ear, with the higher middle ear pressure (Figure 38.2).

The vestibular system is sensitive to pressure changes in the middle ear (Case Report 38.4). Vertigo can be produced by a pressure increase of 60 cm H_2O in one middle ear. The range of

CASE REPORT 38.2

The patient, a certified diver, frequently developed dizziness during descent. She commonly experienced difficulty in equalizing the middle ear spaces and frequently resorted to nasal decongestants. There were no symptoms suggestive of disorientation during ascent, and usually the sensation of dizziness reduced as she remained at a constant depth.

On examination, there was no conventional evidence of any abnormality in ear function; she had normal pure tone audiograms and normal electronystagmography (ENG) to positional and bithermal caloric stimuli.

Dysbaric ENG studies (as described by Edmonds and colleagues was performed with the diver the sitting upright with the eyes closed in a compression chamber. ENG monitoring was continued while the patient was subjected to changes in pressure. The compression was at the rate of 9 metres/min to a depth of 18 metres. The patient was then kept at the depth of 18 metres for 2 minutes and ascended at the same rate. Minor problems were encountered with middle ear equalization during descent, but they did not require cessation or delay of this descent.

The ENG results verified the subject's observation of vertigo associated with compression, which was relieved by maintenance of pressure and absent during decompression. The nystagmus 'saw-tooth' ENG pattern was obvious during and immediately after descent.

Diagnosis: middle ear barotrauma of descent, inducing vertigo.

CASE REPORT 38.3

This subject also had normal hearing and vestibular function demonstrated before having difficulty in equalizing both middle ear pressures during a recompression chamber descent. Because of the inability to achieve this middle ear equalization, the compression was terminated at 4.5 metres. At that time, the electronystagmography monitoring (performed coincidentally for another experiment) demonstrated severe nystagmus associated with the subjective complaint of vertigo. The diver was in the supine position. Vertigo persisted for many minutes after the initial middle ear injury, and nystagmus was demonstrated in a progressively decreasing degree for approximately 12 minutes. The nystagmus 'saw-tooth' pattern was maximal between 3.0 and 4.5 metres during descent, less at 5 minutes and almost absent at 12 minutes.

Diagnosis: middle ear barotrauma of descent, inducing vertigo.

effects is from a transient physiological disorder (Lundgren's alternobaric vertigo) to a pathological entity (Edmonds and Freeman's inner ear barotrauma).

FORCEFUL AUTOINFLATION ('EQUALIZING THE EARS')

Some subjects can produce vertigo merely by performing autoinflation, and it may be presumed that the middle ears are ventilated unequally because of unequal Eustachian tube patency. This is a clinical manifestation of Hennebert's sign. Another proposed mechanism is an abnormally mobile stapes.

Decompression sickness

Although vertigo has often been reported among air-breathing scuba divers with decompression sickness, there is considerable doubt about the frequency of the diagnosis when, as in many of the cases reported, there are no other manifestations

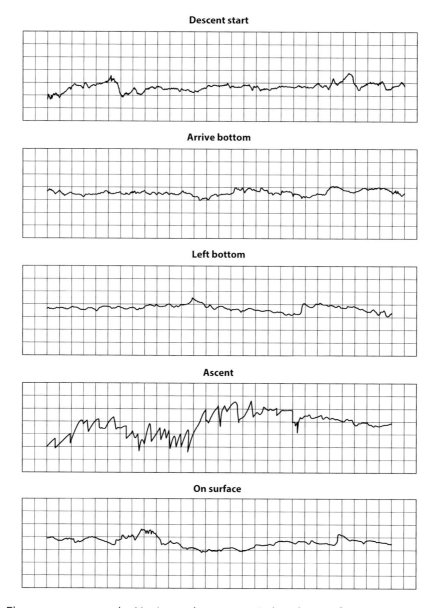

Figure 38.2 Electronystagmography. Vertigo and nystagmus induced soon after commencement of ascent.

of the disease (see Chapters 11 and 12). It is likely that many of the cases of permanent vestibular damage that were originally attributed to decompression sickness were actually caused by inner ear barotrauma. The delay of onset of symptoms is not necessarily a diagnostic feature favoring decompression sickness because it is not uncommon in cases with perilymph fistulae. Vertigo may occur with or without loss of hearing in both diseases.

Even allowing for the misdiagnoses, there are still some patients who presented with hearing loss and/or vertigo probably resulting from decompression sickness. This is especially so with deep diving, using helium as a breathing gas and during change-over between gas mixtures. In these patients, it is necessary to institute recompression therapy to prevent permanent inner ear damage.

CASE REPORT 38.4

In an accidental demonstration of Louis Pasteur's aphorism, 'Chance favours the prepared mind', a medical colleague was compressed to 30 metres in a chamber while testing an improvised electronystagmography (ENG) set-up. He had some difficulty in middle ear equalization because of an upper respiratory tract infection, but this was dismissed as of secondary importance to the experiment. Immediately on commencing ascent, he complained of vertigo, coinciding with classic 'saw-tooth' appearance on ENG. Ascent was continued, and both the symptom and the ENG abnormality cleared. This was the first ever demonstration of Lundgren's alternobaric vertigo (see Figure 38.2).

Diagnosis: middle ear barotrauma of ascent, causing vertigo.

The consequences of vertigo, such as near drowning, vomiting, dehydration, electrolyte disturbances and distress, are more important in a patient who is already seriously ill with decompression sickness. If vertigo is incorrectly diagnosed during ascent (e.g. if the symptoms are attributed to seasickness), then further decompression may result in more damage to the vestibular apparatus.

Recompression therapy, if promptly instituted, should result in cure (see Chapter 13). Objective tests of vestibular function can and should be performed under hyperbaric conditions, when doubt exists regarding clinical management. These investigations include ENG and iced-water caloric tests and are valuable in differential diagnosis, prognosis and response to treatment.

There are also long-term sequelae. With vestibular damage, there is a likelihood that the diver may not be able to continue with his or her occupation and may be restricted from other occupations such as flying or driving.

Miscellaneous conditions

Certain specific medical causes of vertigo are also occupational complications of diving.

Migraine is a typical example, and it is recommended that patients with this disorder should limit their diving (see Chapter 40). *Otitis media* can also be classified both as an occupational disease of divers and as a cause of vertigo. *Benign positional paroxysmal vertigo* may be induced by the diver adopting a position that triggers this response.

TULLIO PHENOMENON

The observation by Tullio early last century, that sound can stimulate the vestibular system, received much attention from the 1930s onwards. Vertigo may be experienced, and nystagmus produced, when subjects are exposed to pure tones ranging from 200 to 2500 Hz at intensities from 120 to 160 dB. Dizziness, nausea and disturbances of postural equilibrium have been correlated with sound stimulation at intensities and frequencies even lower than these (Case Report 38.5).

In diving, the Tullio phenomenon is especially seen with compression chambers that do not have muffling systems over the air inlets and in which there is excessive enthusiasm to 'flush-through' the chamber with the compressed gas – producing very loud noises. This phenomenon may also be observed in helmet divers, caisson workers and aircraft personnel.

UNEQUAL VESTIBULAR RESPONSES

This group includes patients who, under most conditions, would be considered 'normal'. In these people, vertigo is the end result of unequal vestibular responses to equal stimuli (i.e. one vestibular apparatus is more sensitive than the other). Even small differences in the vestibular responses may produce some demonstrable dysfunction when exposed to the stimuli encountered with diving or hyperbaric environments.

In some of these cases, the inequality can be demonstrated by conventional cochlear or vestibular function tests. In some cases, a damaged vestibular apparatus on one side may have been the result

CASE REPORT 38.5

A 35-year-old male diver was subjected to a recompression chamber dive to 9 metres. There were no problems with middle ear equalization during descent. While in the outer lock, and before equalizing the chambers, the diver used the intercom phone system, with the earpiece next to his right ear. The chamber pressures were equalized, and the diver moved from the outer to the inner lock. A 'flush-through' was then performed. This procedure involves the replacement of a large quantity of compressed air in the chamber, exchanging the chamber air and removing carbon dioxide. In this particular case, it was performed by a chamber operator under training, and excessive zeal was used in opening the valves, thus producing a great deal of noise. After approximately 20 seconds, the noise of the 'flush-through' was so intense that 'it knocked me off balance'. There was no obvious change of pressure during this period and therefore no need to perform Valsalva manoeuvres or middle ear equalization. The diver felt severely giddy and disorientated and was unable to stand. His right ear was nearer the inflow of the gas, and when he attempted to use this ear to communicate through the telephone intercom, as he had previously done, he was unable to hear the voice of the surface attendant. He was able to use his left ear for this. He noted that he was falling to the left when he finally got out of the chamber and was feeling off balance through most of that day. He claimed that he was far more sensitive to noise, even though his later audiograms had not changed. Impedance audiometry revealed a tympanic membrane far more mobile on the right side than the left. Electronystagmography demonstrated nystagmus on the vertical tracing in the positional test, even though the caloric test results appeared normal.

Clinical examination of the ear, nose and throat was normal, without any evidence of patulous Eustachian tubes. The tympanic membranes were easily moved with middle ear autoinflation, and there was no evidence of middle ear barotrauma.

Diagnosis: Tullio phenomenon, manifesting with vertigo and dysacusis.

CASE REPORT 38.6

After firing 50 rounds from a .222 rifle, this man developed tinnitus and slight hearing loss. When scuba diving, he developed vertigo and nausea during subsequent ascents that sometimes led to vomiting. Some relief was obtained by stopping ascent and assuming a prone position.

Pure tone audiograms verified the slight hearing loss, but electronystagmograms, both positional and caloric, were normal. Exposure to compression in a chamber verified the development of vertigo during ascent.

Diagnosis: vertigo from unequal barotrauma effects because of inequality of inner ears.

of a previous diving accident, whereas in other cases non-diving aetiologies may be detected. An example of the latter is the inner ear damage that results from gunfire, especially when this damage is unilateral (Case Report 38.6).

The fact that asymmetry cannot be demonstrated in many patients probably reflects the relative crudity of our investigations. As ENG, or computerized positional tests, become more precise, and with accurate and controlled stimuli, marginal asymmetry of vestibular function may be demonstrated.

Caloric responses

A common syndrome of vertigo induced by diving seems explicable only by postulating a greater caloric response from one vestibular apparatus than from the other. There is usually no abnormality evident on otoscopic examination. There is no reason to postulate barotrauma, sensory deprivation, decompression sickness, inert gas narcosis or other conditions. Vertigo is most commonly experienced by divers who have descended without any difficulty in equalizing pressures in the middle ear cavities and have reached a level at which they then perform a horizontal swim. The vertigo normally comes on within 5 minutes of the commencement of the swim and tends to recur when the diver attempts similar dives under similar conditions within the next few weeks. These cases have previously been given the nondescript term 'idiopathic vertigo of divers'.

The belief that this particular syndrome is caused by unequal vestibular response to caloric stimulation is supported by the following:

- The time delay before vertigo is produced, unlike vertigo from barotrauma.
- The spatial orientation of the diver during the swim that is suggestive of caloric-induced vertigo.
- The tendency for this disorder to recur during similar dives and without any otoscopic abnormalities present, thus discounting the likelihood of unequal stimulation.

Barotrauma

Even though the Eustachian tubes may be patent and equal, thus ensuring symmetrical pressure changes in the middle ear cavities, vertigo may result if one vestibular apparatus is relatively hypofunctional. Under these conditions, the vertigo occurs during or immediately following the changes of pressure (i.e. descent or ascent).

Vertigo from barotrauma is more severe when the diver is in the upright position than in the almost horizontal 'caloric' position (see Case Report 38.6).

Gas toxicity

This field has been little explored by otophysiologists. The difficulty of differentiating vertigo from dizziness, lightheadedness and disorientation makes any review of the historical diving literature almost valueless in this context. Because of the interference in cerebral function, the gas toxicities may result in serious disorientation whether or not vertigo is noted or nystagmus is demonstrated.

INERT GAS NARCOSIS (NITROGEN NARCOSIS)

As divers descend beyond 30 metres while breathing air, they become progressively sedated and narcotic from the influence of nitrogen (see Chapter 15). Dizziness has been described by many divers under these conditions, but there is some doubt about whether this proceeds to true vertigo. Whether or not dizziness does represent a true vertigo, like other symptoms of nitrogen narcosis, dizziness should be quickly corrected by reducing the nitrogen pressures (i.e. with ascent).

Nystagmus seems to be accentuated by exposure to high nitrogen pressures, a finding supporting the possibility of nitrogen narcosis as a contributory aetiological factor, in conjunction with the dysbaric and caloric stimuli to which divers are exposed.

HIGH-PRESSURE NEUROLOGICAL SYNDROME

Vertigo, nausea and tremor are some of the symptoms reported with the high-pressure neurological syndrome. The effects are probably either in the subcortical or reticular activating system, are aggravated by too rapid a compression and are relieved within a few hours of reaching depth. It is probably not specifically a vestibular problem.

OXYGEN TOXICITY

Vertigo is a documented symptom of oxygen toxicity when it affects the neurological system. Vertigo may be a warning symptom. It is also precipitated during the reduction from high oxygen pressures (i.e. an 'oxygen off effect'), as well as following oxygen convulsions. These situations are likely only when divers use oxygen, mixed gases or rebreathing equipment, when the safe limits for oxygen pressures and durations are exceeded. Nausea and vomiting are also associated with somewhat lower oxygen pressures (1 to 2 ATA), but whether these symptoms are related to vertigo is unknown.

CARBON DIOXIDE TOXICITY

Disorientation is a characteristic feature of carbon dioxide toxicity, but vertigo is far less definite. It has been reported in association with vomiting by submariners who have become acclimatized to breathing high carbon dioxide pressures and who then revert to breathing air or oxygen. This is known as the 'carbon dioxide off effect'. A similar state occurs clinically in divers using rebreathing equipment with partially ineffective carbon dioxide absorbent systems, when they reduce their high carbon dioxide exposure (e.g. when they rest after an energetic swim).

OTHER GASES

The effect of hypoxia, hypocapnia, carbon monoxide poisoning and so forth may well include vertigo because this is a possible symptom with any factor that disturbs the state of consciousness. In these cases, the effects are analogous to drug effects, although some drugs, such as mefloquine (Larium), can specifically induce vertigo.

Motion sickness

Motion sickness is a complication of certain diving operations (e.g. on the diving boat, while decompressing on a platform or rope underwater or while swimming). One aetiological hypothesis is an excessive and unequal vestibular response to motion, with nausea, vomiting, syncope and vertigo (see Chapter 26).

Sensory deprivation

Sensory deprivation, especially when it involves those senses involved in spatial orientation, is likely to aggravate vertigo and to produce disorientation. Abnormalities of vestibular or cochlear function would not be expected in most of these cases. It is possible that sensory deprivation will serve to decrease the threshold for vertigo and nystagmus. This belief receives support from the techniques aimed at reducing extraneous stimuli, which are used during vestibular testing in otological laboratories. Deprivation produces disorientation.

Blue orb syndromes

Frequently, the diver overcomes the lack of sensory input by visual fixation on objects that are associated with him or her, such as a companion diver, a buddy or surface line or equipment. The syndrome can be prevented by avoiding conditions mentioned earlier and by corrected by swimming to the surface, the sea bed or along ledges (see Chapter 41).

FURTHER READING

Buhlmann AA, Gehring H. Inner ear disorders resulting from inadequate decompression: vertigo bends. In: Lambertsen CJ, ed. *Proceedings of the Fifth Underwater Physiology Symposium*. Bethesda, Maryland: Federation of American Societies for Experimental Biology; 1976:341–347.

Edmonds C. Round window rupture in diving. *Forsvarsmedicin*. 1973;**9**(3):404–405.

Edmonds C. Diving and inner ear damage. *Diving and Hyperbaric Medicine* 2004;**34**:2–4.

Edmonds C, Blackwood F. Disorientation with middle ear barotrauma of descent. *Undersea Biomedical Research* 1975;**2**:311–314.

Edmonds C, Freeman P, Tonkin J, Thomas R, Blackwood F. *Otological Aspects of Diving*. Sydney: Australasian Medical Publishing; 1973.

Elliott E, Smart DR. A literature review of the assessment and management of inner ear barotrauma in divers and recommendations for returning to diving. *Diving and Hyperbaric Medicine Journal* 2014;**44**(4)243-5.

Farmer JC. Otological problems in diving. In: Bennett PB, Elliott H, eds. *The Physiology and Medicine of Diving*. 4th ed. London: Saunders; 1993.

Gempp E, Louge P. Inner ear decompression sickness in scuba divers: a review of 115 cases. *European Archives of Oto-rhino-laryngology* 2013;**270**:1831–1837.

Hunter ES, Farmer JC. Ear and sinus problems in diving. In: Bove AA, Davis J, eds. *Bove and Davis' Diving Medicine*. 4th ed. Philadelphia: Saunders; 2004.

Kennedy RS. *A Bibliography of the Role of the Vestibular Apparatus Under Water and Pressure.* USN MRI M4306-03. 5000BAK9. Report no. 1. Washington, DC: US Navy; 1972.

Kitajima N, Sugita-Kitajima A, Kitajima S. Altered eustachian tube function in SCUBA divers with alternobaric vertigo. *Otol Neurotol*;2014; 35(5):850–6.

Lundgren GEC. Alternobaric vertigo: a diving hazard. *British Medical Journal* 1965;**1**:511.

Molvaer OI, Albrektsen G. Alternobaric vertigo in professional divers. *Undersea Biomedical Research* 1988;**15**(4):271–282.

Money KE, Buckingham IP, Calder IM, *et al.* Damage to the middle ear and the inner ear in underwater divers. *Undersea Biomedical Research* 1985;**12**(1):77–84.

Parker DE, Reschke MF, Tubbs RL. Effects of sound on the vestibular system. In: *AGARD Conference.* No.128. NATO Publication, Washington DC.

Smerz RW. A descriptive epidemiological analysis of isolated inner ear decompression illness in recreational divers in Hawaii. *Diving and Hyperbaric Medicine* 2007;**37**(1):2–9.

Terry L, Dennison WL. *Vertigo Amongst Divers.* Special report 66-2. Groton, Connecticut: US Navy Submarine Medical Centre; 1966.

Tjernstrom O. Alternobaric vertigo. Proceedings First European Undersea Biomedical Symposium, Stockholm, *Forsvarsmedicin* 1973;**9**(3):410–415.

Vorosmarti J, Bradley ME. Alternobaric vertigo in military divers. *Military Medicine* 1970;**135**:182–185.

This chapter was reviewed for this fifth edition by Carl Edmonds.

39

Cardiac problems and sudden death

INTRODUCTION

Sudden death has been observed and described since antiquity. In modern times there is little doubt that the immediate cause of many scuba fatalities is either a myocardial infarction or a cardiac dysrhythmia. This is increasing in frequency, possibly because of the increasing age of the diving population. Cardiac deaths are observed repeatedly in Australian reports on diving deaths, and they accounted at least in part for 6 of 10 breath-hold diving deaths (mainly snorkelling) and 2 of 6 compressed gas divers in 2006[1]. A Divers Alert Network (DAN) investigation into the common causes of scuba diving deaths identified cardiac incidents as the 'disabling factor' in 26 per cent – the third most common such factor after emergency ascent and insufficient breathing gas[2]. On land, ventricular fibrillation is the most common cause, followed by bradyarrhythmias and torsade de pointes. In the water, the ratio is uncertain. Importantly, sudden cardiac death while diving is more complex than the simple development of infarction or dysrhythmia – death while immersed is a result of interrelationships among the diver, the equipment and the environment. These complexities and interrelationships cannot be overstated.

Diving induces a series of stresses that may have an impact on cardiac function via the conducting system, coronary blood supply or efficient muscular contraction. Environmental factors cause reduction of blood volume, tachycardia or bradycardia, hypertension and increased cardiac work[3,4]. These stresses can induce dysfunction even in the absence of disease. During a standard, resting dive in healthy volunteers, for example, Marabotti and colleagues[4] demonstrated an increase in left ventricular volume and diastolic dysfunction, with increases in both end-diastolic and end-systolic left ventricular volumes that were maximal after reaching the surface at the end of the dive (Figure 39.1).

In the presence of such changes, dysrhythmias, including various degrees of heart block, paroxysmal tachycardia and fibrillation, further reduce the efficiency of the heart's ability to supply an adequate blood flow under the heavy physiological demands imposed by the environment.

Exceeding the coronary arteries' ability to supply the myocardium with oxygen may result in myocardial ischaemia, causing sudden death. Although this is possible with normal coronary arteries, it is much more likely when the diver has reached an age at which coronary artery disease has developed. Most myocardial infarctions occur

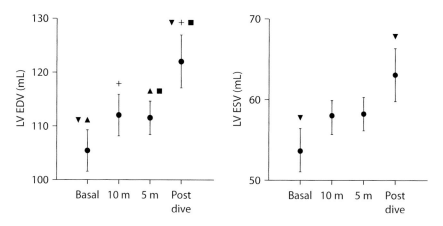

Figure 39.1 Left ventricular end-diastolic volume (LV EDV) and end-systolic volume (LV ESV) in basal conditions, during scuba diving at two different depths (10 metres and 5 metres) and after the dive. Matched symbols indicate statistically significant difference. (Reproduced from Marabotti C, Scalzini A, Menicucci D, *et al*. Cardiovascular changes during SCUBA diving: an underwater Doppler echocardiographic study. *Acta Physiologica* 2013;**209**:62–68; permission pending.)

secondary to rupture of atheromatous plaque with less than 40 per cent coronary stenosis. Because these lesions are not haemodynamically significant, the victim is often asymptomatic before the event. Half of all myocardial infarcts are associated with a triggering event.

Triggers of plaque rupture may be extrinsic or intrinsic. Extrinsic triggers induce a surge in sympathetic activity causing changes in heart rate, blood pressure and coronary blood flow. Intrinsic triggers induce a hypercoagulable state or impair fibrinolytic activity, thus altering coagulation status.

The importance of triggering events is illustrated by the marked increase in myocardial infarction incidence during both natural and human-made disasters.

Accounts of sudden death while diving often identify a substantial number of middle-aged men who suddenly and inexplicably lose consciousness and die – often in cold water. The behaviour of the victims, the ineffectiveness of resuscitation and the timing of the brain damage and death suggest a cardiac dysrhythmia as the underlying cause. Most of the victims either had previous cardiovascular disorders such as hypertension or dysrhythmia or showed significant coronary artery stenosis at autopsy. Physicians conducting diving medical examinations should be aware that minor cardiac

irregularities may preface major problems, particularly in people diving in cold water.

Some victims were described as unusually tired or resting, having previously exerted themselves, or being towed at the time – suggesting some degree of exhaustion. Others acted as if they did not feel well before their final collapse. Some complained of difficulty in breathing only a few seconds before the collapse. Others signalled that they needed to buddy breathe, but rejected the offered regulator. Explanations for the dyspnoea include psychogenic hyperventilation, autonomic induced ventilatory stimulation and pulmonary oedema – the last condition being demonstrated at autopsy. In most cases, there was an adequate air supply available, a finding suggesting that dyspnoea was not related to equipment problems. Some victims lost consciousness without giving any signal to their buddy or an observer. Others requested help in a calm manner.

Many autopsies of such cases reveal moderate stenosis of a coronary artery or evidence of infarction. Pulmonary oedema to a degree frequently associated with left ventricular failure is seen in some cases[1,2].

It is very likely these cases of sudden death are similar to others associated with swimming and cold water immersion. It is probable that they are related to other sudden death syndromes in activities such as squash, other athletics and adultery, although in these particular environments there is much more opportunity to desist and obtain relief from physical stress, and for subsequent resuscitation, than in the water.

This supposition is supported by the research of McDonough and his colleagues[5] showing strikingly higher frequencies of dysrhythmias when scuba diving. These rhythm disorders included both supraventricular and ventricular premature contractions and dysrhythmias[5]. More recently, studies of autonomic activity using heart rate variability confirmed a parasympathetic dominance with increased vagal activity and reduced sympathetic tone during both scuba diving and breath-hold diving – thus presumably increasing the likelihood of escape rhythms[6]. Episodes of sympathetic stress, as during an untoward event, may rapidly increase the oxygen consumption of the myocardium and predispose to both ischaemia and dysrhythmia.

Some of the factors that stress the cardiovascular system in diving are as follows:

- Exercise.
- Psychological factors.
- Cold.
- Immersion.
- Breath-hold diving.
- Reflexes associated with diving.
- Breathing equipment resistance.
- Aspiration.

These triggers are even more likely to provoke a cardiac incident in the presence of underlying cardiac disease, occult or manifest.

CARDIAC STRESS FACTORS

Exercise

Perhaps the most famous example of death resulting from exercise is that incorrectly attributed to the famous athlete Pheidippides (490 B.C.). A young Greek soldier ran 42 kilometres from the battlefield of Marathon to the city of Athens, delivered news of victory over the Persians and then dropped dead. The feat is commemorated by the present day marathon athletic event.

The increased parasympathetic (vagal) tone associated with fitness training may make the fit individual more susceptible to a variety of atrial dysrhythmias. Alternately, fatigue is more likely in unfit individuals and has been shown to be a dangerous factor in those susceptible to dysrhythmias.

Increased cardiac output and heart rate do not produce blood pressure elevation on land because of vasodilatation in the muscles and the skin. Vasodilatation is inhibited when the skin is exposed to cold water. The inclination to perform heavy work with elevated oxygen consumption is enhanced in the sea because the diver rarely feels overheated and uncomfortable.

Vigorous exercise does not usually prevent, and may even intensify, the normal diving bradycardia.

The metabolic acidosis and hypercapnia associated with extreme exercise and the cardiorespiratory effects of diving, which hinder carbon dioxide elimination, aggravate any tendency to cardiac dysrhythmia. Myocardial ischaemia and hypoxia, resulting from inadequate cardiac output and/or coronary narrowing, complicate this condition, and both predispose to myocardial ischaemia and sudden death.

Both clinically and on exercise provocation in the laboratory, dysrhythmias are often observed 5 to 10 minutes after the maximal effort, and they are therefore more likely to occur at the end of a dive.

Personality and psychological factors

It is not the delicate, neurotic person who is prone to angina, but the robust, the vigorous in mind and body, the keen ambitious man, the indicator of whose engine is always set 'full speed ahead'.

William Osler

Anxiety and the sympathetic response may have deleterious effects on cardiac function, especially if there is already cardiac disease. This is appreciated by physicians and is well typified by the demise of John Hunter – the eminent pathologist and surgeon who inoculated himself with syphilis, which he believed to be gonorrhoea, while performing research for his treatise on venereal disease. When confronting a particularly disturbing managerial committee of the hospital, he clutched his heart, stated, 'Gentlemen, you have killed me' and slumped dead over the table.

If the diver perceives a threat, whether it is real or not, there will be an autonomic stress response. During this anxiety state, a massive sympathetic discharge is present, with blood pressure reaching very high levels and causing excessive strain on the heart. Heart rates of up to 180 per minute can be produced and reduce cardiac output, thus diminishing coronary blood flow proportionately.

The sympathetic autonomic response to stress can result in dysrhythmias, myocardial ischaemia and even sudden death in the presence of underlying cardiovascular disease.

Another form of psychic stress is the vagal response, which produces exactly the opposite effects from the foregoing (i.e. hypotension and bradycardia to the stage of cardiac standstill). This is analogous to the syncopal episodes (fainting) of people who respond with an extremely exaggerated reaction to stress (e.g. fainting at the sight of blood or on receipt of tragic news). The vagal parasympathetic response could cause an inappropriate cardiac inhibition in the aquatic environment, with syncope leading to drowning. One such influence is the diving response, which is augmented by exposure to cold (e.g. with cold water on the face), with perhaps concomitant induced breath-holding.

Panic disorder has been reported to produce cardiac ischaemia in the absence of atherosclerosis[6]. Nevertheless, although stress is the trigger, underlying coronary artery disease is usually the substrate.

Cold

Any patient with angina pectoris attests to the deleterious effects of cold in aggravating the condition. In the case reports on exercise stress precipitating cardiac death during scuba diving, a common factor was the association with cold water. Cold can produce a variety of cardiac insults, with various types of responses (see Chapter 28).

During cold water immersion, there is usually an increase in sympathetic activity, as indicated by a rise in circulating noradrenaline, concurrently with or just preceding the release of adrenaline from the adrenal glands. This sympathetic activity is responsible for the increase in heart rate, systolic blood pressure and ventilation. The deleterious effect on cardiac efficiency may be very significant. An increase in the diastolic blood pressure is also possible, but not invariable. It may be overridden by the adrenaline effect, which at physiological doses causes a drop in the diastolic pressure. The sympathetic response is greater in subjects who are physically unfit and who have not adapted to cold water exposure.

The normal bradycardia of immersion is markedly enhanced in cold water. Breath-holding and cold immersion combine to produce such an intense bradycardia that unconsciousness and drowning may ensue – so called 'hydrocution'. Sudden death from a vagal parasympathetic reflex can follow inhalation of water into the nasopharynx and on the glottis. There may also be a reflex following cutaneous stimulation from cold that produces coronary spasm or sudden death in people who are immersed in very cold water. Another cutaneous reflex induces considerable hyperventilation, sufficient to reduce carbon dioxide tension in the arterial blood to levels that have been associated with ventricular fibrillation in both animals and humans.

In general, the degree of 'diving reflex' bradycardia is greater with lower water temperatures. With the development of hypothermia, the myocardium becomes hyper-excitable and is susceptible to episodes of ventricular extrasystoles, tachycardia and fibrillation. This becomes more frequent in the late stages and during rewarming.

Peripheral vaso-constriction results in centralization of blood, with diuresis and associated fluid and electrolyte loss.

Immersion

An immediate reflex from immersion causes a sudden and temporary increase in cardiac output and stroke volume, each by up to 100 per cent, before stabilizing at a lower level.

Immersion counters the effect of gravity and thus expedites venous return from the vessels of the limbs (see Chapter 3). This redistribution of blood increases intrathoracic blood volume by up to 700 ml and right atrial filling pressure by 18 mm Hg. The cardiac output, and thus the work of the heart, is increased by more than 30 per cent. Cold water intensifies these effects. Centralization of blood and the subsequent diuresis may also be associated with an increased susceptibility to syncopal episodes after leaving the water. Negative pressure breathing as a result of immersion the body while breathing from the lower pressure at the surface through a snorkel also increases the diuretic effect of immersion.

Reflexes associated with diving

DIVING RESPONSE

In diving mammals, the diving response is associated with bradycardia and intense peripheral and selective visceral vaso-constriction. The reduced cardiac output is preferentially distributed to the heart and brain. This combination of effects results in maintenance of normal arterial blood pressure, reduction of heat loss and conservation of oxygen for vital organs.

In humans, the reflex is more rudimentary (see Chapters 3 and 61). Although there is diving bradycardia, it is often complicated by the development of idioventricular foci producing ectopic beats. Abnormalities on the electrocardiogram (ECG) are frequent during or after the dive. T-wave inversion, premature ventricular excitation and atrial fibrillation, together with other irregularities and dysrhythmias, are common. They reflect inhibition of vagal rhythms and interference with atrio-ventricular conduction. In 1973, Hong showed an incidence of cardiac dysrhythmias in Korean women divers that increased from 43 per cent in summer (water temperature, 27°C) to 72 per cent in winter (water temperature, 10°C). This and other cold adaptive findings in this group of divers are summarized in a 1991 paper by Park and Hong[7].

The drop in cardiac output noted in diving mammals is seen to only a slight degree in humans. A proportionate drop in cardiac output does not compensate for the intense vaso-constriction of the peripheral vessels resulting when humans are immersed in cold water, and therefore there is a significant rise in arterial blood pressure, only partly attenuated by the accompanying bradycardia.

The diving response may well have some protective value in the drowning situation. It has been used in the treatment of paroxysmal atrial tachycardia. Nevertheless, it is likely that it may contribute significantly to otherwise inexplicable diving deaths.

CAROTID SINUS SYNDROME

This disorder is frequently observed, although often not recognized, by divers whose wetsuit or close-fitting drysuit applies pressure to the carotid bifurcation (see Chapter 42). The neck constriction is especially noted with wetsuit tops, which are pulled over the head. Bradycardia and hypotension are reflexly produced, resulting in a sensation of fainting, dizziness or even convulsions.

The extent of the relationship of the carotid sinus syndrome with sudden deaths in scuba divers is not yet clarified. Certainly, the cardiovascular effects are dramatic, and the disorder is not uncommon among divers who wear tight-fitting 'pullover' wetsuits. The syndrome also increases in frequency and severity with advancing age. Occasionally, divers in great distress are seen pulling the neck of the wetsuit away from the throat, and sometimes this is done before the loss of consciousness. In only 1 of 100 well-documented deaths in one series from Australia and New Zealand was the carotid sinus reflex incriminated, but in other series there were reported complaints of dyspnoea and tight-fitting wetsuits, which could well be related to this syndrome.

OTHER CARDIAC REFLEXES

Various other reflexes influence dysrhythmias. Some have afferent stimuli from skin or mucosal areas (e.g. the pharynx), whereas others are associated with breath-holding, Valsalva manoeuvres and exercise. One French electrocardiogram (ECG) study in experienced breath-hold divers showed the expected bradycardia but also dysrhythmias in 6 of the 10 of the divers. The atrial dysrhythmias were frequently multiple, and the ventricular dysrhythmias were bigeminal. These responses were discussed in detail by Lindholm and Lundgren[8] and by Ferrigno and colleagues[9].

In persons with known coronary artery disease, diving produces a much more powerful coronary vaso-constrictor response than does the clinically used cold pressor test.

Hyperbaric exposure

Pacemaker automaticity, conduction and repolarization are all affected by hyperbaric exposure.

Experiments on subjects with prolonged exposure to hyperbaric air between 1 and 40 metres of equivalent sea water depth in a dry chamber verified that the hyperbaric air caused an increase in parasympathetic tone of sufficient magnitude to induce cardiac dysrhythmias. Hyperoxia is one cause of this, and nitrogen has been incriminated as a cause of beta blockade. Associated with the reduction in heart rate and the increase in QT interval in the ECG, asymptomatic supraventricular dysrhythmias (generally atrio-ventricular nodal escape rhythms) were seen in 10 per cent of the subjects. Oxygen at high partial pressures acts as a vaso-constrictor, increasing blood pressure and reducing heart rate.

Acid-base changes

The influence of exercise on both pH and metabolic biochemical changes can exacerbate the reflex changes discussed earlier. Hypocapnia following cold water stimulation and hyperventilation, diuresis and changes of blood volume from the effects of immersion and the effects of salt water aspiration all ultimately act toward altering the *milieu intérieur*. These effects are aggravated when they are superimposed on pathological changes of age and disease.

Acidosis, produced by the effects of exertion, breathing against a resistance (regulator and increased gas density) and carbon dioxide accumulation, reduces the ventricular fibrillation threshold and depresses myocardial contractility. Underwater exertion, while breathing through scuba regulators, can produce end-tidal carbon dioxide levels of more than 70 mm Hg.

The interrelationships of many of the foregoing factors may lead to either cardiac dysrhythmias or myocardial ischaemia. The dysrhythmia is made more likely by the occurrence of sympathetic and parasympathetic stimuli separately or combined, when there is a potentiation more than merely a summation of effects. The ischaemia may be caused by diminished cardiac output, coronary occlusion or spasm and increased metabolic demands of the myocardium.

Drugs

Certain drugs are likely to increase the possibility of cardiac events during diving. They include:

- Alcohol.
- Nicotine.
- Caffeine.
- Cocaine.
- Sympathomimetic agents.
- Beta blockers.
- Calcium channel blockers.
- Pro-arrhythmic drugs.

Many antihypertensive drugs cause an interference in autonomic regulatory control of the heart rhythms, reduced exercise tolerance, exertional syncope, syncope when climbing from the water and increased restriction of the airways (especially beta blockers).

As demonstrated with quinidine and its derivatives, antidysrhythmic drugs can become pro-dysrhythmic, under certain circumstances[10]. This is especially so with class I/III drugs and is not necessarily dose related (except sotalol). These drugs may affect the original dysrhythmia by increasing its incidence, its frequency or its haemodynamic consequences. They may also induce new dysrhythmias, in response to their effect on re-entrant circuits, or *torsade de pointes*, resulting from marked QT prolongation on repolarization. These drugs may produce more bradycardia and increased ectopic beats, triggering the induction of spontaneous clinical re-entrant dysrhythmias.

Calcium channel blockers and beta blockers have some characteristics in common. They both induce bradycardia, thereby aggravating the reflex and metabolic effects mentioned earlier. A ventricular rhythm breakthrough is then possible. In both cases, the ventricular dysrhythmias are more likely if the diver has coincidental or occult coronary artery disease or conductive abnormalities.

Cocaine is infamous for its ability to cause ventricular dysrhythmias and sudden death, even in young, fit athletes.

PRE-EXISTING CARDIAC DISEASE

In younger divers, the presence of myocarditis (often associated with generalized infections) or undiagnosed hypertrophic cardiomyopathy may predispose to sudden death. Underlying cardiac disease, especially genetic disorders, may be completely asymptomatic and lead to sudden death in apparently young and healthy persons. Inherited long QT syndrome has been noted as a cause of paediatric drowning. Drowning resulting from this and similar abnormalities may be undetected unless specific investigations are undertaken. Persons with Marfan's syndrome are at risk of sudden death secondary to aortic dissection.

A study of sudden death in young competitive athletes revealed hypertrophic cardiomyopathy as the cause in 36 per cent, and coronary anomalies in 19 per cent. Ruptured aorta, myocarditis, dilated cardiomyopathy, mitral valve prolapse, premature atherosclerosis and aortic stenosis were each between 3 and 5 per cent[11]. Structural lesions found at post-mortem examination in cases of sudden cardiac death during occasional sporting activity are summarized in Table 39.1[12].

Undiagnosed endocardial fibrosis was found at post-mortem examination in a 27-year-old scuba diver illustrating the importance of pre-dive medical assessments and also the stresses of diving on a diseased heart[13].

With increased age, there is an increased likelihood of disease, mainly associated with coronary artery disease and hypertension.

The risks of sudden death in apparently healthy men is markedly increased where routine ECGs have detected ST-segment or T-wave abnormalities, especially in association with ventricular ectopic beats or left ventricular hypertrophy.

The rise in heart rate is an integral part of the cardiovascular response to exercise. However, in the transition from rest to exercise, older individuals do not adapt as well, having a less adequate increase in both heart rate and cardiac output. Occasionally, tachycardia may be excessive and result in a decrease in efficiency by interfering with venous return and thereby reducing cardiac output. The reduction in diastolic coronary blood flow may precipitate myocardial ischaemia.

Some divers continue diving despite having known cardiac disease, and these patients are likely to have increased risk of the sudden death syndrome, both from the disease entity itself, aggravated by the dive, and from the drugs taken to treat or control the condition. Following myocardial infarction, the likelihood of dysrhythmias is increased. Underwater swimming has been shown to increase extrasystoles in these patients. Also, awareness of angina is rare underwater, compared with equivalent land exercise, despite similar ST-segment depression. Persons with aortic stenosis are at particular risk of syncope during exercise.

The increased risk of infarction and dysrhythmias following coronary by-pass surgery, angioplasty or stenting is observed even on land.

Table 39.1 Cardiac lesions found after sudden death during sporting activity

Younger group (<30 years old)	Older group (>30 years old)
Hypertrophic cardiomyopathy	Atherosclerotic coronary artery disease
Arrhythmogenic right ventricular cardiomyopathy	Hypertrophic cardiomyopathy
Non-atherosclerotic coronary disease	Bundle of His abnormalities
Dilated cardiomyopathy	Dilated cardiomyopathy
Aortic stenosis	Arrhythmogenic right ventricular cardiomyopathy
Atrial septal defect	Obstructive cardiomyopathy
Bundle of His abnormalities	

Source: Adapted from Tabib A, Miras A, Taniere P, Loire R. Undetected cardiac lesions cause unexpected sudden cardiac death during occasional sport activity: a report on 80 cases. *European Heart Journal* 1999;**20**:900–903.

Skilled history taking, including a search for predisposing factors such as family history, diabetes or hypertension, may identify divers at risk.

Relevant investigations in questionable cases include a standard 12-lead ECG, which may reveal many of the foregoing conditions, including hypertrophic obstructive cardiomyopathy, left ventricular hypertrophy, ischaemic or previous infarction or QT syndromes. A maximal stress ECG, with 24-hour Holter monitoring, and echocardiography, may then follow. Computed tomography angiography may prove to be the best screening test for coronary artery disease.

The chances of surviving a dysrhythmia or infarction are markedly diminished if the event occurs underwater. For assessment of cardiac fitness for diving, see Chapters 52 through 54 and 56.

BREATH-HOLD DIVING

The dysrhythmias identified with breath-hold diving are mainly those of alterations in respiratory patterns, submersion, exercise and cold exposure. Many of these may have implications for scuba diving.

Dysrhythmias are found even in common respiratory manoeuvres, such as deep inspiration, prolonged inspiration, breath-holding and release of breath-holding. The effects of breathing against resistances, 'skip' breathing and the changes in respiratory pattern that occurs with snorkel and scuba diving are presumably related, but they are yet to be investigated.

Submersion (see earlier) increases the central blood volume, elevates arterial pressure and increases stroke volume.

The exercise of swimming fast underwater for 50 metres produces a heart rate of about 55 beats per minute. This requires an oxygen consumption of 5 to 10 times the resting level and would result in a rate of about 180 beats per minute on land.

The bradycardia of breath-hold diving is greatest when exercise is combined with cold water exposure. There are a dozen reports of the bradycardia being 20 beats per minute or less, with half a dozen at 10 or less.

When asphyxia is superimposed on breath-holding apnoea, the stimulation of carotid body chemoreceptors is markedly enhanced and may lead to vagally mediated cardiac arrest.

PULMONARY OEDEMA

Immersion and cold increase the venous return to the heart (increased pre-load). Cold increases the work of the heart (increased after-load) by vasoconstriction. The combination of immersion and cold exposure could therefore be expected to precipitate heart failure in persons with impaired cardiac function. Immersion pulmonary oedema (IPE) is uncommon, but reports are increasing over time as the condition is more widely recognized. Individuals with overt cardiac disease, especially with ischaemic heart disease, left-sided heart failure of any cause or dysrhythmias as described earlier are likely candidates for pulmonary oedema. However, there are reports of otherwise healthy individuals developing pulmonary oedema when swimming or diving[14,15]. Transient myocardial dysfunction is common during IPE. In one series, 28 per cent of 54 patients diagnosed with IPE proved to have transient dysfunction, and this was more likely in those patients who were more than 50 years old, with hypertension or diabetes. Occult hypertension was common[16].

Symptoms range from acute dyspnoea, with or without pink, frothy sputum, to mild dyspnoea with scanty haemoptysis and wheezing. Accentuated vaso-constrictor responses sufficient to lead to cardiac decompensation and pathological exercise-induced increases in blood flow have been postulated as immediate causes. Such people are at increased risk of recurrence and should probably not continue to dive. A case report in Sydney illustrated the danger of returning to diving[17]. The series of Gempp and associates[16] and that of Hampson and Dunsford[18] suggested that the disorder may not be that rare and that very cold water is not always associated.

Additional mechanisms may be involved in swimmers and breath-hold divers. Head-out water immersion increases the cardiac preload because of the increased intrathoracic blood volume. Negative pressure breathing is also increased because of the pressure differential between mouth and thorax. Deep breath-hold dives could reduce lung volume to below residual volume, which is compensated for by a further increase in intrathoracic blood volume. The rise in transpulmonary capillary wall pressure causes fluid to shift into the interstitial space and thus into the alveoli, thus leading to alveolar oedema and haemorrhage.

In some of the reported cases, concurrent use of aspirin was thought to be contributory. Extreme exercise is also associated with pulmonary oedema in non-aquatic sports.

For the differential diagnosis of pulmonary oedema, see Chapter 42.

REFERENCES

1. Lippmann J, Walker D, Lawrence C, Fock A, Wodak T, Jameson S. Provisional report on diving-related fatalities in Australian waters 2006. *Diving and Hyperbaric Medicine* 2011;**41**:70–84.
2. Denoble PJ, Caruso JL, Dear G de L, Pieper CF, Vann RD. Common causes of open-circuit recreational diving fatalities. *Undersea and Hyperbaric Medicine* 2008;**35**:393–406.
3. Bachrach AJ, Egstrom GH. *Stress and Performance in Diving*. San Pedro, California: Best Publishing; 1987.
4. Marabotti C, Scalzini A, Menicucci D, *et al.* Cardiovascular changes during SCUBA diving: an underwater Doppler echocardiographic study. *Acta Physiologica* 2013;**209**:62–68.
5. McDonough JR, Barutt BS, Saffron RN. Cardiac arrhythmias as a precursor to drowning accidents. In: Lundgren CEG, Ferrigno M, eds. *The Physiology of Breathhold Diving*. Washington, DC: Undersea and Hyperbaric Medical Society; 1987.
6. Shattock MJ, Tipton MJ. 'Autonomic conflict': a different way to die during cold water immersion? *Medical Journal of Australia* 2012;**168**:390–392.
7. Park YS, Hong SK. Physiology of cold-water diving as exemplified by Korean women divers. *Undersea Biomedical Research* 1991;**18**(3):229–241.
8. Lindholm P, Lundgren CEG. The physiology and pathophysiology of human breath-hold diving. *Journal of Applied Physiology* 2009;**106**:289–292.
9. Ferrigno M, Ferretti G, Ellis A, *et al.* Cardiovascular changes during deep breath-hold dives in a pressure chamber. *Journal of Applied Physiology* 1997;**83**:1283–1290.
10. Ross DL, Cooper MJ, Chee CK, *et al.* Proarrhythmic effects of antiarrhythmic drugs. *Medical Journal of Australia* 1990;**153**:37–47.
11. Maron BJ, Thompson PD, Puffer JC, *et al.* Cardiovascular preparticipation screening of competitive athletes: a statement for health professionals from the Sudden Death Committee (clinical cardiology) and Congenital Cardiac Defects Committee (cardiovascular disease in the young), American Heart Association. *Circulation* 1996;**94**(4):850–856.
12. Tabib A, Miras A, Taniere P, Loire R. Undetected cardiac lesions cause unexpected sudden cardiac death during occasional sport activity: a report on 80 cases. *European Heart Journal* 1999;**20**:900–903.
13. Obafunwa JO, Purdue B, Bussital A. Endomyocardial fibrosis in a scuba diving death. *Journal of Forensic Sciences* 1993;**38**(5):1215–1221.
14. Pons M, Blickenstorfer D, Oechslin E. Pulmonary oedema in healthy persons during scuba-diving and swimming. *European Respiratory Journal* 1995;**8**:762–767.
15. Weiler-Ravell D, Shupak A, *et al.* Pulmonary oedema and haemoptysis induced by strenuous swimming. *British Medical Journal* 1995;**311**:361–362.
16. Gempp E, Louge P, Henckes A, *et al.* Reversible myocardial dysfunction and clinical outcome in scuba divers with immersion pulmonary edema. *American Journal of Cardiology* 2013;**111**(11):1655–1659.
17. Edmonds C, Lippmann J, Lockley S, Wolfers D. Scuba divers' pulmonary oedema: recurrences and fatalities. *Diving and Hyperbaric Medicine* 2012;**42**(1):40–44.
18. Hampson NB, Dunsford RG. Pulmonary edema of scuba divers. *Undersea and Hyperbaric Medicine* 1997;**24**(1):29–33.

This chapter was reviewed for this fifth edition by Michael Bennett.

40

Neurological disorders of diving

INTRODUCTION

Because of the vulnerability of neurones to ischemia and consequent hypoxia, the nervous system is a primary target in diving accidents. Combined with the nervous system response to heightened environmental stimuli and its sensitivity to gas mixtures other than air, this vulnerability may result in a plethora of effects related to diving.

Scuba diving may result in neurological injury, with both temporary and permanent impairment. Many of these problems are discussed in previous or following chapters including cerebral arterial gas embolism (CAGE; see Chapter 6), neurological decompression sickness (DCS; see Chapter 12), hypoxic encephalopathy (see Chapter 16), nitrogen narcosis (see Chapter 15), the high-pressure neurological syndrome (see Chapter 20) and neuropsychological disorders (see Chapter 41).

Other problems include headaches in diving, brachial plexus lesions, scuba diver's thigh, epilepsy and other neuralgias and nerve lesions.

CEREBRAL ARTERIAL GAS EMBOLISM

Bubbles can enter the arterial circulation either by direct introduction or by shunting from the veins. Both can occur in diving, with bubbles forming from dissolved gas in the veins potentially able to shunt across a patent foramen ovale (see Chapter 10) or bubbles being introduced directly into the arterial circulation by pulmonary barotrauma (see Chapter 6). A significant proportion of any bubbles in the arterial circulation will distribute to the cerebral circulation (see Chapter 6). Large bubbles may obstruct flow and cause infarction in the affected downstream territory, whereas smaller bubbles may pass through the capillaries into the venous system. Bubbles may damage the vascular endothelium during this process of redistribution through the blood vessels and cause activation of white blood cells and inflammatory cascades, as well as damage to the blood-brain barrier. These processes may result in injury to the surrounding tissue.

Serious neurological symptoms referable to cerebral injury that develop immediately after an ascent should usually be treated as CAGE. The manifestations may include loss of consciousness, confusion, aphasia, visual disturbances, lateralized sensory abnormalities, vertigo, convulsions and varying degrees of mono-paresis or hemi-paresis. Early radiological investigation (e.g. computed tomography scan) may reveal bubbles in the cerebral vasculature.

NEUROLOGICAL DECOMPRESSION SICKNESS

The nervous system is frequently involved in DCS (see Chapters 10 and 11). Symptoms of brain involvement range from difficulty with concentration or cognitive function, mild confusion and impaired judgement through to frank confusional states and loss of consciousness. Spinal cord involvement manifests with bladder, motor (typically paraparesis) and sensory disturbance; typically below a spinal sensory level.

Peripheral nerve involvement is a plausible explanation for non-dermatomal sensory disturbances such as paraesthesiae[1], which are a common presentation[2]. Such symptoms may be bilateral and widespread, and they are frequently described by patients as 'patchy tingling'. It is important to differentiate this presentation from cerebral or spinal manifestations, which are more ominous.

SUBCLINICAL NEUROLOGICAL DAMAGE

Some studies have presented evidence of chronic changes in the brains of asymptomatic divers who may not have a past history of DCS when compared with control subjects (see Chapter 44).

The significance of some of these changes is unknown. There are also anecdotal reports suggesting that diving, even in the absence of a gross insult, may cause brain damage and dementia. Reputable studies to support this hypothesis are lacking (see Chapter 41).

HYPOXIC ENCEPHALOPATHY

Hypoxia, most often seen in association with closed or semi-closed rebreather units, may occur as a result of exhaustion of the gas supply, failure of the diving equipment, inadequate flow rates, dilution and increased oxygen consumption (see Chapter 16). It also occurs in drowning. The clinical features are those of hypoxia from any cause and are not unique to divers.

NITROGEN NARCOSIS

'Nitrogen narcosis' refers to the clinical syndrome characterized by impairment of intellectual and neuromuscular performance and by changes in mood and behaviour when nitrogen is breathed at partial pressures greater than approximately 3 ATA. The effects are progressive with increasing depth and reverse completely with ascent to the surface (see Chapter 15).

HIGH-PRESSURE NEUROLOGICAL SYNDROME

The high-pressure neurological syndrome occurs at depths greater than 150 to 200 metres and is one of the important limitations to deep diving (see Chapter 20). Clinical features include the following:

- Tremor.
- Fasciculation.
- Myoclonic jerks.
- Psychomotor performance decrement.
- Dizziness, nausea and vomiting.
- Impaired consciousness.

The onset of this syndrome can be delayed by slowing the rate of compression and introducing small amounts of a narcotic gas (e.g. nitrogen to the oxygen-helium mixture).

NEUROPSYCHOLOGICAL DISORDERS

Because cerebral involvement is present in some major diving accidents, neuropsychological sequelae are possible. They may be evident from the time of the accident or may develop soon after. They may also be persistent and may be associated with abnormal electroencephalograms or psychometric test results.

As with subclinical neurological damage (see earlier), there are anecdotal reports suggesting that diving, even in the absence of a gross insult, may cause neuropsychological problems. However, once again, reputable studies to support this hypothesis are lacking (see Chapter 41).

HEADACHE

Headache is a common symptom in diving, but there are many potential causes, and it is often difficult to determine the cause in cases of recurrent headaches. The following causes are not all inclusive, and the clinical details of each type of headache may be found either in the appropriate sections of this book or in general medical texts. The differential diagnosis depends on a detailed clinical and diving history, a physical examination and (possibly) laboratory investigation.

Anxiety (tension)

The psychological reaction induced in susceptible novice divers exposed to a stressful underwater environment may produce a typical tension headache.

Sinus barotrauma

Sinus barotrauma should always be suspected when pain occurs in the anatomical location of a sinus during changes in pressure (ascent or descent). The pain is caused by distortion of pain-sensitive tissues lining the sinus when pressure within the sinus cavity is less or greater than the ambient pressure, and this in turn occurs when the sinus ostia are obstructed during changes in ambient pressure. Such obstruction is more likely during upper respiratory tract infections, but it may have an anatomical cause, such as an obstructing polyp. Barotrauma of descent affecting the frontal sinus is the most common. It is often relieved by ascent. Ethmoidal sinus pain is referred to the intraorbital area, and maxillary sinus pain may be referred to the teeth. Sphenoidal sinus pain may be referred to the parieto-occipital area (see Chapter 8).

Mucocele or other sinus disease can be produced by diving. Rupture of the cells in the ethmoidal sinus air cells can cause a sudden and explosive headache and result in a small haematoma or bruising below the glabella, at the root of the nose. A similar but rare explosive headache can develop during ascent with rupture of the mastoid air cells that causes a generalized pain later localizing to the mastoid region. Pneumocephalus can follow the sinus rupture (see Figure 40.1). Computed tomography scans demonstrate these lesions with precision.

Infections

Infections in the mastoid cavities or sinuses usually cause pain 4 to 24 hours after the dive and are commonly associated with a preexisting upper respiratory tract infection and/or barotrauma. See Chapter 29 for more detail.

Cold

In some subjects, exposure to very cold water may induce a throbbing pain, particularly over the frontal area but sometimes also including the occipital area. It is probably analogous to the head pain experienced by some people when eating cold food, such as ice cream. The onset maybe rapid after cold water contact, or it may progressively increase in intensity with the duration of exposure. There may be acclimatization to the cold after a period of exposure after which the headache resolves, but it may last the entire dive and resolve only some minutes after the diver has left the water. Whether this is a migraine variant, a neurocirculatory reflex or merely the result of an increase in muscular tone is not known. Prevention is by the use of a protective hood to ensure warmth.

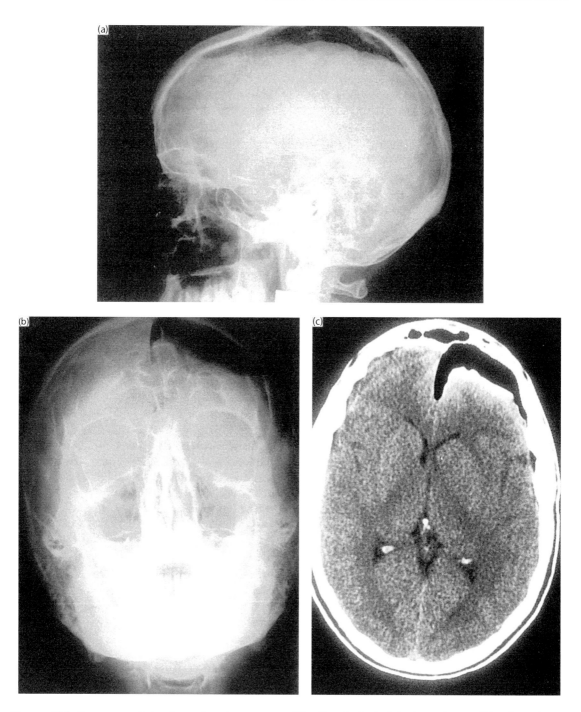

Figure 40.1 Pneumocephalus from sinus barotrauma. The films include **(a)** a lateral view, **(b)** a frontal view and **(c)** a CT scan. (c) There is a pneumocephalus which is loculated on the left and has some 'mass effect' causing depression of the underlying brain on the CT scan. (Courtesy of Dr. R.W. Goldman.)

Salt water aspiration

Headache following aspiration of sea water usually follows a latent period of 30 minutes or more, is usually associated with myalgia and is aggravated by exercise and cold.

Mask tension

Inexperienced divers tend to adjust the face mask straps far too tightly and this may result in a headache not dissimilar to that of a tight hat, ill-fitting spectacle frames etc. due to direct local pressure effects. It is related to the duration of the dive and clears shortly after.

Carbon dioxide

Carbon dioxide (CO_2) toxicity (or, more correctly, 'hypercarbia') may cause a characteristic generalized headache that has a progressive onset during the dive (potentially becoming severe) and gradually declines over several hours after diving. It is not particularly responsive to simple analgesia. This is almost certainly one of the most common and important causes of headache in diving because hypercarbia itself is common and has multiple causes.

The intuitively most obvious cause is failure of the CO_2 scrubber in a rebreather so that CO_2 is rebreathed (see Chapter 62). However, rebreather use is restricted to a very small proportion of the diving population.

Less obvious, but more common (and applicable to both open-circuit and rebreather diving) is a variable tendency to hypoventilate and therefore to retain CO_2 during diving. The crucial points that must be grasped to understand this phenomenon are first, that elimination of CO_2 from the body is directly proportional to lung ventilation and second, that CO_2 levels in the blood are carefully regulated by changes in lung ventilation mediated by the respiratory controller in the brainstem. Rising CO_2 levels stimulate the respiratory controller to increase ventilation to eliminate more CO_2 and *vice versa*.

This control process is readily disturbed by diving. Diving, by various means, increases the work required to breathe. When the work of breathing increases, some individuals respond by increasing their ventilation effort to maintain normal lung ventilation and to keep the arterial levels of CO_2 normal. In contrast, the respiratory controller in other persons seems less inclined to drive extra work to keep lung ventilation normal, and ventilation drifts lower than required to keep the CO_2 at normal levels. This condition is referred to as CO_2 retention. Put simply, the diver is not breathing enough to eliminate the CO_2 he or she is producing. These individuals are vulnerable to developing symptoms of hypercarbia such as headache. This is more likely if the diver is working hard underwater (and therefore producing more CO_2), if the diver is using poorly tuned scuba equipment (which may increase the work of breathing) or if the diver attempts to prolong the air supply by consciously resisting the urge to breathe more (often referred to as 'skip breathing').

A careful history of the circumstances under which headaches arise (e.g. exercise, hunting dives) and a determination of whether the diver is frequently in the position of having more air left in the cylinder at the end of a dive often give clues to the diagnosis. Experimental dives in which habitual hard underwater work is strictly avoided may help prove the case if headaches usually occurring on most dives do not arise on strictly restful dives. The key to avoiding such headaches is to avoid hard work underwater, use high-performance regulators and never 'skip breathe'.

Other gas toxicity

Headaches have also been described with oxygen toxicity, carbon monoxide toxicity and other gas contaminations. These are much less common but remain part of the diving headache differential diagnosis. The simultaneous occurrence of headaches (with or without other symptoms) in multiple divers all using gas from the same source should always raise the suspicion of gas contamination.

Decompression sickness and arterial gas embolism

Headache may be a symptom of DCS or arterial gas embolism (AGE), but its cause and importance in this setting are both uncertain. Headache is such a non-specific symptom with so many potential causes that the diagnosis of DCS or AGE should never be made on the basis of a headache alone. When headache accompanies other symptoms of DCS or AGE, then it may be considered part of the clinical picture, but its prognostic significance is uncertain, and the severity of the case should be based on an appraisal of the accompanying symptoms. For example, a case of DCS manifesting with musculoskeletal pain and a headache can still be considered a 'mild' case, assuming, of course, that the neurological examination is normal and the case meets the other criteria for the 'mild' categorization (see Chapter 11). In contrast, a case in which there is headache accompanied by aphasia and hemi-paresis is without doubt severe. In both cases, it is the accompanying symptoms that inform our view of severity, rather than the headache *per se*.

Migraine

Traditionally, migraine sufferers have been advised not to take up diving, particularly if their events are stereotypically severe or disabling. It is of concern that attacks may be induced by some aspect of diving or the diving environment discussed in this section (e.g. cold, anxiety, oxygen or CO_2 tensions, intravascular bubbles).

Once a migraine attack has commenced during diving, the patient is potentially at risk of interference with consciousness, perception and motor impairment, vertigo, vomiting and psychological complications. Such symptoms may lead to diagnostic confusion with cerebral DCS and/or air embolism. Some divers have had their first migraine episode underwater – although there is usually a positive family history to aid in diagnosis.

Prevention is best achieved either by not diving or by avoiding the specific provoking stimulus (e.g. use of a wetsuit hood if cold is the precipitant or limit of diving exposures to shallow no decompression diving with generous safety margins). Safety techniques such as buddy diving are also very important for those persons with migraine who insist on diving.

Neuromuscular pain

Headache may be induced by exacerbation of certain neuromuscular disorders such as cervical spondylosis. This diagnosis can sometimes be confirmed by cervical spine x-ray studies, which may demonstrate loss of lordotic curvature, narrowing of intervertebral spaces and osteophytosis in the lateral views. Divers who develop this disorder are usually older or have a history of head and neck trauma. They often swim underwater with flexion of the lower cervical spine (to avoid the tank) and their upper cervical spine hyperextended (to view where they are going). This positioning produces C1, C2 and C3 compression and distortion of the cervicocranial relationships, an unnatural posture aggravating underlying disease, which may otherwise be asymptomatic.

The headache is usually occipital and may persist for many hours after the dive. Occasionally, the pain is referred to the top and front of the head, possibly because of fibres of the trigeminal nerve passing down the cervical spinal cord and being affected by damage to the upper cervical vertebrae.

Other conditions

Other factors may be contributory in the aetiology of sporadic headache in divers. These include such diverse factors as alcohol overindulgence, dehydration and glare from the sun.

Some causes of headache in diving are as follows:

1. Anxiety.
2. Sinus barotrauma, sinusitis and other disorders.
3. Cold exposure.
4. Salt water aspiration.
5. Tight face mask straps.
6. CO_2 and carbon monoxide toxicity.
7. DCS.
8. Pulmonary barotrauma.
9. Migraine.
10. Cervical spondylosis.

EPILEPSY

Epilepsy is a total contraindication to diving, and thus seizures resulting from epilepsy would not normally be expected in a diver. However, occasionally an individual's first epileptic convulsion develops underwater, and aspects of the diving environment that can lower the seizure threshold may contribute to such events. Postulated pro-convulsive stimuli encountered in diving include the following:

- Sensory deprivation or disturbance, including unusual vestibular stimulation.
- Hypercarbia or (less commonly) hypocarbia.
- Hyperoxia or (less commonly) hypoxia.
- Nitrogen narcosis (sedation).
- Anxiety.

Other medical seizure-promoting factors that are also of potential relevance include hypoglycemia, cerebrovascular accidents, previous or acute cerebral trauma and tumors.

Management of an epileptic attack underwater poses difficult problems. The confusional state during the aura and post-ictal phases is likely to be unmanageable underwater, and the diver will almost certainly need to be taken to the surface. One possible exception may be the technical diver wearing a full-face mask. The fear of pulmonary barotrauma during ascent, at least in the tonic phase of a seizure when the vocal cords may be closed, has to be weighed against the likelihood of drowning during the clonic and immediate post-ictal phase, when the diver is unconscious. A review of management of a seizing diver concluded that if the mouthpiece is retained, it should be held in place and ascent initiated immediately after the clonic phase of the seizure. If the mouthpiece is not retained, then ascent should be initiated immediately after the diver is located, even if clonic movements continue[3].

Subsequent management includes the exclusion of other causes, appropriate investigations, exclusion from diving and the warning that subsequent episodes may occur on land, even years later.

BRACHIAL PLEXUS INJURY

Brachial plexus injury was related mostly to the use of standard dress diving equipment (now used mainly as a tourist attraction, as opposed to working dress), with which the weight of the helmet is taken directly on the supraclavicular region. This may be from mishandling the helmet or by having inadequate or incorrectly placed padding over the area between the neck and shoulder. It is more likely to be caused out of the water, when the

weight factor is greatest. The standby diver is thus more prone to this disorder.

The middle and lower cervical roots are more likely to be involved (i.e. the fifth to seventh), and this injury may be either temporary or permanent. Patients with minor cases present with paraesthesiae and numbness of the lateral aspect of the arm, forearm, thumb and adjacent fingers. Severe cases result in both motor and sensory damage over the affected nerve distribution. Rigid shoulder harnesses of normal open-circuit scuba can also cause this injury.

SCUBA DIVER'S THIGH (MERALGIA PARAESTHETICA)

The lateral femoral cutaneous nerve is vulnerable to compression neuropathy by pregnancy, tight trousers, pelvic tilt, harnesses and low-positioned weight belts. Meralgia paraesthetica results in numbness over the upper thigh, anteriorly and laterally. It usually clears up in a few months.

NEURALGIAS AND OTHER NERVE LESIONS

Chronic and sometimes severe pain, referable to nerves, nerve roots or nerve plexus, may follow neurological DCS[1]. Spinal cord lesions may also be responsible for some of these cases.

Many of the fish poisons and marine toxins may produce a bilateral peripheral neuropathy. Marine envenomations may produce adjoining localized neuropathies.

Involvement of the trigeminal and facial nerves may follow sinus or middle ear barotraumas (see Chapters 7 and 8).

PARAESTHESIAE

Diving-induced paraesthesiae

The causes of diving induced paraesthesiae include most of the causes of peripheral neuropathy referred to previously in this chapter. Specifically, these would include localized or segmental paraesthesiae associated with DCS, barotrauma-induced neuropathies affecting the fifth and seventh cranial nerves and meralgia paraesthetica.

Paraesthesiae can be anxiety induced, often associated with DCS (either actual or feared) and its subsequent treatment. This often affects younger and possibly less experienced divers, who may have an increased trait anxiety level. It manifests mainly as paraesthesiae affecting the hands, probably related to anxiety-induced hyperventilation, but usually not to a degree causing carpo-pedal spasm.

Anxiety-induced paraesthesiae are usually able to be ameliorated by rebreathing techniques (traditionally into a brown paper bag), but also by breathing carbogen (95 per cent oxygen, 5 per cent CO_2) and by increasing the work of breathing – which occurs with recompression, sometimes giving a misleading impression of DCS 'cure'. It also responds to both reassurance and anxiolytics, although the use of anxiolytic agents is not currently fashionable.

Paraesthesiae may also be induced by a Raynaud's reaction to cold water exposure. This is specially seen in female divers and is associated with a cold, vaso-constrictive response, usually bilateral and affecting the hands, which appear pale.

Other forms of cold-induced paraesthesiae occur in divers predisposed because of pre-existing peripheral neuropathy or drugs. The carbonic anhydrase inhibitors typify the implicated drugs, and they are taken either orally or as guttae (glaucoma treatment).

Some fish poisonings, especially ciguatera, induce paraesthesiae and may be experienced during the diving vacation. Marine venoms, especially those of the coelenterates, but also with other marine stinging incidents, can produce localized neuropathies with paraesthesiae.

Altitude-induced paraesthesiae

Paraesthesiae caused by DCS may be aggravated during altitude exposure (e.g. flight) as a result of expansion of bubbles affecting the cerebral, spinal or peripheral neurological system. It is also plausible that the relative hypoxia associated with altitude exposure may somehow cause recurrence of symptoms emanating from recently damaged neural tissue, although this notion has never been proven.

Paraesthesiae may occur during flight because of hyperventilation associated with the anxiety of air travel (increased if there is a fear of DCS), thus causing hypocapnia and mild alkalosis. This is complicated by the reduction of density of the environmental air. Hypoxia at altitude may also increase respiratory drive. Relief may be obtained by anxiolytic medication, oxygen breathing and rebreathing systems, as described earlier. This disorder is commonly misinterpreted as a recurrence of DCS, and it may be unnecessarily treated by recompression if an anxiety state continues once the diver has returned to sea level.

REFERENCES

1. Edmonds C. Dysbaric peripheral nerve involvement. *South Pacific Underwater Medicine Society Journal* 1991;**21**(4):190–197.
2. Haas RM, Hannam JA, Sames C, Schmidt R, Tyson A, Francombe M, Richardson D, Mitchell SJ. Decompression illness in divers treated in Auckland, New Zealand 1996-2013. *Diving and Hyperbaric Medicine* 2014;**44**:20–25.
3. Mitchell SJ, Bennett MH, Bird N, Doolette DJ, Hobbs GW, Kay E, Moon RE, Neuman TS, Vann RD, Walker R, Wyatt HA. Recommendations for rescue of a submerged unconscious compressed gas diver. *Undersea and Hyperbaric Medicine* 2012;**39**:1099–1108.

This chapter was reviewed for this fifth edition by Simon Mitchell.

41

Psychological and neuropsychological disorders

OVERVIEW

One should avoid the misguided belief that the knowledge of this topic in any way reflects the effort that has been spent investigating and reviewing it. Nevertheless, its importance is unquestioned.

Psychiatric problems can be sub-divided into those that are functional and those that are organic. The organic disorders include both psychoses and the organic brain syndromes.

The *functional disorders* are commonly referred to as psychological, neuroses or 'nervous illnesses'. These are characterized by disturbances of feelings, attitudes and habits severe enough to disrupt the patient's life or to reduce his or her efficiency. They are personalized reactions to stress and so reflect the degree of stress and the susceptibility of the personality. The symptoms are usually those of anxiety and/or depression, but occasionally they encompass hysterical or obsessional features.

Organic disorders range from the psychoses (schizophrenia and mood disorders, including mania, hypomania, endogenous depression and bi-polar states) to acute toxic-confusional states to dementia – and all may be associated with irritability, depression, behavioural and cognitive changes. They are presumed to have a biochemical or physical basis (e.g. damage to the brain from trauma, toxins, abnormal gas pressures, metabolic or neurodegenerative disorders).

By far the most important psychological reaction to diving is panic. It contributes to 39 per cent of recreational diving deaths (see Chapter 45). Other less catastrophic reactions include the psychoneuroses (i.e. personalized reactions to the environment and/or equipment). Post-traumatic stress disorder (PTSD) is encountered after accidents, as is symptomatic depression. Therapists' attitudes and the therapeutic situation itself may contribute to these post-treatment sequelae.

Mild confusional states may accompany many diving disorders. Transitory cognitive changes may result.

Brain damage, with its myriad neuropsychological presentations, may result from some specific diving disorders (decompression sickness [DCS], cerebral arterial gas embolism [CAGE], hypoxia, carbon monoxide toxicity) but is unlikely without such clinical incidents.

BEHAVIOURAL CHARACTERISTICS

With regard to the **psychological traits of divers,** the relationship between personality and diving is complex[1-4]. Successful divers are characterized by an average or below average neuroticism level. The psychological mechanism of denial, in which the subject refuses to react to the hazards, is thought to have adaptive value under some diving conditions. The combination allows professional divers to continue to work despite stress that would be disruptive to many 'normals'. At other times it may lead the diver into danger.

Psychometric profiles show that intelligence is positively correlated with successful diving, as are emotional stability and self-sufficiency.

Divers are, by nature and selection, risk takers. This was more so earlier last century when the risks in diving were extreme. They also approach psychologists and questionnaires with a risk-taking style that may well produce variances between their psychometric results and those of 'normal' controls.

Because divers are risk takers, and physically active individuals, they are more likely to engage in activities that attract attention from law enforcement authorities. In this way they are probably similar to Icelandic seafarers who also have a high incidence of accidents, violence, homicide and suicide.

Suicide was shown to be responsible for 17 per cent of the deaths of professional divers in the United Kingdom. **Accidents** accounted for 48 per cent of their deaths (diving or drowning accidents in 28 per cent and non-diving accidents in 20 per cent), and the death ratio was significantly higher than expected, after correction for age[4,5]. This finding contrasts with the reduced incidence of suicide and murder among recreational divers in Australia.

Some aberrant behaviour of divers may be transitory, occur soon after diving and be caused by the organic disorders referred to later. It may also result from constitutional factors.

PSYCHOLOGICAL DISTURBANCES

Psychoneuroses refer to the abnormal response of the individual to stress, but also normal responses to abnormal and excessive stress – when they may disrupt the diver's life[6-10].

Some psychological disturbances experienced during diving are well known but poorly documented. They include anxiety and panic, phobic anxiety states, somatoform disorders, illusions, post-traumatic stress disorder, compensation disorder and drug use.

Anxiety and panic

Anxiety and panic are often associated with hyperventilation, inducing paraesthesia, dyspnoea, tachycardia and other cardiac-type symptoms, disturbance of consciousness, carpo-pedal spasm and hyperreflexia, globus hystericus and gastrointestinal symptoms. The hypocapnia, which produces many of the symptoms, is corrected by rebreathing and by hyperbaric exposure (a treatment sometimes leading to a false validation of DCS). See Chapter 45 for a detailed account of panic in diving.

Phobic anxiety states

In susceptible people, the normal anxiety induced by diving may be complicated by an overawareness of potential dangers, with a resultant increase in anxiety. Apprehension, palpitations, increased rate of breathing and epigastric sensations are symptoms of anxiety and are interpreted as indicative of 'something wrong'. A vicious circle results. The diver may then develop an actual **phobia** about being underwater or confronting hazards such as marine animals.

Some candidates develop this condition even before attempting a diving course and realize that they would be apprehensive in such an environment. Other motivating factors may temporarily override this fear.

In some cases, there is a history of traumatic exposure to water (e.g. a near drowning incident) or viewing the film *Jaws,* which may initiate the phobic state – especially in susceptible individuals.

People with genuine **claustrophobia** avoid immersion or being confined in a recompression chamber. In the water, this syndrome may manifest only during times of diminished visibility (e.g. murky water, night diving, wearing a face mask) or prolonged exposure.

The **agoraphobic reaction** is also termed the **blue orb** or **blue dome syndrome,** from aviation medicine. It develops progressively, as the diver becomes more aware of his or her isolation and the lack of contact with people or objects. It may be aggravated by nitrogen narcosis at depth and by sensory deprivation (see Chapter 38). The diver is usually alone, without physical or visual contact with the diving craft or the sea bed. The fear is one of isolation in the vastness and depth of the water.

If reassurance, in the form of a companion diver or visual fixation on familiar objects, is not available, then the diver may panic and ascend rapidly. Drowning, DCS and pulmonary barotrauma are possible complications. If the diver regains physical or visual contact with the sea bed, the diving boat or a companion diver (or even focuses on his or her own equipment), the symptoms usually abate (Case Report 41.1).

All phobic anxiety states can be treated by desensitization or deconditioning techniques. They are prevented by avoiding the environmental circumstances that predispose them and also by repeated diving exposures under supportive tuition. The use of sedatives is to be discouraged, but anxiolytics may be of value during the supervised deconditioning process.

Somatoform disorders

These disorders are characterized by symptoms that were originally combined under the term 'hysteria'. A common feature is a complaint that is somatic, but with an origin that is psychological. The aetiology is described in psychological terms, but the symptom (frequently pain) is a means of eliciting care for an individual in distress – one who is otherwise unable to express this need.

As a general rule, this disorder pattern is established before the age of 30 years; otherwise, the symptom is more likely to be based on an organic disorder.

For those clients who develop functional pain, one should always exclude endogenous depression. In this situation, treatment of the depression is integral to removal of the symptoms.

The classical production of **conversion** is a disorder consequent to trauma. An intolerable experience or feeling or memory is overcome by repressing that experience. Concurrently with this a somatic symptom arises. Most of these presenting symptoms

---

CASE REPORT 41.1

AR, a 21-year-old diver with limited open water experience, dived from a boat into clear water, without tidal currents. The water was 70 metres deep, although the diver was no deeper than 15 metres. Approximately 10 minutes after commencing the dive, AR noted a feeling of fear of the deep blue water. His breathing became fast and he started to panic, with an overwhelming desire to return to the safety of his boat. He ascended to the surface, to swim back to it. His anxiety remained until he saw the reef coming into his visual range, 5 metres below him. Once back on board, he felt quite well.

Diagnosis: agoraphobic reaction.

are neurological, but they are functional in origin. There is thus a primary gain achieved by the patient. The secondary gain may be produced by the social environment surrounding the now invalid client.

The essential feature of **hypochondriasis** is a preoccupation with, and a fear of having, a serious disease – usually based on hypersensitivity to or misinterpretation of physical sensations, which are interpreted as evidence of illness. This disorder is frequently seen after divers have been suspected of possibly having DCS and treated accordingly. Some of these patients continue to have recurrences of decompression-type symptoms months or years after the event, despite reassurances and evidence of their well-being.

In such cases, if it is thought necessary to investigate to exclude other causes, then the investigations should be performed as rapidly as possible so that the period of diagnostic uncertainty is reduced to a minimum. Reassurance should be as prompt as possible because continuous interest and concern on the part of the physician can promote and prolong the disorder.

It is for this reason, as well as many others including PTSD, that unnecessary hyperbaric treatments should be avoided. They induce loss of both self-control and self-esteem.

The **Baron Von Munchausen syndrome** may be the basis of false claims related to diving. Some patients have presented with a diving history and clinical symptoms suggestive of a diving disorder, usually DCS. The patient may move from one hyperbaric unit to another for repetitive treatments – presumably either as an attention-seeking device or for the warmth and support that such a therapeutic unit may supply. These cases are the aquatic equivalent of the terrestrial Munchausen syndrome (Case Report 41.2). There is a similar syndrome recorded in caisson workers.

CASE REPORT 41.2

During a flight to Sydney, Miss PH, 30 years old, developed episodes of breathlessness and unconsciousness with a convulsive state. Between episodes she explained to the flight attendant that she had been diving to 50 metres for approximately 35 minutes, 2 hours before the flight.

On examination at a Sydney hospital, she complained of pain on deep inspiration and a slight ache in the right knee exacerbated by movement. Over the next few hours, she had three grand mal convulsions with epistaxis and peri-orbital petechiae. Pain in the right knee had become worse, and there was an overlying area of diminished sensation. A diagnosis of decompression sickness was made, and treatment was arranged at a nearby recompression chamber.

Before recompression she was conscious, rational, and gave a detailed history of the dive. Apart from the area of diminished sensation over the right knee and decreased knee and ankle reflexes, there were no other neurological signs detected. She was placed in the recompression chamber and pressurized to 18 metres on 100 per cent oxygen initially, and she improved symptomatically. During decompression, she had three grand mal epileptic convulsions. Upon recovery, she complained of worsening of her knee and chest symptoms. She was therefore pressurized on air to 50 metres, where she again showed improvement, but again subsequently deteriorated. Following a series of epileptiform seizures, she became unresponsive to vocal and painful stimuli for brief periods. Some hours later, after consciousness had returned, she complained of severe abdominal, chest, right hip and right knee pain.

At this stage, investigations by telephone revealed that she had not, in fact, been diving. She had a long psychiatric history of hysterical symptoms, genuine epilepsy and a recent interest in a *Skin Diver* article on decompression sickness. She stopped her anticonvulsant treatment about 24 hours before presenting for treatment. Because of the long duration of exposure to pressure of both the patient and the attendants, subsequent decompression proceeded at a slow rate. The chamber reached the 'surface' after approximately 48 hours.

Provisional diagnosis: aquatic Baron Von Munchausen syndrome.

Illusions

Sensory deprivation, especially with impaired diving visibility, is likely to aggravate the tendency to misinterpret stimuli. Anxiety associated with diving results in heightened suggestibility (e.g. terror on sighting unexpected objects, mistaking another diver for a shark).

Post-traumatic stress disorder

GENERAL

As with motor vehicle accidents and other catastrophes (war, earthquakes, volcanic eruptions, bush fires, mass shootings, murder, rape and home invasion), PTSD is but one of a number of possible psychological sequelae which may co-exist. The others are as follows:

- Dissociation (hysterical reaction).
- Somatization (conversion of anxiety into a physical disorder).
- Depression and bereavement (especially if loved ones have been involved).
- Anxiety and hyperventilation.
- Compensation neurosis.
- Affect dysregulation (a lack of self-regulation leading to difficulty in controlling anger or producing self-destructive, suicidal or risk-taking behaviour).

PTSD was defined in 1980, but it was known previously as post-traumatic anxiety, shell-shock, battle fatigue, daCosta syndrome and other terms. It is an anxiety disorder that develops in some divers exposed to a severe and usually life-threatening situation.

In a lesser degree, PTSD could have survival value, ensuring that we refrain from situations that had previously been experienced as dangerous.

It has been claimed that there are anatomical and pathological organic cerebral changes with PTSD, with specific changes in neuropsychological functioning, but this view is contentious.

AETIOLOGY

PTSD is more likely to develop in divers who normally have higher levels of trait anxiety (neuroticism) or when the stress has been particularly severe or prolonged. It is less likely to occur in divers who are trained in the emergency situation and who are more prepared for it.

The usual diving provocations are accidents that cause death of a diving companion or involve the diver in a near death situation, usually with the threat of drowning.

Other aggravating situations include the prolonged stress and trauma of medical evacuation and hyperbaric therapies.

Prevention is achieved by the early application of rest, support and the comfort of one's companions. Unfortunately, in diving accidents, as in aviation and many others, there is a tendency to blame and discredit the victim – by instructors, peers and even therapists.

CLINICAL FEATURES

The diver has intense fear that the event may recur and is preoccupied with this thought. It may intrude as vivid memories – in the form of dreams, nightmares or flashbacks.

The diver responds by avoidance behaviour (i.e. avoiding things, situations or people that serve as reminders of the event). He or she may also appear to block out all emotion.

There may be other general factors associated with the increased anxiety level – irritability, insomnia, various aches and pains, panic attacks, globus hystericus, hyperventilation, dyspnoea and/or a choking sensation.

TREATMENT

First aid after the accident should be supportive and reassuring and yet still encouraging the patient to verbalize the experience. This may have some preventive value, although there is little to support the value of the conventional 'counseling de-brief'. Instead, make the victim feel safe, allow rest and provide support. Repeated hyperbaric therapies tend to interfere with this approach.

The disorder is likely to be evident within a week or two of the event. The customary treatment is for psychological intervention in which the client is encouraged to remember the events in a non-stressful situation, but with the emotional memory expressed. Confidence is engendered, and the disorder diminishes.

Unfortunately, PTSD is characterized by avoidance mechanisms, so the victim tends to stay away from the therapeutic situation that will allow venting of the memories and the emotions.

Other treatments that may be required include education about anxiety management, cognitive behavioural therapy, insight-orientated psychotherapy and other techniques.

Medications may be of value, based on the symptoms. Modern antidepressants (e.g. selective serotonin reuptake inhibitors) may stabilize the client, and tricyclic antidepressants may be of value if there is any major sleep disturbance. The anxiolytics are no longer considered the best agents for this indication.

Compensation (occupational) neurosis

This disorder includes a range of presentations from malingering to the exaggeration of genuine symptoms for secondary gain. The lucrative occupation of professional diving and the litigious nature of many societies both encourage this disorder, which often bestows rewards on the adversarial consultants – legal and medical.

Frequently, the claimant becomes obsessed by the procedure, and the ultimate financial recompense is offset by a limitation in life style, a loss of self-esteem and withdrawal from the diving fraternity.

Protraction of the legal proceedings has positive implications for the insurance companies involved.

Drug use

During diving and diving medical examinations (see Chapters 43 and 53 to 59), the influences of drugs have to be considered. This is especially so with recreational drugs and psychotropic agents.

The use of illicit or recreational drugs, or even herbal supplements, may induce problems in their own right, such as with designer drugs, cocaine or Kava use. These substances aggravate cardiac deaths, especially in diving situations. Other medical diseases such as acquired immunodeficiency syndrome (AIDS) and systemic or hepatic infections may be related to illicit intravenous drug use. Complications from nicotine and alcohol are well recognized.

Various prescribed drugs may have harmful side effects (e.g. sedatives, narcotics, other psychotropics, cardiovascular, autonomics, neuroleptics). They may also cause heightened anxiety and impairment of judgement or cognitive function from withdrawal effects that have implications for diving safety.

PSYCHOSES

Psychosis would usually preclude a candidate from diving training. Certain psychoses may result in pathological delusions related to diving, a misuse of the diving environment or false claims related to diving.

Schizophrenia may cause a diver to develop primary delusions centered on the diving activity (e.g. paranoia toward sharks that results in a personal vendetta against them). The development of a complex delusional system regarding international undersea control, radioactivity, diving inventions and so forth has also been observed.

Bi-polar disorders may be dangerous along either psychological axis. The grandiosity and self-assurance in a hypomanic state are as potentially dangerous as the suicidal inclinations during depression, and they may be hazardous to others.

Suicide, although not well recognized, is not a rare event among those who have access to the sea (see earlier). With the more widespread attraction to this sport of a greater range of personalities, the incidence could increase. The aetiology of suicide is not different from that in the general population, but the means may differ considerably.

Swimming into the blue oceanic horizon has a certain flamboyant appeal and has been used by some less prosaic souls. One diver completed the suicide formalities by documenting his intent to free ascend while breath-holding, and he succeeded in bursting his lungs. Others use mundane methods despite the exotic environment (Case Report 41.3).

Unfortunately, **psychotropic drugs,** given for therapeutic reasons, may cause problems. Side effects of psychotropic medications may include decreased epileptic seizure threshold, sedation, cardiac arrhythmias, reduced exercise capability, autonomic nervous system interference and other issues.

CASE REPORT 41.3

FR refilled his scuba cylinder from the local diver shop and hired a boat and diver to take him on a dive. He quietly read a science fiction book on the way out. He then entered the water, surfaced very soon and asked the boat operator to hand him a bag he had brought. That was the last the boat operator saw of him. He was found the next morning by the water police while still wearing his scuba equipment and with a 22-calibre bullet through his brain.

These effects would increase the hazards associated with scuba diving, especially in inexperienced divers.

The influence of drugs on the diving disorders such as stress reactions, dysbaric disease, gas narcoses and so forth are usually not well documented, but they are potential sources of concern (see Chapter 43).

NEUROPSYCHOLOGICAL MANIFESTATIONS

Aetiology

The neurological insults from diving accidents may be many and varied[11–15], and they may summate. There are often neurological signs of cerebral or cerebellar disorders.

Causes of permanent intellectual impairment from compressed gas diving include the following:

- Neurological DCS.
- CAGE from pulmonary barotrauma.
- Severe hypoxia, usually from near drowning.
- Carbon monoxide toxicity.

Ill-defined and unquantified damage from other gas toxicities is possible (e.g. carbon dioxide, nitrogen, oxygen and contaminants). If extreme, high-pressure neurological syndrome (HPNS) and hypothermia have been implicated as causes of central nervous system (CNS) damage.

Organic brain syndromes

DELIRIUM (TOXIC-CONFUSIONAL STATE)

This condition is, by definition, a fluctuating and transitory state, although it can manifest briefly during other organic brain syndromes.

A disturbance of consciousness is the main characteristic, and it can be seen in many diving disorders, but especially hypoxia, carbon dioxide toxicity, hypothermia, cerebral DCS, CAGE, marine animal envenomations, nitrogen narcosis and HPNS.

The more florid delirium, with its extreme alertness, produces sleep disruption, disordered speech, perceptual abnormalities (illusions, hallucinations), disturbances of affect (fear, delusions, paranoia) and disturbances of cognition (especially memory).

Although all these may be present in some of the more florid cases (e.g. patients coming out of coma from a hypoxic near drowning accident), in other cases the disorder may be more subtle. All that may be evident is unaccustomed behaviour, either hyper-activity or hypo-activity, drowsiness, slight bewilderment or lapses of memory and judgement. The hyper-alert state may be evident only as insomnia, and the hallucinations may manifest only as vivid dreams.

It is in such cases that the behaviour of the diver, based on impaired judgement, may be inappropriate (i.e. the diver may deny symptoms or ignore them). The diver may insist on driving his or her vehicle to the recompression chamber. The diver may also forget some of the symptoms he or she had complained of. Instead of gross confusion, there may be only irritability – which can manifest as intolerance to advice or treatment.

These patients must be treated gently and with encouragement, not with criticism and impatience, to maintain their cooperation.

A common mistake made by hyperbaric clinicians is to confuse the behavioural abnormalities of an *acute organic brain syndrome* – as happens with both CAGE and DCS – with hysterical and psychopathic diagnoses. Thus, the obstreperous diver with an illogical reluctance to enter the recompression chamber is the patient who may need it most. The best interpreters of behaviour disorder are the diver's colleagues and family. They will recognize the behaviour as atypical and thus indicate that it may be based on recent brain damage.

Most diving medical facilities have simple clinical psychological testing procedures to record the following:

- Orientation for time, place and person.
- Attention and concentration (e.g. serial sevens, reversal of order).
- Recent memory (three objects or words, recalled 3 minutes later).
- Abstract thinking (e.g. proverbs, differences).
- Speed of responses.

The mini-mental state examination, once practised, is of diagnostic value. Some groups even include formal psychological tests (e.g. Raven's Advanced Progressive Matrices, Digit Symbol, Koh's Block). Such tests may readily demonstrate an abnormality, even though it will not indicate the cause. The same test performed within minutes of an appropriate therapy may demonstrate improvement.

Electroencephalograms (EEGs) and some of the cerebral scanning techniques may also indicate an anomaly.

One of the most common causes of delirium in general medicine is a head injury, and this is not at all dissimilar to the intracerebral vascular trauma of DCS and CAGE. The pathological features of CAGE may develop more slowly, with the emboli-induced vascular damage allowing a diffusion of blood components into the cerebral tissue, for hours after the initiating bubble has passed through the vasculature.

SUB-ACUTE ORGANIC BRAIN SYNDROMES

Between transitory delirium and chronic dementia, there can be a variety of other syndromes, with characteristics of each of the two extreme disorders, in any combination.

Cerebral involvement of the diseases mentioned earlier can produce organic psychiatric syndromes such as confusional states, depressive syndromes and symptomatic depressions that may last for months, often after all neurological signs have cleared.

If *symptomatic depression* remains after hyperbaric therapy, the diver may develop a modification of personality, with anxiety, emotional lability, difficulty in coping, delayed insomnia (waking up in the early hours) and even suicidal ideation. Small doses of sedative antidepressants, taken nightly, may have a beneficial result in a week or two. An organically orientated psychiatrist should be consulted.

Superimposed on the organic brain syndromes there may be specific clinical features related to the anatomical sites affected by the disease.

Dementia

Dementia implies permanent impairment of short-term and/or long-term memory or other brain dysfunction, often with one of the following:

- Impaired abstract thinking and/or intelligence.
- Impaired judgement (personal and social).
- Impaired impulse control.
- Regional cortical dysfunction.
- Personality change significant enough to interfere with work and social relationships.

This disturbance of cognitive function must be demonstrated in the absence of any disturbance of consciousness (e.g. delirium).

These patients are less able to cope with or introduce new ideas, and there is a diminishing of thought, abstract concepts, judgement and insight (the dysexecutive syndrome). Affect or mood changes, especially emotional lability, are characteristic. There can be a dominance of paranoid, hypomanic or depressive features. Patients may attempt to cope with their limited abilities by obsessionality and orderliness.

NEUROPSYCHOLOGICAL IMPAIRMENT FROM DIVING ACCIDENTS

Reports from the 1950s and 1970s claimed that divers and caisson workers who suffered severe neurological DCS were likely to sustain permanent brain damage. Unfortunately, these reports are often inappropriately quoted as evidence that diving, as such, is also a cause of dementia.

In 1959, **Rozsahegyi**[16] in Hungary examined 100 subjects between 2.5 and 5 years after CNS DCS and concluded that more than half had some psychological disorder; 75 per cent had neurological findings on clinical examination. Quiet men would frequently become irritable and uncontrolled after the injury, and pathological drunkenness and alcohol intolerance were common.

Neurological, EEG and psychiatric disturbances were organic. Rozsahegyi concluded that chronic, progressive encephalomyelopathy resulted from repeated decompressions and neurological DCS. Paradoxically, some of his patients improved over years of follow-up.

The observations prompted research into the relationship between the neurological sequelae of DCS and intellectual functioning. Between 1975 and 1977, three **Texas studies**[17-19] reported neurological and psychological problems, with psychometric tests, in a small number of divers who experienced DCS affecting the CNS. Unfortunately, these were mainly cases under litigation, and the same cases were repeated in the three series; they were not three separate series.

A **Norwegian** report[20] in the early 1980s claimed neuropsychological damage after 'near miss' diving accidents. The investigators compared nine divers with some controls. There appeared to be a change in cognitive functioning; most of the divers reported impaired memory capacity as the main problem. In addition, difficulty in concentration, irritability, alcoholism and aphasia were noted.

The foregoing authors used Rozsahegyi's series[16] of CNS DCS cases as evidence for the unsubstantiated hypothesis of chronic progressive encephalomyelopathy resulting from decompressions (without DCS).

Clinical DCS cases among recreational divers from **Hawaii**[21], **Australia**[22] and **Israel**[23], during the following decade, showed an increased proportion of neurological manifestations, compared with the predominance of joint involvement from the earlier navy studies.

In a 1-year follow-up of 25 recreational divers treated in **New Zealand** for DCS in 1987,

Sutherland and associates[13] found that 74 per cent had some degree of morbidity, mostly in the form of personality changes. Impaired cognition was present in 48 per cent. Mood disorders were present in 56 per cent, and these disorders mostly developed after discharge from treatment.

Morris and colleagues[24] in 1991 studied 292 professional divers and showed some impairment of cognitive function in divers who had suffered decompression illness. Any impairment of memory and non-verbal reasoning in those divers without previous decompression illness was predominantly related to age. There was no change in personality attributed to uncomplicated diving exposure. Many psychometric tests were performed, with results that were not very consistent. It appears that there was no obvious dose-response relationship between the quantity of diving and the neuropsychometric results, but there was a relationship between the presence of DCS and some types of cognitive impairment.

There were serious questions raised by **Edmonds and Hayward**[25] about the selection of divers and the matching of controls in most surveys, and there was little consistency in the neuropsychological findings of the various studies on DCS cases.

An investigation by **Gorman and associates**[11] on recreational divers who had been treated for DCS by the Royal Australian Navy demonstrated a large number of neurological, EEG and psychometric abnormalities during the subsequent weeks. This was so even with divers who had no obvious clinical neurological component to their DCS. There was no clinical or investigatory evidence, sought or implied in this series, to demonstrate long-term sequelae. Improvement was demonstrated, and the 48 per cent of divers who had EEG changes the week after a DCS incident was reduced to 17 per cent 1 month later.

EEGs and evoked cortical potentials may be abnormal at the time of such an incident, but these abnormalities are unlikely to persist unless clinical changes are gross[26-28]. Abnormalities in EEGs and neuropsychometric testing[12] are to be expected during illness, or if subjects are not fully alert and cooperative.

A review of various effects of DCS on diving was made by **Shields and colleagues**[29] in 1996.

It was carried out on 31 divers who had DCS, 31 who did not and 31 controls. The following conclusions were drawn.

- Both diver groups had high levels of abnormally long latencies in evoked potential measurement (brainstem auditory evoked potentials, somatosensory evoked potentials, sensory evoked potentials). The DCS diver group had a 14 times higher presence of abnormal P40 latencies (sensory evoked potentials – tibial) than the non-DCS divers and a 7 times higher presence of abnormal P40 latencies than non-diving controls.
- On psychometric assessment, the DCS-diver group had a statistically significant poorer logical memory performance than the non-diving control group on immediate recall and then the non-DCS diver group on delayed recall.
- Although 28 per cent of divers had 99m-technetium hexamethyl-propylene-amine oxime (HMPAO)–single photon emission computed tomography (SPECT) scan results outside normal limits, the absence of an established baseline for the incidence of pattern variants in the standard population made this observation difficult to interpret. The clinical significance is unclear.
- The significance of these findings in terms of a diver's current state of health or quality of life is unclear. More extensive studies are required to shed light on these aspects.

Imaging techniques have been used to demonstrate cerebral damage and perfusion abnormalities after appropriate treatment has been instituted[30-33]. This imaging confirmed the presence of both anticipated and unexpected lesions.

Nevertheless, definite spinal cord disease in divers[33], in excess of that expected from clinical examination, has been demonstrated by some pathologists. To a lesser degree, the same may be claimed for cerebral vascular disease, but a clinical concomitant has not yet been demonstrated.

The **Medical Research Council (MRC) DCS Panel report**[31] in 1988 on the long-term health effects of diving was edited by M. J. Halsey. It was stated that divers' autopsies showed extensive histopathological features of the brain. Dr Ian Calder claimed anecdotally that the pathological features represent about 10 years of aging. It is not clear from the MRC report (or to attendees) whether the pathologists were referring specifically to cases of DCS, deep and helium divers or conventional air-breathing divers. Reference was made to cases of serious DCS with frontal cerebral lesions, causing neuropsychological problems in divers in Hawaii that included apathy, depression and socioeconomic difficulties.

Some informative studies have been carried out, using neuropsychological techniques during or immediately after diving[34] and diving accidents[11,15], and results have shown acute neurological impairments.

The judgement of a brain-damaged patient, especially someone in an influential administrative position, may have implications for other diving units under his or her control. The anecdotal observations of dementia in middle-aged professional divers who had not adhered to established safety regulations and decompression procedures are contentious and deserve clarification.

NEUROPSYCHOLOGICAL IMPAIRMENT FROM DIVING

A more contentious belief has arisen regarding the possible dementia-producing effects of diving *per se,* without sustaining a clinical neurological disease. This hypothesis has triggered a multitude of investigations, desperate for possible associations, employing non-standard research tools and with dubious controls. One is reminded of the economists' dictum that 'if you torture the data long enough, you can force a confession'. Despite the abundance of research, there is little or no consensus.

Diving folklore

In a symposium in Norway in 1983[32], there was apparent acceptance of the neuropsychological complications of diving with compressed air. There was no consensus reached regarding any long-term neuropsychological complications of deeper diving, which had been investigated more fully.

The folklore belief developed among many occupational diving groups that dementia ('diver's dumbness' or the 'punch drunk syndrome') was produced by prolonged compressed air diving. This presumption was supported during the 1980s by media reports of brain damage in divers.

In the United Kingdom, anecdotal observations from the Royal Navy and pilot studies from the University of Lancaster were widely quoted, far more than their scientific value warranted, and heightened concern among divers.

In a report on abalone divers in Australia[35], it was stated that 30 per cent of the divers suffered chronic ear damage, 20 per cent had dysbaric osteonecrosis and 10 per cent had brain damage, but no supporting evidence was cited.

Circumstantial evidence

Some of diverse reports have been used as circumstantial evidence that diving produces neuropsychological damage and, by implication and extrapolation, subsequent dementia.

In Sweden[36], abnormal EEGs were noted in 3.5 per cent of free ascent trainees, a finding suggesting the presence of CAGE.

Kwaitowski[37] investigated 150 professional Polish divers and found abnormal EEGs in 43 per cent, compared with 10 per cent in the general population.

Hallenbeck and Anderson[38] and Hills and James[39] demonstrated that 'silent' bubbles produced during decompression could damage the blood-brain barrier temporarily and produce extravasation of blood constituents and fluid into the cerebral tissue.

Calder[31,33] reviewed neuropathology findings at autopsies on divers. These abnormalities were more extensive than would have been anticipated from the mild or treated DCS previously experienced by subjects. There was, however, more spinal than cerebral damage. There is also some doubt about how clinically free of symptoms and signs some of the patients were[40].

Vascular changes in divers may be related to a higher than normal number of unidentified bright objects (UBOs) in the magnetic resonance imaging (MRI) scan, also referred to as white matter hyperintensity brain lesions (WMHs), but there is no correlation yet demonstrated between these and any neuropsychometric abnormalities. As Hallenbeck[41] noted in 1978, when investigating the possibility of 'diving encephalopathy', even clinically obvious transient ischaemic attacks with definite pathological features usually remit without sequelae.

Psychometric surveys – does diving cause dementia?

Most of the earlier studies[16–20] suffered from gross errors[25], including the following:

- A heavy reliance on anecdotal reporting.
- Ill-defined diagnoses (not differentiating DCS, CAGE, near drowning and hypoxia, gas toxicities, inner ear and life style diseases).
- Statistics. Controls were absent or inappropriate. Search were made for multiple associations without adjusting for this number. Other controls were not matched for previous intelligence quotient [IQ], age, alcohol consumption, head injury or other factors.
- Selection. Some were medico-legal cases or involved in compensation.
- Use of experimental and non-standardized psychometric, neurological and pathological investigations.
- Psychometric tests that were inappropriate or not internationally standardized.
- Support and misquoting from non–peer-reviewed articles or abstracts.
- Extrapolations and overstatements.

Selective reporting and referencing, especially when limited to Internet availability and excluding the comprehensive conferences and texts on this subject, are common. Some reports of possible impaired cognition in divers were retracted by the report authors in follow-up, more comprehensive, surveys[25], but the retractions and reservations are rarely quoted, even though the original reports are still used to support the hypothesis.

Psychometric examinations on divers revealed that divers' personality profiles, and their psychometric test results, are different from those of non-divers[1–3].

These differences need to be appreciated when using controls and drawing conclusions.

US NAVY

Two extensive surveys[7,8] on psychometric disability in US Navy divers demonstrated statistically significant – but divergent – results.

Becker[14], in the US Navy, using conventional and reputable psychometric testing, could find no evidence in six subjects 3 years after an 1800-foot dive to support his previous impression of impairment of cognitive function.

Curley[42] investigated 25 US Navy deep saturation divers with conventional psychometric testing. After a 4-year longitudinal neuropsychological assessment at the Navy Experimental Diving Unit, this investigator did not detect any permanent residual defects in cognitive or CNS functioning in these divers.

AUSTRALIAN 'EXCESSIVE DIVER' SURVEYS

In 1985, multiple investigations[43,44] were performed on Australian abalone divers because of their extremely aggressive diving procedures, excessive diving exposure, the high prevalence of conventional occupational diseases and the alleged presence of a punch drunk syndrome[35]. Prohibition of the transfer of abalone diving licenses meant that this was a closed community at that time.

It was presumed that if damage was present, its specific nature would be especially obvious in this group. Conversely, if this excessive diving group showed no evidence of intellectual impairment, the disorder would be an unlikely or uncommon complication in more conservative air diving groups. An initial pilot survey[43] indicated that these excessive divers may have such a problem.

This excessive diving population of 152 divers had, on average[44]:

- Been diving for more than 16 years.
- Spent 12 years in professional abalone diving.
- Spent more than 5 hours per day on compressed air (hookah) for 105 days each year.
- Reached just over 50 feet (15.25 metres) on a typical day.
- Claimed to have been seriously 'bent' more than four times, but did not count the minor types of DCS.

Routinely, 58 per cent of the excessive divers employed a dive profile that required some time for decompression but was omitted. In this group, 69 instances of DCS were diagnosed and treated by medical evacuation and recompression therapy in a chamber. Of these, at least 39 cases were neurological. Other patients were untreated, given oxygen or treated by in-water regimens.

Multi-disciplinary and special interest researchers independently investigated these excessive divers by using objective standardized psychological, neurological and electrophysiological tests. The purpose was to employ internationally accepted investigations, standardized for the Australian population, to indicate the existence and site of brain damage.

Because of the contradictory findings between the Texan and Norwegian studies on the Wechsler Adult Intelligence Scale, this test was repeated by Edmonds and Coulton[45] on a much larger (n = 67) group of this 'excessive' diving population. A multiple regression analysis was made against all diving co-variants and the 10 subtext scores (verbal IQ, performance IQ, total IQ) and deterioration index ('dementia score'), corrected for age. Apart from minor and clinically unimportant associations, the analysis showed no relationship between the type of diving and these measurements of intellectual functioning, nor was there an abnormal profile or scatter in the divers' results that could have implied brain damage. This investigation indicated that if neuropsychological changes were present, they would be of more subtle than those detected by such conventional test batteries.

Neurobehavioural researchers, who specialized in detection of minor abnormalities among occupational groups exposed to chemicals, heavy metals and toxins, also examined this group of excessive divers. Williamson and colleagues[3,46] reported two such studies.

In the first study, the investigators found that the divers did as well as or better than the controls on some tests (reaction time, some memory and motor tests) and worse than controls on others (visual and short-term memory and some psychomotor learning skills). However, the way in which divers chose to complete their tests differed from the controls, in that they were more likely to take risks and substitute speed for accuracy. This difference in behaviour should be taken into account when interpreting neuropsychological assessments in other surveys.

The second study focussed on neuropsychological functioning and a number of diving-related variables, but the associations found were weak. What it did demonstrate was that the deficits in neurobehavioural tests were in those divers who consistently exposed themselves to gross decompression omissions and experienced more DCS.

Another sub-group of 48 excessive divers was subjected to the more conventional psychometric tests by Andrews and associates[47]. This study compared excessive divers with non-diving fisher controls living in the same locality. These investigators found that the differences were small, and the divers' scores were within normal limits for the general population. Andrews and colleagues also compared the 'abnormal low' performance members from both the diver and control groups, and they found no evidence for a sub-set of divers with abnormal scores. The authors concluded that 'there was no evidence for the accumulation of subclinical insults leading to a dementing process'.

Hjorth and colleagues[48] performed double-blind assessments on EEGs and carried out multiple evoked cortical potentials on 20 excessive divers. Apart from a couple of minor abnormalities in the EEGs, no significant findings were made. Visual evoked cortical potentials and upper and lower limb somatosensory evoked cortical potentials were all normal.

In the Australian 'excessive diver' cross-sectional survey, there was no evidence of diving-related dementia or evidence that diving *per se* caused any cognitive impairment. It was concluded that if divers who were exposed to excessive diving did not show clinical or insidious abnormalities, then there was little likelihood that others, less exposed, would be so affected.

UK AND EUROPEAN REVIEWS AND SURVEYS

A smaller **Norwegian survey**[49] of 'excessive' divers compared 20 construction divers (mean, >4000 dives) with age-matched controls and diving trainees. Various conventional neuropsychometric tests were performed. These investigators were unable to demonstrate any clear evidence of neuropsychological deficit resulting from the extensive diving. The only evident abnormality was a prolonged reaction time.

Two other reviews were carried out in the **United Kingdom.** In the 1990s, Evans and Shields[50] conducted a critical review of the literature of potential neurological long-term effects of diving and reassessed histopathological observations, diagnostic neurological imaging, psychometric testing, electrophysiological studies and retinal angiography. Their considerations and conclusions are worthy of note, if only to demonstrate the current areas of contention.

- The neuropathological studies were cause for concern, but further studies were needed – including assessment of human post-mortem material and animal studies to determine whether histopathological effects of hyperbaria could occur without signs of DCS.
- Diagnostic neurological imaging changes in the CNS in divers presenting with acute DCS were demonstrated. Their reliability in the healthy diver population had yet to be established. Investigations were continuing, particularly regarding cerebral perfusion and positron emission tomography (PET)–mediated assessment of cerebral metabolism, with the potential of detecting subtle neurological changes, if such exist.
- Neuropsychological studies of diving were contradictory; some recorded no apparent deficits, whereas others found positive correlations between diving and poor test performance. Clearly, there was a need for a well-controlled longitudinal study of a cross section of the diving community.
- EEG studies were disappointing. The evidence was often contradictory, with poor correlation between EEG abnormalities and clinical signs. Computer analysis, especially with brain electrical activity mapping, was potentially of interest, but it was still in its infancy, and controversy remained over its use and reliability.
- Evoked potentials were employed, including visual evoked potentials, brain stem auditory evoked potential and somatosensory evoked potentials. As with EEG, measurement of evoked potential in divers proved disappointing, both in the management of acute dysbaric

illness and as a research tool in investigation of long-term sequelae. The field of electrophysiology did not appear to have lived up to its early promise in the identification of subclinical neurological lesions.

- Retinal fluorescein angiography in asymptomatic divers was employed, to demonstrate neurological lesions[33]. The correlations with any clinical sequelae had not been validated.
- In conclusion, it was determined that, in relation to the problem of long-term neurological damage in divers, it had not been determined whether a problem exists. There was difficulty in drawing conclusions from the small number of papers, which were repeatedly quoted but had only a few cases and great difficulty in controlling for confounding variables. There was danger in false-positive findings with powerful and sensitive methods of neurological investigation that may not have clinical implications.

Another excellent review of the long-term health effects of diving was presented by Elliott and Moon[51], in their text *The Physiology and Medicine of Diving* (fourth edition, 1993). Since that publication, and also since the Norwegian publication, *Long Term Health Effects of Diving*[33], of an international consensus conference at Godoysund, Norway in 1993, there have been some additions to the available data on this subject. In general, they have supported most of the conclusions drawn earlier.

A study from Finland[52], evaluating the EEG and MRI investigations after diving and decompression incidents, supported the value of the EEG assessment as a non-specific indicator of CNS damage and its improvement with recompression therapy. The MRI was not a particularly valuable investigation, and these workers were not able to verify evidence of increased CNS lesions in normal divers as compared with non-diving, healthy controls. Some of the divers treated for DCS had hyperintense lesions in the brain and white matter.

Another well-controlled survey, from Germany[53], compared 59 military and commercial divers (with at least 500 hours of diving) with 48 control subjects matched for age, body mass index, alcohol and smoking history, but who had never dived. These investigators could not find any increased prevalence of brain lesions in the divers, with a

fluid-attenuated inversion recovery sequence and T1- and T2-weighted pre- and post-contrast MRI.

A comprehensive review by Dutka[54] illustrated the failure to reach any valid consensus on the value of various screening techniques (computed tomography [CT], MRI, SPECT) in demonstrating long-term abnormalities resulting from diving *per se*. There are relatively controversial and unhelpful results from applying these techniques to acute cases of DCS, but much optimism for the future application with PET and its extensions.

No significant advances have been made over the last decade in the application of neuropsychometric assessments in eliciting long-term effects of diving.

Slosman and associates[55] in 2004 suggested the following:

- Depth of dives had a negative influence on cerebral blood flow and its combined effect with body mass index and age.
- A specific diving environment (more than 80 per cent of dives in lakes) had a negative effect on cerebral blood flow.
- Depth and number of dives had a negative influence on cognitive performance (speed, flexibility and inhibition processing in attentional tasks).
- A specific diving environment had a negative effect on cognitive performance (flexibility and inhibition components).

These investigators concluded that scuba diving may have long-term negative neurofunctional effects when it is performed in extreme conditions, namely cold water, with more than 100 dives per year and at depths greater than 40 metres.

In 2004 in a large, well-controlled study, the ELTHI (*Examination of the Long Term Health Impact of Diving*) project[56], 1540 long-term commercial divers were compared with matched offshore worker controls, with questionnaires, clinical examination and neurological assessments. Health-related quality of life was similar in each group and within normative values. A significant group of divers (18 per cent) complained of 'forgetfulness or loss of concentration', and this was related to their diving experience. This complaint was associated with a significant moderate reduction in group mean quality of life. A random sample of this group had a lower group mean performance on objective tests of cognitive function, most particularly of memory, and structural differences on cerebral MRI. Welding activities had an unexpected amplifying effect in terms of these symptoms. Divers reporting 'forgetfulness or loss of concentration' tended to have had longer diving careers and had done more mixed gas bounce, saturation and surface decompression diving. They were more likely to have suffered DCS. There was a very high prevalence (50 per cent) of objectively determined hearing disorders in both divers and off-shore workers.

Kowalski and associates[57] in 2011 reported on 17 divers who had logged between 150 and 1200 diving hours and 8 very experienced divers logging between 2800 and 9800 diving hours, with no clinically evident DCS. These divers were compared with 23 healthy matched controls for their reaction time. Motor reaction time and decision reaction time were reduced in the 'very experienced' divers, but not in the 'experienced' divers. No increased errors were observed in any of the tasks for either diving group. The findings were said to support the proposal that minimal cerebral lesions occur after diving even without DCS. An alternative hypothesis, that the explanation may lie in peripheral nerve disease, was not explored.

Because this contentious issue has been debated for over half a century with miniscule results, it is no longer credible to publish more reports based on dubious selection procedures and statistics, by employing the rationalization that 'the topic needs to be discussed', nor is it constructive to search for smaller and smaller anomalies based on non-standardized investigations – no matter how technologically innovative they may be.

Two conclusions from the available data can be made:

1. Clinically evident brain damage, verified by neuropsychological testing and standardized neurological imaging techniques, to a degree consistent with dementia, does occur in brain damage from diving accidents, such as decompression illness.
2. There is no substantial evidence of an equivalent disorder (permanent, progressive brain damage or 'encephalopathy') from diving *per se*.

In a related occupational field, in DCS-prone U-2 pilots who are exposed to long-duration high-altitude flights, investigations demonstrated a fourfold number and a threefold volume of WMHs compared with controls[58,59]. The distribution was generalized, and they did not increase with time, unlike the frontal lesions associated with ageing. WMHs were not increased in those pilots with a DCS history, but they were still presumed to be related to the effects of cerebral microemboli or thrombi. There were no associated clinical manifestations, and the pilots were engaged in complex cognitive activities without any suggestion of early dementia.

CONCLUSIONS

The adverse effect of DCS and its treatment on the anxiety and self-esteem of the diver, together with attitudes of both peer and therapist groups, may well have psychological implications, such as symptomatic depression, a psychoneurotic reaction or PTSD. These effects, together with the physiological influences of sleep deprivation, hyperbaric therapy, drug administration and non-cerebral manifestations of DCS, may well complicate the interpretation of psychometric assessments performed soon after the incident.

Some divers tend to be more 'risk taking' than non-divers, both in their life's activities and in their approach to psychometric testing. More carefully controlled studies have failed to substantiate the hypothesis of an insidious development of occult dementia, or even evidence of 'early neurological aging', in conventional divers.

Otological, visual, spinal and peripheral neuropathies from DCS, oxygen toxicity and other diving disorders may also affect neurobehavioural function (and neuropsychological tests) without implying dementia.

There is ample evidence that acute and temporary neurological insults are experienced by compressed air divers and other divers. These insults are not typically translated into evidence of permanent brain damage or dementia.

Earlier studies, confirming that neurological DCS could cause permanent neuropsychological damage, had serious limitations in their diagnostic categories, statistical analysis and misuse of control groups. They were inappropriately used to imply diving-induced brain damage without preceding clinical diseases. There is some relationship between excessive decompression stress and neuropsychological damage, a finding supporting the observations that DCS induces some neuropsychological changes.

Brain damage and dementia can supervene if there is clinically significant cerebral injury (severe hypoxia, carbon monoxide toxicity, CAGE or cerebral DCS). Any long-term effects of the HPNS have yet to be defined, qualitatively or quantitatively.

A plethora of studies in the last few decades, incorporating scanning techniques, especially CT, SPECT, MRI and PET, demonstrated significant, minimal or no abnormalities from diving *per se*. There is no positive consensus at this stage because of the complicating factors of the degree of decompression exposure, varied radiological interpretations, definitions of normality, publication bias, clinical significance of the findings and many of the confusing parameters that bedevilled interpretation of the psychometric studies of the past. A critical review of these scanning applications is eagerly awaited.

The more recent psychometric studies have not validated the suspicion of a clinically significant diving-induced organic neuropsychological syndrome, although this research does hint at the possibility of minimal effects, not necessarily dysfunction, from diving. This also assumes a judicious experimental design, correct matching of controls and an appropriate statistical application.

There is insufficient evidence to conclude that long-term compressed air diving exposure, apart from the well-documented neurological diseases of diving, causes dementia or any other clinically significant organic neuropsychological deficits.

REFERENCES

1. US Navy. *Bibliographical Sourcebooks of Compressed Air Diving and Submarine Medicine.* Vols. 1 to 3. Washington, DC: Department of the Navy; 1948, 1954, 1966.
2. Edmonds C. *The Diver.* Royal Australian Navy (RAN) School of Underwater Medicine report 2/72. Sydney: RAN School of Underwater Medicine; 1972.
3. Williamson A, Edmonds C, Clarke B. The neurobehavioural effects of professional abalone diving. *British Journal of Industrial Medicine* 1987;**44**:459–466.
4. McCallum RI. A study of the mortality of professional divers. In: Long Term Health Effects of Diving. International Consensus Conference, Bergen, Norway. 1994.
5. Buzzacott P, Denoble P. The epidemiology of murder and suicide involving scuba diving. *International Maritime Health* 2012;**63**(4):207–212.
6. Beaumont PJB. *Textbook of Psychiatry.* Melbourne: Blackwell Scientific; 1989.
7. Biersner RJ, Ryman DH. Psychiatric incidence among military divers. *Military Medicine* 1974;**139**:633–635.
8. Hoiberg A, Blood C. Age-specific morbidity and mortality rates among US Navy enlisted divers and controls. *Undersea Biomedical Research* 1985;**12**:191–203.
9. Campbell ES. *Psychological Issues in Diving.* (Including DAN's *Alert Diver*, Sept–Dec, 2000). 2010. http://www.scuba-doc.com/PsychIssues.pdf
10. Bachrach AJ, Egstrom GH. *Stress and Performance in Diving.* Flagstaff, Arizona: Best Publishing; 1987.
11. Gorman D, Beran R, Edmonds C, *et al.* The neurological sequelae of DCS. In: *Ninth International Symposium on Underwater and Hyperbaric Physiology.* Bethesda, Maryland: Undersea and Hyperbaric Medical Society; 1987.
12. Bell D. *Medico-Legal Assessment of Head Injury.* Springfield, Illinois: Charles C Thomas; 1992.
13. Sutherland A, Veale A, Gorman D. Neuropsychological problems in recreational divers one year after treatment for DCS. *South Pacific Underwater Medicine Society Journal* 1993;**23**(1):7–11.
14. Becker B. Neuropsychological sequelae of a deep saturation dive. In: *Eighth International Symposium on Underwater Physiology.* Bethesda, Maryland: Undersea and Hyperbaric Medical Society; 1984.

15. Curley MD, Schwartz HJC, Zwingelberg KM. Neuropsychological assessment of cerebral DCS and gas embolism. *Undersea Biomedical Research* 1988;**15**(3):223–236.

16. Rozsahegyi I. Late consequences of the neurological forms of DCS. *British Journal of Industrial Medicine* 1959;**16**:311–317.

17. Kelly PJ, Peters BH. The neurological manifestations of decompression accidents. In: Hong SK, ed. *International Symposium on Man in the Sea*. Bethesda, Maryland: Undersea Medical Society; 1975:227–232.

18. Levin HS. Neuropsychological sequelae of diving accidents. In: Hong SK, ed. *International Symposium on Man in the Sea*. Bethesda, Maryland: Undersea Medical Society; 1975:233–241.

19. Peters BH, Levin HS, Kelly PJ. Neurologic and psychologic manifestations of decompression illness in divers. *Neurology* 1975;**27**:125–127.

20. Vaernes RJ, Eidsvik S. Central nervous dysfunction after near miss accidents in diving. *Aviation, Space, and Environmental Medicine* 1982;**53**(8):803–807.

21. Erde A, Edmonds C. DCS: a clinical series. *Journal of Occupational Medicine* 1975;**17**:324–328.

22. How J, West D, Edmonds C. DCS in diving. *Singapore Medical Journal* 1976;**17**(2):92–97.

23. Melamed Y, Ohry A. The treatment and the neurological aspects of diving accidents in Israel. *Paraplegia* 1987;**18**:127–132.

24. Morris PE, Leach J, King J, Rawlings JSPR. *Psychological and Neurological Impairment in Professional Divers*. P2050 final report. London: Department of Energy; 1991.

25. Edmonds C, Hayward L. Intellectual impairment with diving: a review. In: *Ninth International Symposium on Underwater and Hyperbaric Physiology*. Bethesda, Maryland: Undersea and Hyperbaric Medical Society; 1987.

26. Moon RE, Camporesi EM, Erwin CW. Use of evoked potentials during acute dysbaric illness. In Elliott DH, Halsey MJ, eds. *Diagnostic Techniques in Diving Neurology*. Workshop of the Long-term Health Effects Working Group of the MRC DCS Panel. London: Medical Research Council; 1987:63–69.

27. Overlock R, Dutka A, Farm F, Okamoto G, Susuki D. Somatosensory evoked potentials measured in divers with a history of spinal cord DCS. *Undersea Biomedical Research* 1989;**16**(Suppl):89.

28. Sedgwick M. Somatosensory evoked potentials in a case of DCS. In: Elliott DH, Halsey MJ, eds. *Diagnostic Techniques in Diving Neurology*. Workshop of Long-term Health Effects Working Group of the MRC DCS Panel. London: Medical Research Council; 1987:74–76.

29. Shields TG, Cattanach S, Duff PM, *et al*. Investigations into possible contributing factors to DCS in commercial air diving and the potential long term neurological consequences. Offshore technology report STO 96953. London: UK Health and Safety Executive; 1996.

30. Hodgson M. Neurological investigative techniques in decompression illness. *South Pacific Underwater Medicine Society Journal* 1993;**23**(1):3–7.

31. Medical Research Council DCS panel report: Long Term Health Effects Working Group. In: Halsey MJ, ed. *Second International Symposium on Man in the Sea*. Honolulu: University of Hawaii; 1988.

32. *Symposium Proceedings. The Long-Term Neurological Consequences of Deep Diving*. In: DH Elliott, ed. EUBS and NPD Workshop. Stavanger, Norway; 1983.

33. Hope A, Lund T, Elliott DH, et al., eds. *International Consensus Conference: Long Term Health Effects of Diving*. Godoysund, Norway: Norwegian Underwater Technology Centre; 1994.

34. Todnem K, Nyland H, Dick APK, Lind O, Svihus R, Molvaer OI, Aarli JA. Immediate neurological effects of diving to a depth of 360 metres. *Acta Neurologica Scandinavica* 1989;**80**:333–340.

35. *Australian Fisheries*. Canberra: Australian Government Publishing Service; 1976.

36. Ingvar DH, Adolfson J, Lindemark CO. Cerebral air embolism during training of submarine personnel in free escape: an electroencephalographic study. *Aerospace Medicine* 1973;**44**:628–653.

37. Kwaitowski SR. Analysis of the E.E.G. records among divers. *Bulletin of the Institute of Maritime and Tropical Medicine in Gydnia* 1979;**30**(2):131–135.

38. Hallenbeck JM, Anderson JC. Pathogenesis of the decompression disorders. In: Bennett PB, Elliott DH, eds. *The Physiology and Medicine of Diving*. 3rd ed. London: Ballière Tindall; 1982:435–460.

39. Hills BA, James PB. Microbubble damage to the blood-brain barrier; relevance to DCS. *Undersea Biomedical Research* 1991;**18**:111–116.

40. Cross M. Diving accident management. In: Bennett PB, Moon R, eds. *41st UHMS Workshop*. Durham, North Carolina: Undersea and Hyperbaric Medical Society; 1990:343.

41. Hallenbeck JM. Central nervous system. In: *Workshop on Long-term Health Hazards of Diving*. Luxembourrg: Commission of European Communities; 1978:2–8.

42. Curley MD. U.S. Navy saturation diving and diver neuropsychologic status. *Undersea Biomedical Research* 1988;**15**(1):39–50.

43. Edmonds C, Boughton J. Intellectual deterioration in excessive diving (punch drunk divers). *Undersea Biomedical Research* 1985;**12**(3):321–326.

44. Edmonds C, ed. *The Abalone Diver*. Morwell, Australia: National Safety Council of Australia; 1986.

45. Edmonds C, Coulton T. Multiple aptitude assessments on abalone divers. In: Edmonds, C, ed. *The Abalone Diver*. Morwell, Australia: National Safety Council of Australia; 1986.

46. Williamson A, Clarke B, Edmonds C. The influence of diving variables on perceptual and cognitive functions in professional shallow-water divers. *Environmental Research* 1989;**50**:93–102.

47. Andrews G, Holt P, Edmonds C, *et al.* Does non-clinical decompression stress lead to brain damage in abalone divers? *Medical Journal of Australia* 1986;**144**:399–401.

48. Hjorth R, Vignaendra V, Edmonds C. Electroencephalographic and evoked cortical potential assessments in divers. In: Edmonds C, ed. *The Abalone Diver*. Morwell, Australia: National Safety Council of Australia; 1986.

49. Bast-Pettersen R. Long term neuropsychological effects in non-saturation construction divers. *Aviation, Space, and Environmental Medicine* 1999;**70**(1):51–57.

50. Evans SA, Shields TG. *A Critical Review of the Literature on the Long Term Neurological Consequences of Diving*. RGIT Hyperbaric Research Unit Surrey, England: RGIT Hyperbaric Research Unit; 1992.

51. Elliott DH, Moon RE. Long-term health effects of diving. In: PB Bennett, DH Elliott, eds. *The Physiology and Medicine of Diving*. Philadelphia: Saunders; 1993:585–604.

52. Sipinen SA, Ahovuo J, Halonen JP. Electroencephalographic and magnetic resonance imaging after diving and decompression incidents: a control study. *Undersea and Hyperbaric Medicine* 1999;**26**(2):61–65.

53. Hutzelmann A, Tetzlaff K, Reuter M, *et al.* MR control study of divers' central nervous system. *Acta Radiologica* 2000;**41**(1):18–21.

54. Dutka AJ. Long term effects on the central nervous system. In: Brubakk AO, Neuman TS, eds. *The Physiology and Medicine of Diving*. 5th ed. London: Saunders; 2003.

55. Slosman DO, de Ribaupierre S, Chicherio C, *et al.* Negative neurofunctional effects of frequency, depth and environment in recreational scuba diving: the Geneva 'memory dive' study. *British Journal of Sports Medicine* 2004;**38**:108–114.

56. Macdiarmid JI, Ross JAS, Taylor CL, *et al. Examination of the Long Term Health Impact of Diving: The ELTHI Diving Study*. Prepared by University of Aberdeen for the Health and Safety Executive. Research

report 230. 2004. http://www.hse.gov.uk/research/rrpdf/rr230.pdf

57. Kowalski JT, Varn A, Röttger S, *et al.* Neuropsychological deficits in scuba divers: an exploratory investigation. *Undersea and Hyperbaric Medicine* 2011;**38**:197–204.

58. McGuire S, Sherman P, Profenna L, *et al.* White matter hyperintensities on MRI in high-altitude U-2 pilots. *Neurology* 2013;**81**(8):729–735.

59. McGuire SA, Sherman PM, M.D. Brown AC, *et al.* Hyperintense white matter lesions in 50 high-altitude pilots with neurologic decompression sickness. *Aviat Space Environ Med.* 2012 Dec;**83**(12):1117–1122.

This chapter was reviewed for this fifth edition by Carl Edmonds.

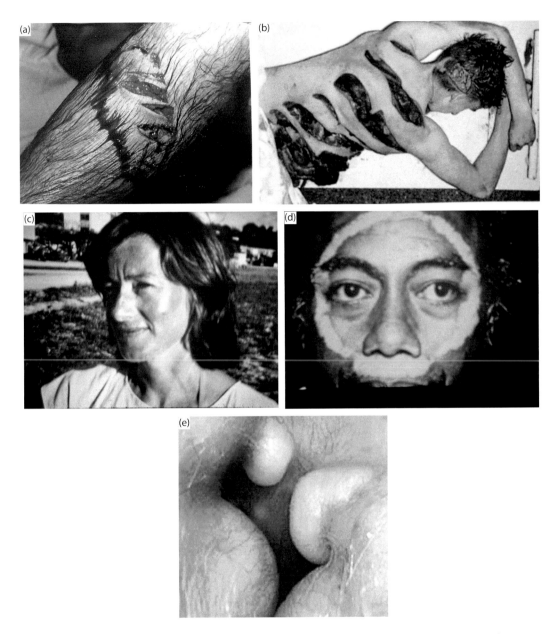

Plate 5, front. Miscellaneous disorders. **(a)** Shark bite. Triangular teeth markings. (Courtesy of Dr C. Barnes.) **(b)** Propeller injuries causing parallel lacerations and injuries in different sites. (Courtesy Dr W. Brighton, from Plueckhahn VD, Cordner SM. *Ethics, Legal Medicine and Forensic Medicine*, 2nd ed. Singapore: Kyodo Printing Co.; 1991.) **(c)** Mask burn – typical. Inflammation around the mask/skin contact. Mild and lasts only a few hours. The conjunctivae are unaffected (compare with mask barotrauma in Plate 2 (b)). (Courtesy of R. Lowry.) **(d)** Mask burn – severe. Using a full-face mask, this South Pacific Islander experienced severe and repeated reactions to the mask that caused blistering, depigmentation and severe scarring, excised by surgery. (Courtesy of Dr C. W. Williams.) **(e)** Exostoses in the external ear.

42

Miscellaneous disorders

This chapter includes many less known or less appreciated disorders or that have not been well defined elsewhere in this text.

CAROTID SINUS SYNDROME

Pressure may be exerted over the carotid sinus by tight-fitting wetsuits, especially when they are of the 'pullover' variety without zippers. Most divers are aware of the unpleasant sensation while wearing these suits and will cut the neckline to release the pressure before other symptoms supervene. Some divers manually hold the collar open to relieve this pressure. Drysuits and some helmets also are incriminated in this disorder.

Some divers may experience a sensation of fainting and have the bradycardia and hypotension that result from pressure on the carotid sinus. This condition may contribute to episodes of falling, convulsions or even the 'sudden death syndrome'.

In all these cases it is necessary to reduce the pressure around the neck. There may be a predisposition resulting from hypersensitivity of the carotid sinus or even disease in the form of carotid plaques.

CAUSTIC COCKTAIL

This disorder occurs when rebreathing equipment is used, such as by technical divers. It is variously termed alkaline cocktail, 'proto cocktail' when Protosorb is the carbon dioxide absorbent used, and 'soda cocktail' when Sodasorb is used.

Exogenous or endogenous water, when mixed with alkaline carbon dioxide absorbent (usually sodium or lithium hydroxide), produces an alkaline solution that may not remain in the absorbent canister. If it travels into the breathing tubing, it may be taken into the mouth and inhaled or swallowed. Severe inflammation, possibly with mucosal ulceration, can result. The extent of these injuries is related to the amount, concentration and distribution of the 'cocktail'.

Traditionally, treatment involves rinsing of the mouth with vinegar or another acidic mixture to neutralize the alkaline cocktail. This therapy may itself be very painful because of the mucosal damage and hypersensitivity and so is detrimental. Rapid irrigation of the area with fresh water or sea water expedites the removal of the irritant material and reduces the symptoms and subsequent damage. Respiratory and gastric involvement is treated according to general medical principles.

COLD URTICARIA

This condition is a predominately localized immunoglobulin E (IgE)–dependent urticarial response to cold – whether it be cold water, ice, wind or volatile fluids. Cold urticaria is usually noticed on the exposed skin, but it may also affect mucosa of the respiratory system (by breathing cold air) or in the mouth and gastrointestinal tract (by swallowing cold drinks). The symptoms may thus vary from skin rash, punctate erythema or urticaria to nasal congestion, swelling of the lips and mouth, cough and dyspnoea, dysphagia and abdominal cramps.

It can often be replicated by placing the hand and forearm in iced water for 5 minutes and observing the development of the skin manifestations over the next 5 to 10 minutes. Occasionally, it can be reproduced by an ice cube.

Generalized symptoms and signs may develop in response to the histamine release and produce headache, flushing, hypotension, syncope and increased gastric secretion. In a highly sensitized patient, swimming in cold water may thus precipitate cardiovascular collapse and death.

Investigations may reveal cold-precipitated plasma proteins, such as cryoglobulin, cold haemolysins and agglutinin, cryofibrinogen and others. There may be elevated IgE and possibly eosinophilia.

The stimulus to tissue damage and mast cell histamine release is the rate of decrease of temperature, more than the exposed temperature. The symptoms tend to develop after the return toward normal temperatures, after the cold-induced vasoconstriction is corrected. The syndrome may develop spontaneously or after some illness of injury (one case followed a jellyfish sting). *Aquagenic urticaria* may be related and has occurred in the same patient, but this may be seen with water of various temperatures (but perhaps carrying allergens).

The response to systematic antihistamines and topical steroids is usually poor (although oral cyproheptadine has received some support). Adrenaline (epinephrine, Epi-Pen) may be needed in severe cases with respiratory or systemic symptoms. Desensitization by gradually increasing the severity of the stimulus from warm, acceptable showers to cold water swimming (under competent supervision) has worked in some cases. The disease tends to clear over some months or years, but it may recur. It is sometimes familial.

DENTAL DISORDERS

Barotrauma (see Chapters 8 and 9) affecting the teeth or sinuses may cause pain referred to the teeth. Subcutaneous and submucosal emphysema may result from barotraumatic pressure gradients permitting gas access to tissues after dental procedures.

Dental electrolysis may be experienced by divers who engage in electric welding. They notice a metallic taste in the mouth adjacent to amalgam fillings. The electrical field set up by the equipment causes the metal in the filling to be released, thus producing both the metallic taste and premature destruction of the fillings.

Dental plates must be secure and not easily displaced during buddy breathing, vomiting, resuscitation or other situations. A candidate who exhales a dental plate while performing lung function tests is just as likely to inhale it while diving. Deaths have been caused by a displaced dental plate.

HYPERTHERMIA

The sea is commonly a heat-extracting environment because of its high conductivity and specific heat and its low temperature (see Chapters 19 and 27). Despite this, hyperthermia has claimed the lives of some divers. It may develop in many ways.

Thermal protection suits, which effectively insulate the diver from low water temperatures, also help to retain the diver's own heat output. Both wetsuits and drysuits, worn before or after immersion, may produce hyperthermia and heat stroke in temperature climates. When these divers also wear their suits at tropical diving resorts, or perform exercise, the danger is increased. The suit may still be worn for mechanical protection, without the diver's realizing its thermal disadvantages. Armoured diving suits, such as the 1-ATA JIM suit, may predispose to hyperthermia because of inadequate ventilation.

Actively produced hyperthermia may result from wearing hot water or other actively heated suits, or by breathing heated gases of high thermal conductivity, such as helium. In deep diving operations, this gas may need to be heated to reduce respiratory heat loss, but the operating range is small, and it is easy to overstep the margins. A further complication is the heat produced by compression of the chamber gas to simulate descent.

Divers with hyperthermia may lose consciousness from postural hypotension when, in their vasodilated state, they are exposed to the effect of gravity – as they emerge from the water onto the dive boat or into the diving bell.

Hyperthermia is a recognized complication of the treatment of hypothermia, by hot water immersion or by active core rewarming.

Hyperthermia is prevented by avoiding the foregoing circumstances. Treatment includes removal of the cause, applying cooling techniques, rehydration and electrolyte replacement.

MUSCULOSKELETAL PROBLEMS

The musculoskeletal problems of **bone cysts** (see Chapter 9), **decompression sickness** (see Chapters 11 and 13), **dysbaric osteonecrosis** (see Chapter 14) and **Irukandji** syndrome (see Chapter 32) are described in other chapters.

Compression (hyperbaric) arthralgia

With the advent of deep and helium diving, a syndrome involving joint noises and sensations was recorded. The noises were described as cracking, creaking or popping, and the sensations varied from discomfort, to a dry and gritty feeling, to a popping or frank pain precipitated by movement. Often the ache is deep and penetrating. Any joint, large or small, can be affected, and even the lumbar spine and xiphisternum have been involved.

The symptoms can appear as early in compression as 30 metres, but they are more common at depths exceeding 100 metres. They are aggravated by fast compression, but they usually improve as the duration at depth continues. Divers show considerable individual susceptibility. This disorder is more likely to be experienced in compression chambers than in water, when fast movements are limited and little mechanical load is placed on the joints. Occasionally, the symptoms can extend into the decompression phase of the dive, but they never commence there.

The current explanation of this disorder involves gas-induced osmosis interfering with joint lubrication and producing cavitation. As the subject is compressed, a relative imbalance is present between the concentration of inert gas in the blood and that in the synovial fluid, and articular cartilage, thus causing a water shift from the joint to the higher osmolarity blood. As equilibration of inert gas develops with a continuation of this exposure to pressure, the original fluid volumes become re-established.

Cramp

Divers and swimmers seem particularly prone to muscle spasms, resulting in temporary pain and disability that may have disproportionately severe complications underwater. Cramp usually develops in muscles that are exposed to atypical exertion (e.g. in physically unfit divers, the use of new fins.) Although the most common sites are the calf of the leg and the sole of the foot, other muscle masses may be affected. These include the thighs (especially hamstrings), upper limbs, abdomen and others. Contributory factors may include cold, dehydration, hypoxia, electrolyte disturbances, hypocalcaemia and exhaustion. Diagnosis is made by observation and palpation of the tight muscle mass. Any previous damage to the neuromuscular system predisposes to muscle cramp.

The immediate treatment consists of slow, passive extension or stretching of the cramped muscle and then a return to safety. Prevention includes maintenance of an adequate standard of physical fitness, constant diving exercise and practice, the fitting of comfortable equipment and fins, avoidance of dehydration and sweating, good nutrition and adequate thermal protection.

Decompression

The musculoskeletal ('bends') pains of decompression sickness are described in Chapter 11. Such symptoms are thought to be caused by tissue distortion from bubbles, and they are relieved rapidly (within minutes) during hyperbaric exposure and less rapidly (hours) to inhalation of 100 per cent oxygen.

There are many less obvious and less well-defined musculoskeletal or arthralgic symptoms that may follow decompression sickness and are possibly attributable to subsequent tissue damage (e.g. in tendons or muscles). Such symptoms may improve somewhat with non-steroidal anti-inflammatory drugs, such as paracetamol, ibuprofen or piroxicam or cyclo-oxygenase 2 inhibitors.

Bubble formation may lead to early injury within the bones – which may or may not progress to dysbaric osteonecrosis. A technetium bone scan may be of value in excluding early and progressive osteoarthrosis. The symptoms usually diminish and gradually disappear over weeks or months.

Sometimes gas develops in synovial joint cavities after long exposures (affecting slow tissues), thus producing loud crunching sounds for a day or two, precipitated by movement (Figure 42.1).

Lumbosacral lesions

Prolonged underwater swimming in an abnormally hyperextended spinal position – such as is

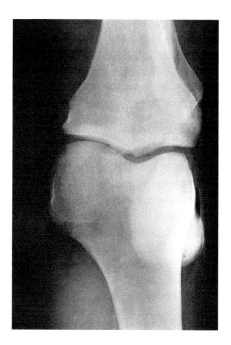

Figure 42.1 Gas in knee joint, from decompression.

employed by shell fishers scanning the sea bed – can aggravate lumbosacral disease. The positioning of the heavy weight belt around the waist may aggravate this condition. Many divers so affected have replaced the weight belt with a much wider weight-containing corset. For cervical spine lesions, see the discussion of headaches in Chapter 40.

Temporo-mandibular joint dysfunction

In the early stages of diving training, a novice may experience apprehension about the air supply. Consequently, the diver is likely to clamp the teeth hard onto the mouthpiece to such a degree that it causes considerable temporo-mandibular joint stress with resultant arthritis. Pain and tenderness are felt just anterior to the ear. Alternative or associated symptoms include trismus, restriction of the ability to open the mouth widely, 'clicking' of the joint and occasionally tinnitus and vertigo. The syndrome is readily relieved by education of the diver and encouraging him or her to relax.

Recurrent problems of temporo-mandibular arthritis and subluxation of this joint are also likely to be aggravated by diving. Apart from the foregoing cause, which is unlikely in experienced divers, there are other stresses placed on the temporomandibular joint that are not normally experienced in non-divers. These include the use of mouthpieces not individually fashioned to the diver's oral and dental configuration, prolonged exposure to a chilling environment and the use of equipment that tends to pull vertically or to one side of the diver's mouth. Most mouthpieces require the diver to hold the mouth open with the mandible protruded, tugging on the mouthpiece – an abnormal position. The symptoms are similar to those described earlier, but in chronic cases, radiological evidence demonstrates the extent of joint damage and dysfunction. The remedy is to avoid the provoking situations (i.e. use well-fitting mouthpieces or an oronasal mask, ensure there is no strain on the demand valve or its hose, and wear a well-fitting hood to avoid cold).

Tank carrier's elbow

In divers, this disorder has been described by Barr and Martin using biomechanical and electromyography studies. It occurs with overuse during dive trips when wrist pronation and dorsiflexion are incurred by lifting tanks by the valve or neck (Figure 42.2). For shorter subjects, this condition is aggravated by the need to flex the elbow to keep the bottom of the tank off the ground. This is a common entity, called 'tennis elbow' in other situations. There is frequently a weakness in grip. Ultrasound may reveal a thickening of the symptomatic common extensor tendon, or even a tear.

The disorder is prevented by ensuring adequate muscular fitness or by carrying tanks horizontally with straps. Treatment is with rest and strapping, but occasionally surgery is needed.

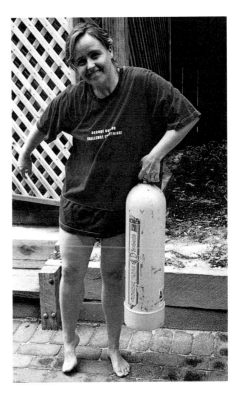

Figure 42.2 Tank carrier's epicondylitis.

CASE REPORT 42.1

A middle-aged man, somewhat unfit, phoned 3 days after a multiple diving exposure and complained of decompression sickness. He had developed pain in the right elbow following the diving, and it had persisted, initially increasing but now constant. There was some weakness in wrist extension.

Pressure with a sphygmomanometer cuff did seem to give relief, when he moved his hand and arm. A Table 6 recompression regimen produced no improvement.

On subsequent examination, there was local tenderness to pressure over the area of the lateral epicondyle. An alternative diagnosis became evident, and it would have been obvious had an adequate history been taken initially.

In fact, he had spent a considerable amount of time during the diving holiday carrying scuba cylinders, and he had developed lateral epicondylitis.

Diagnosis: tank carrier's elbow (tennis elbow).

OCULAR DISORDERS

'Bubble eyes'

Some divers complain of gas bubbling from the inner canthus of the eye. The cause is an excessively patent nasolacrimal duct. This structure frequently has an imperfect valve, formed by the mucous membrane in the nasal cavity. The normal passage of tears from the eye and down the duct is not impeded. Unfortunately, the passage of air up the duct may be expedited when the diver increases nasopharyngeal pressure, such as during the Valsalva manoeuvre. It can be demonstrated by viewing the air bubbling out the lacrimal canal during this manoeuvre. There is a possibility of the spread of organisms from the nasopharynx, with resulting conjunctivitis.

Ocular problems from corneal lenses

When soft contact lenses are used during diving, the corneal microlens is permeable to gas and nutrients. These lenses are therefore safe, except for the likelihood of being lost during such diving techniques as face mask removal, followed by opening the eyes underwater.

Ophthalmologists claim that soft lenses shrink when exposed to fresh water, and they may cling to the cornea and be temporarily difficult to remove. If exposed to sea water, these lenses swell and can float out of the eye. Others have observed that sea water can increase the adherence of soft contact lenses to become stuck to the cornea. Because these lenses are usually enclosed within an air-containing mask, this should not usually cause a problem.

The smaller hard contact lenses are also not very secure in that they cover less of the cornea. Some are less permeable and have the potential of causing problems during decompression. Underneath the hard lenses, small bubbles develop during decompression, in the pre-corneal tear film. They coalesce and expand during decompression and may damage the corneal tissue. Divers may be aware of a sensation of discomfort in the eyes, the appearance of halos with radiating spokes when looking at lights and

also decreased visual acuity. In mild cases, the symptoms last only a few hours.

The symptoms may be prevented by the drilling of a small, 0.4-mm hole in the centre of the hard lens, and this is then termed a fenestrated hard lens. The hole serves as a channel through which the small amounts of tear fluid can pass, carrying the gas with it. These problems are likely to occur especially in deeper or longer dives or during hyperbaric treatments.

The problem of loss of a lens during any diving operation makes these visual aids unacceptable for many professional divers. The increased likelihood of eye infections and the difficulty with eye toilet and lens disinfection procedures, as well as the blurred vision that sometimes accompanies the lens usage, make them a hazard in remote areas and oil rigs.

Fresh water organisms, such as *Acanthamoeba*, which can cause severe infections, corneal ulcerations and blindness, should not be a problem in sea water or inside face masks.

Ocular fundus lesions

The ocular lesions of **infections, barotrauma** and **hyperoxia** are described elsewhere (see Chapters 9, 17 and 29).

Retinal fluorescein angiography demonstrated that the retinal capillary density at the fovea was low, and microaneurysm and small areas of capillary non-perfusion were seen, more often in divers than in non-divers (see Chapters 41 and 44). The prevalence of the fundus abnormality was related to the length of diving history. The changes were consistent with the obstruction of the retinal and choroidal circulations. This obstruction could have been caused either by intravascular bubbles formed during decompression or by altered behaviour of blood constituents and blood vessels in hyperbaric exposures.

These lesions did not appear to have any influence on visual acuity, and there was an increased prevalence of such lesions in divers who had had decompression sickness. Nevertheless, even if one excluded the divers with decompression sickness, this did not abolish the correlation between diving experience and pigment epithelial changes.

The defects in retinal pigment epithelium are indistinguishable from those documented in eyes following choroidal ischaemia.

It is possible, but without specific evidence, that these abnormalities may cause problems in later life. It is also necessary that these observations be verified by other workers.

'Swimmer's eyes' (blurred vision)

Keratitis may cause blurred vision and 'rainbow' or 'halo' effects because of corneal irritation from exposure to suspended particles and hypertonic saline (sea water), chlorine, ammonia and hypotonic water (swimming pools and fresh water). This is less likely with mask-wearing divers than with swimmers, but it is not uncommon when divers use chemical preparations to clean and de-mist the mask's glass face plate.

Underwater welding causes ultraviolet keratopathy. Apart from keratopathy, which is detected on slit-lamp examination, other causes of blurred vision include the following:

- Cerebral involvement with dysbaric disease.
- Displaced contact lens.
- Contact lens problems (see earlier).
- Touching the eye after handling a transdermal patch (scopolamine).
- Delayed delivery pilocarpine preparations, used in glaucoma.
- Oedema and haemorrhages from face mask barotrauma.
- Gas toxicities.

Trauma

Damage to the eyes can result from face mask implosion, from inadequately strengthened glass – during descent or contact with a released anchor as the diver swims down the chain. Dramatic injuries have been caused by spear guns (see later).

It has been demonstrated that divers with radial keratotomy (usually performed for surgical treatment of myopia) may have a weakened cornea and be more susceptible to trauma – with rupture along the lines of the incision. Barotrauma effects in the face mask with descent that cause rupture of

the eyeball are a possibility. For this reason, such patients are usually advised not to dive with the usual (half-face) masks. Alternatives may include gas-filled contact lenses (not easily available), face masks with openings to the water and full-face masks connected to the air supply.

Other disorders

These disorders include **oxygen toxicity** (see Chapter 17), **decompression sickness** (see Chapter 11), **mask barotrauma** (see Chapter 9) and **mask burn** (see later). See Chapters 53 and 54 for discussions of ocular aspects of medical selection for diving.

PULMONARY OEDEMA AND DYSPNOEA

Diving diseases

Pulmonary oedema has been described in a variety of diving diseases. In some cases, it is a consequence of the other diving respiratory disease, such as in the following:

- Drowning syndromes, including salt water aspiration (Chapters 21 to 25).
- Pulmonary barotrauma (see Chapter 6).
- Scuba divers' (immersion) pulmonary oedema (see Chapter 30).
- Decompression sickness (see Chapters 10 to 13).
- Underwater blast (see Chapter 34).
- Some gas contaminants (see Chapter 19).
- Pulmonary oxygen toxicity (see Chapter 17).

These disorders are discussed in their specific chapters.

Asthma provocation

The scuba situation is likely to induce asthma in those so predisposed (see Chapter 55). There are multiple provoking factors, including the following:

- Exercise, especially if swimming against a significant tidal current.

- Breathing against a resistance (the demand valve).
- Breathing cold dry air (decompressed air).
- Breathing dense air (related to depth).
- Salt water spray inhalation provocation.
- Psychological stress and hyperventilation.

Cold urticaria

This disorder is discussed in an earlier section of this chapter.

Deep diving dyspnoea

Cold gas inhalation at depth makes all divers susceptible to dyspnoea at great depths as a result of convective heat loss in the airways and the local response to this loss. It may also precipitate broncho-constriction (see Chapter 55).

Other non-diving disorders may manifest as dyspnoea while diving because of the exceptional physical demands of this activity. Examples include lung disease and drug effects from beta blockers or irritants (e.g. cannabis).

SKIN REACTIONS TO EQUIPMENT

A plethora of dermatological disorders may be found in diving medicine. Some of these (e.g. **decompression sickness, barotrauma**) are discussed in other chapters. There are however, a small group of skin reactions to materials used in the equipment. Other reactions may be related to the direct effect of the equipment, without any specific diving medical illness. A few such disorders are described here, but many others are possible.

Contact dermatitis (mask, mouthpiece and fin burn)

Rubber products may have incorporated in their manufacture an antioxidant or accelerator (e.g. mercaptobenzothiazole and others). This substance acts as an irritant and, because of the minor insult to the skin, may sensitize the diver to further contact. The diver may then observe an irritation with inflammation around the contact area. A similar disorder was seen among surgeons who wore rubber gloves. The three manifestations in diving are mask burn, mouthpiece burn and fin or flipper burn.

MASK BURN

This condition varies from a red imprint of the mask skirt to a more generalized inflammation with vesicles, exudate, crusting and other lesions. It may take weeks before the mask can be worn again, and the disorder will recur if a similar type of mask is used. To overcome this problem, silicone masks are now common (Plate 5).

The treatment is either by soothing lotion, such as calamine, or a steroid preparation, applied regularly until relief is obtained.

MOUTHPIECE BURN

This condition may manifest as a burning sensation on the lips, especially associated with hot drinks, fruit juices or spicy material. There may be inflammation and vesiculation of the lips, tongue and pharynx.

A silicone product similar to that described earlier can replace the rubber mouthpiece. For treatment, hydrocortisone Linguet tablets may be effective.

FIN OR FLIPPER BURN

This condition is a reaction very similar to mask burn and mouthpiece burn, but may be mistaken for more common infections of the feet and has been mistreated as a fungal disease. The disease continues while the fins or flippers are being used. Wearing protective non-rubber footwear under the fins prevents recurrence. The treatment is as described earlier for mask burn.

Angioneurotic oedema (dermatographia)

The effect of localized pressure on one part of the skin that produce a histamine response has been well recorded in other texts and occurs in up to 5 per cent of the population. This condition is occasionally seen among divers when the ridges or seams of the wetsuit push onto the skin. Under these conditions, there are often stripes on the skin, with either erythema or oedema along these lines. The condition can be reproduced by firm local pressure.

The disorder can be confused with an allergic response to the resins and adhesives used in joining the seams of the suit.

It can be prevented either by wearing wetsuits that do not have such internal seams or, alternatively, by using undergarments that protect the skin from the localized pressure of the seams.

Allergic reactions

Unlike the foregoing complaints, there are rare cases of allergy to the wetsuit material, the dyes used in it or the adhesives used in its manufacture. Where this is the case, there is a rash over the contact area.

Burns

Heating systems, so valuable in the cold ocean environment, can sometimes cause problems. Apart from the overheating of some diving suits, thus causing hyperthermia, there are also reports of significant local exothermic reactions causing burns to the skin. Air-activated thermal heating pads can be applied to the hands and torso when diving in cold waters and using drysuits. When the drysuit is inflated with high-oxygen gas, which it often is, the thermal reaction is excessive and can cause severe burns and an emergency situation. The undersuit clothing can even be ignited under these conditions of high oxygen and high pressure causing high temperature. These heating pads should be avoided if oxygen-enriched air is able to be brought into contact with them.

Diaper Rash (nappy rash)

The micturition that follows immersion, exposure to cold and emotional stress may be performed during a normal dive. The urine usually has little effect because it is diluted with water and gradually washed away with the pumping action of the diver's movements of the wetsuit. Unfortunately, if there is excess ammonia present, the diver may react with the equivalent of a nappy rash of children. Sometimes, divers are unaware of the aetiology, and there is some embarrassment when this diagnosis is imparted to them.

With drysuits, sometimes diapers are used for long-duration dives, thereby producing a similar result.

Fin ulcers

Erosion of the hard edge of the fin, on the dorsum of the foot, may initiate an ulcer. It is likely with new or ill-fitting fins and may be prevented by wearing booties as protection. Secondary infection by both marine and terrestrial organisms is common and is aided by softening and maceration of the skin as a result of immersion.

The inflammation, which develops within a few hours of the trauma, may then prevent the subsequent use of fins and endanger the diving operation. A prolonged period out of the water, and the administration of local antibiotics, may be required. The prompt use of these drugs (e.g. neomycin) within an hour or two of the injury and the subsequent wearing of booties with fins may relieve this situation. Chronic ulcers are mainly a problem in the tropics.

TRAUMA

Because divers use motorized **boats** as tenders, and because they use the same environment as other marine vehicles, there is always a risk of boating injuries (e.g. lacerations from propellers). This risk is enhanced by the problem the diver has in locating boats by either vision or hearing. Although the boats are readily heard underwater, the sound waves are more rapid, thus making directional assessment by binaural discrimination very difficult. Usually, by the time the diver sees a boat approaching, it is too late to take evasive action. All diving tenders should have guards over the propellers to reduce the hazard, and divers should employ floats with diving flags if they dive in boating waterways.

The lacerations inflicted by propellers tend to be parallel and linear along one aspect of the body or limb – unlike the concentric crescents on opposite sides, as seen in shark attack. The treatment is along the same general lines as for shark attack.

Head injury from ascending under the boat and hitting the hull is not uncommon (thus the advised technique of holding the hand above the head during ascent), and head injury may also occur as the diver swims alongside the hull (explaining the reason that the diver holds an arm between the head and the boat).

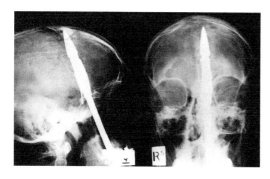

Figure 42.3 Spear in brain. Client survived!

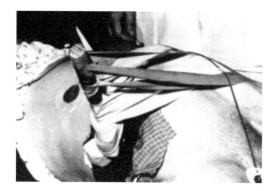

Figure 42.4 Spear in chest, with shaft cut to prevent painful leverage during respiration.

Other causes of trauma are numerous. **Weights** and **scuba cylinders** take their toll of broken toes and metatarsals, as well as subungual haematoma.

Spear guns account for as much morbidity and death as sharks, where spear fishing is allowed (Figures 42.3 and 42.4). Power heads, carbon dioxide darts and other underwater weapons cause a variety of injuries.

Dam outlets and underwater siphons can trap a diver and then plug the outlet with the diver's body – which is then exposed to the full pressure gradient from the weight of water above him or her. This causes massive and grotesque injuries and death.

Other forms of environmental trauma are described in Chapter 5.

FURTHER READING

Anderson GP. Skin burns as a result of using commercial hand warmers in a dry suit using nitrox as a breathing gas [abstract]. In: *Proceedings of the 2005 Scientific Meeting of the Undersea and Hyperbaric Medical Society.* 2005. http://archive.rubicon-foundation.org/1655

Barr LL, Bount D. Martin LR. Tank carriers' lateral epicondylitis: a biomedical rational for injury and prevention. *South Pacific Underwater Medicine Society Journal* 1991;**21**(1):37–41.

Barr LL, Martin LR. Tank carriers' lateral epicondylitis: case reports and a new cause for an older entity. *South Pacific Underwater Medicine Society Journal* 1991;**21**(1):35–37.

Butler FK. Diving hyperbaric ophthalmology. *Survey of Ophthalmology* 1995;**39**:347–365.

Curran JN, McGuigan KG, O'Broin. A case of deep burns while diving the *Lusitania*. *Journal of Plastic, Reconstructive, and Aesthetic Surgery* 2010;**63**:579–581.

Elliott D, Moon RE. Long-term health effects of diving. In PB Bennett, DH Elliott, eds. *The Physiology and Medicine of Diving.* Philadelphia: Saunders; 1993, 585–604.

Fauci AS, Kasper DL, Martin JB, *et al.*, eds. *Harrison's Textbook of Medicine.* 14th ed. New York: McGraw-Hill; 1999.

Fisher AA. *Atlas of Aquatic Dermatology.* New York: Grune & Stratton; 1978.

Hope A, Lund T, Elliott DH, *et al.*, eds. *International Consensus Conference: Long Term Health Effects of Diving.* Godoysund, Norway: Norwegian Underwater Technology Centre; 1994.

Lobbezoo F, van Wijk AJ, Klingler MC, Ruiz Vicente E, van Dijk CJ, Eijkman MA: Predictors for the development of temporomandibular disorders in scuba divers. *J Oral Rehabil*; 2014 Aug;41(8):573–80.

Luong KV, Nguyen LT. Aquagenic urticaria. *Annals of Allergy, Asthma, and Immunology* 1998;**80**(6):483–485.

US Navy Diving Manual Revision 6 SS521-AGPRO-010 (2008). Washington, DC: Naval Sea Systems Command; 2008.

This chapter was reviewed for this fifth edition by Carl Edmonds.

43

Drugs and diving

INTRODUCTION

The *Oxford English Dictionary* defines a drug as 'a medicine or other substance which has a physiological effect when ingested or otherwise introduced into the body'. In this sense, oxygen, carbon dioxide, nitrogen and other inert gases under increased partial pressures may be considered drugs and are important in considering interactions with agents more conventionally regarded as drugs. Therapeutic drugs are given to produce specific responses in the body, but all drugs may also cause **side effects** (any effect of a drug that is in addition to its intended effect, especially an effect that is harmful or unpleasant) and **adverse effects** (side effects plus the consequences of dosing and administration errors).

Many divers do take drugs either routinely or intermittently, both for therapeutic and recreational purposes. A 2002 survey of 709 mostly experienced or professional divers suggested that nearly 25 per cent took at least one therapeutic drug, including pseudo-ephedrine and nasal decongestants to prevent barotrauma, antihistamines to prevent seasickness, antihypertensive agents (8.9 per cent), and asthma drugs (2.8 per cent)[1]. To date, there is limited information on the effects of most drugs under diving conditions.

In the diving context, drugs should be considered in terms of their principal therapeutic effects, their possible side effects in the underwater environment and their interaction with hyperbaria. The most important areas of concern in diving are effects on the central nervous system, autonomic nervous system and cardiovascular and respiratory systems. Many studies have concentrated on the neurobehavioural effects of drugs under pressure, but other effects such as enhancement of cardiac arrhythmias or aggravation of oxygen toxicity may be equally important.

Other aquatic environmental influences, such as cold, sensory deprivation, spatial disorientation, reduced vision, reduced sound localization, vertigo and weightlessness, may also profoundly alter the behavioural effects of certain drugs.

Another largely unresearched area is the effect that drugs may have on the uptake and elimination of inert gas, thereby altering the propensity to decompression sickness (DCS). For example, dehydration has been associated with increases in the incidence and severity of DCS, and diuretics (e.g. alcohol and some antihypertensive agents) may induce dehydration.

Immersion and pressure produce cardiovascular alterations (see Chapter 2), which affect the distribution of cardiac output. Reduced perfusion of gut, liver, and kidney may have an impact on absorption, distribution, metabolism and excretion of drugs.

The significance in diving of certain side effects may not be immediately apparent. For example, the widely used drug aspirin has a profound effect on platelet function and causes increased bleeding tendency. This effect may be crucial in, say, inner ear barotrauma or severe DCS. Aspirin may also cause increased airway resistance in susceptible individuals. It is therefore important that all the effects of a drug be considered.

Some side effects of drugs that may be important in the underwater environment include the following:

- Nervous system: headache, dizziness, acute psychosis, tinnitus, tremor, incoordination, extrapyramidal syndromes, paraesthesiae, peripheral neuropathy (disorientation while immersed; potential confusion with DCS).
- Cardiovascular system: tachycardia, bradycardia, arrhythmias, hypotension (postural), chest pain, oedema (incapacitation; sudden death).
- Blood: anaemia, thrombocytopenia, neutropenia, disturbances of coagulation (susceptibility to infection; bleeding into tissue bubbles).
- Alimentary system: nausea, vomiting, abdominal cramps, heartburn, diarrhoea, altered liver function, liver failure (dehydration; incapacitation; metabolic derangement).
- Renal system: renal failure, electrolyte disturbances, disturbances of micturition (metabolic derangement).

- Musculoskeletal system: myalgia, arthralgia, fatigue (dysfunction; potential confusion with DCS).
- Skin and mucosa: pruritus, rash, angioneurotic oedema, photosensitivity (potential confusion with DCS).
- Eye: glaucoma, photophobia, blurred vision, scintillation (incapacitation; potential confusion with DCS).

There are two possible attitudes to the use of drugs and diving. One advocates that drugs are useful to counteract minor problems (e.g. Eustachian tube dysfunction, seasickness) and that these drugs will make diving easier and safer. The other view is that the diver should not be under the influence of any drugs because of possible side effects. The latter concept would require divers to stop taking some drugs days to weeks before diving. The more conservative physicians would include such drugs as alcohol, nicotine and caffeine in their recommendations. The best approach probably lies in individualizing advice in the clinical and diving context.

As discussed in Chapter 53, a history of drug intake may give important clues to the presence of otherwise undetected organic or psychological disorders.

> As in pregnancy, the safe use of many drugs while diving has not been established.

DRUGS UNDER PRESSURE

Even if the effect of a drug at 1 ATA is well understood, it may be very different at hyperbaric pressures. Physiological influences (e.g. increased hydrostatic pressure, varying pressures of oxygen and nitrogen or other diluent gases) may alter drug **pharmacodynamics** (what a drug does to the body) or **pharmacokinetics** (what the body does to a drug). The functional result of drug-hyperbaria interaction may be negative (pressure reversal of anaesthesia), neutral, additive or synergistic. For example, the addition of some degree of nitrogen narcosis or elevated carbon dioxide may combine with a central nervous system depressant drug (e.g. alcohol, antihistamines or opiates) to produce an unexpectedly severe impairment of mental function or even unconsciousness.

UK Medicines Information[2] produced a good summary of the information sites available about diving while using a wide range of medications, and Rump and associates[3] in 1999 reviewed the effects of hyperbaria and hyperoxia on the disposition of drugs. The relatively few human and animal studies do not show alterations by hyperoxia of the pharmacokinetics of gentamicin, caffeine, lignocaine, pentobarbital or pethidine.

Animal experiments have been carried out on a number of drugs, usually at very great pressures. Such information, albeit valuable in elucidating mechanisms of drug action and pressure interaction, is of limited value in the normal current diving range of pressures. Information in this area comes from a limited number of human and animal studies of the effects of drugs and pressure on behavioural and other physiological functions.

In 1979, Walsh and Burch[4] studied the behavioural effects of some commonly used drugs at air pressures of 1.8, 3.6 and 5.4 ATA. These investigators found that all drugs in the study impaired learning at pressure (i.e. cognitive functioning). Of the drugs, diphenhydramine had the most effect, caffeine and dimenhydrinate (Dramamine) varied widely with individual susceptibility and aspirin and acetaminophen had less effect.

Illustrating the difficulty in interpreting animal experiments, the same authors found that in rats, 5 to 10 times 'normal' doses at pressures of 3, 5 and 7 ATA were required to show performance decrements with diphenhydramine and pseudoephedrine, but with dimenhydrinate no effect was seen.

In animals, amphetamines exacerbate the behavioural effects of hyperbaric air (not ameliorate these effects, as expected). Hyperbaric air and amphetamines combine to produce behavioural changes not seen with either alone. Conversely, hyperbaric nitrogen can decrease the incidence of convulsions initiated by amphetamines.

A clear synergistic relationship between alcohol (2 ml/kg) and pressure (air at 4 and 6 ATA) has been demonstrated in the processing of visual information in humans.

One of the newer non-sedating antihistamines used for allergic rhinitis and nasal decongestion was studied in humans under hyperbaric conditions. Clemastine fumarate was found not to increase the sedative effects of nitrogen narcosis or to increase the development of cardiac arrhythmias[5].

There are isolated anecdotal reports of therapeutic drugs producing unexpected effects on divers at pressure. The effects are usually on judgement, behaviour or level of consciousness and involve paracetamol (32 ATA), dextropropoxyphene (4 ATA), hyoscine (scopolamine), oxymetazoline spray (5 ATA) and phenylbutazone.

Diabetic patients demonstrate reduced insulin requirements while undergoing hyperbaric oxygen therapy, probably because of oxygen effects on insulin sensitivity, but hypoglycaemia may also be problematic while air diving (see Chapter 57).

Some information comes from anecdotal reports of the use of drugs in hyperbaric or saturation diving operations. The finding that drugs have occasionally been used safely in such situations does not mean that they can be regarded as safe for diving.

ANAESTHESIA UNDER PRESSURE

Anaesthesia may be required for operative procedures during decompression and saturation diving operations. Decompression requirements may preclude removing the patient from the chamber.

Nitrogen is an anaesthetic agent, but only at very great pressures (around 12 to 15 ATA), and thus is not a practical option. Other inert gases such as krypton and xenon produce anaesthesia at much lower pressures but have not been used much in practice.

Nitrous oxide (N_2O) requires a partial pressure of greater than 800 mm Hg (1.1 ATA) for surgical anaesthesia[6]. Indeed, in the late nineteenth century, mobile hyperbaric operating rooms were developed in France for the purpose of administering 100 per cent N_2O anaesthesia, and the practice was demonstrated successfully by Paul Bert and others. In retrospect, many of the apparent anaesthetic actions of N_2O at minimal hyperbaric pressures probably resulted as much from hypoxia as from actions of the drug. True N_2O anaesthesia as described by Russell and colleagues[6] in 1990 was associated with signs of increased sympathetic activity (e.g. tachycardia, hypertension and mydriasis). Clonus and opisthotonus developed in some subjects. A stable physiological state was difficult to maintain. The use of N_2O anaesthesia is also complicated by high lipid solubility and tissue uptake, as well as by counterdiffusion problems (see Chapters 2 and 11), thus increasing the risk of subsequent DCS.

Volatile anaesthetics such as halothane and enflurane have been used to about 4 ATA pressure. They reduce the cerebral vaso-constriction of hyperbaric oxygen, an action that may be advantageous for oxygen delivery but may predispose to central nervous system toxicity. The newer volatile agents (e.g. isoflurane and sevoflurane) probably behave similarly but have not been tested. There is little dose-response information at very great pressures, especially regarding organ toxicity if higher doses are required to overcome pressure reversal effects. Pressure reversal of anaesthesia at very great pressure (see Chapter 15) is not of practical significance.

Opiates appear to have similar effects under some saturation diving conditions as at the surface, but respiratory depression would be a possibility in hyperbaric air at depth (because of the additive narcotic effect of nitrogen). The resultant carbon dioxide retention would enhance oxygen toxicity (see Chapter 17).

Neuromuscular blocking drugs are unaltered in effect at low (hyperbaric oxygen therapy) pressures, although they mask an oxygen convulsion.

The use of regional or intravenous anaesthesia is usually preferred to gaseous anaesthesia.

Regional anaesthetic techniques (with care not to introduce gas) have theoretical support, and major procedures may be performed. The minor effects of pressure reversal are not relevant considering the relatively massive doses applied directly to nerves, but effects on toxicity and pharmacokinetics from altered effects on blood flow and tissue binding may be. Conventional doses of lignocaine have been used up to 6 ATA.

Ketamine, in combination with a *benzodiazepine* to prevent psychological phenomena, is a useful anaesthetic in the field because of relative preservation of respiratory reflexes.

> Emergency drugs should not be withheld because of uncertainty about their effects in a hyperbaric environment.

PROPHYLAXIS AND THERAPY OF DIVING DISORDERS

Barotrauma

Divers seek therapy to allow them to enter the water when they may otherwise be unfit. The most common use of drugs is to prevent barotrauma of the middle ear or sinuses. Both topical and systemic vaso-constrictors are employed to shrink nasopharyngeal mucosa to allow pressure equalization through sinus ostia or Eustachian tubes. Taylor and colleagues suggested frequent pseudo-ephedrine use in about 10 per cent of divers and of nasal decongestants in about 3 per cent[1].

Although widespread use of these drugs testifies to their general safety, it is possible these drugs are used inappropriately to overcome incorrect diving techniques, upper respiratory tract infections or allergies. Rebound congestion leading to either barotrauma of ascent or descent (see Chapters 7 and 8) later in the dive with topical vaso-constrictors is also a potential problem.

Pseudo-ephedrine is used alone or as a common component of 'cold and flu' preparations. Side effects may include tachycardia, palpitations, hypertension, anxiety, tremor, vertigo, headache, insomnia, drowsiness and, rarely, hallucinations. Some individuals show a marked intolerance, and there has been a report of one individual suffering severe vertigo and unconsciousness in a dive to 45 metres after having used an excessive amount of oxymetazoline spray before the dive.

Oxygen toxicity and nitrogen narcosis

Drugs have been sought to prevent or reduce the effects of raised partial pressures of these oxygen and nitrogen, but they remain investigational and are of no practical value to the diver (see Chapters 15 and 17). No drug has been shown to overcome nitrogen narcosis in humans.

Diazepam has been used to prevent or treat the convulsions of oxygen toxicity (see Chapter 17). The roles of gamma-aminobutyric acid (GABA) analogues, superoxide dismutase, and magnesium sulphate are under investigation.

High-pressure neurological syndrome

The addition of nitrogen or hydrogen to a helium-oxygen mixture to reduce the onset and severity of this syndrome is an interesting example of the interaction of pressure and a 'drug' (see Chapter 20). Drugs that potentiate transmission at GABA synapses (e.g. the anticonvulsant sodium valproate and flurazepam) protect against high-pressure neurological syndrome in small mammals.

Decompression sickness

PROPHYLAXIS

Researchers have considered the use of drugs to try to prevent or minimize DCS. Drugs that inhibit platelet adhesiveness have been shown to reduce morbidity and mortality from DCS in animals but have not been demonstrated as useful in humans.

Aspirin inhibits platelet aggregation and may prevent aggregation induced by intravascular bubbles. Possible disastrous haemorrhagic effects in, say, the inner ear or barotrauma or spinal DCS have prevented any recommendation for routine use.

More recently, attention has focussed on nitric oxide donors to prevent DCS. In 2006, Dujić[7] showed that nitroglycerine reduced bubble counts in volunteer divers, and statins may have a similar effect[8]. Aerobic exercise before diving is also protective – presumably by the induction of endogenous nitric oxide and the possible elimination of potential nucleation sites for bubbles. Certain other drugs have been suggested because of a possible influence on the blood-bubble interface. Alternatively, drugs may be used to reduce the release of tissue injury mediators from cells.

It has also been postulated that perfluorocarbons (PFCs) may prove useful in absorbing and holding nitrogen that could otherwise come out of solution during decompression. This intriguing prospect has yet to be tested in the field, but it has been successfully reported in animal models.

Finally, drugs, such as isoprenaline (isoproterenol), which enhance cardiac output and cause general vasodilatation, have been shown to shorten time to desaturate slower tissues in rats. Timing the administration of such an agent would be difficult.

None of these drugs is recommended for routine use at the time of writing, but nitric oxide donor agents may be the most promising.

THERAPY

Drugs used as an adjunct to the treatment of DCS are discussed in Chapter 13.

Drugs may be encountered in diving in four ways:

- Prevention of disorders produced by the diving environment.
- Treatment of dysbaric-induced diseases.
- Treatment of concurrent diseases, acute or chronic.
- Drugs taken for 'recreational' or social purposes.

THERAPY OF COINCIDENT ILLNESS

Quite apart from the unknown effect of many therapeutic drugs in the aquatic or hyperbaric environment, it is often the condition for which these drugs are taken that renders diving unwise (see Chapters 52 to 54). For example, the use of a tetracycline antibiotic may be acceptable for chronic acne but not for bronchitis. A thiazide diuretic may be acceptable for mild hypertension but not for congestive cardiac failure. A calcium channel blocker may be tolerable for hypertension but not for paroxysmal supraventricular tachycardia.

Even if the medical condition for which the drugs are taken and the possible interaction with pressure are ignored, many drugs may themselves produce unwarranted risks. This feature is reflected in the denial of flying or driving licences to people who require certain therapeutic drugs. More stringent considerations should apply to the use of drugs in the subaquatic environment.

The mode of administration of drugs is relevant in certain situations. For example, drugs given in depot form may lead to localized scarring and be a nidus for bubble development. Certain implantable infusion pumps, especially those with a rigid casing, are designed to operate under positive internal pressure to deliver the drug and to prevent leakage of body fluids back into the pump. If the external pressure exceeds this, then not only is the drug not delivered, but also body fluids will leak into the pump. On decompression, the increased pressure in the pump may suddenly dispense the contents into the tissues or blood, with potentially disastrous consequences.

Some drugs, or classes of drugs, that may be encountered in the diving population with possible associated risks in diving are discussed here. Some of these drugs are available 'over the counter' (OTC) without a prescription. The diver may be unaware of possible side effects.

Diuretics may cause dehydration, or electrolyte loss, especially in a tropical environmental. This may increase the risk of DCS. Potassium loss may predispose to arrhythmias.

Anti-arrhythmics may themselves, under certain circumstances, provoke arrhythmias. Amiodarone produces photosensitivity and may impair vision. Beta blockers and calcium channel blockers are also used as anti-arrhythmic drugs.

Beta blockers (beta-adrenergic blocking drugs), often prescribed for hypertension, decrease the heart rate response to exercise and reduce exercise tolerance – effects that may be critical in an emergency situation. Bradycardia and other dysrhythmias are possible. These drugs may also cause bronchoconstriction, especially in persons with a history of asthma. Divers may complain of cold hands or even a Raynaud-like syndrome of the fingers on exposure to cold water.

Topical beta blockade for control of glaucoma may be absorbed systemically and cause bronchospasm, bradycardia, arrhythmias or hypotension and decreased stress response. Newer agents such as betaxolol are more specific and have fewer cardiorespiratory effects than, for example, timolol drops. Divers using one of these specific eye drops should have no underlying cardiac disease and no abnormalities on cardiorespiratory assessment.

Peripheral vasodilators including *calcium channel blockers* may produce orthostatic hypotension. This is not a problem underwater but rather at the moment of exit, because of the loss of hydrostatic support. Dizziness or syncope may result.

Angiotensin-converting enzyme (ACE) inhibitors can produce a dry cough and airway mucosal swelling, which may be dangerous or diagnostically confusing in the diving or hyperbaric environment. There are also reports of bronchospasm. These side effects usually appear within the first 2 weeks of treatment. The newer angiotensin II receptor antagonist drugs (e.g. irbesartan and candesartan) are often prescribed to avoid these potential problems, but they may still occur in rare cases. These are probably the preferred agents for the treatment of hypertension in divers.

Psychoactive drugs, including sedatives and tranquillizers, produce varying degrees of drowsiness. Patients who take these drugs are advised to avoid activities such as driving a car or operating machinery where decreased alertness may be dangerous. Diving falls into this category. Potentiation of inert gas narcosis is also possible.

Phenothiazines may produce extrapyramidal syndromes, and some of these drugs used for nausea or motion sickness (e.g. prochlorperazine) may produce oculogyric crises.

Tricyclic antidepressants are known to cause cardiac arrhythmias, and under conditions of increased sympathetic stimulation, this effect may be exacerbated.

Antihistamines are mainly used for their anti-allergy effects (urticaria, hayfever, allergic rhinitis, anticholinergic effects, drying effect with the 'common cold') or as anti-emetics (e.g. motion sickness). The main side effect important in diving is sedation. Newer agents, such as fexofenadine and loratadine, do not appear to cross the blood-brain barrier significantly, so drowsiness is not as much of a problem. These newer drugs are used for allergic rhinitis and not as anti-emetics. Many antihistamines are available OTC.

Anticholinergics, used as antispasmodics for the gastrointestinal and urinary systems, cause dry mouth, blurred vision, photophobia and tachycardia. Decreased sweating may lead to heat stroke in the tropics. Divers may not be aware that anticholinergics such as atropine may be present in OTC anti-diarrhoea preparations.

Antibiotics are probably safe for the diver, while bearing in mind the indication and provided there are no side effects. In the diving context, photosensitivity, especially related to tetracyclines, may be relevant. Many antibiotics also cause nausea and vomiting.

The antiviral drug acyclovir, used not only for human immunodeficiency virus infection but also for oral and genital herpes, may cause headaches, nausea and vomiting.

Antimalarial drugs may be prescribed for divers visiting tropical areas. Divers and their medical advisers should be aware of the side effects of any antimalarials prescribed. Most antimalarial chemoprophylactic regimens must be commenced 1 to 2 weeks before departure to allow time for blood levels to reach a steady state. This also allows adverse reactions to occur, so that medications can be altered before departure. Apart from idiosyncratic adverse reactions, a major concern among the widely prescribed antimalarials relates to *mefloquine* (Lariam). Common side effects include vertigo, visual disturbances, difficulty with coordination and psychosis. Because the drug has a half-life of approximately 3 weeks, these effects can take some time to subside if they occur. Severe neurological symptoms have been reported 2 to 3 weeks after a single dose. This drug has been withdrawn in some countries. Mefloquine can also cause bradycardia, an effect potentiated by concurrent administration of beta blockers. Safer alternatives for divers would include doxycycline, chloroquine and pyrimethamine (Maloprim). Advice should be sought on the appropriate agent to be taken when travelling to specific areas.

With regard to *analgesics,* the problems of aspirin are discussed earlier. Paracetamol is probably safe. *Non-steroidal anti-inflammatory drugs (NSAIDs),* which may be available OTC, may precipitate bronchospasm and commonly cause gastric irritation and heartburn. The newer cyclo-oxygenase-2–specific inhibitors, introduced to avoid the gastric problems, have been associated with serious vascular events (including myocardial infarction) and bronchospasm. Stronger analgesics decrease mental performance and may combine with inert gas narcosis to produce a more marked degree of central nervous system depression, as well as complicating the therapeutic assessment of pressure effects. Nausea is a common side effect.

Insulin and *oral hypoglycaemic agents* may cause severe hypoglycaemia with altered consciousness. The diving environment hinders the early recognition and self-treatment of insulin-induced hypoglycaemia (see Chapters 53, 54 and 57).

Thyroxine may cause tachycardia, arrhythmias, tremor, excitability and headache. Hyperbaric oxygen toxicity is enhanced.

Steroids may produce a wide variety of adverse reactions such as fluid and sodium retention, potassium loss, diabetes, peptic ulceration, avascular necrosis of the femoral or humeral head (see also Chapter 14), thromboembolism and increased susceptibility to hyperbaric oxygen toxicity and infection. Anabolic steroids are widely abused for strength and bodybuilding. Side effects include psychosis, aggressive behaviour and sudden death.

Oral contraceptives, because of their tendency to cause hypercoagulability of the blood, were postulated to cause increased DCS. This is probably not significant with the currently used low-dose agents (see Chapter 60). Some women experience migraine, nausea and increased mucosal congestion.

Bronchodilators are contraindicated because active bronchospasm precludes diving. Many diving physicians now permit diving in patients with well-controlled asthma, and this practice is detailed in an appendix to the South Pacific Underwater Medicine Society diving medical guidelines (see Chapter 55). The need for rescue bronchodilators is a trigger for ceasing diving until control of the condition is regained. Theophylline and derivatives may produce cardiac arrhythmias and also allow bubble transfer through the pulmonary filter. Adrenergic drugs, even beta$_2$-selective drugs, taken orally or more usually as inhaled aerosols, may have a cardiac stimulant effect. Aerosols, while producing marked improvement or prevention of symptoms, may still leave small regional microscopic areas of lung unaffected, leading to localized air trapping.

The anti-neoplastic drug *bleomycin,* used for testicular cancer and reticuloses, renders the patient particularly sensitive to pulmonary oxygen toxicity. Although some investigators have reported series of apparently safe diving after bleomycin, most physicians continue to disqualify such individuals. De Wit and colleagues[9] in 2007 concluded: 'We strongly believe that resuming scuba diving 6–12 months after an uncomplicated series of three or four cycles of BEP is completely acceptable. Caution should only remain for patients who develop clinical signs of pulmonary-function impairment during or shortly after bleomycin treatment. We deem the conservative opinions of many physicians and diving organisations about recreational diving after bleomycin treatment as unnecessary – opinions that we hope to change. Young men affected by testicular cancer should be able to undertake their normal daily life as fully as possibly after treatment with bleomycin'. Nevertheless, any permission to dive in these patients should not be taken lightly.

Histamine H$_2$-receptor blockers, such as cimetidine, ranitidine, famotidine and nizatidine, used for peptic ulceration and reflux oesophagitis, may occasionally produce drowsiness and headache. Nizatidine has a lower incidence of such side effects. The *proton pump inhibitors,* such as omeprazole and pantoprazole, are used for similar indications but do not appear to have caused problems.

Drugs of another widely used class in modern society, the cholesterol-lowering *statins,* do not appear to have any significant side effects, and they have even been suggested to prevent DCS.

RECREATIONAL DRUGS

These drugs, which may be either legal or illegal under various national legislations, are widely consumed (regularly or occasionally) for social or mood-altering qualities. They include tobacco, alcohol, marijuana, sedatives and tranquillizers, hallucinogens, cocaine and opiates (e.g. heroin, morphine, pethidine). These drugs may be taken singly or in combination. A Los Angeles coroner reported that 20 per cent of diving deaths in southern California were associated with the use of drugs.

Tobacco

The acute effects of nicotine include increased blood pressure and heart rate and coronary vaso-constriction. The inhalation of tobacco smoke containing nicotine and tar causes increased bronchospasm, depressed cilial activity and increased mucus production in bronchial mucosa. These effects may lead to intrapulmonary air trapping and increased pulmonary infection. There is therefore an increased possibility of ascent pulmonary barotrauma.

Carboxyhaemoglobin levels in smokers range from 5 to 9 per cent. Significant psychomotor effects from exposure to this level of carbon monoxide have been reported, although this does not seem to be a problem with long-term exposure.

Many studies of smoking and physical fitness show detrimental effects. Increased heart rate and decreased stroke volume are the opposite of the changes with aerobic training. Oxygen debt accumulation after exercise is greater among smokers.

Long-term use may lead to chronic bronchitis and emphysema, with decreased exercise tolerance and eventually marked hypoxaemia. It may also lead to coronary artery disease and peripheral vascular disease. Reduced blood volume and decreased haematocrit develop with long exposure to increased carboxyhaemoglobin.

Nasopharyngeal mucosal congestion may predispose to sinus and middle ear barotrauma.

Alcohol

The acute effects of alcohol are well known, particularly the depressant effects on central nervous system functioning. Alcohol is associated with up to 80 per cent of all drowning episodes in men.

The detrimental effect on intellectual function, judgement and coordination is well known. The addition of hyperbaric air (nitrogen narcosis) has a synergistic action in impairing mental performance.

Studies in pilots have shown significant performance decrements at blood alcohol levels of 0.04 per cent, a permissible level for driving in many countries. Visual tracking performance is reduced at 0.027 per cent. Alcohol also lowers blood glucose, with consequent performance impairment.

Other acute effects of alcohol that are relevant to diving include the following:

- Increased risk of vomiting.
- Peripheral vasodilatation increasing heat loss and thus leading to hypothermia.
- Diuretic effect causing dehydration and increasing the risk of DCS.
- Dose-dependent impairment of left ventricular emptying at rest, probably acting directly on the myocardium.

The long-term overuse of alcohol is associated with damage to the liver, brain and heart, as well as an increased risk of a number of other diseases.

Marijuana

Cannabis intoxication alters perception of the environment and impairs cognitive and psychomotor performance[10]. The 'mind-expanding' experience produces a sensation of heightened awareness even for things that are not physically present. There may be feelings of euphoria, indifference, anxiety or even paranoia. Subjects may experience fears or 'hang-ups' of which they were not previously aware. Nitrogen narcosis can produce similar effects. The notion of combining these effects is 'mind-boggling'.

Impaired judgement and ignoring of routine safety procedures while influenced by cannabis may be major contributory factors in some diving accidents.

Physiological effects include conjunctival injection, tachycardia, increased oxygen consumption and heat loss with decreased shivering threshold. Hypothermia may thus develop insidiously.

Acute toxic psychosis can develop with 'flash-backs', depersonalization and derealization. A high proportion of users occasionally will experience 'bad trips'.

Regular cannabis use is associated with suppression of the immune system and respiratory disease. Heavy smoking can produce respiratory irritation and isolated uvulitis. Heavy use is also associated with schizophrenia and depression.

The adverse effects of cannabis on diving performance are as follows:

- Slowed complex reaction time.
- Space and time distortion.
- Impaired co-ordination.
- Impaired short-term memory.
- Impaired attention, especially for multiple tasks.
- Additive effects with alcohol and other drugs.
- Impaired temperature control.

Caffeine

Caffeine is present in coffee and a variety of cola drinks. Moderate coffee drinking has not been associated with an increased risk of coronary heart disease and is probably safe in most healthy persons. However, consumption does produce a small increase in blood pressure and may induce cardiac arrhythmias or even lethal ventricular ectopic activity in certain susceptible individuals.

Caffeine withdrawal symptoms include headache and fatigue. Less often anxiety, nausea, vomiting and impaired psychomotor performance are seen.

Amphetamine

Methamphetamine, even in lower dose ranges, has been associated with erratic driving, risk taking and increased misadventure rate. Higher doses cause tachycardia, dilated pupils, paranoia and aggressive behaviour. Withdrawal is characterized by fatigue, somnolence and depression. As in driving, methamphetamine ingestion is inconsistent with safe diving.

Sedatives and tranquillizers

These drugs also impair judgement and performance. Interaction with the diving environment produced the following extraordinary case (Case Report 43.1).

Cocaine

The most marked pharmacological effects of this useful topical local anaesthetic and vaso-constrictor

---

CASE REPORT 43.1

DS, a 20-year-old man, dived to a depth of between 45 and 50 metres with companions, all of whom were deliberately under the influence of large oral doses of barbiturates, which were taken while on the way out to the dive site by boat. After an undetermined period under water, the patient lost consciousness at depth and was taken rapidly to the surface by his companion. On returning to shore, he was driven to his companions' apartment, where he remained unconscious, presumably sleeping off the drugs. On regaining semi-consciousness 48 hours later, he found that both legs were partially paralyzed and that he had paraesthesiae below the knees and in the palm of his left hand. He was dizzy and ataxic. He presented to hospital 60 hours after diving. A diagnosis of spinal decompression sickness was made, with possible cerebral involvement from air embolism, although no firm evidence of pulmonary barotrauma was found.

Immediate management was by intravenous infusion of fluids and high doses of steroids* with hyperbaric oxygen (US Navy Table 6). He improved rapidly with recompression (Courtesy of Dr I. P. Unsworth).

  * Note this is no longer recommended.

---

drug are intense sympathetic stimulation, both centrally and peripherally, and euphoria.

Symptoms, which are dose related and rapid in onset, include changes in activity, mood, respiration, body temperature, blood pressure and cardiac rhythm. Morbidity and mortality are mainly associated with its cardiac toxicity, which produces myocardial infarction and cardiac arrhythmias in young people[11]. Sudden cardiac death syndrome in athletes taking cocaine is well known. Alcohol and cocaine are synergistic in producing cardiac damage. Cerebrovascular accidents, pneumomediastinum, rhabdomyolysis with renal failure and intestinal ischaemia have also been described. Death may also ensue from respiratory failure or convulsions.

Cocaine inhalation (snorting) produces intense mucosal ischaemia and may lead to infarction of nasal cartilage. Cocaine smoking has been reported to produce severe reactive airway disease.

Withdrawal symptoms are marked by severe depression.

Opiates

This class of drugs covers opium and its derivatives, including morphine, heroin and synthetic opiates such as pethidine, fentanyl, dextromoramide and dextropropoxyphene.

Although the analgesic effects of morphine have been shown to be little affected at pressure, the behavioural effects of these drugs with hyperbaric air have not been widely investigated.

High doses of these drugs can produce respiratory depression, whereas lower doses can produce alterations of mood, impaired psychomotor performance and constipation. These effects may be altered in an unpredictable way by immersion and hyperbaria.

Other drugs

Other abused drugs with significant effects that may adversely affect diving performance include *hallucinogenics* such as lysergic acid diethylamide (LSD), phencyclidine (PCP) and ketamine.

Performance-enhancing drugs are widespread in sport and may be encountered in certain diving populations. These drugs are a mixed group, including beta blockers (to reduce tremor), amphetamines, anabolic steroids, hormones, diuretics and sympathomimetics.

The development of novel *methods of self-administration* of illicit substances has increased the incidence of pulmonary complications[12]. The reason may be the route of administration, the presence of contaminating foreign material or microbiological pathogens or altered host immune response.

CONCLUSION

There is little information on the effects drugs have on human physiological or psychological performance in the aquatic hyperbaric environment. Conversely, there is more information on the effect of certain drugs on animals under extreme hyperbaric conditions. This research is often designed as much to elucidate mechanisms of drug action and biochemical functions as to define the safe uses of drugs under pressure. There are relatively few research data at conventional scuba depths. More research is needed in this area.

In the meantime, knowledge of both the diving environment and pharmacology including side effects should guide rational advice to divers.

REFERENCES

1. Taylor S, Taylor D, O'Toole K, Ryan C. Medications taken daily and prior to diving by experienced scuba divers. *South Pacific Underwater Medicine Society Journal* 2002;**32**(3):129–135.
2. UK Medicines Information. What information is available on drugs and diving? *Medicine Q&As*. 2013. Q&A 288.3. http://www.evidence.nhs.uk/
3. Rump AF, Siekmann U, Kalff G. Effects of hyperbaric and hyperoxic conditions on the disposition of drugs: theoretical considerations and a review of the literature. *General Pharmacology* 1999;**32**(1):127–133.
4. Walsh JM, Burch LS. The acute effects of commonly used drugs on human performance in hyperbaric air. *Undersea and Biomedical Research* 1979;**6**(Suppl):49.
5. Sipinen SA, Kulvik M, Leiniö M, Viljanen A, Lindholm H. Neuropsychologic and cardiovascular effects of clemastine fumarate under pressure. *Undersea and Hyperbaric Medicine* 1995;**22**(4):401–406.
6. Russell GB, Snider MT, Loumis JL. Hyperbaric nitrous oxide as a sole anaesthetic agent in humans. *Anesthesia and Analgesia* 1990;**70**:289–295.
7. Dujić Z, Palada I, Valic Z, *et al.* Exogenous nitric oxide and bubble formation in divers. *Medical Science of Sports and Exercise* 2006;**38**(8):432–435.
8. Duplessis C, Fothergill D, Schwaller D, *et al.* Prophylactic statins as a possible method to decrease bubble formation in diving. *Aviation, Space, and Environmental Medicine* 2007;**78**(4):430–434.
9. De Wit R, Sleijfer S, Kaye SB, *et al.* Bleomycin and scuba diving: where is the harm? *Lancet Oncology* 2007;**8**(11):954–955.
10. Kalant H. Adverse effects of cannabis on health: an update of the literature since 1996. *Progress in Neuro-psychopharmacology and Biological Psychiatry* 2004;**28**(5):849–863.
11. Loper KA. Clinical toxicology of cocaine. *Medical Toxicology and Adverse Drug Experience* 1989;**4**(3):174–185.
12. Heffner JE, Harley RA, Schabel SI. Pulmonary reactions from illicit substance abuse. *Clinical Chest Medicine* 1990;**11**:151–162.

This chapter was reviewed for this fifth edition by Michael Bennett.

44

Long-term effects of diving

Undisputed causes of diving-related residual sequelae include decompression sickness (DCS), cerebral arterial gas embolism (CAGE), inner ear and other barotrauma and dysbaric osteonecrosis. There is also some evidence suggesting that changes in bone, the central nervous system and the lung can be demonstrated in some divers who have not experienced a diving accident and who have no discernable clinical disease.

INTRODUCTION

Although some diving-related accidents may have long-term sequelae, this chapter is primarily concerned with the development of long-term effects in divers where no obvious precipitating cause can be identified. In relation to some sequelae, this remains a contentious issue despite significant efforts to elucidate the pathological mechanisms, or simply to quantify the epidemiology of any long-term deficit. For other sequelae, the cause and effect are clear.

With the improvement in prevention and treatment of diving accidents over the last few decades, more attention is now focussed on the possible undesirable long-term health effects of diving. This interest has been encouraged by the workplace health and safety aspects of commercial diving, greater attention to worker's compensation and litigation, medical research funding and other financial grants and the proliferation of sophisticated high-technology techniques developed for medical investigation.

Although much of the investigative effort in this field is centered on the professional diver, these concerns are also very real for large numbers of recreational divers.

Long-term effects can be defined as follows:

- Outside the range of normal in an appropriately matched population.
- Causally related to diving.
- Persisting beyond the acute and rehabilitation phase of a diving accident.
- Having no explanatory non-diving pathological; features.
- Producing a demonstrable reduction in the performance or quality of life of the diver.

There is no dispute that some diving accidents may have permanent sequelae. Problems include the following:

- Dysbaric osteonecrosis.
- Neurological DCS.
- Pulmonary barotrauma with CAGE.
- Hypoxia from any cause.
- Hearing loss and vestibular damage.
- Other otological and sinus damage.
- Many gas toxicities, including oxygen, carbon monoxide, carbon dioxide and high-pressure neurological syndrome.
- Some marine animal injuries.

The question we ask here is this: 'Do long-term health effects occur in divers who have not suffered a specific diving accident?'

For many of the postulated long-term effects discussed in this chapter, this is a very difficult question to answer. Where any group of divers appears to have a common set of symptoms and signs related to their previous diving activity, there are a number of physiological and pathological changes that may be implicated. These (non-exclusive) aetiologies include the following:

- Increased environmental pressure (immersed or non-immersed).
- Increased gas partial pressures.
- Oxygen toxicity.
- Gas induced osmosis.
- Asymptomatic bubble development, with local tissue effects, blood-bubble interaction (haematological effects) and blood-brain barrier disruption.
- Barotrauma damage to surrounding tissues.
- Asymptomatic lipid emboli.
- Adaptive effects of diving.

The following is a discussion of individual conditions of interest to either compressed gas workers or divers.

DYSBARIC OSTEONECROSIS

This significant and serious disorder has been reported in divers who have not necessarily suffered DCS. It is essentially a disease of divers exposed to environmental pressures for moderately long durations, and it is therefore more frequent in caisson workers, commercial and scientific divers and others who have prolonged exposures. Dysbaric osteonecrosis is the subject of Chapter 14. The aetiology, diagnosis, prognosis and treatment of this disorder are complex and specialized subjects in their own right and are not discussed further here.

NEUROLOGY

The range of potential neurological injuries as a consequence of diving is large, including injuries secondary to barotrauma (e.g. to some cranial nerves, including the facial, infraorbital maxillary, cochlear and vestibular, and to the ear and respiratory sinuses), hypoxia, DCS, nitrogen narcosis and physical trauma. These disorders are discussed in Chapters 7 to 9, 37, 38 and 40. A history of compressed gas breathing has also been linked to neurological syndromes that are more difficult to define.

Todnem and associates[1] in 1990 compared 156 Norwegian commercial divers with 100 unmatched, non-diving controls and found that divers had a higher incidence of specific neurological symptoms or cerebral dysfunction in non-diving situations (12 per cent versus 0 per cent). There was a history of diving misadventure is some divers, but not all the divers had symptoms (51 per cent of the divers had a history of DCS, 33 per cent had neurological symptoms during decompression and 14 per cent had been unconscious at some time). The divers had more general neurological symptoms and abnormal signs than controls. The abnormalities predominantly involved the distal spinal cord and peripheral nerves. There was an independent correlation between these abnormalities and diving exposure, DCS and age. Electroencephalogram (EEG) abnormalities were also correlated with both saturation diving and previous DCS in a follow-up paper.

In another investigation of 375 North Sea divers, Irgens and colleagues[2] in 2007 found divers to have lower health-related quality of life (SF-36) scores than the Norwegian normative data, and worse still if they gave a history of DCS. Both these studies suggest that deep saturation diving and a history of DCS may predispose divers to long-term neurological deficits. The issue is not settled, however. Ross and associates[3], also in 2007, reported on North Sea divers, but these 1540 divers were operating out of the United Kingdom. In contrast to the Norwegian data, Ross suggests there was no difference between divers and a cohort of non-diving offshore workers in rates of ill-health retirement or sickness benefits. Health-related quality of life (SF-12) was within normal limits for both groups, and divers were less likely to be receiving medical treatment. In contrast, divers were more likely to report 'forgetfulness or loss of concentration' (18 per cent *versus* 6 per cent; odds ratio, 3.8; 95 per cent confidence interval, 2.7 to 5.3), musculoskeletal symptoms and impaired hearing. Overall, Ross and colleagues concluded there was no evidence to suggest any major impact on the long-term health of UK divers.

These conflicting results may be the consequence of differences in methodology, but they are difficult to interpret. One conclusion is that similar effects are found in divers and non-divers in otherwise similar occupations, and that the factors of welding experience, exposure to contaminants and off-shore stress factors are relevant. More work is needed before the true risk of this type of diving exposure can be stated with certainty.

There is no dispute that DCS does leave some individuals with permanent neurological symptoms and signs. Permanent neurological damage is typified by the classical case of spinal DCS with permanent paraplegia. Lesser manifestations may vary from the obvious and debilitating to mild. Mild residual symptoms include paraesthesia and patchy areas of numbness from peripheral nerve involvement. Subjective manifestations such as short-term memory loss and difficulty in concentrating may require formal psychometric testing to identify their presence and quantify their degree. Whether sub-clinical and cumulative lesions can occur in divers who have never experienced clinical DCS is unknown. Similarly, it is not known whether such lesions can develop after complete recovery from DCS. Even if they do occur, it is not at all clear they can be avoided by conservative diving practices.

Central neurological damage may be transient, or it may be permanent and cumulative.

EEG changes after diving accidents or incidents may indicate damage, but the alteration in EEG behaviour is sometimes difficult to interpret. Computed tomography (CT) and magnetic resonance imaging (MRI) scans, as well as evoked cortical potentials, may reveal only gross abnormalities and may miss small multi-focal damage (see Chapters 40 and 41).

Investigators have turned to some of the newer radiological and scanning techniques to assess the neurological effects of diving. Moen and associates[4] in 2010, for example, reported regional functional abnormalities throughout the brain, including large frontal and temporal white matter regions, the hippocampus, and parts of the cerebellum by using diffusion-perfusion-weighted MRI. These investigators concluded that 'the findings may explain some of the long-term clinical symptoms reported among professional divers'[4]. The appropriate interpretation of such abnormalities remains problematic.

Technetium-99m hexamethylpropyleneamine oxime single photon emission computed tomography scanning

Technetium-99m hexamethylpropyleneamine oxime single photon emission CT (^{99m}Tc-HMPAO-SPECT) is a technique used to image regional blood flow. HMPAO is radiolabelled with ^{99m}Tc, and SPECT uses single gamma ray emitting radiotracers, which are detected by gamma cameras to produce three-dimensional images. The ^{99m}Tc HMPAO is injected intravenously and diffuses across the blood-brain barrier. The complex remains bound in the brain tissues for up to 8 hours, thus effectively producing a frozen picture of regional blood flow at the time of injection.

In 1998, Adkisson and associates[5] first reported the use of this technique in diving accident victims. These investigators studied 28 patients within 1 month of presentation with DCS (neurological DCS, 23; CAGE, 4; limb bend, 1). They reported cerebral perfusion deficits in all patients with neurological DCS and CAGE and a high degree of correlation between the clinical picture and the site of the perfusion deficit. The possibility of occult neurological damage was raised by the appearance of cerebral perfusion deficits in divers who showed clinical signs only of spinal cord involvement. The patient with a limb bend had a normal scan.

Subsequent investigations raised doubts about the significance of these findings. Hodgson and colleagues[6] in 1990 compared 10 divers with acute DCS with 10 divers who had been treated for DCS some 3 to 5 years earlier, 10 divers who had never experienced DCS and 10 population controls. Although there was a trend toward a larger number of deficits in individuals with DCS, there were no statistical differences among the groups and no apparent correlation between the sites of the perfusion deficits and the clinical presentation. There was also a higher than predicted number of positive scans in both the divers never treated for DCS and the non-diver controls. These findings therefore do not support the assumption that asymptomatic divers sustain neurological injury because the same deficits were reported in individuals who had never dived. In a similar report, Shields and colleagues[7] in 1997 compared SPECT images in 28 commercial divers with a history of DCI, 26 divers with no such history and 19 non-divers. No association was evident between abnormal findings and a history of either diving or DCI. There was some evidence that divers with more than 14 years of diving experience or more than 100 decompression days per year had sub-clinical perfusion abnormalities. The significance of these deficits and the true incidence in control populations have yet to be determined.

Divers with sub-clinical pathological deficits

In 1981, Palmer and associates[8] reported the autopsy of a male sports diver who had recovered almost completely from an episode of spinal DCS 4 years earlier, but who was subsequently found to have extensive morphological changes in the posterior and lateral columns of the spinal cord.

Palmer and colleagues[9] went on to report on the spinal cords from eight professional and three amateur divers who died accidentally. In all cases bar one, the divers had passed a diving medical examination within the last year. None of the divers revealed a history of DCS and none had documented neurological abnormalities. Tract degeneration was found in the spinal cords of three professional divers, variously affecting the posterior, lateral and, to a lesser extent, anterior columns. In one there was degeneration of afferent fibers within the posterior columns. These features were difficult to recognize in haematoxylin and eosin sections but were clearly shown by the Marchi staining technique. Marchi-positive material does not appear in degenerating myelinated fibers until 7 to 10 days after the initiating lesion and does not appear intracellularly until some 10 weeks after the lesion.

In 1991, Palmer and associates[10] examined the brains of 12 amateur and 13 professional divers, all but 1 of whom had died accidentally. Only 3 subjects had reported a previous episode of DCS. Grossly distended, empty vessels were found in the brains of 15 of 22 divers who died as a result of diving accidents. These findings were presumably caused by gas bubbles (see post-mortem decompression artifact in Chapter 51). The most striking long-term change observed in the brains was that of perivascular lacuna formation found in cerebral and/or cerebellar white matter in 3 amateurs and 5 professionals. Hyalinization of vessel walls was also found in the brains of 3 amateur and 5 professionals. Necrotic foci in gray matter occurred in 7 cases, and perivascular vacuolation of white matter occurred in 7 cases. Palmer proposed these changes arose from intravascular gas bubble formation producing sudden distension and occlusion of small arterial vessels. With passage of the bubble, the vessel returns to its normal size, leaving a surrounding area of degenerated tissue within the lacunae. Hyalinization of the vessel wall may also occur as a consequence of this rise in luminal pressure. In a previously asymptomatic professional diver, there was also unilateral necrosis of the head of the caudate nucleus.

This study provides evidence of chronic changes (lacunae formation and hyalinization of vessel walls) in the brains of asymptomatic divers who did not have a past history of DCS when compared with control subjects. This may be relevant because it is now generally accepted that bubbles are produced with all but the most innocuous dive profiles.

NEUROPSYCHOLOGY

Over the years, anecdotal reports in the literature, combined with an almost folklore belief among many occupational air diving groups, have generated the hypothesis that diving, even in the absence of a gross insult, causes brain damage and dementia in divers. There are no reputable studies to support or refute this hypothesis directly. In one report in the Norwegian 1994 conference on the long-term effects of diving, Curley and associates[11] found no evidence to support a correlation between altered neuropsychometric test results and function with diving exposure in a group of 421 US Navy divers (see Chapter 41).

Behavioural factors

Perhaps one of the most important basic findings, when comparing divers with non-divers, is the difference in their psychological and behavioural characteristics. Chapter 41 contains a description of the psychological factors associated with the *diving personality*.

When it became evident that divers, and especially those who undertook extreme diving activities, perform differently in both psychological testing and behaviour, conclusions were drawn about the possible effects of diving on a 'normal' or 'average' personality.

Not only do divers perform differently on psychological tests, but they also differ in their mode of death. There is a preponderance of traumatic causes of death and of suicides. The incidence of accidental deaths is higher, from drowning and diving accidents. Non-diving accidents (which included murders) comprise 20 per cent and suicides 17 per cent of the deaths of occupational divers.

One must be careful not to conclude immediately that these statistics reflect the effect of diving. They may, instead, reflect the personality of divers.

It is possible, and indeed likely, that divers are not identical to the 'normal' population. They may well be attracted to this occupational activity by their love of adventure, risk-taking behaviour, physical activity and so forth and may well succeed in this occupation because of their reduced innate levels of anxiety (neuroticism, trait anxiety). This combination of factors may to lead to situations in which their love of adventure becomes dangerous or in which their propensity for physical activity may be inappropriate.

It is possible that the higher incidence of violent death and suicide is related to the life style, which includes not only the diving activities, but also exposure to hazardous environments, possible drug and alcohol abuse and other unknown influences.

Alternatively, it is also feasible that the neuropsychological sequelae associated with diving accidents, or some other form of cumulative brain damage, could lead to the behaviour referred to earlier.

HEARING LOSS AND VERTIGO

One of the most obvious long-term sequelae of diving is hearing loss. This discussed at length in Chapter 37, with the less appreciated permanent vestibular damage, as described in Chapter 38. Because hearing loss is more easily recordable and perceived by the subject, it is more frequently documented. Permanent vestibular damage is likely to be compensated by adaptive neurological processes, which may result in the subject's not being aware of any deficit. It may be evident only in provocative situations or with vestibular function testing.

SINUS DISEASE

Although rarely mentioned in this context, sinus disease is a common long-term sequela of diving. It is usually a result of repeated sinus barotrauma (see Chapter 8), with subsequent infections sometimes superimposed on the barotrauma.

The problem of chronic sinus disease is often a cumulative result of inappropriate diving activities, especially when divers persevere despite the evidence of barotrauma and infections. The reduction of the lumen of the sinus ostia or duct results from chronic inflammation and gradual scarring.

In these circumstances, it is frequently the very experienced diver who presents at the latter part of his or her diving career with the development of sinus barotrauma interfering with descent.

Investigations in divers (e.g. MRI of the skull) often coincidentally demonstrate the presence of chronic sinus disease.

OPHTHALMOLOGICAL EFFECTS

Because the eye develops as an extension of the forebrain, it has long been recognized that the fundus may reflect changes occurring within the central nervous system. Lesions of the retina may indicate more widespread changes within the central nervous system. Such disorders include oxygen toxicity, DCS and CAGE.

In 1998, Polkinghorne and colleagues[12] used retinal fluorescein angiography in 84 divers and 23 non-divers to determine whether blood vessel changes are common in the ocular fundi of divers. These investigators proposed that such changes could give an indication of vascular obstruction elsewhere, particularly in the central nervous system. Twelve of the divers had been diagnosed previously with DCS, nine with neurological DCS (none had visual symptoms) and three with joint pain only. The authors reported that retinal capillary density at the fovea was low in divers and both microaneurysms, and small areas of capillary nonperfusion were evident. The divers had significantly more abnormalities of the retinal pigment epithelium than did the comparison group of non-divers. These investigators found a positive correlation between the presence of fundus abnormality and the length of diving history. No subject had any recorded visual loss as a consequence of diving.

These investigators concluded that all changes were consistent with obstruction of the retinal and choroidal circulations and that this obstruction was likely the result of intravascular bubble formation during decompression or the altered behaviour of blood constituents and blood vessels under hyperbaric conditions.

Other investigators have not reproduced these findings. In 1992 Holden and associates[13] performed fluorescein angiography in 26 divers who had used safe diving practices for at least 10 years and in 7 controls. There was no significant difference in the incidence of macular abnormalities between these groups. The authors suggested that adherence to safe diving practices could protect against the effects reported by Polkinghorne and colleagues.

Murrison and associates[14] in 1996 compared the retinal fluorescein angiograms of 55 Royal Navy divers and 24 non-diver servicemen. There were no differences between divers and non-divers, and the prevalence of abnormalities was not correlated with diving experience.

It is difficult to interpret these diverse findings. Military diving is conservative and highly regulated, and therefore the proposal by Holden and associates that safe diving may protect against lesions is credible. However, the lack of correlation of length of diving history in military divers with presence of lesions disputes the accumulative dose effect as proposed by Polkinghorne and colleagues.

Prospective longitudinal studies of recreational, military and professional divers will be required before it can be established whether diving results in these ocular vascular changes. It is not clear that anyone is undertaking this work.

PULMONARY FUNCTION

It has long been believed that some divers are able to tolerate higher levels of carbon dioxide than non-divers. If this is correct, then it is uncertain whether such a physiological anomaly is based on natural selection for diving activities or is a long-term adaptation from diving. It is not clear whether this ability is of value in diving (permitting the diver to tolerate slight variations in carbon dioxide tensions) or hazardous (making the diver more susceptible to carbon dioxide toxicity, oxygen toxicity or DCS).

It is generally accepted that divers have larger vital capacity and total lung capacity than non-divers, although there are some surveys in which this was not evident. It is certainly true of apnoea divers[15]. One major longitudinal study demonstrated an initial adaptive increase in lung volume in divers, followed by a progressive decline, possibly age related.

In 1990, Thorsen and associates[16] demonstrated that divers develop some degree of airflow obstruction as a result of airway narrowing. One aspect of this is an increase in hyperreactivity, demonstrated by histamine provocation testing. Although some of these effects may be related to a cumulative pulmonary oxygen toxicity or repetitive pulmonary gaseous microembolization, the same effect has also been observed in elite athletes. Pulmonary transfer capacity for carbon monoxide is diminished after deep dives and may not be totally reversible.

Lung function appears to be altered by even a single diving exposure. In a report to a 1993 international consensus conference on the long-term effects of diving, Reed[17] summarized these findings:

- The respiratory effects of single deep saturation dives include a reduction in pulmonary diffusion capacity, increase in lung volumes and impairment of exercise performance. There may also be deleterious effects on indices of ventilatory capacity. These changes indicate a peripheral lung lesion affecting gas exchange.
- Both cross-sectional and longitudinal studies relating pulmonary function to diving history have demonstrated loss of function associated with indices of diving exposure.

The underlying aetiology of these changes is uncertain. Proposed mechanisms include lung overdistension, hyperoxia, vascular bubbles, exposure to increased ambient pressure *per se* and gas and particulate contaminants associated with compressors and chambers. The association with diving *per se* may not be causal.

OTHER EFFECTS

Various other possible long-term effects of diving have been suggested. Cardiac hypertrophy has been reported in professional divers and may have sinister implications. It is possible that there are contributions to cardiac disease associated with either intravascular emboli affecting the coronary arteries or damage to the primary endothelium from these intravascular bubbles.

Arthritic disorders may have a higher incidence in divers than in non-divers. One study investigated morbidity and mortality among 11 517 US Navy divers[18]. Increased hospitalization for joint disorders was noted in the 23- to 28-year-old divers, without an obvious explanation.

Many haematological and some vascular changes have been noted with various forms of decompression, but few continue for any length of time after ascent. Fox and associates[19] in 1984 illustrated an increased incidence of chromosomal aberrations in cultured T lymphocytes of divers. The health effects related to these isolated observations are unknown, and there have been no follow-up studies to confirm these findings in divers – although many other occupational groups have shown similar changes, usually related to low-dose radiation exposure (e.g. flight cabin attendants). There have been no permanent haematological vascular changes demonstrated, apart from those referred to earlier.

Investigations suggesting either sub-fertility of divers or a preponderance of female progeny among divers have not been substantiated.

Long-term effects, both physical and neuropsychological, of injuries from marine animal envenomations have been observed. There are few or no documented investigations of these cases, despite the plethora of clinical evidence and case reports of osteomyelitis and even amputation induced by various marine envenomations. Long-term inflammatory responses from foreign body reactions are also well known (see Chapter 32). Very significant neuropsychological sequelae of some of the fish poisons have also frequently been documented (see Chapter 33). All these cases have a specific temporal relationship, continuing from the time of the specific incident.

CONCLUSION

In 1993, an international consensus conference on the long-term health effects of diving was held in Norway[20]. The stated objective of the meeting was to agree on possible long-term health effects of diving based on the knowledge and experience at that time; however, there was a strong bias toward presumed decompression effects. The participants summarized current knowledge and produced the following consensus statement. Little has changed in the more than 20 years since that conference.

The consensus in part states: "The changes are in most cases minor and do not influence the diver's quality of life. However, the changes are of a nature that may influence the diver's future health.

The scientific evidence is limited, and future research is required to obtain adequate answers to the questions of long-term health effects of diving."

REFERENCES

1. Todnem K, Nyland H, Kambestad BK, Aarli JA. Influence of occupational diving upon the nervous system: an epidemiological study. *British Journal of Industrial Medicine* 1990;**47**:708–714.
2. Irgens Å, Gronnin M, Troland K, *et al.* Reduced health-related quality of life in former North Sea divers is associated with decompression sickness. *Occupational Medicine* 2007;**57**(5):349–354.
3. Ross JAS, Macdiarmid JI, Osman LM, *et al.* Health status of professional divers and offshore oil industry workers. *Occupational Medicine* 2007;**57**:254–261.
4. Moen G, Specht K, Taxt T, *et al.* Cerebral diffusion and perfusion deficits in North Sea divers. *Acta Radiologica* 2010;**51**(9):1050–1058.
5. Adkisson GH, Macleod MA, Hodgson M, *et al.* Cerebral perfusion deficits in dysbaric illness. *Lancet* 1989;**2**:119–121.
6. Hodgson M, Smith DJ, Macleod MA, Houston AS, Francis TJR. Case control study of cerebral perfusion deficits in divers using ⁹⁹Tcᵐ hexamethylpropylene amine oxime. *Undersea Biomedical Research* 1990;**18**(5–6):421–431.
7. Shields TG, Duff PM, Evans SA, *et al.* Correlation between 99Tcm-HMPAO-SPECT brain image and a history of decompression illness or extent of diving experience in commercial divers. *Occupational and Environmental Medicine* 1997;**54**(4):247–253.
8. Palmer AC, Calder IM, Mccallum RI, Mastaglia FL. Spinal cord degeneration in a case of 'recovered' spinal cord decompression sickness. *British Medical Journal* 1981;**283**:888.
9. Palmer AC, Calder IM, Hughes JT. Spinal cord degeneration in divers. *Lancet* 1987;**2**:1365–1366.
10. Palmer AC, Calder IM, Yates PO. Cerebral vasculopathy in divers. *Neuropathology and Applied Neurobiology* 1992;**18**:113–124.
11. Curley MD, Wallick MT, Amerson TL. Long-term health effects of US Navy diving: neuropsychology. In: *Long term health effects of diving: an International Consensus Conference.* Hope A, Lund T, Elliott DH, Halsey MJ, Wiig H (eds). Bergen Norwegian Underwater Technology Centre 1994;209–226.
12. Polkinghorne PJ, Sehmi K, Cross MR, Minassian D, Bird AC. Ocular fundus lesions in divers. *Lancet* 1988;**2**:1381–1383.
13. Holden R, Morsman G, Lane CM. Ocular fundus lesions in sports divers using safe diving practices. *British Journal of Sports Medicine* 1992;**26**(2):90–92.
14. Murrison AW, Pethybridge RJ, Rintoul AJ, Jeffrey MN, Sehmi K, Bird AC. Retinal angiography in divers. *Occupational and Environmental Medicine* 1996;**53**(5):339–342.
15. Ferretti G, Costa M. Review: diversity in and adaptation to breath-hold diving in humans. *Comparative Biochemistry and Physiology* 2003;**136**:205–213.
16. Thorsen E, Sedegal K, Kambestad B, Gulsvic A. Divers' lung function: small airways disease? *British Journal of Industrial Medicine* 1990;**47**(8):519–523.
17. Reed JW. Effects of exposure to hyperbaria on lung function. In: Hope A, Lund T Elliott DH, Halsey MJ, Wiig H, eds. *Long Term Health Effects of Diving: An International Consensus Conference.* Bergen, Norway: Norwegian Underwater Technology Centre; 1994.
18. Hoiberg A, Blood C. Age-specific morbidity and mortality rates among US Navy enlisted divers and controls. *Undersea Biomedical Research* 1985;**12**:191–203.
19. Fox DP, Robertson FW, Brown T, *et al.* Chromosome aberrations in divers. *Undersea Biomedical Research* 1984;**11**:193–204.
20. Long term health effects of diving: consensus document. In: Hope A, Lund T, Elliott DH, Halsey MJ, Wiig H, eds. *Long Term Health Effects of Diving: An International Consensus Conference.* Bergen, Norway: Norwegian Underwater Technology Centre; 1994.

This chapter was reviewed for this fifth edition by Michael Bennett.

PART 8

The Diving Accident

45

Stress responses, panic and fatigue

INTRODUCTION

Although compressed air diving was possible for most of the twentieth century, it became popular only following development of scuba equipment in the late l940s.

At that time, only those who sought excitement and had a genuine love of the sea would embrace the sport of diving. Natural selection dictated that these would be aquatic people, with skills and personality suited to this and other water activities – the 'waterperson' concept. Diving was merely an extension of this overall interest and ability.

In the l960s, these 'natural' divers commercially exploited their talents and became instructors. They required of their trainees a level of water skills often in excess of that possessed by most. Few trainees took up this challenge. Those who did were required to show personality characteristics that could tolerate extremes of physical discomfort, environmental hazards and inadequate equipment.

During the l970s, with the availability of more user-friendly equipment and the change in societal attitudes away from the hunter-killer male chauvinistic approach, there was a movement toward the ecologically perceptive diver, equipped with a camera and not a catch bag.

Thus, the tough male stereotype of the pre-l960s was supplanted by the sensitive and sociable diver of the post-1980s. The belief that diving should be available to all even resulted in a number of handicapped groups entering the scuba diving world. These included paraplegic divers and blind and deaf divers, as well as the introduction of 'friends of divers' (i.e. children, members of the diver's family, other peer groups).

Some of the people now undertaking scuba diving are probably more accident prone – or at least less able to cope with demanding situations – than those of the earlier years. New types of disorders are arising apart from the traditional diseases. The stress syndromes of diving are typical examples of these newer disorders. Diving trainees of the new millennium reflect the general population, with a wide range of physical, medical and psychological limitations. The various psychological reactions of divers are described in Chapter 41.

The ocean environment can be unforgiving, and it may not make allowance for the personality of the new divers. Also, the user-friendly equipment may expedite diving but promote new difficulties and dependency.

PERSONALITY FACTORS

The early divers were somewhat like the early aviators. They were adventure seekers, and they often carried out their activities because of necessity. These included such groups as explorers, treasure hunters (salvage) and military divers.

With the increasing sophistication of equipment and the greater complexities of deep diving, the commercial divers of this century are far more careful, obsessional, regulation-following and conscientious than their forebears.

The personality characteristics required for a recreational diver, who can choose the dive conditions and vary the dive duration, are quite different from those of the professional diver, who may have to remain isolated in the underwater environment and be able to use underwater habitats for days or weeks at a time.

This chapter summarizes some of the expert observations that have been made on divers.

Traditional beliefs

Yarborough, in 1955, stated that the diver not only had to have an absence of physical defects, but also should possess a stable psyche and a phlegmatic personality. The possession of a temperament free of alarmist characteristic was essential. This requirement was later validated by the progressively increasing numbers of divers who died as a result of 'panic'.

Dr Harry Alvis in 1957 stated that divers were not the most normal of normal people. A special type of personality was required. Divers are risk takers.

Sir Stanley Miles, in 1962, stated in the first sentence of his seminal text on *Underwater Medicine,* 'It is most important, right at the outset, to realize that the problems of man's adaptation to a watery environment are primarily those of temperament'.

Bowen and Miller, in 1967, stressed the hazardous nature of diving activities. Danger ('and drowning') was always one breath away. Co-operation was imperative for safety, and yet the diver was necessarily a lonely person, dependent more on his or her own quick actions for personal safety.

Caille, 1969, stated that of all divers, the greater physical and mental demands were made on military and naval personnel who fulfilled a combat role. There was only a small margin underwater for deviations from normal health. No one could predict when and in what circumstances a candidate would be exposed to excessive stress (danger).

Research observations

Many psychometric studies have been performed on divers, but because each group has different operational requirements, the results do not have widespread relevance. In general, comprehensive psychometric assessments probably do not have a predictive value that is commensurate with the time and cost of the investigations.

In most of the diving training during the 1950s and 1960s, there was a consistent 50 per cent failure rate in **professional diving** courses. This selection meant that some standards were being applied. In comparison, there is little or no failure rate in many of the current recreational diving courses – suggesting that few or no standards are being applied, other than the ability to pay.

Ross, in 1950, conducted an investigation into **Australian Navy divers** and found that the major characteristic required appeared to be sufficient self-control to face threatening situations without inducing disabling anxiety. He also noted the importance of an 'adventuresome approach, diligence in performing work, self-reliance, tolerance of discomfort and an indifference to minor injuries and illnesses'. Physical attributes such as stamina, athletic fitness and an affinity for strenuous effort were important.

In the training of the underwater demolition teams from the US Navy, **psychometric testing** revealed that mechanical and arithmetical comprehension was more highly correlated with success than were other characteristics, such as clerical ability.

Psychological tests on some groups of divers, such as **underwater demolition teams,** showed traits that were quite different from those seen on the tests performed on other diving groups. Nevertheless, some characteristics continued to be present among most divers. These included objectivity, low neuroticism (trait anxiety), aggression and self-sufficiency. Fear and anxiety were not acceptable characteristics.

Edmonds, in l967, carried out a prospective assessment of **500 diving candidates,** who were undergoing a diving course that had a 41 per cent pass rate. A statistical analysis of the results showed that the diver was a psychologically stable, medically and physically fit individual who was not overtly worried by diving hazards and who had both the desire and ability to perform in the water environment. In comparison with the unsuccessful candidates, the diver was usually more mature, motivated by love of water sports (but not by adventure or comradeship), not fearful of the hazards likely to be encountered, physically fit, thick-set (low Cotton's Index of Build or body mass index), a non-smoker and free of medical disorders, very capable of breath-holding and swimming, intelligent, self-sufficient, non-neurotic, simple and practical.

Physical fitness and especially aquatic fitness were important characteristics for successful diving. A failure to complete a 200-metre swim in less than 5 minutes, without swimming aids, was an indicator of poor aquatic fitness and failure of the course.

After 3 years of detailed investigation, Edmonds had merely confirmed the anecdotal views of Yarborough and Ross, expressed many years previously.

Comparisons of divers with non-divers in the US Navy revealed that divers had less hospitalization for stress-related disorders, but more hospitalization for environmentally induced disorders. The interpretation that they did more but thought less is possibly an oversimplification.

Different personality characteristics are required for different types of professional diving. In saturation diving, the divers have to work together within a small enclosed area where an affinity and ability for teamwork and tolerance are needed. An abalone diver, who works in isolation for many hours each day, does not require such social skills (and often does not possess them). A navy diver who detonates or defuses underwater explosives needs good mechanical aptitude. Technical divers need increased conscientiousness and obsessionality because of the narrower margin for error.

Divers performed quite differently on psychometric testing from their non-diving controls. Professional abalone divers, even in the l980s, tended to be risk-taking types, and this was demonstrated in their attitude to, and results of, psychometric tests.

Similarly, the range of skills required for recreational divers varies with the type of diving. Nevertheless, self-reliance and freedom from neuroticism (low trait anxiety) seem common among all diving groups.

Within any occupational group, because the requirements are the same, male and female group members will probably have similar personality profiles.

Morgan and his colleagues verified that **anxiety** (trait anxiety, neuroticism) was likely to predispose to panic responses. **Introverted** people are more concerned with the exercise demands of diving – becoming more susceptible to exhaustion and fatigue – than extroverts. These investigators demonstrated that **panic** was a frequent problem, even among experienced divers, and it was observed in 54 per cent of recreational divers (64 per cent in females, 50 per cent in males). Male divers tended to report this later – when the event became life threatening – than did female divers.

STRESS RESPONSES

Stress responses assist in the survival of the species, but they are of value to the individual only if they are not excessive. The stress response acts through the autonomic nervous system. This prepares the animal for 'fight or flight'. The respiratory and circulatory systems are stimulated, and there are biochemical and haematological changes to support this hyper-alert state. The animal is then ready for action in a condition of high physiological excitation.

The stress responses in diving can be understood only by having an appreciation of the complex interaction of humans, their technology and the environment in which they use it.

The reason that stress responses are ignored in most diving texts is that they are psychologically complex and ill-defined and do not lend themselves readily to academic study or pathological scrutiny.

They include three of the most common causes of accidents and deaths from scuba diving (see Chapter 46):

- **Panic** – a psychological stress response, related to anxiety.
- **Fatigue** – a physiological stress response to exceptional exertion.
- **Sudden death syndrome** – a pathological stress response of the heart (see Chapter 56).

The induction of panic in the anxious diver, fatigue in the physically unfit and cardiac death in the medically unfit are more clearly understood when one considers specific equipment problems (see Chapter 4) and environmental demands (see Chapter 5).

Training in appropriate behaviour and learning how to recognize and reduce the development of stress disorders – how to avoid them and how to ameliorate them – are major factors in promoting diving safety. Repetition of skills related to equipment and experience of different environments are the mainstays of instruction.

It is not uncommon for less astute divers to indulge in a type of self-deceit that causes them to risk injury rather than admit they are facing a new challenge for which they are ill-equipped or ill-prepared. And yet, 60 per cent of recreational divers indicated that they had experienced trouble and required assistance at least once in the previous 3 years. Stress situations are inevitable in diving.

PANIC

Panic is a psychological response to stress and is probably the most common single contributor to death in scuba diving. It is an extreme form of anxiety identified by unreasoning fear and loss of control. It is produced when an animal perceives or experiences a threat (the stressors). The threat may be real (environmental or physiological) or imaginary (psychological). An imaginary threat can be as intense a stimulus in producing the stress response as the more obvious physical causes.

The psychological response of the diver to actual or perceived problems and hazards is based on his or her innate susceptibility (neuroticism). The diver must be aware of problems to be able to create an anxiety state of sufficient magnitude to be termed 'panic'. Under identical conditions, different divers react in different ways, and those with a tendency to high anxiety are more likely to react with panic.

Neuroticism (trait anxiety) is an indication of the individual's tendency to break down under stress. It is mainly inherited and can be assessed by various personality tests or by monitoring the physiological responses to stress. However, there are some divers who have specific anxieties (state anxiety) to aquatic threats (e.g. drowning, claustrophobia, sharks), even with normal neuroticism levels.

Panic commences as a loss of confidence. The diver then experiences a loss of control over the situation, thereby producing a vicious circle in which further loss of confidence is experienced. Inappropriate behaviour very rapidly takes over, with the diver reaching a state in which self-preservation is threatened. Panic was implicated as a significant factor in more than 80 per cent of scuba diving fatalities surveyed in Los Angeles County in 1970. It contributed to at least 39 per cent of the deaths in the Australian survey of recreational diving fatalities, probably 37 per cent of recreational scuba drownings and 58 per cent of recreational scuba near drownings.

Anxiety is often induced by certain diving tasks, especially those of mask clearing, buddy breathing, free ascent training, open ocean diving, diving alone, diving with sharks and other situations, and it is known that the autonomic nervous system responses are exaggerated, before, during and after these experiences. As in all other diving techniques, repeated non-stressful diving training and experiences promote confidence and reduce the degree of state anxiety.

Specific fears or **phobias** associated with the diving and aquatic environments are also reduced by acquiring relevant experience. This is achieved by considerate and repetitive training under those environmental conditions. It is referred to by behavioural psychologists as 'desensitization' or 'deconditioning'. A diver who is exposed to certain environmental conditions repeatedly, and with good intuition and with preparation for emergencies, is less likely to act irrationally or to panic when he or she is subsequently faced with those conditions.

Sensory deprivation is referred to as the **blue orb syndrome** and is described in Chapter 41. Both this and excessive sensory overload act by disrupting psychological equilibrium and predispose divers to panic. Panic can be influenced in either direction, depending on the thought processes (cognitive and appraisal) of the victim. The beneficial influence of low neuroticism is affected by such intangibles as volition, self-confidence, exertion, experiences and aquatic skills.

> It takes as long to die of panic as it does to assess the situation rationally and initiate effective and corrective action.

The sympathetic nervous system responses to fear produce a terror-stricken facial appearance, pallor, dilated pupils, shallow rapid respirations, rapid jerky movements and irrational behaviour. The diver focusses excessive attention on either the equipment or the surface. All these features can be observed by companion divers. The affected diver would add dyspnoea, palpitations and a sensation of panic to the symptom complex. The physiologist would include hypertension, increased cardiac output, arrhythmias, increased circulation to muscles, adrenal and steroid hormonal secretions and cerebral excitation. Fear alone, without the addition of any other stress, may cause death.

Surveys of divers indicate that most trainees consider that they are not adequately acquainted with the frequency and importance of anxiety symptoms induced by diving or with the recognition and treatment of these symptoms.

Addressing this problem requires classroom discussion and repeated practical experiences and supervised training in skills to cope with both equipment and environments. The usual basic open water certification course is inadequate for this purpose, and it explains the high overrepresentation of novice divers in the recreational diving fatality statistics (7 per cent of the fatalities occur on the first open water dive and 23 per cent on an early dive).

Morgan noted that terms such as panic, stress and fatality are rarely mentioned in diving courses, texts or manuals.

There are many factors, any one of which can lead to a panic situation. Table 45.1 lists some of these factors (see also the later discussion of fatigue). They basically all lead to a diver's inability to cope with the equipment or the environment. They tend to relate to each other. For example, if one looks at the first cause in each column, it will be evident that a diver who is swimming against a tidal current will be more likely to become fatigued if he or she has reduced efficiency by being overweighted. In some cases, one factor predominates, whereas in others, a combination produces the same eventual result. There are some circumstances in which any and all divers would panic. The art lies in recognizing and

Table 45.1 Contributors to panic

Personal factors	Equipment problems	Environmental hazards
Fatigue	Buoyancy	Tidal currents
Physical unfitness or disability	Snorkel	Entry and exit techniques
Previous medical disorders	Face mask	Cold
Seasickness and/or vomiting	Weight belt	Surf
Alcohol or drugs	Wetsuit	Kelp
Inexperience	Scuba cylinder	Caves, wrecks
Inadequate dive plan	Regulator	Ice and cold water
Techniques (buddy breathing)	Other equipment	Deep diving
Psychological neuroticism and anxiety	Reliance on equipment	Dangerous marine animals
Sensory deprivation	Loss of equipment	Poor visibility
Vertigo and/or disorientation	Misuse of equipment	Explosives
Diving accidents	Entrapment – lines	Boat accidents

CASE REPORT 45.1

(This is a composite report, with many unwitting contributors.)

Nick was a recently qualified diver who was not using all his own equipment and was diving in an unfamiliar area. He borrowed a wetsuit, but it was a bit tight around the chest and restricted his breathing. He decided to overweight himself by two extra 1-kilogram lead weights because he felt that he could have some difficulty with descent under ocean conditions.

It was one of his first open ocean dives, and there had been some question regarding whether the conditions were suitable for diving. Even before entry into the water, he was not entirely happy with himself.

Initially, the dive was uneventful, other than Nick's being a little apprehensive regarding his ability to outlast his companions.

Note: One of the more serious marine hazards is the diver who aims to dive deeper or longer, using less air than his companions – thereby setting up a competitive situation and placing everyone in jeopardy, including the diver.

In this particular dive, Nick was convinced that he was using more air than his companions. This tended to aggravate his apprehension, and he wondered whether he was running out of gas. There was unfortunately no way to confirm this because he was not wearing a contents gauge on the scuba regulator, and he felt that he was probably a long way from either the boat or the shore.

A mixture of inexperience and misplaced pride prevented him from surfacing to clarify his position, and he noticed that he was becoming rather more anxious. His breathing rate increased, and, as if to confirm his worst fears, he noticed a resistance in his regulator. He then concentrated on his breathing and noted that both it and his heartbeat seemed to be fairly rapid. He considered the possibility of turning on his emergency reserve and finally decided to do this, to see whether it would have any effect on the respiratory difficulty. It did not.

A thought flashed through his mind that he was not enjoying this dive. He had spent a disproportionate amount of time looking at his equipment, at his buddy or at the surface. He did not inform his companion that the reserve valve had been activated, hoping against hope that his companions would be equally short of gas. Another fear was that he was not making very much headway against the current, and he thought that he was probably still a long way from completing the dive. He was now becoming far more apprehensive, and there was greater resistance from the demand valve. He decided to leave his weight belt on for the moment and argued that perhaps he could last a little longer. He was becoming very anxious, with increased respiration and greatly increased breathing resistance.

In fact, and putting it in its simplest terms, he was not getting enough air. The situation was serious. He decided to surface fast. During ascent, which was rapid but not rapid enough for Nick's peace of mind, he could see the surface, but despite previous assurances to the contrary, he did not get more air as he ascended. He reached the surface just in time to wrench off his face mask and regulator; he felt about to 'black out'. By expenditure of considerable effort, he managed to keep his head above water for a few terrifyingly precious seconds before one of the small waves sloshed over him. Some water got into his mouth and caused him to cough. He struggled hard to maintain his head above water. Unfortunately, he was becoming very fatigued – exhausted – and wondered how long he could keep this up. Then strength and determination seemed to recede.

His 'buddy' realized that Nick had disappeared, and after delayed reconnaissance of the area, he decided to ascend. By the time the buddy reached the surface, Nick was no longer to be seen. Nick's body was subsequently found within a few metres of where he had sunk (despite the tidal currents), with his weight belt still fastened, his buoyancy vest uninflated, ample air in his scuba cylinder – and at a distance so close to shore that he could well have swum under almost any conditions, using mask, snorkel and fins.

Autopsy diagnosis: drowning.

True diagnosis: death from panic. Rereading this case history will reveal that anxiety and panic explain every facet, and drowning explains only the final result.

avoiding these circumstances as much as possible and in ensuring that the diver's capabilities are not exceeded by the limitations of the equipment and the demands of the environment.

Respiratory control, by encouraging divers to learn to breathe slowly and deeply through the regulator, has been advised by many diving instructors. It has some experimental backing both in reducing the resistance to breathing and as a technique to control the cyclical aggravation of anxiety and hyperventilation. Some divers have automatically adapted their respirations along these lines. In a near panic situation, all divers should adopt this approach by reducing activity and controlling respiration.

'A contented man is one who knows his limitations'. —Old man in a pub

'Know your limitations and dive within them' is a venerable admonition given to new divers. Every diver has certain limitations, and apprehension is felt when he or she perceives that these limitations are being exceeded. Then the first seeds of panic are sown.

FATIGUE

Fatigue is a common contributor to diving deaths (28 per cent) and accidents, resulting from personal, equipment or environmental problems that impose excessive demands on physical effort and result in exhaustion.

Personal factors

Adequate physical fitness is essential in diving activities, which invariably, sooner or later, impose considerable physical demands. Fitness to undertake aquatic activities can be evaluated by reference to both past performance and present capabilities (e.g. swim speeds, breath-holding ability). Age is associated with a reduction of physical fitness (see Chapter 58).

In some situations, even unfit divers are not at risk. In others, even very vigorous, fit divers are sorely tried.

Personality factors are also important. Given the same physical fitness and exercise load, the extrovert diver has more ability to ignore the environmental and physical demands, whereas an introvert is likely to be aware of the development of fatigue earlier. A neurotic diver, or one with high trait anxiety, is more susceptible to fatigue earlier than the more stoic diver.

Many other factors may influence the diver's fitness. Examples include the use of alcohol or drugs, development of seasickness, medical disorders, diving accidents such as decompression sickness, vertigo or disorientation, salt water aspiration and hypothermia.

Equipment

The scuba cylinder, buoyancy compensator and other equipment cause excessive drag with normal swimming. Regulators limit respiration. Protective suits limit chest movement. Greater swimming effort is needed to overcome negative buoyancy. Even experienced divers without assistance who are supporting a 5-kg negative buoyancy (weights held above the water) can remain on the surface for less than 10 minutes before submerging (see Chapter 4).

Environment

Most tidal currents in excess of 1 knot are beyond the capability of many divers for more than a few minutes. Cold exposure and hypothermia aggravate fatigue (see Chapter 5).

FURTHER READING

Bachrach AJ, Egstrom GH. *Stress and Performance in Diving.* San Pedro, California: Best Publishing; 1987.

Edmonds C. *The diver.* Royal Australian Navy (RAN) School of Underwater Medicine report 2/72. Sydney: RAN School of Underwater Medicine; 1972.

Edmonds C. *The Abalone Diver.* Morwell, Australia: National Safety Council of Australia; 1987.

Edmonds C, Walker D. Scuba diving fatalities in Australia and New Zealand. Part 1. *South Pacific Underwater Medicine Society Journal* 1989;**19**(3):94–104.

Egstrom GH. Diving equipment. In: Bove AA, Davis JC, eds. *Diving Medicine.* 2nd ed. Philadelphia: Saunders; 1990.

Egstrom GH, Bachrach AJ. Diving behavior. In: Bove AA, Davis JC, eds. *Bove and Davis' Diving Medicine.* 4th ed. Philadelphia: Saunders; 2004.

Kraft IA. Panic as the primary cause of diving deaths. *Undercurrent* 1977;**May**:8–12.

Morgan WP. Anxiety and panic in recreational scuba divers. *Sports Medicine* 1995;**20**(6):398–421.

Morgan WP, Raglin JS. Psychological considerations in the use of breathing apparatus. In: Lindgren C, ed. *Proceedings of Undersea and Hyperbaric Medical Society Workshop. Physiological and Human Engineering Aspects of Underwater Breathing Apparatus.* Bethesda, Maryland: Undersea and Hyperbaric Medical Society; 1989.

Raglin JS, O'Connor J, Carlson N, Morgan WP. Response to underwater exercise in scuba divers differing in trait anxiety. *Undersea and Hyperbaric Medicine* 1996;**23**(2):77–82.

Reseck J. *SCUBA Safe and Simple.* Englewood Cliffs, New Jersey: Prentice Hall International; 1975.

US Department of the Navy. *Bibliographical Source Books of Compressed Air Diving and Submarine Medicine.* Vols. 1 to 3. Washington, DC: US Department of the Navy; 1948, 1954, 1966.

This chapter was reviewed for this fifth edition by Carl Edmonds.

46

Why divers die: the facts and figures

INTRODUCTION

Despite inherent risks, diving is a relatively safe activity as long as certain conditions are satisfied. These include the following:

- Adequate medical, physical and psychological fitness.
- Appropriate and adequate training.
- Suitable and reliable equipment.
- Adequate experience and preparation.
- The ability to manage prevailing environmental conditions.
- Common sense.

To some extent, the type of diving activity influences the causes of diving fatalities. For example, the risk profile for deep oil rig divers is different from that of navy clearance divers, technical rebreather divers and open-circuit recreational divers. Health issues transcend all divisions.

The following discussion focuses on fatalities in recreational divers.

Historically, participants in recreational diving were mainly experienced breath-hold divers who were generally comfortable in the water and who possessed reasonably sound water survival skills. However, as the greater community has become more aware of the attractions of the underwater world and training has been targeted at a broader sub-set of the population, there has been an increase in the number of divers with relatively poor aquatic skills and sometimes poor health and fitness. In addition, some of the earlier divers who have continued diving have developed medical conditions that may render diving less safe. Unless this situation is carefully managed by appropriate and adequate participant screening, training, supervision and accident management systems, it can be a recipe for unnecessary morbidity and mortality.

As with most activities, whether recreational or occupational, there are many more non-fatal incidents than deaths. For example, a 12-year analysis of recreational dive-related incidents in the United Kingdom recorded a total of 4799 incidents, of which 197 were fatalities[1]. Although the fatality numbers are believed to be reasonably accurate, it is likely that the non-fatal incidents are significantly under-reported because many divers will not take the time to complete such a report. These non-fatal incidents are potentially a far richer source of information, not only because of the greater volume, but also because the protagonist can often provide valuable information, unlike in a fatality. Divers Alert Network (DAN) Asia-Pacific, DAN America and the British Sub-Aqua Club (BSAC) are three of the organizations that collect data on non-fatal recreational diving incidents, as well as fatalities.

DIVING FATALITY DATA COLLECTION

Various organizations and individuals have collected data on diving fatalities. The BSAC has reported diving accidents in the United Kingdom since 1965 and provides annual reports on incidents and fatalities. These reports reveal that 648 dive-related fatalities were recorded between 1965 and 2013 inclusive. This number includes a few snorkellers, but most were scuba divers. John McAniff from the National Underwater Accident Data Centre (NUADC), University of Rhode Island, reported diving fatalities in US waters and of US citizens worldwide from 1970 to 1990. From 1990 to 1994, the reports were compiled and published in collaboration with DAN America, which thereafter took on the responsibility of reporting on recreational diving deaths. The current DAN America reports highlight the deaths of US and Canadian citizens worldwide. There were 4212 reported deaths between 1970 and 2012 inclusive.

In Australia, the publication of diving fatality reporting was formally begun by Bayliss in 1969 and continued with the introduction of Project Stickybeak by Dr Douglas Walker, who single-handedly reported snorkelling and compressed air diving fatalities until 2003, at which time this author (JL) and DAN Asia-Pacific took over responsibility for the project, in collaboration with Dr Walker. Between 1970 and 2013, there were 373 reported scuba diving fatalities (including 11 in rebreather divers). The Australian data also include snorkelling deaths, of which there were an additional 311 during the same period.

Figure 46.1 shows the comparative data for reported scuba deaths from 1970 to 2013 inclusive. There appears to have been an initial downward trend in the United States but no obvious trend thereafter. The fatality rates in the United Kingdom and Australia appear to have been relatively stable (other than in 1972 to 1973 in the United Kingdom, with what appear to have been highly unusual circumstances [or a reporting error]).

WHAT IS THE LIKELIHOOD OF A DIVING FATALITY?

Various researchers have tried to estimate the risk of a diving death. In some places, where fatality reporting is reliable, it is relatively easy to know the number of divers who died during a particular period. However, a risk estimate requires that

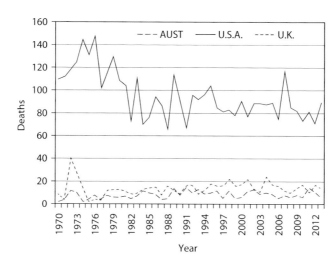

Figure 46.1 Scuba fatalities in the United States, United Kingdom and Australia from 1970 to 2013.

one also knows how many active divers there were during that same period or how many dives were conducted (i.e. the denominator of exposure), and reliable reports of these numbers are usually very difficult to obtain. Some estimates are based on diver activity sample surveys, and these vary in reliability. Some are based on actual recorded activity in a particular locality (e.g. tank fills or actual dives conducted), and these should be more reliable. Some potentially reliable estimates are based on insurance data where the denominator is the number of divers insured and the numerator is the number of deaths among these insured. However, it is possible that insured divers are atypical in that they are often older, among other factors.

Some of the published estimates are shown in Table 46.1[2]. Risk estimates vary from place to place, not only based on the methodology, as described earlier, but also influenced by the diver population (resulting from factors such as age and health), local conditions (i.e. water temperature, currents, tidal movements) and other factors such as local training and standards of diving practice.

Various comparisons are circulated by different parties, but some, possibly more reliable data, indicate that the risk of a recreational scuba diving fatality may be comparable to that of driving a motor vehicle and jogging. However, any such estimate must be used cautiously because of differing measures of exposure.

DIVERS ALERT NETWORK FATALITY REPORTING

In 2008, DAN America introduced sequential analysis ('root cause analysis') for the investigation of diving fatalities, by dividing the cause of each accident into a chain of four sequential events[3]. These are defined as follows:

- *Trigger:* The earliest identifiable event that appeared to transform an unremarkable dive into an emergency.

Table 46.1 Scuba Annual Fatality Rates (AFR)

Group	Denominator	Time period	Rate (95% CI)	
			AFR (per 100,000 divers)	per 100,000 dives
USA, DEMA study (Monaghan 1989)	Estimated	1986	3.4 to 4.2	
Finland (Sipinen 1990)	Measured	1986, 1987	62 (7–117) (1 in 1,600)	
USA (National Safety Council 2004)	Estimated	1989	16.7	0.8 to 1.6
Ontario, Canada (Heinicke 2008)	Survey	1986–95	12.2	
Victoria, Australia (Lippmann 2008)	Tank fill count	1993–94		2.5
Orkney, Scotland (Trevett *et al.* 2001)	Measured	1999–2000		3 to 6
BC, Canada (Ladd *et al.* 2002)	Tank fill count	1999–2000		2.04
Australia (Lippmann 2008)	Survey	2000–06	3.57 (1 in 28,000)	0.57
Japan (Ikeda & Ashida 2000)	Tank fill count			1.0 to 2.4
BSAC (Cumming 2006)	Measured	2000–06	14.4 (10.5–19.7)	0.45[a]
DAN America insured (Denoble et al. 2008)	Measured	2000–06	16.4 (14.4–19.0) (1 in 6,000)	0.7[b]
DAN Europe insured (unpublished)	Measured	1995–2008	71 (59–82) (1 in 4,000)	

Source: Reprinted with some modifications from Denoble PJ, Marroni A, Vann RD. Annual fatality rates and associated risk factors for recreational scuba diving. In: Vann RD, Lang MA, eds. *Recreational Diving Fatalities. Proceedings of the Divers Alert Network 2010 April 8–10 Workshop.* Durham, North Carolina: Divers Alert Network; 2011:73–83.
[a] Average number of dives per member estimated by survey: 32 (Cumming 2006).
[b] Average number of dives per member estimated by survey:25 (Dear 2000).

- *Disabling agent:* A hazardous behaviour or circumstance that was temporally or logically associated with the trigger and perhaps caused the disabling injury.
- *Disabling injury:* An injury directly responsible for death or incapacitation followed by death from drowning.
- *Cause of death:* The cause of death was specified by the medical examiner and could be the same as the disabling injury, or it could be drowning secondary to injury.

The disabling injury is determined using the following (or similar) criteria:

- *Asphyxia:* Asphyxia with or without aspiration of water and with no indication of a prior disabling injury.
- *Cerebral arterial gas embolism (CAGE):* Gas in the cerebral arteries with or without evidence of lung rupture.
- *Cardiac:* Acute episode of chest discomfort signalled by the diver, distress without obvious cause, history of cardiac disease or autopsy findings.
- *Trauma:* Witnessed trauma, traumatic findings at autopsy.
- *Decompression sickness:* Signs or symptoms, autopsy findings.
- *Other:* Stroke, cerebral haemorrhage and other disorders.
- *Unknown:* Body not recovered, no autopsy available, no indications of disabling injury at autopsy.

The use of such a sequential analysis can be illustrated by the following example: A diver runs out of air, makes a rapid ascent to the surface, suffers (CAGE), loses consciousness in the water and subsequently drowns. In this incident, the trigger could be recorded as exhaustion of breathing gas, the disabling agent was a rapid ascent, the disabling injury was CAGE and the cause of death was drowning. Often the disabling injury can be more relevant to the assessment of a diving fatality than the cause of death. The cause of death, in this case drowning, does not provide as accurate an insight into the accident as the fact that the diver suffered from CAGE before drowning.

Such an analysis can often be difficult to perform accurately for several reasons. First, it can sometimes be difficult, albeit impossible, to determine the trigger and/or disabling agent accurately, especially if the incident was unwitnessed. This can lead to some differences in interpretation and classification of events. There could be several triggers. In the foregoing example, the diver may have been suffering from nitrogen narcosis, and this could have been a factor in his running out of air and could be considered an alternative trigger or a co-trigger. Running out of air could potentially be classified as a disabling agent, rather than a trigger.

In addition, the standard of autopsies and the level of diving medical knowledge of forensic pathologists or other medical examiners vary greatly and are often poor. Therefore, important clues to, and sometimes strong evidence of, the disabling injuries and subsequent causes of death are often missed. However, despite these limitations, the sequential analysis, if sensibly considered, can provide a useful tool in the analysis of diving-related deaths.

Application of the sequential analysis

The following discussion provides an overview of the victims and their activity at the time of the incident. These data are based on 947 scuba deaths reported by DAN America (1992 to 2003)[3], 351 compressed gas deaths reported by DAN Asia-Pacific from 1972 to 2005[4] (mostly recreational scuba but including 62 surface supply and 1 case where the equipment was unknown) and 140 deaths reported by BSAC (1998 to 2009)[1]. Initially, summaries of the sequential analyses from the United States and Australia are presented, followed by a discussion of the various factors associated with these analyses and those identified in the UK data.

TRIGGERS

In the US report, triggers were identified in 346 of the incidents (37 per cent). These were reported as insufficient gas (41 per cent), entrapment (20 per cent), equipment problems (15 per cent), rough water (10 per cent), trauma (7 per cent), buoyancy trouble (5 per cent) and inappropriate gas (2 per cent).

In the Australian study, the triggers identified in 292 cases were classified as equipment related (18 per cent), gas supply related (18 per cent), rough water (16 per cent), anxiety/ stress (11 per cent), exertion (11 per cent), buoyancy trouble (5 per cent), other and unknown (the latter two were combined for the analysis and contributed to 21 per cent of the total). This information is shown in Figure 46.2.

When one compares the two series, there are some differences in the classification. For example, trauma in the Australian series (usually from shark attack or boat propeller injury) was classified as a disabling agent rather than a trigger.

DISABLING AGENTS

The disabling agents identified in 332 deaths in the US series included emergency ascent (55 per cent), insufficient gas (27 per cent) and buoyancy trouble (13 per cent). Those disabling agents identified in 313 cases in the Australian series were gas supply related (26 per cent), ascent related (21 per cent), cardiovascular disease or other medical condition (19 per cent), buoyancy related (12 per cent), entrapment (11 per cent), trauma (3 per cent) and other (8 per cent).

DISABLING INJURIES

Disabling injuries were identified in 590 incidents (62 per cent) in the US report and in 311 of the deaths in Australia (89 per cent). A comparison of these injuries is shown in Table 46.2.

Asphyxia (defined as a condition arising when the body is deprived of oxygen, thus causing unconscious or death) was the most common disabling injury reported in both data sets. Unsurprisingly, triggers associated with this included insufficient gas, entrapment, equipment problems, rough water and buoyancy problems. The higher proportion of asphyxia identified in the Australian series may result in part from the 20 years of earlier data included in this set. As evidenced in the Australian report, earlier deaths involved a higher incidence of equipment problems or lack of appropriate equipment, younger divers with fewer cardiac issues and possibly an increased likelihood of forensic pathologists in the past to assume that a death in the water was primarily caused by asphyxia/drowning (a belief that is still common in many places).

CAUSES OF DEATH

Although the causes of death as certified by the forensic pathologists or medical examiners were

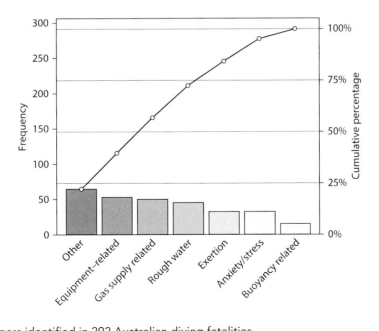

Figure 46.2 Triggers identified in 292 Australian diving fatalities.

Table 46.2 Comparison of disabling injuries (per cent) from US and Australian data

Disabling injury	USA (%)	Australia (%)
Asphyxia	33	49
CAGE	29	25
Cardiac	27	18
Trauma	4	5
DCS	2.5	1
Inappropriate gas	2.5	not reported
Other	2	2

not included in the US report (likely because the disabling injury was seen as more relevant by the researchers, as explained earlier), these causes were provided in the Australian report on the basis of 315 cases and were drowning (56 per cent), CAGE/pulmonary barotrauma (21 per cent), cardiac (16 per cent), trauma (4.5 per cent), decompression sickness (1 per cent) and others (1.5 per cent). The difference between 56 per cent drowning and 49 per cent asphyxia as the disabling injury may reflect cases where drowning was assessed in the study to have been secondary to an injury such as CAGE.

RISK FACTORS FOR DIVING FATALITIES

Numerous risk factors for diving deaths are identified through sequential analysis and various other means of reporting. Some of these are discussed in the following paragraphs and include personal factors, as well as factors directly related to the dive itself and equipment used.

Personal risk factors

AGE

The median age reported in the US series was 43 years, and in Australia it was 34 years (with a mean of 35.8). Sixteen per cent of the Australian fatalities between 1972 and 2005 occurred in divers 50 years old or older. The age of these victims increased steadily at a rate of about 0.5 years per calendar year during this period, from a mean of

around 25 years in 1972 to just over 40 years by 2005. However, more recent data show that, from 2001 to 2009 inclusive, the proportion of victims who were more than 50 years old had risen to more than 35 per cent[5]. This no doubt partly reflects the ageing of existing divers and the enlistment of older divers, but it may also indicate an increased risk for older divers who are well represented in cardiac-related fatalities, as discussed later.

The BSAC study calculated the ratios of the age of the victims to the number of divers in the general diving population in that age range, as identified in an earlier diving activity survey. This showed an increased risk for divers more than 50 years old, and the risk rose very substantially for divers more than 60 years old.

An analysis of DAN America insurance data indicated that 31 per cent of the fatalities in insured members occurred in divers 50 years old or older, and the fatality rates on a per diver basis increased with age for both genders[6].

GENDER

In the Australian series, 88 per cent of the victims were male and 12 per cent female, but the proportion of female deaths increased from 7 per cent in 1972 to 22 per cent in 2005. This was very likely a reflection of the increased participation of women in the sport. According to more recent Professional Association of Diving Instructors (PADI) certification ASDD "data"[7] and DAN America diving activity data[8], approximately one third of divers are women.

The analysis of the DAN America insurance data revealed that the relative risk for male divers in their 30s was six times greater than for female divers in the same age range. This difference diminished with increasing age and, by the age of 60 years, the death rates in both genders were similar.[6]

HEALTH FACTORS

Various medical, physical and psychological conditions have been shown to, or are believed to, increase the risk of an accident while scuba diving (and snorkelling). These are discussed in detail elsewhere in this book but include cardiac conditions, diabetes, respiratory, neurological and cerebrovascular conditions and conditions affecting a diver's mobility in the water.

The reality is that many divers continue to dive with known or occult medical conditions. For example, DAN Asia-Pacific membership records for 2012 indicated that in excess of 10 per cent of its members are diving despite admitted histories of asthma, diabetes, cardiac disease, hypertension and a broad range of other conditions. This information was provided for insurance purposes and is likely significantly underreported.

A 2003 survey of 346 Australian divers indicated that 10.4 per cent had past or current asthma, the same percentage had hypertension or coronary artery disease and one fourth reported past or current psychological symptoms[9].

A 2007 survey, which included 550 certified divers in the United States, found that one third of the respondents reported having a pre-existing medical condition (for which more than one third of these did not seek diving medical advice)[10]. The conditions included hypertension (42 per cent), asthma (18 per cent), diabetes (7 per cent), musculoskeletal disorders (3 per cent), heart disease (3 per cent) and epilepsy (1 per cent), among others. Interestingly, no significant differences were observed in reported injuries in this group based on pre-existing medical conditions. The respondents had a mean age of 44 years and mean dive experience of 12.6 years, and, as with many surveys, there is a risk of selection bias.

Despite the increasingly apparent incidence of medical conditions in divers, most fatality reports show comparatively little evidence of deaths directly attributable to such conditions other than those that are cardiac related. There have certainly been reports of fatalities caused by conditions such as the following: epilepsy; stroke; respiratory conditions such as asthma, chronic obstructive pulmonary disease, the presence of lung cysts or scarring; and, more recently, immersion pulmonary oedema because it has been better recognized. However, despite the concern about these conditions, verified deaths attributable directly to these disorders do not appear to be common, likely in part because of the difficulty of detection and/or indicating causality at autopsy.

Somewhat an exception to this is a series of 100 scuba diving deaths in Australia and New Zealand that was published in 1990[11]. The researchers had access to detailed information about the fatalities, generally including autopsy reports, witness reports and medical histories. Table 46.3 provides a summary of some of the medical conditions that were thought to have been 'probable' or 'likely' contributors to these deaths. However, some of these assertions (e.g. the contribution of asthma as a causative factor in the deaths of some of the victims with a history of asthma) have been questioned and remain the subject of debate.

Autopsy data for the victims included in the US fatality series revealed the presence of pre-existing medical conditions, as shown in Table 46.4. Some victims had multiple conditions. Medical conditions included those that were previous, current or indicated by reported medications. Conditions were reported only if positive indications existed, and this stipulation was believed to have led to underreporting. In many cases, no causal relationship was evident, especially with conditions that were not cardiac related.

Cardiac-related fatalities

Although fatalities involving various other medical conditions are not commonly reported, deaths identified as having primary cardiac-related causes have been increasingly cited, especially in more recent years. Just over 26 per cent of the deaths reported in the US study appeared to have been precipitated by a cardiac condition. Although the long-term Australian study reported an overall incidence of 18 per cent between 1972 and 2005, this incidence had risen steadily throughout the study period. Australian data from 2004 to 2009 inclusive indicate that between 28 and 38 per cent of the deaths during that period appear to have been caused by a cardiac incident[5].

The BSAC data indicate that the deaths of 36 of the 140 victims were believed to have been caused by pre-existing medical conditions, which included 'a few strokes' but were mainly cardiac related.

Diving involves potential cardiac stressors, including unaccustomed exertion, anxiety, breathing resistance and restriction from equipment,

Table 46.3 Some medical contributors to
100 deaths

Condition	Pre-existing (%)	Fatal dive (%)
Panic	—	39
Fatigue	—	28
Vomiting	1	10
Narcosis	—	9
Drugs	8[a]	7
Severe lack of physical fitness	4	4
Severe disability	3	3
Severe visual loss	3	3
Alcohol	—	2
Motion sickness	2	2
Gross obesity	8[a]	2
Carotid sinus reflex	—	1
Salt water aspiration	—	37
Pulmonary barotrauma	—	13
Cardiac disease	3	12
Asthma	9	8
Respiratory disease (non-asthma)	5	7
Hypothermia	—	3
Hyperthermia	8[a]	2
Ear problems	2	2
Diabetes	1	1
Epilepsy	1	0

Some divers had multiple conditions.
Source: From Edmonds C, Walker D. Scuba diving fatalities in Australia and New Zealand: 1. The human factor. *South Pacific Underwater Medicine Society Journal* 1990;**19**(3):94–104.
[a] Not considered as contributing factors, but included because other co-related disorders coexisted.

Table 46.4 Medical history of victims in the United States: 1992 to 2003

Condition	Incidence (%)
Cardiovascular disease	27
Diabetes	4
Asthma	3
Respiratory	3
Seizure history	1

autonomic cardiogenic reflexes as part of the diving reflex, the effects of cold and pulmonary and cardiac reflexes triggered by inhalation of, or immersion in, water. Most of the divers who died of cardiac causes were men more than 40 years old, and the deaths were generally 'silent'. Sometimes there was evidence of an infarct, but often the deaths were believed to have been a result of a cardiac dysrhythmia. Although there is no direct evidence of dysrhythmias at autopsy, the diagnosis was generally made on the basis of the presence of substantial coronary disease, witness reports, history and lack of evidence of other possible causes (see Chapter 39).

STRESS RESPONSES, PANIC AND FATIGUE

There has been little research on the relationship between various mental disorders and diving. However, it seems obvious that conditions affecting cognition and decision making have the potential to compromise diving safety.

Some of the disorders of concern include anxiety, phobias, panic disorders, depression, schizophrenia, bipolar disorder and narcolepsy. These are discussed in Chapter 41. However, in addition to concerns about the possible impact of the disorders themselves, various medications are used to treat these conditions, and, therefore, the potential effects of these medications, singly, or in combination, have raised additional concerns, as discussed in Chapter 43.

The stress syndromes can be based on psychological and physical unfitness, drug intake, medical problems and inadequate training and inexperience.

Anxiety can be readily provoked in the diving environment and can easily lead to panic, which is often associated with diving accidents and fatalities.

Panic is a psychological stress reaction evolving from anxiety. The threat of death is a reasonable cause of anxiety. Under selected circumstances, anyone will panic. In diving-related deaths, difficulty in obtaining air and the inhalation of water are often associated with panic.

Panic also occurs when a diver finds himself or herself in unfamiliar circumstances, such as greater than customary depth, compromised air supply, buoyancy problems, being left alone, poor visibility and/or disorientation, strong water movement, challenging surface conditions or equipment malfunction or perceived malfunction such as overbreathing a regulator or snorkel.

The consequences include rapid ascents and inappropriate actions, such as abandoning a regulator, snorkel or mask, and a failure to respond appropriately, such as by ditching weights or inflating buoyancy compensator devices (BCDs).

Panic was reported in approximately one fifth of the deaths involving emergency ascents in the US series, and it sometimes caused aspiration or increased gas consumption. In the Australian series, anxiety/stress was believed to have been a trigger in 11 per cent of the cases. Interestingly, there was a positive association between female gender and the anxiety/stress-related trigger.

Fatigue is a physiological stress reaction to muscular effort that was often underestimated by the victims. With sufficient physical demand, anyone can become fatigued. Salt water aspiration, panic and cardiac disease all occurred more frequently than would be expected in these cases.

Fatigue often develops when a diver is cold or overweighted or during an attempt to swim against a current. The last situation is especially noticed when the victim swims against the equipment drag, if overweighted and with an inflated BCD. Fatigue is more likely in, but certainly not restricted to, those who are physically unfit or disabled. Panic, water aspiration, cardiac disorder and asthma may be precipitated (Case Report 46.1)[18].

EXPERIENCE

There is little doubt that experience plays an important part in a diver's ability to make appropriate judgements and take suitable actions to prevent or deal with an incident. Frequent exposure helps to maintain a diver's skills and comfort. However, even highly experienced divers sometimes come to grief after making errors, thus exceeding their abilities or equipment or health capabilities.

In the US accident reports, diving experience was characterized according to case report estimates of the number of dives in the past year, the total reported lifetime dives and the annual diving frequency. A 'novice' diver was defined as having fewer than 20 lifetime dives, an 'occasional' diver as having more than 20 lifetime dives but fewer

than 20 in the past year and a 'frequent' diver as having more than 50 lifetime dives and more than 20 in the past year. The resultant data are shown in Table 46.5.

Unfortunately, the fatality reports on which the Australian review was based did not use an objective measure to record the experience of the victim. Instead, their level of experience was based on statements by the buddy or family. This made the determination of experience highly subjective and difficult to compare, except for those divers who had no experience.

In the UK study, in 9 per cent of deaths, inexperience was considered the primary causal factor.

Deaths during training

In the Australian series, 16 per cent of the victims died on their first dive, under instruction, alone or with a friend. In a 2010 paper, PADI reported that, over a 20-year period, there was a death rate of 1.765 per 100000 divers during diver training[12]. Some injuries and deaths during training are inevitable because individuals of unknown compatibility with diving are pitted against, and learning to adapt to, the potentially hostile environment. Unforeseen circumstances, medical factors, human error, carelessness, ignorance and occasionally negligence can intervene, and a student comes to serious harm.

It is incumbent on the instructor to make every effort to make this experience as safe as possible for the student. Training agencies have standards that their instructors are obliged to adhere to, and these include guidelines on training, ratios, equipment and various other factors. Ratios are set for ideal conditions and should be reduced accordingly if conditions are less than ideal (e.g. low visibility or current). There are tragic reports of the consequences of failure to do so (Case Report 46.2).

Dive-related risk factors

DIVE PURPOSE

The reports reviewed are mainly for recreational diving, although the Australian data also included some working divers, such as abalone divers. They also include some instructors who died while leading dives.

CASE REPORT 46.1

This victim was a 50-year-old man who had certified as a diver 5 years earlier and had logged approximately 75 dives, mostly shore dives in temperate waters. He also held Advanced Open Water and Nitrox certifications. The victim suffered from lumbo-sacral spondylosis as a result of a work injury and was being treated for hypertension and proteinuria, managed with telmisartan. He was taking rabeprazole sodium for gastro-oesophageal reflux. He also suffered from idiopathic lymphoedema and had been hospitalized on three occasions for cellulitis in his legs. He had given up smoking 2 years earlier and now went to the gymnasium about four times a week to help manage his spondylosis, swam regularly and appeared to be relatively fit although 'solid looking and carrying a bit of fat'. An electrocardiogram taken after an episode of chest pain a year earlier indicated 'normal tracing other than bradycardia' (48 beats/minute). He had been certified fit to dive 3 months earlier by a doctor trained in dive medicine. This medical examination was sought because the diver was planning to upgrade his diving qualifications and was keen to become an instructor eventually.

He was now enrolled in a Rescue Diver course and was participating in some surface rescue drills. The group consisted of an instructor, an assistant instructor and four students. It was windy (gusts of up to 40 knots), but they dived from the shore in an area sheltered by a long breakwater and where the water was relatively calm. The victim was wearing a mask, snorkel and fins, a semi-drysuit, hood, boots and gloves, buoyancy compensator device with cylinder, a regulator with 'octopus', dive computer and gauge and a weight belt with six weights (weight unreported). The water temperature was 12°C. The group was in the water approximately 50 metres from shore and had been doing surface rescue tows for about 20 minutes. The depth was 2 to 3 msw. The victim had acted as both the rescuer (required to tow another diver about 30 metres) and the rescuee, which was the last role he had undertaken. He had not submerged at any time during the exercise. Shortly after completing a briefing, the instructors heard thrashing in the water and realized that it was from the victim, who was about 2 metres distant and floating on his back. One of the other students turned to him and asked if he was 'OK', which he said he was. However, he then began thrashing and turning over in the water before becoming motionless, face-down. When one of the instructors went to him and rolled him over, the victim was unresponsive with froth coming from his mouth, although he appeared to be breathing. While the instructors and another diver towed the victim toward the rocks, he appeared to have a seizure and became apnoeic and cyanotic. One of the rescuers commenced mouth-to-mask rescue breathing as they towed the victim.

Once they reached shore, the instructors began basic life support while one of the students went to call an ambulance. When the ambulance arrived 16 minutes later, the paramedics initially had considerable trouble drying the victim's chest sufficiently for the defibrillator pads to adhere. When this was achieved, the victim was found to be asystolic. An intravenous line was established, and he was intubated and given 5 mg of adrenaline intravenously (5 × 1 mg). After about 15 minutes, a shockable rhythm appeared, and he was given three shocks and transported to hospital, where he was later pronounced dead. When tested, his equipment was found to be functioning correctly, his cylinder was full and the air met appropriate purity standards.

Autopsy: The heart weighed 498 g (normal range [NR], 400 ± 69 g) and had a normal external contour. There was an area of congestion in the posterior basal left ventricular wall. The left ventricular myocardium and right ventricular myocardium measured 16 mm (concentrically) and 6 mm in thickness, respectively. There was severe atherosclerosis with up to 80 per cent stenosis of the left anterior descending coronary artery, 90 per cent stenosis of the first diagonal branch and 90 per cent stenosis of the left circumflex coronary artery. The right coronary artery showed mild atheroma. The upper and lower airways were free of debris and foreign material. The lungs were congested. The right lung and left lung weighed 914 g and 647 g, respectively (NR, 663 ± 217 g, 569 ± 221 g). The brain weighed 1365 g (NR, 1423 ± 161 g) and was normal. The right kidney and left kidney weighed 157 g and 141 g, respectively (NR, 169 ± 37 g, 174 ± 35 g) and appeared unremarkable macroscopically. Histology of the heart showed widespread vacuolation of the myocytes but no acute infarction or fibrosis. Renal histology showed occasional sclerosed glomeruli, a patchy interstitial lymphocytic infiltrate and slightly hypercellular intact glomeruli consistent with the history of previous renal disease. The cause of death was given as ischaemic heart disease (likely cardiac arrhythmia). *Toxicology:* alcohol undetected (<10 mg/100 mL).

Comments: It is likely that the substantial exertion of the rescue exercises triggered an arrhythmia in this susceptible diver. What this case highlights is that even those middle-aged divers who ostensibly have a good exercise tolerance and who exercise regularly can have occult severe coronary disease. The role of screening tests in divers of this age remains controversial because of the high false-positive rates and complications of the invasive investigations. One hopes that technologies such as magnetic resonance imaging angiograms may enable non-invasive evaluation of the coronary vessels in individuals such as this. The rescuers acted swiftly and appropriately, unfortunately to no avail.

Summary: history of spondylosis, hypertension, proteinuria, reflux, idiopathic lymphoedema and cellulitis; experienced diver; exercised regularly; recent dive medical examination; doing rescue training on surface; suffered seizure and became unconscious; cardiac death.

Sequential analysis: trigger: exertion; disabling agent: cardiovascular disease; disabling injury: cardiac incident; cause of death; cardiac-related.

From Lippmann J, Lawrence C, Wodak T, Fock A, Jamieson S. Provisional report on diving-related fatalities in Australian waters 2009. *Diving and Hyperbaric Medicine* 2013;**43**(4):194-217.

Table 46.5 Experience of diving victims (United States and Australia)

Experience level	Per cent (%)	Experience level	Per cent (%)
United States		**Australia**	
Frequent	18	Experienced	44
Occasional	22	Inexperienced	37
Novice	28	None	16
Unknown	32	Unknown	3

CASE REPORT 46.2

This victim was a 20-year-old female, apparently healthy, foreign national who was studying in Australia. She was described as an 'inexperienced swimmer'. She and some friends booked an introductory scuba dive. At the dive shop, she completed the required paperwork and did not declare any medical conditions. She was fitted with a wetsuit.

A dive briefing (in English) was given during the 20-minute boat trip to the dive site. Once at the site, the victim was in a group of four with her friends, under the supervision of one of two instructors.

The 'students' entered the water and floated on the surface supported by their buoyancy compensator devices (BCDs) and holding onto a rope at the boat's stern. The victim was wearing a mask, snorkel, fins, a 5-mm wetsuit and reportedly a weight belt with 9.5 kg of weights.

The group swam on the surface to shallow water near the shore of a small island, where they were taught basic skills while standing or swimming in water of a depth of around 1.5 msw. The sea was reportedly choppy, and waves disrupted the training from time to time. The visibility was reported to have ranged from 1 to 1.5 metres, described as 'cloudy from recent rains', and there was a current. When satisfied with their skills, the instructor led the group into deeper water to a depth of around 2.5 msw. The students 'crawled along the bottom' in a line, with the instructor just ahead, reportedly checking them regularly. The instructor could see the faces of the students but not their entire bodies. After one check, the instructor noticed that the victim was missing and ascended to the surface with the rest of the group. The instructor then called to the boat driver that a diver was missing, told the students to swim to the shore and then began a search.

Before the group surfaced, witnesses saw the victim surface alone, call for help and then apparently sink. The lookout jumped into the water to find her but was unable to see her in the cloudy water. The other instructor located the victim on the sea bed about 40 minutes later. She was unconscious and apnoeic, with the regulator still in her mouth. He brought her to the surface and onto a police boat, where basic life support was performed by police for 15 to 20 minutes on the way to the boat ramp. There, ambulance paramedics took over resuscitation and continued en route to hospital, where the victim was pronounced dead on arrival. On inspection, the regulator mouthpiece was found to be perforated, thus potentially enabling water aspiration.

Autopsy: unavailable.

Comments: This was likely a very avoidable tragedy. Although the standards under which the instructor was operating allow a maximum ratio of four students to one instructor on this programme, the instructor is advised to reduce this ratio in the event of adverse conditions, including poor visibility, rough water and/or current. Had this instructor done so, it would have been easier to monitor fewer students. The conduct of such a dive with the instructor swimming in front of the students can increase the likelihood of separation. Introductory dives are better conducted with participants holding hands, linking arms or swimming in formations that enable the instructor to see all the divers at all times. It appears that the student was likely to have been overweighted, and this would have made it difficult for her to remain on the surface without inflating her BCD and/or ditching her weight belt, something that she would have had little or no training in. Even if she had been told about weight belt ditching, it might well not have been absorbed, given all else that was happening, possibly magnified by a language problem.

Although the actual timings were unavailable to these reviewers, it would be interesting to know how much time was spent in the shallows learning and practising the basic skills before setting off on the actual dive. It seems that it may have been minimal. It is important to provide adequate time to enable the students to learn and practise the essential skills and to feel comfortable enough to participate further. Language difficulties may also have affected the briefing and training adversely in this instance. Finally, if the perforation in the mouthpiece caused the victim to aspirate water, it would likely have increased anxiety.

Summary: apparently healthy; weak swimmer; introductory scuba dive; some chop and current and poor visibility; ratio of four students to one instructor; relatively little training/orientation time; overweighted; perforation in mouthpiece; separation; probable drowning or cerebral arterial gas embolism.

Sequential analysis: trigger: unknown; disabling agent: unknown; disabling injury: unknown; cause of death: unknown.

From Lippmann J, Lawrence C, Wodak T, Fock A, Jamieson S. Provisional report on diving-related fatalities in Australian waters 2009. *Diving and Hyperbaric Medicine* 2013;**43**(4):194-217.

In the US series, the main activities were sight-seeing (45 per cent), training (14 per cent), hunting and harvesting seafood (13 per cent) and wreck diving (12 per cent). Five per cent were reported to be working at the time of their death.

In the Australian series, 54 per cent of the deaths were recorded as during recreation, 16 per cent while collecting seafood (most of these involved shark attacks while collecting abalone, crayfish or scallops), training (8 per cent), cave diving (4 per cent) and resort diving (2 per cent).

GAS SUPPLY

Despite the improvements in equipment, the almost universal use of contents gauges and redundant second stages, gas supply emergencies remain common. This is often a result of lack of attention, often through inexperience, sometimes at depth where gas supply is consumed more quickly and attention may be impaired by narcosis. Other causes include poor dive planning and equipment failure. Additionally, entrapment by weed, lines or nets or in a cave or wreck often leads to exhaustion of gas supply unless help is readily at hand.

Occasionally, a diver dies as a result of failing to open the cylinder valve sufficiently, or at all, before entering the water. This is often because the valve had been opened earlier and then closed with pressure remaining in the lines and indicated on the contents gauge.

Insufficient gas accounted for 41 per cent of the triggers in the US series and 27 per cent of the disabling agents and, as expected, was highly associated with drowning and CAGE. Inappropriate gas (e.g. hyperoxic, hypoxic and carbon monoxide) was reported as a causative factor in 1 per cent of the deaths in that series.

Gas supply problems were believed to have been the trigger in 18 per cent of the Australian deaths and included exhaustion of supply, contamination, supply interruption and inappropriate gas. They were also cited as the disabling agents in 26 per cent of cases. Figure 46.3 shows the remaining gas for these divers.

Running out of gas was determined to be the primary cause in 8.5 per cent of the UK diving fatalities.

EQUIPMENT

Problems with equipment can arise from a torn mask or fin strap, a sticking BCD inflator-deflator, regulator malfunction, cylinder O-ring 'blow-out', burst hose, or scrubber failure in a rebreather, among a variety of other causes. Some of these problems can be easily overcome by adequate training and preparedness, including equipment redundancy, but others can be catastrophic, especially in the less experienced diver or one without appropriate equipment redundancy or relatively easy access to the surface.

Many divers have come to grief as a result of panic after breaking a mask strap, or failure to cope with the loss of a fin resulting from a torn or disconnected strap. Adequate checking and

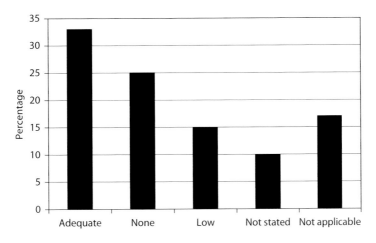

Figure 46.3 Remaining gas status (Australia).

maintenance of equipment are essential to safe diving. This applies to all equipment, but it is especially important when using equipment such as a rebreather, in which correct sensor and scrubber functions are vital. It can pay to be obsessive when using these devices.

Equipment problems were thought to be the trigger for 18 per cent of the Australian accidents. These included sticky BCD inflators, broken mask and fin straps, drysuit blow-up, tank slippage and weight belt detachment. Equipment faults appear to have contributed to the deaths of 12 per cent of the victims in the United Kingdom.

In the United States, equipment trouble was reported to have contributed to 11 per cent of the fatalities in the following proportions: BCD, 3 per cent; breathing apparatus, 2 per cent; diving suit or dress, 1 per cent; gas supply, 1 percent; mask or fins, 1 per cent; and multiple problems, 3 per cent.

The US series does not specify the type of breathing apparatus used by the victims. However, DAN America annual reports for fatalities in 2005 and 2006 indicate that the majority of victims in those years had been using open-circuit systems (92 per cent and 88 per cent, respectively), and rebreather users comprised 8 per cent and 10 per cent, respectively[13,14].

In the United Kingdom, 14 per cent of the victims were using rebreathers, and there were 11 deaths reported in rebreather users in the Australian group (3 per cent). The fatality rate in rebreather users is increasing over time with the increase in usage. A 2013 review of the 181 reported deaths in recreational divers using closed-circuit rebreathers that occurred worldwide from 1998 to 2010 inclusive estimated that the fatality rate for closed-circuit rebreather users was about 10 times that of recreational divers using open-circuit systems. The author of the review also suggested that closed-circuit rebreathers have a 25-fold increased risk of component failure compared with mani-folded twin-cylinder open-circuit systems. It was suggested that this risk could be partly offset by carrying a redundant 'bail-out' system[15].

BUOYANCY

Control of buoyancy and appropriate weighting are very important parts of diving and are often not taught and/or learned adequately during initial training. Some instructors intentionally overweight students during training in the hope that this will prevent them from floating mid-water and so enable better control for the instructor. However, this can create bad habits for the diver and also can make it extremely difficult for a panicking diver, student or otherwise, to reach or remain on the surface if required. This overweighting has certainly led to fatalities during training and thereafter.

Being overweighted creates extra drag and consequent exertion, increases breathing gas consumption and, if the diver is swimming near the bottom, can reduce visibility. Lack of appropriate buoyancy control can also cause disorientation in the water; it often leads to barotrauma of descent and sometimes uncontrolled ascent, with the risk of pulmonary barotrauma and the possibility of CAGE. Problems with drysuit inflation and loss of buoyancy control secondary to deployment of a surface marker buoy are not uncommon, and inadvertent release of a weight belt or integrated weights sometimes occurs, with potentially serious consequences.

In the US analysis, buoyancy trouble was reported in 31 per cent of cases, with 11 per cent being negative, 1 per cent positive, 4 per cent variable and 15 per cent unspecified. The Australian study cited buoyancy problems as triggers in 5 per cent of deaths and as disabling agents in 12 per cent. The British study reported that in about 13 per cent of the cases, poor buoyancy control was the primary causal factor in the incident (about half of the divers were too light and the rest too heavy).

Weights management

In Chapter 48, the importance of an unconscious diver's reaching the surface quickly or remaining on the surface is highlighted. This means that the diver needs to attain sufficient positive buoyancy by inflating the BCD and/or ditching weights, and ditching weights is the only alternative if the gas supply is exhausted. Although usually mentioned during training, ditching weights is often not practised sufficiently, if at all.

Almost three fourths of the divers who died in Australia were found with their weights in place. This finding highlights the ongoing problem that divers are reluctant, or unable, to ditch their weights when they get into trouble. It is likely that, on many occasions, by the time a stricken diver recognizes the need to ditch the weights, he or she may be too incapacitated to do so, especially if this is not an embedded reaction from training and practice. On some occasions, the diver was unable to ditch the weight belt because it was positioned underneath, or entangled with, other equipment.

Table 46.6 shows the BCD management of the victims in Australia. The high percentage of divers who were not wearing BCDs is mainly from the earlier part of the reporting period, when fewer divers wore these valuable devices. In fact, the proportion of victims not wearing BCDs declined from 80 per cent in 1972 to 10 per cent in 2005, although half of the victims in 2005 had not inflated their BCDs. Overall, 36 per cent of the victims failed to inflate their BCDs.

DEPTH

Deeper diving appears to be increasing in popularity, partly because of the flexibility enabled by use of dive computers, the increase in technical diving and greater access to potentially deeper sites. Deeper diving undoubtedly carries higher potential risks with associated increased breathing gas consumption and narcosis, among other factors. A report on dive accidents within the US Navy indicated that the accident rate (not just fatalities) for dives between 30 and 61 metres (101 to 200 feet) was more than double the rate between 15 and 30 metres (50 to 100 feet), and it was nine times that of shallow dives[16]. Although this report

Table 46.6 Buoyancy compensator device management

BCD	Per cent (%) occurrence
Not inflated	36
Not worn	32
Inflated	9
Part inflated	6
Faulty	4
Buddy inflated	3
Not applicable	1
Not stated	9

BCD, buoyancy compensator device

is relatively old and is not based on recreational diving, it provides some sobering reflection. However, recreational dive accidents often occur in relatively shallow water, especially with less experienced divers, and many accidents occur at the surface.

The 2008 DAN America diving activity data reveal that 30 per cent of reported dives were to depths greater than 27 metres (90 feet), an increase from 20 per cent in 2004. Of the 48 reported fatalities that year, 27 per cent occurred at depths greater than 36 metres (120 feet), in itself providing no clear indication of increased risk. The median depth for fatal dives was 18 metres (60 feet)[14].

In the Australian series, half of the victims appear to have gotten into trouble in the first 10 metres (33 feet), with 27 per cent of the total incidents occurring at the surface. In contrast, the BSAC data for 140 deaths indicate that 38 per cent occurred at depths deeper than 40 metres (132 feet), whereas, according to its earlier activity survey, only 11 per cent of diving takes place in this range. The higher incidence in the United Kingdom is probably largely the result of the more challenging diving conditions with cold water, poor visibility and often rough surface conditions. Nitrogen narcosis was reported to be the primary causal factor in 5 of 140 deaths (3.5 per cent).

BUDDY STATUS

Some divers choose to dive solo, preferring the solitude and freedom from considering the needs of, or monitoring, a companion. This may well be fine unless a serious problem develops. Although diving with a buddy does not guarantee that assistance will be at hand, the presence of a buddy has the potential to increase the likelihood of help when required and reduce the time to rescue and first aid management. However, in reality, the 'buddy system' often fails, and divers often separate before or when a problem develops (Case Report 46.3). Separation can occur for a variety of reasons, including buoyancy problems, poor visibility, gas supply problems where one diver is forced to ascend without being able to communicate with the buddy, distraction, the need to monitor multiple buddies rather than a single diver and subsequent confusion about who is monitoring whom or simply lack of attention. When one buddy is leading another,

CASE REPORT 46.3

This victim, a 48-year-old man, was a non-drinker and non-smoker, had no known health conditions and played golf regularly. He had been certified as a diver for many years but dived infrequently. In this case he had not been diving for between 6 and 18 months before his accident. He had previously been a snorkel and lifesaving instructor, so he was presumably a competent swimmer.

At about a 10-msw depth during descent, one of the victim's fins came off and floated to the surface. His buddy ascended to retrieve the fin and then brought it to him. While he was trying to replace the fin, the victim's other fin came off, and the victim then indicated that he would surface and replace the fins there. The buddy then descended to join the other divers.

Some 10 minutes later, the driver of the boat saw the victim surface and wave a fin to attract attention. However, the victim soon submerged again and was out of sight, with no visible bubbles. He was later found at a depth of 21 msw, unconscious, with his regulator displaced. A cable from a fishing net was tangled around his waist, and his weight belt was in place. When brought onto the boat, the victim was unconscious and apnoeic. Cardiopulmonary resuscitation was commenced but proved unsuccessful.

Autopsy: There was blood-stained frothy fluid in the nostrils and in the trachea. The lungs (right, 698 g; left, 632 g) were congested and oedematous. The heart (417 g) showed borderline left ventricular hypertrophy (15 mm). There was a 5-mm segment of myocardial bridging (the artery dives into the myocardium for a distance of 5 mm before returning to the surface) at the middle part of the left anterior descending branch. More significantly, there was a focal atheromatous stenosis at the proximal end of the bridging, up to about 60 per cent occlusion and focal myocardial scarring. The cause of death was drowning, based on the history and findings of the lungs.

Comments: Coronary narrowing of 75 per cent is generally used as the best statistical break point for attributing death to coronary artery stenosis. However, a lesser stenosis may cause sudden cardiac death during exertion or in the presence of left ventricular hypertrophy.

The presence of a 60 per cent focal stenosis of the left anterior descending coronary artery just proximal to the start of the short segment of myocardial bridging and associated scarring of the myocardium led the pathologist reasonably to suggest that a cardiac arrhythmia could have preceded the drowning.

It is possible that this accident could have been averted or reduced in severity had the victim and his buddy remained together to replace the fins. It is also unfortunate that the victim failed to inflate his buoyancy compensator device and/or release his weight belt, thus enabling him to remain on the surface. It is possible that he suffered a cardiac arrhythmia, causing him to become unconscious, sink and drown, although this is speculative. He may also have aspirated water while trying to stay on the surface with no fins or buoyancy aid. It is not clear from the reports whether he was likely to have become entangled before or after losing consciousness.

Sequential analysis: trigger: loss of fins (equipment related); disabling agent: buoyancy related? cardiovascular disease?; disabling injury: asphyxia? cardiac related?; cause of death: drowning.

From Lippmann J, Lawrence C. Diving-related fatalities in Hong Kong Waters, 2006–2009. *Undersea and Hyperbaric Medicine* 2012;**39**(5):895–904.

the diver in front can easily lose contact with the follower unless he or she checks regularly. Once separation has occurred, the immediate benefit of having a buddy is gone. However, separation may well alert a more conscientious buddy to a problem and initiate a search and possible rescue or recovery faster than it would otherwise occur.

Figure 46.4 shows the buddy status of the victims included in the Australian series. Sixty-five per cent were alone at the time of the incident,

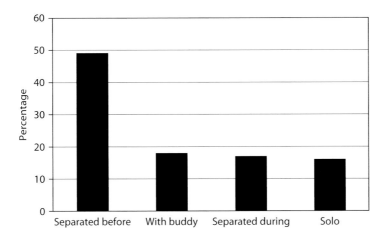

Figure 46.4 Buddy status of 351 dive accident victims in Australia.

whereas an additional 17 per cent separated from their buddy during the incident.

In the UK series, 13 per cent of the overall deaths were in intentional solo divers, a percentage thought likely to be higher than the general proportion of solo divers. In almost 39 per cent of the studied cases, separation had occurred before the incident. Nineteen per cent of fatalities were in divers who dived with a group of three or more, and almost three fourths of these had separated from the group.

WATER CONDITIONS

Adverse sea conditions often play a part in diving incidents. Choppy surface, high swell, surge, current, poor visibility and cold water temperature can provide challenges to the diver, sometimes beyond his or her ability to deal with them. Such challenges can be both physical and psychological. Relevant experience and preparedness are the best defences.

Although the most vulnerable are inexperienced divers, sometimes the unexpected can occur, and this can prove too much for even the highly experienced diver, especially if hampered by poor health or lack of fitness. Rough water was cited as a factor in 22 per cent of the US fatalities and as the trigger in 16 per cent of the fatalities in Australia.

Several deaths were caused when divers were sucked against water inlets in dams or elsewhere and were unable to escape. A small percentage, albeit regular, of deaths occur in caves where

Table 46.7 Causes of trauma to divers in United States and Canada (n = 30)

Cause	Frequency
Contact with rocks in surf zone	9
Boat propeller	9
Boat or Jet-ski	4
Shark	2
Electric shock	2
Struck by large fish/marine mammal	2
Alligator	1
Pre-dive trauma	1

divers become disorientated from poor visibility, usually as a result of silting, and/or failing to have appropriate training or equipment.

TRAUMA

A diver can suffer severe trauma during a dive for a variety of reasons, which include the following: propeller injury or impact with a boat (sometimes the dive boat but often other vessels) or Jet Ski; bites from marine animals such as sharks, crocodiles, moray eels, barracuda and sometimes even aggressive triggerfish, among others; injuries from creatures such as stingrays, sailfish and stonefish; and forceful contact with rocks or reef, usually as a result of surge or surf.

Table 46.7 shows the cause of the 30 cases (5 per cent) of trauma in the US series.

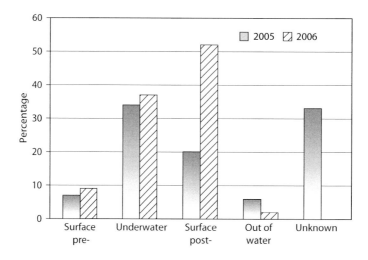

Figure 46.5 Phase during which divers become unconscious: 2005 (n = 89) and 2006 (n = 46).

In Australia, from 1972 and 2005, 5 per cent of the deaths were a direct result of trauma. These included 10 shark and 1 crocodile attacks, 3 deaths from boat propellers and 2 from divers hitting their heads on rocks.

The British series included three trauma-related deaths. One diver struck his head against a rock in rough seas, another was killed by a boat propeller and the third fell under the trailer while recovering the dive boat.

LOSS OF CONSCIOUSNESS

A variety of conditions, including asphyxia, cardiac events, stroke, diabetes, epilepsy, gas contamination, hypoxic or hyperoxic breathing gas, among others, can cause a diver to become unconscious in the water. Figure 46.5 is based on DAN America data for 2005 and 2006 and shows, where known, the phase of the dive during which the divers lost consciousness[13,14].

PREVENTION

The only way to eliminate the possibility of a dive-related accident is to refrain from diving. This is the path that most people, who have not developed a more than passing interest in, or become smitten by, the underwater world have chosen. However, for those who dive, or intend to do so, accident minimization strategies can certainly reduce the risk of an accident to an acceptable level. Some of these strategies or suggestions are discussed in the following section.

Adequate medical, physical and psychological fitness

The issues relating to psychological fitness have been highlighted earlier.

Many divers, or potential divers, fail to understand the difference between physical fitness and medical fitness to dive. Physical fitness is required for many sporting activities and incudes sufficient aerobic capacity, strength and dexterity to deal with the physical demands of the sport. In the case of scuba diving, this usually involves the carrying of heavy equipment, the ability to swim effectively, potentially against a strong current; and (usually) the ability to visualize and manipulate equipment. Unlike in earlier years, many participants who are now attracted to diving are older, more are likely overweight and with a lower level of aquatic skills, all potentially affecting the diver's ability to meet the required physical demands.

Medical fitness for diving entails the absence, or adequate control, of medical diseases that are incompatible with safe diving. Some divers with significant medical contraindications (e.g. epilepsy) are highly physically fit, and this is often not appreciated by the divers and by many medical practitioners.

To this end, it is important that both prospective and existing divers are adequately screened for medical contraindications to diving. Until recently in Australia and New Zealand, every new diver was required to undergo a dive medical examination before certification. However, this requirement disappeared relatively recently because the certification agencies withdrew their support for it. Future research will be important to determine whether or not this change has any measurable impact on morbidity and mortality of divers.

In most places (now including Australia), a short self-reporting medical questionnaire is used for this purpose, and only those people with positive responses are advised to seek medical assessment. This procedure is supported by the diving industry and by many divers, mainly because it is quick and easy, incurs no cost and so provides minimal barriers to training or continuance of diving. However, the disadvantage is that it relies on the dive professionals and the potential divers to fully understand the questions, the reason behind these questions, the possible implications of failing to declare a required condition (whether intentionally or because of inadequate explanation or misunderstanding as a result of language difficulty or poor comprehension) and the reason that it is important to discuss this with a doctor, preferably one who has training in diving medicine.

The increase in knowledge and experience in diving medicine, together with the changing medico-legal environment in which fitness-to-dive assessments are conducted, have led to changes in the criteria for determining whether a person is considered fit to dive. Previously, there was a variety of absolute contraindications, which included asthma, diabetes, previous myocardial infarct and epilepsy, among others. Current fitness-to-dive assessments often involve the doctor's identifying the risks and thoroughly explaining these to the candidate. The candidate then, to a large extent, makes his or her own decision about risk acceptance, based on information and advice provided. As shown in the data highlighted previously, these changes have enabled many individuals with a variety of chronic or previous medical conditions that would have formerly excluded them from diving to take up, or continue, the activity. Most of these persons manage to dive without significant incidents; others are not so fortunate.

Appropriate and adequate training

Unlike in the early days of diving, almost all divers now receive some diver training, usually from a certified instructor, rather than from just a 'friend' who is a diver. There is no doubt that such training has reduced the accident rate in divers.

The requirements for training and certification have changed over the years, and there has been some debate about whether all the changes have been for the better. Diver training and certification is governed by a variety of international training organizations, each having its own standards and procedures. There are external standards such as those propagated by the International Standards Organization (ISO), the World Recreational Scuba Training Council (WRSTC) and some national standards. Such standards are created by interested parties and should represent acceptable practice. However, as with many such standards, they can be influenced to varying degrees by commercially driven imperatives, and they may be somewhat pragmatic, rather than representative of ideal practice.

Using Australia as an example, there have been substantial changes to training requirements over time. At Open Water level, a requirement for a minimum logged underwater time of 4 hours was progressively replaced to become a current minimum of 80 minutes. Although there appear to be no data that directly indicate that the reduction in underwater time has had an impact on safety in Australia, and other factors in training have changed, some arguably for the better and some for the worse, time spent underwater with an instructor is likely an important contributor to safety.

One way to extend instructor supervision is through specific further training programs to extend a diver's knowledge and skills. Such courses include the (arguably poorly named) Advanced Open Water Diver, buoyancy control, rescue, night diving and deeper diving, among many others. It is valuable for a diver to extend experience through further training supported by appropriate independent experience.

Two key training-related aspects that arise regularly in fatality reports are poor buoyancy control and failure to release weights when necessary. Training agencies and instructors should ensure that adequate time and focus are spent in teaching and practising these important skills during training. Emergency drills such as ditching weights need to be practised repeatedly to embed the skill. Certified divers need to continue to practise these skills periodically, as well as additional skills such as air-sharing and mask clearing. A recent positive development has been the inclusion of more buoyancy control training and the introduction of weight belt ditching in the revised PADI Open Water course.

Suitable and reliable equipment

All equipment used for diving is potentially life-support equipment and should be considered and treated as such. As discussed earlier, apparently minor failures such as a torn mask or fin strap can prove catastrophic in some situations with certain divers. The type and amount of equipment required depend on the diving activity planned and also on the training and experience of the diver.

A simple piece of equipment such as a snorkel (often now abandoned by some technical divers) can be a lifesaver in a situation where a diver needs to remain on the surface without access to his or her other breathing gas supply. The presence of a snorkel and possession of adequate snorkelling skills have saved many divers from disaster.

It is evident that breathing gas supply problems remain common precipitants for diving fatalities. The introduction of 'octopus' regulators revolutionized the management of out-of-air emergencies when a buddy was close at hand, a vast improvement on alternatives such as 'buddy breathing' or 'free ascent'. However, these alternatives remain valuable back-up skills. The 'octopus' should be functioning adequately and positioned where it is easily accessed by the wearer and/or the buddy.

Redundant gas supplies are essential for divers who dive deep and/or who do not have direct access to the surface. These supplies have saved many lives, but occasionally have contributed to an incident, usually as a result of the diver's unfamiliarity with the system and/or error in accessing the supply through task loading. Systems should be configured as simply as possible to avoid confusion when required.

All scuba divers must ensure that their cylinder valves are opened fully (or almost so) before entering the water. If the valve is opened after attaching the regulator and then closed for any reason (e.g. boat transit to site), it is a good idea to bleed the lines. In this way, if the diver forgets to open the valve, this will become immediately obvious when taking a breath and/or checking the contents gauge before entering the water.

Contaminated breathing gas remains a problem and can be avoided by correct use and appropriate maintenance of compressors, as well as care and ongoing vigilance of the positioning of the air intake (see Chapter 19). Incorrect breathing mixtures can arise through inadequate monitoring and subsequent checking at, or after, the filling stage and before use. It can also occur when a diver incorrectly selects the wrong gas during a dive as a result of stress or carelessness. Equipment failure (e.g. scrubber or sensor failure in a rebreather) is another cause. The keys to avoid this are, again, familiarity with equipment and appropriate maintenance. Contamination of the gas supply is becoming an increasing concern in some developing countries where funds are scarce, there is no strict regulatory framework to ensure compliance to relevant standards and litigation may be difficult. Travelling divers should be aware of this issue. Some relatively cheap and portable devices are available to detect carbon monoxide and certain other contaminants.

BCD inflator-deflator mechanisms are common causes of buoyancy control problems because poorly maintained mechanisms often jam. Poor design of such mechanisms where the inflator and deflator buttons are close together and/or easily confused have also caused errors and subsequent buoyancy-related accidents. Careful choice of and familiarity with such a device help to minimize problems.

In addition to taking appropriate care of and maintaining of their regulators, divers need to ensure that their cylinders are in good condition. Occasionally, a diver is seriously injured or killed as a result of a cylinder explosion. It is important to ensure that cylinders are visually and hydrostatically inspected at sufficiently regular intervals, and that this inspection is conducted by a reputable service agent. Travelling divers should be vigilant with the cylinders provided to them in certain destinations, especially in remote areas where access to appropriate testing facilities may not be so readily available.

Adequate experience and preparation

Relevant training provides some preparation for particular types of diving. However, nothing replaces experience. Frequent exposure to particular situations generally creates both confidence and competence in dealing with such circumstances. A diver who has been frequently exposed to conditions such as swell, surge, poor visibility and colder waters is usually more comfortable in such an environment than one who has dived only in relatively clear, calm and warm tropical waters, even if he or she has undergone further training.

Dive accident reports often include cases where the victims went diving in very unfamiliar conditions and were inadequately prepared for them. These cases often result from challenging sea conditions. In some places, there are not infrequent reports of inexperienced, ill-equipped divers who became lost in caves and died as a result. In contrast, despite occasional mishaps, trained, experienced and well-equipped cave divers often venture great distances and depths in relative safety because they are well prepared for the dive at hand.

Recent experience is also important. Deaths of experienced divers who have not dived for several years are not uncommon. It is always important in such circumstances to ensure the equipment is functional and to refresh skills in relatively unchallenging circumstances before returning to normal diving.

Environmental hazards

Diving takes place in a variety of environments, which include the ocean, bays, lakes, dams, rivers, under ice, in caves and on and in wrecks. Each such environment has some common, but also some unique, factors that can be challenging to

those who dive there, especially if these divers are inexperienced in that environment.

Potentially adverse environmental factors include rough conditions, poor visibility, currents, cold water temperature, entrapment hazards, boating hazards and dangerous marine life.

Divers often encounter poor surface conditions in the ocean or bays, and factors such as swell, chop and surge are frequently implicated with deaths, often directly by drowning but also from drowning secondary to trauma caused by impact with rocks or other hard surfaces or from cardiac events precipitated by the conditions.

Strong currents can be present in the sea and in rivers, and these routinely take their toll on divers. Most currents run horizontally across the earth's surface, and divers can and do get lost at sea as a result of these currents. Other divers drown after exhaustion from trying to swim against these currents or as a result of a cardiac incident precipitated by the exertion. However, the currents that can often present the greatest risk run downward or upward and are caused when a horizontal current hits an underwater wall and is forced to flow downward, or upward. The diver can be dragged down to great depth and/or dragged rapidly toward the surface. Local knowledge about the prevalence, strength and timing of such currents is important when planning to dive in such locations.

Diving in colder water increases the potential for hypothermia unless the diver is adequately insulated. A hypothermic diver progressively loses dexterity, strength and mental clarity, including the awareness of danger and the desire and ability to deal with it. Appropriate insulation is essential when diving in cold water.

As shown in the accident data, entrapment is a common factor in diving deaths. This occurs as a result of entanglement with various lines or hoses (sometimes from the diver himself), fishing nets, seaweed and reef. Prior knowledge about the likely presence of such hazards can help reduce the risk. A sharp and easily accessible dive knife and shears can be invaluable tools to free oneself from entanglement; as can the presence of a buddy.

Entrapment also occurs when a diver becomes disorientated and lost inside a cave or wreck and cannot find an exit point. Sometimes such an exit point is close at hand but invisible as a result of silting. The best way to avoid such a situation is through relevant training, which would include the use of guidelines, and other appropriate equipment, and pre-knowledge of the site gained by discussion with others and/or studying maps of the site, if available. Once again, divers need to try to gain local knowledge about the potential for such problems.

Finally, various sites play host to a variety of potentially dangerous marine creatures, and it is sensible for a diver to seek local knowledge about these. Such creatures and their habits and interactions with divers are discussed in Chapters 31 and 32. Many members of the general community believe that we divers are crazy to dive because of the perceived high risk of shark attack. To put this risk into perspective, records kept in the Shark Attack File at the Florida Museum of Natural History indicate that between 1820 and 2012, there were 218 reported shark attacks on divers, including at least 41 per cent of on scuba divers[17]. Despite the high likelihood of underreporting, this remains a very, very small number compared with the number of scuba dives performed each year.

Common sense

The final ingredient in the recipe for safe diving is common sense. A diver can be healthy, well-trained, experienced, generally prepared and then simply make a stupid decision that leads to his or her demise. As we all know, this is not confined to diving and routinely occurs on our roads, at work and in other aspects of our lives.

Ensuring that one is clear-headed before diving is part of good preparation. Some victims have made poor decisions while under the influence of drugs, both therapeutic and recreational, some make poor decisions as a result of stress and/or task-loading and many others are reluctant to abort a dive when indicated because of the amount of effort or expense taken to get there, despite circumstances or conditions beyond their experience and/or capabilities. Many victims of both fatal and non-fatal incidents made poor decisions to descend deeper to view a marine creature or take one last photograph, even though these divers are low on breathing

gas and close to, or beyond, planned decompression limits.

To maximize safety, a diver needs to begin the dive clear headed and prepared, remain fully alert and focused on the surroundings, equipment function, gas supply and decompression obligation and use common sense when making safety-related decisions.

CONCLUSION

Dive fatalities usually involve a cascade of events, culminating in the diver's becoming incapacitated. Such events arise from problems with a diver's health, inadequate training and/or experience or preparation for the dive undertaken, equipment malfunction, inability to deal with adverse conditions, unpleasant interaction with a marine creature or boat, diver error or a combination of these factors.

The major purpose of most of the dive fatality reporting projects is to detect, examine and report the accidents of the unfortunate victims, to learn from their misfortunes and so minimize the likelihood that others will follow the same paths. Such reports are available as specific reports published by DAN America, DAN Asia-Pacific and the BSAC, among others. Detailed reports are also published in diving medical journals (e.g. *Diving and Hyperbaric Medicine* and *Undersea and Hyperbaric Medicine*), as well as periodically in the general medical literature. Summarized reports are also released to various diving media to publish as desired.

However, such reports are valuable only if they are carefully read and absorbed by divers, dive professionals, training agencies and medical professionals, and the insights derived from these are used to change practice. Frustratingly, it is clear that divers continue to make the same mistakes, and similar scenarios are played out repeatedly. Far more education and dissemination of information are required to reduce diving-related mortality.

In addition, there needs to be a greater willingness of the diving community to report dive accidents that are witnessed or heard about, to increase data capture and so facilitate the accuracy of reporting.

REFERENCES

1. Cumming B, Peddie C, Watson. A review of the nature of diving in the United Kingdom and of diving fatalities (1998–2009). In: Vann RD, Lang MA, editors. *Recreational Diving Fatalities. Proceedings of the Divers Alert Network 2010 April 8–10 Workshop.* Durham, North Carolina: Divers Alert Network; 2011:99–117.

2. Denoble PJ, Marroni A, Vann RD. Annual fatality rates and associated risk factors for recreational scuba diving. In: Vann RD, Lang MA, eds. *Recreational Diving Fatalities. Proceedings of the Divers Alert Network 2010 April 8–10 Workshop.* Durham, North Carolina: Divers Alert Network; 2011:73–83.

3. Denoble PJ, Caruso JL, Dear G de L, Vann RD. Common causes of open-circuit recreational diving fatalities. *Undersea and Hyperbaric Medicine* 2008;**35:**393–406.

4. Lippmann J, Baddeley A, Vann R, Walker D. An analysis of the causes of compressed gas diving fatalities in Australia from 1972–2005. *Undersea and Hyperbaric Medicine* 2013;**40:**49–61.

5. Divers Alert Network Asia-Pacific. *Diving-Related Fatality Database and Cumulative Register.* http://danap.org

6. Denoble PJ, Pollock NW, Vaithiyanathan P, Caruso JL, Dovenbarger JA, Vann RD. Scuba injury death rate among insured DAN members. *Diving and Hyperbaric Medicine* 2008;**38**(4):182–188.

7. Professional Association of Diving Instructors. *Statistics Report.* http://www.padi.com/scuba/about-padi/PADI-statistics/default.aspx

8. Divers Alert Network. *Annual Diving Report: 2008 Edition.* Durham, North Carolina: Divers Alert Network; 2013.

9. Taylor D McD, O'Toole KS, Ryan CM. Experienced, recreational scuba divers in Australia continue to dive despite medical contra-indications. *Wilderness and Environmental Medicine* 2002;**13**(3):187–193.

10. Beckett A, Kordick MF. Risk factors for dive injury: a survey study. *Research in Sports Medicine* 2007;**15**(3):201–211.

11. Edmonds C, Walker D. Scuba diving fatalities in Australia and New Zealand: 1. The human factor. *South Pacific Underwater Medicine Society Journal* 1990;**19**(3):94–104.

12. Richardson D. Training scuba divers: a fatality and risk analysis. In: Vann RD, Lang MA, editors. *Recreational Diving Fatalities. Proceedings of the Divers Alert Network 2010 April 8–10 Workshop.* Durham, North Carolina: Divers Alert Network; 2011:63–71.

13. Divers Alert Network. *Annual Diving Report: 2007 Edition.* Durham, North Carolina: Divers Alert Network; 2007.

14. Divers Alert Network. *Annual Diving Report: 2008 Edition.* Durham, North Carolina: Divers Alert Network; 2013.

15. Fock A. Analysis of recreational closed-circuit rebreather deaths 1998–2010. *Diving and Hyperbaric Medicine* 2010;**43**(2):78–85.

16. Weathersby, PK; Survanshi, SS; Hays, JR; MacCallum, ME. *Statistically Based Decompression Tables III: Comparative Risk Using U.S. Navy, British and Canadian Standard Air Schedules.* Naval Medical Research Institute report NRMI 86–50; Bethesda, Maryland: Naval Medical Research and Development Command; 1986.

17. Florida Museum of Natural History. International Shark Attack File. *1820–2012 Statistics of Shark Attacks on Divers Worldwide.* http://www.flmnh.ufl.edu/fish/sharks/scuba/All2.htm

This chapter was reviewed for this fifth edition by John Lippmann.

47

Unconsciousness

INTRODUCTION

Normal cerebral function depends on a steady supply of oxygen and glucose to the brain. Impairment of cerebral circulation and/or a fall in blood oxygen or glucose will rapidly cause unconsciousness. Cerebral function may also be altered by the toxic effects of gases, drugs and metabolites.

Unconsciousness during or after a dive can have many causes, and it must be treated as an emergency. Some of the causes require prompt action beyond simple first aid.

Drowning is the most likely result of unconsciousness in the water. It may be the final common pathway of a number of interactive situations related to environment, equipment, technique or physiology. Many accidents in the water are fatal, not because of the cause, but because there is no one to rescue the unconscious victim. In the water, unconsciousness from whatever cause may result in loss of a respirable medium and aspiration of water. This secondary effect may be the fatal one and may obscure the original cause of the 'blackout'.

Should the diver survive an episode of unconsciousness, attempts should be made to elucidate the specific factors involved. Otherwise, this situation is likely to recur, but with more tragic results, in a subsequent and similar dive exposure.

This chapter summarizes the various causes of unconsciousness and relates them to the type of diving equipment used. Repeated reference to Table 47.1 is recommended in the consideration of such cases.

More detailed discussions of the diagnosis and management of the specific diseases peculiar to diving are found in the appropriate chapters.

CAUSES

A scheme showing the causes of unconsciousness in divers is shown in Table 47.1. This list does not signify either incidence or relative importance.

Causes possible in all types of diving

HYPOCAPNIA FROM HYPERVENTILATION

Unconsciousness resulting from hypocapnia is a theoretical possibility that is self-correcting on land. It is observed in an anxiety or panic situation and has been suggested as a cause of unconsciousness in divers.

Hyperventilation can produce dizziness and altered consciousness. Unconsciousness is rare, is usually short-lived and manifests as syncope (fainting). The postulated mechanisms are cerebral

Table 47.1 Causes of unconsciousness in diving

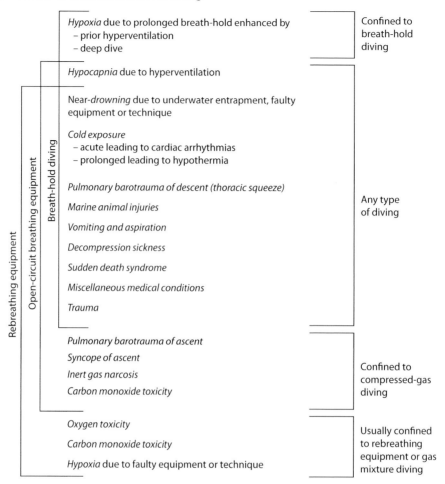

Rebreathing equipment	Open-circuit breathing equipment	Breath-hold diving	*Hypoxia* due to prolonged breath-hold enhanced by – prior hyperventilation – deep dive	Confined to breath-hold diving
			Hypocapnia due to hyperventilation	
			Near-*drowning* due to underwater entrapment, faulty equipment or technique	Any type of diving
			Cold exposure – acute leading to cardiac arrhythmias – prolonged leading to hypothermia	
			Pulmonary barotrauma of descent (thoracic squeeze)	
			Marine animal injuries	
			Vomiting and aspiration	
			Decompression sickness	
			Sudden death syndrome	
			Miscellaneous medical conditions	
			Trauma	
			Pulmonary barotrauma of ascent	Confined to compressed-gas diving
			Syncope of ascent	
			Inert gas narcosis	
			Carbon monoxide toxicity	
			Oxygen toxicity	Usually confined to rebreathing equipment or gas mixture diving
			Carbon monoxide toxicity	
			Hypoxia due to faulty equipment or technique	

vasoconstriction and reduced cerebral blood flow as direct effects of hypocapnia.

Hypocapnia is an uncommon event in diving because any tendency to overbreathe it is countered by the following:

1. Breath-holding (leading to an inexorable rise in carbon dioxide tension from metabolic activity).
2. The resistance of the breathing apparatus and increased gas density at depth (promoting hypoventilation).
3. Oxygen breathed at higher pressures (both depressing the respiratory response to carbon dioxide and interfering with the transport of carbon dioxide in the blood, thus increasing tissue carbon dioxide tension).

4. Increased dead space with closed or semi-closed rebreathing apparatus (increasing rebreathing and thus elevating carbon dioxide tension).

If hyperventilation does cause unconsciousness during diving, it is likely only near the surface or with an excessive supply of gas. In breath-hold diving, hyperventilation may lead to syncope at the surface, but a graver danger of hyperventilation is hypoxia toward the end of the dive (see later).

NEAR DROWNING

Near drowning is one of the most common causes of unconsciousness (and subsequent death) in divers (see Chapter 22). It may follow salt water aspiration (see Chapter 24). Analysis of the contributing factors is vital if recurrence is to be prevented (see Chapter 25).

COLD

Sudden exposure to cold water may cause reflex inhalation. In some people, cold water in the pharynx may stimulate the vagus nerve and cause reflex sinus bradycardia or even asystole.

Prolonged exposure to cold sufficient to lower the core temperature to less than 30°C causes unconsciousness and the possibility of cardiac arrhythmias. A fall in core temperature to 33°C to 35°C may lead to an insidious onset of confusion and decreased mental and physical function. In this hypothermic state, the diver is likely to drown (see Chapters 27 and 28).

Cold urticaria causing unconsciousness is described in Chapter 42.

PULMONARY BAROTRAUMA OF DESCENT (THORACIC SQUEEZE)

In the breath-hold diver, pulmonary barotrauma of descent is likely only when descent involves a pressure change ratio greater than that between the initial lung volume, or total lung capacity with maximum inspiration, and the residual volume (see Chapter 6). Most barotrauma with deep breath-hold diving is less dramatic and is detected by haemoptysis after surfacing. Hypoxia on ascent is a far more common cause of unconsciousness in this situation.

In the scuba diver, thoracic squeeze is unlikely except when the diver is grossly overweighted and sinks rapidly or first loses consciousness from some other cause and then sinks. In both situations, loss of the air supply before the descent makes the diagnosis more tenable.

The diver supplied with gas from the surface is at greater risk. Thoracic squeeze is possible if the increase of gas pressure does not keep pace with the rate of descent or if the gas pressure fails (e.g. severed gas line) in equipment not protected by a 'non-return' valve.

MARINE ANIMAL INJURIES

Unconsciousness may result from the bite of the sea snake or blue-ringed octopus, the sting from coelenterates such as *Chironex* or the injection of toxin from cone shells, fish or stingrays (see Chapter 32).

The casual snorkeller is as likely to be a victim as is the experienced scuba diver.

Accurate diagnosis depends on awareness, knowledge of geographical distribution of dangerous marine animals, the clinical features and, most important, identification of the animal.

VOMITING AND ASPIRATION

Vomiting and aspiration may result from seasickness, aspiration and swallowing of sea water, gastrointestinal barotrauma, unequal vestibular caloric stimulation (e.g. perforated tympanic membrane) and middle or inner ear disorders. Causes unrelated to diving itself include overindulgence in food or alcohol, gastroenteritis and other illnesses.

Aspiration of vomitus from the mouthpiece is a possibility in the inexperienced diver. Vomitus ejected into a demand valve may interfere with its function, or it may damage the absorbent activity in rebreathing sets. If the diver removes the mouthpiece to vomit, he or she may then aspirate sea water during the subsequent reflex inhalation. In severe cases, unconsciousness may result from respiratory obstruction and resultant hypoxia.

DECOMPRESSION SICKNESS

This disorder is extremely unlikely in breath-hold divers, although it has been described in native pearl divers (in whom it is known as Taravana) and submarine escape training instructors who have a very short surface interval between deep breath-hold dives (see Chapter 61).

Unconsciousness during or immediately after compressed gas diving is occasionally caused by cerebral or cardiovascular decompression sickness (see Chapter 11) or cerebral arterial gas embolism from pulmonary barotrauma of ascent (see Chapter 6).

MISCELLANEOUS MEDICAL CONDITIONS

The diver is as prone to the onset of sudden incapacitating illness as are active people on land. Diagnoses such as myocardial infarction, cardiac arrhythmia (see Chapter 39), syncope, cerebrovascular accident, diabetes with hypoglycaemia or hyperglycaemia or epilepsy, for example, should be considered. The metabolic disturbances of renal failure, liver failure or adrenal failure can affect cerebral function, but these disorders would be infrequent in divers.

Drugs, either legal or illicit, may depress central nervous system function, enhance carbon dioxide retention (e.g. opiates), affect cardiac performance (e.g. some antihypertensives) or alter blood glucose (insulin or oral hypoglycaemic agents). This topic is discussed in more detail in Chapters 39, 43, 56 and 57.

TRAUMA

A diver could be rendered unconscious by a blow to the head or chest. Underwater explosion is discussed in Chapter 34.

> Diagnosis of the cause of unconsciousness in a diver includes the following:
>
> - Type of equipment and breathing gases.
> - Depth and duration of this and other recent dives.
> - Environmental factors.
> - Clinical history and physical signs.

Causes confined to breath-hold diving

The main causes, hyperventilation and breath-holding–induced hypoxia, are discussed in Chapters 16 and 61, as is hypoxia of ascent.

Causes usually confined to compressed gas diving

PULMONARY BAROTRAUMA OF ASCENT

Cerebral arterial gas embolism (see Chapter 6) is the provisional diagnosis to be excluded in the diver who surfaces and rapidly becomes unconscious.

Tension pneumothorax may also cause unconsciousness secondary to hypoxia or cardiovascular disturbance.

SYNCOPE OF ASCENT

Syncope of ascent causing unconsciousness or altered consciousness may result from partial breath-holding during ascent. This condition is thought to be caused by an increase in intrathoracic pressure interfering with venous return and

thus reducing cardiac output. Unless it proceeds to pulmonary barotrauma or drowning, it is rapidly self-correcting with the resumption of normal respiration.

POSTURAL HYPOTENSION

Postural hypotension causing syncope may develop as the diver leaves the water, and it is caused by a loss of hydrostatic circulatory support. This is more likely in the dehydrated or peripherally vasodilated diver, from whatever cause. It is common after prolonged immersion and was first recognized during the rescue of ditched aviators in the Second World War. Postural hypotension is also aggravated by many drugs.

INERT GAS NARCOSIS

In deep dives, unconsciousness may result from the narcotic effects of nitrogen in compressed air (see Chapter 15). At less profound depths, narcosis can be associated with irrational behavior, poor judgement and drowning. An unconscious diver on the surface is not suffering from nitrogen narcosis because the narcosis is reversible on reduction of the environmental pressure.

Unconsciousness resulting from inert gas narcosis is likely at depths greater than 90 metres, breathing air, but variable degrees of impaired consciousness may be seen from 30 metres onward. This is especially so if other factors contribute (e.g. carbon dioxide accumulation, oxygen pressures).

CARBON MONOXIDE TOXICITY

Carbon monoxide toxicity is often proposed as a cause of unconsciousness in scuba divers (see Chapter 19). Diagnosis is made by examining compressor facilities and is confirmed by estimations of carbon monoxide in the gas supply and the victim's blood.

Causes more likely with technical diving and rebreathing equipment

OXYGEN TOXICITY

Central nervous system oxygen toxicity becomes more likely if the partial pressure of oxygen in the inspired gas exceeds 1.6 ATA, especially with heavy exercise (see Chapters 17 and 63). High inspired oxygen is possible at any depth on a rebreather set because the diver carries 100 per cent oxygen and the gas in the breathing loop may be mismanaged. Closed-circuit oxygen sets are particularly dangerous because of the combined potential for hypercarbia.

CARBON DIOXIDE TOXICITY

The most common cause of unconsciousness in divers using rebreathing equipment is a build-up of carbon dioxide (see Chapters 4, 18 and 63).

The possibility exists that some compressed air divers, under conditions of increased gas density at depth and heavy exercise, may retain carbon dioxide. The carbon dioxide produced as a result of the work of breathing may exceed the amount expelled with ventilation, resulting in a rising arterial carbon dioxide tension despite the best efforts of the individual. Resultant carbon dioxide toxicity may impair consciousness and exacerbate either oxygen toxicity or nitrogen narcosis.

HYPOXIA RESULTING FROM FAULTY EQUIPMENT OR TECHNIQUE

Hypoxia may be produced by insufficient oxygen in the inspired gas mixture, dilution, ascent, excess oxygen consumption or incorrect gas mixture for the set flow rate (see Chapters 4, 16 and 63). The manifestations are those of hypoxia from any cause. Provided the hypoxia is rapidly corrected, prompt recovery can be expected.

> A rapid recovery is expected in uncomplicated cases of transient hypoxia, carbon dioxide toxicity, syncope of ascent and oxygen toxicity – after the patient is removed from the offending environment.

CONTRIBUTORY FACTORS

Several factors, although not direct causes, may contribute to the development of unconsciousness underwater. The *inexperienced diver* is more likely to be involved in such an episode.

The role of *psychological factors* in causing unconsciousness has often been postulated. The anxious diver may be more prone to cardiac arrhythmias related to sympathetic nervous system stimulation.

Cardiac arrhythmias have been postulated as a cause of otherwise unexplained collapse or death in the water (see Chapter 39).

A vigorous *Valsalva manoeuvre* may increase the likelihood of syncope secondary to reduced venous return and hence decreased cardiac output. This situation is less likely in the water because the hydrostatic support reduces peripheral pooling of blood.

The *overheated diver* may develop heat exhaustion with mild confusion, but heat stroke with coma and/or convulsions is unlikely.

The *diver exposed to cold* may have a higher incidence of equipment (and absorbent) failure, dexterity reduction and cardiac reflexes.

A fall in plasma glucose may result from fasting or high physical activity. In the normal individual, the degree of *hypoglycaemia* is not enough to produce symptoms. Alcohol, by inhibiting gluconeogenesis, may contribute to significant hypoglycaemia in the fasted (greater than 12 hours) diver. Long-term alcohol abuse damages liver glycogen storage, and hypoglycaemia may develop after a shorter fast.

Some cases of unconsciousness are particularly difficult to explain, even with recourse to multiple imaginative factors.

'SHALLOW WATER BLACKOUT'

The term *'shallow water blackout'* was used initially by the British to refer to carbon dioxide toxicity with rebreathing equipment, whereas the term has more recently been used to describe unconsciousness toward the end of a breath-hold dive where hyperventilation preceded the dive. This term has therefore created much diagnostic confusion and should be avoided (see Chapter 3).

Attempts to define specific causes of unconsciousness should always be made. Nomenclature should then follow this specific cause (e.g. syncope of ascent, dilution hypoxia, carbon dioxide toxicity, oxygen toxicity).

MANAGEMENT

The first steps in management of all cases are the establishment and maintenance of respiration and circulation. The administration of 100 per cent oxygen at I ATA will do no harm, even in central nervous system oxygen toxicity, and is of great benefit in most other cases. If breathing is not spontaneous, positive pressure respiration will be required. Positive pressure ventilation should not be withheld in any case of respiratory arrest or significant hypoventilation, despite the argument that it may be detrimental in cases of pulmonary barotrauma. External cardiac massage may also be necessary. Divers suspected of having cerebral arterial gas embolism or decompression sickness require rapid recompression as well (see Chapters 6, 13 and 48 to 50).

The most common causes of unconsciousness in divers are as follows:

1. *Breath-hold* – hyperventilation followed by breath-holding, leading to hypoxia.
2. *Compressed air equipment* – drowning as a result of faulty equipment or technique.
3. *Rebreathing equipment* – carbon dioxide toxicity.

Maintenance of adequate circulation and ventilation may be all that is required in cases of near drowning, pulmonary barotrauma of descent and marine animal envenomations.

Patients with carbon dioxide toxicity, oxygen toxicity, nitrogen narcosis and temporary hypoxia from whatever cause, uncomplicated by aspiration of sea water, usually recover rapidly with return to normal atmosphere.

Miscellaneous medical conditions, hypothermia, aspiration of vomitus, trauma and others are managed along general medical principles.

The medical assessment should encompass the following:

- A clinical and social history.
- A diving history and profile.
- Physical examination and investigation.
- Examination of the equipment and gas used.
- An appreciation of the environmental factors.

Valuable information, including the sequence of events leading to unconsciousness, may be obtainable only from the diver's companion or other observers.

FURTHER READING

Acott CJ. Extraglottic airway devices for use in diving medicine–part 3: the I-Gel™. *Diving and Hyperbaric Medicine* 2008;38(3):124–127.

Caruso JL. Pathology of diving accidents. In: Brubakk AO, Neuman TS, eds. *Bennett and Elliott's Physiology and Medicine of Diving. 5th ed.* London: Saunders; 2003:729–743.

Leitch DR. A study of unusual incidents in a well-documented series of dives. *Aviation, Space and Environmental Medicine* 1981;52:618–624.

Mitchell SJ, Bennett MH, Bird N, *et al.* Recommendations for rescue of a submerged unresponsive compressed gas diver. *Undersea and Hyperbaric Medicine* 2012;39(6):1099–1108.

This chapter was reviewed for this fifth edition by Michael Bennett.

48

First aid and emergency treatment

INTRODUCTION

This chapter deals with the immediate management of diving accidents. Specific diseases are discussed in greater detail elsewhere in this book, but an overview is presented here for easy reference.

Despite the best-laid plans, diving accidents will occur. Frequently, they result from a chain-reaction sequence, often originating from a failure to follow simple safeguard procedures. Prevention of injury is paramount, and individual divers have a responsibility to themselves and to those who dive with them to ensure that they are medically, physically and psychologically fit to dive. They should also be, appropriately trained and/or experienced for the planned diving with due respect for the prevailing conditions (e.g. depth, current, temperature). Additionally, they need to ensure that they have appropriate, adequate and functional equipment and suitable and sufficient breathing gas for the planned dive. Before entering the water, all divers should have discussed alternate exit routes, if any. They should also ensure they are carrying an appropriate personal locator device

(whistle, light, strobe, safety sausage or surface marker buoy, electronic position-indicating radio beacon) and have discussed emergency procedures with their companions.

When a diving accident occurs, the dive organizer should be able to identify the symptoms and signs of this illness or injury and implement an emergency action plan. Such a plan should include the following:

- The number for the appropriate diving emergency hotline (e.g. Divers Alert Network [DAN]).
- The local contact numbers for emergency services and a means of contacting them (e.g. radio or mobile telephone).
- The location and contacts of the nearest medical facility.
- The location and contacts of the nearest recompression facility.

The plan should also include the ready availability of suitable oxygen administration equipment (i.e. capable of delivering near 100 per cent inspired oxygen) and adequate supply, an appropriate first aid kit and the location of and contact for the nearest automated external defibrillator (AED).

FIRST AID

There are two aspects to first aid – the rescue and the specific first aid treatment.

Rescue

In one report on a series of diving fatalities, only 20 per cent of victims were rescued within 5 minutes of the incident. In almost 70 per cent of the deaths, the victim was submerged for more than 15 minutes between the accident and the rescue. With such a long period of submersion without breathing, the likelihood of survival, especially without substantial neurological dysfunction, is extremely low. Therefore, in many cases, there is a progression from unconsciousness to death that could possibly have been prevented by prompt recovery from the water.

A Canadian series of 37 deaths highlighted the importance of the diver's reaching the surface, unconscious or otherwise, rather than having to be searched for, and retrieved from, underwater. Twenty-two of the 25 divers who reached the surface survived. In contrast, none of the 12 divers for whom underwater search and recovery were required survived.

Undoubtedly, equipment redundancy and the ability to implement self-rescue techniques are important for all divers. However, the practice of buddy diving is arguably the single most important factor in rescue. Ideally, it requires that each diver is responsible for the welfare and safety of his or her companion. This infers a reliable method of communication between the divers, close observation of each other, a practised rescue technique and basic resuscitation skills.

The best way to minimize the time a diver spends unconscious underwater is to have an effective buddy system. A 34-year review of Australian diving deaths indicated that 65 per cent of the victims were alone at the time of their accident, whereas an additional 17 per cent separated from their buddy during the accident (see Figure 46.4 in Chapter 46.).

In another Australian analysis of 100 diving deaths, in 25 per cent of the cases, the victim was not discovered to be missing until all other divers had completed the dive. In most of these cases, the subsequent body search by members of the diving group was unsuccessful.

There has been ongoing debate about the effectiveness of performing in-water rescue breathing (expired air resuscitation) and/or in-water external chest compressions. Some studies implied that adequate compression force may be created on a mannikin in the water. However, in reality, there is very likely little benefit in attempting in-water chest compressions, given the difficulty in generating adequate cerebral and cardiac perfusion in a person positioned horizontally on a hard surface, much less an unconscious diver hanging near-vertically in the water. In-water compressions are therefore not recommended.

On the other hand, there is both experimental and anecdotal evidence that rescue breathing can be delivered effectively and may prevent cardiac arrest if it is provided early and effectively. A study that examined the outcome of a large series of swimmer rescues by lifesavers concluded that in-water rescue breathing appeared to increase the likelihood of survival if the submersion time was less than 15 minutes.

As part of a broad overview of diver rescue protocols, the Diving Committee of the Undersea and Hyperbaric Medical Society (UHMS) published some recommendations for in-water rescue breathing that were based largely on those of the International Lifesaving Federation. In reality, the particular circumstances dictate the most appropriate course of action. However, the guiding principles are to support ventilation and remove the diver from the water with minimal delay.

Whether diving from shore or from a vessel, there should be a proven and exercised system for retrieving an unconscious diver from the water, ideally in a horizontal position.

First aid treatment

Once the diver is out of the water, appropriate airway management, assessment and resuscitation can be implemented. Resuscitation of the diver should follow the guidelines issued by the relevant national resuscitation peak body (e.g. American Heart Association, European Resuscitation Council, Australian Resuscitation Council). These guidelines should ideally be derived from the evidence-based recommendations of the International Liaison Committee on Resuscitation (ILCOR). However, if the airway is compromised by the presence of water and/or stomach contents, the diver should be quickly placed into the recovery position to facilitate clearing the airway before being repositioning on his or her back for the commencement or continuation of resuscitation.

POST-RESCUE MANAGEMENT

All recreational divers should be encouraged to acquire first aid skills and maintain competence in airway management, cardiopulmonary resuscitation, haemorrhage control and delivery of 100 per cent oxygen. They should also be aware of basic warming techniques for hypothermia and methods of managing marine animal envenomation, including pressure and immobilization and the use of vinegar and heat as appropriate.

Importantly, divers should recognize their own limitations when dealing with diving emergencies and seek expert diving medical advice promptly and emergency medical support as necessary. DAN provides diving emergency advisory hotlines that are available around the clock to any diver, diving companions or medical professionals (see later).

Positioning

A diver suspected of suffering cerebral arterial gas embolism (CAGE) should immediately be placed in a horizontal posture. Previously, a head-down position was recommended in patients suspected of having CAGE to prevent re-embolization. Unfortunately, patients were transported in this position, often for many hours, and this resulted in deteriorating cerebral function as a consequence of cerebral oedema. It is now generally advised that a horizontal posture is the best early position for most victims of decompression illness (DCI). Divers who are suspected of having CAGE should

be discouraged from sitting or standing until advice has been obtained from a diving physician.

If CAGE is suspected, testing of balance or gait should ideally be left to the diving physician at the treating recompression chamber. Spontaneously breathing patients with an altered mental state or who are at risk of aspiration should be placed in the recovery position. Divers with vestibular symptoms and/or hearing loss should be kept as still as possible and should avoid straining manoeuvres (e.g. Valsalva's manoeuvre), which could further damage their inner ear and/or encourage shunting through a patent foramen ovale, if present.

Oxygen first aid

Surprisingly, there are few studies to support the efficacy of oxygen therapy for most illnesses and injuries, even though oxygen therapy has been an integral part of the standard of care for many medical conditions for decades. In fact, there has been debate about possible adverse effects of providing very high-concentration oxygen after resuscitation and for patients with stroke or myocardial infarction. However, there is some evidence and many anecdotes to support the delivery of oxygen to victims of DCI.

Breathing high-concentration oxygen increases the rate of inert gas elimination from tissues and bubbles and helps to reduce any associated hypoxia. A retrospective study analyzing more than 2000 dive accident cases concluded that oxygen first aid increased recompression efficacy and decreased the number of recompression treatments required if the oxygen was given within 4 hours after surfacing.

> All dive sites should be equipped with an oxygen delivery system capable of administering near 100 per cent oxygen to a spontaneously breathing diver and as close as practicable to 100 per cent oxygen to unconscious, non-breathing victims.

The delivery of near-100 per cent oxygen to a diver who is breathing spontaneously is not difficult, even for the minimally trained lay first aid provider. However, the delivery of near-100 per cent oxygen to an unconscious, non-breathing diver can be problematic. The equipment most commonly used for

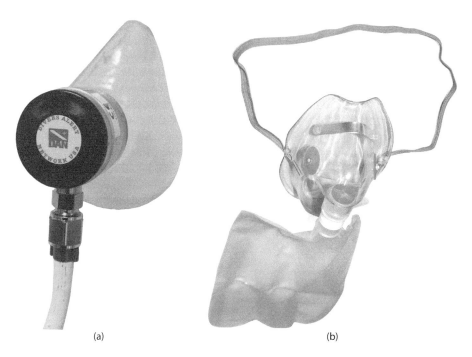

(a)   (b)

Figure 48.1 **(a)** Medical oxygen demand valve and tight-sealing oronasal mask. This system is capable of providing 80 to 100 per cent oxygen to a breathing patient. **(b)** Non-rebreather mask. This mask is capable of providing up to 95 per cent inspired oxygen to a breathing patient with an adequate flowrate and seal. However, in the field, the inspired oxygen concentration is more likely to be 70 to 80 per cent. The mask is fitted with a one-way valve to prevent expired breath from entering the reservoir while enabling the oxygen in the reservoir to be inhaled and two lateral one-way valves to prevent air entrainment while allowing expired breath to be vented to the atmosphere. ((a) Courtesy of Divers Alert Network.)

this is a bag-valve-mask with reservoir. Such devices are valuable in trained, skilled and well-practised hands but can be ineffective and potentially harmful in the hands of occasional users (Figure 48.1). An alternative device that can deliver 100 per cent oxygen is a manually triggered oxygen-powered resuscitator. These devices are somewhat easier to use than bag-valve-masks, but they still require appropriate training and regular practice, are more expensive and require ongoing maintenance, especially when they are used in an aquatic environment.

The recreational dive industry has been pragmatic about this situation, and recreational dive professionals are usually trained to ventilate a non-breathing diver by using a resuscitation mask with oxygen-supplemented expired breath because this procedure is far easier to perform by those with minimal training. This technique can deliver an inspired oxygen concentration of around 50 per cent with an oxygen flow rate of 15 lpm.

The volume of oxygen needed is often substantial, and a good 'rule of thumb' for the provision of appropriate oxygen first aid is that the supply should be sufficient for delivery to at least one diver for the duration of the retrieval to the nearest medical facility where there is an adequate further supply. In remote places, injured divers may need to breathe high-concentration oxygen for up to 24 hours, or sometimes longer, until a medical evacuation team arrives. It is essential that dive operators and divers understand the importance of this and plan accordingly. Thought should be given to the potential need to have additional equipment and/or oxygen supply in the event that another diver may need oxygen simultaneously.

One hundred per cent oxygen should be administered continuously to all diving accident victims until diving physician advice is received (Figure 48.2). Formerly, it was advised that first aid

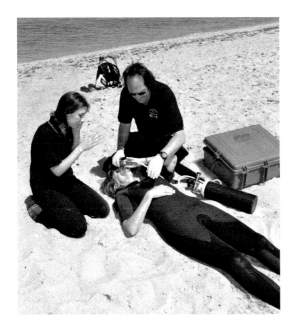

Figure 48.2 Administering oxygen for aid to an injured diver.

oxygen administration be regularly interrupted to give short air breaks, to reduce the likelihood of pulmonary oxygen toxicity. However, this is generally unnecessary with normobaric oxygen administration in the field. The reality is that the concentration of oxygen delivered is often far lower than 100 per cent because of the type of delivery device used, less than optimal function of the device, insufficient flow rate and/or poor a mask seal. In addition, air breaks occur when the patient eats, drinks and toilets.

Prompt, high-concentration and adequate oxygen first aid will often prevent, reduce or sometimes eliminate symptoms of DCI. However, even if symptoms disappear with oxygen first aid, if oxygen administration is ceased prematurely, these symptoms will often return. It is not uncommon for dive operators to provide oxygen to one of their clients with suspected decompression sickness (DCS) for 15 to 60 minutes with initial resolution of symptoms, only for the symptoms to return with a vengeance several hours later. Therefore, it is important that diving medical consultation is sought as early as possible. Periods of oxygen breathing, the mode of delivery and the patient's response should be recorded and reported.

In remote locations, periods of at least 4 to 5 hours of continuous high-concentration oxygen breathing are commonly advised to relieve symptoms of mild DCS while further action is contemplated or being prepared. In many cases, this proves adequate to eliminate symptoms and prevent recurrence. However, the decision on whether or not evacuation to a recompression facility is required should be made by a diving physician. One factor that requires consideration is the level of confidence the doctor has in the reliability of information provided by the patient or the patient's companions in the common absence of the ability to have a reliable neurological assessment performed.

Fluids

Intravenous fluids should be administered to all seriously injured divers. One reasonable regimen is 1 litre as fast as possible followed by 1 litre over 4 hours of normal saline alternating with Hartmann's solution. This regimen may need to be varied if clinical parameters such as urine output and blood pressure are low. Urinary catheterization may be required if urine output is low. Cerebral injury may be exacerbated by hyperglycemia, and therefore glucose-containing solutions should be avoided unless the patient is hypoglycemic.

Consideration may be given to the administration of suitable oral fluids (e.g. water or readily available isotonic drinks) as long as the patient is fully conscious, does not suffer from nausea and vomiting and is able to urinate. The administration of oxygen will be interrupted if the patient is given oral fluids, and it is preferable for these interruptions to be kept to a minimum.

Drugs

There is no indication for the use of aspirin or steroids in the first aid management of a diving accident victim with DCI. If the patient has significant pain and analgesics are required, it is advisable first to discuss this issue with the treating hyperbaric specialist. Response of symptoms to recompression forms the basis of the selection of an appropriate treatment table, and analgesics may mask symptoms, thus making this decision more difficult than needed.

This being said, there is evidence that the provision of non-steroidal anti-inflammatory drugs (NSAIDs) before, together with, or after treatment may accelerate recovery. Therefore, an increasing number of dive physicians advise divers with musculoskeletal symptoms of DCS to take NSAIDs to help reduce symptoms before, during or after treatment. This approach can be particularly useful if the diver is remote and it will be many hours before he or she would reach a recompression facility. Nitrous oxide (or a nitrous oxide-oxygen mixture [Entonox]) must never be used in divers following diving exposure because nitrous oxide may diffuse into and expand the bubbles, thereby aggravating the clinical effect.

LOCAL MEDICAL TREATMENT

The local physician may be able to play a role in the prevention of diving accidents by the appropriate medical screening of diving candidates and in the provision of advice on safe diving practices, if indeed this knowledge and training are possessed. The local physician is responsible for primary care, such as a thorough neurological examination, oxygen and intravenous fluid administration, correction of electrolyte disturbance and advanced life support.

In many cases, the local physician can work as a liaison between the divers and a diving medicine specialist, especially when recompression therapy is required. The physician is also important in integrating the patient's transport and medical evacuation needs, if these are required. This physician should be able to communicate directly with a specialist in diving medicine, so that the appropriate measures can be instituted. This communication can be achieved via a diving emergency and/or advisory hotline or through consultation with a diving medical officer at a local hyperbaric unit.

Prompt assessment and early consultation with a specialist diving physician are recommended to maximize the likelihood of full recovery from disorders such as DCS and CAGE.

TRANSPORT

The need for prompt recompression in both CAGE and neurological DCS is well accepted. In many circumstances, the facilities may not be immediately available for formal recompression therapy. Therefore, a decision has to be made about whether the patient is to be transported to a recompression chamber, have a recompression chamber transported to him or her (which is now relatively rare) or recompressed by descent in the water, a technique increasingly used by some technical divers and in some remote diving fishers communities.

Retrieval

In some remote places where diving is popular, there may be a recompression chamber available to treat divers (Figure 48.3). These chambers can be very valuable if they are well run and maintained, which is, unfortunately, not always the case. Many of these chambers, even some of the better-managed ones, are unsuitable for treating a seriously ill diver, who often needs to be evacuated to a facility that can provide a higher level of care. Such evacuations can be difficult and very expensive, costing tens of thousands of dollars or, sometimes, several hundred thousand dollars.

The decision to transport an injured diver suspected of having DCI should be made as early as possible to reduce the inevitable delay. Extended delays to recompression, especially in the presence of serious symptoms and the absence of appropriate first aid, could contribute to a poorer outcome and should be avoided where possible.

Whatever mode of transport is used, appropriate resuscitation such as oxygen and intravenous fluid administration must not be compromised.

The decision on mode of transfer should be made in conjunction with the receiving hyperbaric unit and often also with dive accident insurer if the patient has such coverage. Road transport may be preferable if long distances and ascent to altitude (mountain ranges) are avoided. Transport by boat is the appropriate and/or only option available in some circumstances.

The use of aircraft (fixed-wing and rotary) often poses a problem of additional altitude stress unless the aircraft cabin can be pressurized to 1 ATA, which is the ideal. A helicopter flight skimming the surface of the ocean adds little further altitude stress; however, even limits of 300 metres over land and 600 metres at night or in bad weather

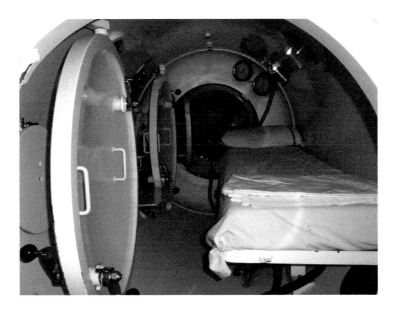

Figure 48.3 A small chamber used to treat divers in a remote location.

may make road transfer a better option. A maximum altitude of 300 metres is generally considered reasonable when transporting an injured diver, although the appearance or recurrence of symptoms after recompression has been reported at lower altitudes than this. It has been suggested that vibration characteristics of both rotary and fixed-wing aircraft may negatively affect the clinical condition of the injured diver. Although some research is under way, there are currently no data available to quantify this clinical impression.

In some circumstances, a commercial aircraft (cabin pressure equivalent to altitude of 2400 metres) is the only available option, and it has often, but not always, been used without significant exacerbation of the diver's symptoms. In such cases, the continuous administration of 100 per cent oxygen is highly desirable but not always possible. A risk assessment needs to be made by the diving physician based on the severity, duration and evolution of the patient's symptoms, the availability of oxygen and other local support, the duration of the flight or flights and the availability of treatment options on arrival.

The diver who has had stable or remitting minor symptoms for more than 24 hours is not likely to deteriorate. In contrast, the diver who surfaces with symptoms of spinal DCS or CAGE is likely to

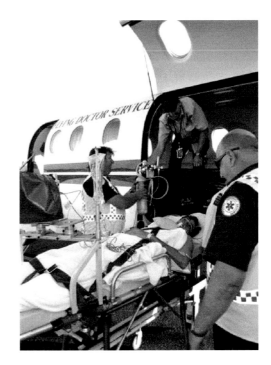

Figure 48.4 Evacuation of a diver with cerebral arterial gas embolism.

deteriorate and has a worse prognosis; therefore, the need for proper assessment and prompt recompression is greater (Figure 48.4).

Any gas-filled space expands with ascent to altitude, so special care should be taken in patients suspected of having a pneumothorax.

The reality is that delays to evacuation are often unavoidable, and even substantial delays are not necessarily detrimental. A 2010 report, which included 60 evacuations for DCI, found that in such evacuations where the median time between injury and arrival at a facility was 16 hours, time did not appear to influence outcome.

Suitable evacuation aircraft are not always immediately available. The same may apply to flight crew and medical personnel. The time of the flight can also be affected by the weather conditions, the light conditions and availability of a suitable landing strip (with landing lights for night time evacuation). If national borders need to be crossed, immigration and customs requirements have to be managed, and this can sometimes cause long delays, depending on the countries involved. Air safety is also a serious consideration. Occasionally, evacuation aircraft have accidents, so there is always a small risk associated with these activities that needs to be balanced against the risks of not evacuating the injured diver.

Portable recompression chambers

An alternative to transporting the injured diver to a hospital-based recompression chamber is to bring a small portable recompression chamber to the diver. The logistics of such an operation, the specialized procedures for transporting the chamber, the lack of sophisticated patient monitoring equipment within the chamber and the need to ensure the availability of adequate supplies of air and oxygen make this option less desirable, and it is now rarely used.

If portable chambers are used, they should be large enough to accommodate a medical attendant as well as the diver, and ideally they should have a transfer-under-pressure capability with other chambers. Once you commit a diver to a treatment in most of these small chambers, you have no means of introducing additional medical personnel into them until the therapeutic table has been completed. To surface the chamber mid-treatment exposes the medical attendant to DCS and induces clinical deterioration in the patient.

In-water recompression

In an attempt to initiate early therapy, many divers (usually diving fishers) have been recompressed on air in the water. Both mechanical and physiological problems are encountered. Requirements for diver support include a sufficient supply of compressed air, tolerable weather conditions, a full-face mask or helmet to prevent aspiration of water, adequate thermal protection and a constant attendant.

The problems often encountered during in-water air recompression therapy include seasickness, drowning, hypothermia, panic and the aggravation of the illness by subjecting the patient to a further uptake of inert gas in the tissues, thus compounding the problem on subsequent ascent. In many cases, the regimen has to be terminated prematurely because of adverse weather conditions, equipment failure, sharks, physiological issues and, finally, psychological difficulties. Even when the treatment does give relief, it often needs to be supplemented with the conventional recompression therapy carried out in a chamber soon after the patient has left the water.

A much more effective approach to in-water recompression therapy uses 100 per cent oxygen, at a maximum of 9 metres, and is relatively short in duration. This regimen, which has been particularly valuable in remote localities, is described in Chapter 13 and in Appendix C. It usually involves a 30- to 90-minute stay at 9 metres, and ascent at the rate of 12 minutes/metre. It has the advantages of not aggravating the disease by adding more inert gas, being of short duration, avoiding any problem of nitrogen narcosis and being suited for shallow bays and off wharves, protected from the open sea.

DIVING MEDICAL KIT

Diving support boats should be equipped for likely accidents. No checklist can contain materials needed for all situations, but as a general guide, the following items should be considered:

- Airways for use in resuscitation.
- Oxygen therapy and resuscitation unit capable of proving near 100 per cent oxygen to a breathing diver, whether conscious or unconscious, and at least 50 per cent oxygen

(preferably 100 per cent) for oxygen supplemented resuscitation. There needs to be at least one person available who is trained, qualified and practised in the use of this equipment.

- An adequate oxygen supply.
- Suction system that is preferably not reliant on potentially scarce oxygen supplies.
- Topical antibiotic or antiseptic for skin injuries.
- Motion sickness tablets and injections.
- Bandages and wound dressings.
- Preparations to prevent and treat common otological problems and cold, sun or wind exposure.

Treatment for dangerous marine animal injury depends on the fauna of the expected dive site, but it may include the following:

- Wound dressing and bandages to manage severe bleeding.
- Tourniquet to be used in the event that other haemorrhage control methods prove ineffective.
- Elastic bandages (sea snake, blue-ringed octopus, cone shell envenomation).
- Local anesthetic ointment for minor stings.
- Local anesthetic injection without adrenaline (scorpion fish, stonefish, stingray, catfish).
- Vinegar for box jellyfish stings (at least 1 litre).
- Appropriate antivenoms (sea snake, box jellyfish, stonefish).

If DCI is possible, consider the following (which may not be practical or appropriate, depending on the setting):

- Intravenous infusion system (e.g. physiological saline).
- Urinary catheter.
- An on-site portable two-person recompression chamber if possible.
- Medical kit required for the recompression chamber.
- Equipment for in-water recompression for remote areas.

Special circumstances will require supplementation of the foregoing medical kits. In remote localities, diagnostic and therapeutic equipment varying from a thermometer to a thoracotomy set may be appropriate. Ear drops to prevent and/or treat external ear infections are especially necessary in the tropics. Broad-spectrum antibiotics are also needed. The use of these depends on the clinical training of the attendants.

A laryngoscope and endotracheal airway or laryngeal mask may be of use if trained medical assistance is available. It is important that diving support boats have radio communications to obtain expert medical advice on the treatment of difficult or unexpected problems. Frequently, medical personnel and paramedical personnel are available coincidentally.

DIVING EMERGENCY HOTLINES

In an emergency, specialist diving medical advice can be obtained from DAN:

- Americas: DAN America: 1-919-684-9111.
- Asia-Pacific: DAN Asia-Pacific Diving Emergency Service (DES): 1800-088-200 (within Australia); +61-8-8212-9242 (from outside Australia).
- Japan: DAN Japan: +81-3-3812-4999.
- Europe: DAN Europe: +39-06-4211-8685.
- Southern Africa: DAN Southern Africa: +27-10-209-8112.

See Appendix F for more information.

FURTHER READING

Bennett M, Mitchell S, Dominguez A. Adjunctive treatment of decompression illness with a non-steroidal anti-inflammatory drug (tenoxicam) reduces compression requirement. *Undersea and Hyperbaric Medicine* 2003;**30**(3):195–205.

Edmonds CE, Walker D, Scott B. Drowning syndromes with scuba. *South Pacific Underwater Medicine Society Journal* 1997;**27**(4):182–197.

Harpur GD. Hypoxia in out-of-air ascents: a preliminary report. *South Pacific Underwater Medicine Society Journal* 1994;**14**(14):24–28.

Harpur GD. Ninety seconds deep scuba rescue. *NAUI News* 1975;**5**(1):17–21.

Lippmann J. In-water rescue breathing. *Alert Diver Asia-Pacific* 2008;**Jan–Mar:**6–10.

Lippmann J. *Oxygen First Aid*. Asia-Pacific ed. Melbourne: Submariner Publications; 2011.

Lippmann J. *The DAN Emergency Handbook*. 7th ed. Asia-Pacific ed. Melbourne: Submariner Publications; 2013.

Longphre JM, Denoble PJ, Moon RE, *et al*. First aid normobaric oxygen for the treatment of recreational diving injuries. *Undersea and Hyperbaric Medicine* 2007;**34**(1):43–49.

Mitchell SJ, Bennett MH, Bird N, Doolette DJ, Hobbs GW, Kay E, Moon RE, Neuman TS, Vann RD, Walker R, Wyatt HA. Recommendations for rescue of a submerged unresponsive compressed-gas diver. *Undersea and Hyperbaric Medicine* 2012;**39**(6):1099–1108.

Szpilman D. Near-drowning and drowning: a proposal to stratify mortality based on the analysis of 1,831 cases. *Chest* 1997;**112:**660–665.

Vann RD, Butler FK, Mitchell SJ, Moon RE. Decompression illness. *Lancet* 2011;**377:**153–164.

Zeindler PR, Freiberger JJ. Triage and emergency evacuation of recreational diver: a case series analysis. *Undersea and Hyperbaric Medicine* 2010;**37**(2):133–139.

This chapter was reviewed for this fifth edition by John Lippmann.

Oxygen therapy

PHYSIOLOGY

Despite some suggestions that administering high concentrations of oxygen (O_2) during resuscitation and following myocardial infarction can result in worse outcomes[1], it remains prudent to suggest that O_2 should be used in almost all serious scuba diving accidents, and there are some data to support this approach.

To understand the requirements for effective O_2 delivery systems, we need to understand a little of the cardiorespiratory physiology discussed in Chapters 2, 16 and 39.

Breathing dry air at 1 ATA results in an inspired O_2 pressure (PIO_2) of approximately 160 mm Hg. The O_2 pressure (PO_2) is diluted somewhat by the 'dead space' of the respiratory passages, the continual absorption of O_2 from the lungs and humidification, resulting in an alveolar PO_2 (PAO_2) of approximately 100 mm Hg (Table 49.1). In healthy individuals, the arterial PO_2 (PaO_2) reaches about 673 mm Hg, if 100 per cent O_2 is breathed at 1 ATA. These and subsequent numbers are approximations and vary with many factors, such as ventilation perfusion ratio, haemoglobin concentration, pH, exercise and carbon dioxide (CO_2) levels.

The normal PaO_2 is about 105 mm Hg, and there is a 65 mm Hg pressure gradient driving O_2 across the alveolar wall into the pulmonary capillaries (where the pulmonary venous PO_2 is about 40 mm Hg). Diffusion is rapid, and the normal PaO_2 is about 100 mm Hg.

Breathing air at 1 ATA, about 97 per cent of the O_2 is transported in combination with haemoglobin in the red cells, with the remaining 3 per cent dissolved in plasma (Figure 49.1). In fact, only 0.003 ml of O_2 is dissolved in each 100 ml of blood for each millimetre of mercury of oxygen tension (Henry's Law). In contrast, 1 g of haemoglobin can bind 1.34 ml O_2, and therefore at a normal haematocrit of 150 g/litre, 100 ml of blood can transport about 20 ml O_2 in combination with haemoglobin. In venous blood, the PO_2 is 40 mm Hg, and the saturation of haemoglobin is about 75 per cent.

Although the primary determinant of ventilation is the arterial CO_2 tension ($PaCO_2$), the rate of CO_2 production during exercise is roughly equal to the consumption of O_2. Thus, although the increased ventilation serves to 'normalize' $PaCO_2$, there is also an increased volume of O_2 available to meet the increase in metabolic demands. With a basal O_2 consumption of 200 ml/minute, the

Table 49.1 Examples of oxygen tensions at different ambient pressures breathing air and 100% oxygen

Pressure	PO$_2$ (air)	P$_A$O$_2$ (air)	P$_A$O$_2$ (100% O$_2$)	Dissolved O$_2$ (ml) (air)	Dissolved O$_2$ (ml) (100% O$_2$)
1 ATA	0.21	102	673	0.32	2.09
2 ATA	0.42	262	1433	0.81	4.44
3 ATA	0.63	422	2193	1.31	6.80

* Breathing gas noted in parenthesis.

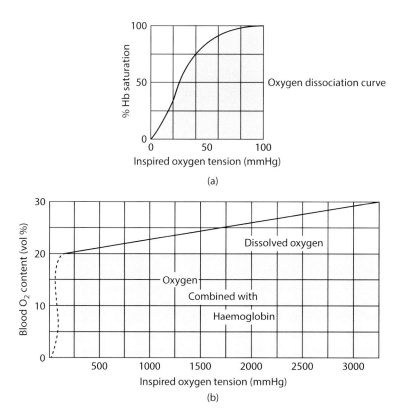

Figure 49.1 The oxygen-carrying capacity of blood (a) while breathing air at 1 ATA and (b) while breathing 100 per cent oxygen from zero to 3500 mm Hg (4.6 ATA). The curve in (a) is the usual oxygen-haemoglobin dissociation curve and is represented in (b) by the dotted portion of the curve.

ventilation rate may be 4 litres/minute (lpm). At an extreme consumption of 1000 ml/minute of O$_2$, the ventilation may rise to 20 lpm to eliminate the approximately equal amount of CO$_2$ produced. At the same time, delivery of O$_2$ to the tissues is enhanced by increasing cardiac output by as much as six or seven times.

The ability to increase O$_2$ delivery to the tissues by administering O$_2$ depends extensively on the starting arterial O$_2$ saturation (SaO$_2$). With normal cardiorespiratory function, the SaO$_2$ is usually around 97 per cent. Only a small amount of extra O$_2$ can be transported bound to haemoglobin (the 3 per cent of unoccupied binding sites), and an even smaller amount of extra O$_2$ is dissolved in the plasma. If, however, the SaO$_2$ is low (e.g. 70 per cent because of impaired diffusion secondary to poor lung function as a result of sea water aspiration), then increasing the inspired O_2 concentration may have profound effects on the delivery of O_2 – again the contribution of O_2 dissolved in the plasma is small.

If we wish to increase the delivery of O_2 to the tissues when the SaO_2 is already high, the only recourse is to increase greatly the amount of O_2 dissolved in the plasma. The only way to achieve this is to inspire hugely increased pressures of O_2 in a compression chamber. At 2.8 ATA (the equivalent of 18 metres underwater), breathing 100 per cent O_2 may result in a PaO_2 of 1800 mm Hg, with similarly impressive increases in the tissues. When treating decompression sickness (DCS), it is this high PO_2 that provides the 'window' to reduce the tissue pressure of nitrogen rapidly and consequently to eliminate nitrogen bubbles (see Chapter 13). Hyperbaric physicians also use similarly high PO_2 values to achieve a myriad of therapeutic effects in the tissues.

At 3 ATA breathing 100 per cent O_2, 6 ml of O_2 is carried dissolved in the plasma – equivalent to the resting O_2 requirement. This was experimentally confirmed by Boerema in pigs, following which he famously wrote that he had demonstrated that under these conditions one could have 'life without blood'[2].

This is not achieved without consequences. Approximately 20 per cent of the CO_2 generated in the tissues is normally transported bound to deoxygenated haemoglobin. Although some excess CO_2 is buffered in the red cells and plasma, there is nevertheless a rise of about 5 to 6 mm Hg of PCO_2 in venous blood ($PvCO_2$) when breathing high O_2, which is compensated over a short time by an increase in the minute ventilation.

For a thorough review of the equipment and techniques discussed earlier, see Lippmann's *Oxygen First Aid: A Guide to the Provision of Oxygen in First Aid and Emergency Care*[3].

PATHOPHYSIOLOGY

The potential effects of hyperoxia are as follows:

1. Reduction in the transport of CO_2 bound to haemoglobin.
2. Depression of ventilation resulting from a suppressive effect on the carotid and aortic bodies (of practical importance only in patients with severe cardiorespiratory impairment).
3. Washout of nitrogen from the alveoli, with increased likelihood of atelectasis as the O_2 is later absorbed.
4. Bradycardia producing a decreased cardiac output and decreased cerebral blood flow. A reflex response to vaso-constriction of peripheral vessels (see the next list item).
5. Vaso-constriction of peripheral vessels of most organs, with increased peripheral resistance. The vaso-constrictive effect of hyperbaric O_2 becomes significant somewhere between 1.5 and 2 ATA. It can be seen as a regulatory mechanism to protect the healthy tissues from exposure to excessive O_2 pressures.
6. Increased free radical production. Breathing oxygen at greater than 1 ATA O_2 increases production of reactive O_2 species (ROS)[3], and this is critically important because it is the molecular basis for several therapeutic mechanisms[4].
7. Angiogenesis and increased fibroblastic activity. Although useful in wound healing, these effects are not always desired, as in the retrolental fibroplasia causing blindness in premature infants who are treated with high O_2 concentrations.
8. Neurological and pulmonary O_2 toxicity (see Chapter 17).
9. Respiratory failure in patients with chronic obstructive airways disease. In this disease – rare in the active diving population – the administration of O_2 may be detrimental because respiration can be dependent on a hypoxic drive. Once this hypoxia is corrected, respiratory failure is possible.

PRACTICAL OXYGEN DELIVERY

The requirements of O_2 delivery systems vary according to circumstance. Very different systems are required to supply O_2 effectively to spontaneously breathing patients and to patients who require artificial respiration, for example. Some of these issues are explored in this section.

Spontaneously breathing divers

SURFACE OXYGEN SYSTEMS

Masks

There are loose fitting masks or devices (e.g. nasal prongs) that simply supplement the diver's normal respiratory air with various amounts of O_2. The effect varies with the type of mask or device, its fit on the diver, the flow rate of O_2 employed and the respiratory minute volume of the diver. These devices are usually recommended for use with modest flow rates (2 to 8 lpm) and provide only moderate levels of supplementation with an upper limit of about 45 per cent O_2 for a nasal cannula or a simple 'Hudson' mask.

Venturi masks have a series of different colour-coded connectors that deliver known fraction of inspired O_2 (FIO_2) at the prescribed flow rate. Up to 60 per cent oxygen is possible with the green connector at a flow rate of 12 lpm. As with all fixed-flow devices, however, the actual FIO_2 achieved greatly depends on the inspiratory flow rate because the O_2 is mixed with air entrained from around the mask.

None of the foregoing masks are adequate for treatment of diving casualties because the inspired O_2 concentration delivered is too low.

The most effective masks have a reservoir that fills with O_2 during expiration and partially overcomes the problem of air dilution. These masks should also be fitted with three one-way valves to reduce air entrainment and prevent expired breath from entering the reservoir. At a flow rate of 15 lpm, these 'non-rebreather masks' can deliver around 80 per cent O_2 and more if they are well-fitting (Figure 49.2). In practice, more than 80 per cent is difficult to achieve.

The Divers Alert Network includes a mask in its O_2 units for use by breathing divers who cannot tolerate a demand valve or for use as a secondary delivery option.

Airtight masks

Rather than plastic, these masks are usually made of polyvinyl chloride or silicone, soft enough to mold to the diver's (or aviator's) face. The O_2 source must be capable of providing low-resistance breathing up to the maximum inspiratory flow rate

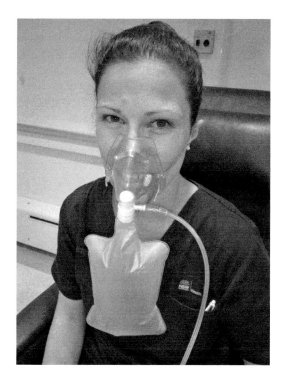

Figure 49.2 A non-rebreathing mask. Note the reservoir bag and one-way valves. (Photograph by M. Bennett.)

or the user will not tolerate the system, as well as an exhalation valve to avoid mixing exhaled and inspiratory gas.

Demand flow devices

One way of achieving high inspiratory O_2 is a demand valve regulated from a high-pressure source (performing the same function as the first and second stages of a diving regulator) combined with an airtight mask. These systems can achieve 100 per cent O_2, in both conscious and spontaneously breathing unconscious patients (Figure 49.3). A further adaptation allows use in unconscious patients who are not breathing, with the addition of a demand valve fitted with manual positive pressure capability. These devices, also known as manually triggered O_2-powered ventilators, require significant skill and practice to use safely and effectively.

Divers are, of course, used to demand systems, and a mouthpiece may be substituted for the oronasal mask to provide O_2 to a conscious patient. When a mouthpiece is used, it is prudent to employ

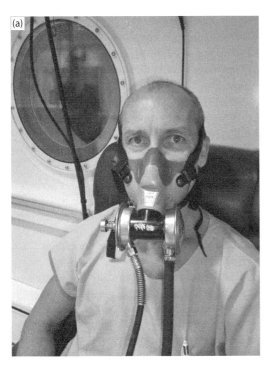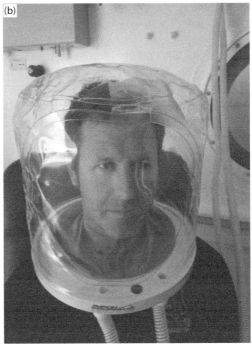

Figure 49.3 One hundred per cent oxygen delivery devices. **(a)** A demand system for use in a chamber (Scott mask). **(b)** A hood for use during hyperbaric oxygen therapy. (Photographs by M. Bennett.)

a nose clip; otherwise, some admission of air is likely through that orifice. Nevertheless, most divers are fully aware of how to block off their nose, and if necessary this can be done by donning their normal airtight half-face mask. Divers are used to breathing with this system and may prefer it.

Helmet systems

Lightweight, transparent plastic hoods are often employed in hyperbaric chambers (see Figure 49.3). These hoods use neck seals and high flow rates (usually well in excess of 20 lpm) to eliminate rebreathing.

The simplest and most effective way to provide near 100 per cent O_2 to a breathing diver is with a demand valve system. If the diver is not breathing, positive pressure ventilation is needed, either by a demand flow device with manual positive pressure capability or with the anaesthetic-type *bag-mask* unit. With the bag-mask unit, there is high O_2 flow to a breathing bag, which is then attached to the mask – the addition of a reservoir bag increases the FIO_2. Inhalation is from the

bag, and exhalation is through a one-way valve. Caution is needed with both devices if pulmonary barotrauma is suspected.

These are all *open-circuit* systems and usually require large volumes of O_2. Demand valves require a minute volume of 5 to 10 lpm, if the patient is relaxed and at rest. Very high O_2 concentrations can usually be achieved if a reservoir is used with a bag-valve-mask system and a flow rate of 15 lpm or higher.

Rebreathing systems

CO_2 absorbent can be used in a semi-closed-circuit or closed-circuit system. In this situation, a lower-flow O_2 supply can be used (e.g. 2 to 4 lpm in a resting patient), with a small but constant and equivalent exhaust system to ensure that there is a no nitrogen build-up. The absorbent removes the CO_2 produced. Problems with such systems include the greater maintenance involved and the higher level of training required for safe use.

There have been a few rebreathers with an absorbent canister filled with potassium superoxide, which gives off O_2 as it absorbs CO_2. This is of considerable value when there are limitations of space or restrictions regarding transport of high-pressure O_2 cylinders. The disadvantages are cost and availability.

Assisted respiration

In the unconscious patient, ventilation can be taken over either manually (bag-valve-mask) or by using gas-powered (usually O_2-powered) ventilators. Ventilators can also be employed to assist respiration when this is present but impaired.

Many different ventilators are available, both pressure cycled and volume cycled. Their use is a specialized field, and use by untrained personnel is not recommended. Some of these ventilators are suitable for use in hyperbaric chambers.

O_2 may also be administered in the underwater situation (see Chapter 13), in recompression chambers (with the same variety of methods described earlier) and during medical evacuation (see Chapter 48).

Hyperbaric oxygen therapy

Hyperbaric O_2 therapy (HBOT) is often employed for a variety of non-diving therapies. Hyperbaric O_2 can assist in relieving tissue hypoxia and oedema. There is evidence that it may reduce the disastrous effect of leucocyte adherence to damaged endothelium, which plays a pathological role in acute decompression illness[5].

A single 45-minute exposure to a PO_2 tension of 2.8 ATA inhibits the activation of leucocytes, a mechanism of central importance in microvascular dysfunction and ischaemia reperfusion injury. This effect lasts at least 24 hours[6].

In the treatment of chronic ischaemic wounds, a series of HBOT exposures is associated with significant angioneogenesis, collagen formation and macrophage function, resulting in significantly improved healing[7].

Poor perfusion and decreased PO_2 tension increase the likelihood of infection in animal experiments. Deep, contaminated tissue injuries can be associated with necrotizing infections, the best known of which is gas gangrene. Hyperbaric O_2 inhibits the germination of clostridial spores and

the production of the alphatoxin that destroys cell membranes and promotes oedema through increasing capillary permeability. Both lead to further falls in tissue PO_2 and rapidly spreading infection. HBOT, along with appropriate surgical and antibiotic therapy, can limit the tissue loss.

For a general review of the mechanisms of and indications for HBOT, please see Neuman and Thom's *Physiology and Medicine of Hyperbaric Oxygen Therapy*[8].

DROWNING SYNDROMES

O_2 supplementation is of enormous value in overcoming the hypoxic effects, including encephalopathy, that often follow the ventilation-perfusion anomalies and blood shunting in the lungs of the victim of near drowning. Although ventilation in these patients tends to increase to reduce the elevated CO_2 levels, this response may not be adequate to overcome the hypoxia.

Supplementary O_2, and especially positive pressure respiration, may reduce the degree of hypoxia and allow time for the diver to recover.

Indeed, one can gradually titrate and reduce the positive pressure of the assisted respirators, and subsequently the O_2 percentages, as the PaO_2 increases.

DECOMPRESSION

Decompression procedures have been developed to allow the safe elimination of inert gas (usually nitrogen) through expiration. O_2 breathing is an effective means of removing the inert gas from the inspiratory gases, thus permitting much more rapid elimination of nitrogen down a steeper pressure gradient from tissue to alveolus. This effect greatly magnifies the usual state of 'inherent unsaturation' that results from the metabolic consumption of O_2. This has been called the 'O_2 window' – a term first used by Behnke in 1967. The O_2 window is the difference between the PaO_2 and the tissue PO_2 (PtO_2)[9].

The O_2 window can be used both when breathing O_2 on the surface (the final decompression stop) or by breathing O_2-enriched gas at depth. In this situation it is not so much the presence of O_2 but the absence of inert gas that is of value.

Hyperoxia-induced vaso-constriction reduces tissue perfusion, somewhat counteracting the benefits the O_2 window and resulting in a slowing of the nitrogen washout. Breathing 100 per cent O_2 at 2.0 and 2.5 ATA in a hyperbaric chamber (beyond safe diving O_2 limits) has been shown to result in 8.9 and 16.9 per cent reductions in perfusion, respectively, compared with controls at 0.2 ATA. It is not clear this is a practical concern in divers, who are usually vaso-constricted from the effects of cold and relative dehydration when they are immersed.

BUBBLE DISEASE

Paul Bert described the value of O_2 with decompression sickness and noted that the animals so affected did not deteriorate while breathing this gas.

When the inert gas bubble phase has developed, it is important to remove the inert gas as rapidly as possible, so that the bubble will diminish and collapse. Unless this is achieved, the tissue around the gas is likely to undergo histological changes resulting in stabilization of the bubble through the deposition of blood constituents around the bubble-tissue interface or the bubble-blood interface.

Bubbles can be reduced in size by using both pressurization (recompression) and enhancing diffusion of gas out of the bubble by increasing the bubble to tissue gas pressure gradient as described earlier (increasing the O_2 or heliox window) (see Figure 10.3).

The use of O_2 is relevant in both DCS, in which there are gas bubbles within vessels or tissues, and some barotrauma accidents, such as pulmonary barotrauma (mediastinal emphysema, pneumopericardium, pneumoperitoneum, air embolism, pneumothorax) and localized surgical emphysema from a variety of causes (see Chapters 6, 8 and 9). It may even be of some value in inner ear barotrauma, where air has passed into the perilymph. When used in suspected DCS, surface O_2 reduces clinical symptoms and the number of sequelae following treatment[10].

GAS TOXICITIES

O_2 may be added to air (nitrox) and used to reduce or avoid the effects of nitrogen narcosis and DCS by reducing the pressure of inspired N_2 (PIN$_2$) at any given depth.

It is also used to overcome or bypass some of the effects of carbon monoxide toxicity and the influence that this has, in a competitive manner, on O_2 transport.

DANGERS

These dangers can be divided into logistical problems and those associated with fire and/or explosion.

The logistical difficulties are similar to those with any compressed gas system. Similar, if not more stringent, care must be taken to ensure that there are adequate supplies of the gas to fulfill the various treatment regimens.

Inside a decompression or recompression chamber, O_2, whether from a cylinder or from the exhaust gases of a diver undergoing treatment, can accumulate such that the internal O_2 concentration rises. High-O_2 environments support vigorous combustion and are to be strictly avoided by the use of monitoring, overboard dump systems or high flush rates. O_2 equipment must be specifically designed for this use, and this is a specialist area.

Specifically designed O_2 regulators reduce the likelihood of spontaneous combustion, especially as the cylinder valve is 'cracked' (turned on). O_2 regulators require special lubricants because of the danger of explosion associated with carbon-based lubricants in the presence of high O_2 pressures. Even the adhesive tape that divers commonly apply to protect the outlet and O-ring of the scuba cylinder, and to signify that it has been filled, should not be used on O_2 cylinders. Maintenance must be undertaken according to the manufacturer's instructions and in an 'O_2-clean' environment. Cleanliness is vital.

When administering O_2, the equipment should be turned on and tested before use. In the case of a demand system, the cylinder is turned on and the valve purged before it is offered to the diver. Although it is rare for the O_2 to be replaced by flame, this situation is worth avoiding.

O_2 cylinders for use in therapy should be of large volume because high flows may be required to deliver adequate PIO$_2$. The sizes, pressure ratings and colour coding of O_2 cylinders vary among countries. In Australia, C size is 490 litres, D is 1640 litres, E is 4100 litres and G is 8280 litres. Even the smallest of these cylinders is not easily carried in some dive boats, where ideal stowage and stability may conflict with cleanliness and produce other problems with boat handling. It is, however, of great importance that O_2 is readily available wherever diving is conducted.

In some instances, O_2 resuscitation devices are fitted with small cylinders for short-term emergencies – inadequate for O_2 therapy over more than a few minutes. Specialized O_2 adapters have been developed to supplement this inadequate supply with that from a larger cylinder. These adapters must be O_2 clean and compatible.

O_2 should be used only in well-ventilated areas, and any obvious source of ignition must be kept well away. In some instances (e.g. the confined cabins of boats or aircraft), great care must be applied to ensure that the exhaled O_2 is ventilated overboard.

Attention must be given to the storage of cylinders, by ensuring that these are adequately shut following use and with positive pressure still within the cylinders (to prevent ingress of water). This is especially so with O_2 because of its increased corrosive properties. The remainder of the distribution system (e.g. regulators, hoses) should be stored after depressurization, as with scuba equipment.

As a rule of thumb, any O_2 cylinder less than half-full should be replaced, although this depends on the size of the cylinder, the availability of other O_2 supplies and the likely period of required O_2 administration. The cylinder valve should not be left on because of the possibility of O_2 escaping and the fatigue it will cause to the O_2 regulator.

The valve should be fully turned off on any empty cylinders to prevent moisture and contaminants from entering.

Before a medical O_2 cylinder is refilled, it is emptied, inspected and, if required, cleaned. Occasionally it may be necessary to use industrial O_2 when medical O_2 is not available. Although the O_2 used to fill such cylinders is very pure, the industrial O_2 cylinder is frequently not properly evacuated and cleaned with each refill, so contaminants may accumulate if the cylinder was left open. Given that industrial cylinders are often used in situations in which environmental and industrial pollutants may be present, care should be exercised. Despite this caution, testing of industrial O_2 by the suppliers does ensure that it is of an extremely high quality, and there should be no hesitation in employing it, if it is the only available source.

REFERENCES

1. Kilgannon JH, Jones AE, Parrillo JE, et al. Relationship between supranormal oxygen tension and outcome after resuscitation from cardiac arrest. *Circulation* 2011;**123**:2717–2722.
2. Boerema I, Meyne NG, Brummelkamp WH, et al. [Life without blood.] *Nederlands Tijdschrift voor Geneeskunde* 1960;**104**:949–954.
3. Lippmann J. *Oxygen First Aid: A Guide to the Provision of Oxygen in First Aid and Emergency Care.* Melbourne: JL Publications; 2011.
4. Thom SR. Hyperbaric oxygen therapy. *Journal of Intensive Care Medicine* 1989;**4**:58–74.
5. Thom SR. Hyperbaric oxygen: its mechanisms and efficacy. *Plastic and Reconstructive Surgery* 2011;**127**(Suppl 1):131S–141S.
6. Buras JA, Reenstra WR. Endothelial-neutrophil interactions during ischemia and reperfusion injury: basic mechanisms of hyperbaric oxygen. *Neurology Research* 2007;**29**(2):127–131.
7. Kranke P, Bennett MH, Martyn-St. James M, et al. Hyperbaric oxygen therapy for chronic wounds. *Cochrane Database of Systematic Reviews.* 2012;(4):CD0041234.
8. Neuman TS, Thom SR, eds. *Physiology and Medicine of Hyperbaric Oxygen Therapy.* Philadelphia: Saunders; 2008.
9. Behnke AR. The isobaric (oxygen window) principle of decompression. Transcript of the Third Marine Technology Society Conference, San Diego. The new thrust seaward. Washington DC, Marine Technology Society 1967.
10. Tikuisis P, Gerth W. Decompression theory. In: Brubakk AO, Neuman TS, eds. *Bennett and Elliott's Physiology and Medicine of Diving.* 5th ed. Philadelphia: Saunders; 2003:425–427.

This chapter was reviewed for this fifth edition by Michael Bennett.

50

Investigation of diving accidents

INTRODUCTION

This chapter should be read in conjunction with Chapter 51. The collection and analysis of data and their contribution to the accident or death investigation are similar:

- Personal and past medical history.
- Environmental conditions.
- Dive profile and history.

These components are equally relevant to non-fatal and fatal diving accidents. For non-fatal accidents, the presence of a first-hand witness, the patient, makes the data more complete and subject to interrogation. A clinical examination of the accident victim is analogous to the autopsy on the deceased (see Chapter 51), and equipment testing for this is more demanding.

In the remainder of this chapter, the approach is mainly from the viewpoint of practical divers or paramedics encountering an accident once first aid and medical treatment have been initiated. This chapter deals more with the diving equipment – giving the non-expert an appreciation of how equipment assessment contributes to

the accident investigation and how anomalies can be interpreted. The actual testing of such equipment is conducted by others – diving technicians and experienced dive accident investigators.

Although attention is appropriately directed to the victim, he or she may merely be the 'canary in the coal mine'. Injury may be caused by incorrect gases, faulty equipment, harsh environments and inappropriate diving practices, shared by others. Thus, others may also be at risk.

Probably the most valuable contribution to the investigation of diving accidents is the early and complete documentation of the events (dive profile and accident) as recorded from the victim and witnesses, together with observations of the state of the victim, the environment and the equipment.

PERSONAL AND MEDICAL HISTORY

Personal data may be relevant in the understanding of the diving accident. First and foremost is the presence of diseases likely to predispose to the diving accident, and reference should be made to Chapters 46 and 52 to 59.

The experience of the diver and his or her companions is of relevance and should be compared with the situation encountered in the eventful dive. Inexperienced divers tend to:

- Misuse or fail to use equipment.
- Use inappropriate equipment.
- Mishandle and damage equipment.
- Fail to undertake proper maintenance and repairs.
- Not recognize early malfunctions.
- Fail to appreciate potential environmental hazards.
- Take inappropriate rescue actions.

Accidents are more likely with the inexperienced diver, and especially during the first open water dive.

Any history of previous diving accidents should be sought. Many problems experienced by divers in the past are repeated under similar conditions. These include hypoxia from breath-holding after hyperventilation by free divers, panic with hyperventilation, salt water aspiration, scuba divers' pulmonary oedema, alternobaric vertigo, barotraumas and especially pulmonary barotrauma, nitrogen narcosis, syncope of ascent, decompression sickness (DCS), oxygen toxicity and carbon dioxide toxicity with rebreathing equipment.

The diver's log book may indicate the type of diving performed and thus may indicate accident potential. So may witnesses, relatives, dive buddies, dive leaders and decompression computers. A pre-dive medical examination may well detect and record relevant factors whose significance may not be evident to non-diving physicians.

Alcohol and drug history may be very relevant, with both illicit and legal drugs contributing to accidents.

> ## Personal and past medical history
>
> - Pre-existing diseases.
> - Past diving experience and training.
> - Previous diving accidents.
> - Drug and alcohol use.

ENVIRONMENTAL CONDITIONS

Environmental factors have contributed to 62 per cent of recreational diving deaths (see Chapters 5, 45 and 46).

Dive information should include the weather and water conditions prevailing at the time of the accident. There may be exceptional stress in the form of impaired visibility, seasickness, tidal currents, cold and other factors. Local hazards may include areas of entrapment (e.g. fishing lines, kelp), the presence of marine animals (e.g., sharks, Irukandji), trauma from boats, surf, explosives and other divers and an inability to surface (e.g. under ledges, in caves, wrecks, dam outlets).

The temperature of the water influences hypothermia, manual dexterity, DCS and also the functioning of various pieces of diving equipment. Carbon dioxide absorbents are less effective under cold conditions. With temperatures approaching freezing point, regulators may freeze.

> ## Environmental conditions
>
> - Wind and weather.
> - Reduced visibility with sediment, night diving and other conditions.
> - Adverse water conditions, waves, rips, currents and 'white water'.
> - Water temperature.
> - Caves, ledges, kelp, fishing nets.
> - Dangerous marine creatures.

DIVE PROFILE AND HISTORY

With fatalities and legally significant accidents, information is collected by the dive accident investigators, as are details of the equipment and gases employed by the diver and his or her associates. This information is complemented by dive computer data.

With most recreational diving accidents, information initially comes from the diver or his or her companion, instructor or rescuer. It is important to let the victim and witnesses tell their stories independently, without interruption, and preferably without a third person present. Then question them to clarify any unclear aspects.

Not only may the diver be exposed to an increased risk of injury during entry to or exit from the water, but also during the dive there may be limitations on both diver and equipment performance.

The depth is of importance in nitrogen narcosis and its influence on divers' behaviour and also in other gas toxicities, such as carbon dioxide and oxygen toxicities. DCS, increased gas consumption, cold, panic and rescue procedures can be adversely influenced.

The speed of ascent, if excessive, can contribute to pulmonary barotrauma, DCS, syncope of ascent and dilution hypoxia with rebreathers. Some recreational divers have been timed to exceed 60 metres per minute in their 'routine' ascents.

Exercise performed during the dive is often relevant. Exertion is required when swimming against currents or being incorrectly weighted. A diver who has to battle a 1-knot current frequently requires excess gas flow. With *scuba* diving, there are problems from increased exertion. First, there is an increased consumption of gas, and this may not be appreciated by the diver who is not wearing or observing a contents gauge to indicate the supply. Second, there is the problem of increased resistance to breathing with resultant dyspnoea and physical exhaustion. Panic and fatigue are then common sequelae.

Exercise is even more influential with *rebreathing equipment* (see Chapter 62). With strenuous exercise, the increased oxygen requirement may be in excess of that supplied by the flow rate and gas mixture chosen, resulting in hypoxia. With increased oxygen consumption there is also increased carbon dioxide production, placing an added load on the absorbent system. Thus, the chances of both hypoxia and carbon dioxide toxicity are increased.

Frequently dive computers can be downloaded to produce not only a detailed dive profile, but also documentation of other recent dives. Dive computer data are best downloaded by a diving technician from the specific computer manufacturer. More frequently, the data come from the injured diver.

The history of recent dives is of great importance when considering the possibility of DCS, and

it may be equally relevant in cases of pulmonary barotrauma, salt water aspiration, scuba divers' pulmonary oedema, hypothermia and other disorders.

Dive profile and history

- Recent dives – log book and companion divers.
- Depth and duration – dive recorder or computer.
- Entry, exit.
- Speed of descent, ascent and stoppages.
- Pre-, during and post-dive exercise.
- Alcohol, drug or food consumption.
- Problems – seasickness, stress, exertion, illness and other disorders.
- Environmental stressors.
- Rescue, first aid and resuscitation attempts.

Accidents frequently involve panic and a rapid ascent. Under these conditions, information of interest may not be remembered clearly. The out-of-air situation and the measures used to counteract it are particular hazards, often resulting in a desperate rapid ascent.

Probably the most neglected information relevant to any accident, and also to the interpretation of the clinical or autopsy findings, is that involving the **first aid and resuscitation** methods employed. Such activities as rescue procedures, re-immersion, recompression, resuscitation, oxygen administration and so forth should be recorded in detail because they influence investigations and interpretations of the diving accident.

CLINICAL EXAMINATION

Often the clinical examination may contribute information that is not evident or appreciated by the patient. Aggravating factors to the accident can vary from pre-existing disorders such as mild asthma, cardiac disease or allergies to specific problems such as an oxygen-induced epileptic convulsion (indicated by a bitten tongue) or an unnoticed marine animal sting.

Vital signs may indicate hypothermia and respiratory and cardiac disorders. Surgical emphysema implies barotraumas with air extension.

Skin lesions may indicate marine animal injuries, DCS, cold urticaria and other conditions.

Examination or investigation may indicate unrecognized upper or lower respiratory tract barotraumas, as well as many of the lesser-known illnesses described in this text.

The combination of the personal and medical history, the environmental factors, the dive profile and the clinical examination will lead to a differential diagnosis that, in turn, dictates the investigations and treatment required.

DIVING EQUIPMENT

After an accident, it is important that no interference occurs with the equipment, except to seal it and close the cylinder valves – to retain the breathing gas for analysis. In doing this it is important to record the readings on any gauges and the number of turns needed to close the valve or valves. In particular, one needs to be on guard against the well-intentioned but ignorant would-be investigator. For example, an attempt to view a carbon dioxide absorbent not only negates the opportunity to test the set for leaks but also contaminates the gas samples with air.

The proper authority for investigating the accident should be identified. In some countries, several groups are involved. The water police and police divers have skills and knowledge of diving equipment. Normally, the equipment is assessed by them. If the diver was employed, the workplace and safety inspectors will be involved to consider any possible fault by the employer. A work-related accident, and accidents where there was possibly a criminal or negligent act, will require professional and expert investigations. The possibility that a student or his or her relatives will litigate against the dive school should also be considered. Under all these conditions, equipment examination should be left to the specialized dive accident investigators.

In most recreational diving accidents, there is no such obligation, and the investigation of the cause is left to the victim, the dive club or the dive instructor – none of whom are usually adept at this task. This is unfortunate because there is a maxim in diving medicine that 'any diving accident that is not adequately explained and then prevented, will recur – but with greater severity'.

Equipment should be protected against interference. The presence or absence of equipment should be documented, and photographs of any possibly contributory equipment should be taken. The performance of similar diving equipment used by other divers may be informative, as may a cylinder containing air from the same source. Assessment needs modification depending on the equipment used and facilities available.

It may be necessary to consult the rescuer and any resuscitators to identify any item that may have been affected or removed by the accident or during rescue. One should look for damage to protective clothing, the diving set and accessories, the face mask and its strap, the buoyancy vest and counterlung integrity or damage. The lugs of the mouthpiece may be bitten during a convulsion. Vomitus may be present on the equipment or on the mouthpiece, and this could be a cause of the accident, a contributor aggravating the situation or the result of vomiting that occurred during resuscitation efforts.

Other points of possible significance include the ease with which the weight belt and other harnesses can be released, and whether this was done. The protective suit, its thickness and its integrity are relevant to both buoyancy and hypothermia. The clothing may be cut off the body at the time of resuscitation, but it should be retained for assessment.

The presence or absence of emergency equipment, such as electronic and other signaling devices, may be significant. The state of inflation of the buoyancy vest may be relevant. A knife is important to overcome entanglements in ropes, fishing lines, kelp and so forth.

A dive computer may have data available on its screen, and these data should be recorded before the computer is turned off. If a dive computer is not available, other monitoring equipment such as a depth gauge, watch or contents gauge on the gas cylinder may be available (see Chapter 51).

Investigation of compressed air sets

This investigation is best performed by a diving technician. Before any connection is disturbed with a compressed air set (scuba or surface supply), it is informative to attempt to inhale gas from the mouthpiece with the gas supply turned off. If air can be inhaled, there is a leak in the system, and the set could have supplied the diver with a water aerosol. This can cause salt water aspiration, depending on the severity and duration of the leak. For hygienic reasons, it may be necessary to sponge the mouthpiece clean, but the demand valve should not be immersed or washed because this may dislodge the cause of the leak, if it is under the exhaust valve. The other causes of leaks that have been seen include perforations in the diaphragm, corrosion of the seat and loose fittings that allow water entry. If there is likely to be air remaining in the cylinder, it may be turned on briefly to check the reading on the contents gauge and to look for leaks in all parts of the set.

The cylinder could then be disconnected and the air analyzed for oxygen, carbon dioxide, carbon monoxide, water vapour and oil content. Odour is an indicator of contamination. It may be appropriate for this analysis to be done by a qualified analytical chemist, rather than by a less well equipped laboratory with inaccurate gas detector tubes. The chemist normally has access to gas chromatography, which can detect a wide range of substances in a small sample. With appropriate equipment, it is possible to analyze the gas in a cylinder that has been emptied. Some of the remaining gas is withdrawn with a syringe and is injected into the column.

In some cases, the cause of the accident is obvious from the analysis. Low oxygen supports a diagnosis of hypoxia. A higher oxygen content than expected, in an air or nitrox mixture, needs to be considered along with the depth reached, and this may suggest oxygen toxicity. A high solids reading should lead to a microscopic examination of the solids. Some accidents have been caused by asthma triggered by pollens.

The functioning of all parts of the equipment should ideally be tested by a qualified and experienced diving technician, who notes the following:

- Whether the demand valve gives a free, controlled release of gas.
- Whether the purge button operates.
- Whether any reserve supply system was operated. The technician also checks that any low-pressure warning system operates at the correct pressure.
- Whether the buoyancy compensator inflates and dumps. A faulty system can lead to either no buoyancy or an uncontrolled ascent and pulmonary barotrauma.
- The accuracy of dive parameter monitors, depth and cylinder contents gauge. Faulty contents gauge readings can lead to unplanned gas exhaustion. A faulty depth gauge can lead to DCS because of incorrect decompression.
- Whether the weights are appropriate for the maintenance of neutral buoyancy and the release mechanism is functional. Excess weight leads to an excessive amount of air in the buoyancy compensator and possible loss of buoyancy control, poor trim and unnecessary exertion. Some buoyancy compensator–weight combinations are appropriate. Some assist in keeping a victim's head out of the water – others are more likely to drown the victim.
- Dive computer assessment (see Chapter 51).

Diving equipment

- Face mask, snorkel, buoyancy vest, depth gauge, watch, contents gauge on cylinder, buddy line, knife, weights and others – presence, absence or condition.
- Protective clothing.
- Functioning demand valve and reducer.
- Cylinder condition, valve position (number of turns to close).
- Position of any reserve gas supply mechanism.

If there is access to the appropriate equipment, the dynamic performance of the gas supply system should be assessed at depth with a simulated breathing machine, or even a diver in a recompression chamber. This may demonstrate a gas supply failure that is not obvious in tests at 1 atmosphere. For example, a restriction in the first stage reducer may be obvious only at simulated depth in a recompression chamber. Some buoyancy compensators take an unacceptable time to inflate at depth.

Investigation of mixed gas sets

With technical divers, the possibility of confusing gas mixtures should be considered. Are the demand valves readily distinguishable? Is the gear likely to cause excessive drag? Such observations can be made on inspection.

For accidents involving the use of more complex equipment, such as a rebreathing set or technical diving equipment with multiple gas mixtures, the investigation can be more difficult. Often the critical question is: What was the diver breathing at the time of the accident? If a rebreathing set has been sealed at the time of the accident, this can be determined by analyzing the gas in the inhalation hose. Samples can normally be drawn from the hose with a fine needle and syringe without causing a leak. Provided the sample can be drawn soon after the dive, the carbon dioxide reading is often close to the correct reading even if the mouthpiece cock has not been shut. With longer delay there will be a fall in carbon dioxide by diffusion to the absorbent even if the mouthpiece has been shut. Oxygen readings may remain helpful for weeks if the set was sealed promptly. In general, the more serious the accident, the less likely it is that the set will be sealed promptly and so the less helpful will be the gas analysis.

With a rebreathing set, a leak test should be performed after the samples have been drawn and before any part of the set is dismantled. If there is gas remaining in the cylinder, the gas can be turned on, the gauge read and the leak test conducted before any part of the set is altered. This is normally conducted by filling the counterlung of the set and then immersing it in a tank of water. Compression of the counterlung, to raise the pressure in the set, often reveals leaks that were not previously observed. If the gas supply is exhausted, the set can be inflated via the mouthpiece.

With a demand set, where fresh gas flow is triggered by a negative pressure, a leak can sometimes be demonstrated by sucking the gas from the set with the cylinder turned off. A leak has been demonstrated if more gas can be sucked from the set a few minutes later. If the set leaks in these circumstances, it is probable that water leaked into it during the dive. This is likely to be significant because a set with wet absorbent has a reduced capacity to

remove carbon dioxide and may give the user a caustic cocktail.

After leak testing, the set can be stripped and defects noted. Valves in the mouthpiece should be examined closely. A perished valve can allow enough gas to escape scrubbing so that carbon dioxide toxicity could occur. On one occasion, a small piece of grass stem in the valve seat caused the same problem. The packing of the canister needs to examined. On occasion, sets have been used for diving with no absorbent. More commonly, there has been some water entry, and carbon dioxide toxicity has occurred because of preferential flow through the reduced dry absorbent.

In a semi-closed circuit set, the flow of gas should be checked several times over a period equal to the dive of interest. During this time, the set should be shaken and moved into several orientations that it could have been in during the dive. One hypoxic incident was caused by salt drying in the reducer housing and remaining as a dust that blocked the reducer jet after the set was shaken.

The composition of the gases must be tested. Accidents where the wrong gas has employed are not rare. The effects of pressure on the performance of the reducer should be checked. In most cases, this can be done with the maker's test equipment.

Testing absorbent activity is by chemical analysis, and it can indicate that the absorbent is 'out of date' or less effective than required.

Specialized testing equipment

With some equipment, it may be necessary to conduct the test in a **recompression chamber**. This is especially so when the equipment (e.g. buoyancy compensators, regulators and gauges) can be influenced by depth (pressure). It also may be necessary to subject the victim to a recompression chamber dive to elicit specific symptoms and validate a diagnosis or increased susceptibility to certain disorders. This has been used to variable effect in demonstrating inert gas narcosis, oxygen toxicity, alternobaric vertigo and other conditions.

Another investigation to test the adequacy of breathing sets is a **simulated breathing machine**. This device is designed to test the various diving sets and allows for a variation in respiratory demands placed on the set. Thus, one can simulate a dive and test various functions such as resistance to breathing from the set and other factors. This machine is available in many research units, and its value depends on the flexibility of the parameters imposed (e.g. temperature, spatial orientation, respiratory volumes and rates). It is not really equivalent to the stressors placed on the diver because divers respond differently to the varying parameters (e.g. divers can panic, or they increase their respiration according to the carbon dioxide concentration), unlike the machine. These machines are more effective in comparing different diving sets than in interpreting the pathophysiology of diving accidents. Nevertheless, they are sometimes of value in clarifying problems with respiratory diving equipment, especially rebreathers.

A test of the performance of carbon dioxide absorbents is needed for rebreathing sets. This test can be done in some military laboratories and firms or departments that test other breathing equipment such as mine rescue apparatus. With this test, it should be possible to establish whether faulty absorbent or inappropriate packing of the canister contributed to the incident. With the set connected to the breathing simulator machine, carbon dioxide is injected into the breathing loop of the set while it is cooled by immersing it in water. The absorbent should continue to absorb the carbon dioxide until the total of the dive time and the test time about equals the expected endurance of the set. If the results suggest that the absorbent was defective, the possibility of a faulty batch of absorbent should be considered and a fresh sample tested to prevent the absorbent causing another incident.

It can be helpful to test the performance of the companion's set. In one case examined, the set used by the diver of primary interest was flooded, and it was not possible to test the absorbent. Testing the companion's set showed that the victim's absorbent was unlikely to have caused the incident.

Perhaps the most technically complex investigation of diving equipment is in the **re-enactment of the incident**. This is fully described in Chapter 51 and is applicable only in serious cases.

CONCLUSIONS

The investigation of diving accidents is a specialized activity. Information can be found in the various diving manuals of the Royal Navy, US Navy, the US National Oceanic and Atmospheric Administration and others see the Further Reading list and Appendix D. The *Encyclopedia of Underwater Investigations* by Robert G. Teather is a useful general reference but has even less detail on the equipment aspects of accident investigation than has been provided earlier. Most of the information provided in this chapter has come from discussions with colleagues working for the Royal Australian Navy, the Royal Navy, the US Navy and the Defence and Civil Institute of Environmental Medicine in Canada.

In Chapter 51, the more sophisticated medical investigations required for diving fatalities are discussed.

FURTHER READING

National Oceanic and Atmospheric Administration. *NOAA Diving Manual.* 5th ed. Washington, DC: US Government Printing Office; 2013. 9781930536630.

Teather RG. *Encyclopedia of Underwater Investigations.* Flagstaff, AZ: Best Publishing; 2013.

US Navy Diving Manual Revision 6 SS521-AG-PRO-010 (2008). Washington, DC: Naval Sea Systems Command; 2008.

This chapter was reviewed for this fifth edition by Carl Edmonds.

51

Investigation of diving fatalities

> Full fathom five thy father lies
> Of his bones are coral made.
> Those are pearls that were his eyes:
> Nothing of him that doth fade
> But doth suffer a sea-change
> Into something rich and strange.

Shakespeare, The Tempest

INTRODUCTION

The causes of diving deaths were extensively reported and investigated over the latter half of the twentieth century, since the advent of scuba diving as a popular sport (see Chapter 46). These reports highlight the importance of early liaison among diving experts, technicians, diving clinicians and pathologists to avoid inappropriate conclusions. Interpretations may be problematic if the autopsy is performed in isolation from the other sources of diving data.

To maximize the value of the post-mortem examination, procedural modifications are recommended for autopsies on divers. Some of the techniques previously proposed for diving autopsies have been superseded or are now inadequate or irrelevant. Interpretations were often misleading or incorrect. Some autopsy techniques that previously appeared to have potential have slipped into disuse because of difficulty in performing them or problems with their interpretation. These situations are mentioned later, together with more constructive developments such as the use of dive computer data, re-enactments of diving incidents, post-mortem whole body computed tomography (CT) scans and the analysis of intravascular and extra-alveolar gas detected by these scans.

The investigation of diving fatalities has changed markedly over the last few decades, more than many conventional pathologists and diving physicians have appreciated. The nineteenth-century caisson physicians who investigated the dysbaric causes of death demonstrated the value of autopsy diagnoses. Later, diving pathologists were not as fortunate – having to cope with the delayed recovery of an often damaged body, as well as the supervening complication of drowning, marine animal trauma, decomposition, post-mortem decompression artefact (PMDA) and resuscitation effects. Drowning was the autopsy diagnosis in about 80 per cent of cases, with about 10 per cent of cases attributed to gas embolism from pulmonary barotrauma. A review of the techniques used to investigate diving fatalities, including the interpretation of autopsy findings, was indicated. A fully annotated description of these fatalities, and the reasons for these deaths, has been published in the forensic pathology literature. A summary of these changes is presented here for diving physicians.

When the first edition of the *Diving and Subaquatic Medicine* text was printed in 1976, the autopsy, which had been the gold standard for post-mortem diagnosis, was being complemented by assessments from the clinical and diving data. This approach focussed on clinical interpretations, the dive profile and equipment testing. A more recent approach to diving accident situations has also been introduced, with an influence on fatality assessments (see Chapter 46).

The investigation of diving deaths has followed the following documented protocol:

1. Recovery, handling and observations associated with the body and all related equipment.
2. Witness and other informed statements.

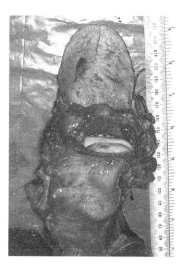

Figure 51.1 Dental plate swallowed during dive and detected at autopsy.

3. Formal autopsy for immersion victims. Techniques for aberrant gas identification and some procedural modifications are recommended for autopsies on divers, to maximize the value of the post-mortem examination.
4. Technical assessments of the functioning of the diving equipment.
5. Gas analysis by reputable laboratories.
6. Coronial or other enquiries.

Under witness and other informed statements, there is a plethora of information that is ascertained by other means, including police interrogations. One item frequently omitted is the previous medical history. Not only past and present disorders may be ascertained, but also a pre-dive medical examination may well have detected and recorded relevant factors whose significance may not be evident to non-diving physicians (Figure 51.1)

Relevant information is discussed in Chapters 5, 45, 46 and 50. Details of the specific diving disorders are found in their appropriate chapters.

RECOVERY OF THE BODY

Following a diving accident, information regarding the likely location of the diver's body is of relevance during the rescue and recovery phases.

In both instances, the rescue or recovery divers are frequently misled into searching for the victim 'down current' or 'out to sea', when the body is much closer to the site of the accident. The reasons for this include the progressively increasing negative buoyancy of the victim with descent and entrapment or snagging of the body or equipment on the sea bed.

A human body, sinking to a depth of 5 metres or more, either without diving equipment or equipped with neutral buoyancy on the surface, becomes negatively buoyant. This is partly so because water replaces some of the diver's gas spaces (especially the lungs) and partly because of the contraction of the gas spaces in the diver's body and equipment, as a result of Boyle's Law during descent. The apparent weight increases with the depth or descent.

A series of relevant observations was made from diving accidents:

- If a rescue diver can effectively swim against the current, it is unlikely that a submerged victim will be far removed from the site at which the incident occurred.
- It should not be assumed that the body of the victim has drifted away from the 'last seen' point until that area has been searched and found to be clear.
- A body, during its descent in water conditions tolerable for divers, drifts no more than a metre horizontally for every metre it descends vertically, and this horizontal drift is reduced with increasing depth. Also, the current is usually much less strong near the sea bed, where the body settles, than near the surface.
- If a marker buoy is dropped into the area where an observer has last seen the diver, the body is most likely to be found near that site. The marker buoy is very valuable in assisting others who may come to the site, after the original observers have left or drifted away.
- The fatality usually follows quickly after the loss of buddy diver contact.
- The major exception to the foregoing is when the diver has maintained positive buoyancy and remained on the surface. Then the effects of tidal currents are very considerable, and the body may be found

kilometres distant from the site of the accident, depending on how soon the search is commenced.

If the body is not in the vicinity of where the diver was last seen, then the location is often able to be predicted by the last known activity of the diver (i.e. if the diver's purpose was diving from point A to point B, the likelihood is that the body will be along that trajectory).

For snorkellers, the body is likely to be found in water in which the sea bed can be viewed from the surface – because snorkellers usually feel uneasy about swimming in water where this is not visible.

Apart from the search procedure, which is not described here because it is performed by rescue and police divers, other techniques are sometimes available for the location of the body. These include sonar systems and remotely operated underwater vehicles with video capability.

On discovering the body, and if there is no likelihood of resuscitation, observations should be recorded regarding its position, the existence of equipment and any evidence of entanglement or tethering. If possible, underwater photographs or videos should be taken. The positioning of the body may explain the presence of 'travel abrasions' because often the forehead, nose, forearms, backs of the hands, knees and tops of the toes may be scraped along the sea bed with water movement of the body. The condition of the face mask and regulator, and any substances within them, should be noted.

The body can usually be brought to the surface by removal of the weights (preferable) or use of the buoyancy compensator. Although the body may feel somewhat heavy initially as it starts to ascend, the ascent rate will increase rapidly because of Boyle's Law effects on gases. These effects may be increased by the natural development of gas in the tissues or by the actions of the recovery team. If a buoyancy compensator is inflated, then care should be used to ensure that the ascent is not rapid (i.e. air may have to be released as it expands during the ascent).

A body left underwater, if it is not entrapped, usually floats to the surface within a few days as a result of decomposition (see later).

Once death has been determined, it is important that no further interference occurs with the body, its clothing or the equipment, except for sealing the equipment, closing cylinder valves (recording the number of 'turns' needed) to retain the breathing gas for analysis, photographing all equipment and securing all the equipment associated with the accident (the victim's and others).

The body should be transferred to the mortuary as soon as practical, both because early refrigeration to around 4°C slows the decomposition that may complicate the interpretation of autopsy findings and to perform scanning, investigation and autopsy.

PERSONAL AND PAST MEDICAL HISTORY

The diver's personal history and past medical history are discussed in Chapter 50.

ENVIRONMENTAL CONDITIONS

Environmental conditions are covered in Chapter 50.

DIVE PROFILE AND HISTORY

Dive profile and history are discussed in Chapter 50.

DIVING EQUIPMENT

Frequent modifications of diving equipment and diving techniques (rebreathing sets, technical diving, varying dive profiles and newer decompression algorithms) require constant updating of test procedures and are thus beyond the scope of this text.

Information about diving equipment is discussed in Chapters 4, 46 and 50. Gas analysis is performed by specialist laboratories, and results are supplied to the diving physician and pathologist. In some circumstances it may be necessary to have a provable chain of custody, and so unauthorized interference with the equipment is prevented.

Dive computer data

Frequently, the description of a fatal dive is vague, sanitized and inaccurate, especially from the diving companions and dive operators, who often have a conflict of interest in the results of an investigation. Also, often the deceased was alone before or at the time of the incident, thus denying the investigator relevant diving data.

Most divers now wear dive computers that accurately depict the details of the fatal dive. Accurate depths, dive durations, ascent rates, the number of ascents, decompression staging and decompression stress, dive profiles (reverse or forward, multi-level or repetitive), water temperature, gas pressures and gas consumption are all informative and accessible by downloading with suitable computer software. If the dive computer is gas integrated (i.e. the changing breathing gas pressure is being recorded and integrated into the data base), then with a knowledge of the scuba tank size, the diver's respirations (rate, volume and gas consumption) can be extrapolated.

This information allows an assessment of the likelihood of pulmonary barotrauma, decompression sickness (DCS), scuba divers' pulmonary oedema (SDPE), panic, fatigue, aspiration, gas toxicity, cold effects and other conditions.

Because previous diving data are also stored in the dive computer, these earlier data may imply a predisposition to diving accidents. They may indicate the diver's inexperience, propensity to rapid ascents, inadequate decompression, deep diving, 'low-on-air' situations and other issues. The dive computer data, from the deceased diver, the diver's companions and rescuers, are downloaded by an impartial and competent technician using appropriate software.

As well as the dive computer worn by most open-circuit or scuba divers, similar information, together with gas analysis data and oxygen pressures, is available for technical and rebreather divers.

POST-MORTEM IMAGING (COMPUTED TOMOGRAPHY)

Post-mortem CT (PMCT) and other imaging techniques such as magnetic resonance imaging are becoming more common as adjuncts, or even replacements, for traditional plain radiographs and formal autopsy. These images are used to detect the site and volume of abnormal gas spaces in the body, as well as other disorders of the brain and respiratory tract. For detecting gas spaces they are more reliable, more sensitive, less invasive, less time consuming and less offensive to various cultural and ethnic groups than a formal autopsy. Ideally, the PMCT should then be complemented by the traditional autopsy to validate the PMCT and to extract and analyze the composition of the detected gas, where possible.

To detect gas, and identify its cause, whole body PMCT should be performed as soon as possible, preferably within hours of the incident (to reduce the influence of decomposition gas) and before the formal autopsy (which can introduce gas artefacts). A delayed PMCT is preferable to no PMCT.

General information

Evidence of pulmonary interstitial oedema is seen with the drowning syndromes (aspiration, near drowning and drowning), cardiac disease and SDPE. SDPE has now been identified as a cause of diving deaths, but with an unknown incidence and lung pathological features similar to drowning.

On PMCT, a 'ground glass' appearance may be observed with all these diagnoses. Sub-glottic fluid in the trachea and main bronchi is also frequent, but this finding is not specific to drowning because it is also present in cardiac deaths. Frothy airway fluid is usually present in drowning and SDPE. The formal autopsy more clearly demonstrates the hyper-expanded lungs of drowning and overweighted lungs in all three disorders (if the autopsy is performed early).

High-attenuation particles, indicating sand or other sediment, may be present in any of the drowning or aspiration syndromes, in the airways and para-nasal sinuses. However, any descent underwater draws fluid and sediment into these contracting gas spaces and may similarly explain the high-attenuation particles that have been detected in drowning cases. These particles may also be observed in near drowning or aspiration, or they may merely be a consequence of descent in an unconscious diver, whether breathing or not. They have not been reported in deaths from SDPE *per se*.

Frequently, haemorrhage or effusion is detected in the middle ear with PMCT. Some reports still imply that this is a sign of drowning. The presence of such middle ear or sinus mucosal congestion or haemorrhage is a frequent observation in clinical diving medicine, and it is often confirmed with radiological scanning (see Chapters 7 and 8). Symptoms usually limit the conscious diver from descending further, but when the victim is unconscious and descending and while there is still circulatory activity, barotrauma is to be expected. Thus, this observation may simply imply descent while the diver is unconscious, but not drowning as such. This explanation of middle ear and sinus barotraumas of descent is far more feasible than an unexplainable indicator of drowning *per se*.

Scans may demonstrate bone lesions and dysbaric osteonecrosis in the shoulders, hips and knees.

In the case of marine animal injuries, there may also be evidence of bone damage and foreign bodies (e.g. shark teeth, fish spines).

Perhaps the most valuable but controversial aspects of PMCT are the observation and interpretation of extraneous gas spaces in the diver's body.

Gas in the whole body post-mortem computed tomography scan and the diving autopsy

The interpretation of gas detected radiologically and with newer scanning techniques has been mired in controversy. Some authors have embraced the newer technologies with enthusiasm, whereas others have denigrated them as being not only valueless, but sometimes misleading. Nowhere is this more so than in the interpretation of extraneous gas in divers at autopsy.

The techniques developed to demonstrate abnormal gas in the diving autopsy were based on the logic that gases are dominant in the causes of death from diving and hyperbaric exposure – from gas embolism induced by pulmonary barotrauma and DCS. Unfortunately, the presence of gas from processes that are not related to the cause of death has complicated this interpretation.

It is often concluded that gas embolism from pulmonary barotrauma caused a diver's death, yet the diver was in a situation where this development was impossible. In 12 of 13 diving fatalities examined by autopsy at the New South Wales

Institute of Forensic Medicine in Australia, intravascular gas was detected. In some cases, the history and autopsy findings were inconsistent with cerebral gas embolism as a cause of death.

The interpretation of abnormal gas in the tissues, (e.g. intrapleural, intragastric, intrahepatic, intramuscular or intravascular gas) following diving exposure requires a knowledge of infrequently accessed literature and an understanding of the processes that cause gas formation – DCS, PMDA, pulmonary barotrauma, drowning, resuscitation or trauma and putrefaction. This knowledge is available from archival reports of both caisson and diving cases and from more recent animal experiments simulating human dives. Interpretation requires an understanding of the whole dive profile and the post-dive exposure and activities. The potential causes of gas are PMDA, DCS, pulmonary barotrauma, resuscitation artefacts, putrefaction or decomposition and drowning.

> ## Aberrant or extraneous gas in the body, post mortem
>
> - Post-mortem decompression artefact.
> - Decompression sickness.
> - Pulmonary barotrauma.
> - Resuscitation artefacts.
> - Putrefaction/decomposition.
> - Drowning.

POST-MORTEM DECOMPRESSION ARTEFACT (POST-MORTEM 'OFF-GASSING')

Boycott, Damant and Haldane in 1908 warned that 'the presence of bubbles *in vivo* must be inferred from their discovery post mortem with considerable caution. The super saturation of the body may be such that the separation of the gas bubbles may take place after death'. In their discussion of diving accidents, Hanson and Young reiterated that post-mortem gas bubbles are of no significance if a diver died under pressure.

The bubbling is mainly from inert gas previously breathed by the diver and then dissolved in the blood and tissues (Figure 51.2). PMDA can develop if the diver dies at depth or soon after ascent and the tissues remain supersaturated with gas at the time of death. After death, the cessation of circulation means that the gas has no normal avenue of escape, and so it comes out of solution into the bubble phase. From deep and/or prolonged dives, such gas can produce extensive surgical emphysema, be present in all tissues and replace blood from both venous and arterial vessels ('gas angiograms') and occupy both sides of the heart.

A PMCT scan should extend to the thighs to demonstrate gas in the intramuscular fascial layers. There are few other explanations for this observation, especially if decomposition is excluded.

Well-controlled animal experiments across different species validate and quantify the concept of PMDA or post-mortem 'off-gassing'. Animals that die at sea level and are then exposed to pressure do not subsequently develop PMDA, nor do those that die immediately after exposure to pressure. Only those animals exposed to pressure while still alive and thus having a functioning circulation and an ability to dissolve high pressure gases into their tissues are so affected after surfacing.

The depths and durations used in these animal experiments were designed to simulate typical no-decompression profiles of human compressed air divers. The development of PMDA revealed a latent period of about an hour until the PMDCA became evident and then a progression of this effect over the subsequent 1 to 8 or more hours.

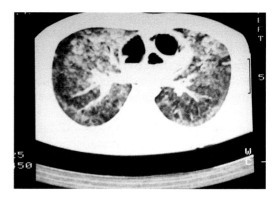

Figure 51.2 Post-mortem decompression artefact. Computed tomography scan showing gas in cardiac chambers.

Thus, the animal experiments confirmed our clinical observations – but were in disagreement with a popular belief that deep diving, in excess of 40 msw, may be necessary for PMDA to develop. Excessive depths were not reached in most of the animal experiments described in the previous paragraphs, nor were they reached by human divers and caisson workers with PMDA, described by earlier authors.

Logically, one can understand that, although a deep or decompression dive is not required to initiate this phenomenon, the amount, extent and speed of development of PMDA are consequences of both depth and duration of the hyperbaric exposure. This phenomenon also depends on which tissues were supersaturated (fast tissues such as blood from short deep dives, slow tissues such as fat from longer shallow dives).

DECOMPRESSION SICKNESS

Although uncommon nowadays, death can occur from DCS, with gas bubbles developing within the tissues. The causes are excessive exposure to pressure (depth) and too rapid an ascent.

In the first half of the twentieth century, DCS-induced deaths were far more frequent, and the disorder was not usually complicated by resuscitation – which may cause local gas artefacts and redistribution of intravascular gas.

Hoff reported on autopsies performed on divers and caisson workers. His conclusion was that the less acute DCS cases tended to have gas in the right ventricle of the heart, whereas victims who died very soon after decompression or from explosive decompression had gas in both arterial and venous systems with widespread gross gas distribution through many tissues. This latter group would have had DCS complicated by the effects of PMDA and/or pulmonary barotrauma causing gas embolism.

Sir Leonard Hill, in his literature review, noted that Von Schrotter observed gas in the vascular system in 11 of his 18 well-described autopsies on DCS victims. Keays described it in 8 of his 12 cases. Paul Bert showed in animal experiments that gas from decompression collected in the venous system and the right side of the heart and also that the composition of this gas reflected tissue gas pressures.

Hill described further autopsies on DCS cases. His caisson workers were exposed to depths equivalent to 19 to 34 msw for over 3 hours, then had a very slow ascent – and so pulmonary barotrauma was an unlikely complication. In these cases, with typical DCS symptoms preceding death, the gas was observed in the venous system at autopsy, collecting in the right side of the heart in 7 of 10 cases. Arterial and left-sided heart gas involvement was not reported in the cases of victims who died after a delay of some hours, when PMDA was less likely.

Patients with DCS who succumb very soon after ascent are also susceptible to supervening PMDA. Of relevance, but not specifically addressed by Hill, were the excessive volume and widespread extent of the gas in four victims who died of DCS within an hour of surfacing. In these cases, there was also gross gas in the arterial system, the left side of the heart, the viscera, subcutaneous tissues, the thighs and even the cerebral ventricles.

In cases of DCS causing death, the major sites of bubbles are blood vessels and lipid-rich structures, such as subcutaneous tissue and myelin sheaths of nerve cells. The histological signs in lipid tissues are haemorrhage, tissue inflammation or necrosis around the gas bubbles, but these findings may take some hours to develop and are frequently not sought by pathologists. These signs may differentiate the DCS bubbles from the PMDA bubbles, that cause no such reaction. Lipid precipitation in the blood may develop if the decompression is rapid, and this was referred to as fat emboli in the older texts. In cases with DCS causing intravascular bubbles, blood analysis may reveal biochemical or coagulation abnormalities.

EXTRANEOUS GAS FOLLOWING PULMONARY BAROTRAUMA

Gas embolism is initially observed as air (nitrogen–oxygen) or gas bubbles in the systemic arterial system (see Chapter 6). It arises from lung rupture, thus allowing air to pass into the pulmonary veins, then to the left side of the heart and the arterial system. Because gas emboli are redistributed partly by buoyancy in the larger vessels, they tend to travel to the brain in the ascending diver and in the erect posture after surfacing. Some of the emboli may obstruct the smaller arterioles or involve multiple generations of arterioles.

Many, however, pass through to the venous system and thus to the right side of the heart and pulmonary capillary filter. This occurs if there is continuing circulation, including effective resuscitation efforts. If the volume of gas is large enough, arterial bubbles may persist and obstruct the arterial tree, especially in small arteries (e.g. the circle of Willis), and validate the pathological diagnosis (Figures 51.3 and 51.4).

Gas also accumulates as pulmonary interstitial emphysema from lung rupture. 'Lymphatic air embolism' may then develop with bubbles moving into the lymphatic system of the lungs, and thence the thoracic duct, from where it passes into the venous system and the right side of the heart.

Other gas pockets develop when the alveolar gas ruptures into the interstitial tissue and tracks through the lungs into the mediastinum and cervical tissues, where the gas manifests clinically as surgical emphysema, and/or rupturing into the pleural or peritoneal cavities, where the gas causes pneumothorax or pneumoperitoneum. All this is detected easily by PMCT, but formal autopsy proceedings, including aspiration, are necessary to analyze the gas involved.

The association of lung damage, pneumothoraces and mediastinal emphysema is strongly supportive of a pulmonary barotrauma origin of the embolism (Figure 51.5), as is a history of rapid ascent followed by unconsciousness.

RESUSCITATION-INDUCED GAS (ARTEFACT)

Resuscitation efforts may include invasive events such as intravenous cannulation, endotracheal intubation and external cardiac compression, any of which may admit small volumes of gas into the venous system or cause local subcutaneous emphysema over the affected sites. This rarely simulates the large volumes seen with PMDA, DCS or pulmonary barotrauma.

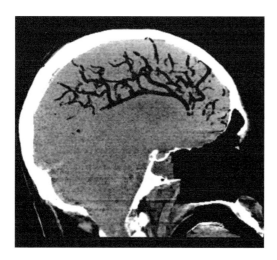

Figure 51.3 Cerebral gas angiogram from arterial gas embolism.

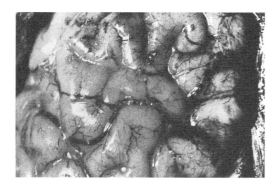

Figure 51.4 Bubbles in cerebral vessels, from arterial gas embolism, post-mortem decompression or autopsy artefact.

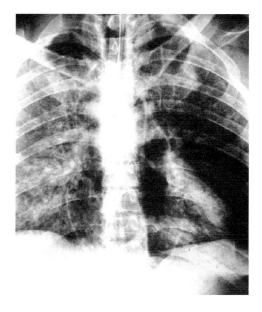

Figure 51.5 X-ray study. Pre-mortem left pneumothorax from pulmonary barotrauma and gas in cardiac ventricles, probably from that or post-mortem decompression artefact.

Knowledge of the resuscitation situation and the usually small amounts of gas, as well as the location of gas, should suffice to exclude this factor as a contributor to death in non-traumatized patients, but it may show up in the PMCT image.

Shiotami and colleagues, using PMCT, quantified the effect of cardiopulmonary resuscitation (CPR) on gas introduction. Of 228 non-traumatic patients who were exposed to CPR, 71 per cent had cardiovascular gas, compared with 0 per cent in the non-CPR controls. The bubbles were very small, mostly grade 1 (less than 5 mm diameter). The gas was found in the systemic venous system and the right side of the heart in most cases. The incidence of cerebral gas was much less (7.5 per cent of 387 cases and 0 per cent in the non-CPR controls). The cerebral gas that was detected was mostly in the venous system. Cerebral venous gas can develop from retrograde flow to the brain against the flow of blood, during CPR and as a result of the thoracic pump effect.

Resuscitation resulting in a viable circulation may occasionally redistribute intravenous gas (e.g. from DCS) into the arterial system, through intrapulmonary shunts or a patent foramen ovale (PFO). It may also help redistribute arterial gas embolism from pulmonary barotrauma into the venous system.

The use of oxygen during resuscitation may reduce the ultimate volume and number of gas bubbles.

PUTREFACTION (DECOMPOSITION)

This process is well described in general medical texts. Putrefaction is evident after about 24 hours if the body is not refrigerated, although the onset varies from 3 to 72 hours, depending on the environmental conditions and the gas volumes detected. Putrefaction produces a foul-smelling gas initially evident in the gastrointestinal tract, the portal veins and the liver. Hydrogen, carbon dioxide, hydrogen sulphide and methane may be present. Because divers who die underwater are exposed to environmental cooling influences, it is likely that putrefaction may be somewhat delayed (see later).

DROWNING

In addition to aspirating fluid, drowning often results in the swallowing of air and water into the gastrointestinal tract, thus explaining the tendency of near drowning victims to vomit, especially during resuscitation. Ascent may increase the volume of gas, as a result of Boyle's Law, and this increased gas volume distends the stomach and also induces vomiting.

On radiology in the upright position, Wydler's sign is a three-layer separation of foam, fluid and solids in the stomach. The gases (usually nitrogen and oxygen) are in approximately the same proportions as in the air or other gases being breathed.

AUTOPSY PROCEDURE

General information

Except for an increase in deaths attributed to cardiac disease in our ageing diver population, factors contributing to a fatal diving accident have not altered greatly over the decades, and they should be known to diving medicine clinicians and forensic pathologists.

An average of 100 diving related fatalities occur in Australia and North America each year. In the majority, an autopsy is performed and the cause of death is determined to be drowning. However, for diving-related deaths, drowning is an unrewarding explanation, especially if contributing factors are not recorded. This incomplete explanation is inadequate for the diver's family and associates, the training agencies, investigators and researchers wishing to prevent future mishaps. Divers carry their own compressed gas life support system with them, and so there must be other reasons why they are separated from this system, inhale water and then drown.

An autopsy on a diver who has died as a result of a diving accident should be undertaken by a pathologist who has had experience in these investigations. The presence of a diving physician is a requirement unless the pathologist is also a specialist in this field. Otherwise, the investigation may be incomplete and misinterpreted.

The most important innovation in the diving autopsy over the last decade is the instigation of a delay in drawing conclusions until all possible diving information is known and integrated by the diving physician. This avoids many inappropriate diagnoses of gas embolism in cases where such an eventuality was clinically impossible.

Site and time of the autopsy

Conducting the autopsy at depth in a hyperbaric environment, which is possible under certain saturation diving conditions, avoids the disruptive influence of PMDA, described earlier. Such an autopsy location would be logistically and technologically problematic for the pathologist, even though some may argue that it should be the 'gold standard' in identifying gas-related diving diseases. In most diving fatalities, the diver is either already at the surface or is brought to the surface with the hope that resuscitation will be effective. Pressurizing the body back to depth is not only impractical but also fails to eliminate the artefacts.

The results of the autopsy must be assessed in relation to the time between the diving accident and the diver's death and also between the death and the time of autopsy. If there has been a substantial period of time between the diving incident and the time of death, then many of the blood gas and biochemical changes will have been nullified, even though the disease progressed to a fatal termination. Thus, the electrolyte changes of drowning and the gas composition with DCS and pulmonary barotrauma may be countered. The pathological lesions demonstrated hours or days later may reflect only the previous existence of the disease. A prolonged time (days) between death and autopsy may induce some changes, such as; electrolyte shifts, gas pressures, reduced lung weights and fluid content, pleural effusions, putrefaction and alcohol production.

Timing of the clinical features is relevant. Extra-alveolar gas from gas embolism, pneumothorax and mediastinal emphysema derived from pulmonary barotrauma occur almost immediately. DCS usually takes some minutes or up to an hour to develop, but then it increases over the next few hours. PMDA is slower, usually developing over the first few hours, but it is faster with extreme exposures. Putrefaction may be detectable by its odour and usually takes more than 24 hours to become clinically evident.

The PMCT scan and then the autopsy should be performed as soon as practical because of these changes.

Decomposition and putrefaction

Bacterial action accelerates after death because of the absence of the natural defences of the living body. These bacteria digest the soft tissues and reduce them to a fluid consistency. A by-product of this may be a complex mixture of foul-smelling gases. This may develop within the various organs of the body, but especially the gastrointestinal tract. The body becomes distended and swollen. There are different implications for submerged bodies, compared with those on land. Buoyancy resulting from this gas may increase and often brings the body to the surface, usually 3 to 7 days after the incident.

The speed of putrefaction depends on the environmental temperature. When the water is near freezing, the body may be preserved indefinitely. In water of 20°C, putrefaction may only take a couple of days. In 30°C water, 12 hours may be sufficient. The process is more rapid with obesity, increased in polluted and stagnant water, and affected by the time and contents of the last meal. Factors that inhibit putrefaction include saponification and the previous ingestion of antibiotics (often taken as antimalarials).

The chronology of decomposition varies, but a typical sequence in 20°C water is as follows.

- 12 to 24 hours: The skin changes colour from normal to light blue to almost green, initially in the lower body, around the pelvis and groin.
- 24 to 36 hours: Discolouration becomes pronounced, and a marbled pattern develops on the skin. Hydrogen sulphide production causes a characteristic dark green or almost black discolouration, and the blood seeps from the vessels to give the body a general purplish-black colour.
- 36 to 48 hours: Face and body swell noticeably, with the characteristic 'bloated' appearance. Where the skin is loose it may become dramatically swollen, such as around the lips, eyelids and scrotum. Crepitus may be noted.
- 60 to 72 hours: Putrefaction is now widespread, even to the fingers and toes. The entire body has now changed colour, and the facial features are unrecognizable.

- 4 to 7 days: Hair, nails and skin become loose and are easily lost. Pockets of foul-smelling gas form under the skin and escape through tears. Malodorous, coloured liquids may escape from the body's natural orifices.
- 2 weeks and longer: The soft tissues are reduced to a grey, greasy, unrecognizable mass. Eventually, only skeletal remains indicate the presence of the body.

The composition of this gas is different from the inert gas bubbles of PMDA, DCS and pulmonary barotrauma, by having higher concentrations of carbon dioxide, hydrogen, hydrogen sulphide and methane. Decompositional gas tends to be first seen radiographically in the hepatic and portal circulation; therefore, care should be taken when interpreting gas present only in the liver.

The autopsy examination

SUPERFICIAL EXAMINATION

The deceased is examined before cleaning or removal of foreign bodies or clothing. Photographs of all lesions should be taken. Damage may result either from the cause of the accident (e.g. shark attack or propeller injury) or from the search and recovery (e.g. grappling hook or line).

Disruption of the skin and subcutaneous tissues is likely to result from post-mortem trauma (during the rescue and recovery), putrefaction and water logging that cause detachment during rescue or ingestion from marine animals. Skin examination may show the duration of exposure (cutis anserine or 'goose flesh'), haemorrhagic or Tardieu's spots of asphyxia or signs of DCS (see Chapter 11). Trauma to the skin from marine animals either may be caused after death or may be instrumental in the death. Small crustaceans and 'sea lice' may cause extensive loss of soft tissues in water within a day or two of death. If there are marine animal lesions, these are usually easy to identify.

Shark bites cause multiple crescentic teeth marks, and tearing wounds illustrate the direction of the attack and the size of the animal (see Plate 5 (a)). Teeth particles in the wound assist in identifying the species of shark. Barracuda bites are clean-cut excisions. Post-mortem feeding by predators is common and is indicated by the absence of haemorrhage and inflammatory response in the surrounding tissues (i.e. circulation had ceased).

Coelenterate injuries may be recognizable by the number and distribution of the whip-like marks, which partly fade after death. An accurate identification of the type of coelenterate or jellyfish is possible by taking a skin scraping for examination of the nematocysts by a marine biologist. Nematocyst identification from jellyfish injury on the skin may remain possible for many days, even though the initially florid lesion may have faded post mortem.

Although serological and immunoglobulin assessments to identify injuries from venomous marine animals have theoretical value, these tests have not reached the international acceptability that was once predicted. Immunoglobulin titres to coelenterate venoms may take several days to develop and are rarely available. In the appropriate setting, morbid anatomy and histology of skin and tissue wounds, as well as microscopic identification of nematocysts, are still of value.

Fish spines can be demonstrated macroscopically and on histological examination. Cone shells may leave a tiny harpoon puncture. Blue-ringed octopus bites appear as a small, angular nick or a single haemorrhagic bleb. The sea snake bite shows two or more fang marks with surrounding teeth impressions. Where an octopus has held a victim, multiple bruising from round sucker pads is seen along the extent of the tentacle contact. Squid and cuttlefish may leave similar circular marks and incisions.

The skin of the fingers may show the effects of immersion (i.e. pale and wrinkled, with the so-called 'washerwoman's skin'; Figure 51.6).

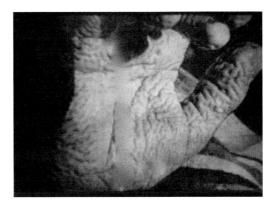

Figure 51.6 Washerwoman's skin.

There may be lacerations from where the diver attempted to clutch barnacles, coral or other sharp objects. Injury inflicted by aquatic animals in the early post-mortem period is especially seen on protuberances (e.g. fingers, nose, lips, eyelids), if these were not protected by equipment.

There is often evidence of vomitus, which may be either causative or an important part of the sequence of events. In cases in which sea water was aspirated while the diver was still alive, there may be white, pink or blood-stained foam in the nose and mouth. Water that enters the airways after death does not usually have this foamy consistency. In cases in which the patient was brought to the surface following significant exposure at depth, there may also be distension of the gas spaces within the body resulting in a distended abdomen and in faecal and respiratory fluid extrusions.

External evidence of barotrauma is important in ascertaining the sequence of events. An unconscious diver, or one who was not able to equalize his or her physiological or equipment gas spaces during submergence, has evidence of barotrauma, as described earlier. Thus, there should be an examination for evidence of mask or face squeeze with haemorrhage into the conjunctiva, ear barotrauma with haemorrhage or perforation of the tympanic membrane and suit squeeze with long, whip-like marks underneath the folds of the protective clothing. Total body squeeze may occur when a surface-supplied helmet is being used. Middle ear haemorrhage, long considered a sign pathognomonic of drowning, is merely evidence of descent while alive. It is verified by otoscopy.

Pulmonary barotrauma of ascent may be inferred by evidence of subcutaneous emphysema localized to the supraclavicular and cervical areas. If this finding is generalized over most of the body, then it is more likely to be caused by the liberation of gas following death (i.e. PMDA). It should not be confused with clinical DCS or putrefactive changes. Where the diver has suffered from DCS, there are often reddish or cyanotic discolourations of the skin (see Chapter 11).

Gas is often implied by a swelling of the body, when the pathologist feels the body, or later when the pathologist cuts into tissues and small gas pockets hiss out at him or her.

GAS SAMPLING

Modifications in autopsy techniques allow for the collection of gas in atypical sites, such as the cardiac chambers, vessels, pleura and peritoneal cavities and in other tissues. This collection can be achieved by opening these sites underwater or by perfusing vessels with inserted gas traps. These techniques are not always easy or reliable, but they allow for the collection and analysis of the gas, which may indicate its source. PMCT is now recommended for demonstration and localization of gas before diving autopsies.

Specific organs

BRAIN

If PMCT is not available, the advantages of opening the skull underwater far outweigh the technical difficulties. A technique to demonstrate air emboli is of paramount importance in the investigation of diving accidents. The circle of Willis and its distribution arteries are the areas to be examined meticulously for evidence of significant gas embolism.

Incision of the scalp and removal of the calvarium, or dissection of the neck, may introduce artefactual 'air bubbles' into the superficial cerebral veins and venous sinuses, and these are not of diagnostic importance.

The customary technique is to perform the craniotomy and cervical incisions underwater, with a constant flushing of the water, thus avoiding the introduction of artefactual air during this procedure or during dissection of the neck. If bubbles are found, they should be photographed *in situ,* or after clamping the carotid arteries and cutting proximal to the clamp, to obtain a better exposure.

Alternatively, the head may be submerged and suspended into a mortuary sink with the body resting on shelving. The scalp is first incised above the water and is then reflected underwater. The head is again elevated, and the skull is cut with a vibrating saw, with care taken not to damage the dura. The head is then submerged for a second time, the calvarium is dislodged, the dura is incised and the brain is removed underwater. The brain may then be placed directly into a formalin container. No air enters the cerebral circulation during the removal of calvarium and brain under these conditions, and so any gas bubbles present when the brain is examined after fixation would have been present at the time of death. Histological sections from the brain should include the 'watershed' area of the frontal cortex 2.5 cm from the midline.

SPINAL CORD

Spinal cord removal may be indicated for examination after fixation. Ante-mortem bubble formation may produce microscopic haemorrhages and infarcts, which are most easily recognized in the spinal cord. After fixation, a transverse section of the spinal cord should be taken from each segment and parasagittal longitudinal sections between each transverse section. Air may enter the spinal venous plexus during removal of brain, abdominal and thoracic organs, so finding gas bubbles in this area in the final stages of the autopsy may not be significant.

Some neuropathologists use the Marchi stain to demonstrate less obvious lesions.

TEMPORAL BONES

The temporal bone and its associated middle ear and mastoid air cell cavities are of special importance in diving accident investigation. Not only does haemorrhage occur in this area, as a result of barotrauma of descent, but also there are specific disorders causing disorientation that may be instrumental in the diving accident. These include such injuries as tympanic membrane perforation, middle ear barotrauma of descent and inner ear disturbances either from barotrauma (haemorrhage or labyrinthine window rupture) or DCS. It is important to record the appearance of the tympanic membrane on otoscopy and the presence of any fluid within the middle ear cavity. A histological examination of the temporal bones, ear and mastoid cavities should be performed by a specialist pathologist (Figure 51.7).

CARDIOTHORACIC SYSTEMS

Various techniques have been established for demonstrating a gas-induced death. PMCT before autopsy is most useful in this regard, but low-penetration X-ray studies taken with the deceased in an upright position could be employed. Gas samples can be collected for analysis at autopsy.

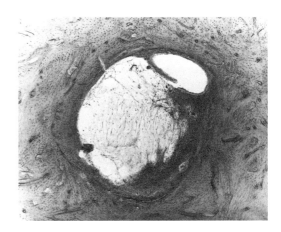

Figure 51.7 Temporal bone with round window fistula.

Some pathologists elevate the chest with a block under the shoulder and carefully open the chest between the major neck vessels. The pericardial sac is opened, and then blood (and gas) is aspirated from the superior point in each of the four chambers and is measured and analyzed. Aspirations must be performed using an 'airtight' technique.

The chest can be opened beneath water in the bath or a water-filled space, so that small amounts of gas in the pleural cavities may be detected. Similarly, the pericardium can be opened and gas sought in the pericardial space and visceral pericardial vessels. The heart is removed, and each chamber is opened underwater. Unless the procedure is carried out underwater, intracardiac gas can be missed.

This procedure can be performed without the necessity of having the whole body immersed by immersing only the heart and lungs. It is achieved by performing a neck incision extending down the midline from the sternal notch to the midpoint between the xiphisternum and umbilicus, and then to each of the antero-superior iliac spines. The skin and the muscles over the chest and the skin over the abdomen are then widely reflected by undercutting, and the trough between the body and the skin is filled with water. The cavities can then be opened, noting the presence of any abnormal gas collection. Some pathologists may not relish performing any procedures underwater because the impaired visibility may increase the risk of personal injury and infections.

Blood samples can be taken from the vena cava and the pulmonary veins. Routine blood analyses should always be taken for haematological and biochemical estimations, either from subclavian vessels or from femoral veins. Blood can be taken from the right and left ventricles and analyzed specifically for chloride levels. Although the interpretation of this technique is controversial, in unresuscitated salt water drowning it may produce indicative results. Vitreous chloride levels may also be of value in drowning cases (see Chapter 21).

Evidence of marine foreign bodies, diatoms and so forth should match those of the area where death occurred. This verifies the site of immersion, not necessarily a cause of death. Diatom identification from various parts of the body, the airways and the incriminated water environment, despite having some potential value, has serious limitations and is rarely undertaken.

Similarly, strontium, chloride, haemoglobin and other biochemical analyses have not achieved widespread acceptance and use.

In drowning, the lungs are often heavier than normal, partly filled with foam, sometimes pink from haemorrhage. They may be distended, crossing to the midline ('emphysema aquosum'), and there may be particles of sediment, sand or marine organisms along the airways. In fresh water drowning, if sufficient time has elapsed between rescue and death, the lungs may appear 'dry' because fresh water can be absorbed into the pulmonary circulation.

There is no single pathognomonic sign of drowning. Pulmonary oedema may also occur in other disorders (DCS, pulmonary barotrauma, SDPE and cardiac failure).

In pulmonary barotrauma, the voluminous lungs may bulge out of the thoracic cavity, and there may be interstitial emphysema, sub-pleural blebs and mediastinal emphysema. Rupture of alveolar walls may be associated with widespread but patchy intra-alveolar haemorrhages. Interstitial emphysema recognized in sections of lung and acute intra-acinar emphysema may be seen. Pneumothorax or pneumoperitoneum is supportive evidence, as is cerebral arterial gas embolism – once other causes have been excluded.

Pulmonary barotrauma may be identified at post-mortem examination by demonstrating an air leak from the lungs to pleura, interstitial tissue or blood vessels. The lungs are inflated using compressed air or oxygen and a cuffed endotracheal tube, to a pressure of 2.5 kPa (25 cm of water), thus producing slight overinflation. With the tube clamped, the lungs are then submerged beneath water, by using a coarse transparent plastic cover to produce complete submersion. With an inverted water-filled glass measuring cylinder, some estimate should be made of the volume of air escaping per minute into veins or from pleura. The tube is then removed; the lungs are then separated, weighed, re-inflated at similar pressure with buffered formalin and retained for examination after fixation.

The pathological cause of the barotrauma (e.g. pleural scarring, evidence of chronic asthma) may also be detected. Acute effects of asthma, although of great importance clinically, may not be evident pathologically within 24 hours. Mucous secretion and eosinophils are usually present in longer-lasting disease, with basement membrane thickening in chronic asthma. The apex of the lung is a common site for unrecognized bullae, which may predispose to pulmonary barotrauma.

With severe DCS (the 'chokes'), the lungs may be engorged and distended with blood and intravascular gas. They are then very heavy and uninflatable.

The presence of a PFO may indicate death from 'paradoxical' emboli derived from DCS. Gas is off-loaded into the venous system and then bypasses the pulmonary filter through the PFO to enter the left side of the heart and ultimately the brain.

In cases of underwater blast, the tissues with a gas-fluid interface are most affected, with shredding and haemorrhages along the airways.

ABDOMEN

Apart from the foregoing observations, it is necessary to inspect the inferior vena cava and descending aorta for gas bubbles and to examine the gastrointestinal tract for haemorrhages and infarcts. These may be related to gas emboli from pulmonary barotrauma or DCS. Pneumoperitoneum may also result from pulmonary barotrauma. In cases of underwater blast, most of the haemorrhages occur in a gas and fluid interface, and the abdomen and gastrointestinal tract are especially involved.

Under these conditions, there are seldom any external signs of violence on the skin or subcutaneous tissue despite severe haemorrhages within the bowel itself.

HISTOLOGY

Routine specimen blocks should be taken from the brain, spinal cord, heart and abdominal viscera. After re-inflation and fixation, sections should be taken from the pleural surface of each lung lobe, as well as sections across each segmental bronchus, including adjacent lung parenchyma. Samples should be taken and kept, even if the pathologist does not intend to examine them personally. They may be valuable in future investigations.

Temporal bone studies and those for dysbaric osteonecrosis are specialized investigations and are often referred to a specialist pathologist. The results may indicate recent or past diving accidents.

OTHER INVESTIGATIONS

Laboratory examinations

Alcohol and drugs may contribute to the diver's death, and blood samples should be appropriately screened. The alcohol level must be considered in light of the post-mortem environment and intervals, to assess the putrefactive neo-formation of this substance.

Perhaps the more important estimation is that of carboxyhaemoglobin because this is a definite indicator of carbon monoxide toxicity – a significant factor in diving deaths (see Chapter 19). Evidence for ante-mortem intravascular blood coagulation and fibrinolysis may occur when there has been intravascular bubble formation. Urine samples may be tested for drugs and fibrin degradation products.

Some authorities compare blood from the vena cava and pulmonary veins to apply various hypotheses that may indicate drowning, on the assumption that aspirated fluid alters the constitution of blood perfusing the pulmonary alveoli. Such tests as osmolarity, specific gravity, chlorides (Gettler's test) and strontium still have some adherents. Haemoglobin and haptoglobin levels may also be assessed.

Other authorities will pursue diatoms, comparing those of the aquatic environment in which drowning allegedly occurred with the same organisms in the victim's lungs, kidneys, bone marrow and other tissues, thereby indicating an active circulation at the time of aspiration.

Various assays may indicate marine animal toxins, with some immunoglobulin analyses already available in specialized laboratories – if death has been sufficiently delayed.

Bacteriological cultures may be indicated. A time delay between the dive and death from encephalitis resulting from *Naegleria* is expected in divers who have exposed themselves to contaminated fresh water areas. Culture for organisms, such as marine *Vibrio* species, should also be performed in a conventional culture medium, as well as in hypertonic saline. Unfortunately, many bacteriologically positive results may reflect contamination, as opposed to actual aquatic infection.

Gas analysis

Unfortunately, analysis of the extraneous gas in the body (e.g. heart, arterial system, pneumothorax, pneumoperitoneum, bowel) is too rarely performed – usually because of the pathologist's omission in collecting it. In general, gas from pulmonary barotrauma reflects the inspired gas, usually air. Resuscitation-induced gas varies with its mode of entry and the resuscitation gas being used. Gas from both DCS and PMDA is composed of inert gases with tissue metabolic gases represented. Putrefaction gas includes hydrogen, carbon dioxide, methane and hydrogen sulphide. Ingested gas in the stomach replicates the gas inhaled from the diving equipment.

RE-ENACTMENT OF A DIVING INCIDENT

This term does not refer to the **testing of diving equipment,** which is performed routinely by dive experts after a diving accident or death (see Chapter 50 for this and other equipment testing), usually by police divers or equipment technicians, at arm's length from the diving operators involved. **Simulated breathing machines** are also available to test the equipment functioning under laboratory conditions. A **re-enactment** is a more recent and totally different concept, more holistic and integrated.

Routine testing of equipment determines that it meets certain performance criteria and that it can be used as intended. It does not imply that it did not contribute to the death. Thus, a diving regulator may be functional under normal conditions, with an experienced diver breathing gently in an upright position, from a regulator producing a watertight seal and with an adequate air supply.

Under different conditions, the diving regulator may malfunction. Such conditions include excessive air consumption from extreme exertion, anxiety, negative buoyancy, swimming against strong currents, being towed, being at great depths, concurrently using air from other outlets and low tank pressure, as well as when the diver is in a different spatial orientation. Problems such as these may be elicited only during a re-enactment, which can also detect hazards such as other equipment problems, potential entrapments, dangerous environments, technique difficulties and excessive personal demands.

Re-enactment of diving fatalities was introduced in 1967 following the unexplained deaths of two rebreather divers. It was designed for internal use by experts in the Royal Australian Navy, the primary organization that investigated such accidents at that time.

The concept, which has become more widespread and is now often employed by police divers, is designed for the situation in which a death has occurred but where there is no convincing explanation for the fatality. The purpose is to identify the presence of adverse situations that had previously not been evident and that may help to clarify the fatal incident or prevent future ones. It is carried out only after all the other dive investigations (including the autopsy) are complete. A re-enactment of the incident requires the following:

- A detailed and accurate knowledge of the dive plan, dive profile, breathing gas composition and volume, environmental characteristics, buoyancy status and equipment used (i.e. conditions that could have contributed to the unexplained death) is necessary.
- An accurate replication of the foregoing is made by expert divers of a similar stature to the deceased, using the same or equivalent equipment and performing a similar dive in similar circumstances. Sample ports allowing for repeated gas sampling and analysis may be added when rebreathing equipment is involved.
- The diver needs to have access to redundant emergency equipment, to be used if necessary.
- Diving physicians, full resuscitation facilities and a rescue dive team must be available on site. It can be a problematic exposure, and attention must be paid to the ethical issues.
- Observer divers record the re-enactment with underwater video equipment. Full documentation of the experiences and observations is made independently by each participant, and this complements the video records.
- The fatal dive profile is repeated, but it is terminated if difficulties arise.
- If more than one potential situation is present for the fatal dive, then more than one re-enactment may be required. In this event, any findings may not represent the actual situation existing at that time of the fatality and should be considered only as possibilities – not actualities.

A variety of observations may clarify the original assessments. These observations include very demanding conditions, entrapment, water aspiration, disorientation, resistance to breathing, equipment inadequacy and gas toxicities (e.g. carbon dioxide, hyperoxia, hypoxia, narcosis).

ACKNOWLEDGEMENTS

Acknowledgements in the review and contributions to this chapter are made to Dr Christopher Lawrence, Director of Statewide Forensic Medical Services, Tasmania and to Dr James Caruso, Chief Medical Examiner/Coroner, Denver, Colorado.

FURTHER READING

Causes of recreational diving deaths

Divers Alert Network. *Reports on Decompression Illness and Diving.* Durham, North Carolina: Divers Alert Network; 1998–1996.

Edmonds C, Walker D. Scuba diving fatalities in Australia and New Zealand: the human factor. *South Pacific Underwater Medicine Society Journal* 1989;**19**(3):94–104.

Edmonds C, Walker D. Scuba diving fatalities in Australia and New Zealand: the environmental factor. *South Pacific Underwater Medicine Society Journal* 1990;**20**(1):2–4.

Edmonds C, Walker D. Scuba diving fatalities in Australia and New Zealand: the equipment factor. *South Pacific Underwater Medicine Society Journal* 1991;**21**(1):2–5.

Accident investigation and autopsy protocol

Caruso JL. Pathology of diving accidents. In: Brubakk AO, Newman TS, eds. *Physiology and Medicine of Diving.* 5th ed. Philadelphia: Saunders, 2003.

Edmonds C, Caruso JL. Recent modifications to the investigation of diving related deaths. *Forensic Science, Medicine, and Pathology* 2014;**10**(1):83–90.

Edmonds C, Caruso J. Diving fatality investigations: recent changes. *Diving and Hyperbaric Medicine* 2014;**44**(2):91–96.

Findley TP. An autopsy protocol for skin and scuba-diving deaths. *American Journal of Clinical Pathology* 1977;**67**(5):440–443.

Hanson RG, Young JM. Diving accidents. In Bennett PB, Elliott DH, eds. *The Physiology and Medicine of Diving and Compressed Air Work.* 2nd ed. Baltimore: Williams & Wilkins; 1975:545–556.

Hayman JA. *Post Mortem Technique in Fatal Diving Accidents.* Broadsheet No. 27. ???: Royal College of Pathologists of Australasia; 1987.

Lawrence C, Cooke C. *Autopsy and the Investigation of Scuba Diving Fatalities. Guidelines from the Royal College of Pathologists of Australia.* 2003. http://www.rcpa.edu.au/getattachment/128c3690-fa49-4456-817a-ee29e49bc524/Autopsy-and-the-Investigation-of-Scuba-Diving-Fata.aspx

Plattner T, Thali MJ, Yen K, *et al.* Virtopsy: postmortem multislice computed tomography (MSCT) and MRI in a fatal scuba diving incident. *Journal of Forensic Sciences* 2003;**48**(6):1–9.

Zhu BL, Quan L, Li DR, *et al.* Postmortem lung weight in drownings: a comparison with acute asphyxiation and cardiac death. *Leg Med (Tokyo).* 2003 Mar;**5**(1):20–26.

Body detection and decomposition underwater

Teather RG. *Encyclopedia of Underwater Investigations.* 2nd ed. Flagstaff, Arizona: Best Publishing; 2013.

Dive computer and re-enactment of the incident

Edmonds C, Caruso J. Diving fatality investigations: recent changes. *Diving and Hyperbaric Medicine* 2014;**44**(2):91–96.

Edmonds C. *Reappraisals of a Diving Disaster.* Royal Australian Navy School of Underwater Medicine Report 4/68. Sydney: Royal Australian Navy School of Underwater Medicine; 1968.

Edmonds C. A forensic diving medicine examination of a highly publicised diving fatality. *Diving and Hyperbaric Medicine* 2012;**42**(4):224–230.

Decompression sickness and post-mortem decompression artefact

Boycott DM, Damant GCC, Haldane JS. The prevention of compressed air illness. *Journal of Hygiene* 1908;**8**(3):342–443.

Hill L. *Caisson Sickness and the Physiology of Work in Compressed Air.* New York: Longmans, Green and Co.; 1912.

Hoff EC. Decompression sickness: pathological lesions, post-mortem findings.

In: *A Bibliographical Source Book of Compressed Air, Diving and Submarine Medicine.* Vol. 1. NAVMED 1191. Washington, DC: US Department of the Navy; 1948:142–162.

Gersh I, Catchpole HR. Decompression sickness: physical factors and pathological consequences. In: Fulton JF, ed. *Decompression Sickness.* Philadelphia: Saunders; 1951:165–181.

Giertsen JC, Sandstad E, Morild I, Bang G, Bjersand AJ, Eidsvik S. An explosive decompression accident. *American Journal of Forensic Medicine and Pathology* 1988;**9**(2):94–101.

Post-mortem computed tomography

Edmonds C, Caruso JL. Recent modifications to the investigation of diving related deaths. *Forensic Science, Medicine, and Pathology* 2014;**10**(1):83–90.

Levy AD, Harcke HT, Getz JM, Mallak CT, Caruso JL, Pearse L, Frazier AA, Galvin JR. Virtual autopsy: two- and three-dimensional multidetector CT findings in drowning with autopsy comparison. *Radiology* 2007;**243**:862–868.

Plattner T, Thali MJ, Yen K, *et al.* Virtopsy: postmortem multislice computed tomography (MSCT) and MRI in a fatal scuba diving incident. *Journal of Forensic Sciences* 2003;**48**(6):1–9.

Resuscitation effects

Shiotami S, Kohno M, Ohashi N, *et al.* Cardiovascular gas on non-traumatic postmortem computerised tomography (PMCT): the influence of cardiopulmonary resuscitation. *Radiation Medicine* 2005;**23**(4):225–229.

Shiotami S, Ueno Y, Atake S, *et al.* Nontraumatic postmortem computed tomographic demonstration of cerebral gas embolism following cardiopulmonary resuscitation. *Japanese Journal of Radiology* 2010;**28**:1–7.

This chapter was reviewed for this fifth edition by Carl Edmonds.

PART 9

Medical Standards for Diving

52

Medical standards for snorkel divers

STATISTICAL DATA

All medical standards for an activity should be based on knowledge of the risks of the activity and the likelihood of reducing these risks by imposing medical limitations (see Chapter 61).

The reported causes of death from snorkelling are as follows:

- Cardiac: 30 to 45 per cent.
- Surface drowning: 25 to 45 per cent.
- Hypoxia from breath-holding, leading to drowning: 15 to 20 per cent.
- Trauma: 8 per cent.

The reported hypoxic drownings were often in younger, experienced free divers whose predisposing factors were hyperventilation before breath-holding, negative buoyancy and diving alone.

The surface drownings and near drownings were often in older, aquatically inexperienced, physically unfit tourists who engaged in commercial reef-snorkelling trips or solo swimming. Frequently, medical disorders– (e.g. epilepsy, asthma or other respiratory disease, salt water aspiration and vomiting) made them more vulnerable. Overall, the physical unfitness and aquatic inexperience that led to panic and aspiration dominated these situations. Many of these snorkellers rejected the use of buoyancy aids, whereas others employed no fins and wore ineffective 'life vests'.

The same stresses were often present in the cardiac deaths. These occurred in the older snorkellers, many of whom were aquatically inexperienced and physically unfit and had previous cardiovascular disease and medications. Swimming against currents and struggling to keep their heads above water were frequent observations among the fatalities. Old, unfit and poorly equipped tourists do not cope well with this situation. Salt water aspiration, panic and fatigue often result in snorkellers with poor aquatic skills. Survival then often depends on the surveillance and skills of others.

Snorkellers who rarely leave the surface still expose themselves to the hazard of drowning and cardiac death. Contributing to the deaths are the personal inadequacies of the snorkeller, environmental hazards and inadequate equipment. Chapters 5, 41 and 61 are relevant.

Reliable data on morbidity in snorkellers are not available, but copious experience with them does lead to reasonable recommendations (see the medical check list, later). Some diving disorders are more frequent with this group than with scuba divers, especially the upper respiratory tract barotraumas and some marine animal injuries.

GENERAL INFORMATION

All prospective divers should first become adept at snorkelling. This expedites the swimming to and from the dive site, and it also extends the distances that a surface swimmer may achieve with greater ease.

Snorkelling acts as an emergency system to be used when more complex diving equipment fails, by allowing the diver to remain on the surface, breathing relatively easily.

Snorkelling is much more widespread, less expensive, less complex and a less regulated activity than compressed air/gas diving. This does not mean that snorkelling is safe.

Problems with basic equipment are dealt with in Chapter 4, the ocean environment in Chapter 5, specific medical problems in Chapter 61 and general problems elsewhere. Because many snorkellers are children, Chapter 58 may also be relevant.

As in scuba diving, there are reasonable standards of physical and medical fitness that should be achieved, but these are usually ascertained by completing a basic questionnaire. Even those who 'fail' the questionnaire can still snorkel after medical approval, under more restricted conditions and with supervision.

Ensuring that the potential snorkeller is capable of physical exertion and possesses aquatic skills sufficient to survive is axiomatic. Also, there should be no increased likelihood of impairment of consciousness – which is far more dangerous at sea than in terrestrial environments. If the snorkeller intends to submerse himself or herself, then the increased risks of barotraumas and breath-holding become relevant.

A typical questionnaire, presented in *Diving Medicine for Scuba Divers* (see www.divingmedicine. info) was designed for schoolchildren who wished to experience snorkelling, but it is now used by commercial dive boat operators who take tourists to the Great Barrier Reef.

MEDICAL CHECK LIST FOR SNORKELLERS

Have you ever had:

1. Any cardiovascular disease (heart, blood pressure, etc.)?	YES	NO	
2. Any lung disease (asthma, wheezing, collapsed lung, tuberculosis, etc.)?	YES	NO	
3. Any fits, epilepsy, convulsions or blackouts?	YES	NO	
4. Any serious disease (e.g. diabetes)?	YES	NO	
5. Serious ear, sinus or eye disease?	YES	NO	
6. Any neurological or psychiatric disease?	YES	NO	

Over the last month have you had any:

7. Operations, illnesses, treatment?	YES	NO
8. Drugs or medications?	YES	NO
9. If female, are you pregnant?	YES	NO

Can you:

10. Swim 500 metres without aids?	NO	YES
11. Swim 200 metres in 5 minutes or less?	NO	YES
12. Equalize your ears when diving or flying?	NO	YES

Name: (If less than 16 years old, guardian to sign)
Date of birth:
Address:

QUESTIONNAIRE FOLLOW-UP

If the candidate indicates an answer in the left hand column of the medical check list, then further investigation or action (limitation) is required before snorkelling is considered as safe. This evaluation must be done by a diving medical qualified physician. It should be performed as described for scuba divers (see Chapter 53). The same high standards should be employed except for those related to pulmonary barotrauma or decompression sickness – illnesses not likely to be encountered by snorkellers.

FURTHER READING

Edmonds C. Snorkel diving: a review. *South Pacific Underwater Medical Society Journal* 1999;**29**(4):196–202.
Edmonds C, McKenzie B, Thomas R, Pennefather J. *Diving Medicine for Scuba*

Divers. 5th ed. 2013. Free download at www. ivingmedicine.info

Edmonds C, Walker D. Snorkeling deaths in Australia. *Medical Journal of Australia* 1999;**171**:591–594.

Lippmann JM, Pearn JH. Snorkeling-related deaths in Australia,1994–2006. *Medical Journal of Australia* 2012;**197**(4):230–232.

Walker DG. The investigation of critical factors in diving related fatalities. Published annually in the *South Pacific Underwater Medicine Society Journal* 1972–1989.

This chapter was reviewed for this fifth edition by Carl Edmonds.

53

Medical standards for recreational divers

INTRODUCTION

All recreational diving candidates are required to undergo some form of medical evaluation before participating in a training course. The 'traditional' approach to this process was for the diver to undergo a 'medical' with a doctor who would exclude the candidate if any contraindications to diving were found. In most jurisdictions, this was a voluntary standard; few places have had any legislated requirement for recreational diving candidates to undergo a medical examination before training. In this regard, two important trends have emerged in recent times.

First, the recreational diving training organizations in many countries and jurisdictions have adopted a policy of asking candidates to complete a questionnaire designed to screen for important and relevant health issues. If there are no positive responses on the questionnaire, the candidate is allowed to proceed to diver training with no further medical evaluation. This is not universal, but it is becoming more common. The screening questionnaire currently recommended by the

Recreational Scuba Training Council is shown at Figure 53.1. If there are positive responses, then the candidate is required to see a doctor for a 'medical'. This has been a controversial development, particularly in Australia and New Zealand, where there is a long tradition of requiring formal medical examinations. Critics highlight the potential for diver candidates to lie on their questionnaire response, and supporters respond with the observation that determined candidates can lie just as successfully in a more formal medical examination. There have been studies suggesting that the questionnaire screening system is efficient in detecting relevant medical problems[1,2] and others demonstrating that it can fail[3].

Second, whereas in the past a medical examination with a doctor was often an exercise in checking for nominal 'contraindications' (e.g. 'asthma') and excluding affected candidates based often on little more than the disease label, a substantial degree of discretionary decision making has become a contemporary trend. Modern diving doctors frequently see themselves as risk

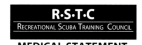

R·S·T·C
RECREATIONAL SCUBA TRAINING COUNCIL

MEDICAL STATEMENT
Participant Record (Confidential Information)

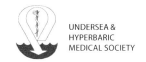

UNDERSEA &
HYPERBARIC
MEDICAL SOCIETY

Please read carefully before signing.

This is a statement in which you are informed of some potential risks involved in scuba diving and of the conduct required of you during the scuba training program. Your signature on this statement is required for you to participate in the scuba training program offered

by _____ and
Instructor

_____located in the
Facility

city of _____, state/province of _____.

Read this statement prior to signing it. You must complete this Medical Statement, which includes the medical questionnaire section, to enroll in the scuba training program. If you are a minor, you must have this Statement signed by a parent or guardian.

Diving is an exciting and demanding activity. When performed correctly, applying correct techniques, it is relatively safe. When

established safety procedures are not followed, however, there are increased risks.

To scuba dive safely, you should not be extremely overweight or out of condition. Diving can be strenuous under certain conditions. Your respiratory and circulatory systems must be in good health. All body air spaces must be normal and healthy. A person with coronary disease, a current cold or congestion, epilepsy, a severe medical problem or who is under the influence of alcohol or drugs should not dive. If you have asthma, heart disease, other chronic medical conditions or you are taking medications on a regular basis, you should consult your doctor and the instructor before participating in this program, and on a regular basis thereafter upon completion. You will also learn from the instructor the important safety rules regarding breathing and equalization while scuba diving. Improper use of scuba equipment can result in serious injury. You must be thoroughly instructed in its use under direct supervision of a qualified instructor to use it safely.

If you have any additional questions regarding this Medical Statement or the Medical Questionnaire section, review them with your instructor before signing.

Divers Medical Questionnaire

To the Participant:

The purpose of this Medical Questionnaire is to find out if you should be examined by your doctor before participating in recreational diver training. A positive response to a question does not necessarily disqualify you from diving. A positive response means that there is a preexisting condition that may affect your safety while diving and you must seek the advice of your physician prior to engaging in dive activities.

Please answer the following questions on your past or present medical history with a **YES** or **NO**. If you are not sure, answer **YES**. If any of these items apply to you, we must request that you consult with a physician prior to participating in scuba diving. Your instructor will supply you with an RSTC Medical Statement and Guidelines for Recreational Scuba Diver's Physical Examination to take to your physician.

_____ Could you be pregnant, or are you attempting to become pregnant?

_____ Are you presently taking prescription medications? (with the exception of birth control or anti-malarial)

_____ Are you over 45 years of age and can answer YES to one or more of the following?
• currently smoke a pipe, cigars or cigarettes
• have a high cholesterol level
• are currently receiving medical care
• high blood pressure
• diabetes mellitus, even if controlled by diet alone

Have you ever had or do you currently have ...

_____ Asthma, or wheezing with breathing, or wheezing with exercise?

_____ Frequent or severe attacks of hayfever or allergy?

_____ Frequent colds, sinusitis or bronchitis?

_____ Any form of lung disease?

_____ Pneumothorax (collapsed lung)?

_____ Other chest disease or chest surgery?

_____ Behavioral health, mental or psychological problems (Panic attack, fear of closed or open spaces)?

_____ Epilepsy, seizures, convulsions or take medications to prevent them?

_____ Recurring complicated migraine headaches or take medications to prevent them?

_____ Blackouts or fainting (full/partial loss of consciousness)?

_____ Frequent or severe suffering from motion sickness (seasick, carsick, etc.)?

_____ Dysentery or dehydration requiring medical intervention?

_____ Any dive accidents or decompression sickness?

_____ Inability to perform moderate exercise (example: walk 1.6 km/ one mile within 12 mins.)?

_____ Head injury with loss of consciousness in the past five years?

_____ Recurrent back problems?

_____ Back or spinal surgery?

_____ Diabetes?

_____ Back, arm or leg problems following surgery, injury or fracture?

_____ High blood pressure or take medicine to control blood pressure?

_____ Heart disease

_____ Heart attack?

_____ Angina, heart surgery or blood vessel surgery?

_____ Sinus surgery?

_____ Ear disease or surgery, hearing loss or problems with balance?

_____ Recurrent ear problems?

_____ Bleeding or other blood disorders?

_____ Hernia?

_____ Ulcers or ulcer surgery?

_____ A colostomy or ileostomy?

_____ Recreational drug use or treatment for, or alcoholism in the past five years?

The information I have provided about my medical history is accurate to the best of my knowledge. *I agree to accept responsibility for omissions regarding my failure to disclose any existing or past health condition.*

_____   _____   _____   _____
        Signature   Date   Signature of Parent or Guardian   Date

Figure 53.1 The Recreational Scuba Training Council pre-participation screening form for recreational divers. (Courtesy of the Recreational Scuba Training Council.)

evaluators and educators rather than as 'gatekeepers', and there is latitude for candidates to choose to dive as informed risk acceptors, provided the risk to them and third parties (e.g. diving instructors and future dive buddies) is not deemed excessive. An associated trend is an aversion to use of the categorical declaration that a candidate is 'fit to dive'. In application of the discretionary approach to evaluating the significance of medical problems in diving, it is more common to use more guarded language when approving a candidate for diving. For example, on the current Recreational Scuba Training Council evaluation form, the doctor signs a statement stating that he or she finds no medical conditions considered incompatible with diving (Figure 53.2). This leaves open the possibility that there are relevant medical conditions, but an evaluation of the risk they represent suggests that they are not 'incompatible with diving'. There is also an opportunity for the physician to record any discussion about risk mitigation in a remarks section (see Figure 53.2).

The authors of this text believe that properly designed questionnaire screening systems can work and that a discretionary 'risk assessment' approach to dealing with any positive responses is appropriate, adaptable and sensible. The risk assessment approach has the advantage of encouraging honesty because the candidate knows that mere mention of a particular health issue will not result in an automatic disqualification. It also ensures that the candidate participates in a discussion with an expert about the risks and benefits of diving applicable to the candidate's particular set of circumstances. If the doctor's final determination is that the candidate should not dive, at least the candidate will understand the basis for that decision. Any subsequent decision on the candidate's part to 'doctor shop' or lie about his or her condition will at least be 'informed'. The disadvantages are that the interaction with a diving doctor can be time consuming, and successful application of this approach requires a significant level of knowledge of both medicine and diving on the part of the doctor.

As part of this paradigm for evaluation of recreational diving candidates, an analytical approach is encouraged in which three questions are asked in respect of any relevant medical condition:

1. Will the condition make a diving disease more likely?
2. Will diving exacerbate the condition?
3. Will the condition prevent the diver from meeting the functional requirements of recreational diving and therefore decrease safety in the water?

Addressing the first two questions requires knowledge of pathology, diving and diving pathophysiology. Thus, by way of examples, in evaluating a pulmonary bulla in relation to question 1, the physician must understand that such lesions trap gas and that, in diving, gas trapping during ascent

---

PHYSICIAN

This person is applying for training or is presently certified to engage in scuba (self-contained underwater breathing apparatus) diving. Your opinion of the applicant's medical fitness for scuba diving is requested. There are guidelines attached for your information and reference.

Physician's Impression

☐ I find no medical conditions that I consider incompatible with diving.

☐ I am unable to recommend this individual for diving.

Remarks _____
_____
_____

Figure 53.2 Physician determination section of the Recreational Scuba Training Council form. Note the absence of any pronouncement of 'fit to dive'. (Courtesy of the Recreational Scuba Training Council.)

can lead to pulmonary barotrauma. In evaluating epilepsy in relation to question 2, the physician must understand that an epileptic seizure can be precipitated by many things, and diving involves exposure to various epileptogenic stimuli (e.g. a markedly elevated inspired oxygen tension) that are not normally encountered in everyday life. Addressing the third question requires a definition of the 'functional requirements of diving'. Interestingly, this matter had not been formally addressed until an attempt at a definition was made in a book published in 2008[4].

The remainder of this chapter describes this previously published definition of the functional requirements of diving with some minor contemporary modification and then considers common physical characteristics and organ system problems in relation to evaluating suitability for diving. It is germane to mention that entire textbooks are dedicated to this subject, and a full treatment is not possible in this short chapter. Practitioners interested in evaluating divers are advised to consult more comprehensive reference material and to complete one of the many courses available that address the important issues.

A FUNCTIONAL ANALYSIS OF DIVING

The following represents a suite of capabilities that a candidate should possess to be capable of learning to dive safely:

- Acquiring and applying a relevant diving theory knowledge base.
- Working as a team and adhering to pre-agreed systems and a dive plan.
- Tolerating the psychological stress of total submergence in water well beyond 'standing depth'.
- Holding an open-circuit regulator in the mouth and sealing the lips around the mouth-piece so that water leakage is prevented.
- Having sufficient corrected visual acuity over short distances to read diving instruments and over long distances to recognize entry and exit points.
- Lifting and carrying individual items of diving equipment on land (a standard set

of single cylinder scuba equipment weighs approximately 23 kg).
- Standing from sitting and walking 30 metres (without fins) in standard scuba equipment.
- Ascending a 1-metre vertical ladder from the water wearing standard scuba equipment.
- Swimming underwater at 0.5 knot for 30 minutes wearing standard scuba equipment adjusted for neutral buoyancy.
- Swimming underwater at 1.2 knot (or making slow progress against a 1-knot current) for 5 minutes.
- Insufflating the middle ears via the Eustachian tubes.
- Towing another diver wearing scuba equipment 30 metres at the surface.

Setting the 'bar' for some of these capabilities is inevitably arbitrary, and there has been considerable controversy over the exercise capacity parameters. These have usually been discussed in the literature as requirements in metabolic equivalents (METs) and an often cited recommendation is for a 12-MET peak exercise capacity. The authors of this text prefer to express exercise requirements in practical terms because this is more likely to resonate with candidates and examining doctors. There is little doubt that to dive the candidate needs to be able to swim underwater wearing scuba gear at about 0.5 knot (the typical speed during gentle underwater swimming) for at least 30 minutes. This corresponds to a work output of about 3 to 4 METs. The recommendation that the candidate should be able increase the effort to swim at 1.2 knots briefly simply reflects the occasional requirement to work hard to 'get out of trouble' such as if caught in a current or being too close to a reef with considerable surge. Swimming underwater at this speed probably requires a work output of about 10 METs. It is has been demonstrated that many divers struggle to reach a peak capacity at this level, and this recommendation can therefore be seen as one of the most 'flexible' of those included in the functional description. If a doctor had minor uncertainty about peak capacity in an otherwise suitable candidate, application of the discretionary approach would involve discussion of the related risks with the individual and for provision of advice to improve fitness and to avoid intentionally exposing himself or herself to potentially strenuous diving situations. Alternatively, if there was significant concern, especially in the presence of risk factors for ischaemic heart disease, the practitioner could defer giving an opinion until an exercise stress test was completed. This can give an objective indication of work capacity and may unmask subclinical cardiac ischaemia.

Perusal of the various capabilities in the analysis of the functional requirements for diving quickly reveals several that are beyond the capacity of a doctor to assess in an office consultation. Indeed, at least some are not likely to be adequately assessed until the candidate actually begins training and his or her performance and behavior is observed in the water. Not only does this add weight to the argument that doctors should not be categorically pronouncing 'fitness to dive', but also it highlights the pivotal role of the diving instructor in the process of determining suitability for diving. This is not a message that diving instructors or their parent training organizations are fond of hearing, but it is a simple logical fact. In many important respects, the diving instructor is much better positioned to act as a gatekeeper on the candidate's path into diving than the diving doctor, and instructors should be paying careful attention to some of the capabilities listed previously. Where a candidate is significantly deficient, he or she should not pass the course and should not be certified.

PSYCHOLOGICAL AND PSYCHIATRIC CONSIDERATIONS

A full psychiatric assessment is impossible to perform in the limited time of a routine diving medical examination, but some clues can be gleaned. Someone with a personality characterized by a tendency to introversion, neuroticism and global mood disturbance is more likely to panic. Useful insight may be gained by direct questions regarding the motivation to dive. A history of claustrophobia or fear of the water may raise concerns. To respond appropriately during a diving emergency, the candidate will need to display emotional maturity and stability.

Freedom from gross psychiatric disorders is essential. There should be no evidence of: anxiety states, major depression, psychoses or any organic cerebral syndromes.

A history of antidepressant, tranquilizer or other psychotropic drug intake is important both as an indication of psychopathology and because of possible interactions of the drug with diving (see Chapter 43). The frequent use of selective serotonin reuptake inhibitors (SSRIs) in the modern context for treatment of 'dysthymic' conditions causes significant confusion in consideration of suitability for diving. The drugs themselves are probably of little significance in diving, although they may cause drowsiness, and (especially in large doses) may reduce the seizure threshold. If the patient is not being treated for a major psychiatric disorder, the doses are normal, the patient has no obvious risk factors for abnormal drug elimination and the patient has used the drug for at least a month with no significant side effects, then the use of SSRIs is not necessarily a reason to discourage diving. The candidate with a history of alcohol or other drug abuse should be assessed critically.

AGE

Diving by young children is controversial. To a large extent, this controversy arises from the emotional and potential medico-legal issues that arise around keeping children safe, rather than from any evidence that diving is dangerous when compared with many other adventurous activities undertaken by children. This, of course, is not to suggest there are no concerns. Children may be trained in diving techniques, but they may not have the physical strength or psychological stability to cope with the physical demands and mental discipline required for safe diving. Conversely, diving can provide an intellectually stimulating and exciting activity that can be shared with parents and that teaches teamwork, discipline and environmental awareness.

Any involvement of children in diving should be conducted strictly according to the age group recommendations and rules imposed by the diver training organizations. For example, at the present time, Professional Association of Diving Instructors (PADI) instructors may offer highly supervised scuba experiences in shallow pools to children 8 years old or older. A child 10 years old or older can train as a junior open water diver but must be supervised on all dives by a PADI professional (even after training). The supervision responsibility is relaxed and devolved to any certified responsible adult from age 12, and at age 14 children can receive full open water diver certification.

Children should be fit and well to undertake diving, and diving should not be used as a vehicle to teach discipline to children with obvious behavioural problems. Parents must be involved in any process of evaluating children for diving, and they need to be explicitly informed that just as with many other activities (e.g. riding a bicycle or swimming), diving carries a small risk of injury or death. Indeed, it should be made clear that the doctor's role is simply to ensure there are no obvious 'medical' reasons that a particular child should not dive. Any notion that the doctor who appropriately discharges this task should be held responsible for any subsequent diving mishaps is ludicrous. The final responsibility for allowing a child to dive resides with the parents.

No upper age limit applies, provided the candidate meets all medical standards. Although physiological age is more important than chronological age, for divers more than 40 years old, it is recommended that regular re-examinations be carried out to detect medical abnormalities that may interfere with efficiency and safety in the diving environment. In particular, in the absence of a clear history of good exercise capacity without cardiac symptoms, consideration should be given to undertaking investigation for myocardial ischaemia in male divers older than 45 years and in female divers older than 55 years, especially if there are any risk factors[5]. This approach recognizes the important role played by myocardial events in diving fatalities revealed in recent research; 27 per cent of diving fatalities among insured Divers Alert Network (DAN) members had a myocardial event as the disabling injury[6]. The stress electrocardiogram is less sensitive than other investigations, but it is cheaper and readily available, and it does provide some valuable information on exercise capacity.

It is widely believed that with increasing age, allowance must be made for a more conservative approach to diving activity, as well as restricting the decompression schedules. One arbitrary recommendation that appeared in previous editions of this text was that older divers reduce their allowable bottom time (no decompression limits) by 10 per cent for each decade after the age of 30 years. On this basis, with the release of this edition, it has now reached the stage where Dr Edmonds is barely able to undertake no-decompression diving.

The issues around age and diving are discussed in more detail in Chapter 58.

WEIGHT

Obesity, usually defined as a body mass index greater than 30, may be associated with reduced functional capacity and comorbidities such as ischaemic heart disease and diabetes. It is controversial whether obesity is a risk factor for decompression sickness (DCS); several studies have drawn conflicting conclusions. For sport diving, it is permissible to allow diving with obesity that would not be accepted in professional or military diving. As with the previously noted allusion to diving more conservatively at advanced age, similar advice has been given to obese divers, but no strategies have been validated and their necessity is uncertain. It is probably appropriate for the diving doctor to inform obese candidates of the theoretical existence of higher risk of DCS in obesity and to recommend conservative practice in use of dive tables and computers.

OCCUPATION

The candidate's occupation may give some indication of his or her physical fitness, but it may also be important in increasing the relevance of diving hazards (e.g. aviators or air crew should be advised of the flying restrictions imposed after diving). Sonar operators and musicians may not wish to be exposed to the possible otological complications of diving that may prejudice their professional life.

DRUGS

A medication history is important in that it may give a clue to the presence and/or severity of otherwise unreported but significant diseases, such as hypertension, cardiac arrhythmia, epilepsy, asthma or psychosis. Also, the effects of drugs may influence a diver's safety and predispose to diving diseases. Both therapeutic and 'recreational' drugs should be considered. These possibilities are discussed more fully in Chapter 43.

CARDIOVASCULAR SYSTEM

As previously mentioned, a myocardial event was the disabling injury in 27 per cent of deaths among insured DAN members. Thus, cardiac disease is an important consideration in selection of recreational diving candidates. A summary of the consensus discussion on cardiac disease at the DAN fatalities workshop in 2010 lists the following cardiac conditions as automatic exclusions from diving[5]:

- Untreated symptomatic coronary artery disease.
- Dilated or obstructive cardiomyopathy.
- Long QT syndrome (or other channelopathies if reported).
- Arrhythmias causing impairment of exercise tolerance or consciousness.
- Poor functional capacity of presumed cardiac origin.
- Severe cardiac valvular lesions (and lower-grade stenotic lesions).
- Complex congenital cardiac disease, including cyanotic heart disease and unrepaired atrial septal defect.
- Presence of an implantable cardiac defibrillator.

Treated asymptomatic coronary disease may be acceptable for recreational diving if exercise capacity is good and there is no inducible myocardial ischaemia on investigation. Similarly, arrhythmias successfully treated by pathway ablation procedures may also be acceptable, but such patients deserve careful consideration by an experienced diving physician.

Cardiac issues in diving are discussed in more detail in Chapter 56.

RESPIRATORY SYSTEM

Respiratory disease is the major cause for disqualification of diving candidates. Divers must not only be able to tolerate moderate physical exertion that requires good respiratory function, but should also have homogeneous compliance throughout the lung parenchyma to minimize the risk of barotrauma in the presence of any rapid changes in lung volumes and transmural pressures.

A history of **spontaneous pneumothorax** is generally considered to preclude diving because of the existence of underlying predisposing lesions, the resulting high incidence of recurrence and the significant danger of developing fatal tension pneumothorax during ascent if pneumothorax develops at depth. Spontaneous pneumothorax is predominantly a disease of young male patients, with the peak incidence being between 16 and 25 years and a second peak in patients more than 40 years old with pre-existing lung disease. These older patients with pre-existing lung disease are usually disqualified on the basis of their respiratory status. Primary spontaneous pneumothoraces are believed to result from the rupture of apical, subpleural blebs that have probably filled with alveolar air dissecting from splits in local small airways[7]. Approximately 50 per cent of these patients have a recurrence, usually on the ipsilateral side. However, recurrences are infrequent after an interval of 2 years[7]. This disorder is not considered familial and is not fatal in most cases, except when recurrence is provoked by such activities as scuba diving, with transformation into tension pneumothorax.

Some liberal diving physicians now believe that if no recurrence of the spontaneous pneumothorax occurs within this 2-year period, candidates can be permitted to commence or resume diving. Other diving physicians express concern with this approach because this presupposes that the cysts somehow disappear after these 2 years. The lack of credible autopsy data to support either argument is a consequence of these individuals' being excluded from diving in the past. These authors continue to believe that a history of spontaneous pneumothorax should result in a diver or diving candidate being advised not to dive. This applies even if a pleurodesis procedure has been undertaken to prevent recurrence. Although pleurodesis reduces the chance of a large tension pneumothorax, it does not resolve the underlying lesions that can predispose to barotrauma that could manifest in other ways (e.g. arterial gas embolism). In one case, hemiplegia from cerebral arterial gas embolism developed in the first dive after pleurodesis. The resultant adhesions and decreased distensibility of the lung from pleurodesis or pleurectomy may also predispose to other episodes of pulmonary barotrauma.

Traumatic pneumothorax is different in that it does not indicate pre-existing lung lesions. Some diving physicians (including several of these authors) take the view that a history of traumatic pneumothorax does not necessarily disqualify a candidate from diving, provided the causative injury has not produced any detectable risk factors for pulmonary barotrauma (e.g. parenchymal scarring, air trapping or pleural adhesions). The usual approach to investigation is to perform a high-resolution computed tomography (CT) scan. If this scan is clear, it is reasonable to warn the candidate or diver of the small (and largely theoretical) risk that remains from an undetected lesion and to allow the candidate to make an informed decision about diving. The same principles can be applied to evaluation of candidates or divers who have suffered a penetrating chest injury or who have undergone surgery on the chest.

A history of **asthma** needs careful consideration, and this problem is given its own chapter elsewhere in this text (see Chapter 55).

Cystic lung lesions, chronic bronchitis, chronic obstructive pulmonary disease and emphysema and active or chronic respiratory infections (e.g. tuberculosis, histoplasmosis, mycotic infections and their sequelae) are usually considered contraindications to diving. Sarcoidosis is also a contraindication because pulmonary involvement is usually greater than suspected clinically.

The history of respiratory disorders is complemented by the physical examination. High-pitched expiratory rhonchi, which may be elicited only during hyperventilation, indicate airway obstruction and should preclude diving before further investigation. Thus, auscultation should be performed during hyperventilation through a wide-open mouth.

The benefit of performing spirometry as a screening test for risk of pulmonary barotrauma in subjects with no relevant respiratory history is uncertain and definitely not proven. Although one could intuitively predict that results suggesting a tendency to obstruction, such as an FEV_1 per cent (the ratio of forced expiratory volume in 1 second [FEV_1] to forced vital capacity [FVC]) below some arbitrary threshold, may predict pulmonary barotrauma, this has not proved the case in studies involving naval submarine escape trainees. Indeed, the only spirometric parameter that appears predictive of barotrauma in this setting is a FVC lower than predicted. This suggests that low-volume or low-compliance lungs may be more vulnerable, but no clear normative values for low risk have been established. Various 'standards' for defining acceptable spirometric variables in diver evaluation are arbitrary and of uncertain value. Thus, 'abnormal' spirometry results *per se* are rarely a valid basis for discouraging a candidate from diving, but they may constitute a valid reason for further investigation to identify pulmonary disease. This somewhat nihilistic view of the value of spirometry as a routine screen does not extend to its use in investigating bronchial hyperreactivity in which it can be extremely useful (see later).

Another controversial investigation in the context of a routine diving medical is the full-plate postero-anterior chest x-ray study, which may be taken in inspiration and expiration, in an attempt to demonstrate air trapping. Combined with a lateral view, the yield may be increased, but it certainly does not exclude significant degrees of air trapping. It is generally agreed that unless there is some aspect of the diver's respiratory history that warrants further investigation, a chest x-ray study is not required. Moreover, if investigation is indicated by some aspect of the history, consideration should be given to using a more sensitive technique such as CT scan. Although the benefit of a routine chest x-ray study is debatable, there remain some conservative physicians who would still request an x-ray study in an attempt to screen for cysts, bullae, fibrotic lesions and other abnormalities.

In cases where the clinical history is equivocal or spirometry yields unexpected or borderline results, further pulmonary function testing may be valuable, such as bronchial provocation testing with exercise or hypertonic saline, chest CT scanning, static lung volumes, compliance testing, carbon monoxide diffusion studies and (rarely) carbon dioxide tolerance. These tests may also be of value in further assessing the veteran diver (e.g. after pulmonary barotrauma).

The most common dilemma is to establish whether there is a relevant tendency to bronchial hyperreactivity in a diving candidate with an equivocal history of 'asthma'. For example, a candidate may present with a history of very occasional seasonal wheeze that he or she treated a few times with a bronchodilator, and baseline spirometry results may be normal. These authors have found pulmonary function testing before and after exercise or ultrasonically nebulized hypertonic saline inhalation very useful (as well as being a dramatic demonstration to the previously doubting candidate). A 15 per cent reduction in FEV_1 after 15 ml 4.5 per cent saline or after a 10-minute period of hard exercise is considered to suggest clinically significant asthma, and it would provide a sufficient basis to advise against scuba diving. Sometimes a reversal of this decrease by administration of inhaled salbutamol is used to support the asthma diagnosis.

Upper respiratory tract

Disorders of the upper respiratory tract comprise the greatest cause of morbidity in divers. A history or physical signs of chronic or recurrent pharyngitis, tonsillitis or sinusitis may predict problems with diving, particularly with respect to Eustachian tube function. Allergic rhinitis may affect sinus aeration or Eustachian tube function, as well as arousing the suspicion of bronchial hyperreactivity. Acute disorders of the ears, nose or throat may temporarily disqualify the diving candidate.

Sinus and nasal polyps may produce obstructions during ascent or descent and result in barotrauma. A deviated nasal septum may also result in abnormal airflow and nasal mucosa, thus influencing the patency of sinus ostia and the Eustachian tubes. Whenever obstruction or restriction of the upper respiratory airways occurs, barotrauma risk is increased. If infection is present, it may be aggravated and spread by diving.

A break in the anatomical boundary of gas-filled spaces is a potential danger in diving that allows access of gas into surrounding tissues.

Such breaks may be caused by trauma (e.g. nasal injuries, dental extractions).

The larynx is vital in protecting the airways, and any significant disorder in this region precludes diving.

THE EAR

Outer ear

Diving should be avoided in the presence of acute or chronic otitis externa. These disorders are discussed in Chapter 29. Cerumen does not need to be removed unless its presence has resulted in complete blockage of the external canal. Inspection should be made for the presence of exostoses, and these should not be of such size as to block the external auditory canal or lead to occlusion by superimposed cerumen or infection.

Middle ear

The diver must be able to equalize volume in the middle ear. A healthy tympanic membrane, intact and mobile, is a prerequisite for diving. Evidence of otitis media should preclude diving until the candidate is fully recovered. Chronic otitis media or cholesteatoma should be successfully treated before diving. Candidates with a tympanic membrane perforation or ventilation tubes should not dive. Obviously, it would be unwise to submit a tympanic membrane that has been weakened by a thin atrophic scar to pressure changes involved in diving. However, a healed perforation that left the tympanic membrane normal in strength and mobility would be quite acceptable. A tympanoplasty is not necessarily a contraindication to diving, if healing has been completed. A retracted and immobile tympanic membrane indicates Eustachian tube dysfunction, and this would preclude diving.

Otosclerosis surgery, with the use of an ossicle prosthesis, or stapedectomy, predisposes to spontaneous or provoked oval window rupture and therefore precludes diving. Patients who have undergone extensive mastoid surgery may experience a strong caloric response and severe vertigo.

The Eustachian tube must function normally (i.e. inflation of the middle ear must be accomplished voluntarily and without excessive force).

The tympanic membrane is observed through the otoscope to move outward as the subject performs the Valsalva manoeuvre. Alternatively, if the view is poor, autoinflation can be confirmed by the subject's own reporting of ear 'popping' verified by a marked shift in the recorded trace in tympanometry performed immediately before and immediately after the Valsalva manoeuvre ('dynamic tympanometry'). The ability to autoinflate at any one point in time does not exclude the possibility of Eustachian tube obstruction at another time. The function of the Eustachian tube depends on normal nasal function, and this requires careful assessment, especially in candidates with such conditions as allergic or vasomotor rhinitis, cleft palate or bifid uvula (see Chapter 35).

Inner ear

COCHLEAR FUNCTION

Ideally, divers should have normal cochlear and vestibular function, but moderate changes in auditory acuity may be acceptable. If auditory acuity is particularly important to the candidate in a non-diving context (e.g. in a musician), it is appropriate to inform the candidate of the potential for cochlear injury to occur in diving.

Loss of cochlear function may be associated with loss of vestibular function. If the vestibular portions of the inner ear respond to stimuli unequally, then vertigo may result, especially when visual fixation is poor, as frequently occurs in diving (see Chapter 38).

Audiograms are usually not part of a 'routine' diving medical examination for recreational diving, although it could be argued that a baseline audiogram is valuable, and a thorough diving physician and an engaged candidate may choose to have one performed. Threshold hearing for divers should ideally be 20 decibels or less at the frequencies between 500 and 4000 Hz using audiometers calibrated to International Organization for Standardization standard. Tested frequencies should extend to 6000 and 8000 cycles/second even though these frequencies may be affected by noise damage. They are also the frequencies most commonly affected by diving.

An ear-bone audiogram is useful for separating conductive from sensorineural hearing loss and should be part of any evaluation of a diver with obvious middle ear barotrauma who is also suspected of suffering hearing loss secondary to inner ear barotrauma (which is much less common). Such suspicion may be aroused if a diver with hearing loss and middle ear barotrauma has a negative Rinne test result (hearing is not enhanced with bone conduction when the tuning fork is placed on the mastoid), and a Weber test (tuning fork on the forehead in the midline) where the sound is best heard on the unaffected side.

VESTIBULAR FUNCTION

It may be wise to recommend that those individuals whose vestibular function is not normal and equal on each side do not dive. A history of Ménière's disease or other chronic vestibular disorder is probably best considered a contraindication to diving. Divers who have inner ear damage from DCS or barotrauma may fall into this category. This is a grey area with no illuminating data. The vestibular organs do compensate well for asymmetry after injury to one of them, and many divers have made a successful return to diving without apparent problems after recovery from inner ear DCS. Return to diving after inner ear barotrauma is more controversial because it may be more difficult to mitigate the risk of future events.

The sharpened Romberg test may detect vestibular abnormality and seems very sensitive to vestibular or other neurological dysfunction in DCS or inner ear barotrauma. It is very useful to establish a diver's normal performance (not everyone can perform it even when well) during a diving medical examination as a baseline for future evaluations.

Procedure for the sharpened Romberg test

1. Wear flat shoes, or bare feet, on a solid flat surface.
2. Stand heel to toe with arms crossed over the chest.
3. Eyes are closed when the candidate is ready (at which point the examiner starts a stop watch), and the candidate attempts to

remain upright for 60 seconds. A degree of 'wobbling' is normal, but if the feet move, the arms are uncrossed, or the eyes open, the timing is stopped.

4. Up to 4 attempts may be made, but if the candidate reaches 60 seconds on any attempts, the test is over and the score is 60.
5. The score is the stable time out of 60 on the best attempt.
6. Scores less than 30 seconds are considered 'abnormal' based on surveys of normal subjects and subjects diagnosed with DCS[8].

THE EYE

Good vision is needed underwater to avoid dangerous situations and, after surfacing, when the diver may have to identify other divers, landmarks, floats, boats and other objects. Distant vision should not be less than 6/18 for both eyes, with 6/24 for the worse eye (corrected or uncorrected).

Myopia is the most common deficiency requiring correction. The use of a corrective lens in the face mask or the use of soft contact lenses is of value in reducing the danger of reduced visual acuity.

In **ocular surgery** the cornea is slow to heal. In radial keratotomy, the cornea never attains full strength if the operation is successful. Mask squeeze or blunt trauma may lead to corneal rupture, usually along the surgical incisions. Patients who have undergone radial keratotomy are usually advised to avoid contact sports thereafter. Ophthalmic surgeons may be unaware of the pressure imbalance that develops between the mask and the eye surface, especially in novice divers. Experienced divers may be permitted to continue diving with special precautions to avoid pressure imbalance in the face mask. Newer procedures such as excimer laser keratotomy do not involve such deep incisions, and generally divers undergoing these procedures are fit to dive once full recovery from the procedure has occurred.

Similar considerations apply to the person who has undergone corneal grafting. In addition, the risk of corneal abrasive trauma must be considered because the cornea has no sensory nerve supply for at least 3 months postoperatively and then only partially recovers.

Patients with sulphur hexafluoride (SF6) in the globe after surgery for retinal detachment must not dive until the surgeon verifies that all gas is gone and exposure to pressure change is no longer hazardous.

Ocular problems are discussed further in Chapter 42.

NERVOUS SYSTEM

Many neurological abnormalities increase risk in diving, as well as complicating the management of neurological disorders resulting from diving such as cerebral or spinal DCS, air embolus from pulmonary barotrauma and oxygen toxicity (see Chapter 40).

Untreated cerebrovascular disorders (e.g. intracranial aneurysm and arteriovenous malformation) carry the risk of sudden death or coma. A cautious return to diving could be considered for patients fully recovered after aneurysm clipping or coiling or after ablation of an arteriovenous malformation as long as a seizure disorder was not part of the presentation as it often is in arteriovenous malformation.

Migraine occurs commonly in the general population. Few people who have migraine see a doctor and even fewer are disabled, although many take drugs that may be relevant. In diving, migraine may be precipitated by: elevated arterial carbon dioxide tension (see Chapter 18), cold water exposure, psychological stress, glare; intra-arterial bubbles (DCS, cerebral arterial gas embolism) and possibly increased oxygen pressure (hyperbaric oxygen therapy). There is also an association between migraine (particularly with aura) and the presence of a patent foramen ovale, which may be a risk factor for the development of certain forms of DCS (see Chapters 10 and 12).

As with 'asthma', diving physicians should consider the individual candidate and not the label when evaluating someone who suffers from 'migraine'. Whether migraine sufferers are advised against diving depends on the frequency, severity and clinical features of their events. A candidate who suffers frequent unpredictable and severe migraines with a neurological aura should probably be advised not to dive. In contrast, a candidate who suffers infrequent events that are not accompanied by other neurological symptoms can dive so long as diving does not prove to be a precipitant.

Epilepsy is an absolute contraindication to diving. Apart from the risk of drowning, there is the risk of pulmonary barotrauma if the diver is returned to the surface when unconscious and not ventilating. Epilepsy, which is usually diagnosed after two or more definite seizures in the absence of any other disorder to explain them, occurs in 0.5 per cent of the population. Salient points in history include the following: 34 per cent of patients with childhood epilepsy have a recurrence after withdrawal of medication; 50 per cent of people who have had one seizure will have another; and patients with 'controlled' epilepsy are 2.5 times more likely to be involved in motor vehicle accidents. Epilepsy should not be confused with the febrile convulsions of infants, which do not have the same ominous sequelae.

In the diving environment, glare, sensory deprivation, unfamiliar vestibular stimulation, narcosis, stress, elevated inspired oxygen tension and hyper-ventilation or hypo-ventilation may be possible 'triggering' factors. Some divers have their first epileptic attack underwater.

A history of head injury may be important because of both the risk of seizure and the effect on cognitive functioning. In assessing the severity of such an injury, one or more of the following points indicate a high risk of post-traumatic epilepsy[9]:

1. Brain contusion (based on findings during surgery or the presence of focal neurological symptoms).
2. Intracranial haematoma.
3. Loss of consciousness or post-traumatic amnesia for more than 24 hours.

In one large and well-conducted study, the risk of new seizures was 6 per cent over the first post-injury year if any of these factors were relevant, which was ~95 times the expected rate for the general population[9]. In contrast, in mild head injuries (defined by an absence of a skull fracture and by loss of consciousness or post-traumatic amnesia lasting less than 30 minutes), the risk was 0.2 per cent over the first post-injury year, which was ~3 times the expected rate. The risk of developing epilepsy remains elevated for severe injuries in perpetuity, but for mild injuries the risk is only twice normal after 1 year, and it becomes indistinguishable from background by 5 years. The authors of this text recommend that a victim of severe head injuries never dives but recognize that the absolute risk after 1 year in the context of mild head injury is small. A risk averse candidate may choose to wait 5 years after mild injury.

Spinal cord injury or disease is important because, in addition to the limitation exposed by the primary neurological deficit, there may also (in theory) be an increased vulnerability to spinal DCS and/or further injury. The vulnerability may be caused by the exhaustion of spinal cord redundancy (e.g. in myelopathies resulting from DCS or poliomyelitis), or it may reflect altered inert gas kinetics. A retrospective observational study suggested that divers with untreated spinal canal stenosis at cervical and thoracic levels (often from disc herniation) may be at higher risk of spinal DCS[10]. Candidates with trauma or disease of the spinal cord should not dive if there are any residual manifestations. Diving needs very careful consideration even if there are no clinically detectable residual deficits (e.g. after surgery to correct spinal stenosis). In the last situations, a highly motivated diver may decide that the benefit of diving outweighs the theoretical risk.

Some neurological handicaps (e.g. traumatic paraplegia, muscular dystrophy) may be 'accepted' for special diving circumstances, such as the specialized handicapped diver program (see Chapter 63). However, such candidates require close supervision and support, and the scope of their diving must be very limited. As well as the obvious limitations, the candidates may also exhibit poor heat and cold tolerance.

Peripheral neuropathy may cause diagnostic confusion in assessing possible DCS, and sensory loss may lead to trauma and delayed wound healing. The underlying cause, however, usually precludes diving.

ENDOCRINE SYSTEM

Diabetes mellitus has traditionally been regarded as a disqualifying condition for several reasons. The most obvious is the risk of hypoglycaemia in a patient with insulin-dependent diabetes. Some diabetic patients have little warning of such events, and the early warning signs may be masked by the underwater environment which also interferes with taking remedial action. However, in the presence of increasing evidence that focussed groups of diabetic patients have developed methods for minimizing risk in diving, and indeed, have been diving safely, the diving medicine community has softened its stance on diving by diabetic patients. In 2005, DAN held a workshop on diving by diabetic patients that developed a consensus agreement on appropriate procedures for selection and training of diabetic divers and detailed guidelines for management of blood glucose levels on the day of diving[11]. These issues are discussed in more detail in Chapter 57.

Thyroid disorders may be missed clinically but are important because of the profound effects they may have on cardiac and neurological function if these disorders are untreated. With good control of hyperthyroidism or hypothyroidism, verified by thyroid function tests, recreational diving may be undertaken. Significant goiter could preclude diving until corrected because of possible airway compression.

GASTROINTESTINAL SYSTEM

Dental health is important because cracked or unstable fillings can result in dental barotrauma. If dentition was so poor as to impair retention of the scuba mouthpiece, then diving would not be safe. Dentures need to be considered in the same way.

Abdominal wall hernias (inguinal, femoral, umbilical, and incisional) that potentially contain bowel may cause problems with the variation in gas volumes during changes of depth. As well as restricting the diver's physical capabilities, there is the potential for incarceration incurred by lifting heavy scuba equipment. Surgical repair is recommended in these circumstances.

The presence of a hiatus hernia may lead to underwater reflux or regurgitation, especially with the head-down position of descent. During ascent, reflux is also possible, as is gastrointestinal barotrauma secondary to expansion of gas in the stomach (see Chapter 9). After surgical repair of hiatus hernia, the candidate should be able to eructate, thus indicating the ability of gastric gas

to escape during ascent. Otherwise, gastric rupture is possible. Similarly, the presence of obstructive lesions anywhere in the gastrointestinal tract should be carefully assessed for their potential to cause barotrauma.

Inflammatory bowel diseases, such as Crohn's disease or ulcerative colitis, are not necessarily a bar to recreational diving during periods when the condition is in remission. The possibility of flare-up at a remote diving location should be borne in mind. Ileostomy or colostomy should present no great problem with diving.

MISCELLANEOUS CONDITIONS

Space prevents discussion of all possible disorders that diving candidates may present to the examining physician. The application of the 'three question approach' articulated at the beginning of this chapter, along with experience of diving and a sound knowledge of diving medicine, should facilitate sensible assessment of suitability for diving in virtually any clinical situation. Nevertheless, certain 'miscellaneous' problems are mentioned here.

Bleeding disorders, such as haemophilia and von Willebrand's disease, are grounds to discourage diving because of the risk of trauma and the unknown effect of expanding intravascular or tissue bubbles. There is some evidence that DCS of the spinal cord or inner ear may be exacerbated by hemorrhage.

The candidate with sickle cell disease should be advised not to dive. Candidates with asymptomatic sickle cell trait may also be at risk, with severe hypoxia or with local tissue hypoxia secondary to DCS.

Polycythaemia causes disadvantageous changes in blood rheology that may complicate embolic injury to critical tissues such as the brain or spinal cord. It may also alter tissue perfusion and thereby change inert gas kinetics in unpredictable ways. Candidates with polycythaemia should be discouraged from diving. Candidates with leukaemia in remission would require careful assessment.

Human immunodeficiency virus (HIV)-positive candidates who are clinically stable are probably at low risk in diving. However, a sufferer of the full-blown acquired immunodeficiency syndrome (AIDS) likely has a greatly increased risk of infection, particularly of the lung and brain, and probably should avoid diving.

A significant musculoskeletal problem limits the diver's physical capabilities and may complicate DCS assessment. A significant history of back injury or recurrent back pain is a contraindication to professional diving, although a recreational candidate may consider diving after appropriate advice, provided there is no neurological deficit and canal stenosis is not present.

Pregnancy is a contraindication to diving and is discussed further in Chapter 60.

Motion sickness is a dangerous disorder to have while diving from boats or in rough water. Vomiting underwater is a problem, especially if the diver vomits into the regulator. The psychological manifestations of motion sickness may also result in injudicious decisions (e.g. to surface without completing adequate decompression stops; see Chapter 26).

Smoking is detrimental because of its specific effect on upper and lower respiratory function that increases the chance of ear, sinus and pulmonary barotrauma. There is also an increased risk of coronary artery and peripheral vascular disease. However, although smoking should be discouraged, it cannot (of itself) be considered a contraindication to diving. Other recreational or social drugs also need to be assessed (see Chapter 43).

Any acute illness is usually a temporary bar to diving.

DIVING HISTORY

Knowledge of previous hypobaric (aviation), hyperbaric and aquatic accidents may be valuable in assessing the likelihood of potential future problems. Specifically, a history of barotrauma, DCS, dysbaric osteonecrosis, nitrogen narcosis, gas toxicities and unconsciousness or near drowning should be sought.

Divers who have suffered mild DCS should undergo thorough follow-up (see Chapter 13). In any case, they should not dive for at least 4 weeks following the episode. If there are no sequelae, diving may be recommended.

Neurological sequelae after DCS are not uncommon and may infer a subsequent predisposition to more accidents of a similar nature. Divers with a persisting neurological deficit after DCS should be discouraged from diving.

Divers who have had pulmonary barotrauma are often regarded as permanently unfit for further diving (see Chapter 6).

CONDITIONAL RECOMMENDATIONS

To the uninformed, recommending that a potential diver with a medical condition confines his or her diving to shallow water may seem to offer a level of protection. However, because the greatest proportionate volume changes occur within the shallow depth range, the diver is at greatest risk of barotraumatic injuries close to the surface. In general, the authors of this text discourage the use of conditional recommendations, although there may be circumstances where they are appropriate.

This does not prevent the diving physician from discussing safety strategies with the diver. Examples include additional safety stops and limiting bottom times in individuals with risk factors for DCS.

REFERENCES

1. Glen S, White S, Douglas J. Medical supervision of sport diving in Scotland: reassessing the need for routine medical examinations. *British Journal of Sports Medicine* 2000;**34**:375–378.
2. Glen S. Three year follow up of a self certification system for the assessment of fitness to dive in Scotland. *British Journal of Sports Medicine* 2004;**38**:754–757.
3. Meehan CA, Bennett MH. Medical assessment of fitness to dive: comparing a questionnaire and medical interview-based approach. *Diving and Hyperbaric Medicine* 2010;**40**:119–124.
4. Mitchell SJ, Bennett MH. Clearance to dive and fitness for work. In: Neuman TS, Thom SR, eds. *The Physiology and Medicine of Hyperbaric Oxygen Therapy.* Philadelphia: Saunders; 2008:65–94.
5. Mitchell SJ, Bove AA. Medical screening of recreational divers for cardiovascular disease: consensus discussion at the Divers Alert Network fatality workshop. *Undersea and Hyperbaric Medicine* 2011;**38**:289–296.

6. Denoble PJ, Caruso JL, Dear G de L, Pieper CF, Vann RD. Common causes of open-circuit recreational diving fatalities. *Undersea and Hyperbaric Medicine* 2008;**35**:393–406.

7. Francis TJR, Denison DM. Pulmonary barotrauma. In: Lundgren CEG, Miller JN, eds. *The Lung at Depth.* New York: Marcel Dekker; 1999.

8. Fitzgerald B. A review of the sharpened Romberg test in diving medicine. *South Pacific Underwater Medicine Society Journal* 1996;**26**:142–146.

9. Annegers JF, Hauser WA, Coan SP, *et al.* A population-based study of seizures after traumatic brain injuries. *New England Journal of Medicine* 1998;**338**:20–24.

10. Gempp E, Louge P, Lafolie T, *et al.* Relation between cervical and thoracic spinal canal stenosis and the development of spinal cord decompression sickness in divers. *Spinal Cord* 2014;**52**:236–240.

11. Pollock NW, Uguccioni DM, Dear G de L, eds. *Diabetes and Recreational Diving: Guidelines for the Future.* Proceedings of the Undersea and Hyperbaric Medical Society/Divers Alert Network 2005 Workshop, Las Vegas, NV, USA. Durham, North Carolina: Divers Alert Network; 2005:86–100.

This chapter was reviewed for this fifth edition by Simon Mitchell.

54

Medical standards for commercial divers

INTRODUCTION

Commercial and professional diving activity encompasses a broad range of divers including the military diver, the off-shore oilfield saturation diver, the recreational diving instructor, the photojournalist, the scientific diver and the police diver. Although their scope of diving varies markedly, what they do have in common is that they are employed and receive financial gain from their diving. The position of divers (e.g. dive masters or science students) who frequently assist commercial operations but do not accept direct financial gain is more difficult to define.

All commercial divers should receive appropriate training in order for them to carry out their task, be capable of dealing with emergencies involving themselves or their buddy and be able to operate in the presence of demanding environmental conditions. The diver who is paid to do a job does not have the luxury of deciding when he or she will dive. The professional diver is often only one part of a team. This diver must be able to replace, and be replaced by, other members as the task demands.

Most deviations from the norm make for complications. A diver less physically strong than the others will sooner or later be exposed to conditions which he or she will be unable to handle. The professional diver must be able to perform all the diving tasks expected of the team as a whole and not have any specific restrictions or limitations imposed on him or her or on the diving practice.

When assessing a candidate's fitness for commercial diving, the doctor is usually constrained by governmental regulations or by commercially agreed standards (Table 54.1). The doctor has to consider the position of the employer as well as the diver and has less scope for including the potential candidate in a discussion of risk factors. The doctor must also consider any legal aspects or compensation liabilities that may arise in the future.

In most industrialized countries, workplace regulations dictate that the employer has a duty of care to ensure that all diving carried out is as safe as is reasonably practicable. The diver also has a responsibility to declare if his or her fitness to dive is compromised for any reason.

Anti-discrimination laws now require statistically sound scientific evidence to support the exclusion of a worker from a particular occupation on medical grounds. It is therefore important that the medical practitioner who undertakes

Table 54.1 Commercial diving regulators in various jurisdictions

Country	Regulation
United Kingdom	Health and Safety Executive. UK Diving Regulations. The Medical Examination and Assessment of Divers (MA1) (April 2008)
France	Hyperbaric Work. Health and Safety Act (1990)
Norway	Manned Underwater Operations (Norwegian Petroleum Directorate [1990])
United States	Association of Diving Contractor Standards (2004)
Australia and New Zealand	Australian Diving Contractors Association (Model Work Health and Safety Draft 2010; AS/NZS 2299.1 [2007])

commercial diving medical examinations has an in-depth knowledge of the particular workplace and environmental conditions under which the diver will operate.

In general, the minimum standards for commercial divers are similar to those that apply to recreational divers and are outlined in Chapter 53. This chapter discusses the additional specific fitness requirements for commercial divers. Because these medical examinations are required at regular intervals, usually annually, the original or baseline data – both clinical and investigatory – allow for comparison with the current assessment and the detection of adverse health effects.

PHYSICAL FITNESS

Physical fitness standards are often contentious and have effectively excluded women from military diving. Professional diving is arduous and involves heavy equipment. One of the rebreather units used by many of the world's navies weighs 29 kg on land when fully charged. Not many women – and not all men – are capable of lifting and carrying this type of load on land. Fitness tests have long been defined in terms of aerobic performance (i.e. a 2.4-km run in less than 10 minutes) and tests of upper body strength (push-ups or chin-ups). However, these types of test give no indication of an individual's ability to do a specific occupational task.

Fitness tests should be performance based, reflect the nature of the activity, and be job specific. For example, if the job requires the diver to climb into a small boat while wearing a 30-kg set, the test should be exactly that. Swimming ability should be assessed as opposed to running speed. Professional

divers also need to have sufficient physical reserves to respond to changing environmental conditions and emergencies.

AGE

Most authorities agree on 18 years as the minimum age for entry into the commercial diving world. This is also realistic when considering the time required for the prerequisite training for bell divers or the age limits in place for enlisting in the military or police forces. It is unlikely that a scientific diver will have the necessary educational qualifications at less than 18 years of age. These general limits on entering the workforce exist to ensure that the potential employee has sufficient emotional and physical maturity to accept the responsibility of the job.

There is no upper limit of age for professional divers, but as for recreational divers, the risks of cardiovascular disease with ageing must be considered. Physical fitness declines with age, along with the ability to recover from injury. The medical practitioner must make some assessment of the ageing diver's pulmonary and cardiovascular reserves and the ability to continue to perform all required tasks. As the diver ages, his or her experience may be of more use in a diving supervisory role.

SKIN

Saturation divers may spend days to weeks at depth, living in a habitat at or close to their working depth. These habitats are often hot and humid and can be an incubator for bacterial skin infections. Divers often share equipment such as wetsuits and regulators. Wet skin can promote the spread of bacteria normally confined to intertriginous zones. Common fungal infections such as tinea pedis require treatment to prevent the entire diving team from becoming infected. *Molluscum contagiosum,* because of its high infectivity, requires treatment before a diver is declared fit to dive. Herpes simplex is relatively common in the general community and does not harm the diver. However, if oral lesions are so widespread and painful that holding a mouthpiece becomes difficult, then the diver should be made temporarily unfit to dive. Herpes zoster infections make the diver unfit to dive until he or she is no longer infectious and the pain and lesions have settled.

Allergic contact dermatoses occur in divers. Antioxidants and glues used in the manufacture of Neoprene wetsuits and drilling muds have been implicated and require assessment by a dermatologist. Because all future exposure to the allergen must be avoided, this can have serious effects on the diver's future.

Aquagenic urticaria is an absolute contraindication to a professional diving career.

VISION

Commercial divers often work in such low-visibility environments that they use their hands to 'see'. However, the diver must be able to read gauges, watches and decompression tables. Contact lenses may be used to correct vision, although hard lenses should be avoided because of the risk of corneal ulceration secondary to the formation of bubbles beneath the lens. This risk is reduced if fenestrations are drilled through the lenses.

Color vision is not essential to diving, although there are some exceptions (e.g. military explosive ordnance divers who require normal color vision to distinguish between the red and the green wire).

EAR, NOSE AND THROAT

Exostoses are particularly common in persons who spend extended time in cold sea water. The diver is rendered temporarily medically unfit by the presence of acute or chronic otitis externa, which is particularly troublesome in chamber operations (see the earlier discussion of skin).

Round window fistula secondary to inner ear barotrauma (see Chapter 7) in the past resulted in an automatic disqualification from diving. There is no doubt that individuals who have persistent labyrinthine symptoms such as vertigo, dizziness and loss of balance should not resume diving. However, in divers who have made a full recovery (with either conservative or surgical management), some diving physicians would consider them fit to dive. This requires careful consideration based on the audiological outcome, and detailed and informed advice must be provided to the diver. Forceful autoinflation must be avoided at all times.

Hearing

The commercial diver must be able to communicate and understand verbal instructions. Most commercial diving standards require an annual audiogram covering the frequency range from 250 to 8000 Hz.

It had been considered for many years that professional divers suffered from an accelerated form of hearing loss. However, many of these studies failed to take into account the diver's exposure to workplace noise in addition to the diving exposure. For example, naval divers were exposed to gunfire and engine room machinery noise. With advances in the management of industrial noise exposure, the diver should not be at increased risk of hearing loss from these extraneous causes.

Diving exposure may result in hearing loss as a consequence of inner ear barotrauma and inner ear decompression sickness. There is also some experimental evidence of cochlear degeneration in animals that have been subjected to accepted compression and decompression schedules. Therefore, the appearance of hearing loss (particularly unilateral loss) should be evaluated carefully. At the time of the annual medical examination, it is also appropriate to provide specific advice to the diver on the importance of using appropriate hearing protection in designated high-noise areas.

NERVOUS SYSTEM

A detailed examination of the nervous system is mandatory, and results should be normal. The presence of any neurological disease is grounds for rejection, especially progressive, relapsing or intermittent conditions. The exception to this rule is any well-documented, non-progressive abnormality (e.g. a patch of anesthetic skin), provided generalized disease is excluded.

RESPIRATORY AND CARDIOVASCULAR SYSTEMS

The minimum standards for the professional diver are the same as those for the recreational diver and are discussed in Chapter 53.

There is no requirement for an annual chest x-ray study in the commercial diving population. A chest radiograph may be indicated in divers who have suffered an intercurrent respiratory illness or a pulmonary injury or as follow-up of a previously documented abnormality.

GASTROINTESTINAL SYSTEM

The commercial diver is often required to work in remote areas and in the absence of qualified medical support. A perforated peptic ulcer is a medical emergency at the best of times, but it is a life-threatening emergency on an isolated diving platform or during a saturation dive. Similarly, treatment of an acute exacerbation of inflammatory bowel disease may cost a company dearly if a saturation dive has to be aborted on medical grounds. Serious consideration must be given to the continued fitness to dive of a commercial diver with chronic gastrointestinal disease.

DIABETES

Diabetes requiring medication is usually considered a contraindication to commercial diving.

SCREENING FOR DYSBARIC OSTEONECROSIS

In the past, most diving medical standards required all professional divers to undergo annual long bone x-ray studies as a screening test for dysbaric osteonecrosis (see Chapter 14). This is no longer required because the incidence of the disease is low, the diver is exposed to a significant radiation dose and the yield of positive results is low. It is recommended that long bone screening be carried out on only those divers who are considered to be at increased risk of dysbaric osteonecrosis. These baseline x-ray studies should be performed once on entry to the profession and be retained for at least the career lifetime of the diver.

If dysbaric osteonecrosis is suspected, a further series of radiographs should be taken, as guided by the clinical presentation. The films must be comparable, and it is recommended they be performed in accordance with the procedural guidelines laid down by the UK Medical Research Council Decompression Sickness Registry. Alternatively, magnetic resonance imaging is more informative and carries less risk.

RETURN TO DIVING AFTER ILLNESS OR INJURY

A careful assessment of dive fitness is required in any diver who suffers an illness or injury. It is important to consider whether or not the condition affects dive safety and whether the diver can continue to perform his or her job. Workplace legislation requires employers to undertake reasonable and practical steps to provide a safe working environment for all. The diver who suffers a traumatic amputation of one or more fingers may still be able to handle heavy and bulky underwater tools, act as a standby diver and tend lifelines. If the individual can still demonstrate proficiency in all these tasks, continued diving may be possible.

The diving medical practitioner must understand the specific job requirements of particular diving operations to be able to provide informed judgements on diving fitness. The diving supervisor can assist the medical practitioner by delineating exact job descriptions. It is equally important to assist the diver who is permanently unfit to dive to understand and accept the reasoning behind the decision.

FURTHER READING

AS/NZ 2299.1:2007. *Occupational Diving Operations. Part 1: Standard Operational Practice.* Melbourne: Standards Australia; 2007.

Joiner JT, ed. *NOAA Diving Manual: Diving for Science and Technology.* 4th ed. Washington, DC: US Department of Commerce National Oceanic and Atmospheric Administration; 2001.

SS521-AG-PRO-010 0910-LP-106-0957. *US Navy Diving Manual Revision 6 (2008). Vol. 2: Air Diving Operations.* Naval Sea Systems Command. http://www.usu.edu/scuba/navy_manual6.pdf.

SS521-AG-PRO-010 0910-LP-106-0957. *US Navy Diving Manual Revision 6 (2008).* Vol. 3: Mixed *Gas Surface Supplied Diving Operations;* and Vol. 4: *Closed-Circuit and Semi-Closed Circuit Diving Operations.* Naval Sea Systems Command. http://www.usu.edu/scuba/navy_manual6.pdf.

Wendling J, Elliott D, Tor N, eds. *Fitness to Dive Standards. Guidelines for Medical Assessment of Working Divers.* 2013. European Diving Technology Committee – Medical Subcommittee. http://www.edtc.org/EDTC-Fitnesstodivestandard-2003.pdf.

This chapter was reviewed for this fifth edition by Michael Bennett.

Asthma

PATHOPHYSIOLOGY

Epidemiology

As of 2011, 235 to 330 million people worldwide were affected by asthma, and approximately 250 000 people died each year of the disease. Rates varied among countries, with prevalences between 1 and 18 per cent. Asthma is more common in developed countries. Within developed countries asthma is more common in those who are economically disadvantaged, whereas in developing countries it is more common in the affluent.

Global rates of asthma increased significantly between the 1960s and 2013. They have plateaued in the developed world since the mid-1990s, with more recent increases primarily in the developing world. Asthma affects approximately 7 per cent of the population of the United States and 5 per cent of people in the United Kingdom, whereas Canada, Australia and New Zealand have rates of about 14 to 15 per cent. Asthma also varies with the definitions applied.

Often diving candidates may have a history of asthma as a child, so the implications of this need to be considered when applying statistical correlates of morbidity.

Wheezing as a child

Wheeze is common in infants[1]. Its prevalence in the first year of life may be as high as 60 per cent (United States) and as high as 32 per cent in the first 5 years of life (United Kingdom). It is caused by a restriction of airflow and is frequent in infants probably because they have proportionately smaller airways.

The three most common causes are as follows:

1. Recurrent wheeze related to abnormal airway mechanics, maternal smoking during pregnancy and genetic factors. Male infants are affected more often, with an increased risk of developing chronic obstructive pulmonary disease after the age of 60 years.
2. Episodic viral wheeze is unrelated to lung function at birth, and there is normal bronchial hyperresponsiveness. Most children are asymptomatic by the age of 10 years.
3. Asthma. The risk is increasingly related to atopy and bronchial hyperreactive response as age increases. Both genetic and environmental factors are present, with a peak prevalence between 5 and 10 years of age.

Other causes of wheeze include abnormalities of the tracheo-bronchial tree, cystic fibrosis, inhaled foreign bodies and chronic lung disease of prematurity.

Often wheezing children are inappropriately labeled as asthmatic. Even so, only 25 per cent of children with asthma at the age of 7 years will have asthma in adult life. This makes the automatic presumption from childhood asthma to adult asthma a dubious one.

Asthma as an adult

Asthma is caused by a hyperresponsiveness of airways to stimuli that do not affect normal subjects[2-4]. The obstruction results from smooth muscle contraction, airway inflammation and oedema and mucus hypersecretion and impaction. Airway lability and episodic airway obstruction are hallmarks of asthma.

Airway inflammation is often present even in asymptomatic asthmatic patients. Eosinophilia and neutrophils are present in the airways and lumen.

The functional consequences of airway narrowing in asthma are a slowing of the rate of expiratory airflow in both small and large airways and an increase in expiratory effort. There is a propensity for small intrapulmonary airways to close prematurely at normal lung volumes.

The increase in total lung capacity and residual volume as asthma progresses requires the asthmatic patient to hyperventilate to maintain alveolar patency, with increased work of breathing. Compliance is reduced with increasing resistance to airflow, thus reducing alveolar ventilation and making the lungs stiff. Increasing ventilation with exercise increases these effects and results in dyspnoea at a lower exercise level than in persons who do not have asthma.

Although some subjects can estimate the degree of the obstruction, this is problematic. Others may not be able to detect even considerable changes in airway function. Thus, relying entirely on symptoms to assess the clinical status of subjects with asthma is not advisable. Asthma is diagnosed by both clinical features and lung function assessments, neither of which is adequate on its own.

There is a classification for asthmatic patients. The first category is mild intermittent asthma.

In these cases, the patient is usually asymptomatic with normal or near normal (within 80 per cent) pulmonary function, and the treatment of choice includes inhaled corticosteroids and intermittent short-acting beta-agonists. Other categories are mild persistent asthma, moderate persistent asthma and severe persistent asthma.

With the increase in clinical severity, the lung function tests are progressively impaired, even between episodes. With this increasing severity, the forced expiratory volume over 1 second (FEV_1) is more reliable than the peak expiratory flow (PEF). The maximum mid-expiratory flow (FEF_{25-75}) is an even more accurate measure of this small airway obstruction. The PEF correlates mainly with flow in larger airways.

Over many years, persistent airway inflammation may cause fixed airway narrowing with a reduced response to broncho-dilating agents (i.e. chronic obstructive airways disease). In older adults, although typical asthma symptoms may still occur, many notice only a reduced exercise tolerance and intermittent chest tightness. They may believe that they do not have asthma because they do not 'wheeze'. They progressively modify their life style to accommodate this loss of pulmonary efficiency. The FEV_1 reduces by an average of 38 ml/year in asthmatic patients compared with 22 ml in normal subjects. The underlying causes of asthma are not known. A combination of genetic factors (especially atopy) and allergen exposure influences sensitization and airway inflammation. Although allergens initiate and sustain airway inflammation, irritants may also trigger this airway narrowing.

Sensitizers include allergens (house mites, moulds, dust and animal dander, especially that of cats and dogs that live indoors). Chemicals include timber preparations, formaldehyde, paint fumes, perfumes, varnishes containing polyvinyl chloride, glutaraldehyde, latex and fumes from soldering.

Trigger factors include exercise, cold, mouth breathing, food (metabisulphite, monosodium glutamate, salicylates) medications (aspirin, nonsteroidal anti-inflammatory drugs, beta-blockers) and irritants (pressurized aerosols, fire smoke, environmental tobacco smoke, soap powders, air conditioning, solvents, household and hobby glues).

ASTHMA IN DIVERS

Respiratory disease is a major reason for medical unfitness of diving candidates[3-14]. Divers must be able not only to reliably undertake severe physical exertion, which implies good respiratory function, but also to tolerate rapid changes in lung volumes and pressures with equal and normal compliance throughout the lung. Any local airway restriction, fibrosis, cyst, or other condition may result in pulmonary barotrauma, with a tearing of lung tissue and subsequent complications, including air embolism (see Chapter 6).

A history of asthma is important because asthma recurrence will result in increased pulmonary airway resistance (predisposing to pulmonary barotrauma and impaired respiratory performance) and also may require the use of adrenergic drugs. Neither is acceptable in diving operations, recreational or professional.

At present many organizations that train recreational divers, as well as the US Navy and commercial diving operators, are reluctant to accept candidates for training or employment who have a history of asthma beyond 12 years of age. This reluctance is based on the belief that these candidates may develop airway obstruction under conditions associated with diving. It is presumed that airway obstruction developing under water would predispose to pulmonary barotrauma because of the impaired ability to empty the lungs during rapid ascent. The risk may be aggravated by greater inspiratory reserve volumes used to keep their airways open, air trapping, interference with the elastic properties of the lung, greater resistance to exhalation and the occasional association of cystic changes[3-5].

Some clinicians[6,7] have documented the association of asthma with diving accidents, including pulmonary barotrauma with minimal provocation (Case Reports 55.1 and 55.2).

Hyperventilation at depth causes divers to consume their air supply more rapidly. The rapid shallow pattern of ventilation in persons with asthma further increases the dead space–ventilation ratio, decreases alveolar ventilation and increases resistance and the work of breathing the denser gas mixtures inspired at depth.

The symptoms and sequelae of asthma may lead to rapid uncontrolled ascent, panic, fatigue and drowning (Case Reports 55.3 and 55.4).

CASE REPORT 55.1

AB, age 43 years, was an experienced diver who previously had asthma as a child and who still had high-pitched rhonchi on auscultation that were exacerbated during hyperventilation.

A professor of respiratory medicine informed him that his lungs had quite adequate function for scuba diving, and the lung function test results were normal. This advice was refuted by members of a Diving Medical Centre, but academic brilliance won out.

At a depth of 18 metres while exploring a wreck, he suddenly became aware, as he floated up over the deck, of a pain in the left side of his chest. He then attempted to ascend, but took more than half an hour to reach the surface. During this time there was a continual pain in the chest, aggravated if he tried to ascend more rapidly. With extreme courage, and commendable control over his breathing gas consumption, he reached the surface – although in great discomfort. He was then given oxygen and was transferred to hospital.

The clinical and x-ray evidence verified the diagnosis of left pneumothorax, and a thoracentesis was performed. He returned to the professor of respiratory medicine, to be reassured that on statistical grounds it was unlikely to happen again, presumably on the 'lightning does not strike twice' theory. The Diving Medical Centre physicians assured him that not only would it happen again but that, with the lung disease, the recent lung damage and the surgical treatment received, it was more than likely to happen again and that it should not have been allowed to happen in the first place. He decided, this time, to take our advice.

Diagnosis: pneumothorax with minimal provocation, asthma.

CASE REPORT 55.2

NZ, age 20 years, had been certified fit to dive despite an asthma history. Before the dive there were no symptoms, but he still used a salbutamol inhaler.

In his first deep dive, after 8 minutes at 30 metres, he took 23 minutes to ascend to 15 metres. Then a burning pain in his chest caused him to make a rapid ascent. He was pulled out semi-conscious and apnoeic. He had four grand mal seizures and was given oxygen. There were no neurological defects, other than disorientation, on examination. After 6 hours, during which time he had another three seizures, he was recompressed to 18 metres on oxygen and was treated with anticonvulsants. There was no evidence of pneumothorax, and he was eventually treated on an air table at 50 metres, having continued to convulse while on oxygen at 18 metres. He survived but has subsequently stopped scuba diving.

Diagnosis: asthma, pulmonary barotrauma, cerebral arterial gas embolism.

Summarized from Pulmonary barotrauma in an asthmatic diver. *South Pacific Underwater Medicine Society Journal* 1982;**12**(3):17–18, courtesy of Dr David Clinton-Baker.

CASE REPORT 55.3

A 46-year-old man had a lifelong history of asthma and was a certified diver. He made an uneventful dive to 9 metres for 30 minutes and surfaced, apart from the group. On the surface he began to struggle, and those who assisted him stated that he was noticeably wheezing. By the time he was brought into the boat, he was in cardiopulmonary arrest, and resuscitation efforts were unsuccessful. The forensic pathologist described the death as 'status asthmaticus'. His usual treatment included theophylline and albuterol (Ventolin).

From Divers Alert Network. *Annual review of recreational scuba diving injuries and deaths*, 1998 ed. Durham, NC: Divers Alert Network; 1998: record no. 1196.

CASE REPORT 55.4

DMcM, age 23 years, was a very fit and courageous athlete who had mild asthma and was advised against scuba diving. Unfortunately, his father, who was a professor of medicine, succumbed to family pressure and wrote a fit-for-diving certificate.

This patient suffered two very similar episodes. In neither case had he had any evidence of active asthma before the dive, and with the second episode he had actually used a prophylactic salbutamol spray before the dive. These episodes occurred in similar sites, at depths of less than 10 metres. On the first occasion, after 30 minutes, he had developed dyspnoea and attempted to return to shore. He had informed his buddy that he was returning to get a salbutamol spray, but he appeared panicky and inhaled sea water. He was then rescued in a comatose state and eventually recovered after a week in intensive care. The treatment was for near drowning.

The second episode was very similar, except that he did not recover. The autopsy revealed evidence of drowning, with mild asthma.

Diagnosis: asthma, panic, near drowning, drowning.

The combination of a number of trigger factors in the scuba environment may explain the provocation of asthma by scuba diving. These factors include the following:

1. Exertion.
2. Hypertonic saline (sea water) inhalation.
3. Breathing cold, dry hyperbaric air.
4. Increased inspiratory effort, from regulator resistance and increased gas density.
5. Hyperventilation or increased respiration.
6. Air trapping increased with immersion.
7. Cold-induced trigeminal nerve reflexes.
8. Stress.

The exertion with diving is especially likely after swimming against a strong current or during rescue attempts while towing a companion. Excessive drag and resistance are caused by scuba equipment and an inflated buoyancy compensator.

Sea water is a hypertonic saline solution, which provokes bronchospasm in some asthmatic patients. It is even used as an asthma provocation test akin to histamine, methacholine or exercise challenge.

Scuba divers typically breathe air with a low relative humidity, higher density and lower temperature than at the surface. Cooling of the airways results from warming inhaled air to body temperature and the heat of vapourization needed for humidification of this air. The extent of airway cooling depends on the level of ventilation (usually increased), temperature of the air (decreased with de-pressurization through the regulator) and the reduced humidity of the inspired air (during compression its water vapour is extracted). Breathing through the mouthpiece of the demand valve circumvents the normal warming and humidification from nasal breathing.

The asthmatic diver already suffers from increased resistance to breathing, but this is increased further by the resistance from the regulator, aggravated when the cylinder pressure is low, the increased gas density with depth and the hyperventilation with asthma and exercise (Case Report 55.5).

Many of the diving accidents in asthmatic divers have been preceded by use of a 'preventive puffer'.

The recommendation that an asthmatic diver take a bronchodilator before the dive has little to commend it. It ignores the following:

1. The asthma-inducing stressors of diving compete effectively with the anti-asthma medications.

CASE REPORT 55.5

DW, age 20 years, was a fit young diver who carried out 30 scuba dives to a maximum of 30 metres, without incident, before he was examined by an experienced diving physician. There was a past history of asthma for which he had used steroid inhalers. On examination, there was no evidence of bronchospasm, and the ratio of forced expiratory volume in 1 second to vital capacity (FEV_1/VC) was 3.9/4.5 without bronchodilators. The chest x-ray study was normal. He was advised that he would be medically fit to dive provided he was free of asthma and if he took an inhalation of fenoterol (Berotec) before each dive.

After undertaking in-water rescue and resuscitation exercises, to a maximum of 5 metres, he developed dyspnoea on the surface. He informed the instructor that he was suffering from asthma and was towed 30 metres back to shore. By then he was cyanosed with wheezing on inspiration and expiration. He then lost consciousness and required expired air resuscitation (by two novice divers but experienced internists). He suffered a grand mal seizure and then gradually improved following oxygen inhalation. He responded to treatment of his asthma with aminophylline over the next few days.

There was no evidence of cerebral arterial gas embolism, and the seizure was considered to be the result of cerebral hypoxia. In retrospect, a history of a mild asthmatic episode 4 days previously was elicited. It was later ascertained that the asthma, which developed on the surface, followed the aspiration of sea water, exertion and exposure to cold.

Diagnosis: asthma, near drowning.

2. The aerosol bronchodilator is more likely to reach and relieve proximal, as opposed to distal, areas of airway resistance.

3. The aerosol may be effective in allowing the person to descend while breathing relatively normally, but it is less effective at the end of the dive, when the dive stressors have been influential.

4. Most sympathomimetic drugs have cardiac arrhythmogenic effects, aggravating an appreciable hazard that already exists in the diving environment (see Chapter 39).

5. Sympathomimetic drugs cause pulmonary vasodilation and reduce the beneficial effect of the pulmonary filtering of venous gas emboli, thereby increasing the risk of arterial bubbles and severe decompression sickness (Case Report 55.6).

Other less appreciated, but well-described, complications experienced more by immersed asthmatic divers include the respiratory reflexes initiated by cold exposure to the trigeminal nerve distribution (both cold water contact and cold air inhalation) and immersion-induced air trapping[8].

The combination of two asthmatic triggers was well demonstrated in the following experiment at the Colorado State University[15] (Figure 55.1). Ten subjects, with exercise-induced bronchospasm over the previous year, were compared with 10 normal controls before and after exercise (5 minutes at 80 per cent of age-predicted maximum levels). They were then all subjected to another comparison of breathing ambient air and breathing through a well-respected commercial scuba regulator. The non-asthmatic subjects had no significant or discernable change in their FEV_1 after exercise and/or breathing through a scuba regulator. The patients with exercise-induced asthma reduced their FEV_1 by 15 per cent following exercise, with a significant further reduction to 27 per cent when they were breathing through

---

CASE REPORT 55.6

FG was a 42-year-old man. This diver completed his course with some difficulty, being physically unfit, somewhat obese, mildly diabetic (not insulin dependent) and not an aquatic person. He also had complained of difficulty with breathing produced by exertion on land, and he had lung function tests suggestive of mild asthma.

He took a 'puffer' before his first open water dive – to 15 metres for 18 minutes. This was followed by a sudden and unexplained death, attributed to a cardiac arrhythmia.

Explanation: The use of sympathomimetic drugs, such as the albuterol (Ventolin) 'puffer', many decongestants and stimulants, is thought to increase the likelihood of ventricular fibrillation – the sudden death syndrome of scuba diving. This is now one of the most common causes of death in recreational diving.

CASE REPORT 55.7

JJM, age unknown. This reply, from a physician, was published in the *British Medical Journal* in response to a published recommendation that asthmatic patients could be allowed to scuba dive.

'I have extremely mild asthma, which manifests perhaps once every 3 years for a brief time during a respiratory tract infection. As I did not encounter any asthmatic symptoms during strenuous high altitude mountaineering I thought it would be reasonable to try scuba diving. I learnt to dive in a warm shallow swimming pool and experienced no difficulties during this or my first sea dive. During my first deep sea dive, however, I had an extremely severe and sudden attack of bronchospasm at a depth of 30 metres. I barely made it to the surface, where my obvious distress and lack of speech caused my partner to inflate my life jacket, thus compromising my respiration further. It was a frightening experience and I have not dived since'.

From Martindale JJ. Scuba divers with asthma [letter]. *British Medical Journal* 1990;**300**:609.

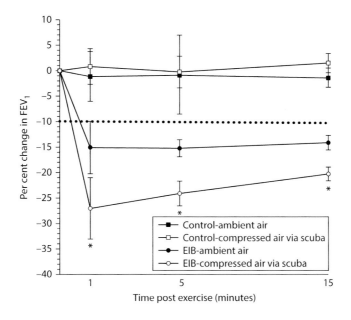

Figure 55.1 Reduction in forced expiratory volume in 1 second (FEV₁) with exercise and breathing through a scuba regulator, in controls and in subjects with exercise induced bronchospasm (EIB).

a scuba regulator. These experiments were based on very moderate stimuli and did not even have the added exposures to immersion or cold.

Treatment

Great difficulty is experienced in treating asthmatic scuba divers who are rescued and survive until recompression. They may suffer a difficult clinical complex comprising unconsciousness from near drowning and/or probable cerebral gas embolism, respiratory impairment from near drowning and/or asthma.

The problems of combining respiratory support and recompression therapy (restricted to 18 metres because of the need for 100 per cent oxygen in the presence of arterial hypoxia), the dangers from arrhythmias and the possible arterialization of trapped pulmonary air emboli with sympathomimetic drugs all make these cases very demanding (Case Report 55.8). Deeper recompression, even though the patient is not responding, may well be a death sentence, and ultimate decompression is daunting with an arterial oxygen tension less than 50 mm Hg. Some successes are doubtful achievements, with residual hypoxic brain damage

(Case Report 55.9). It is the personal belief of the authors of this text, not validated by experimental evidence, that heliox is a less problematic gas than air or even oxygen in hyperbaric treatments in asthmatic divers.

Even accepting that the case reports are incomplete (especially regarding previous medical history), it seems evident from the Divers Alert Network (DAN) data that the risks of arterial gas embolism and severe decompression sickness are significantly greater in divers with current asthma, with an odds ratio of 4.16. The exact degree of increased risk is a matter of controversy.

Other risks have been observed. Unexplained unconsciousness at depth is one of these (see Case Report 18.1).

There is no specific disadvantage to the use of inhaled steroids in divers, taken in moderation, and the hope is that some of the new anti-asthmatic drugs now under development will totally block the hyperreactive and bronchoconstrictive effects of asthma. When this is achieved, then the specific provoking factors associated with scuba diving may be blocked, and, if no lung damage has occurred, the optimistic hopes of safe diving for asthmatic patients may be realized.

CASE REPORT 55.8

MB, age 25 years, was a very fit, mildly asthmatic sportsman. He had been diving for 4 months when he went to 18 metres for 20 minutes. Without an obvious reason, he performed a rapid ascent and developed dyspnoea and confusion on the surface and left-sided hemiplegia within a few minutes. He was taken by helicopter to the Royal Australian Navy recompression chamber. He was initially compressed to 18 metres on oxygen, but because he did not regain consciousness, he was then taken to 50 metres.

After a 3-day vigil in which the patient was subjected to vigorous attempts to treat him, he died, still under pressure. During that time, he was treated conscientiously for his asthma, which was evident on auscultation, impaired ventilation and cerebral arterial gas embolism (CAGE). He was given steroids and anticonvulsants (for his repeated epileptic episodes), with measures to counter possible cerebral and pulmonary oedema, as well as maintenance of his electrolyte and pH levels. It was a therapeutic quandary and nightmare.

The autopsy revealed mild cerebral oedema, congestion of the meningeal vessels and ischaemic cell damage in the right frontal lobe and the right thalamus. There was a tear on the posterior section of the upper lobe of the right lung, with intra-alveolar haemorrhages and rupture of alveolar septa. The basal membranes were thickened and muscles showed hypertrophy, consistent with asthma.

Diagnosis: asthma, pulmonary barotrauma, CAGE.

Courtesy of Royal Australian Navy Submarine and Underwater Medicine Unit.

CASE REPORT 55.9

WD, age 33 years, had been a qualified diver for 4 years, despite having known, but very mild, asthma. He was classified as fit by a doctor who claimed experience in diving medicine. The doctor also gave a prescription for salbutamol and advised him to take it before diving. He followed this advice. He even had a pocket sewn in his wetsuit to hold the inhaler.

He descended to 9 metres for 20 minutes, before an ascent to take his bearings. On returning to his companion, he appeared distressed and then did a further rapid ascent to the surface. There he appeared to be confused and removed the regulator from his mouth. He inhaled some sea water and then lost consciousness and had an epileptic convulsion.

He was rescued by his companion, and within 30 minutes he reached the Navy recompression chamber by helicopter. He was comatose, with brainstem spasms, bronchospasm and very inadequate air entry bilaterally. He was compressed to 18 metres on oxygen. Despite endotracheal intubation and 100 per cent oxygen at 18 metres, with positive pressure respiration, the arterial partial pressure of oxygen (PaO_2) level remained at 50 to 70 mm Hg. The arterial partial pressure of carbon dioxide levels were usually above 100 mm Hg, and the pH remained below 7.0.

Mainly because of the death of an almost identical asthmatic diver, just previously, after a descent to a much greater depth, it was decided to surface this patient over a period of approximately 5 hours, while attempting to maintain as high an oxygen pressure as possible. The problem was in the combination of diagnoses, including cerebral arterial gas embolism (CAGE; the initial incident), asthma (as detected by the significant bronchospasm) and near drowning (caused during the surface difficulties and rescue of the patient).

A decision to go deeper, to overcome the effects of the air embolism, would be complicated by prejudicing the PaO_2 level. The greater depth and increased density of the gases would probably interfere with adequate ventilation, carbon dioxide exchange and acidosis. Aminophylline could cause arterialization of pulmonary emboli. The coincidental hypothermia (33 to 35°C) was not considered a definite problem and could even be advantageous – if it was not for the effect that sympathomimetic drugs, required for asthma, could have on cardiac arrhythmias. Steroids were given for rather indefinite but multiple reasons (asthma, cerebral damage, near drowning).

Initially, the chest x-ray films verified gross pulmonary oedema, consistent with the combined effects of asthma and near-drowning. Subsequent chest x-ray studies revealed a persistent right lower lobe opacity, clearing up over the next month.

With attention to the respiratory status, the brain damage and the fluid and electrolyte status, the patient gradually improved over the next few weeks and regained consciousness. The result was a severely brain-damaged young man, continually incapacitated by myoclonic spasms, almost certainly post-hypoxic but possibly contributed to by CAGE. There was residual dysarthria, left hemiparesis, an ataxic gait and myoclonic jerks. The electroencephalogram was consistent with hypoxia, and the computed tomography scan was normal.

Diagnosis: asthma, CAGE, near drowning.

CONTROVERSY

There is still controversy regarding the medical fitness for asthmatic patients to scuba dive. This arises historically because of a variety of different mind sets employed in the diving medical community. They can usually be recognized as follows.

1. A rigid approach whereby all persons with asthma and previous asthma are automatically unfit, based on both the beliefs and experiences of diving physicians of the distant past, often from the military. Most medical problems that are intermittent and that could incapacitate divers are unacceptable in military and occupational diving teams. This is related to the non-voluntary nature of diving activities in these organizations.
2. Diving physicians with long 'hands-on' involvement in diving activities. These physicians have taken detailed histories of divers encountering problems because of asthma, the treatment of divers with asthma in recompression chambers and subsequent autopsies. These clinicians have described the aggravating and precipitant trigger factors of asthma during diving and the consequences to the diver. Such observations are depicted in the case reports provided earlier in this chapter.
3. Recommendations of diving organizations. There is a wide range of such surveys, varying from the fatality statistics based on newspaper articles to the more extensive – but still incomplete – analyses of diving fatality investigations (see Chapter 46). With rare exceptions, diving fatality surveys have not sought the diver's medical history from the family and/or the family physician. The fatality investigators may not even realize the importance of this factor in their assessments. Thus, the asthma history may be underestimated. Nowadays, medicolegal and privacy aspects make this accurate history taking more difficult to acquire.
4. The *avant-garde* physician, often desperate to obtain or retain a reputation in a fringe field of medicine, not requiring academic expertise or critical peer review.
5. The would-be academic, who can come from any of the previous groups, searching for a *cause célèbre*.
6. A scientist, genuinely searching for an answer from the available but inadequate data.

POPULATION STATISTICS

It has been estimated that 4 to 7 per cent of the world's population has clinical asthma. The incidence in Australia and New Zealand is higher[2].

In one symposium[13] on asthma and diving, Professor Des Gorman referred to an 'infamous UK epidemiological survey which I believe is a role model of how not to do such studies'. Unfortunately, most of the other population 'statistics' available are no better, do not warrant any extrapolations and probably would not pass adequate peer (epidemiological) review.

The incidence of asthma in divers is not known. Self-selecting surveys (e.g. those asking a large population about a disease X) automatically select disproportionately more responses from people with disease X. Such surveys often also suffer from a very low response rate and are virtually valueless or misleading in determining prevalence figures. There have been a number of such surveys reported.

Questionnaires sent out in a skin diving magazine with a response rate of less than 5 per cent indicated that 3.3 per cent of the respondents currently had asthma[14].

Surveys with a higher percentage of respondents among divers still have the disadvantage of screening a survival population (i.e. those who have not died or retired from diving because of the illness under question, or from prudence).

A UK prevalence of asthma of about 4 per cent (31 of 813) of divers was deduced from a survey of selected diving physicians[16]. Details were not available to identify whether these responses were based on historical (childhood) or current adult data.

Some authors[3,4,10] assume against all logic and even their own statistics[14], that the diving population (trainees or experienced) have the same prevalence of asthma as the normal population. One would expect that many asthmatics would not wish to even contemplate the possibility of scuba diving, because of increased respiratory difficulties. One review[10] that is frequently quoted claims a prevalence of asthma in divers as 5 to 8 per cent, but this is not evident from the references cited.

Most of the current statistics are contaminated by selection of the data, or not discriminating between a past history of asthma and current asthma. Frequently these reports of population statistics are in the form of abstracts (no paper available), or unaccompanied by details of the questionnaire employed.

A more comprehensive UK survey[17] was also less biased as it did not selectively focus on asthma and analyzed 2240 responses (21 per cent). It indicated an asthma prevalence of 1.7 per cent in divers.

A DAN survey[11] indicated that 13 of 696 respondents were currently asthmatic (defined as having an attack within 1 year or using broncho-dilators). This equates with a 1.9 per cent incidence. There was a 5.3 per cent incidence of respondents with a past history of asthma.

An analysis of the DAN membership survey in a 1989 report by Wachholz[18] indicated that only 1.2 per cent of the 2633 respondents had active asthma, and 3.9 per cent had a history of asthma. The DAN survey had an 11 per cent response rate and was multifactorial, avoiding specific self-selection of respondents for asthma.

In Australia, where pre-diving medical examinations were mandatory for scuba training, 68 of 2051 (3.3 per cent) candidates admitted to a history of asthma – some of which were childhood cases. Only 1.4 per cent gave a history of asthma since childhood. Of those who gave a history of childhood asthma only, 50 per cent were ultimately considered fit to dive. The survey by Parker[19] verified not only the sometimes innocuous nature of the asthma history, but also that diver trainees did not reflect the normal adult population.

DEATH STATISTICS

Again, these statistics are not comprehensive. Although some authors quote the large US fatality statistics, based originally on University of Rhode Island surveys, in fact the compilation of these data allowed hardly any conclusions regarding such contributing factors as asthma. Because most of the information was obtained from newspapers, the likelihood of a documented medical history was close to nil. This has not prevented some authors from quoting these figures and ignoring the statistical adage that absence of evidence is not evidence of absence. Reviewing fatality documents and then assuming that if asthma was not specifically recorded then it did not exist make most of the 'fatality statistics' either an underestimate or misleading.

The statistics used to illustrate the contribution of asthma to diving fatalities are conflicting and inadequate. They are reported here only to illustrate the range of conclusions drawn.

In US fatalities from the DAN database, it was attempted to record a past medical history. This was admitted to be not very successful, but some medical history was available in about half the cases. In one DAN database[20], a survey of 4 of the 60 cases was recorded as having asthma (see Case Report 55.3). In the fatality statistics available from DAN (1998), of the cases on which information was available, 7 per cent were taking medication for asthma.

Most recent DAN reports indicate that the incidence of asthma in diving accidents and fatalities is around 3 per cent, the same as the incidence in the general and diving population. Unfortunately, it is usually not clear from the statistics whether they refer to current or past asthma and to what extent the asthma contributed to the deaths.

One series of 100 consecutive recreational diving deaths was recorded in Australia[21], and a determined effort was made to obtain the full medical history of all the divers, together with an assessment of the various factors contributing to the diving death. It revealed that 8 (of the 49 cases in which a full medical history was available) had asthma as a likely contribution to the death. One other case clearly had asthma, but because it had never been diagnosed as such, it was recorded merely as a 'respiratory disease contribution'. This would suggest that a minimum of 9 per cent of the deaths were in divers who had asthma as a contributing factor in this series. In 51 of the cases, the past medical history was unavailable for a variety of reasons, including medico-legal. Thus, the true incidence of the contribution of asthma to diving deaths was probably greater than the 9 per cent claimed.

In comparing the Australian data on diving deaths with the presumed incidence of active asthma in the Australian diving population (see earlier), it was concluded that the asthma cases were more highly represented than they should have been by chance alone. This is also consistent with the individual clinical cases demonstrating the actual existence and effect of the asthma.

The death statistics highlight the difficulty in obtaining precise information and also the time-consuming nature of this quest.

A microcosm of the problem is evident in the New Zealand reports. Those who denigrate the contribution of asthma to diving deaths quote a figure of 1 out of 11 cases[22]. Those who are more impressed with its relevance quote 5 out of 20[23]. The difference in the statistics is likely a reflection of the thoroughness with which the medical history is sought.

Reliance on autopsy data to implicate asthma has been suggested. The first pathological sign of an acute episode of asthma is eosinophilic infiltration of the mucosal lining of the lungs[24]. It usually takes some 24 hours to develop. An acute attack initiated during diving would therefore not likely be detected at autopsy unless the diver survived for this time. Evidence of chronic asthma effects, albeit indicative of the disease, does not necessarily imply that this disease has contributed to the death, nor does the presence of current asthma. This contribution can be concluded only from a careful and complete case analysis.

Prospective surveys of asthmatic patients who do dive have been under way since the 1990s[25]. Since 2005 there have been a dozen or so reports proposing a more tolerant approach to diving in patients with asthma. Unfortunately, these reports are based on the same statistical misinterpretations made by their predecessors – selection bias in survival surveys of current divers, thus suggesting a high rate of asthmatic divers and failure to ascertain the complete medical history in diving fatalities.

For most of the often quoted surveys, it was not possible to differentiate those divers and diving fatalities with a current history of asthma from those with only a distant past history, nor was it possible to assess the contribution of asthma to the deaths. It is for this reason that many diving physicians prefer to rely on well-documented cases, rather than conflicting population statistics, to draw conclusions.

INVESTIGATORY TESTS

These tests can be subdivided into basic expiratory spirometry, performed in most clinicians' offices, flow volume curves and the more sophisticated pulmonary function tests performed in lung function laboratories, bronchial-provocation tests, chest x-ray studies and scanning techniques.

Lung function tests

Expiratory spirometry[2,3,13,26–28] is now performed readily and cheaply, using either the traditional Vitalograph or more sophisticated digital expiratory spirometers that not only record the volume and the flow data, but also convert this into a percentage of the predicted level according to the age, sex and height of the diver.

Expiratory spirometry

FEF_{25-75} or MMEF – maximum mid-expiratory flow.

FEV_1 – forced expiratory volume over 1 second.

MEF_{25} or FEF_{75} – maximum expiratory flow at 25 per cent of vital capacity.

MEF_{50} or FEF_{50} – maximum expiratory flow at 50 per cent of vital capacity.

MEF_{75} or FEF_{25} – maximum expiratory flow at 75 per cent of vital capacity.

PEF – peak expiratory flow.

VC or FVC – vital capacity.

The use of the peak expiratory flow meter has now been relegated from the clinician's office to the patient. Repeated measurements of the peak expiratory flow, showing not only the actual flow rate but also its variation, can indicate the need for treatment. It should not be used as a single diagnostic test.

Expiratory spirometry, readily available since the 1970s, measures the forced expiratory volume, usually over a 1-second time period (FEV_1), and VC (i.e. the maximum amount of air able to be exhaled). The ratio of these two, the FEV_1/VC, was an estimate of overall lung efficiency, and if it was more than 2 SD (standard deviation) below the mean, then it was considered abnormal.

Previously, a reduction in the FEV_1/VC ratio to less than 75 per cent was thought to indicate a probable degree of airways obstruction, and this is usually so. However, elite athletes with extremely high VC volumes could, because of the latter, reduce the FEV_1/VC percentage level. Thus, this ratio should be treated with caution to ensure that a low figure is not the result of the large lungs seen in these athletes.

Investigations of submariners exposed to free ascent training compared the results of the FEV_1/VC measurements with the incidence of pulmonary barotrauma[29]. The investigators concluded that there was not a relationship between a low FEV_1/VC ratio

and this disorder, but there was an association with a low VC. Because this paper has been used to discredit the value of the FEV_1/VC ratio as a criterion for selecting out those predisposed to pulmonary barotrauma, it should be remembered that all these candidates were carefully selected beforehand to exclude lung disease. Thus, it is a survey of demonstrably normal healthy submariners. These candidates not only had no medical history or clinical examination suggestive of lung disease, but also were subjected to much more sophisticated lung function tests, including provocative testing with exercise and lung volumes with helium dilution and gas transfer analyses, when required, to ensure their normality.

It is not surprising, in this study, that a reduced FEV_1/VC ratio had poor predictive value for pulmonary barotrauma. All the cases that would have been picked up by this ratio were already screened out or were verified to have no disease. Regarding the relationship with low VC, Harries[13] noted that 'anything that might affect some one's vital capacity, forced or otherwise, would tend to make it small rather than large', and therefore the occasional candidate with lung pathology who did manage to slip through the selection net could have been picked up by the lower VC.

In an unselected population, such as those wishing to undertake recreational diving activities, the FEV_1/VC measurements and ratio should still be performed, to detect the occasional trainee with lung disease.

The mid-expiratory flows, as measured by the FEF_{25-75} or the maximum mid-expiratory flow (MMEF), give an excellent indication of obstruction to airflow. The MEF_{75}, MEF_{50} and MEF_{25}, respectively, give a measurement of obstruction to the large, medium and smaller airways. A value 2 SD below the predicted would be considered abnormal.

An obstruction to airflow would be expected to indicate a propensity to pulmonary barotrauma. Investigation of pulmonary function in divers who developed pulmonary barotrauma demonstrated reduced compliance at maximum inspiratory pressures[30]. This, hyperinflation and increased airway closure with immersion, are characteristic of asthmatics.

A later valuable survey, performed by German diving clinicians[28], supported this concept. These workers analyzed 15 consecutive cases of pulmonary barotrauma and investigated clinical, radiological and lung function data. These cases were compared with 15 cases of decompression sickness. A comparison of the pre-dive lung function between the groups showed a significantly lower MEF_{50} and MEF_{25} in the patients with pulmonary barotrauma (P <0.05 and P <0.02, respectively).

Of the 15 patients with pulmonary barotrauma, 2 had a past history of asthma. Because all the divers had passed medical examinations for fitness, and some were professional divers, this group would have to be considered as selectively excluding some divers with previous lung damage or asthma.

These investigations support the use of lung function tests in selection of divers to reduce the risk of pulmonary barotrauma.

In assessing divers to ensure that their lung function is normal, a reduction of the expiratory spirometry levels below 2 SD (or at the fifth percentile level) was recorded by Neuman and colleagues[3,13] as follows: forced vital capacity (FVC) below 75 per cent of predicted, FEV_1 below 80 per cent, FEV_1/VC below 85 per cent and FEF_{25-75} below 65 per cent. Above these predicted levels, the results could be considered normal.

Bronchial provocation and dilator tests

Some tests[24,27,31] provoke asthma in those so inclined by inducing hyperresponsive activity of the airways. These are diagnostic tests.

Pharmacological stimuli – methacholine and histamine – act directly on the airways to induce bronchial hyperreactivity.

Physical stimuli induce airways drying and changes in osmolarity. These are achieved by exercise and hyperventilation. Because the major effect is in the evaporation from the airways, the dryness of the inhaled air and the degree of ventilation are the major determinants. Hypertonic saline inhalation has a similar result.

Exercise inducing a (dry air) ventilation of about 20 times the total volume, for 6 to 8 minutes, will produce a 10 per cent drop in the FEV_1 in asthmatic patients 10 to 20 minutes later. Isocapnoeic hyperventilation with cold dry air has a similar effect, and it is a less unpleasant investigation. Non-isotonic aerosol sprays, such as hypertonic saline, provoke a similar response in patients with asthma.

Mannitol has been demonstrated to be a stable and predictable provoking substance that can be used in consulting rooms, with good reliability.

The reduction in flow rates using these provocation tests is detected by serial measuring of the FEV_1 or MMEF.

The chemical challenges were found to be more sensitive than the physical stimuli and had more false-positive results.

The hyperventilation provocation with dry air has some face validity for scuba. The increased density of the breathed gas with increased depth, together with the increased ventilation with exercise and anxiety, will have a comparable effect in dehydrating the airways and triggering asthma.

In the air-conditioned clinic, with the patient breathing cold, dry air, exercise-induced asthma can be verified by repeating expiratory spirometry tests while the candidate undergoes a reasonably strenuous exercise such as bicycling at 900 kpm/minute for 5 to 6 minutes or exercising at 80 per cent of the maximal oxygen uptake. These activities are roughly equivalent to a 1-knot swim, which most divers encounter during diving. Subsequent detection of rhonchi on auscultation (more obvious with hyperventilation) or a progressive reduction in lung function (MMEF, MEF_{50}, MEF_{25}) should give sufficient indication that the candidate is hyperresponsive and should not proceed with a diving course.

Another clinical test for asthma is by using a rapid-action beta$_2$-agonist such as salbutamol and observing a change in expiratory spirometry 15 minutes later. An increase in FEV_1 by 15 per cent is considered a positive result.

CONSENSUS CONFERENCES

There have been many committees formed from prestigious organizations with multi-disciplinary input to consider the assessment of asthmatic patients' fitness to dive. These organizations included the Diving Medical Centres of Australia[7] (1991), the Thoracic Society of Australia and New Zealand[32] (1993 and 2004), the British Thoracic Society[33] (1993), Medical Seminars Inc and the Undersea and Hyperbaric Medicine Society[13] (1995) and the South Pacific Underwater Medical Society Recommendations (2010).

There is little substantial difference in these recommendations, but all are obliged to rely on grossly inappropriate and often misleading diving population statistics. The latest of these recommendations is reprinted here, in full, but with the qualification that pathological effects of asthma are far more significant in their consequences to divers than to terrestrial athletes – and far more likely to be induced with compressed gas diving.

Guidelines for assessment of the diver with asthma

South pacific underwater medical society recommendations: 2010

INTRODUCTION

Asthma is a chronic inflammatory lung disorder characterised by wheezing, cough, shortness of breath and chest tightness. Inflammatory changes cause the bronchial smooth muscle to be hyper-responsive to a variety of stimuli including exercise and dry air. The narrowed airways, combined with the production of thick dry mucus, mean airflow may be severely limited and threaten life if not promptly treated. Prevalence depends greatly on how asthma is defined and may be as much as 30% in Australia and even higher in New Zealand.[1,2]

Importantly for diving physicians, a resolution of asthma during adolescence may be more apparent than real, suggesting it may be unwise to assume that once clinically resolved, asthma will not pose a future threat to health in a young diving candidate.[3]

ASTHMA AND DIVING

There are several reasons why divers with asthma may be at greater risk of misadventure than those without asthma:

1. Bronchial hyper-responsiveness may lead to air trapping during ascent, overpressure within the lung units involved, and therefore increase the risk of pulmonary barotrauma (PBT) and cerebral arterial gas embolism.
2. Even in the person with well-controlled asthma, an exacerbation may be provoked in response to exercise (submerged or on the surface), salt water aspiration or breathing dry, cold air. Such an exacerbation is difficult to treat while submerged and may restrict the ability of a diver to safely complete or abort the dive.
3. A diving regulator may produce a fine mist of seawater (hypertonic saline with added biological material) which may provoke bronchoconstriction.
4. Bronchial constriction, added resistance in the regulator and increased gas density at depth will increase the work of breathing, further exhausting an individual with acute bronchospasm.
5. There is a possibility that bronchodilators may provoke the passage of bubbles across the pulmonary filter and therefore predispose an asthmatic to DCI [decompression illness].
6. There is some evidence that breathing through a diving regulator increases airway resistance in people with asthma compared with those who do not have asthma.[4]

Prospective divers with asthma may be so well controlled by the current generation of inhaled corticosteroids (ICS) and long-acting bronchodilators that their lungs are no longer reactive to stimuli such as exercise and salt water. Such 'well-controlled' individuals may have risks from diving that are close to those without asthma. If this is so, then the implication is that people with asthma who are asymptomatic and show normal lung function on testing with spirometry and bronchial provocation may be able to dive with an acceptable level of risk.

ASTHMA THERAPY

The emphasis is on the administration of long-term modulation of airway inflammation with inhaled corticosteroids (ICS), combined with long-acting beta-2 agonists (LABA). These two classes of agents complement each other by acting on the two major components of asthma – inflammation and bronchoconstriction. The general approach to pharmacological therapy is to step up medication until control of symptoms is achieved. Current guidelines for treatment are published by the National Asthma Council Australia and can be found online through their website at <www.nationalasthma.org.au>. This organisation publishes an evidence-based guide to managing asthma that is available without cost in hard copy or electronic format (The Asthma Management Handbook).[2] These comprehensive guidelines emphasise the importance of an established doctor-patient relationship within which adequate attention can be paid to education, joint goal-setting, monitoring, review and the identification of risk factors.

Any consideration of the suitability for a candidate to undertake diving should start with the assurance that such an arrangement is in place.

ASSESSING A CANDIDATE WITH ASTHMA FOR DIVING

These candidates should have simple spirometry including measurements of forced vital capacity (FVC), forced expiratory volume in the first second (FEV_1), the ratio of FEV_1/FVC and peak expiratory flow (PEF). A single-breath flow-volume loop is recommended (by referral to a pulmonary laboratory, if necessary) as the information obtained (particularly changes in mid-expiratory flow rates and in the response to bronchodilators or to exercise) provides better evidence of small airways disease than an FEV_1/FVC ratio alone. The best of three attempts should be accepted.

Those who indicate a history of asthma in the last ten years, exhibit signs of wheezing or an unexplained cough, but have normal spirometry, should have bronchial provocation testing. The SPUMS recommended definitions of abnormal spirometry are one or more of: FVC < 80% of predicted, FEV_1 < 80% of predicted, FEV_1/FVC ratio < 75% predicted or PEF < 80% of predicted.

For a more thorough discussion of lung function testing, please refer to the joint American Thoracic Society and European Respiratory Society document.[5]

BRONCHIAL PROVOCATION TESTING

These tests should be performed in an appropriate laboratory in order that both challenge and response are measured in a standardised way. The role of testing was reviewed in 2004 by the Thoracic Society of Australia and New Zealand (TSANZ).[6]

Indirect methods including dry-air hyperpnoea, exercise and hypertonic challenges (saline or mannitol) are more specific for identifying individuals with current airways inflammation because they cause release of mediators from inflammatory cells in the airways, probably via an osmotic effect. The choice of which test to use will depend partly on local resources, but both exercise and 4.5% saline have the benefit of exposing the diver to stimuli that may actually be encountered during scuba diving. Another advantage is that treatment with ICS will reduce bronchial hyper-responsiveness over several weeks, making these tests useful indicators of the response to therapy.[7]

In general, most authorities accept a reduction in FEV_1 of greater than 15% as a 'positive response' to indirect challenges. The same implication is derived from demonstrating more than a 15% improvement with the administration of a bronchodilator. A positive response should lead to a recommendation against undertaking diving, but does not preclude re-testing and reassessment after asthma control has been established. A proposed schema for dealing with an asthmatic patient is contained in Figure 1.

ADVICE TO THOSE WHO 'FAIL' BRONCHIAL PROVOCATION

Diving is inadvisable for any person with asthma who fails bronchial provocation testing by an indirect method. These candidates should be counselled with regard to the theoretical dangers discussed above and the implications of their response clearly pointed out.

Candidates may be re-tested when control has been established by stepwise escalation of therapy. Current data suggest that normalisation of response with treatment is possible, and these candidates may be able to dive at some future time provided asthma control is maintained. These individuals should be re-assessed annually.

Figure 1 suggested schema for dealing with asthmatics who present for an assessment for fitness to dive. See text for a discussion of appropriate advice. [†]Assess these candidates with a low threshold for provocation testing if there is any doubt about possible symptoms of exercise-induced bronchospasm.

ADVICE TO CANDIDATES WHO 'PASS' BRONCHIAL PROVOCATION TESTING

There are two groups of candidates who do not demonstrate bronchial hyper-responsiveness: those not taking medication do not require follow-up unless they develop symptoms; those taking anti-asthma medication should be re-assessed annually or sooner if they develop any symptoms.

All current divers with controlled asthma are strongly encouraged to monitor their peak flow twice daily during diving periods, with the recommendation to refrain from diving if PEF is more than 10% below their best value.[8] SPUMS strongly advises divers against diving when symptomatic.

Medical review is required after the development of any symptoms related to asthma.

CONCLUSIONS AND RECOMMENDATIONS

- Asthma may place an intending diver at increased risk of drowning, pulmonary barotrauma, and/or arterial gas embolism.
- Those with asthma who are symptomatic or display hyper-reactivity of airways to indirect stimuli should be advised against diving due to the potential risk from pulmonary barotrauma and an exacerbation of their disease either underwater or on the surface.
- Spirometry should be performed in all intending divers with any respiratory symptoms or a history of significant respiratory disease. Peak flow meters are of limited use in assessing respiratory function for diving fitness, but may be useful for day to day monitoring of status. Spirometry should be a single-breath flow-volume curve, if possible.
- Divers with controlled asthma who are cleared for diving are advised to have annual review of their diving fitness.
- All risks should be explored fully in discussion with the candidate, and the diving physician should satisfy themselves that the candidate appreciates these risks. Written guidelines should be provided and the individual should accept responsibility for following these guidelines. The consultation should be carefully documented.

REFERENCES

1. Ross Anderson H, Gupta R, Strachan DP, Limb ES. 50 years of asthma: UK trends from 1995 to 2004. *Thorax* 2007;**62**:85–90.
2. Guidelines Committee. *Asthma Management Handbook 2006.* National Asthma Council Australia Ltd, Melbourne, Australia. http://www.nationalasthma.org.au, 2006 [cited 03 July 2011] Available from: http://www.nationalasthma.org.au/cms/images/stories/amh2006_web_5.pdf
3. Taylor DR, Cowan JO, Greene JM, Willan AR, Sears MR. Asthma in remission: can relapse in early adulthood be predicted at 18 years of age? *Chest* 2005;**127**:845–850.

4. Gotshall RW, Fedorczak LJ, Rasmussen JJ. Severity of exercise-induced bronchoconstriction during compressed-air breathing via scuba. *South Pacific Underwater Medical Society Journal* 2004;**34**:178–182.
5. Miller MR, Hankinson J, Brusasco V, Burgos F, Casaburi R, Coates, *et al.* Standardisation of spirometry. ATS/ERS Task Force: Standardisation of lung function testing Series (2). *European Respiratory Journal* 2005;**26**:319–338.
6. Anderson SD, Wong R, Bennett M, Beckert L. Summary of knowledge and thinking about asthma and diving since 1993. Discussion paper for the Thoracic Society of Australia and New Zealand, November 2004. *Diving and Hyperbaric Medicine* 2006;**36**:12–18.
7. Koskela HO, Hyvarinen L, Brannan JD, Chan HK, Anderson SD. Responsiveness to three bronchial provocation tests in patients with asthma. *Chest* 2003;**124**:2171–2177.
8. British Thoracic Society Fitness to Dive Group: British Thoracic Society guidelines on respiratory aspects of fitness for diving. *Thorax* 2003;**58**:3–13.

From South Pacific *Underwater Medicine Society. Guidelines for Assessment of the Diver With Asthma.* 2010. http://www.spums.org.au/story/spums-medical.

The South Pacific Underwater Medicine Society, in 2010, created a flow chart as a guide to establishing the acceptability of asthmatic patients to dive (Figure 55.2).

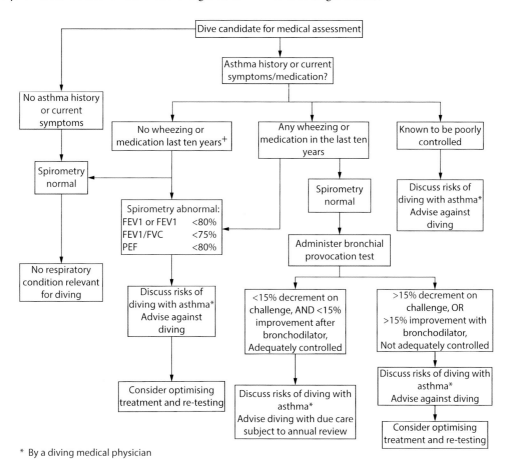

* By a diving medical physician

Figure 55.2 Assessment of a possible asthmatic patient for recreational scuba diving. South Pacific Underwater Medicine Society guidelines. (Courtesy of the South Pacific Underwater Medicine Society.)

CONCLUSION

There is no universal consensus on which, if any, asthmatic patients are safe to dive. If a patient has a past history of asthma, but no clinical or laboratory evidence of it or its sequelae over the last 5 years, most physicians would accept the candidate as fit. The increased likelihood that asthma may recur in a patient who had asthma in the past may indicate more frequent periodic medical checks and monitoring.

Most experts argue that the respiratory impairment in patients with current asthma is unacceptable, with the known but unpredictable and excessive environmental demands on pulmonary function during diving.

The conservative experts – and the authors of this text are of this group – are strongly influenced by the clinical experiences of asthmatic divers who have not survived or who withdraw from diving because of their asthma, as shown in the case reports earlier in this chapter.

Physicians who advise asthmatic patients not to dive frequently support the candidates' snorkeling and swimming interests because these activities are usually carried out in an atmosphere that does not provoke asthma – breathing 100 per cent humidified air and not exposed to pulmonary barotrauma.

ACKNOWLEDGMENT

Acknowledgment for reviewing the original chapter is given to Professor David M. Dennison, Emeritus Professor of Clinical Pathology, Royal Brompton Hospital and National Heart and Lung Institute, London.

REFERENCES

1. Freezer N. Wheeze in young children. *Australian Doctor* 1998;**Dec:**i–vii.
2. Jenkins CR, Woolcock AJ. Asthma in adults. *Medical Journal of Australia* 1997;**167**:160–167.
3. Neuman TS, Bove AA, O'Connor RD, Kelsen SG. Asthma and diving. *Annals of Allergy* 1994;**73**:344–350.
4. Bove AA. Observations on asthma in the recreational diving population. *South Pacific Underwater Medicine Society Journal* 1995;**25**(4):222–225.
5. Edmonds C. Asthma and diving. *South Pacific Underwater Medicine Society Journal* 1991;**21**(2):70–74.
6. Weiss LD, Van Meter KW. Cerebral air embolism in asthmatic scuba divers in a swimming pool. *Chest* 1995;**107**:1653–1654.
7. Edmonds C, Lowry C, Pennefather J. *Diving and Subaquatic Medicine.* 3rd ed. Oxford: Butterworth-Heinemann; 1992.
8. Leddy JJ, Maalem T, Roberts A, Curry T, Lundgren CEG. Effects of water immersion on pulmonary function in asthmatics. *Undersea and Hyperbaric Medicine* 2001;**28**(2):75–82.
9. Martindale JJ. Scuba divers with asthma [letter]. *British Medical Journal* 1990;**300**:609.
10. Van Hosen KB, Neuman TS. Asthma and scuba diving. *Immunology and Asthma Clinics of North America* 1996;**16**(4):917–928.
11. Corson KS,. Dovenbarger JA, Moon RE, *et al.* A survey of diving asthmatics [abstract]. *Undersea Biomedical Research* 1992;**19**(Suppl).
12. Wells JH, Moon RE. What is the risk of pulmonary barotrauma (PBT) due to asthma in scuba divers? *Journal of Allergy and Clinical Immunology* 1993;**91**:172.
13. Elliott DH. *Are Asthmatics Fit to Dive?,* Maryland Undersea and Hyperbaric Medical Society; 1996.
14. Bove AA, Neuman T, Kelson S, *et al.* Observation on asthma in the recreational diving population [abstract]. *Undersea and Biomed Research* 1992;**19**(Suppl):5.
15. Gotshall RW, Fedorczak LJ, Rasmussen JJ. Severity of exercise induced bronchoconstriction during diving with compressed air, breathing via scuba. *South Pacific Underwater Medical Society Journal* 2004;**34**(4):178–182.
16. Farrell PJ. Asthmatic amateur divers in the UK. *South Pacific Underwater Medicine Society Journal* 1995;**25**(1):22.

17. Dowse MStL, Bryson P, Gunby A, Fife W. *Men and Women in Diving*. Fort Bovison, United Kingdom: DDRE; 1994.

18. Wachholz C. *Analysis of DAN Member Survey*. Divers Alert Network; 1989.

19. Parker J. The relative importance of different parts of the diving medical in identifying fitness to dive and the detection of asthma. *South Pacific Underwater Medicine Society Journal* 1991;**21**(3):145–152.

20. Divers Alert Network. *Annual review of recreational scuba diving injuries and deaths*, 1998 ed. Durham, NC: Divers Alert Network; 1998.

21. Edmonds C, Walker D. Scuba diving fatalities in Australia and New Zealand. *South Pacific Underwater Medical Society Journal* 1989;**19**(3):94–104.

22. Walker D. New Zealand diving related fatalities 1981–82. *South Pacific Underwater Medicine Society Journal* 1984; **14**:12–17.

23. Sutherland AFN. Asthma and diving. *South Pacific Underwater Medicine Society Journal* 1992;**22**(3):86.

24. Reed CE, ed. Changing views of asthma. *Triangle: The Sandoz Journal of Medical Science* 1988;**27**(3).

25. Farrell PJ, Glanvill P. Diving practices of scuba divers with asthma. *British Medical Journal* 1990;**300**:609–610.

26. Clausen J. Pulmonary function testing. In: Bordow RA, Moser KM, eds. *Manual of Clinical Problems in Pulmonary Medicine*. 4th ed. Boston: Little, Brown; 1996.

27. Chatham M, Bleecker E, Smith P, Rosenthal R, Mason P, Normal P. A comparison of histamine, methacholine and exercise airway reactivity in normal and asthmatic subjects. *American Review of Respiratory Diseases* 1982;**126**:235–240.

28. Tetzlaff K, Reuter M, Leplow B, Heller M, Bettinghousen E. Risk factors for pulmonary barotrauma in divers. *Chest* 1997;**112**:654–659.

29. Brooks GO, Pethybridge RJ, Pearson RR. *Lung Function Reference Values for FEV1, FVC, FEV1:FVC ratio, and FEF25-75 Derived From the Results of Screening 3788 Royal Navy Submariners and Royal Navy Submarine Candidates by Spirometry*. EUBS paper no. 13. Aberdeen, United Kingdom: European Undersea Biomedical Society; 1988.

30. Colebatch HJH, Smith MM, Ng CKY. Increased elastic recoil as a determinant of pulmonary barotrauma in divers. *Respiratory Physiology* 1976;**26**:55–64.

31. Anderson SD, Brannan J, Trevillion L, Young IH. Lung function and bronchial provocation tests for intending divers with a history of asthma. *South Pacific Underwater Medicine Society Journal* 1995;**25**(4):233–249.

32. Jenkins C, Anderson SD, Wong R, Veale A. Compressed air diving and respiratory disease. *Medical Journal of Australia* 1993;**158**:275–279.

33. British Thoracic Society Fitness to Dive Group. British Thoracic Society guidelines on respiratory aspects of fitness for diving. *Thorax* 2003;**58**:3–13.

This chapter was reviewed for this fifth edition by Carl Edmonds.

56

Cardiac and peripheral vascular disease

INTRODUCTION

The existence of significant cardiovascular disease largely excludes a candidate from being declared fit to dive. Diving is an unpredictable sport, and a diver must have sufficient cardiovascular reserve to cope with the physical stresses of swimming against a strong current or providing assistance to a buddy who is in trouble. Psychological stresses such as panic and anxiety also place demands on the cardiovascular system.

The existence of serious cardiovascular disease also disqualifies the candidate from diving because of the risk of sudden collapse or decreased exercise tolerance (see Chapter 39). A Divers Alert Network (DAN) investigation into the common causes of scuba diving deaths identified cardiac incidents as the 'disabling factor' in 26 per cent – the third most common such factor after emergency ascent and insufficient breathing gas[1].

> Any congenital abnormality that interferes with the exercise capacity of the individual, induces arrhythmia or reduces the cardiac response to exercise precludes diving activity. This would be the case with such disorders as coarctation of the aorta.

HYPERTENSION

The Heart Foundation in Australia defines high blood pressure as an arterial pressure greater than 140 mm Hg systolic or 90 mm Hg diastolic, although 'normal' blood pressure is defined as up to 120/80 mm Hg. Intermediate pressures are classified as 'normal to high' and should be monitored regularly. Although it is generally accepted that the young trainee diver's blood pressure should not exceed 140 mm Hg systolic and 90 mm Hg diastolic, there is some flexibility for the older recreational candidate. The South Pacific Underwater Medicine Society (SPUMS) 2010 *Guidelines on Medical Assessment for Recreation Diving* suggests that the resting blood pressure should not exceed 150/95 mm Hg[2]. It is perhaps more appropriate to suggest the blood pressure should be within the normal range for the age of the candidate.

In assessing the hypertensive diver, the following should be considered: the aetiology (e.g. coarctation, endocrine disorders, idiopathic), severity (end-organ damage), drug therapy and the increased risk of coronary artery disease (CAD) and stroke.

It is unreasonable to condone diving if there are end-organ manifestations of chronic hypertension, such as retinal changes, left ventricular hypertrophy or dysfunction or abnormal renal function. These candidates usually have sustained blood pressure elevation, with diastolic values higher than 100 to 110 mm Hg. These individuals should be advised not to dive and should be referred for diagnosis and treatment.

Antihypertensive drugs may alter the capability of the cardiovascular system to respond to stress and exercise. Care should be taken to assess the potential impact of any of these agents fully. At best, the blood pressure may be controlled by diet, weight loss and exercise. Divers with continuing moderate and severe hypertension should be advised against diving.

The UK Sports Diving Medical Committee lists approved treatments as 'dietary measures including salt restriction, diuretic therapy (when being used to treat hypertension but not if also being used to treat cardiac failure) and low doses of mild vasodilators (e.g. amlodipine or ACE [angiotensin-converting enzyme] inhibitors)'[3]. ACE inhibitors (e.g. enalapril, captopril) are the preferred agents in hypertensive patients with type 2 diabetes, but they cause a persistent cough in some patients (1 to 3 per cent) that would preclude diving. Many physicians would add the related angiotensin II receptor antagonists (e.g. irbesartan, candesartan) to the list of acceptable agents. These are often used to avoid the side effects of ACE inhibitors.

Thiazide diuretics do not appear to compromise the circulation, and with long-term therapy the cardiac output remains normal, the peripheral resistance decreases, plasma renin activity decreases and there is a persistent deficit in extracellular water and plasma volume. Associated hypokalemia must be treated.

Beta-blockers are generally not appropriate agents for use in divers. They are associated with reduced exercise tolerance and autonomic nervous system blockade, with the added danger of cardiac deaths if diving is carried out while taking these drugs (see Chapter 39). Beta-blockers may also have other side effects, such as bronchospasm. Calcium channel blockers may have negative inotropic effects and may be arrhythmogenic. Occasionally, a physician may approve the use of a low dose of a beta-blocker (preferably cardioselective) or calcium channel blocker. In such cases, the diver should demonstrate the ability to attain a heart rate that is at least 90 per cent of maximum (220 minus the diver's age in years) beats per minute. If beta-blockers are used, there must be no evidence of bronchospasm, preferably assessed by lung function tests performed on and off treatment.

Individual judgement must be exercised in each case, possibly permitting restricted recreational diving.

The maximal stress exercise electrocardiogram (ECG) is useful in evaluating patients with borderline hypertension. The stress simulates the physical activity required in diving, and the recording of the blood pressure during the test allows an assessment of how the individual will respond to some of the diving stresses. The hypertensive individual shows a marked elevation in systolic pressure and a small rise in diastolic pressure. The normal individual shows a rise in systolic to a lesser degree and a slight fall in diastolic pressure. The stresses associated with diving other than exercise may aggravate this hypertensive response. Individuals with labile hypertension and marked elevations of systolic blood pressure during exercise must be considered with some reservation for diving.

For patients whose hypertension is not associated with end-organ damage, whose hypertension is adequately controlled by drugs (without any evidence of the foregoing side effects) and who have no excessive risk factors (see Table 56.1), diving may be permitted.

ISCHAEMIC HEART DISEASE

CAD is a potentially lethal, but often asymptomatic, disease that may be present from the mid-30s onward. Evidence for the presence of CAD should be sought before medical approval for diving. With CAD, the myocardium is susceptible to ischaemia whenever there is an excessive load placed on it from physical activity or stress. These loads may produce an elevation in blood pressure and can be initiated by such factors as cold, anxiety, and real or imagined threats. Asymptomatic CAD can be difficult to detect and physical activity or elevation of the blood pressure may be required before the disease becomes manifest. Significant disease may be present despite normal physical examination findings.

Table 56.1 Absolute risk of major cardiovascular events

Other risk factors and disease history	Blood pressure (mm Hg)		
	Grade 1 (mild hypertension) SBP 140–159 or DBP 90–99	Grade 2 (moderate hypertension) SBP 160–179 or DBP 100–109	Grade 3 (severe hypertension) SBP ≥180 or DBP ≥110
No other risk factors	Low risk	Medium risk	High risk
1–2 risk factors	Medium risk	Medium risk	Very high risk
3 or more risk factors or target-organ damage or diabetes	High risk	High risk	Very high risk
Associated clinical conditions	Very high risk	Very high risk	Very high risk

DBP, diastolic blood pressure; SBP, systolic blood pressure.

Risk factors include smoking, hypertension, a family history and raised serum cholesterol or triglycerides. These factors should be sought and can be collated into an overall estimate of risk (see Chapter 53). If in doubt, resting and maximal exercise ECGs should be performed and should not show evidence of abnormal arrhythmias or ST-segment depression. SPUMS recommends that an exercise ECG be considered for any diver in whom there is clinical suspicion of CAD, and particularly divers more than 45 years old, on at least a 5-yearly basis[2]. ECG stress testing may also include echocardiography to visualize heart wall motion and contractility.

Risk factors for cardiovascular disease

- Used for risk stratification.
  - Levels of systolic and diastolic blood pressure (grades 1 to 3).
  - Men >55 years.
  - Women >65 years.
  - Smoking.
  - Total cholesterol >6.5 mmol/L (250 mg/dl).
  - Family history of premature cardio-vascular disease.
- Target organ damage.
  - Left ventricular hypertrophy (electrocardiogram, echocardiogram or radiogram).
  - Proteinuria and/or slight elevation of plasma creatinine concentration (1.2 to 2.0 mg/dl).
  - Ultrasound or radiological evidence of atherosclerotic plaque (carotid, iliac and femoral arteries, aorta).
- Heart disease.
  - Myocardial infarction.
  - Angina.
  - Coronary revascularization.
  - Congestive heart failure.
- Renal disease.
  - Diabetic nephropathy.
  - Renal failure (plasma creatinine concentration >2.0 mg/dl).
- Vascular disease.
  - Dissecting aneurysm.
  - Symptomatic arterial disease.
  - Advanced hypertensive retinopathy.
  - Hemorrhages or exudates.
  - Papilloedema.
  - Generalized or focal narrowing of the retinal arteries.
- Other factors adversely affecting prognosis.
  - Reduced high-density lipoprotein cholesterol.

(Continued)

- Raised low-density lipoprotein cholesterol.
- Microalbuminuria in diabetes.
- Impaired glucose tolerance.
- Obesity.
- Sedentary life style.
- Raised fibrinogen.
- High-risk socioeconomic group.

- High-risk ethnic group.
- High-risk geographic region.
- Associated clinical conditions.
  - Cerebrovascular disease.
    - Ischaemic stroke.
    - Cerebral hemorrhage.
- Transient ischaemic attack.

Myocardial ischaemia may have several manifestations. Symptoms of chest pain or discomfort, dyspnoea or syncope on exercise should be actively sought. Angina pectoris associated with exercise may or may not be associated with a history of myocardial infarction, and it is likely to proceed to this condition in the event of severe exercise. A large infarction may result in sudden death.

The resting ECG shows abnormalities only when there is interference with the conduction system, or when significant damage has already been caused to the cardiac tissue. A maximal stress test produces demands comparable to that which is likely to be experienced in the diving environment. During this stress test, there may be several important findings:

1. The blood pressure response may be abnormal.
2. The cardiac rhythm may show exercise-induced abnormalities, with conduction disorders, premature ventricular or atrial beats.
3. The ECG may suggest the presence of myocardial ischaemia, with ST-segment or T-wave changes (Figure 56.1).

Although there are occasional false-positive results with such investigations, it would be unrealistic to subject an individual at high risk to any form of diving without ensuring that there was no demonstrable CAD. Those candidates with a genuinely positive stress test result should be advised against diving.

False-positive results may be seen when there is ventricular hypertrophy associated with extreme athletic activity, in other causes of left ventricular hypertrophy or with the use of digitalis derivatives. Either of the last two situations would result in exclusion from diving. Beta-blocking drugs may render the exercise ECG unreliable. Occasional premature ventricular and atrial beats are found on the ECGs of many asymptomatic individuals with no known heart disease. These findings do not preclude diving. However, if the arrhythmia becomes predominant with exercise, it may have far more significance.

Serum cholesterol and triglyceride levels, serum enzyme levels, glucose estimations and other biochemical tests have been suggested by various authorities for professional diving and may also

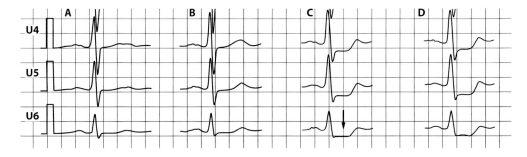

Figure 56.1 Stress electrocardiogram of a patient with coronary heart disease. ST-segment depression (arrow) indicates myocardial ischaemia at 100 watts of exercise: A, at rest; B, at 75 watts; C, at 100 watts; D, at 125 watts.

be useful in assessing the older recreational diver, especially if other coronary risk factors exist.

Some physicians allow experienced divers who have had a myocardial infarction to return to non-strenuous recreational diving after a year or more, if there were no sequelae and a normal exercise stress ECG without evidence of ischaemia or arrhythmia on exercising to at least 13 METS. This is a fairly stiff test. Even so, most physicians believe that this is poor advice because this disease has a high incidence of recurrence and increased propensity to arrhythmias. The role of further investigations (e.g. echocardiography, or even computed tomography coronary angiography) is unclear and a matter of personal interpretation. The reader is reminded that it is virtually impossible to make entry-level diving activity non-stressful or non-strenuous.

An experienced diver who has undergone coronary artery revascularization and has a normal stress test causes problems because he or she has an increased risk of myocardial infarction and arrhythmias. Also, not all obstructions may be overcome, and the re-stenosis rate is high. With internal mammary artery grafting, the pleural cavity is usually invaded, leading to the probability of adhesions and thus also precluding diving.

PERIPHERAL VASCULAR DISEASE

Peripheral vascular disease limits aquatic exercise capability. Cold water may precipitate Raynaud's phenomenon in susceptible individuals. Peripheral vascular disease has a strong association with concomitant CAD, cerebrovascular disease and diabetes. These disorders all require investigation in their own right when assessing a candidate's fitness to dive.

Varicose veins are hydrostatically supported in the water, and the main problems would be trauma causing haemorrhage and infection if skin changes are present. These complications are preventable with protective clothing.

HEART FAILURE

Individuals with significant left ventricular dysfunction are at increased risk of developing pulmonary oedema when diving. This condition may be aggravated by the increased venous return associated with immersion and the cardiovascular stresses associated with physical activity and psychological stress. Heart failure should be considered a contraindication to diving.

VALVULAR DISORDERS

Valvular heart disease is usually a contraindication to diving. In many cases, the abnormal valve produces chronic overload on the work of the heart, and this may be aggravated by the effects of stress with increased cardiac demand. Valvular regurgitation or stenosis influences the capacity of the heart to respond to stress or exercise with increased cardiac output. Turbulence may also increase gas phase separation (generate bubbles).

Some authorities believe that the asymptomatic patient with mild aortic or mitral valve regurgitation, which does not limit exercise tolerance, may be approved for recreational diving. The prospect that turbulence across the valve may increase gas phase separation has not been investigated. Nevertheless, patients with aortic or mitral stenotic lesions should never dive because of the reduced fixed output and the likelihood of central blood shifts precipitating pulmonary oedema. Aortic stenosis is also associated with syncope and death on exertion.

Patients who have prosthetic valves and/or who are taking anticoagulant drugs should also be excluded. Apart from the potential cardiac abnormalities, anticoagulation is generally regarded a contraindication to diving. Anticoagulated patients are at serious risk of bleeding with middle or inner ear barotraumas and into the spinal cord with neurological decompression sickness (DCS). Coral cuts and minor trauma may also place the anticoagulated patient at risk of uncontrollable hemorrhage. Of particular concern is subdural bleeding from minor head trauma while submerged.

Mitral valve prolapse is found in about 7 to 10 per cent of the general population (it is twice as common in girls and women), with clinical evidence (systolic auscultatory click) in only one in seven. Diagnosis is usually made by echocardiography. In some patients, mitral valve prolapse is associated with arrhythmias, chest pain and sudden death. The prolapse itself may be of little consequence, but associated arrhythmias are relevant.

Detection may require Holter monitoring. The totally asymptomatic diver with a normal ECG (normal QT interval), no arrhythmias and no redundant valve leaflets on echocardiography may be permitted to dive.

ARRHYTHMIAS

Arrhythmias, whether from CAD or other disease, are a cause of sudden death. Especially ominous are any dysrhythmias resulting in a reduction of cardiac output (e.g. ventricular tachycardia). These individuals are in danger of sudden death with any severe stress or exercise.

Patients with paroxysmal atrial or supraventricular tachycardia are susceptible to cardiac symptoms that cannot be tolerated in scuba diving (see Chapter 39). Although the diving reflex is one of the treatments for supraventricular tachycardia, it can also precipitate it.

Wolff-Parkinson-White syndrome, characterized by a short PR interval and a 'slurred' upstroke on the QRS complex, is associated with paroxysmal atrial tachycardia and sudden death. These individuals can move rapidly into a shocked state. When left-sided accessory pathways are ablated, an interatrial, transseptal puncture may be used, which may create a right-to-left shunt and predispose the individual to an increased risk of DCS.

Sinus bradycardia at a rate of less than 60 beats/minute must also be investigated. The bradycardia associated with athletes responds to exercise with an appropriate increase in rate, and this differentiates it from the more serious bradycardias caused by ischaemia or conduction defects affecting the sinoatrial node, which respond inadequately or inappropriately to exercise. Common causes of bradycardia in a general population are drugs such as beta-blockers.

Conduction defects need to be assessed. Isolated right bundle branch block in an asymptomatic individual with no other heart disease evident is acceptable, although a few of these patients have an associated atrial septal defect, and this may need to be excluded. Left bundle branch block is also occasionally found in the normal population, but it is more likely to be associated with CAD. If, following adequate cardiac assessment, there is no evidence to believe that the left bundle branch block is other than benign, then the individual may be allowed to dive.

First-degree atrioventricular (AV) block is sometimes a normal finding. If there is no evidence of cardiac disease either in the patient's history or the examination, and if there is a normal ECG response to exercise, the individual should be allowed to undertake diving.

Second-degree AV block is much less likely to be benign and usually excludes diving activities. It is sometimes a normal finding in athletic young adults with a high vagal tone; during sleep or at rest, and it is vagally induced. The second-degree block of Mobitz type 2 is especially ominous and often precedes the onset of complete heart block. If the conduction abnormality disappears with a mild degree of exercise, the heart rate response is appropriate and there is no underlying disease or drug causing the rhythm disturbance, then the individual can be approved for diving. Complete AV block is a contraindication because of the inability of the heart to respond appropriately to exercise stress.

PACEMAKERS

The presence of a pacemaker usually implies the presence of an underlying cardiac disease, which in itself disqualifies the patient from diving. Pacemakers vary in their ability to withstand pressure, and in rate-responsive pacemakers, the rate response is often lost at depth, only to return on surfacing as long as the pacemaker has not been taken so deep as to cause permanent damage[4]. There are considerable differences in the depths to which pacemakers have been tested: Vitatron Collection II and Vita pacemakers are tested to a pressure equal to 11 msw, Medtronic recommends that Thera, Prodigy, and Elite II pacemakers should not be exposed to pressures greater than that of 30 msw and the Intermedics Dash 292-03 has been tested to 60 msw[4]. It is best to consult the manufacturer when considering the fitness to dive of a patient with an implantable pacemaker.

There have even been anecdotal reports of individuals diving with implantable defibrillators. Few physicians would find this acceptable.

INTRACARDIAC SHUNTS

Congenital heart disease should be carefully assessed. Atrial or ventricular septal defects, even though diagnosed as having left-to-right shunts, are often bi-directional in diastole or under positive intrathoracic pressure (e.g. during a modified Valsalva maneouvre). This could allow bubbles returning to the right side of the heart from the periphery to pass into the left side of the heart and thus the systemic circulation, bypassing the normal pulmonary filter.

In approximately 33 per cent of the population, the foramen ovale does not seal at birth, and blood from the right atrium may pass directly to the left atrium through the patent foramen and into the systemic circulation. In 1989, Wilmshurst and associates[5] and Moon and colleagues[6] suggested that the presence of a patent foramen ovale (PFO) is a risk factor for the development of DCS, and in particular serious neurological DCS occurring early (within 30 minutes of exiting the water) and with symptoms and signs out of proportion to the dive stress. The size of the PFO also appears to be important, with larger defects being more positively associated with serious DCS. In a blinded case-control study, Wilmshurst and Bryson[7] in 2000 found a medium to large PFO in 52 per cent of 100 consecutive divers with a history of neurological DCS versus 12.5 per cent of 123 control divers (P < 0.001). When detected, small PFOs cause considerable anxiety among divers, but they may not substantially increase the risk of DCS. For example, Cross and associates[8] in 1992 reported 26 divers (10 professional divers logging 650 dives over 13 years, 16 recreational divers logging 236 dives in an average of 7.5 years) with an easily demonstrable foramen ovale who never experienced DCS.

The evidence should be interpreted in the overall context of the risk of DCS. The incidence of DCS in divers is about 2.28 per 10 000 dives. Given that most of these DCS episodes are not serious neurological cases, and that about one third of divers have a PFO, the risk of developing DCS in the presence of a PFO remains small. At this time, there is no justification for the routine screening of entry-level dive candidates for PFO.

Balestra and associates[9] cautioned divers to refrain from strenuous arm, leg or abdominal exercise (e.g. dive cylinder handling or boarding the boat fully geared up) after diving because these activities have been demonstrated to cause sufficient changes in intrathoracic pressure to promote the shunting of blood through a PFO.

Transcutaneous closure of a PFO is now a routine procedure using one of a number of devices (Figure 56.2). This option is increasingly being offered to divers with a history of 'undeserved' or skin DCS in whom a PFO has been identified on subsequent investigation by bubble contrast echocardiography. This test involves the injection of bubbles into the venous circulation and should not be performed acutely after diving when a nitrogen load remains.

The place of PFO closure was reviewed by Calvert and colleagues in 2011[10]. Closure is associated with a number of adverse events, including thrombus formation, cardiac tamponade, stroke and failure to close the defect. Following closure, the diver requires a period of anticoagulant therapy during which diving should be forbidden.

Consensus remains elusive, and divers are increasingly seeking both PFO testing and closure

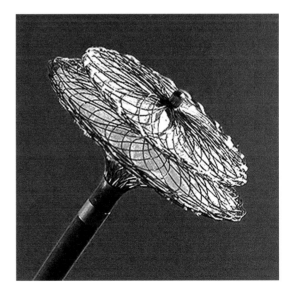

Figure 56.2 An Amplatzer device used for percutaneous closure of a patent for amen ovale (PFO). The device is deployed (as shown), after being partially introduced through the PFO.

under circumstances that may not be in their best medical interest.

REFERENCES

1. Denoble PJ, Caruso JL, Dear G de L, Pieper CF, Vann RD. Common causes of open-circuit recreational diving fatalities. *Undersea and Hyperbaric Medicine* 2008;**35**:393–406.
2. South Pacific Underwater Medicine Society. *Guidelines on Medical Risk Assessment for Recreation Diving.* 2010. http://www.spums.org.au/story/spums-medical
3. United Kingdom Sports Diving Medical Committee (UKSDMC). *Hypertension and Diving.* 2014. http://uksdmc.co.uk/
4. Wilmshurst PT. Cardiovascular problems in divers. *Heart* 1998;**80**(6):537–538.
5. Wilmshurst PT, Byrne JC, Webb-Peploe MM. Relation between interatrial shunts and decompression sickness in divers. *The Lancet* 1989;**2**:1302–1306.
6. Moon RE, Camporesi EM, Kisslo JA. Patent foramen ovale and decompression sickness in divers. *The Lancet* 1989;**1**:513–514.
7. Wilmshurst P, Bryson P. Relationship between the clinical features of neurological decompression illness and its causes. *Clinical Science (London)* 2000;**99**:65–75.
8. Cross SJ, Evans SA, Thomsen LF. Safety of subaqua diving with a patent foramen ovale. *British Medical Journal* 1992;**304**(6825):481–482.
9. Balestra C, Germonpre P, Marroni A. Intrathoracic pressure changes after Valsalva strain and other maneuvers: implications for divers with a patent foramen ovale. *Undersea and Hyperbaric Medicine* 1998;**25**(3):171–174.
10. Calvert PA, Rana BS, Kydd AC, Shapiro LM. Patent foramen ovale: anatomy, outcomes, and closure. *Nature Reviews Cardiology* 2011;**8**(3):148–60.

This chapter was reviewed for this fifth edition by Michael Bennett.

57

Insulin-dependent diabetes mellitus

INTRODUCTION

Since 2000, opinion within the diving medical community has swung decisively toward a consensus that under carefully selected, controlled and monitored conditions, persons with insulin-dependent diabetes mellitus (IDDM) may safely undertake scuba diving[1–3].

In Australia and New Zealand, the South Pacific Underwater Medicine Society (SPUMS) published a revision of their *Guidelines on Medical Risk Assessment for Recreational Diving* in 2010[2] with an appendix outlining a detailed position on diving with IDDM (attached at the end of this chapter, with permission from SPUMS, as Appendix A). This position was developed following the 2005 workshop on diving with diabetes in Las Vegas Nevada, hosted jointly by the Divers Alert Network (DAN) and the Undersea and Hyperbaric Medical Society (UHMS)[1]. The result of that workshop was a radical change in the official positions of most of the major diving medical organizations.

This chapter summarizes the arguments for and against diving with IDDM and outlines the findings of the 2005 workshop. In addition, an appendix (Appendix B) offers advice to the diabetic diver.

HISTORY

The 'traditional' view of all major diving medical organizations has been to deny persons with IDDM from access to dive training on the basis of several legitimate concerns. These concerns are outlined in Table 1 in Appendix A. In general, it was believed that the combined threat of both hypoglycaemia and hyperglycaemia, the pathophysiology of end-organ damage and the potential confusion of the signs and symptoms associated with diabetes mellitus (DM) with those of decompression illness (DCI) absolutely contraindicated diving for these individuals. Unsurprisingly, epidemiological data of diving morbidity and mortality were unhelpful in supporting or refuting this position, given that divers with IDDM were very uncommon – and if there were such divers they were likely to be operating covertly.

In fact, before 1975, the situation in the United Kingdom (the monarchist oppressors of the would-be Republic of Australia) was somewhat different. Until that year, certain diabetic persons, whether dependent on insulin or not, were allowed to dive, provided their diving physicians passed them as medically fit. Unfortunately, in that year a diabetic diver on a wreck in British waters completed a dive to 30 metres, ascended normally within the no-stop times according to the British Sub-Aqua Club (BSAC)/Royal Navy Physiological Laboratory (RNPL) 1972 tables and signalled 'OK' to the boat, but was then observed to have difficulty in swimming to the boat. He had to be dragged on board, where he collapsed. His problems were put down entirely to his having DM, *and a diagnosis of DCI was not considered.* Consequently, he was not recompressed for many hours, by which time he had become permanently paralyzed from the waist down. Later, he committed suicide as a result of his depression at being confined to a wheelchair.

The medical committee of the BSAC of the time then banned all persons with newly diagnosed DM from diving with the BSAC, a ban that was later extended to most of the existing diabetic divers already diving with the club. The United Kingdom had fallen into line with the general consensus. Following the growing understanding of the role of a patent foramen ovale (PFO) in divers, however, the case was re-examined. The diabetic diver's symptoms, which had appeared within minutes of surfacing from the dive, suggested strongly that a PFO could be found in the diver. As fortune would have it, the diver's heart had been well preserved. A large PFO was indeed found, and expert opinion was given that *cerebral arterial gas embolism from bubbles passing through the PFO* was a much more likely cause of the problems suffered by the diver.

A conference held in Edinburgh in 1994 discussed the medical assessment of fitness to dive. It was clear that the majority of diving physicians present believed that diabetic persons should not be allowed to dive[4,5]. No data were presented at the conference to support this view. At this meeting, notice was given of a prospective data collection on diabetic divers by Edge and colleagues[6]. A similar plan was outlined at the UHMS conference that year.

Meanwhile, largely outside the mainstream diving medical community and operating on a small scale, several organizations and individuals continued to train people with IDDM to dive[7,8]. In the United Kingdom, Edge and associates continued to collect data on active diabetic divers. Given these initiatives, and with a growing body of opinion and experience that individuals with IDDM could dive safely, the stage was set for the 2005 workshop.

PATHOPHYSIOLOGY

In DM, the fundamental defect is in insulin secretion and/or action. In the classical young-onset form of the disease (type 1), there is near total insulin deficiency, with inevitable widespread metabolic changes. Almost invariably, this means the diabetic person must inject insulin at regular intervals to counteract the deficit – thus giving rise to the term IDDM.

In the type 2 form of DM, there is resistance to secreted insulin. This condition leads to hyperglycaemia and hyperinsulinaemia and is closely associated with obesity, hypertension and dyslipidaemia. When this form of DM is treated by controlling the diet alone or by means of diet control and oral medication a diabetic person is said to have non–insulin-dependent disease (NIDDM). Diving with NIDDM is outside the scope of this chapter.

The chronic complications of DM are all considered to be caused by the development of

DM-specific microvascular problems. These problems do not occur without long-standing hyperglycaemia. Subjects with IDDM (or NIDDM) are susceptible to microvascular complications, although patients with NIDDM are usually older at presentation and may die of macrovascular disease before microvascular disease is advanced. However, it is worth noting that more than 40 per cent of subjects with IDDM survive for more than 40 years, and half of these persons never develop significant microvascular complications.

There are two chronic complications of DM that are of particular concern to scuba divers. These are diabetic neuropathy (particularly autonomic neuropathy) and cardiovascular disease. Both are discussed here.

DM commonly affects the autonomic nervous system, and up to 50 per cent of diabetic patients demonstrate some *diabetic neuropathy*[9]. Autonomic symptoms are uncommon in young diabetic patients, but more abnormalities are found in older patients and in those with DM for more than 20 years. The prevalence of autonomic abnormalities (defined as abnormal tests of autonomic function, usually based on cardiovascular tests, in the absence of clinical symptoms) is similar in IDDM and NIDDM, a finding suggesting that the metabolic consequences of hyperglycaemia, rather than the type of DM, lead to autonomic nerve damage.

Cardiovascular disease in patients with DM causes an increase in mortality as compared with the non-diabetic population, and there is a large excess of cardiovascular deaths in patients with proteinuria. This increased risk of death is shared by those with impaired glucose tolerance. Symptoms of angina pectoris may be masked in diabetic patients by autonomic neuropathy, and breathlessness may be the only sign of silent, reversible ischaemia.

PHARMACOLOGY

The only effective therapy for IDDM is, unsurprisingly, insulin administration. Ideally, administration should mimic endogenous insulin production with low resting secretion and an appropriate response to the ingestion of carbohydrates to maintain tight homeostasis, to promote the ingress of glucose into the cells where it is available for metabolic activity and to boost the production of glycogen as an energy store. In practice, this goal is difficult to achieve.

The first preparations of insulin were impure and short acting. Later preparations were purified to improve efficacy and tolerance. Their form was altered to lengthen duration of action, analogues were synthesized and insulins with the human amino acid sequence were manufactured. Today, most insulin used is pure 'human' insulin, manufactured using recombinant DNA technology, although highly purified pork and beef preparations are still available. Several preparations have been developed, including short-acting, intermediate-acting, and long-acting forms. Short-acting (soluble) insulins are absorbed after subcutaneous injection at a rate that is a function of the time for dissociation of the hexameric pharmaceutical insulin to single (monomeric) units. This is necessary before absorption into the circulation can occur. The longer-acting preparations are intended to supply basal insulin to control blood glucose concentration between meals, but absorption still varies greatly and there is no homeostatic mechanism, so glucose concentrations fluctuate widely in many patients.

It is increasingly common to improve control of DM with the use of continuous subcutaneous insulin administration via a pump, adding 'top-up' doses of short-acting insulin to deal with rising blood glucose after eating. This is, however an expensive option not available to all patients. An emerging alternative is islet cell transplantation, although this option is not without problems and is usually reserved for more 'brittle' diabetes[10].

There are theoretical concerns about the absorption and utilization of insulin and, to a lesser extent, the oral hypoglycaemic and biguanide agents when the patient is either under pressure or exposed to a higher partial pressure of oxygen. One particular concern expressed is the effect of pressure on a depot injection of long-acting insulin. The studies of diabetic subjects in the hyperbaric chamber and in open water would indicate that from a practical viewpoint this does not appear to be a problem.

POTENTIAL RISKS FOR DIVING WITH INSULIN-DEPENDENT DIABETES MELLITUS

The major potential problems that may arise for divers specifically as a consequence of diabetes are summarized in Table 1 in Appendix A, taken from the SPUMS guidelines[2] and based on the discussions at the 2005 workshop[1].

Hypoglycaemia

Periods of significant hypoglycaemia are common, and perhaps inevitable, in individuals with tight diabetic control. Low blood glucose is characterized by symptoms related both to the lack of sugar directly and the adrenergic response this elicits. The most common signs are generalized weakness, light-headedness, trembling, sweating, hunger, disorientation and irritability. In some people, there are minimal or absent prodromal signs, and unconsciousness may occur without warning (hypoglycaemic unawareness).

Hypoglycaemia may be precipitated by stress, cold and exercise during diving, with potentially catastrophic consequences if impaired mentation or unconsciousness ensues before the blood glucose level can be corrected. Early signs of hypoglycaemia may go unnoticed while a diver is submerged and may later be confused with the symptoms of DCI, hypothermia or seasickness.

Hyperglycaemia

Poor blood glucose control is associated with periods of significantly high blood glucose, and this condition may be associated with acute dehydration. Coupled with the tendency for dehydration during and after diving as a consequence of the central blood shift, divers with DM may be significantly dehydrated and consequently at high risk of DCI.

The diver with poorly controlled IDDM, when not diving, may be relatively hypoinsulinaemic, and exercise may aggravate hyperglycaemia and ketonaemia. The effect of exercise on persons with IDDM and NIDDM has been extensively researched[11].

Coronary artery disease

Vasculopathy is common as an expression of end-organ damage in patients with diabetes. Coronary artery disease impairs exercise tolerance and increases the likelihood of myocardial ischaemia or infarction. As discussed in Chapters 39 and 56, these cardiovascular disorders are increasingly common causes of sudden death in divers.

Hypoglycaemic unawareness

Repeated episodes of hypoglycaemia may result in a resetting of the homeostatic mechanism. The adrenergic response to low glucose may be reduced or absent, so that the individual is not 'warned' of impending neuro-glycopaenia (low glucose levels in the brain). These individuals may suffer profound and dangerous hypoglycaemia without warning.

The diver with well-controlled IDDM, when not diving, is almost invariably hyperinsulinaemic. Thus, during exercise, the increased peripheral glucose uptake is not compensated for in the normal way by an increase in the hepatic release of glucose, so that hypoglycaemia is more likely.

Peripheral neuropathy

Another expression of end-organ damage is peripheral neuropathy including the autonomic nervous system. Although sensory neuropathy may be confused with DCI, the inability to mount an adrenergic response to falling blood glucose levels is a further reason for hypoglycaemic unawareness, and it is of more grave significance.

Peripheral vascular disease

Poor arterial supply to the periphery, particularly the lower limbs, may result in reduced exercise capacity and the tendency to develop wounds that do not heal and that may then become sites of infection – including osteomyelitis.

Renal impairment

The kidney is another end organ to suffer the effects of this disease. DM is associated with significant renal impairment and the loss of the ability to maintain the internal milieu. Proteinuria is common. Patients so affected may present with either polyuria or oliguria, metabolic acidosis and other electrolyte disturbances.

Visual impairment

Diabetic retinopathy may significantly impair vision such that the affected individual cannot read his or her own gauges or dive computer and may perhaps be unable to locate a dive vessel on surfacing.

STUDIES IN DIABETES MELLITUS AND SCUBA DIVING

The studies reported by Prosterman, Vote, Edge, Dear and others all lend support to the idea that people with DM may be able to dive safely, provided certain conditions are met[7,12–15]. However, all studies can be criticized from the point of view that the diabetic divers were closely monitored throughout. The divers all entered the water with a blood glucose level as low as 4.4 mmol/litre but that was stable or rising before the dive.

These studies are not able to answer the question as to whether a diabetic diver, diving in open water away from medical facilities, can dive safely, but they do permit a detailed examination of the blood glucose and other hormonal profiles of divers during a typical diving period.

The answer to that question was addressed directly in the long-term study carried out in the United Kingdom by the Diving Diseases Research Centre (DDRC)[3]. Analysis suggested that such diving may be safe. Over a series of 8760 dives undertaken by 323 divers, only 3 incidents were reported during diving – 1 an episode of hypoglycaemia underwater that was managed successfully. Two deaths were reported, both in individuals with NIDDM, 1 in a diver who had a myocardial event while submerged.

PRACTICAL ASPECTS OF TRAINING CANDIDATES WITH INSULIN-DEPENDENT DIABETES MELLITUS TO DIVE

It is generally agreed that persons with DM who are prone to acute complications (e.g. hypoglycaemia) or who have chronic complications that could significantly affect diving safety should be advised against diving. Similarly, the progressive nature of many complications of diabetes suggests that there should be longitudinal health surveillance and periodic reassessment of suitability over the period of a diabetic person's participation in diving. The following discussion is made in general reference to Appendix A – the SPUMS guidelines on diving with diabetes. Readers should refer to that document online for the most up-to-date modifications and if their immediate interest is in NIDDM.

Which diabetic candidates can be safely trained to dive?

The approaches adopted by several groups have a great deal in common and were summarized very well in the report of the UHMS/DAN workshop[1]. The most important common features are as follows: close attention to the quality of diabetic control, both historically and during diving activity; a proscription against diving in the presence of clinically significant secondary complications; and a requirement for medical assessment that is more comprehensive than that required of non-diabetic diving candidates.

Admission criteria for recreational dive training for a diabetic candidate

1. The candidate must be 16 years or older. (Some would argue that these 'special' dive candidates should be legally adults to accept the risks and constraints involved.)
2. At least 1 year has passed since the initiation of treatment with insulin. (the reason is to establish good control of DM with a change in regimen.)

3. No hypoglycaemic episodes requiring intervention from a third party have occurred for at least 1 year, and there has been no history of "hypoglycaemia unawareness"(see the earlier discussion of potential complications).

4. Glycosylated haemoglobin (HbA1c) is less than or equal to 9 per cent when measured no more than 1 month before initial assessment and at each annual review. (This upper limit is higher than normally recommended for good DM control and carries the potential risk of increased end-organ damage. These are guidelines for diving, not best practice management.)

5. No admissions or emergency visits to hospital occurred for any complications of DM for at least 1 year.

6. The candidate has no known retinopathy (worse than 'background' level), significant nephropathy, neuropathy (autonomic or peripheral), coronary artery disease or peripheral vascular disease.

7. Before the first diving medical assessment and each annual evaluation, a review must be conducted by the candidate's personal diabetologist who must confirm that:
   - Criteria 3 to 6 are fulfilled.
   - The candidate demonstrates accurate use of a personal blood glucose monitoring device.
   - The candidate has a good understanding of the relationship among diet, exercise, stress, temperature and blood glucose levels.

8. Before commencing diving for the first time and at each annual review, a diving medical examination must be completed by a doctor who has successfully completed a postgraduate diving medical examiners course. (The diabetologist's review report must be available. This examination includes appropriate assessment of exercise tolerance, and for candidates over 40 years should include an exercise electrocardiogram.)

9. As part of the assessment by the diving medical examiner, the candidate must acknowledge (in writing) his or her understanding of, and intention to dive in accordance with, the recommended guidelines.

10. Steps 2 to 9 of this protocol must be fulfilled on an annual basis. (Where possible, the same diabetologist and diving medical officer should be used for these annual reviews.)

Scope of diving

Most diving physicians accept that some forms of diving are likely to be unsuitable for divers with IDDM. SPUMS has recommended the following as appropriate definitions for the scope of diving:

1. Diabetic divers are suitable for recreational diving only. This does not include occupational activities such as diving instruction and dive guiding ('dive-mastering').

2. Diabetic divers should not undertake dives deeper than 30 metres of sea water; dives longer than 1 hour, dives that mandate compulsory decompression stops or dives in overhead environments. These practices all hamper prompt access to surface support.

3. Diabetic divers do not undertake more than two dives per day and use a minimum surface interval of 2 hours. Diving can be a physically demanding activity and fatigue is common following a 'normal diving day', even for non-diabetic divers.

4. Diabetic divers must dive with a buddy who is informed of their condition and aware of the appropriate response in the event of a hypoglycaemic episode.

5. Diabetic divers should avoid combinations of circumstances that may be provocative for hypoglycaemic episodes such as prolonged, cold dives involving hard work.

Managing blood glucose on the day of diving

The following recommendations are based on the published experience of several established diabetic diving programmes[1].

1. On every day on which diving is contemplated, the individual must assess himself or herself in a general sense. If he or she is uncomfortable, unduly anxious or unwell in any way

(including seasickness), or if blood glucose control is not in its normal stable pattern – **diving must not be undertaken**.

2. The diabetic diver should establish a blood glucose level of at least 9 mmol/litre and ensure that this level is either stable or rising before entering the water. Measurements should be taken three times before diving at 60 minutes, 30 minutes and immediately before gearing up. Diving should be postponed if blood glucose level is less than 9 mmol/litre or if there is a fall between any two measurements.

3. Individually tailored reductions in doses of insulin on the evening before or on the day of diving may assist in complying with these parameters. Initial testing of individual protocols should be conducted under very controlled circumstances. Where relevant, a regimen of incremental glucose intake to correct inappropriate pre-dive levels or trends may assist in complying with these parameters.

4. Attempts to comply with the requirements at point 2 in this list should not result in a blood glucose level greater than 14 mmol/litre, and diving should be cancelled for the day if levels are higher than 16 mmol/litre at any stage. Prescription of a strict upper limit is somewhat arbitrary, but 16 mmol/litre approaches the renal threshold for glucose, and there is some evidence that persons with DM who are involved in diving do dehydrate more readily than do persons without DM.

5. Diabetic divers must carry oral glucose in a readily accessible and ingestible form at the surface and during all dives. We strongly recommended that parenteral glucagon is available at the surface. If premonitory symptoms of hypoglycaemia are noticed underwater, the diver must surface, establish positive buoyancy, ingest glucose and leave the water. An informed buddy should be in a position to assist with or initiate this process.

6. Blood glucose levels must be checked at the end of every dive. The requirements for blood glucose status outlined at point 2 remain the same for any subsequent dive. Because of the recognized potential for late decrements in blood glucose levels following diving, blood glucose levels should be checked 12 to 15 hours after diving.

7. Diabetic divers are strongly recommended to drink between 1000 and 1500 ml of extra water over a period of several hours before their first dive of the day.

8. Diabetic divers must log all dives, associated diabetic interventions and results of all blood glucose level tests conducted in association with diving.

CAN DIABETIC DIVERS BECOME SCUBA INSTRUCTORS?

As divers who were diabetic when they started their recreational scuba diving training progress through the personal training levels, it is inevitable that a few will wish to develop their instructional skills. Currently, the position of all diver training agencies throughout the world is that no diabetic diver can become an instructor. However, there are undoubtedly diabetic divers who have trained as instructors before they became diabetic. Should these divers retain their instructor status, or should they continue to dive but be prevented from teaching?

The diving instructor has a general duty of care to the person or persons he or she is instructing. All recreational diving agencies take this duty of care seriously, with compulsory courses and examinations for the various levels of instructor grading that they offer. For the diabetic diving instructor, there is an added level to this duty of care, which is that he or she must not become hypoglycaemic at any stage during a dive, thereby necessitating rescue either by the diver under instruction or by another diver or member of the surface cover. For a novice diver under instruction, the responsibility for rescuing the instructor may be too great, depending on the skill of the novice and the level at which he or she has competence to deal with the situation. The chance of a hypoglycaemic attack occurring in the instructor will be greater if the instructor is a relatively inexperienced diver and as the duration of the dive becomes longer.

At present, the SPUMS guidelines prohibit persons with diabetes from being declared medically fit for the purpose of instruction. BSAC, the Sub-Aqua Association (SAA) and the Scottish Sub-Aqua Club (SSAC) are considering recommendations proposed by the United Kingdom Sport Diving Medical Committee (UKSDMC) that recreational scuba diving instructors who are diabetic should have to provide evidence that they have been able to avoid disabling episodes of hypoglycaemia, both on shore and in the water, for a continuous period of not less than 2 years. This is a compromise between two views:

1. If a diabetic diver has proved that he or she can dive safely throughout the training, then this person should be allowed to instruct, provided he or she is able to attain the necessary skill level.
2. No diabetic diver should ever be allowed to instruct because of the increased risk in the water as a result of being diabetic.

It is unwise to draw any firm conclusions concerning the fitness of diabetic divers to become instructors from the small numbers of diabetic diving instructors in the industry. The industry is likely to proceed cautiously.

NOTES OF CAUTION

Any handicapped individual can be subjected to diving with a relatively low risk, if the diving conditions can be meticulously controlled, supervised with adequate safety precautions and include specialized procedures for rescue and first aid.

A similar situation exists for the underaged diver, whereby a diving 'experience' is able to be enjoyed, while the child is otherwise medically fit, under the full control of a diving instructor – extending from dive planning to an environmental assessment and then total dive supervision.

Live-aboard diving boats are a different environment with the effects of seasickness, high temperatures (in the tropics), variable catering, unhygienic conditions and a physically demanding and unpredictable diving environment. One would expect that these factors must increase chance of both hypoglycaemia and hyperglycaemic (ketoacidotic) events.

Diving in the United States, Australia and much of the world is much less regimented than the well-disciplined BSAC (club diving) of the United Kingdom or of the Caribbean Camp DAVI

(Diabetes Association of the Virgin Islands)[7] with its specialized diabetic instructor, physician and nurse.

The physical stresses of diving and its risks cannot be equated with those of other sports. Unlike the athlete on the track or the tennis court, the ocean does not always permit the diver to take 'time off'. It has been suggested that any certification should be based on a handicapped scuba model, not an open water certification[17].

When the YMCA introduced a protocol for training divers with IDDM in 1995, Hill pointed out some inherent difficulties in the protocol[17]:

- The mandate that the diabetic diver must have an 'informed dive buddy' was unrealistic among the diving population, who knew little about DM, glucose testing, differential diagnosis or treatment of IDDM.
- The recommended time and frequency limitations, being between 20 and 30 minutes, may cause problems with group diving, particularly drift diving, and this, together with the restriction of two dives per day, would likely not be observed.
- There seemed to be no restriction regarding other certifications being given (e.g. junior or advanced qualifications). Juvenile diabetic divers were less compliant with DM management and less likely to be stable. Increased risks were likely in deep, wreck, ice or cave diving – and leadership certifications would be of concern.
- Modifying or omitting prescribed medications, to undertaking diving activities, was to be devised with the assistance of the diabetic diver's physician. This physician would usually have little or no experience in diving physiology or medicine.
- No prevention is 100 per cent successful, and the treatment of these diabetic complications during the dive would require extreme knowledge and skill.
- There is a difficulty in diagnosis if the diver becomes symptomatic or unconscious.
- The significant problem of hyperglycaemia in patients who have reduced their insulin dosage to prepare for a presumed or possible excess effort is more than a theoretical concern.

Perhaps what these comments highlight is that diabetic divers comprise a very specialized group. They require specialized and individual training by very knowledgeable dive instructors, working with conscientious and disciplined clients. Once training has been completed, these divers need to continue to dive with knowledgeable and probably trained buddies. It does not imply that these divers equate with the normal certified diver in terms of risk exposure or routine precautions.

From the report of Edge and colleagues in 2005[3], one could get the impression that hypoglycaemic episodes have not been reported in association with diving, except for a single case. Of the 241 divers with IDDM in the UK survey, there were 45 reports of hypoglycaemia during the survey period; 41 of these were 'not dive related' (at least 24 hours after diving). On investigation, 3 of the remaining 4 cases were incorrectly coded initially and were not in fact episodes of low blood glucose. This survey presumably includes *all* episodes of hypoglycaemia and compares very favourably with the rates of *severe* hypoglycaemic episodes per 100 years among patients with IDDM (requiring assistance and treatment) as recorded in an extensive, multi-centre survey of 1441 patients with IDDM in 1993[18]. One would have to presume either that the subjects in the UK divers' trial had extraordinarily well-controlled DM or that the reporting was unreliable and perhaps subject to reporting and recall bias.

Also, in an early report of the Virgin Islands experience[19], rarely referred to now, 4 per cent of 50 divers experienced hypoglycaemic episodes underwater (2 episodes per 50 diver vacation weeks).

In the previously described UK experiments, ostensibly demonstrating the effect of exercise, the authors described the exercise load as 'equivalent to an arduous swim'. Perusal of the original report[13] does not support this. In fact, 6 minutes of 'work' spread over a 16-minute period could possibly be considered demanding by some indolent divers, but it would certainly not be equivalent to a near maximum oxygen uptake exertion induced by a long swim, against a current greater than 1 knot or while rescuing a companion diver. No reports to date have subjected diabetic divers to an arduous exercise task.

In a survey published in an un-refereed journal from DAN[20], 55 per cent of diabetic divers claimed to have experienced hypoglycaemic episodes while exercising and 15 per cent while diving. Low blood glucose after diving was reported in 20 per cent. The investigators concluded 'hypoglycaemic episodes [in IDDM] are common...with diving'.

Although the specific range of blood glucose levels is not always available in the foregoing reports, those ranges that were given seemed to vary from potentially hypoglycaemic to clinically hyperglycaemic (ketoacidotic) levels. The results available do not reassure doubting physicians that DM-related accidents are unlikely.

CONCLUSION

The main reason advanced by diving physicians for not allowing persons with IDDM that is controlled with medication to dive is that there is a risk (the level of which is undefined) that the diver may become hypoglycaemic while diving and drown. Sufficient evidence has been gathered from the studies under medically supervised conditions and the study of diabetic divers in a normal diving environment that, in well-controlled and well-educated diabetic subjects who follow the guidelines, this risk is minimal. The risks of experiencing mild hypoglycaemic attacks underwater are small, but they are not negligible. However, the problems arising as a result of a hypoglycaemic attack while diving are decreased when the diabetic diver carries glucose paste in a form that can be ingested underwater. Furthermore, the risk of hypoglycaemic attacks while diving can be further decreased by ensuring that the blood glucose is measured immediately before going diving and again immediately after returning to the boat or shore (whichever is first). The advent of personal, portable, calibratable glucometers has made these measurements much less of a problem than they were a few years ago.

A greater problem would appear to be the risk of sudden death underwater as a result of an increased tendency for the development of coronary atheromata in the diabetic diver. This risk is higher in those diabetic divers who have NIDDM, whether they are taking medication or controlling the disease with diet only. However, there are insufficient data to be able to say whether the risk of sudden death underwater is increased over that present in the non-diabetic population, and it must be remembered that 'absence of evidence is not evidence of absence'.

The studies have not shown whether the diabetic diver is increasing his or her risk of developing long-term complications of DM as a result of diving or whether the severity of any complications that do develop is worse as a result of diving.

In light of the evidence presented in this chapter, it is believed that a ban on all diabetic divers is unsupportable. If a diabetic person conforms to the guidelines presented, there appear to be no significantly increased risks to that person's health and well-being over that of a non-diabetic diver. However, diabetic divers must continue to dive with a degree of caution that is over and above that required by their non-diabetic counterparts. It is known that various diabetic divers will not wish to follow the guidelines, and that is of course their right, but they are not allowed to dive within the club system in the United Kingdom, and their activity is not condoned by SPUMS. Whether a diabetic diver can go on to become an instructor is more debatable, but at present there is no evidence that a well-motivated individual with well-controlled DM could not do so.

REFERENCES

1. Pollock NW, Uguccioni DM, Dear G de L, eds. *Diabetes and Recreational Diving: Guidelines for the Future. Proceedings of the Undersea and Hyperbaric Medical Society/Divers Alert Network 2005 June 19 Workshop.* Durham, North Carolina: Divers Alert Network; 2005.
2. South Pacific Underwater Medicine Society. *Guidelines on Medical Risk Assessment for Recreational Diving.* 2010. http://www.spums.org.au/story/spums-medical
3. Edge CJ, St. Leger Dowse M, Bryson P. Scuba diving with diabetes mellitus: the UK experience 1991–2001. *Undersea and Hyperbaric Medicine* 2005;**32**(1):27–37.
4. Cali-Corleo R. Special medical problems in recreational divers: diabetes. In: Elliott DH, ed. *Medical Assessment of Fitness to Dive.* Ewell, United Kingdom: Biomedical Seminars; 1994:44.
5. Seyer J. Recreational diving legislation and medical standards in France. In: Elliott DH, ed. *Medical Assessment of Fitness to Dive.* Ewell, United Kingdom: Biomedical Seminars; 1994:62–65.
6. Edge CJ, Douglas J, Bryson PJ. Diabetic diver assessment. In: Elliott DH, ed. *Medical Assessment of Fitness to Dive.* Ewell, United Kingdom: Biomedical Seminar; 1994:59–61.
7. Prosterman SA. Insights of a diving instructor teaching and managing diabetes. In: Pollock NW, Uguccioni DM, Dear G de L, eds. *Diabetes and Recreational Diving: Guidelines for the Future. Proceedings of the Undersea and Hyperbaric Medical Society/Divers Alert Network 2005 June 19 Workshop.* Durham, North Carolina: Divers Alert Network; 2005.
8. Scott DH. A diving with diabetes program: the YMCA experience. In: Pollock NW, Uguccioni DM, Dear G de L, eds. *Diabetes and Recreational Diving: Guidelines for the Future. Proceedings of the Undersea and Hyperbaric Medical Society/Divers Alert Network 2005 June 19 Workshop.* Durham, North Carolina: Divers Alert Network; 2005.
9. Nicolucci A, Carinci T, Cavaliere D, et al. A meta-analysis of trials on aldose reductase inhibitors in diabetic peripheral neuropathy. *Diabetic Medicine* 1996;**13**:1017–1026.
10. Srinivasan P, Huang GC, Amiel SA, Heaton ND. Islet cell transplantation. *Postgraduate Medical Journal* 2007;**83**(978):224–229.
11. Choi K-L, Chisholm DJ. Exercise and insulin-dependent diabetes mellitus (IDDM): benefits and pitfalls. *Australian and New Zealand Journal of Medicine* 1996;**26**:827–833.
12. Vote DA, Doar PO, Stolp BW, Dear G de L, Moon RE. Measurement of plasma glucose under hyperbaric oxygen conditions. *Undersea and Hyperbaric Medicine* 1999;**26**(Suppl):53.
13. Edge CJ, Grieve AP, Gibbons N, O'Sullivan F, Bryson P. Control of blood glucose in a group of diabetic scuba divers. *Undersea and Hyperbaric Medicine* 1997;**24**:201–207.
14. Lerch M, Lutrop C, Thurm U. Diabetes and diving: can the risk of hypoglycemia be banned? *South Pacific Underwater Medicine Society Journal* 1996;**26**:62–66.

15. Dear G de L, Pollock NW, Uguccioni DM, et al. Plasma glucose responses in recreational divers with insulin-requiring diabetes. Undersea and Hyperbaric Medicine 2004;31(3):291–301.

16. Bryson P, Edge C, Gunby A, St. Leger Dowse M. Scuba diving and diabetes; collecting definitive data from a covert population of recreational divers: interim observations from a long-term on-going prospective study. Undersea and Hyperbaric Medicine 1988;25(Suppl):51–52.

17. Hill RK, Jr. Sugar wars. Sources Magazine 1995;September/October:60–61.

18. The effect of intensive treatment of diabetes on the development and progression of long-term complications in insulin-dependent diabetes mellitus. The Diabetes Control and Complications Trial Research Group. New England Journal of Medicine 1993;329:977–986.

19. Dear G de L, Uguccioni DM. Diabetes and diving. Alert Diver 1997;Jan–Feb:34–37.

20. Dovenbarger J, Dear G de L. The DAN diabetes survey. Alert Diver 1996;Jan–Feb:22.

APPENDIX A: SUGGESTED ASSESSMENT FOR THE DIABETIC DIVER

The South Pacific Underwater Medicine Society Guidelines on Medical Risk Assessment for Recreational Diving

Introduction

Among diving medical physicians, diving by people with diabetes has been one of the most controversial issues in debates over 'fitness to dive' for several decades. There are several valid concerns that seemed reason enough for diving physicians to take a conservative stance[1-3]. Recently, there has been a softening of attitudes, culminating in joint Undersea and Hyperbaric Medical Society/Divers Alert Network (UHMS/DAN) recommendations on diving with diabetes, and several studies demonstrating the feasibility of safe blood glucose management by diabetic persons who dive[4-6]. Notwithstanding the potential for bias in the relevant surveys, people with diabetes appear to be diving with an incidence of problems similar to that recorded among populations of non-diabetic divers[7].

Table 1 Acute and chronic complications or associations recognized in diabetes, and their potential interactions with diving

Complication	Potential interaction with diving
Hypoglycaemia	May be precipitated by stress, cold and exercise during diving.
	Potentially catastrophic consequences from impaired mentation and consciousness underwater.
	Impending symptoms may be less likely to be noticed during diving.
	Potential for confusion with symptoms of decompression illness (DCI) or other possible problems such as hypothermia or seasickness.
Hyperglycaemia	May augment dehydration stress; a possible risk factor for DCI.
	May worsen outcome in neurological DCI[8].
Coronary artery disease	Impairment of exercise tolerance.
	Possibility of myocardial ischaemic event.
Resetting of hypothalamic glucose control	Release of adrenaline during hypoglycaemia occurs after neuro-glycopenia and patient may become incapacitated before noticing hypoglycaemic symptoms: a phenomenon known as 'hypoglycaemia unawareness'[9].
Autonomic neuropathy	Blunting of adrenaline release expected when blood glucose falls, thereby worsening potential for hypoglycaemia[8].
Peripheral neuropathy	Possible confusion with signs of DCI.
Peripheral vascular disease	Impairment of exercise tolerance.
Renal impairment	Multiple possibilities depending on severity.

Diabetic persons prone to acute complications (e.g. hypoglycaemia) or suffering chronic complications that could significantly affect diving safety should be advised against diving. Similarly, the progressive nature of many complications of diabetes suggests there should be longitudinal health surveillance and periodic reassessment of suitability over the period of a diabetic person's participation in diving.

Which diabetics should dive?

The approaches adopted by several groups have a great deal in common and have been summarized very well in the report of the UHMS/DAN workshop[4]. The most important common features are close attention to the quality of diabetic control, both historically and during diving activity, a proscription against diving in the presence of clinically significant secondary complications and a requirement for medical assessment that is more comprehensive than that required of non-diabetic candidates.

The following criteria are appropriate for recreational dive training for a diabetic candidate:

1. Age 16 years or more.
2. At least 6 months since the initiation of treatment with oral hypoglycaemic agents (OHAs) or 1 year since the initiation of treatment with insulin. An established diver using OHAs who is started on insulin should wait at least 6 months before resuming diving.
3. No hypoglycaemic episodes requiring intervention from a third party for at least 1 year and no history of 'hypoglycaemia unawareness'.
4. Glycosylated haemoglobin (HbA1c) up to 9 per cent when measured no more than 1 month before initial assessment and at each annual review. This upper limit is higher than normally recommended for good diabetic control and carries the potential risk of increased end-organ damage.
5. No admissions or emergency visits to hospital for any complications of diabetes for at least 1 year.
6. No known retinopathy (worse than 'background' level), significant nephropathy,

neuropathy (autonomic or peripheral), coronary artery disease or peripheral vascular disease.
7. Before the first diving medical assessment (see 8) and each annual evaluation, a review must be conducted by the candidate's personal diabetologist, who must confirm that:
   - Criteria 3 to 6 are fulfilled.
   - The candidate demonstrates accurate use of a personal blood glucose monitoring device.
   - The candidate has a good understanding of the relationship among diet, exercise, stress, temperature and blood glucose levels.
8. Before commencing diving for the first time and at each annual review, a diving medical examination must be completed by a doctor who has completed a post-graduate diving medical examiner's course. The diabetologist review report must be available. This examination will include appropriate assessment of exercise tolerance, and for candidates over 40 years should include an exercise electrocardiogram.
9. As part of the assessment by the diving medical examiner, the candidate must acknowledge (in writing):
   - Receipt of and intention to use the recommended diabetic diving protocol (see later).
   - The need to seek further guidance if there is any material that is incompletely understood.
   - The need to cease diving and seek review if there are any adverse events in relation to diving suspected of being related to diabetes.
10. Steps 2 to 9 of this protocol must be fulfilled on an annual basis. We strongly advise that where possible the same diabetologist and diving medical officer should be used for these annual reviews.

Scope of diving

1. Diabetic divers are suitable for recreational diving only. This does not include occupational activities such as diving instruction and dive guiding ('dive-mastering').
2. Diabetics should not undertake dives deeper than 30 metres of sea water; dives longer than 1 hour, dives that mandate compulsory

decompression stops or dives in overhead environments. These practices all hamper prompt access to surface support.

3. Diabetic divers do not undertake more than two dives per day and use a minimum surface interval of 2 hours. Diving can be a physically demanding activity and fatigue is common following a 'normal diving day', even for non-diabetic divers.

4. Diabetic divers must dive with a buddy who is informed of their condition and aware of the appropriate response in the event of a hypoglycaemic episode.

5. Diabetic divers should avoid combinations of circumstances that could be provocative for hypoglycaemic episodes such as prolonged, cold dives involving hard work.

BLOOD GLUCOSE MANAGEMENT ON THE DAY OF DIVING

The South Pacific Underwater Medicine Society (SPUMS) recommendations are based on the published experience of several established diabetic diving programmes.[5,7,11]

1. On every day on which diving is contemplated, the diabetic diver must assess himself or herself in a general sense. If he or she is uncomfortable, unduly anxious or unwell in any way (including seasickness), or if blood glucose control is not in its normal stable pattern – **diving must not be undertaken**.

2. The diabetic diver should establish a blood glucose level of at least 9 mmol/litre and ensure that this level is either stable or rising before entering the water. Measurements should be taken three times before diving at 60 minutes, 30 minutes and immediately before gearing up. Diving should be postponed if blood glucose is less than 9 mmol/litre, or there is a fall between any two measurements.

   Where relevant, strategic and individually tailored reductions in doses of OHA medication or insulin on the evening before or on the day of diving may assist in complying with these parameters. Initial testing of individual protocols should be conducted under very controlled circumstances. Where relevant, a regimen of incremental glucose intake to correct inappropriate pre-dive levels or trends may assist in complying with these parameters.

3. Attempts to comply with the requirements at point 2 in this list should not result in a blood glucose level greater than 14 mmol/litre, and diving should be cancelled for the day if levels are higher than 16 mmol/litre at any stage. Prescription of a strict upper limit is somewhat arbitrary, but 16 mmol/litre approaches the renal threshold for glucose, and there is some evidence that diabetic persons involved in diving do dehydrate more readily than non-diabetic divers[6].

4. Diabetic divers must carry oral glucose in a readily accessible and ingestible form at the surface and during all dives. We strongly recommended that the diabetic diver also have parenteral glucagon available at the surface. If premonitory symptoms of hypoglycaemia are noticed underwater, the diver must surface, establish positive buoyancy, ingest glucose and leave the water. An informed buddy should be in a position to assist with or initiate this process.

5. Blood glucose levels must be checked at the end of every dive. The requirements for blood glucose status outlined at point 2 remain the same for any subsequent dive. Because of the recognized potential for late decrements in blood glucose levels following diving, blood glucose levels should be checked 12 to 15 hours after diving.

6. Diabetic divers are strongly recommended to drink between 1000 and 1500 ml of extra water over a period of several hours before their first dive of the day.

7. Diabetic divers must log all dives, associated diabetic interventions and results of all blood glucose level tests conducted in association with diving.

   This protocol should be combined into an information package to be given to the diabetic diver by the examining doctor on completion of their diving medical examination. Other ancillary information and tips and tricks that are not sufficiently critical to be specified in the protocol can be incorporated in this package. For example, a pro-forma for a diabetic dive log could be included, as could advice about simulated 'dives trips' to swimming pools as 'dress rehearsals' in glucose management.

The following pro-forma statement is to be added to the certificate in the SPUMS Guidelines to Medical Practitioners, for use when counselling diabetic candidates about diving.

Statement regarding diabetes and diving

I, ………………………………………, hereby acknowledge my understanding and acceptance of the following issues:

1. Altered consciousness, heart attack or exhaustion during diving may lead to drowning and other life-threatening complications.
2. A history of diabetes implies a greater risk of these events.
3. Diving itself may make these events more likely in a diabetic patient by precipitating hypoglycaemia or imposing high physical demands in certain situations.
4. That because of the issues described at 1 to 3, diabetic persons are frequently considered unfit to dive.
5. That the extra risk in diving for a diabetic diver who meets certain criteria for selection as a diver and who practises appropriate diabetic diving technique is likely to be relatively small. Unfortunately, this risk cannot be exactly quantified.
6. That any decision for a diabetic person to dive must be based on the perceived benefit weighed against the potential risk.

Having decided to proceed with diver training, I acknowledge:

1. That Dr ………………………'s assessment of my risk in diving has been based in part on my own reports of blood glucose control and my general state of health. I acknowledge my responsibility for the accuracy of those reports.
2. That if the pattern of my diabetes changes significantly, or if I suffer any adverse diabetes-related event in which I require assistance or medical consultation at any time, then the risk of diving may be increased and

I should cease diving and discuss the issue with Dr……………………… again.
3. That I should not dive during any period likely to be associated with worsening of my glycaemic control, such as during a cold or other illness.
4. That if I find diving precipitates any problems in relation to my diabetes, I should cease diving forthwith and seek review with Dr…………………………
5. That I understand the necessity to more closely monitor and adjust my glucose levels on diving days, in accordance with the diabetic diving guidelines.
6. That I have read, understood and had an opportunity to ask questions about the diabetic diving guidelines.
7. That I understand the necessity to inform my dive buddy and dive group about my diabetes.
8. That I must undergo annual review with Dr……………………… or another diving doctor as long as I continue to dive.

Finally, I understand that:

being informed of the above issues, having had my questions answered, and having been counselled about my risk in diving I accept that I am responsible for my decision to dive. I hold no one else responsible for any adverse consequences of this decision.

Signed: …

Dated: …

References

1. Taylor L, Mitchell S. Diabetes as a contraindication to diving: should old dogma give way to new evidence? *South Pacific Underwater Medicine Society Journal* 2001;**31**(1):44–50.
2. Thomas R, McKenzie B. *The Diver's Medical Companion.* Sydney: Diving Medical Centre; 1981:137.
3. Betts JC. Diabetes and diving. *Pressure* 1983;**June:**2–3.
4. Pollock NW, Uguccioni DM, Dear G de L, eds. *Diabetes and Recreational Diving: Guidelines for the Future.* Proceedings

of the Undersea and Hyperbaric Medical Society/Divers Alert Network 2005 Workshop. Durham, North Carolina: Divers Alert Network; 2005.

5. Lerch M, Lutrop C, Thurm U. Diabetes and diving: can the risk of hypoglycemia be banned? *South Pacific Underwater Medicine Society Journal* 1996:**26**(2):62–66.

6. Dear G de L, Pollock NW, Uguccioni DM, Dovenbarger J, Feinglos MN, Moon RE. Plasma glucose responses in recreational divers with insulin requiring diabetes. *Undersea and Hyperbaric Medicine* 2004;**31**(3):291–301.

7. Edge CJ, St. Leger Dowse M, Bryson P. Scuba diving with diabetes mellitus: the UK experience 1991–2001. *Undersea and Hyperbaric Medicine* 2005;**32**(1):27–38.

8. Moon RE. Fluid resuscitation, plasma glucose and body temperature control. In: Moon RE, ed. *Report of the Decompression Illness Adjunctive Therapy Committee of the Undersea and Hyperbaric Medical Society*. Bethesda, Maryland: Undersea and Hyperbaric Medical Society; 2003:119–128.

9. Braatvedt G. Hypoglycemia in adult patients with diabetes mellitus. *New Ethicals* 2000;**April:**53–60.

10. Seckl J. Endocrine disorders. In: Elliott DH, ed. *Medical Assessment of Fitness to Dive*. Ewell, United Kingdom: Biomedical Seminars; 1995:172–176.

11. Kruger DF, Owen SK, Whitehouse F. Scuba diving and diabetes. *Diabetes Care* 1995;**18**(7):1074–1075.

From South Pacific Underwater Medicine Society. *Guidelines on Medical Risk Assessment for Recreational Diving.* 2010. http://www.spums.org.au/story/spums-medical.

APPENDIX B: ADVICE TO THE DIABETIC DIVER

Pre-dive advice

The diabetic diver should be as fit and mentally prepared to dive as his or her non-diabetic buddy. The diabetic diver should be especially careful with regard to being adequately hydrated because there is some evidence that the level of hydration affects the chances of experiencing decompression illness. The dive master should be aware that the diver is diabetic and should also be informed of the profile of the dive (plan the dive, dive the plan). The diabetic diver's buddy should be a person who is either:

1. A regular diving partner and who is familiar with the diabetic person and the problems he or she is likely to experience.
2. A trained medic or paramedic who is familiar with the problems of diabetes and the practical management of divers with diabetes.

The diabetic diver should carry the following in his or her dive kit:

1. Oral glucose tablets or a tube of glucose paste.
2. Emergency intramuscular injection of glucagon.
3. Glucose oxidase sticks together with the necessary glucometer kit and *clear* instructions for use of such a kit.

It is essential that there is at least one person in the dive party of the diabetic diver who is able to use and administer the glucose tablets and an intramuscular injection of glucagon.

A diabetic diver should dive no deeper than 30 metres until considerable experience of diving and its associated problems have been gathered by the UK Sport Diving Medical Committee. He or she should remain well within the tables and always have immediate access to the surface (including no-decompression diving only).

He or she should not dive with another diabetic diver as a buddy.

Safety equipment must be carried (e.g. marker buoy, flag, flares). Long-term build-up of nitrogen in the tissues must be avoided by ensuring that no more than 3 consecutive days' diving are undertaken, with no more than two dives to be done each day.

It would seem sensible for the diabetic diver to ensure that he or she has a slightly high blood sugar level before the dive by consuming glucose in whatever form is preferred (see Appendix A).

Post-dive advice

On arrival back at the boat (or on shore if a shore dive), the diabetic diver should check his or her glucose level and, if necessary, correct it in the appropriate manner. Any adverse symptoms or signs should immediately be reported either to the diving buddy or to the dive master and should not be passed off as merely 'part of diving'.

It is important to realize that the symptoms of low blood sugar may mimic those of neurological decompression illness or a gas embolism and vice versa (e.g. confusion, unconsciousness, fits). In this situation, give first aid therapy to the casualty as if he or she had both conditions. Give oxygen therapy and treat for possible low blood sugar.

Treatment of a possible low blood sugar attack

In the event of an incident in the water or on the boat, the diabetic diver should be brought to the boat or shore as soon as possible. The blood glucose should be measured using the equipment in the diabetic emergency kit if this can be swiftly performed. Oral glucose should be administered to the diver with low blood sugar if the diver is conscious; otherwise, an intramuscular injection of glucagon (1 mg) should be given. Medical attention and recompression facilities should be sought as soon as possible.

This chapter was reviewed for this fifth edition by Michael Bennett.

58

Age and diving

PROFESSIONAL DIVING

The age range for the initial training of professional navy divers varies from 20 years at one extreme to 35 years at the other. In adulthood, age is of limited value in success prediction for achieving diving skills, but the most successful age is in the early 20s. Most professional diving schools prefer to select divers 22 to 29 years old. Candidate older than this age range will have a more limited life as a working diver, whereas those who are less than 22 years old are usually not experienced enough in their basic work skills and also perhaps not as reliable, responsible or mature. Failure rates in the training of professional diving candidates who are less than 19 years old makes this practice commercially unprofitable.

The incidence of decompression sickness (DCS) – which is very relevant to deep or commercial diving – is probably related to advancing age. Although not evident in all surveys, most observers have noted this association. One investigator believed that DCS rates double in divers who are 28 years old, compared with those who are 18 years old; however, most observe the association only

after the age of 40 years, with a linear relationship after that. Bubble production is increased with age. Altitude DCS has a similar relationship.

The incidence of death from cardiac disease is much greater after the age of 45 to 50 years, when it is second only to drowning as the cause of death. It has been shown that the incidence of dysbaric osteonecrosis is related to age (but this may be aggravated by greater hyperbaric exposure with age), as is scuba divers' pulmonary oedema.

Beyond the age of 35 years, apart from an appreciable increase in susceptibility to these diving illnesses, there is a probable reluctance to persevere with demanding environmental and social conditions. There is also an increased incidence of general medical problems. In an Australian survey, the incidence of medical disorders causing failure to comply strictly with the Australian Standards for Professional Divers was 45 per cent in divers who were more than 35 years old. This finding compared with a 20 per cent incidence in the candidates in their 20s, thus illustrating the high medical standards required but not always achieved, as well as the adverse effects of age.

THE AGED DIVER

The British Sub-Aqua Club compared the fatality rate of divers of different ages with their frequency in the diving population in the decade to 2009. The divers who were less than 30 years old were underrepresented in the fatality statistics (ratio of <1). Divers more than 50 years old were overrepresented (ratio >1), and by the 60s decade, the ratio was 3.5:1. Combining the data from the various Divers Alert Network organizations showed that the annual fatality rates were 10 per 100 000 divers for divers up to age 25 years and nearly 35 per 100 000 for divers at age 65 years. Old divers die more frequently while diving.

In recreational diving, there is no upper age limit. Especially with experienced divers, recreational divers can often modify their diving activities to take into account the limitations imposed by ageing.

There is also a tendency for much older people, and especially those associated with yachting, to take up diving as part of their marine lifestyle. Thus, we now have people starting to dive who have retired from their normal occupation. This puts an added burden on the medical examiner, but diving is often a valuable contribution to the quality of life of these people.

There are still the same hazards as mentioned earlier, but because the diving activities can be tailored to the individual, greater tolerance can be allowed in recreational than professional diving – if the diver is appropriately informed and dives accordingly. Nevertheless, recreational diving often does not have the same logistical support and safety procedures as professional diving.

With increasing age, there is increasing infirmity and a greater use of medications, both of which can reduce diving safety. Of special note is the prevalence of the following:

- Arthritis and musculoskeletal disorders.
- Cardiovascular disorders.
- Diabetes or obesity.
- Cerebrovascular disease and dementias.
- Ocular problems.
- Neoplasia.

The reduction in physical fitness, involving both cardiac and respiratory function, as well as muscular strength, is likely to restrict considerably the environmental demands that can be met safely.

Reduced physiological reserves attributed to ageing may also be related to genetically determined disorders or to disuse. Preconceived attitudes may reduce the expectations of performance, thereby leading to disuse.

Physical fitness and physiological factors

Maximum oxygen consumption reduces approximately 1 per cent per year. In sedentary individuals, the decline is greater in early adulthood, and the curve is less steep in later life. With regular exercise, this decline can be halved. It is caused by both cardiorespiratory and musculoskeletal factors.

Swimming without fins, at a speed of about 30 metres per minute (a 1-knot current speed) requires a metabolic equivalent (MET) unit of 10.0. One MET unit is defined as consumption of 3.5 ml O_2/kg body weight/minute.

In the **cardiovascular system,** there is an increase in arterial stiffness with ageing, leading to an increase in systolic blood pressure and left ventricular hypertrophy. The exercise-induced rise in heart rate declines by 3.2 per cent per decade.

In terms of age-related **respiratory function,** there is a decrease in elasticity of the lung parenchyma, an increase in fibrous tissue and greater resistance to airflow. By the age of 70 years, the vital capacity reduces by 30 to 50 per cent, and the residual volume increases by 40 to 50 per cent. These changes result in breathlessness at lesser workloads.

Maximum **muscle strength** is achieved by the third decade, levels off until about the age of 60 years and then declines by 10 to 15 per cent per decade.

Psychological factors

Listing the physiological decrements associated with age would ignore the considerable individual variation, and so assessment must be performance based on each case.

Diving concerns specific to ageing

If the aged diver is able to continue to achieve a standard of physical fitness commensurate with diving safety, then he or she should cope with the multiple theoretical and practical physiological decrements. Thus, irrespective of age, the diver (either trainee or experienced) should still be able to perform a 1-kilometre swim in less than half an hour, or a 200-metre swim in less than 5 minutes, unaided by equipment. If the diver, aged or otherwise, is unable to achieve such a basic standard of physical fitness and aquatic skill, then much diving activity would be unacceptably hazardous.

Certain diving illnesses are more likely to develop with age. The most important of these is cardiac disease, which is now probably the most common medical cause of death in recreational diving (drowning reflects only the medium in which the accident occurs). The strenuous exercise required to swim against tidal currents and to rescue other divers is such that a sub-clinical obstruction to a coronary artery, 80 per cent or greater, could be converted into a clinical case report of the sudden death syndrome.

Although physiological age is more important than chronological age, for divers more than 40 years old it is recommended that regular re-examinations be carried out to detect medical abnormalities that may interfere with efficiency and safety in the diving environment. Cardiac stress testing during maximal exercise may be recommended as part of each 5-year medical examination after this age, especially if other cardiac risk factors are present.

DCS is more common with increasing age and becomes a considerable handicap beyond the age of 40 years. With increasing age, a more conservative allowance must be made – restricting the decompression schedules. The authors of this text arbitrarily recommend that older divers reduce their allowable bottom time by 10 per cent for each decade after the fourth. Scuba divers' pulmonary oedema is also more common in middle-aged and older divers.

One of the most common problems of the ageing diver is presbyopia. This interferes with the diver's ability reading the meters, gauges and camera settings. It can be overcome by the use of a convex lens, stuck onto the lower rim of the face mask.

Increased sensitivity to cold can be partly countered by limiting diving to warmer waters or the use of thermal protective clothing. Aged persons are more susceptible to temperature changes.

There are suggestions that repetitive and excessive diving may produce some form of cerebral impairment that increase the effects of ageing. There is little evidence to support such a concept. Indeed, the anecdotal evidence for such a situation is countered by equivalent anecdotal evidence implying that old divers are an exciting, innovative and socially active group (see Chapter 41).

There are positive aspects to age, including the accumulated knowledge both of diving and other related activities, more prudence and care in dive planning and the choice of diving sites and possibly more mature judgement. The aged diver is less likely to be swayed by social, peer, financial or ego pressures.

Many very old divers arrange for a personal dive guide to assist in suiting up, carrying tanks, donning gear, managing entrances and exits from the water and accompanying them during the dive. The problem comes in getting older divers to recognize when the time comes to ask for help.

Many divers have continued diving into their 80s, and the social value of diving should not be underestimated. In Australia, there was even a Sub-Aquatic Geriatric Association, to which this author has received (junior) honorary membership.

CHILDREN

So far, the youngest child to die while scuba diving was 7 years old, but there have been many accidents and deaths between the ages of 10 and 15 years.

The most prudent advice to parents is to encourage children to acquire aquatic and snorkelling skills at this age, to consolidate the basic capabilities needed later for scuba training.

There is a common belief that children should not exceed 9 metres of depth until their bones have reached osteogenic maturity (i.e. when the epiphyses have fused). There is very little evidence that DCS or dysbaric osteonecrosis has influenced bone growth in young animals. Nevertheless, that possibility causes some hesitation in contemplating diving in excess of this depth because of our limited knowledge.

Official recommendations

Most reputable scuba training organizations make 15 years the minimum age for certification of recreational diving, although they may train younger children in water skills. The more commercial agencies qualify younger children to dive. The usual rationalization is this: 'If a child under 12 is physically, mentally and emotionally able to handle the skills and understand the knowledge needed to scuba dive, he or she should be able to get certified'. The problem with this response is in the first word, 'if'.

The South Pacific Underwater Medicine Society Committee on Medical Standards for Recreational Diving met in 1990 and carefully considered this subject. They recommended a minimum age of 16 years for scuba diver training. The decision was based purely on safety factors.

The Australian Standards reduced the recommended age to 14 years, to comply with diving instructor agencies' demands. The Australian Standard 4005.1 of 1992 stated that the selection criteria required that the trainee shall comply with the following:

- Be at least 14 years of age.
- But, persons less than 14 years of age may in some cases be eligible to train for conditional certification that allows the young person to dive with a certified diver, with consent of parents or guardians.
- Under the medical section of the Australian Standards AS 4005.1, it is stated: 'Children under the age of 16 shall only be medically examined after consultation by the doctor with the parent or guardian to establish the child's physical and psychological maturity. Between the ages of 16 and 18 it is preferable to consult with the parent or guardian before medically examining the child'.

The Australian Surf Life Saving Association, whose judgement is not influenced by commercial factors but that is very committed to children's involvement, does not allow active lifesaving responsibilities until the age of 16 years, and even then only under the supervision of a patrol leader who is 18 years old or older.

Attitudes

The physicians, who are probably more concerned with safety than some instructor bodies, recommend a minimum age of 16 years, with parental informed consent and approval necessary between the age of 16 and 18 years.

Unfortunately, the Australian Standards were not prepared by diving physicians. Although there was a representative present, he was greatly outnumbered by the industry and diving training organization representatives. They have different agendas and different motivations from the physicians. There was no one present with pediatric and psychological training.

If one looks at the Australian Standards' document, it is implied that even they have some concern regarding the child's safety, until the age of 18 years. Off-loading the responsibility to parents who have no practical knowledge of the risks of scuba diving was a reprehensible act.

It is surprising that some commercial organizations have accepted a diver who is less than 14 years old to 'dive with a certified diver'. This is inadequate because it allows one young 'conditionally qualified' child to dive with another diver who may be equally inexperienced.

The corollary is this: Would you allow a 12- to 14-year-old child to:

- Fly an airplane?
- Drive a motor vehicle?
- Take out a financial loan?
- Be legally responsible for decisions made?
- Make medical and health judgements?
- Make life-threatening decisions for himself or herself and others?

If one agreed that 12- to 14-year-old children should be restricted in this way, then it would be interesting to compare this decision with that of a child of similar age who is undertaking scuba diving.

Often the aim of the parent is to share a life experience with a child. Certainly, the deaths or disabilities that have eventuated, either in the psychologically ill-equipped child or a medically compromised parent, have led to the most intense agony and guilt in the survivor.

The legal aspects, which must be considered, are dealt with later in this chapter.

Psychological maturity

Psychological maturity is the main reason that the authors of this text recommend that children not to be given diving certification.

Certification implies that the diver can make informed judgements about dive planning, environmental conditions, equipment usage and the interrelationships of all these factors. For a dive to be safe, informed judgement is sometimes essential. It is related to maturation and experience, not just intelligence.

A child may have no difficulty handling the intellectual content of the diving course, but he or she will have difficulty with its application. Unfortunately, children do not have the same appreciation of mortality (death) and the implications of morbidity (disease or accidents) as an adult.

Children are more immature. That is what makes a child. They tend to be more immediate in their gratification needs and have a shorter attention span. They are not as good at long-term planning as adults. Unfortunately, sometimes the long-term planning will not be needed if the child dies or suffers significant damage.

Materialistic factors also come into play. Children are less likely to abort a dive if they have already committed themselves financially or logistically. With age, judgement does come. Older people see death more clearly.

Psychological reactions are also different in children. Children react with behaviour that, in adults, would be abnormal. They are far more likely to display anxiety or hysterical reactions, and the control of these reactions is part of the maturing process.

The appropriate response to a life-threatening situation, or even one that is perceived to be life-threatening, is not to burst into tears. Unfortunately, this is a child's natural reaction, and it is often very effective in obtaining adult assistance. Tears are not easily seen through a face mask and, in any case, tend simply to add to the large ocean environment. They do not have the same power underwater as they do on land, with mummy watching.

Children's reactions are certainly rapid, but they are not always appropriate for long-term health and safety.

Endurance and perseverance are characteristics that develop with age. These take over when panic and tantrums have been controlled. Imagination is an endearing characteristic, but it makes children susceptible to fear and terror.

Children are dependent. They slowly mature to become independent and then act responsibly. They are more likely to rely on the statements and decisions of others, as opposed to assessing what they themselves can cope with. This may be appropriate for a trip to the zoo, but it is not good in open ocean diving. In the latter environment, divers have to be self-reliant and to recognize their own limitations, but they also have to be able to act accordingly. They are responsible for the safety and rescue of their companion. Would you really want a 12-year-old child to be responsible for your safety or for your other children's safety?

Children are suggestible and very easily impressed. They can be influenced directly by others and also by the encouragement and enthusiasm that their parents may exhibit. Thus, the child may well continue an activity, such as scuba diving, to please mum or dad, to impress their parents and peers and to gain attention. These are not prudent motivations for scuba diving. Children are very easily intimidated, and, for the sake of the child, I would prefer to see an indifferent parental reaction than an enthusiastic one.

Physical maturity

The requirement for properly fitting equipment implies the need to upgrade this equipment regularly during the growing years.

There is the likely problem, sooner or later, that the child will have to swim against unexpected tidal currents to return to safety. Some children may have this physical ability, but they may not have the psychological endurance in such an emergency. Others will have neither.

A small child could have great difficulty in coping with the rescue of a larger 'buddy'.

With physical immaturity, there is also the problem of increased dangers from certain diving medical disorders. These include such issues as hypothermia, gas toxicities, susceptibility to marine venoms and barotraumas.

Medical aspects

The reason that children suffer 'glue ears' is that their Eustachian tubes are narrower and smaller. So are the sinus ostia. Children's upper and lower respiratory passages are narrower by comparison with the air cavities associated with them. That is the reason why children have more trouble with barotraumas in aviation as well as in diving exposures.

Some diseases (e.g. asthma) are more likely to occur in young childhood than in late adolescence, when the airways have grown relative to the lung volumes. That is one reason why children sometimes seem to 'grow out' of asthma.

Many experts have questioned the safety of exposing children to diseases such as pulmonary barotrauma and arterial gas embolism (one cause of acute decompression illness), especially in children where there is still growth of organs (i.e. where a bubble can do more damage than it would in a full-sized adult). Damaged tissues that could be so affected include the brain, inner ear, bone and coronary artery, among others. The worry here is that, for the same degree of bubble development, there could be much greater ultimate damage.

When should children dive?

It is the opinion of the authors of this text that children less than 16 years old should have 'dive experiences' only under the following, moderately safe, conditions:

1. They want to, without parental or peer pressure.
2. They are medically fit to do so.
3. They dive to a maximum depth of 9 metres, to prevent some of the problems referred

to earlier. The 9-metre depth will certainly not prevent a child from developing pulmonary barotrauma, cerebral arterial gas embolism or any of the other respiratory tract barotraumas. It will, however, usually prevent DCS.
4. They are trained and taken by a qualified instructor and under the personal and total control of that instructor (i.e. not three or four trainees together). A buddy line between the child and the instructor is prudent, to prevent unexpected and uncontrolled ascents.
5. All dives are to be carried out only in calm water and good environmental conditions and with the same controls as referred to in items 1 to 4 of this list, with an experienced diver of instructor standard taking absolute control.

Giving a diving certificate to children who are less than 16 years old, other than a certificate that stipulates diving under the foregoing very special conditions, is irresponsible.

Legal implications

There are many complicated legal and financial implications that may subsequently overtake the grief aspects associated with the death or disability of a child or the child's companion diver, and these eventually are quantified financially.

The *statute of limitations* varies according to the local jurisdiction, but usually damage to a child will be legally actionable until the child is into his or her mid-20s. The financial recompense will cover educational needs, social and occupational limitations, emotional pain and medical treatments. By this time, the child may already be engaged in his or her own law career tuition.

Duty of care is applicable to the parents or guardian who signed permission for diver training to commence, the trainer and the diving organization and the physician who verified fitness. This fitness encompasses physical and psychological criteria, including the child's ability to understand and comprehend, then make mature judgements, as well as the ability to take appropriate actions. It is difficult to comprehend how a child can reasonably take care and responsibility in a hazardous environment for another child or a parent who may be his or her companion diver.

Insurance companies may not cover the behaviour of the physician, by postulating that the physician has not acted within an area of his or her expertise – as a diving medical expert. In this regard they may be justified. The diving organizations are treated more leniently because they are a continuing source of premiums.

The outcome of any court case is likely to reflect judicial sympathy for grieving parents or a disabled child no longer able to engage in adventuresome activities, more than for an affluent physician – and with this the authors of this text are in agreement. For this and the foregoing reasons, most cases are settled out of court. Diving organizations customarily settle out of court so that they can quote 'no convictions' to their future trainees.

FURTHER READING

Bennett and Elliott. *The Physiology and Medicine of Diving*. 5th Ed. London: Saunders; 2003.

Bove AA. Diving in the elderly and young. Chapter 20 in Bove and Davis' *Diving Medicine*. 4th Ed. Philadelphia: Saunders; 2004.

Cali-Corleo R. The diver over the age of forty. In: Elliott D, ed. *Medical Assessment of Fitness to Dive*. Biomedical Seminars (University of Surrey): Guilford, United Kingdom; 1994.

Caruso JL, Uguccioni DM, Ellis JE, Dovenbarger JA, Bennett PB. Diving fatalities involving children and adolescents, 1989–2002. Underwater and Hyperbaric Medical Society Abstract. May, 2004. Available at: http://archive.rubicon-foundation.org/1599.

Cumming B, Peddie C, Watson J. A review of the nature of diving in the UK and of UK diving fatalities, 1998–2009. In: *Diving Fatalities Conference*. Durham, North Carolina: Divers Alert Network; 2010. Available at https://www.diversalertnetwork.org/files/Fatalities_Proceedings.pdf.

Edmonds C. *The Diver*. A Royal Australian Navy School of Underwater Medicine Report 2/72. Sydney: Royal Australian Navy publication; 1972.

Edmonds C. Scuba kids. *South Pacific Underwater Medicine Society Journal* 1996;**26**(3):154–157.

Edmonds C. Children and diving. *South Pacific Underwater Medicine Society Journal* 2003;**33**(4):206–211.

Hills BA. *Decompression Sickness*. Vol. 1. New York: John Wiley; 1977.

Ogle S, Gwinn T. The older athlete. In: Sherry E, Wilson S, eds. *The Oxford Handbook of Sports Medicine*. Oxford: Oxford University Press; 1998.

Mebane YG. Recreational diving medical standards. In: Elliott D, ed. *Medical Assessment of Fitness to Dive*. Biomedical Seminars (University of Surrey): Guilford, United Kingdom; 1994.

Schwartz K. Age and diving. *Alert Diver* 1996;**Sept**:36–39.

Walker R. How old is enough? *South Pacific Underwater Medicine Society Journal* 2003;**33**(2):78–80.

This chapter was reviewed for this fifth edition by Carl Edmonds.

59

Diver selection

INTRODUCTION

Advertisements suggest that everyone can be taught to scuba dive and that furthermore, scuba diving is a fun, safe and easy recreational activity. But what makes a good diver, and more importantly, are there particular individuals who should not dive? What is the role of medical standards and medical examinations?

Recreational diving is frequently not physically demanding, but it can be so at times, and this complicates the process of setting pragmatic selection standards. As discussed in Chapter 53, there is little evidence-based guidance available on the essential criteria that a recreational diving candidate should possess to dive independently and safely. Occupational or professional diving is more often physically demanding, and this arguably mandates a different set of standards. Thus, in considering selection criteria, it is necessary to consider the qualities required for both professional and recreational divers.

THE PROFESSIONAL DIVER

There are relatively few data in the scientific literature on diver selection; however, most that exist deal with professional navy divers. These divers are subjected to an arduous physical fitness program and operate under extreme conditions. They are commonly seen as the elite of the navy.

Biersner[1] found successful military divers to have a greater incidence of conduct disorder behaviours (e.g. truancy, arrests) than their non-diving counterparts. He also found that a significant proportion of divers demonstrated antisocial personality traits[2], and divers were more likely to be individualistic, unsympathetic and aggressive. Other investigators[3] have found a positive relationship between mechanical aptitude and success as a diver.

Beckman and colleagues[4] evaluated navy divers (who had successfully passed their diving course) and found that they were best described as optimistic, independent, self-serving, analytical and tending toward social aggressiveness. This personality style appears most closely to resemble the non-pathological antisocial personality. Beckman and associates also went on to say that this personality style may be quite adaptive, considering the unique nature of the employment. Yet an antisocial personality potentially creates problems in team building, team activities and discipline-oriented organizations.

Although most navies require their diving course recruits to undergo a formal psychological screening test, they do not specifically deny entry to a candidate who is somewhat introspective and pessimistic. The screening tests are used to exclude those candidates with increased anxiety and depression levels, as well as gross psychopathology. Generally, the best candidates are conscientious, open to experience (and this generally reflects intelligence levels), low on neuroticism and socially adjusted. Teamwork is most important, along with adjustment to military life and authority.

Professional divers must be able to operate under conditions of stress and do not have the luxury of diving only when they feel like it. Aquadro[5] stated that the following tendencies militate against the ability to withstand stress: below average intelligence, tendencies to claustrophobia, unhealthy motivations, history of past personal ineffectiveness, difficulties in interpersonal relations and lack of adaptability.

However, despite the foregoing, it is not possible to select only successful candidates before the commencement of the diving course. Professional diving courses still have failure rates of up to 30 per cent. Candidates often say they feel uncomfortable or it was not what they expected. Previously unrecognized claustrophobia may become evident. Poor visibility, strong currents, hard work, heavy equipment, cold and obvious risk do not equate with the often glamorous but misconceived perception of professional diving.

THE RECREATIONAL DIVER

Recreational divers require a level of physical and psychological fitness to undertake sports diving. It can be argued that these divers can pick and choose when they wish to dive and under what environmental conditions; however, a certain level of intelligence and the knowledge of water conditions are required to exercise this judgement. Even then, the ocean is not always predictable.

Motivation for undertaking a diving course should be considered, and perhaps the most important selection criterion should be that the individual is a willing volunteer. Spousal pressure can be enormous. It is important to identify the scared, reluctant candidate whose only reason for undertaking the course is his or her partner's insistence. These candidates are at risk of being bullied by their partner, concealing their true anxieties and ending up as a diving statistic. This individual may not feel able to refuse the partner's request; however, if the alert doctor or diving instructor recommends against diving, this is often acceptable to the dominant partner.

In the latter regard, it may be appropriate for doctors and diving instructors to advise couples not to form a buddy pair during their training course. The male partner is often more proactive and may put his partner's equipment together and generally take charge. This often has the effect of making the female partner feel inadequate for not understanding the activity, but she then is too embarrassed to ask questions. The couple may not always dive together, and both individuals must have confidence in their own individual general diving ability and their ability to cope in the event of difficulty.

Diving candidates should feel comfortable in the water, and in one study poor swimming ability was a major factor in diving course failure. Any recreational activity is usually undertaken for the pleasure it provides. The candidate who is uncomfortable in the water, is a poor swimmer or who is physically unfit is less likely to pass the course or enjoy diving and more likely to have a higher risk of accidents.

The recreational diving training agencies can legitimately point to data suggesting that diving is a relatively safe sport, but the existence of risk should never be denied. Evidence supports panic behaviour as one of the major influencing factors for injuries and fatalities. Individuals with raised anxiety trait levels, in comparison with divers in general, are more likely to experience symptoms of state anxiety and panic episodes when they are confronted with various stresses while diving[6]. When identified, such individuals should be discouraged from diving.

Although the ideal diving candidate has not been identified, intelligence, adaptability, physical fitness, water skills, low anxiety trait levels, strong motivation and social adjustment have all been recognized as contributing to the production of a good diver.

The diving medical selection process (see Chapters 53 and 54) aims to ensure that diving candidates meet appropriate standards, but it must be clearly understood that this process is not over when the candidate completes the pre-participation questionnaire or the consultation with a doctor. The diving medical physician does not have the time or (usually) the experience to conduct an in-depth psychological assessment on all diving candidates. The diving instructor is perhaps in a much better position to assess these aspects of the candidate during the practical evolutions of the course. Diving instructors have an important role in ensuring that candidates who are unsuitable in this regard not proceed to certification.

REFERENCES

1. Biersner RJ. Social development of Navy divers. *Aerospace Medicine* 1973;**44**:761–763.
2. Biersner RJ, Dembert ML, Browning MD. The antisocial diver: performance, medical and emotional consequences. *Military Medicine* 1979;**144**(7):445–448.
3. Wise DA. *Aptitude Selection Standards for the US Navy's First Class Diving Course.* United States Navy Experimental Diving Unit Report 3-63. Panama City, Florida: Navy Experimental Diving Unit; 1963.
4. Beckman TJ, Lall R, Johnson WB. Salient personality characteristics among Navy divers. *Military Medicine* 1996;**161**(12):717–719.
5. Aquadro CF. Examination and selection of personnel for work in underwater environment. *Journal of Occupational Medicine* 1965;**7**:619–625.
6. Morgan WP. Anxiety and panic in recreational scuba divers. *Sports Medicine* 1995;**20**(6):398–421.

This chapter was reviewed for this fifth edition by Simon Mitchell.

PART 10

Specialized Diving and Its Problems

60

Female divers

INTRODUCTION

The era when scuba diving was considered a male-dominated macho sport is long past. Female divers account for some 28 per cent of all recreational diving certifications issued[1], and women are employed worldwide in recreational, scientific, occupational and certain specific military diving operations. Notwithstanding this welcome trend, it remains a fact that some gender-related physiological differences are relevant to diving. Although the importance of some of these differences was probably overemphasized in the past, it remains relevant to consider them.

HISTORY OF WOMEN IN DIVING

With a history going back some 2000 years, the original shell divers of Asia were both male and female. This changed approximately 400 to 500 years ago, some say because of the better tolerance to cold exhibited by women, whereas others attribute it to the folklore that diving affects male virility.

The female Ama divers of Korea and Japan have been famous for their breath-hold diving capability. These women adapted well to their diving activities in various ways, such as by increasing their basal metabolic rate, at least during the colder months, up to 30 per cent above normal. This meant that they used more food to produce heat and energy to allow them to endure the cold water. To conserve heat, they developed increased body tissue insulation, about 10 per cent above normal, a reduction in their blood flow to the skin (30 per cent less than normal) and an ability to tolerate a lower water temperature before the shivering developed.

In Western society, there were both cultural and legal restrictions on the aquatic activities of women. In the early part of the twentieth century, it was customary to expect female swimmers to be bedecked in a full blouse and skirt, long dark-coloured hose, rubber bathing slippers and a bathing hat. Presumably, only a very competent swimmer would attempt to cope in the ocean with those restrictions.

In the 1940s, Simone Cousteau joined her illustrious husband, Jacques Cousteau, in using and becoming adept with the scuba apparatus called the Aqualung.

Lottie Hass proved her expertise at diving and underwater photography, despite discouragement from her husband, the famous Hans Hass. She inspired others with her success in both roles and in her autobiography *Girl on the Ocean Floor*.

In Australia, Valerie Taylor and Eva Cropp led a group of very enterprising and capable women who captured the admiration of the public with their skills and abilities at handling marine animals. The work of these women was immortalized in film and television productions. Dee Scarr demonstrated the same skills in the Caribbean.

Some female scientists excited the diving world. Eugenie Clark became known as the 'shark lady' because of her brilliant work in this field, and Sylvia Earle, in 1969, led the first all-women team of aquanauts in the Tektite II habitat experiments. These women stayed underwater for 2 weeks in the Tektite habitat and were acclaimed for their diving and scientific professionalism.

Kati Garner was the first woman to graduate from the US Navy Diving School, which she did in 1973. Many hundreds of women have successfully followed her.

In more recent times, with the popularization of free diving and technical diving, some women have truly made their mark. Arguably the most famous of the female free divers is Tania Streeter from the United Kingdom who, incredibly, held the depth record for no limits free diving for both male and female divers for a period. She still holds the no limits record for female divers (see Chapter 3). Jill Heinerth is a technical diver from Florida who has become famous for her outstanding photography and for her role as an educator and outspoken advocate for rebreather diving safety and the environment.

Perhaps the most important contribution of women to diving has been in the instructional area. Many male instructors used the training period as an ego trip for themselves, by denigrating the trainees' apprehensions and relating stories to demonstrate their own prowess. With the increase in the number of women instructors, there has been a removal of the old 'bravado' image of the instructor. Instead of a glib and depreciating response to questions, diving trainees are now far more likely to be listened to and have their questions considered and answered in a non–point-scoring way.

About 1 in 3 of the current trainees is a woman. The ratio of female divers in the diving death statistics is 1 in 10. Women divers seem less likely to die than men divers, but to make the figures more meaningful, the actual number of dives performed by members of each gender would be required.

ANATOMICAL DIFFERENCES

Compared with men, women typically produce less power or speed and have a lower work capacity and less stamina. Despite fitness training, women possess a higher percentage of body fat. A 20-year-old sedentary woman has approximately 25 per cent body fat, a trained woman has 10 to 15 per cent fat and a trained man has 7 to 10 per cent fat. Of total body mass, trained men have relatively more muscle: 40 per cent compared with 23 per cent muscle in a comparatively fit woman[2]. This means that a woman may find it more difficult to swim against a strong current and tire more easily than her male buddy. Nevertheless, these generalizations are unlikely to be relevant in all but the most demanding diving situations (e.g. being caught in a current) or activities (e.g. some aspects of military diving).

The female diver may also experience difficulty in lifting and carrying her dive equipment. A fully charged standard dive cylinder with a buoyancy compensator device and regulator weighs around 23 kg on land, whereas the mixed gas rebreather set used by many of the world's navies weighs 29 kg when fully charged. The buoyancy on entry into the water alleviates this load.

Women may be able to conserve energy more efficiently than men. Their increased body fat provides better insulation from heat loss and increased buoyancy. Women have a lower basal metabolic rate, thus reducing their caloric need. Women have fewer sweat glands, and sweating begins at a higher core temperature, thereby conserving heat. However, the converse is also true, and this increases a woman's susceptibility to heat stress. Overall, women are more susceptible to thermal stress than men because of an increased conductive heat loss resulting from their slightly higher ratio of surface area to volume and their smaller muscle mass and less metabolically active tissue to generate heat during activity[2].

The ability to cope with cold water exposure is partially adaptive (i.e. it can be improved with repeat exposures). This was substantively demonstrated by the Korean Ama, who proved that women are able to adapt. It is noteworthy that since 1976 and the introduction of wetsuits, these adaptations have been lost[3]. The likelihood in our culture is that women will expose themselves less to cold water and therefore be more sensitive during the diving course. This sensitivity can easily be managed by careful attention to selection of high-quality wetsuits of the correct size, so that water circulation through the suit is minimized, and of the correct thickness for the environmental conditions. In very harsh conditions, a drysuit may be recommended.

The effect of these physiological differences on recreational divers is relatively minor. On beginning diving, it is possible that the average woman will be unable to match the physical performance of her average male counterpart; however, with training she will soon adapt. Sports divers should plan their dives to avoid conditions requiring sustained maximal aerobic endurance and should learn to dive within their own physical limitations. Modern diving equipment with properly fitting wetsuits or drysuits should ameliorate the cold disadvantage, and if overheated on the boat, the female diver can remedy this condition by immersion. For the professional female diver, individual characteristics and capabilities are more important than alleged gender disadvantages.

MENSTRUATION

Whether a woman dives during her menstrual period depends on how she feels. Over the 3 to 5 days, she is likely to lose between 50 and 150 ml of blood and cellular debris. This is an insignificant amount physiologically, but there has been a great deal of fear that even this small amount may attract sharks. There is no support for this belief, and in fact female divers appear to experience a lower incidence of shark attack than do male divers.

For most healthy, active women, changes associated with their menstrual cycle are negligible and cause minimal interruption to their lives. Although the menstrual cycle may have some psychological and physiological effects, examination of the statistics in the Olympic Games during the 1970s showed no significant performance decrement at any specific stage of the menstrual cycle. Brown[4] compiled a small survey of female divers and found that 89.9 per cent of women dive while menstruating without any physical or psychological problems. Of those who did not dive, 4.8 per cent were menopausal or had not had the opportunity to dive while menstruating.

Another disorder that sometimes has a marked increase in incidence during the menstrual cycle is migraine. If divers suffer from this condition, especially in the pre-menstrual period, it is worthwhile either avoiding diving or ensuring that they do not do anything that can aggravate or precipitate a migraine-type syndrome.

At pre-menstrual and menstrual periods, there may be a congestion of the mucosal membranes, possibly associated with the oedema and fluid retention. When this happens, it may be more difficult to equalize the middle ears (because of the Eustachian tube swelling), and this mucosal congestion may also predispose to sinus barotrauma.

There is mounting evidence that the risk of decompression sickness (DCS) in women is highest during the first week of the menstrual cycle. The first study specifically designed to address this issue examined the relationship between the phase of the menstrual cycle and the occurrence of DCS in US Air Force (USAF) personnel undertaking hypobaric exposures[5]. This study demonstrated a clear correlation between the incidence of DCS and the time since the start of the last menstrual period. A higher number of subjects developed DCS earlier in the menstrual cycle (0 to 4 days), and the study concluded that women were at higher risk of developing altitude DCS during menses, with the risk decreasing linearly as the time since the last menstrual period increases. The study did not address the likely mechanisms for the findings or its application to female divers.

However, since that time there have been several studies of both altitude-induced and diving-related DCS that all drew the same conclusion[6]. Although these studies suffer from small size and some methodologic issues, the unanimity of the findings is compelling evidence that there is indeed an increase in risk of DCS early in the menstrual cycle. The reasons for this increase remain unclear.

These findings suggest that it may be prudent for female divers to add some safety margin to their decompression staging requirements during the week before menstruation and while menstruating. Susceptible women would be prudent to avoid diving or modify their diving if they have psychological or physiological problems during this time, such as anxiety, tension, depression, malaise and muscle cramps, nausea and vomiting or a propensity to seasickness.

ORAL CONTRACEPTION

Oral contraceptive pills are known to be associated with an increased risk of thromboembolism because they accelerate blood clotting and increase platelet aggregation and are associated with an increased blood concentration of some clotting factors[7]. There is, however, no evidence to suggest that oral contraceptives increase a woman's susceptibility to DCS, and the risk of becoming pregnant is far greater. There is some preliminary evidence that taking an oral contraceptive may ablate the cycle-related difference in DCS risk described earlier[6], but this is uncertain.

DECOMPRESSION SICKNESS

There has been a common perception that women have an increased susceptibility to DCS, perhaps because of their increased body fat percentage. However, studies examining this hypothesis are conflicting.

Bassett[8] looked at the incidence of altitude DCS in the USAF from 1966 to 1977. Of these 104 cases, 32 (31 per cent) occurred in women. Statistically, women were 4 times more susceptible to altitude DCS than were men, and women had more cutaneous symptoms, more rapid onset of DCS pain and more recurrences and more lasting effects of DCS compared with men exposed to the same altitude exposures. These women also gave a history of vascular or migraine headaches. The application of these results to hyperbaric exposures is uncertain.

Bangasser[9] conducted a retrospective study of 649 female divers by questionnaire comparing the reported incidence of DCS in female and male diving instructors. Her results suggested a 3.3-fold greater incidence of DCS in female diving instructors. However, there were several major weaknesses associated with this study. It was retrospective, no controlled criteria existed to determine whether DCS actually occurred and the diagnostic evaluations were based solely on the respondent's replies. It is unlikely that divers incapacitated by accidents or those suffering from fatalities were accounted for in this study.

Zwingleberg and associates[10] compared women with men in a review of DCS in deep diving operations. The investigators concluded that women divers are at no greater risk of developing DCS under similar bounce dive exposures, but these investigators also cautioned against extrapolation of the results to all dive exposures. The dives in these exposures were of short duration and thus may not reflect repetitive, computer-based, multi-level, prolonged and/or technical diving. Moreover, the study was almost certainly underpowered for female subjects to enable a valid comparison.

A retrospective survey[11] looking at men and women in diving showed that men had a higher rate of DCS than did women. Although men and women dived the same depths, men dived more aggressive profiles. These investigators concluded that their study showed no evidence that women are more susceptible to DCS than men, and that any physiological effects of gender are likely to be masked by gender-related differences in diving behaviour.

Arguably the most carefully conducted prospective experiment compared the incidence of DCS between genders in a series of 961 hypobaric exposures[12]. There was no gender-based difference in incidence. It must be observed that although this study is highly relevant, it was conducted using hypobaric rather than hyperbaric exposures.

It is probably correct to say that we still do not have definitive data on the influence of gender on risk of DCS in diving exposures. However, it seems probable, based on the current state of knowledge, that any differences are unlikely to be large and that even if a physiological difference favouring men does exist, it is likely to be more than compensated for by the inherently more conservative approach that many women bring to their diving. No evidence exists in the literature of a difference in susceptibility to pulmonary barotrauma or cerebral arterial gas embolism between the sexes, and the incidence of patent foramen ovale is equal.

PREGNANCY

Diving during pregnancy is a controversial subject. Questions such as the following remain definitively unanswered: 'Does diving increase the risk of foetal abnormality? 'What is the incidence of foetal DCS?' Medical ethics prevents performance of prospective studies. Much of the available data come from animal studies and from extrapolation from our knowledge of other situations that may influence the health of the mother and foetus.

Although only approximately 35 per cent of the current diving population consists of women, these women are mostly in the childbearing age group, and many are such diving enthusiasts that a 9-month interruption is not appreciated. For those women whose career involves diving, the 9-month interruption is sometimes very disruptive.

Potential problems of the pregnant diver

The following list is adapted from Lanphier[13].

- Maternal factors.
  - Morning sickness and motion sickness.
  - Reduced respiratory function.
  - Circulatory competition with placenta.
  - Altered sympathetic response.
  - Reduced fitness and endurance; unusual fatigue.
  - Size – fit of suit, harness, and other equipment; clumsiness leading to injury.
  - Effects of lifting heavy weights.
  - Increased fat and fluid – increased susceptibility to DCS?
  - Mucous membrane swelling – difficulty in equalizing middle ear and sinus spaces.
- Foetal factors.
  - General factors.
    - Hypoxia from various mishaps.
    - Hyperoxia – closure of ductus arteriosus? haemoglobin breakdown? consumptive coagulopathy?
    - Exercise hyperglycemia; post-exercise hypoglycemia.
    - Exercise hyperthermia.
    - Physical injury.
    - Leaking membrane – infection.
    - Marine animal envenomation – direct or indirect damage.
    - Decompression – bubbles – altered placental flow.
  - Early pregnancy.
    - Malformation related to maternal DCS.
    - Teratogenic effects of pressure – oxygen? nitrogen? dive-related medications? bubble formation? other effects?
    - Recompression treatment – exceptional exposure to hyperbaric oxygen.
    - Decompression – bubbles – birth defects.
  - Late pregnancy.
    - Premature delivery.
- Decompression – stillbirth.

Perhaps the greatest concern of any mother is that some behaviour or activity in which she indulges may harm the foetus. Many women may dive unaware that they may be pregnant (i.e. before their first missed period), and it is this early stage when vital organogenesis is occurring.

Maternal factors

During the first trimester, and especially between the sixth and twelfth weeks, there is a variable but definite increased incidence of nausea, vomiting, gastric reflux and a propensity to seasickness. These conditions may contribute to diving accidents and deaths (see Chapter 46).

From the fourth month onward, there tend to be fluid retention and mucosal swelling, thereby making the middle ear and sinus equalization process more difficult and potentially predisposing to barotrauma.

During pregnancy, there is a progressive interference with respiratory function. The pregnant uterus pushes upward, impairing the downward excursion of the diaphragm, reducing functional residual capacity and reducing overall compliance of the respiratory apparatus. The mother's basal metabolic rate and oxygen consumption are higher than in non-pregnant women, thereby resulting in greater carbon dioxide production and mandating greater respiratory minute volumes to eliminate the carbon dioxide. This is largely achieved through a significant increase in respiratory rate. These respiratory changes may reduce the woman's ability to cope with strenuous activity.

There are also significant changes in cardiovascular function, with blood volume and cardiac output progressively increasing through pregnancy. This hyperdynamic circulation may alter the perfusion of some organs and, along with fluid retention, may change inert gas uptake and elimination kinetics. This factor, along with the hypercoagulability that accompanies pregnancy, may increase the risk of DCS in the mother, but this is entirely speculative. Uterine blood flow may be compromised during periods of increased exercise and increased sympathetic activity, both of which occur during diving.

The change in shape of a pregnant woman may have unfortunate implications. The wetsuit must be altered to ensure that there is not an increase in abdominal tension, which will push the diaphragm even further up into the thoracic cavity and aggravate the respiratory difficulties. The weight gain and the change in posture cause the woman to be more unbalanced. Weight belts are difficult to position, and exits from the water are more difficult.

During the last 3 months, some pregnant women 'leak' through the membranes of the foetus into the vagina without being aware of it. They presume that this slight discharge is normal. Unfortunately, should sea water gain entry to the womb, it would carry the danger of infection and/or premature labor.

Effects on the foetus

The effects of bubble formation on the foetus have not been completely elucidated, with conflicting results in animal experiments. Long-standing opinion[14] is that bubbles are less likely to form in the foetus than in the mother, but foetal bubbles have been found in the absence of maternal DCS. In other words, the absence of DCS symptoms in the mother does not exclude formation of bubbles in the foetus. Bubbles in the foetus are likely to be more ominous than in the mother because of differences in foetal anatomy and physiology.

The lungs in an adult act as an effective bubble filter, whereas in the foetus most of the blood circumvents the lungs by passing through the ductus arteriosus and patent foramen ovale. Therefore, any bubbles in the foetal blood may pass directly to the cerebral circulation. Animal studies have shown an increased rate of foetal loss when the mother is exposed to a decompression insult. The impression is this – the closer to term, the greater the risk.

Investigation of the Ama, the free diving women of Korea, suggested that both hypoxia and bubble production were potential problems for the foetus under certain conditions[15]. The breath-holding Ama divers who dived up until a few days before childbirth had a 44.6 per cent incidence of prematurity, with an infant weighing less than 2.5 kg (compared with 15.8 per cent in the non-diving women from the same district)[15]. The rate of stillbirth, however, was lower among the Ama.

In 1977, Susan Bangasser[16] followed up a group of women who were pregnant when they were diving. Approximately 72 women were questioned, and it was found that more than one third stopped diving during the first trimester (when they found out they were pregnant) and more than one third stopped in the second trimester mainly because of their increased size, but 20 per cent continued diving. Most were very seasoned and competent divers. The deepest dive was 55 meters, and 5 decompression dives were performed. All babies delivered were normal; however, there were some complications: 1 premature birth, 1 septic abortion, 2 miscarriages and 2 caesarian sections.

Bolton[17] conducted a retrospective survey of 208 female divers of whom 136 dived in pregnancy. The average depth of dives was 13 meters, and 24 women dived to 30 meters during the first trimester of pregnancy. The frequency of birth defects was significantly greater in pregnancies during which females dived (5.5 per cent compared with 0 per cent), but this incidence was still within the range of the normal population. The data were also not analyzed with reference to maternal age, a known factor contributing to birth defects.

Turner and Unsworth[18] reported the case of a mother who dived 20 times in 15 days during the end of the first trimester of pregnancy. Most dives were 18 meters or less, but 3 were to 30 meters, and 1 dive was to 33 meters. There were no diving accidents, although there was a single episode of rapid ascent. The only medication used was pseudoephedrine on 2 or 3 occasions. The foetus had unusual malformations, and the embryopathic timetable would suggest that the damage was done around day 40 to 45. She dived between the fortieth and fifty-fifth days. Abnormalities in the foetus included a unilateral ptosis (drooping eyelid), a small tongue, micrognathia (a small lower jaw) and a short neck. The penis was adherent to the scrotum. The fingers were in fixed flexion with webbing between them, and the thumb was abnormal. The hip joints were dysplastic and had a reduced range of movement. One hip was dislocated. There were flexion deformities of the knees and other abnormalities of the feet. Arthrogryposis was present and presumed to result from either muscle disease or abnormalities of the cells forming the anterior root ganglion, so the same embryopathic timetable may be applicable.

A Scandinavian study by Bakkevig and colleagues[19] was conducted on 100 pregnancies in divers, 34 in which diving was continued and 66 in which it was not. The diving exposures were associated with 5 birth defects, and the non-diving exposure was associated with 1 birth defect. The incidence of infant anomalies was thus 15 per cent in the diving group and 1.5 per cent in the non-diving divers. None of the divers had DCS, and the incidence of other pregnancy-related problems was the same in each group.

Another potential problem for the foetus is oxygen toxicity. Diving on compressed air exposes the foetus to an increased partial pressure of oxygen, and the mainstay of treatment regimens for diving accidents is recompression on 100 per cent oxygen. In the foetus, ductus arteriosus blood flow decreases dramatically when the oxygen tension in the pulmonary circulation increases. The foetal pulmonary bed is hypersensitive to oxygen tension and responds with vasodilatation when the oxygen tension rises. There is consequently a shift from a foetal to a neonatal blood flow pattern[1]. This shift reverses when the oxygen tension falls, but it is unknown whether this has long-term sequelae for the foetus. Hyperbaric oxygen therapy (HBOT) in pregnancy has been used liberally in Russia, although the outcomes of such therapy are not

well reported. In the Western world, HBOT has been used in the treatment of carbon monoxide poisoning in pregnant women without reported complications.

There are no reports in the diving literature of air embolism affecting a pregnant diver. Taylor[2] reported 15 cases of air embolism from sexual encounters, all occurring in young women in their second or third trimester in whom air was forcibly blown into the vagina. In 12 of the 15 cases, there was maternal and foetal death. One patient was treated with HBOT for 39 hours, with resultant moderate neurological defects in the mother and a stillborn infant. It was concluded that air embolism of the uteroplacental bed appears lethal.

Marine envenomation carries undefined foetal toxic effects, and specific antitoxins may also hold risks for the foetus.

Post-partum factors

There are no contraindications to women diving while breast feeding. However, it is generally recommended that women not dive until 6 weeks post partum, to avoid intrauterine infection.

Recommendations

In 1978, the Undersea Medical Society held a workshop on this subject, and it was recommended that, until further studies were made, women who are or who may be pregnant should be discouraged from diving.[20] The conclusion, supported in the Society's symposium on women in diving in 1986,[21] was as follows:

- Diving can increase the incidence of birth defects.
- Foetal resistance to bubble formation (DCS) is offset by the dire consequences of this.
- Maternal DCS late in pregnancy entails a higher risk of stillbirth. The risk may be increased by recompression.

There are insufficient hard data to state unequivocally that diving will produce danger to the foetus, but there is some evidence suggesting that this could be so. A 9-month respite from diving seems a small price to pay for improved certainty of a healthy child. Alternately, a birth defect possibly caused by diving would be a heavy burden, outweighing any benefit that diving in pregnancy could possibly confer. With this said, a history of diving during an undiscovered pregnancy is not an indication for termination of pregnancy. The woman should be advised to cease diving henceforth and reassured that most pregnancies in women actively diving are normal.

MAMMARY IMPLANTS

Vann and associates[20] exposed mammary implants to various simulated dive profiles, followed by altitude exposures to simulate aircraft travel. The implants were observed for bubble formation and volume changes. Minimal volume changes occurred after each dive, although numerous bubbles formed, reaching their maximal size in 3 hours. When the implants were exposed to high altitude following a dive, significant volume changes occurred. The volume changes were least for saline and greatest for gel saline implants. The investigators concluded that bubble formation in breast implants may occur after shallow saturation diving, but it is unlikely to result in tissue damage. However, prolonged deep saturation diving followed immediately by flying in an unpressurized aircraft at 30 000 feet (a highly unlikely situation) should be avoided because the resultant bubble formation may be of sufficient magnitude for tissue trauma to occur.

REFERENCES

1. Richardson D. Training scuba divers: a fatality and risk analysis. In: Vann RD, Lang MA, eds. *Recreational Diving Fatalities. Proceedings of the Divers Alert Network 2010 April 8–10 Workshop*. Durham, North Carolina: Divers Alert Network; 2011:119–164.
2. Taylor MB. Women and diving. In: Bove AA, Davis JC, eds. *Diving Medicine*. 2nd ed. Philadelphia: Saunders; 1990.
3. Park YS, Lee KS, Paik KS, *et al*. Korean woman divers revisited: current status of cold adaptation. *Undersea Biomedical Research* 1981;**1**(Suppl):25.
4. Brown E. The Michigan Sea Grant Program. Women diver survey: preliminary results. In: *Proceedings PADI Women in Diving Seminar*. Santa Ana, CA: Professional Association of Diving Instructors; 1977.
5. Rudge FW. Relationship of menstrual history to altitude chamber decompression sickness. *Aviation, Space, and Environmental Medicine* 1990;**61**:657–659.
6. Lee V, St. Leger Dowse M. Decompression illness and the menstrual cycle. In: Fife CE, St. Leger Dowse M, eds. *Women and Pressure*. Flagstaff, Arizona: Best Publishing; 2010:69–80.
7. Murad F, Haynes RC. Estrogens and progestins. In: Gilman AG, Goodman LS, Rall TW, Murad F, eds. *Goodman's and Gilman's The Pharmacological Basis of Therapeutics*. 7th ed. New York: Macmillan; 1985.
8. Basset BE. Safe diving equals fun diving: prescriptions for diving women. *South Pacific Underwater Medicine Society Journal* 1979;**9**(1):9–14.
9. Bangasser S. Decompression sickness in women. In: Fife W, ed. *Women in Diving*. UHMS workshop no. 35. Kensington, Maryland: Undersea Hyperbaric Medical Society; 1987.
10. Zwingelberg KM, Knight MA, Biles JB. Decompression sickness in women divers. *Undersea Biomedical Research* 1987;**14**(4):311–317.
11. Dowse MSt.L, Bryson P, Gunby A, Fife W. Men and women in diving: a retrospective survey. Rates of decompression illness in males and females. In: Marroni A, Oriani G, Wattel F, eds. *Proceedings of the International Joint Meeting on Hyperbaric and Underwater Medicine*. Milan, Italy: European Underwater Biomedical Society; 1996.
12. Webb JT, Kannan N, Pilmanis AA. Gender not a factor for altitude-induced decompression sickness risk. *Aviation, Space, and Environmental Medicine* 2003;**74**(1):2–10.
13. Lanphier EH. Pregnancy and diving. In: Fife W, ed. *Women in Diving*. UHMS workshop no. 35. Kensington, Maryland: Undersea Hyperbaric Medical Society; 1987.

14. Fife CE, Fife WP. Should pregnant women scuba dive? A review of the literature. *Journal of Travel Medicine* 1994;**1**:160–165.

15. Harashima S, Iwasaki S. Occupational diseases of the Ama. In: Rahn H, Yokoyama T, eds. *The Physiology of Breathhold Diving and the Ama of Japan*. National Academy of Sciences publication 1341. Washington, DC: National Academy Press, 1965.

16. Bangasser S. Pregnant diver update. *South Pacific Underwater Medicine Society Journal* 1978;**8**(3–4):86–87, 98.

17. Bolton ME. Scuba diving and fetal well-being: a survey of 208 women. *Undersea Biomedical Research* 1980;**7**(3):183–189.

18. Turner G, Unsworth I. Intrauterine bends? *The Lancet* 1982;**1**(8277):905.

19. Bakkevig MK, Bolstad G, Holmberg G, Ornhagen H. Diving during pregnancy. In: *Proceedings of the 15th Annual Meeting of the EUBS*. Eilat, Israel: European Underwater and Baromedical Society; 1989.

20. Kent MB (ed). Effects of Diving on Pregnancy. 19th Undersea and Hyperbaric Medical Society Workshop. UHMS Publication Number 36(EDP)1-31-80. Kensington, MD: Undersea and Hyperbaric Medical Society; 1978.

21. Fife W (ed). Women in Diving. 35th Undersea and Hyperbaric Medical Society Workshop. UHMS Publication Number 71(WS-WD)3-15-87. Kensington, MD: Undersea and Hyperbaric Medical Society; 198119871987.

22. Vann RD, Riefkohl R, Georgiade GS, Georgiade NG. Mammary implants, diving and altitude exposure. *Plastic and Reconstructive Surgery* 1988;**81**(2):200–203.

This chapter was reviewed for this fifth edition by Simon Mitchell.

61

Breath-hold diving

INTRODUCTION

Breath-hold diving is also called snorkel diving and free diving. The illnesses mentioned here are described in much greater detail in other specific chapters of this text, and Chapter 52 deals with the medical standards usually applied.

Traditional breath-hold divers include the female shell divers of Japan (Ama) and Korea (Hae-Nyo), the sea-men (Katsugi) of Japan, the sponge divers of Greece, the pearl divers of the Tuamotu archipelago and Bahrain and the underwater warriors of Persian King Xerxes in the fifth century BC. More recently, the abalone and paua divers of the United States and New Zealand, spear fishers worldwide and submarine escape tank attendants of the United States, Europe and Australia illustrate the diversity and dangers of this type of diving.

The number of professional breath-hold divers in Korea and Japan has remained steady at about 20 000. The numbers of abalone and paua divers have remained fairly constant, probably only a few hundred, because of the dwindling supply of this natural resource. The pearl divers of the Tuamotu Archipelago, the Middle East and the Torres Strait, as well as the sponge divers of Greece, no longer have a viable existence. Compressed air diving, including scuba and surface supply, have dominated the occupational activities associated in the past with breath-hold diving.

The recreational snorkellers of Australia are now a major part of the tourist industry of the Great Barrier Reef. Similar explosions of population are seen in the Caribbean, Indo-Pacific Islands and the Mediterranean.

Recreational snorkelling became one of the most widely embraced sports of the latter part of the twentieth century, and thus the risks associated with this type of diving are becoming better appreciated.

A small group of adventurers have extended the depths, as well as the techniques and parameters, of deep breath-hold diving. Sometimes, the descents and/or ascents are assisted by weights or floats. Sometimes, the breathing gases or techniques are modified. With these complexities come added risks, outside the scope of this text.

FATALITY STATISTICS

There are few well-documented series. Walker[1] described 90 snorkelling deaths between 1972 and 1987, although many had no forensic assessment. Edmonds and Walker[2] described 60 between 1987 and 1996, all of which had coroners' inquiries and/or autopsy investigations. Lippmann and Pearn[3] described 130, up until 2006.

The causes of death were as follows:

- Cardiac – 30 to 45 per cent
- Surface drowning – 25 to 45 per cent
- Hypoxia from breath-holding, leading to drowning – 15 to 20 per cent
- Trauma – 8 per cent

These three series were compared. There was a change in the demographical factors in that the later snorkellers were significantly older, with a higher proportion of women than previously. The three major causes of death were drowning, cardiac disorders and hypoxia from hyperventilation and/or ascent producing drowning. Other causes included deaths from marine animals and trauma.

Tourists were overrepresented in both the surface drowning and the cardiac groups. Inexperience, medical and physical unfitness, equipment and environmental factors contributed to the deaths in these two groups. Adverse environmental factors (e.g. currents and choppy surface conditions) were contributors in 15 per cent of the deaths. The absence of fins in 40 per cent made coping with aquatic conditions much more difficult.

The surface drowning cases usually occurred in situations in which supervision was inadequate and therefore rescue and resuscitation were delayed.

The snorkellers with cardiac-related cases often died very quietly in calm, still water, and these deaths were frequently predictable from the cardiovascular history and the physical and aquatic unfitness of these snorkellers.

The deaths in younger, fitter, experienced divers were more related to the production of cerebral hypoxia after hyperventilation and breath-holding, often occurring during ascent and associated with spear fishing or underwater endurance attempts (see Chapter 16).

MARINE ENVIRONMENTS

Like all other divers, breath-hold divers are susceptible to the hazards of the marine environment. These include injuries from marine animals, infections and envenomations. They include exposure to water currents, water temperatures less than thermoneutral (35°C) and the various drowning syndromes, including salt water aspiration, near drowning and immersion pulmonary oedema. Motion sickness is a common problem, as are trauma (e.g. from ocean currents, rocks, boats) and entrapment (see Chapters 5, 21 to 24, 26 to 28, 31 and 32).

EQUIPMENT PROBLEMS

Some hazards are related to the equipment worn by the free diver (e.g. mask, snorkel, fins), together with the problems of entrapment and the use of spear guns, floats and boats. These hazards are no different in principle from those encountered by scuba divers, but the disadvantage for the free diver is that a supply of air is not available to the diver underwater in his or her attempt to overcome the problems. This is especially so with the increased danger from entrapment and entanglement in lines (e.g. floats, spears). Some of the modern mono-filament fishing lines cannot be snapped or even cut by a knife. A scuba diver has much more time to cope with such difficulties.

The most common equipment problems include the absence of fins, flooding of the face mask and restriction from snorkel breathing with exertion. The reduction in maximum voluntary ventilation and the increase in the work of breathing produce dyspnoea when the respiratory demands are great (see Chapters 3 and 4).

DYSBARIC DISEASES

Barotrauma

Barotraumas of descent are more common in free divers than in scuba divers because of the rushed nature of this activity. Free divers have so little time that they have to descend more rapidly and often without as much attention to the early symptoms that indicate barotrauma. They also experience more ascents and descents, thereby producing more barotraumas.

Following barotrauma of descent, there is often an associated barotrauma of ascent. This is especially seen in otological, sinus, dental and gastrointestinal barotraumas. Ascent cannot be delayed, or even slowed, and so the manifestations cannot be diminished – as with scuba (see Chapters 7 to 9).

Pulmonary barotrauma of descent (lung squeeze) is rare, but it is mostly seen in breath-hold divers (see Chapter 6).

More recently, the practice of 'lung packing' or glossopharyngeal insufflation, used by free divers to prolong their underwater endurance or increase their depth capability, has been associated with pulmonary barotrauma and arterial gas embolism.

Decompression sickness

Decompression sickness has also been postulated as a sequel of intensive free diving.

Perusal of Cross's original report[4] would indicate that many of the cases could have been caused by a variety of other disorders (e.g. inner ear barotrauma, salt water aspiration, near drowning causing hypoxic encephalopathy and drowning).

The reason that decompression sickness can develop with breath-hold diving is that the nitrogen pressure in the lungs increases with depth, and with the greater depths there is a greater nitrogen partial pressure, with nitrogen diffusing from the lungs into the bloodstream and thence to the tissues. If the surface interval is inadequate to eliminate this nitrogen, then the nitrogen will accumulate with repeated dives throughout the day.

Paulev[5], a Danish submarine escape tank diver in the Norwegian Navy, performed 60 breath-hold dives to 20 metres in 5 hours, each lasting about 2.5 minutes, with surface intervals of less than 2 minutes. He developed symptoms consistent with decompression sickness. Other submarine escape instructors have suffered similar problems in both Norway and Australia. Unfortunately, many of these divers were also exposed to compressed air breathing – either in chambers or air pockets in the escape tanks – while they waited for the submarine escape trainees to emerge.

Taravana

Cross[4] described an illness called Taravana (*tara,* to fall; *vana,* crazily) in the pearl divers of the Tuamotu Archipelago. The dives were to 30 to 40 metres, lasting 1.5 to 2.5 minutes each, over a

7-hour period, with 20 per cent of divers developing symptoms. The illness, which was characterized by vertigo, nausea, hypoaesthesias, paresis, unconsciousness and death, could have been caused by decompression sickness in some of the cases.

There is no doubt regarding the possible cerebral damage that can be produced by multiple breath-hold dives, possibly with short surface intervals. Although still open to question, there is a possibility that these cases may reflect release of gas from supersaturation, thus producing decompression sickness, arterial gas embolism from pulmonary barotrauma or other causes of hypoxia. Taravana is popularly believed to be the result of acute decompression illness, even though venous bubbles are not readily detected following breath-hold dives. The symptoms are especially cerebral in nature and may involve multiple sites – as demonstrated clinically and by magnetic resonance imaging.

HYPOXIC BLACKOUT

Hypoxic blackout, which encompasses the contributions of hyperventilation and then breath-holding, exertion and the hypoxia of ascent, is fully described in Chapter 16.

Despite this traditional cause of hypoxia, probably the most common cause in free divers is panic or the aspiration of salt water, resulting in near drowning and drowning states (see Chapters 21 to 24).

CARDIAC DISORDERS

Human breath-hold divers produce dramatic bradycardia from the diving reflex. It reaches its maximum effect in 20 to 30 seconds, usually to two thirds the pre-dive level, but sometimes to less than 10 beats/minute in experienced divers. It bears a linear relationship with the water temperature below 15°C and a non-linear relationship at higher water temperatures. The bradycardia may well allow for other arrhythmias to develop. The arterial blood pressure seems to increase with the diving reflex in humans, and the diving response is augmented by fear.

In humans, unlike most of the other diving mammals, free diving is associated with significant cardiac arrhythmias. These arrhythmias can also occur with related respiratory manoeuvres such as deep inspiration, prolonged inspiration, breath-holding, release of breath-holding and the Valsalva manoeuvre.

In a study of Korean women divers, the incidence of cardiac arrhythmias was 43 per cent in the summer (water temperature, 27°C) as compared with 72 per cent in the winter (water temperature, 10°C).

There is a high frequency of arrhythmias from immersion breath-holding, even without diving.

The head-out immersion position increases the workload on the heart because of the negative pressure effect (the intrapulmonary pressure remains at 1 ATA, whereas a negative pressure, needed to inhale, is approximately –20 cm H_2O). There is a reduction in the functional residual capacity of the lungs, an increased work of breathing and an increase in the intrathoracic blood volume, with a corresponding dilatation of the heart, especially the right atrium. The immersion diuresis and associated loss of sodium may perpetuate cardiac problems.

With deep breath-hold dives, the peripheral circulation replaces some of the residual volume of the lungs because of the effect of Boyle's Law, contracting the total lung volume to less than the residual. Then up to a litre of extra blood can fill the pulmonary circuit and the heart. The distension of the right atrium may be a major cause of arrhythmias taking over from sinus rhythm.

The relatively high incidence of cardiac deaths during snorkelling (and scuba diving) activities may be partly related to the foregoing physiological changes and partly caused by the excessive workload experienced by novice snorkellers. This excessive workload eventuates when they attempt to overcome the stressful influences of panic, adverse tidal currents and negative buoyancy (see Chapter 56).

PULMONARY DISORDERS

The most common lung disease is the aspiration of sea water. This either produces the drowning syndromes (see Chapters 21 to 24) or provokes asthma in those so inclined.

The changes in lung volumes with the head-out position are described earlier, with the pooling of blood in the thorax, thus reducing respiratory capability.

Pulmonary oedema has been described in association with immersion, as have other causes of dyspnoea including coronary artery disease, cardiac arrhythmia, cold-induced hypertension and cold allergy (see Chapters 30, 42 and 56).

GASTROINTESTINAL PROBLEMS

The pressure gradients associated with the head-out immersion position, commonly experienced in free divers between dives, causes an increased gastroesophageal pressure gradient, from 6 mm Hg in air to 16 mm Hg during immersion. This predisposes to gastric reflux in those susceptible to it and with an inadequate oesophageal sphincter.

This also increases the tendency to vomiting, which can be aggravated by other factors such as alcohol intake, seasickness, salt water aspiration, otological and gastrointestinal barotrauma and Valsalva manoeuvers performed in the inverted position.

REFERENCES

1. Walker DG. The investigation of critical factors in diving related fatalities. Published annually in the South Pacific Underwater Medical Society Journal 1972–1989.
2. Edmonds C, Walker D. Snorkeling deaths in Australia. *Medical Journal of Australia* 1999;**171:**591–594.
3. Lippmann JM, Pearn JH. Snorkeling-related deaths in Australia 1994–2006. *Medical Journal of Australia* 2012;**197**(4):230–232.
4. Cross ER. Taravana: diving syndrome in the Tuamotu diver. In: Rahn H, Yokoyama T, eds. *Physiology of Breath-Hold Diving and the Ama of Japan.* National Academy of Sciences publication 1341. Washington, DC: National Academy Press; 1965:207–219.

5. Paulev P. Decompression sickness following repeated breath-hold dives. In: Rahn H, Yokoyama T, eds. *Physiology of Breath-Hold Diving and the Ama of Japan.* National Academy of Sciences publication 1341. Edited by H. Rahn. Washington, DC: National Academy Press; 1965:211–226.

FURTHER READING

Cross ER. Taravana: diving syndrome in the Tuamotu diver. In: Rahn H, Yokoyama T, eds. *Physiology of Breath-Hold Diving and the Ama of Japan.* National Academy of Sciences publication 1341. Washington, DC: National Academy Press; 1965:207–219.

Edmonds C. Snorkel diving: a review. *South Pacific Underwater Medicine Society Journal* 1999;**29**(4):196–202.

Edmonds C, McKenzie B, Thomas R, Pennefather J. *Diving Medicine for Scuba Divers.* 5th ed. 2013. Free download at www.divingmedicine.info

Edmonds C, Walker D. Snorkeling deaths in Australia. *Medical Journal of Australia* 1999;**171**:591–594.

Lippmann JM, Pearn JH. Snorkeling-related deaths in Australia 1994–2006. *Medical Journal of Australia* 2012;**197**(4):230–232.

Hayward JS, Hay C, Mathews BR, Overweel CH, Radford DD. Temperature effects on the human dive response in relation to cold-water near drowning. *Journal of Applied Physiology* 1984;**56**:202–206.

Hickey DD, Lundgren CEG. Breath-hold diving. In: Shilling CW, Carlstrom CB, Mathias RA, eds. *The Physician's Guide to Diving Medicine.* New York: Plenum Press; 1984:206–221.

Hong SK, Wong SH, Kim PK, Suh CS. Seasonal observations on the cardiac rhythm during diving in the Korean Ama. *Journal of Applied Physiology* 1967;**23**:18–22.

Hong SK. Breath-hold diving. In: Bove AA, Davis JC, eds. *Diving Medicine.* 2nd ed. Philadelphia: Saunders; 1990.

Hong SK. Hae-Nyo, the diving women of Korea. In: Rahn H, Yokoyama T, eds. *Physiology of Breath-Hold Diving and the Ama of Japan.* National Academy of Sciences publication 1341. Washington, DC: National Academy Press; 1965:99–111.

Kohshi K, Katoh T, Abe H, Okudera T. Neurological diving accidents in Japanese breath-hold divers: a preliminary report. *Journal of Occupational Health* 2001;**43**:56–60.

Kohshi K, Wong RM, Abe H, Katoh T, Okudera T, Mano Y. Neurological manifestations in Japanese Ama divers. *Undersea and Hyperbaric Medicine* 2005;**32**:11–20.

Lamb LE, Dermksian G, Sarnoff CA. Significant cardiac arrhythmia induced by common respiratory maneuvers. *American Journal of Cardiology* 1958;**2**:563–571.

Lin Y-C. Physiological limitations of humans as breath-hold divers. In: Lin Y-C, Shida KK, eds. *Man in the Sea.* Vol. 2. Honolulu, Hawaii: University of Hawaii Press; 1990.

Lundgren C. Physiological challenges of breath-hold diving. *UHMS Annual Meeting*, Boston. 1999.

Park YS, Shiraki K, Hong SK. Energetics of breath-hold diving in Korean and Japanese professional diving. In: Lin Y-C, Shida KK, eds. *Man in the Sea.* Vol 2. Honolulu, Hawaii: University of Hawaii Press; 1990.

Paulev P. Decompression sickness following repeated breath-hold dives. In: Rahn H, Yokoyama T, eds. *Physiology of Breath-Hold Diving and the Ama of Japan.* National Academy of Sciences publication 1341. Edited by H. Rahn. Washington, DC: National Academy Press; 1965:211–226.

Rahn H, Yokoyama T, eds. *Physiology of Breath-Hold Diving and the Ama of Japan.* National Academy of Sciences publication 1341. Washington, DC: National Academy Press; 1965.

Sasamoto H. The electrocardiogram pattern of the diving Ama. In: Rahn H, Yokoyama T, eds. *Physiology of Breath-Hold Diving of the Ama of Japan.* National Academy of Sciences publication 1341. Washington DC: National Academy Press; 1965:271–280.

Scholander PF, Hammel H, LeMessurier H, Hemingsen E, Garey W. Circulatory adjustment in pearl divers. *Journal of Applied Physiology* 1962;**17:**184–190.

Shilling CW, Werts MF, Schandelmeier NR. Man in the ocean environment. In: Shilling CW, Werts MF, Schandelmeier NR, eds. *The Underwater Handbook.* New York: Plenum Press; 1976.

Tamaki H, Kiyotaka K, Shuichi S, *et al.* Breath-hold diving and cerebral DCI. *Undersea and Hyperbaric Medicine* 2010;**37:**7–11.

This chapter was reviewed for this fifth edition by Carl Edmonds.

62

Technical diving

INTRODUCTION

Arguably the most significant trend in recreational diving practice to have emerged since the 1980s is the growth in the use of so-called 'technical diving' methods. A description of technical divers' motivations, 'language' and methods will provide medical personnel with a good platform for more productive interactions, and this is what this chapter attempts to provide. It must be understood, however, that this chapter is not intended to be a technical diving manual, nor is it a detailed educational resource for trained technical divers.

There has been much debate over which diving techniques should be referred to as 'technical diving' and which should not. This is because techniques such as diving using nitrox have now become so mainstream that some technical divers no longer consider they deserve the 'technical' designation. For the purposes of this chapter, however, we consider technical diving to include dives that *intentionally breach no-decompression limits ('decompression diving'), use gases other than air (including nitrox) or use equipment other than single-cylinder open-circuit scuba.*

LIMITATIONS OF RECREATIONAL SCUBA AIR DIVING

Single-cylinder scuba air diving as taught to entry-level recreational divers imposes limitations on depth and duration that have fueled the trend toward the development and use of technical diving methods. These limits are the breathing gas supply, no-decompression limits, cold, nitrogen narcosis, oxygen toxicity and the work of breathing.

Breathing gas supply

Conventional scuba diving is conducted with a single cylinder of air. More specific examples are discussed later, but typically these cylinders have internal volumes of around 12 litres, and they are filled to pressures around 200 ATA. If we assume that a diver consumes about 20 litres of air per minute during 'normal' finning at the surface, then the time the diver could spend finning at 90 metres

(10 ATA), irrespective of air's unsuitability at this depth for other reasons (see later), is given by the following equation:

$$\text{Duration} = \text{Volume of gas carried (litres)} \div \text{Gas consumption (litres/minute)}$$

$$= (200 \text{ ATA} \times 12 \text{ litres}) \div (20 \text{ litres/minute} \times 10 \text{ ATA}) = 12 \text{ minutes}$$

This calculation does not account for descent and ascent time, and it assumes that the diver is happy to breathe the cylinder down until it is essentially empty, which is clearly not the case. The point is that single-cylinder air diving significantly limits the duration of deeper dives.

No-decompression limits

No-decompression limits become progressively shorter as depth increases, to the point where beyond about 40 metres it is virtually impossible to perform no-decompression dives. Deeper dives require planning for decompression and therefore become 'technical'.

Cold

Depending on the water temperature, and the quality of the thermal protection employed, cold may become a limiting factor on dive duration.

Nitrogen narcosis

The narcotic effect of the nitrogen in air becomes increasingly prominent at depths beyond 30 to 40 metres (see Chapter 15).

Oxygen toxicity

As depth increases, the inspired partial pressure of oxygen (PIO_2) in the respired air increases. If this rises much above 1.3 ATA, then there is a rapidly increasing risk of cerebral oxygen toxicity (see Chapter 17). Frequently, the first manifestations are loss of consciousness and a seizure, which will often lead to death by drowning. We can calculate

the ambient pressure at which an air-breathing diver will be breathing 1.3 ATA of oxygen by dividing 1.3 by the fraction of oxygen in air:

$$1.3 \div 0.21 = 6.2 \text{ ATA } (= 52\text{-metre depth})$$

Thus, if the maximum PIO_2 is 1.3 ATA, then the maximum operating depth (MOD) for air is 52 metres, and its use should be limited to depths no greater than this.

Work of breathing

At all depths, air must be supplied by the regulator at ambient pressure to facilitate breathing. Air supplied at greater pressure is denser by definition, and it does not flow as freely through the tubes and orifices of the regulator, or through the lungs for that matter. It follows that the work required of the respiratory muscles to initiate and maintain normal air flow (the 'work of breathing'), increases as depth increases. Because air is a 'heavy' gas, this can become very noticeable at extreme depth. Indeed, it would become exhausting to perform significant work at extreme depths while breathing air.

TECHNICAL DIVING TECHNIQUES

Individual technical diving techniques have evolved to address one or more of the foregoing limitations. Some of these techniques are primarily intended to enhance duration, whereas others are specifically targeted at extending the depth range. Most often, several of the techniques discussed here are combined to facilitate longer dives beyond the recreational depth range. Such dives would be dangerous at best, or simply impossible, if they were performed using conventional single-tank scuba air diving.

Nitrox diving

Nitrox diving is probably the most widely used technical diving method, although, as intimated earlier, its use is so widespread that many divers no longer refer to it as 'technical'. The term 'nitrox' refers to mixtures of oxygen and nitrogen in which there is more oxygen than found in air. For this reason, nitrox is often referred to as 'enriched air' or 'enriched air – nitrox' (EANx). By convention, the mix is described by reference to its oxygen content. Thus, if a nitrox mix contains 36 per cent oxygen, then it is referred to as 'nitrox 36' ('Nx36') or 'EANx36'. The use of nitrox confers several advantages.

REDUCED UPTAKE OF NITROGEN

Because the amount of nitrogen taken up into the diver's blood and tissues during a dive is proportional to the inspired partial pressure of nitrogen (PN_2), any reduction in the inspired fraction of nitrogen (FN_2) will reduce the amount of nitrogen absorbed. This can be illustrated by consideration of Table 62.1, which compares the approximate PN_2 breathed by an air diver and a diver using nitrox 40 over a range of depths. A striking feature of these data is that the nitrox 40 diver is breathing the same PN_2 (2.4 ATA) at 30 metres as the air diver at 20 metres (see shaded cells). It follows that with respect to nitrogen absorption, the nitrox 40 diver at 30 metres is at an 'equivalent air depth' (EAD) of 20 metres.

This reduction of nitrogen absorption during nitrox diving is an advantage that can be used in one of two ways.

First, the nitrox diver can use the reduced absorption of nitrogen to increase allowable dive time by using the EAD to derive the no-decompression limit for the dive or as a basis for calculating decompression. This approach allows longer dives and shorter decompression. Alternatively, the nitrox diver can ignore this potential for increasing duration and assume that he or she is using air for the purposes of bottom time calculation. This has the advantage of widening the safety margin for avoiding decompression sickness (DCS). Some occupational diving groups such as diving instructors or aquaculture divers, whose work involves potential risk factors for DCS such as multiple ascents, use nitrox in this way.

Another often reported advantage of nitrox diving presumed to be associated with reduced nitrogen uptake is a reduced level of post-dive fatigue. However, in the only evaluation of this phenomenon in which fatigue was objectively measured and the divers were blinded to the gas they were breathing, no difference between nitrox and air diving was found[1].

ACCELERATED ELIMINATION OF NITROGEN

In addition to reducing nitrogen uptake at depth, nitrox breathing also hastens nitrogen elimination during decompression (in comparison to air) because a steeper gradient for nitrogen elimination between body tissues and the lungs is established if more oxygen is breathed. This phenomenon is useful for reducing the length of decompression stops during decompression diving, and the discussion returns to this subject later.

Table 62.1 Inspired pressures of nitrogen at various depths when breathing air and nitrox 40[a]

Depth	Ambient pressure (ATA)	PN_2 in air (ATA) (FN_2 = 0.8)	PN_2 in nitrox 40 (ATA) (FN_2 = 0.6)
Surface	1	0.8	0.6
10 metres	2	1.6	1.2
20 metres	3	**2.4**	1.8
30 metres	4	3.2	**2.4**

[a] Inspired pressures of nitrogen at various depths when breathing air and nitrox 40. Note 1: for simplicity, the % of nitrogen in air is rounded to 80% and the fraction of nitrogen (FN_2) in air therefore equals 0.8. Note 2: The inspired partial pressure of oxygen using Nx40 at 30 m would equal 1.6 ATA and most training agencies would not recommend this because of concerns about oxygen toxicity. Nitrox 40 is used here as a mathematically convenient illustration of the potential effect of different on nitrox mixes on the PN_2 breathed at depth.

POSSIBLE REDUCTION IN NITROGEN NARCOSIS

It is frequently argued that because the degree of nitrogen narcosis is directly proportional to the PN_2 breathed, then any reduction in the inspired FN_2 should reduce the narcotic effect. From Table 62.1 one could therefore predict that a nitrox 40 diver at 30 metres would be experiencing the same amount of narcosis as the air diver at 20 metres. A counter argument holds that oxygen may be just as narcotic as nitrogen and that replacing nitrogen with oxygen confers no benefit in this regard. There is evidence that supports both viewpoints to some extent.

Oxygen is more soluble in lipid and therefore has a higher theoretical narcotic potency than nitrogen at an equivalent partial pressure. However, because oxygen is metabolized, its partial pressure in tissues and cells does not rise significantly when it is breathed within the pressure range that can be safely tolerated during diving by humans. Thus, whereas oxygen is theoretically more narcotic than nitrogen, its partial pressure in tissues may not rise sufficiently for this narcotic effect to be apparent, even when more oxygen is substituted for nitrogen in a nitrox mix.

Not surprisingly, then, for mixes containing only nitrogen and oxygen, decreasing the nitrogen-to-oxygen ratio (while remaining within a safe PO_2) does seem to decrease the narcotic effect somewhat, although perhaps by not as much as may be predicted if oxygen is assumed to be completely non-narcotic. For these reasons, although there may be a narcotic difference between nitrox and air, the difference may be too small to notice reliably.

DISADVANTAGES OF NITROX DIVING

Because nitrox contains a higher fraction of oxygen, it actually cannot be safely used for diving as deep as with air. Its advantage in deep diving is as a decompression gas after a helium-containing gas (see later) is used for the deeper phase of the dive. The concept that the PIO_2 limits the depth at which a particular gas may be used arises time and again throughout any discussion of technical diving. Clearly, one of the key aspects, if not *the* key aspect, of nitrox diving is correct planning to ensure that a safe PIO_2 is not exceeded. Calculation of the MOD for a nitrox mix is achieved using the following formula:

$$MOD = ([PO_{2max} \div FO_2] - 1) \times 10$$

Where PO_{2max} = the maximum tolerable PO_2 in ATA and FO_2 = the fraction of oxygen in the mix.

If we use this equation to calculate the maximum depth for use of nitrox 40 so that we avoid exceeding a PIO_2 of 1.3 ATA, then we get:

$$MOD\ metres = ([1.3\ ATA \div 0.4] - 1) \times 10$$
$$= 22.5\ metres$$

Similarly, if we know the depth you want to visit, we can calculate the maximum safe FO_2 in the nitrox mix to be used from:

$$Maximum\ safe\ FO_2 = PO_{2max} \div P_{amb}$$

Where PO_{2max} = the maximum tolerable PO_2 in ATA and P_{amb} = the ambient pressure in ATA.

If we use this equation to plan a dive to 30 metres with a PO_{2max} of 1.3 ATA, then we get:

$$Maximum\ safe\ FO_2 = 1.3\ ATA \div 4\ ATA = 0.325$$

Thus, nitrox 32 is the ideal mix for this dive, to minimize the risk of oxygen toxicity while also minimizing nitrogen absorption.

MANAGING THE OXYGEN EXPOSURE

The foregoing calculations are used to ensure that the maximum safe PIO_2 is not exceeded during diving. Unfortunately, even the chosen 'safe' PO_{2max} becomes less safe the longer it is breathed. Thus, in addition to avoiding exceeding a PO_{2max}, divers must also monitor the duration of exposure in managing the risk of cerebral oxygen toxicity. The higher the PO_2 breathed, the shorter the 'safe' duration over which it can be breathed. There are no guidelines that can claim to be validated against extensive outcome data, but the most extensively used limits are those promulgated by the National Oceanic and Atmospheric Administration (NOAA) for single and 24-hour cumulative exposures. These limits are given in Table 62.2.

Table 62.2 National Oceanic and Atmospheric Administration exposure limits (minutes) over a range of partial pressures of oxygen

PO$_2$ (ATA)	Single exposure (minutes)	24-hour exposure (minutes)
1.6	45	150
1.5	120	180
1.4	150	180
1.3	180	210
1.2	210	240
1.1	240	270
1.0	300	300
0.9	360	360
0.8	450	450
0.7	570	570
0.6	720	720

PO$_2$, partial pressure of oxygen.

These limits are useful in providing some guidance to entry-level technical divers who should minimize risk in their planning. However, extensive experience has shown the limits to have poor positive predictive value for problems if they are exceeded by a resting diver during decompression. This is a common situation on very deep, long technical dives. It must also be observed that seizures have occurred by divers who are clearly diving within the recommended limits. The unfortunate truth is that cerebral oxygen toxicity is very difficult to predict reliably.

MANAGING DECOMPRESSION STATUS

The concept of EAD was introduced earlier when it was deduced from Table 62.1 that it would be valid for the nitrox 40 diver at 30 metres to use the air diving no-decompression limit for 20 metres given that the PN$_2$ breathed in both situations was the same. The EAD can be calculated for any depth and any nitrox mix by using the following formula:

$$EAD \ (m) = ([FN_2 \times \{depth + 10\}] \div 0.79) - 10$$

Where EAD = equivalent air depth in metres, FN$_2$ = the fraction of nitrogen in the nitrox mix, depth = the depth (metres) at which the nitrox is being used and 0.79 = the fraction of nitrogen in air.

Consider, for example, a nitrox 40 dive at 20 metres. The EAD is given by:

$$([0.6 \times \{20 + 10\}] \div 0.79) - 10 = 13 \ metres$$

Therefore, for the purposes of calculating the no-decompression limit, the diver using nitrox 40 at 20 metres can assume that he or she is diving at 13 metres. This results in a significant no-decompression limit advantage. There are various proprietary software packages and computers that factor gas mix characteristics into the decompression plan and produce suitable procedures for any combination of gas, depth and duration of bottom time. Decompression from deeper technical dives is discussed later.

NITROX ANALYSIS

Nitrox is frequently made by blending appropriate proportions of air and oxygen, or by oxygen concentrators that remove some nitrogen from air as cylinders are filled. These are not exact processes, and it is crucial that divers confirm for themselves the mix they are breathing before using it. Analysis for oxygen content is performed using devices with a galvanic cell as the central component. These cells produce an electrical current that, within the range of interest to gas blenders, is linearly proportional to the percentage of oxygen in the gas to which they are exposed. The current is measured and electronically processed, and the result is displayed as a percentage of oxygen content. The galvanic cells themselves cannot be turned off, and they last between 1 and 2 years. The analyzer should be calibrated regularly against air and a known source of 100 per cent oxygen.

Configuration of equipment for longer dives

Both nitrox diving and the other technical diving methods that are yet to be discussed may involve much longer underwater durations than would be possible with the single-cylinder configuration employed by most scuba divers. Therefore, before moving on to a discussion of other techniques, it is logical to consider briefly the changes in equipment configuration used by technical divers to extend their underwater duration.

OPEN-CIRCUIT CYLINDER CONFIGURATIONS

There is a range of cylinders made from both aluminium and steel, with various internal volumes and pressure ratings. Discussing the entire range is beyond the scope of this chapter. However, high-capacity steel cylinders with a slightly higher pressure rating than the most frequently encountered aluminium recreational cylinders are popular with technical divers. Steel cylinders with a working pressure of 232 ATA and water capacity of up to 18 litres are readily available. The compressed gas capacity of such cylinders is therefore 232 ATA × 18 litres = 4176 litres. This compares with the typical aluminium cylinders (working pressure of 207 ATA and water capacity of 11.2 litres), which hold 2318 litres of compressed gas.

With respect to cylinders, a Deutsches Institut für Normung (DIN) cylinder valve into which the regular first stage is screwed (rather than clamped) is popular with technical divers because it allegedly provides increased protection against O-ring failure.

Technical divers frequently use two back-mounted cylinders instead of the conventional single cylinder. Each cylinder has its own regulator and independent submersible pressure gauge, and typically the twin cylinders are 'manifolded'. This means that the two cylinders are linked by a manifold so that they potentially form one large common gas supply. There are three isolation valves in the system: a pillar valve on each cylinder and an isolation valve in the middle of the manifold. In this arrangement, turning off the pillar valve on one of the cylinders isolates the regulator on that side, not the gas in the cylinder. Thus, if the left-hand pillar valve is turned off, the left-hand regulator is isolated and cannot be used, but the right-hand regulator still draws gas from both cylinders. If the manifold isolation valve is closed, then the system is effectively reduced to two separate scuba sets. The reason for this arrangement is to maximize redundancy while coping with common scuba system failures (which usually involve the regulators).

Twin sets effectively double the volume of gas that can be carried conveniently on the back. In some technical diving situations, this still may not be sufficient, or alternatively, different gas mixtures may be carried to allow accelerated decompression (see the later discussion of decompression diving). With the capacity for carrying back-mounted gas fully used, the next option is to use sling tanks.

Sling tanks are usually single scuba cylinders, each with its own independent regulator and submersible pressure gauge. Perhaps the most important issues with respect to the use of sling tanks are clear labeling (with gas mix and MOD) and consistent positioning; especially where the sling tanks are used to carry different gases for different purposes as described in the later section on decompression diving. Many technical diving accidents have occurred as a result of divers' mistakenly using inappropriate gases (usually too oxygen rich) for the depth where they are.

REBREATHERS

The use of rebreather underwater breathing apparatus is another strategy to extend gas supply and improve duration, as discussed later.

EXTENDING THERMAL DURATION

There is little use in carrying sufficient gas for prolonged dives if thermal protection is inadequate to allow that gas supply to be fully exploited. The anticipated temperature and the selection of appropriate thermal protection are important aspects of technical dive planning.

Wetsuits may be adequate in some tropical situations, but drysuits coupled with an appropriate undergarment are frequently used for long technical dives. Divers operating in very cold conditions may also use battery-powered heating vests under the drysuit, especially during long decompressions.

Gas for drysuit inflation must be drawn from one of the cylinders carried by the diver. If the dive involves the use of helium mixtures (see Mixed gas diving), then a mix containing helium should not be used for drysuit inflation because helium readily conducts heat and reduces the efficiency of the drysuit. Air is a good choice, and some divers even carry a small cylinder of argon for drysuit inflation because it has good insulating properties. Controlled studies of this strategy have failed to demonstrate a significant advantage, however. High FO_2 mixes should be avoided in the drysuit, especially if an actively heated undergarment is used. Incidents involving burning undergarments have occurred under these circumstances.

One problem of an extended period in a drysuit is urination. Solutions to this potentially unpleasant problem include the wearing of adult-size absorbent nappies and the use of so-called 'pee valves' that allow urination to the external environment during diving.

Decompression diving

At depths below 40 metres, it becomes virtually impossible to perform dives that do not require decompression stops. To state the obvious, the moment decompression stops become necessary, the option of ascending 'directly' to the surface in a reasonably timely manner has been removed. It follows that the essence of decompression diving is in the planning and safe execution of decompression stops. If these stops are not conducted properly, the risk of DCS rises in proportion to the degree of omitted decompression. In electing to perform decompression dives, the diver must therefore commit himself or herself to a new level of meticulous planning and preparation to minimize the chances of complications.

PLANNING DECOMPRESSION DIVES

The process of planning a decompression dive is a complex business even if mixed gases are not involved (see later). Most plans start with a target depth and desired duration and build from there. By way of a relatively simple example, one may plan a dive to 40 metres for 30 minutes bottom time with air used as the bottom gas with a switch to Nx50 during ascent to accelerate nitrogen elimination and therefore shorten the decompression time. The final stop at 3 metres would be on 100 per cent oxygen for the same purpose.

The first part of any plan like this would be to check that air at 40 metres results in an acceptable PIO_2, and to determine what depth would be appropriate for the switch to Nx50. The PIO_2 at 40 metres using air is 0.21×5 ATA = 1.05 ATA, which is less than the widely adopted maximum of 1.3 ATA. Once again, assuming a maximum acceptable PIO_2 of 1.3 ATA, then the MOD for Nx50 is ([1.3 ATA ÷ 0.5] − 1) × 10 = 16 metres, and the diver would plan to make the switch from air to Nx50 at that depth or the next shallowest decompression stop; 100 per cent oxygen breathed at 3 metres (1.3 ATA) obviously gives a PIO_2 of 1.3 ATA.

The next step would be to enter this time, depth and gas plan into a decompression planning software package. There is a reasonably detailed discussion about the theoretical advantages and disadvantages of different classes of predictive algorithms used in these packages in Chapter 12, and this issue is not revisited here. The decompression planner produces a decompression profile that prescribes the stops required for adequate outgassing during ascent to the surface. One example for this dive, calculated using the Buhlmann ZH-L16 limits with 40-70 gradient factors (see Chapter 12), is given in Table 62.3.

The next step in planning is to calculate the gas requirements for the dive based on the plan for 30 minutes spent at 40 metres and the depths and times of the prescribed stops. Technical divers are taught to plan gas consumption based on their surface air consumption (SAC) during typical diving activity, which they usually measure in a pool exercise early in their training. This must be corrected for the ambient pressure at depth. For example, if a diver has an SAC of 20 litres/minute, then the air requirement for the 30-minute period at 40 metres (5 ATA) is given by:

30 minutes × 20 litres/minute × 5 ATA = 3000 litres

Table 62.3 Decompression calculation for a 40-metre dive for 30 minutes bottom time, derived using the Buhlmann ZH-L16 limits with 40–70 gradient factors

Depth (metres)	Duration (minutes)	Run time (minutes)	Gas
40	30	30	Air
40–15	3 (travel)	33	Air
15	2	35	Nx50
12	3	38	Nx50
9	5	43	Nx50
6	6	48	Nx50
3	12	59	100% oxygen

Nx, nitrox.

Similar calculations must be made for each stop for air, Nx50 and oxygen, and the quantities are totaled for each gas. It is usual to add a reserve fraction of at least 30 per cent in case of unexpected variation from the calculation parameters or the need to share gas with a buddy. Once the required gas volumes are established, then the cylinder configuration can be planned. For a dive of this nature, the air would typically be carried on the back, and the Nx50 and oxygen would be carried in sling tanks on either side. A diver wearing a similar configuration to this is shown in Figure 62.1.

Decompressions almost always take place on a natural wall, or a 'down line' to the dive site. This gives reference to the divers who are trying to control their depth precisely. Alternatively, divers learn to 'shoot a bag' or, more correctly, send a surface marker buoy (SMB) to the surface by using a reel and line, and the diver subsequently 'hangs' under the buoy. This allows the surface support to keep track of where the diver is, which, in open ocean where there are currents, is critically important. On dives with large numbers of divers using a single down line, it is common for a decompression station to be constructed to accommodate multiple divers on the long, shallow decompression stops (Figure 62.2).

Mixed gas diving

We have yet to discuss how to overcome the barriers that impede dives to depths beyond the recreational air diving range. In particular, how can divers ameliorate the debilitating effects of nitrogen narcosis, the toxicity of oxygen and the high gas density that would be encountered if they took

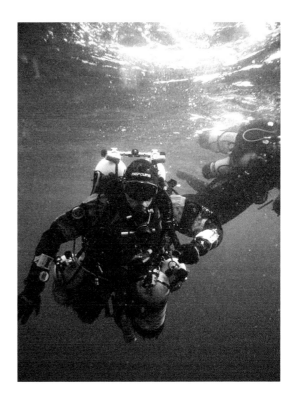

Figure 62.1 Diver wearing a typical cylinder configuration for a decompression dive using open-circuit scuba. See text for explanation.

air deeper and deeper? The answer is that they must introduce a lighter and less narcotic gas into the respired mix to replace at least some of the nitrogen, and they must reduce the amount of oxygen in the mix below that found in air. The use of gases crafted in this way is referred to as 'mixed gas diving'.

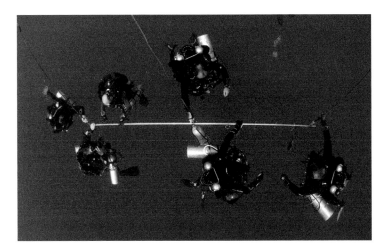

Figure 62.2 Decompression station with bars at strategic depths (such as 9, 6 and 3 metres) designed to accommodate multiple divers on decompression stops.

INTRODUCING ANOTHER 'DILUENT' OR 'CARRIER GAS' TO REPLACE NITROGEN

Mixed gas diving usually involves the introduction of helium into the breathing gas. Helium has some very relevant properties. First, it is much less narcotic than nitrogen. Indeed, it can be breathed at extreme depths with almost no narcotic effect at all. Second, it is very light, and it is much easier to breathe than nitrogen at high pressures. The work of breathing is markedly reduced by helium at extreme depths.

Helium may be used to replace the nitrogen completely, thus leaving helium and oxygen only ('heliox'). Heliox is used most commonly by the military and commercial sectors because the complete absence of nitrogen narcosis means that delicate tasks (e.g. defusing a mine) can be completed safely. In deep recreational diving, it is more common to replace only some of the nitrogen and to leave a mix of helium, nitrogen and oxygen, commonly known as 'trimix'. There are three reasons for this choice:

First, helium is very expensive (especially in countries outside the United States), and so using no more than necessary makes economic sense, especially in open-circuit diving.

Second, most decompression algorithms penalize the use of helium by imposing longer decompression stops. This is based on assumptions about helium kinetics that will not be detailed here, but that predict the need for such longer stops. Experimental comparisons of helium and nitrogen kinetics in animals have cast doubt on the perceived kinetic differences, but they are assumed to exist by modern algorithms, and so some technical divers respond by minimizing helium in their mixes[2].

The third reason for leaving some nitrogen in a gas mix for very deep dives is amelioration of the high-pressure neurological syndrome (see Chapter 20).

REDUCING THE FRACTION OF OXYGEN BELOW THAT FOUND IN AIR

Most trimix dives involve the use of so-called 'hypoxic' mixes; in other words, mixes containing less oxygen than air. In this regard, it is worth noting that the minimum FO_2 in a mix that can safely be breathed at the surface is around 16 per cent (a PO_2 of 0.16 ATA). A dive should not be started on a mix that contains less oxygen than this.

To plan the composition of a trimix gas for a deep dive, the first step is to decide on the depth and the target PIO_2. For example, if a dive is planned to 90 metres where the pressure is 10 ATA and the target PIO_2 is 1.3 ATA then:

Ideal FO_2 in the mix = 1.3 ATA ÷ 10 ATA = 0.13

Thus, the plan would be to use a mix with 13 per cent oxygen for breathing at 90 metres.

HOW MUCH NITROGEN?

The usual aim is to use the minimum amount of helium in the mix to reduce the amount of nitrogen narcosis to an acceptable level. Determination of an 'acceptable level' of narcosis is a somewhat personal issue, but, for example, a diver may be prepared to accept a level of narcosis equivalent to what he or she would experience when breathing air at 40 metres. A useful descriptive expression for this is to say that the diver is prepared to tolerate an 'equivalent narcotic depth' (END) of 40 metres. Expressed more quantitatively, this is equivalent to breathing 3.95 ATA of nitrogen (calculated by multiplying the FN_2 in air by the ambient pressure at 40 metres: 0.79×5 ATA = 3.95 ATA).

Continuing with the 90-metre (10-ATA) dive example, and assuming that the END is to be 40 metres (3.95 ATA nitrogen if breathing air):

Ideal FN_2 in the mix = 3.95 ATA $\div$ 10 ATA = 0.4

So, the bottom mix should contain 40 per cent nitrogen, and the balance fraction of helium needed after addition of the 13 per cent oxygen calculated earlier would be 47 per cent. By convention, trimix gases are designated by their oxygen and helium content, so this mix would be 'trimix 13:47'.

PLANNING OF MIXED GAS DIVES

The process of planning a deep mixed gas dive is similar to that for the air-nitrox-oxygen decompression dive example given earlier (see Table 62.3). A target depth and time are chosen, the ideal bottom gas is identified and decompression gases are chosen. It is customary to switch to mixes with less or no helium and more nitrogen and oxygen (e.g. nitrox) as decompression proceeds. The final shallow stop is typically undertaken while breathing 100 per cent oxygen, as in the previous example. The time, depth and gas plan is entered into a decompression planning software package, and the decompression plan is calculated. Once this is known, it facilitates calculation of the required supplies of all gases in the manner previously described.

Rebreather diving

None of the techniques described to this point have addressed the fundamental issue that often limits duration on dives in which a self-contained breathing apparatus is used; that is, the inherent gas supply inefficiency of open-circuit systems that vent exhaled gas to the water. This is where rebreathers have a distinct advantage. They recycle the breathing gas so that much less gas is used, and the cost of expensive gases such as helium is vastly reduced.

REBREATHER BASICS

A rebreather is a circle circuit analogous to those used in an anaesthesia machine. The diver exhales through a carbon dioxide (CO_2) absorbent into a 'counterlung' (analogous to the bag on an anaesthesia machine) and then inhales back out of the counterlung. One-way valves in the mouthpiece ensure unidirectional flow around the circuit. There is invariably some sort of gas addition system to maintain a safe PIO_2 in the circuit ('loop'). This *breathing loop with a counterlung, CO_2 scrubber and gas addition system* is the fundamental constituent of all rebreather systems.

GENERIC COMPONENTS OF ALL REBREATHER SYSTEMS

Breathing hoses

The breathing hoses appear, on the face of it, to be relatively simple components: usually two corrugated rubber hoses (one for inhalation and one for exhalation) with a mouthpiece in the middle. However, appropriate use and care of the hoses are vital for several reasons. First, the mouthpiece contains one-way check valves to ensure that flow through the loop is only in one direction. If these were malfunctioning, it could result in highly dangerous rebreathing of unscrubbed and poorly oxygenated gas. Second, the hoses represent arguably the most vulnerable component of an otherwise well-protected loop system. A rupture or disconnection of the hoses would result in an unrecoverable flood of the loop, and the diver would have to 'bail-out' onto another gas supply. Finally, and in relation to this second point, the mouthpiece has a valve system that must be closed to prevent flooding of the loop when the mouthpiece is removed in the water. The diver cannot simply remove and replace the mouthpiece underwater as with an open-circuit scuba.

An increasingly popular modification to the rebreather mouthpiece is the incorporation of an open-circuit regulator, with a switching system that allows an instant transfer to open-circuit breathing without the need to remove the rebreather mouthpiece in making the transfer. This is commonly known as a bail-out valve (BOV). There are increasing numbers of reports of rebreather divers developing CO_2 toxicity and failing to make the transfer to open circuit bail-out even though open-circuit systems were carried for that purpose. Invariably, these divers subsequently remark on the fact that the CO_2 made them so short of breath that they could not bring themselves to take the rebreather mouthpiece out for fear of drowning. With an integrated rebreather/open-circuit mouthpiece, the transfer can be made with the mere 'flick of a switch'. The extra complexity (and cost) of a BOV therefore seem justified.

Carbon dioxide scrubber

The scrubber assembly consists of a canister with one or more inlet and outlet holes to allow gas flow through the medium contained within. There are many designs and characteristic flow paths, referred to by such terms as 'axial' and 'radial', but they are all designed to expose the gas to the scrubber material efficiently. The aims are to ensure that gas flow is evenly distributed around that material and to prevent so-called 'channeling' where gas flows through low-resistance pathways that bypass proper contact between gas and scrubber material.

The most common absorbent materials are sodium hydroxide/calcium hydroxide compounds that react with CO_2 as follows:

$$CO_2 + 2NaOH \rightarrow Na_2CO_3 + H_2O + heat$$

Then:

$$Na_2CO_3 + Ca(OH)_2 \rightarrow 2NaOH + CaCO_3$$

Thus, the sodium hydroxide reacts with the CO_2, and the calcium hydroxide is used to regenerate the sodium hydroxide, being converted to calcium carbonate in the process. This continues until all the calcium hydroxide is consumed. The reaction liberates heat and water, and the consequent warming and humidification of the breathing gas are clear advantages of diving a rebreather in cold water. Not surprisingly, a given amount of absorbent can remove only a finite amount of CO_2, and a newly charged scrubber canister has a 'duration' that is typically 2 to 4 hours, depending on the amount of absorbent held. The actual effective duration is somewhat context sensitive. Several factors such as hard work (producing more CO_2), very cold temperatures and extreme depth are all factors that may reduce useful life or efficiency of the equipment. CO_2 scrubber failure can have catastrophic consequences. If CO_2 levels in the inhaled gas are allowed to rise, then the diver may suffer CO_2 toxicity and its unpleasant and dangerous symptoms such as headache, shortness of breath, disorientation, impaired cognition and, ultimately, unconsciousness. It is also notable that high CO_2 levels are a significant risk factor for cerebral oxygen toxicity.

With this in mind, several rebreather manufacturers have introduced CO_2 analyzers into the inhale limb of the loop to detect CO_2 breaking through the scrubber. Some units incorporate so-called 'temperature stick' devices in the scrubber. These devices track the active front of maximal chemical interaction between CO_2 and scrubber material by measuring the temperature through the scrubber material stack. The scrubber material tends to expire first where the exhaled gas enters the canister and then progressively through the stack toward the gas exit portal or portals. As this occurs, the temperature front moves in the same direction. Monitoring the progress of the front through the scrubber canister is akin to a fuel gauge in a car and is potentially a good warning of the likelihood of CO_2 'breaking through' the scrubber. However, temperature sticks are not actually measuring CO_2 in the inhaled gas, and the presence of some chemical activity on the temperature stick cannot guarantee that break-through is absent.

Counterlung

The counterlung is essentially a bag that provides capacitance to the loop so that the diver can freely inhale and exhale without any ingress or egress of gas from outside.

The counterlung is positioned differently in various rebreathers. These positions can be broadly classified as on the back, on the chest, and over the shoulder. These various positions affect the breathing characteristics of the rebreather according to the counterlung's position relative to the lungs.

In the *horizontally* swimming diver with the counterlung on the back, the counterlung is actually at a slightly lower pressure than the lungs (a negative static lung load), thus making exhalation feel easy but inhalation feel slightly more difficult. The opposite is true for the counterlung located on the chest (a positive static lung load). There is some evidence that a positive static lung load is better tolerated by divers working hard underwater, and this design is favoured for rebreathers designed for attack swimming by military divers. A detailed explanation of this and other relevant issues is given elsewhere[3].

SPECIFIC REBREATHER TYPES

Rebreathers are usually classified according to their design and operating mode. The most common are so-called 'closed-circuit rebreathers' (CCRs), and these are discussed in detail here.

Some units used by the military are 'oxygen rebreathers' where the only gas used is 100 per cent oxygen, so the content of the loop is known, and these simple devices require no gas monitoring. The depth range in which they can be used is usually limited to 0 to 6 metres because of an escalating risk of oxygen toxicity at greater depths.

Another type used by recreational divers is the so-called semi-closed unit. In this type, gas with a known oxygen content (higher than air, such as nitrox) is introduced to the loop at a constant rate designed to ensure that a safe loop PO_2 is maintained across a range of plausible exercise levels. For obvious reasons, this modality is associated with considerable potential for the PIO_2 to vary according to exercise levels (and oxygen consumption), and oxygen monitoring is highly desirable in these units.

Closed-circuit rebreathers

If a diver uses mixed gas (heliox or trimix) to advance into deeper, extended-duration dives, then carriage of the required gas volume in open-circuit scuba may impose some limitations, and the helium used will be very expensive. Although CCRs are not just for deep diving, there is no doubt that they provide huge advantages in this endeavour by conserving expensive gas.

It is the gas addition system that makes a CCR unique. Indeed, the gas addition system in a CCR is a big step ahead of even the semi-closed-circuit rebreather in its sophistication and gas efficiency. Whereas a semi-closed-circuit rebreather adds oxygen to the loop at a constant rate in premixed nitrox, a CCR has independent cylinders of two gases: pure oxygen and a '*diluent*' gas (named so because it is used to dilute the oxygen in the loop). Oxygen and the diluent are added to the breathing loop *separately* to form an appropriate mix, and only enough oxygen to meet the metabolic requirements of the diver is used.

The diluent gas is chosen according to the nature of the dive. If a dive within the normal recreational diving range (<40 metres) is planned, then it is very common to use air as the diluent. In this setting, the rebreather blends air and oxygen in the loop to make nitrox. If a deep dive is contemplated, air is no longer a suitable diluent for the same reasons that it is not suitable for deep diving on open circuit. In this case, the diver will fill the diluent cylinder with either heliox or trimix, and the rebreather will blend it with oxygen to produce an appropriate mixed gas. The choice between these diluent gases is based on the same principles applied when using them on open circuit. Military divers often choose heliox (no nitrogen) because no narcosis can be tolerated when defusing a mine. Technical divers usually choose trimix. In CCR diving, this is mainly because of the shorter decompressions that usually result (see earlier), rather than any concerns over consumption and cost of helium.

The diluent contains some oxygen because most CCRs usually have a means of breathing it using an open-circuit regulator should the need arise (e.g. rebreather failure). The amount of oxygen needs to be chosen carefully. The diluent is primarily there to dilute oxygen in the rebreather loop so that the PO_2 can remain within safe limits at the planned depth. It will be no use if the diluent itself contains sufficient oxygen that the loop PO_2 would exceed the maximum safe limit at that depth even if it contained only diluent. For example, if a dive is planned to 90 metres (10 ATA) and the diver wishes to avoid a PO_2 of more than 1.3 ATA, the oxygen fraction in the diluent cannot exceed 0.13 (13 per cent).

Gas addition system

The key feature of CCR operation is a gas addition system that blends the diluent and oxygen to

Table 62.4 Fraction of oxygen in the loop required to produce an inspired partial pressure of oxygen of 1.3 ATA at various depths[a]

Depth (metres)	Ambient pressure (ATA)	FO₂ in loop	Loop PO₂ (ATA)
Surface	1.0	0.7[b]	0.7[b]
3	1.3	1.0	1.3
10	2.0	0.65	1.3
20	3.0	0.43	1.3
30	4.0	0.33	1.3
40	5.0	0.26	1.3
50	6.0	0.22	1.3
90	10.0	0.13	1.3

FO_2, oxygen fraction; PO_2, partial pressure of oxygen.

[a] Note how the diver's inspired mix will change at different depths.

[b] Note also that it is impossible to achieve a loop PO_2 of 1.3 ATA at the surface, where ambient pressure is 1 ATA. The shallowest depth at which a 1.3 ATA PO_2 set-point can be achieved is 1.3 metres. Most closed-circuit rebreathers have a surface mode in which the set-point is an achievable PO_2 of 0.7 ATA (or similar), so that the rebreather does not continually add oxygen in a futile attempt to achieve a loop PO_2 of 1.3 ATA.

maintain a constant PO_2 in the loop. The expression 'constant PO_2' is used a little reservedly because it is not quite constant during all phases of the dive; especially the descent. However, for the most part, the CCR maintains the PO_2 in the loop at a constant 'set-point' that is selected by the diver. Obviously, to achieve this, the FO_2 in the mix must change as the depth (and therefore ambient pressure) changes. By way of example, the FO_2 in the loop to produce a PIO_2 of 1.3 as deep as 90 metres is shown in Table 62.4.

Constant PO_2 is a significant advantage because it means that the diver is breathing the optimal safe level of oxygen throughout the dive, and this in turn minimizes inert gas uptake at depth and maximizes inert gas elimination during decompression.

In all CCRs, diluent is introduced into the loop when the counterlung volume falls. The most obvious and important requirement for diluent addition is during the descent when the counterlung is compressed and gas must be added to restore its volume. CCRs have an automatic diluent addition valve (ADV – Figure 62.3), which is opened automatically as the loop volume falls, thus allowing inflow of diluent gas to restore volume in the loop.

In broad terms, oxygen addition can be handled in two ways: either by an electronically

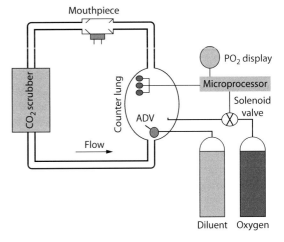

Figure 62.3 Stylized layout of a typical closed-circuit rebreather. For convenience, the oxygen sensors (black circles) are depicted as located in the counterlung, but this is never the case. See text for further explanation.

operated and essentially automated system or by the divers themselves (i.e. manually). In either case (and virtually always in the manual units), manufacturers may include a constant mass flow valve to add oxygen continuously at a rate slightly higher than basal metabolic requirements, with the extra oxygen required to achieve the set-point added either by electronic systems or manually. Because the most prevalent CCRs are of the electronic type without a constant mass flow valve, their operation is described in a little more detail here.

In electronic CCRs ('eCCRs'), oxygen is added through an electronically operated solenoid valve that opens when the PO_2 in the loop falls below the set-point selected by the diver (see Figure 62.3). There are typically three oxygen sensors. These are galvanic fuel cells that produce an electronic current proportional to the PO_2 to which they are exposed. The sensors are 'consuming' and have a finite but poorly predictable 'life', after which they fail. This property mandates multiple sensors and a need for discipline in replacing them periodically according to manufacturers' recommendations (typically 18 months after manufacture).

The sensor data are interpreted by a microprocessor that averages the readings from all three sensors. If one deviates by more than a certain threshold, a 'voting logic' algorithm will result in its being ignored. When addition of diluent, consumption of oxygen or a decrease in ambient pressure causes the averaged PO_2 reading to fall below the set-point, the solenoid valve opens intermittently, letting oxygen into the loop until the PO_2 set-point is restored. All CCRs have at least one display that allows the user to read the actual PO_2 in the loop. The layout of the gas addition system in electronic CCRs that facilitates these functions is shown in Figure 62.3.

TRACKING DECOMPRESSION STATUS

Since 2000, a proliferation of dive computers and software packages that implement both bubble model and gradient factor algorithms (see Chapter 12) for constant PO_2 diving has occurred. These systems are generally successful, although there is a significant but unmeasured incidence of 'unexpected' DCS after deep rebreather dives (and technical dives in general). Occasionally, such cases can be severe and even life-threatening, even though the diver has adhered to the protocol prescribed by the computer. In addition, and at the risk of stating the obvious, the long decompression obligations that accumulate in deep technical dives raise the potential for significant omitted decompression (and severe DCS) if divers are forced to

surface prematurely because of events such as gas toxicity or equipment failure.

REBREATHER PROBLEMS

Rebreathers, and particularly CCRs, are complex devices, and their use introduces hazards that are either absent or less likely to arise in the use of open-circuit scuba equipment. Most prominent among these hazards is the development of PO_2 values in the loop that are either too high or too low. Either extreme can be disastrous. A high PO_2 can induce a seizure without warning, whereas a low PO_2 can result in unconsciousness, also without warning. There are numerous ways that either state can be induced. A comprehensive discussion of the failure modes of rebreathers is beyond the scope of this chapter, but it is worthwhile to consider the following examples.

In a CCR, hypoxia could arise because the diver exhausts the oxygen supply, forgets to open the oxygen cylinder, forgets to turn the rebreather electronics on or makes an ascent at sufficient speed that the solenoid valve cannot add oxygen quickly enough to maintain the PO_2, or hypoxia could result from a solenoid failure or electronics failure. An excessively high PO_2 could occur if an oxygen-rich mix was mistakenly added to the diluent cylinder, if the solenoid or manual oxygen injection valves jam open or if the diver makes a rapid descent when already diving at an established high PO_2 set-point (e.g. 1.3 ATA).

A particularly dangerous cause of high PO_2 is the simultaneous failure of two oxygen sensors to the extent that both read close to the set-point, but only when the loop PO_2 is dangerously high. The third sensor may be accurately reflecting the true loop PO_2, but the CCR will ignore it because it is the 'odd man out' in the voting logic algorithm. If the diver also ignores it (which has happened), then there is a high likelihood of a fatal event.

All rebreathers are prone to scrubber failure if the scrubber is incorrectly packed or the scrubber material is used for too long, thus allowing CO_2 'break-through' and rebreathing. This can result in CO_2 toxicity. Rebreathers are also prone to catastrophic loop floods, for example, caused by ripping of one of the breathing hoses. If the loop floods, the rebreather is completely unusable.

Perhaps not surprisingly, there is emerging evidence for a disturbingly high fatality rate in the use of CCRs by recreational technical divers[4]. It must be conceded that, especially with respect to eCCRs, the devices facilitate a level of complex diving that was hitherto out of the range of most divers. Some of the deep long dives being conducted with these devices are inherently risky in their own right, irrespective of the breathing system used. Nevertheless, the fatality rate seems high, and the exact reasons for this are unknown. Mechanical problems or failures with the rebreathers themselves are rarely identified, and errors in the use of these complex devices are more frequently found. These errors often pertain to very basic procedures, such as failure to change CO_2 scrubber material in a timely fashion, the use of oxygen cells beyond their recommended life or after they show signs of failing and ignoring or responding inappropriately to alarms during the dive.

The rebreather community is aware of these problems, and some generic mitigation strategies are widely used. For example, most technical divers using rebreathers for deep diving carry open-circuit bail-out gas supplies so that if the rebreather fails for any reason, the diver can complete the decompression and surface safely on open circuit. All the divers in Figure 62.2 can be seen wearing a sling tank of open-circuit bail-out gas. Although the necessity to carry this open-circuit bail-out gas negates some of the advantages of the rebreather, the risk of not doing so is widely considered to be too high. A consensus conference on rebreather safety identified several strategies deserving of emphasis to improve safety. These included encouraging the use of pre-dive and post-dive checklists, scrupulous attention to proper procedure around the use of oxygen sensors and maintenance of high standards of training.[5]

LIMITS OF TECHNICAL DIVING

Technical divers have collectively recorded some remarkable achievements, which are too numerous to describe here. Suffice it to say that the history of many previously 'lost' ship wrecks has been illuminated by their discovery and identification, and much more is known about many underground waterways following their exploration.

The authors of this text are fundamentally opposed to depth records in technical diving for their own sake, and we subscribe to the view that the risks involved in very deep diving should, at least to some extent, be justified by a tangible goal (e.g. the identification of an historic wreck). Nevertheless, for completeness we mention that technical divers using open-circuit equipment and trimix gas have reached depths near 320 metres, and rebreathers have been taken to around 290 metres on technical bounce dives. It is germane to point out that none of the relevant dives achieved anything other than reaching a very great depth; the divers simply turned immediately and began their decompression.

Of much greater practical relevance are the remarkable dives that have been undertaken in support of cave exploration and to identify wrecks. For example, cave divers in Florida recently explored more than 11 km of cave over a 7-hour period at around a 90-metre depth. This was followed by a decompression that took some 15 hours. The logistics involved in dives of this nature are staggering. At a more mainstream level, cave dives involving long penetrations and/or deep depths are now relatively common, and ocean dives to reefs or wrecks in depths down to 100 metres are also frequent.

The factors that limit very deep diving are primarily physiological and include high-pressure neurological syndrome and the respiratory limitations imposed by high gas density. The factors that limit duration of dives to more modest depths are more logistical, such as cost (for helium if an open-circuit system is used), decompression length (it can be both boring and physically exhausting) and thermal protection.

REFERENCES

1. Harris RJ, Doolette DJ, Wilkinson DC, Williams DJ. Measurement of fatigue following 18 msw dry chamber dives breathing air or enriched air nitrox. *Undersea and Hyperbaric Medicine* 2003;**30**:285–91.

2. Doolette DJ, Mitchell SJ. Recreational technical diving. Part 2. Decompression from deep technical dives. *Diving and Hyperbaric Medicine* 2013;**43**:96–104.
3. Doolette DJ, Mitchell SJ. Hyperbaric conditions. *Comprehensive Physiology* 2011;**1**:163–201.
4. Fock A. Analysis of recreational closed circuit rebreather deaths 1998–2010. *Diving and Hyperbaric Medicine* 2013;**43**:78–85.
5. Vann RD, Denoble PJ, Pollock NW, eds. *Rebreather Forum 3 Proceedings*. AAUS/DAN/PADI: Durham, NC; 2014

FURTHER READING

Gurr K. *Technical Diving From the Bottom Up.* 2nd ed. Penzance, United Kingdom: Periscope Publishing; 2010.

Mitchell SJ, Doolette DJ. Recreational technical diving. Part 1. An introduction to technical diving. Diving and Hyperbaric Medicine 2013;43:86–93.

Mount T, Dituri J, eds. *Exploration and Mixed Gas Diving Encyclopaedia: The Tao of Underwater Survival.* Miami, Florida: IANTD Publishing; 2008.

This chapter was reviewed for this fifth edition by Simon Mitchell.

63

Divers with disabilities

INTRODUCTION

Limitation resulting from disability is as much a political question as it is a physiological one. Attitudes to personal rights and freedoms may conflict with clinical judgement and risk assessment. Thus, the views expressed here are reflections of personal prejudices as much as experience and reason.

The medical assessment of a fully able or disabled diver should be identical. Informed assessment of any disability, the effect of the disability on the independence of the diver in the water and the ability of the disabled diver to render assistance to his or her dive buddy are mandatory for unqualified medical fitness to dive. Not all disabled divers are successful in attaining an unlimited open water certification; however, under certain conditions the disabled diver will still be likely to enjoy a supervised and supported 'diving experience'.

Most diving trainer organizations do not accept medically imposed diving restrictions, thus making medical approval an all-or-none entity. This limits the flexibility of the diving physician to indicate the additional conditions that would make many diving trainees with disabilities acceptable for open water qualification.

The considerable positive aspects to diving for the person who has a disability include proof of an ability to engage in an exciting, physically active, intellectually stimulating social activity. The gravity-free liberation of movement is an added thrill for those so limited in their terrestrial environment. The improvement in their self-esteem and quality of life can be substantial.

DEFINITION

An individual with a disability can be defined as an individual with a disadvantage or impairment that limits fulfillment of a normal role. Impairment describes the loss or abnormality of physiological, psychological or anatomical structure or function, whereas disability is defined as the restriction or lack of ability to perform in a normal manner or range as a result of an impairment.

It has long been recognized that rehabilitation programs should address both the physical and the psychological needs of the individual who has a disability. The mastery of a recreational sporting activity usually associated with the physically fit goes a long way to improving self-esteem and a sense of competence. Can an individual with a disability successfully learn to scuba dive?

The answer is 'of course'; but this does not necessarily mean that this person can become a fully certified independent diver. Both the single amputee and the person with high-level quadriplegia are classified as having a disability, yet the degree of their disabilities and their ability to undertake a scuba diving course differ greatly.

TRAINING OPTIONS

Worldwide, there are two different approaches to the question of teaching divers with disabilities to scuba dive. The first approach is to offer no special training for disabled persons and require them to undertake the standard open water course like everyone else. Most of the entry-level courses do not teach buddy rescue skills, a problem for many disabled divers, and many individuals with disabilities are able to complete the course successfully. A perceived difficulty with this approach is that the disabled diver may require more intensive instruction and assistance than is available during the standard weekend courses.

Since the 1990s, various training organizations have emerged that cater to scuba diver training of people who have disabilities. Some of these are non-profit organizations, and others are off-shoots of the commercial training agencies. This second approach is one of providing an independent training and certifying agency for divers with disabilities (e.g. the Handicapped Scuba Association [HSA]).

Not only is there specialized and individual training for the candidate, but also there is extended training for instructors and for volunteer companion divers. These instructors and volunteers all need an understanding of the degree of disability, as well as an appreciation of the generic disability and its influence on diver activity and safety.

Each instructor acquires medical information through lectures on specific disabilities – what they are and how they relate to diving – followed by a series of confined and open water exercises, designed to simulate disabilities. By "acting out" these disabilities, instructors actually experience what it is like to be a mobility-impaired or sight-impaired diver, a sensitizing, often surprising revelation even for instructors who have been training divers for many years.

Open water certification of the diver who has a disability stipulates the number and quality of diving companions that are required for safety, specialized diving equipment indicated, environmental restrictions and safety equipment and techniques needed.

The HSA, founded in 1981, offers different levels of certification based on degrees of functionality in the water:

Level 1: The candidate has successfully met all standards, can take care of himself or herself, help another diver in distress and perform a rescue. This diver is certified to dive with another certified companion.

Level 2: The candidate has demonstrated an ability to handle emergency situations and, in general, care for himself or herself while scuba diving. This diver is unable to help another diver in distress. This diver should dive with two able-bodied certified dive buddies.

Level 3: The candidate has demonstrated an ability to dive safely but needs considerable assistance and would not be able to respond to an emergency, such as self-rescue. This diver must dive with two able-bodied, certified buddies, one of whom is trained in scuba rescue.

Most instructor agencies would agree that training a severely disabled person is staff and time intensive, with at least initially a 1:1 student-instructor ratio and constant attention to safety. The British Sub-Aqua Club[1] believes that the integrated approach with mainstream divers is more beneficial in the long term.

MEDICAL FITNESS

Disabled divers require the same medical examination as non-disabled divers. In Australia, Australian Standard AS4005.1-1992 stipulates the minimum requirements for the training and certification of recreational divers and describes in detail the medical criteria to be used. The standard requires that 'a full examination of the central nervous system must show normal function, but localized minor abnormalities such as patches of anesthesia are allowed, provided that generalized nervous system disease can be excluded', thus effectively ruling out the paraplegic person or the victim of childhood polio.

Yet, experience has shown that some such individuals can become proficient divers.

Fleming and Melamed[2] reported in 1977 the results of a training course for six severely disabled persons with paraplegia and double leg amputees. These investigators concluded 'that self-contained diving training is an excellent rehabilitatory activity for disabled people with the following limitations: no paraplegic should dive in the sea with a lesion above T5, no paraplegic whose injury was caused by the bends should dive at all and no disabled diver should undertake decompression dives'. These conclusions were based on their practical experiences.

Patient A, paraplegic (T4) after a gunshot wound, was permitted to dive in the pool only. The other five candidates successfully completed an open water dive. Patient A performed most of the requirements correctly in the pool, but short bursts of intense exercise caused a difficulty in breathing because his diaphragm was his sole muscle of respiration. This situation proved critical, whereas the pupil with a T6 lesion was considered safe.

Fleming and Melamed believed that this loss of respiratory reserve secondary to the loss of the normal muscles of respiration should require careful assessment of individuals with lesions above T8.

These investigators also pointed out to individuals with partial spinal lesions of whatever cause that there is a possibility that diving could make the lesion complete.

Williamson and associates[3] reported on the medical and psychological aspects in the selection and training of disabled persons for scuba diving. Sixteen individuals with a wide range of disabilities underwent a formal scuba diving course. Subjects' disabilities ranged from brainstem injury, congenital deafness, congenital blindness and paraplegia to bilateral amputation. Nine of the 16 candidates completed the open water training program. The medical assessment differed significantly from the norm in the following ways:

1. No selection of applicants occurred on the basis of previous athletic achievement or independence of mobility.
2. No preconceptions existed that full, unrestricted diving certification of the 'successful' candidates was a necessary end point of their training.

3. The group included a range of medical disabilities hitherto regarded as being at least relative contraindications to diving, such as brainstem damage, myelitis, impaired bladder and bowel control and blindness.

One of the candidates (who had poliomyelitis, L2) developed symptoms of spinal decompression sickness (DCS). He had completed eight open water dives over a period of 3 days, all within the limits of the US Navy diving tables. He required five recompression chamber treatments and was left with residual paraesthesia in the left leg and an area of enlarged numbness on the inner aspect of the left thigh. In view of this case, these investigators acknowledged the reservations of others with regard to the increased hazards in individuals with partial spinal cord lesions.

Follow-up psychological test results revealed an improvement in the subjects' physical self-concept sub-scale that was considered the result of their diving experience.

These investigators reported an initially higher incidence of ear problems and coral cuts and found that incomplete bladder and bowel control was not a disability.

Both studies reflect the need for the medical assessment of disabled divers to be performed by experienced diving physicians with knowledge of diving training and who can relate this knowledge to the individual's disability. Particular hazards to consider include the risk of trauma and coral cuts in the paraplegic diver with loss of sensory input and the risk of pressure ulcers from sitting for prolonged periods on the boat. The loss of muscle control may cause the paraplegic diver's legs to float; this can be counteracted by the use of leg weights. The diver with a lower limb amputation has no use for fins, but in divers with use of their arms, webbed gloves may help forward propulsion. The diver with a double lower limb amputation may also experience difficulty in maintaining positional control when swimming. The loss of upper limb function in some ways is more serious because this causes problems with buoyancy control and mask clearing. Stroke victims with weak facial muscles may have difficulty holding the regulator within the mouth.

Perhaps the greatest difficulty faced by disabled divers is gaining access to dive boats, pools and dive shops. Wheelchair access to these facilities is often limited, and the disabled diver may well need assistance to carry his or her equipment. Fear of falling or injury while transferring to a dive boat or in transit to the dive site should not be underestimated. Consideration should also be given to the safety of the disabled diver in the event of a boating accident that could result in the boat's sinking.

Blind divers need assistance with navigation. Profoundly deaf divers have difficulty in responding to an emergency recall alarm, but they are superior at communicating with each other underwater, by hand signals.

In assessing fitness to dive, the medical practitioner should always consider whether the underlying medical condition will predispose the individual to a diving-related illness such as pulmonary barotrauma and DCS. Madorsky and Madorsky[4] argued that because reduced circulation in paralyzed limbs may increase the time it takes for nitrogen to escape from the tissues, it is recommended that dive tables be used extremely conservatively. Williamson and colleagues[3] recommended that a specially modified set of decompression tables be used by disabled divers, based on the assumption that disabled divers are predisposed to the development of DCS because of their pre-existing disorders. It seems reasonable advice to suggest that disabled divers introduce a 'safety' factor when planning their dives.

It is important that disabled divers with neurological conditions have their impairment fully documented and that their condition be stable before they learn to dive. The individual with progressive multiple sclerosis poses major diagnostic difficulties if he or she develops neurological symptoms after the dive. Are the symptoms the result of neurological DCS or a progression of the disease? The diver with a below knee amputation who has a discrete, well-demarcated area of numbness on the stump secondary to nerve resection is far easier to assess.

Novice divers are more likely to have pulmonary barotrauma and resultant cerebral arterial gas embolism. Non-disabled divers find buoyancy control difficult to master, let alone the disabled diver with reduced upper limb control. This difficulty may increase the risk of pulmonary barotrauma

and neurological impairment in an individual who already has a disability. The great variety of disabilities and the often unpredictability of the ocean environment makes assessment of fitness to dive extremely complex. The equipment needs, potential risks, limitations and required safety precautions are a challenge. Assistance is available from the publications referred to previously, and through organisations such as PADI (Robinson and Fox[5]) and NOAA[6].

LEGAL IMPLICATIONS

The Americans with Disabilities Act became effective July 1992 in the United States and is applicable to businesses that employ 15 or more persons. The Act prohibits employers from discriminating against qualified persons with disabilities and charges them with the responsibility of making reasonable accommodation to allow and assist the worker to do the job. Reasonable accommodation may not be required if it creates undue hardship for the employer or if there is a reasonable medical judgement that there is a high probability of substantial harm to the disabled individual. This reasonable medical judgement must be based on sound scientific evidence and established data.

In the United Kingdom, Australia and New Zealand, the test of foreseeability is applied when considering fitness for an occupation. If it is reasonably foreseen that, because of a certain disease or disorder, injury could be sustained to either the person or others, then this exposure should be avoided if at all possible.

The emphasis should be on the candidate's ability in determining what is safe to undertake, not so much on the disability.

SUMMARY

The medical assessment of a disabled diver should not be different from that of a fully able person. Consideration should be given to the nature of the disability, the effect of that disability on the diver's ability to operate independently in the water and on the diver's ability to provide assistance to his or her buddy. Additional personnel, equipment, retrieval and first aid facilities may be indicated. Increased risk to dive companions should be considered and incorporated into dive planning.

The examining doctor must fully understand the etiology of the disorder and be competent to assess whether a diving-related illness such as DCS could result in progression of the symptoms and signs of the diver's disability.

Many disabled divers are not able to fulfill the certification requirements demanded by mainstream training agencies. However, with appropriate supervision and training they may be able to undertake a 'diving experience' with resultant positive psychological benefits.

CONTACT ORGANIZATIONS

Campbell E. *Diving With Disabilities*. 2010. Scubadoc's Diving Medicine Online: http://www.scuba-doc.com/divdis.htm
Handicapped Scuba Association International (1104 El Prado, San Clemente, California 92672): http://www.hsascuba.com
International Association for Handicapped Diving: http://www.iahd.org/index

REFERENCES

1. Dive training for the disabled: what is it worth? *Diver* 1997;**Aug**.
2. Fleming NC, Melamed Y. Report of a scuba diving training course for paraplegics and double leg amputees with an assessment of physiological and rehabilitation factors. *South Pacific Underwater Medicine Society Journal* 1977;**7**(1):19–34.
3. Williamson JA, McDonald FW, Galligan EA, Baker PG, Hammond CT. Selection and training of disabled persons for scuba-diving: medical and psychological aspects. *Medical Journal of Australia* 1984;**141**:414–418.
4. Madorsky JGB, Madorsky AG. Scuba diving: taking the wheelchair out of wheelchair sports. *Archives of Physical and Medical Rehabilitation* 1998;**69**:215–218.
5. Robinson J, Fox AD. *Scuba Diving With Disabilities*. Champaign, Illinois: Kinetics Publishers; 1987.
6. NOAA Diving Manual on-line (Appendix A covers Diving with Disabilities) http://www.ndc.noaa.gov/rp_manual.html or National Oceanographic and Atmospheric Administration. *NOAA Diving Manual*. 5th ed. Washington, DC: US Government Printing Office; 2013.

This chapter was reviewed for this fifth edition by Carl Edmonds.

Submarine medicine

INTRODUCTION

Submarines are the silent enemy, operating in often hostile waters. The nature of the environment in which they operate offers a great advantage in warfare; however, if disaster befalls the boat this environment can quickly become a tomb. This chapter introduces the reader to the submarine environment and the medical aspects of submarine escape and rescue.

The first recorded submarine military success relates to the *Seadiver,* a hand-propelled submarine built by Bavarian artilleryman Wilhelm Bauer. In 1850, the Danish fleet blockaded the port of Kiel, and the very appearance of the *Seadiver* was enough to scatter the Danes in panic. By 1851, the Danes had regrouped, and the *Seadiver* attempted to repeat her success. Unfortunately, she sank to the bottom in 18 metres of water, and Bauer and his two crewmen, working from first principles, devised and carried out the first successful submarine compartment (or rush) escape. This method, albeit with

modification and refinement, is still taught today. Although submarines became more sophisticated, it took the success of the German U-boats during World War I to spark the interest of many nations.

The experience of most nations' involvement with submarines is exemplified by that of Australia. Australian submarine operations date back to World War I. The *AE1* was commissioned in 1913 and was lost with all hands on approximately 14 September 1914 off New Britain. The submarine failed to return from patrol, and the cause of its loss remains unknown. No trace of the *AE1* has been found. The *AE2* was commissioned in June 1913 and was lost as a result of enemy action in the Sea of Marmora on 30 April 1915. The *AE2* was the first allied warship to penetrate the Dardanelles and saw 5 days of action in these waters before being sunk by enemy fire. The entire crew survived. The *AE2* has been found and dived in approximately 70 metres of depth, and salvage operations have been discussed. Australia became an active diesel submarine nation in the 1960s with the purchase of Royal Navy Oberon class boats, and during the 1990s the Royal Australian Navy (RAN) commissioned the new Collins class submarines.

The world's first nuclear powered submarine, the USS *Nautilus* was launched by the US Navy (USN) in 1954. The development of the nuclear propulsion plant was a result of the combined efforts of USN, government and contract engineers led by Captain Hyman G. Rickover. Nuclear power enabled a submarine to operate as a true submersible, capable of staying submerged for a prolonged period without the need to surface or 'snorkel' to run diesel engines and recharge batteries.

The USN submarine force of today comprises multi-mission nuclear Attack class submarines (SSN) and Ballistic Missile submarines (SSBN). The SSN submarines are designed to seek and destroy enemy submarines and surface ships, conduct intelligence collection and facilitate special force troop or diver delivery for anti-ship or land-based operations. The SSBNs are armed with long-range strategic missiles. Although the missiles have no pre-set targets, they can be rapidly targeted using secure and constant at-sea communications links. Their sole role is to provide strategic deterrence, and this class of submarine provides the United States' most survivable and enduring nuclear strike capability.

THE SUBMARINE ENVIRONMENT

Submarine patrols, where the boat remains submerged and undetected, may last for 14 days for conventionally powered boats and for up to 90 days for nuclear powered boats. Environmental conditions on board submarines are constantly improving, and maintaining a respirable atmosphere is one of the most important tasks for the crew. Even so, it is said that a submariner could always be detected by the lingering aroma of diesel. Some submariners continue to conserve shower water even when ashore.

The submarine internal environment operates at 1 ATA pressure. When submerged, the shipboard air may be exchanged with the external environment via the 'snorkel' (an air pipe to the surface). The 'snorting' time required to replenish the boat with clean air free of contaminants is directly proportional to the internal volume of the boat and is inversely proportional to the ventilation flow rate. If the rate of air leaving the boat is greater than the flow of fresh gas into the boat, a partial vacuum can be drawn. When snorting, oxygen is replenished, and contaminants such as carbon dioxide, carbon monoxide, hydrocarbons, refrigeration gases and bacteriological aerosols are eliminated.

If for operational reasons 'snorting' is not possible, oxygen can be generated by burning oxygen candles, from high-pressure or liquid oxygen stores, or via an oxygen generator that produces oxygen through the electrolysis of water. Carbon dioxide is absorbed by soda lime or lithium hydroxide scrubbers (a non-reversible process, and therefore large stores of absorbent material are required) or by passing the submarine air through a regenerative scrubber. Monoethanolamine absorbs carbon dioxide when cold and releases it when heated. The liberated carbon dioxide is then dumped overboard. Hydrogen and carbon monoxide are removed through a catalytic oxidative process, and aerosols and vapours are separated from the atmosphere by filters and adsorption onto activated charcoal.

Monitoring systems provide a constant readout of principal atmospheric constituents (e.g. oxygen, carbon dioxide and some fluorocarbons) and activate an alarm if abnormal readings are detected. For substances not measured routinely, other gas detection methods are available (e.g. detection tubes). On nuclear submarines, radiation levels are routinely monitored at multiple locations, both inside and outside of engineering spaces. The crew members wear personal dosimeters that provide individual exposure information for radiation health surveillance, and portable radiation monitoring equipment is available for detection of contaminants and for use in the case of accidental exposure or system failure.

SUBMARINE SINKINGS

There have been more than 170 recorded peacetime submarine sinkings in the world since 1900. It is said that the most likely situation for a submarine accident is at times of transit through ports, channels and fishing grounds, with collision and grounding the most likely mechanisms. The basic underlying premise for survival is that once a submarine becomes disabled, at least one compartment remains intact or can be secured long enough for survivors to decide on and carry out a course of action. This may involve either escape or rescue.

If a submarine is disabled and sinks, the means by which the crew member is evacuated back to the surface depends on a number of factors, including the following:

- The internal pressure of the submarine.
- The internal atmosphere of the submarine.
- The weather conditions.
- Whether or not rescue forces on the surface are available.

There are two methods of *escaping* from a disabled submarine. One is where the survivors leave the submarine through an escape hatch and make an ascent to the surface through the water. This ascent may be done through a submarine escape tower (SET), where the submariner spends the least time exposed to ambient environmental pressure. The other is from a flooded compartment that is in direct contact with the outside environment. This is known as compartment escape and is less desirable because of the longer period the individuals are exposed to raised ambient pressure.

The escaping submariners wear a specially designed submarine escape immersion suit (SEIS). An SET escape wearing an SEIS has been proven to be possible from a depth of at least 180 metres, whereas a compartment escape is thought to be survivable only from a depth of 60 metres.

The second escape method is active *rescue*, which involves the use of a submersible to transport the survivors to the surface where, if required, subsequent decompression can be undertaken. The depth of the stricken submarine and the operating capability of the rescue craft generally limit rescue.

Another form of rescue is by salvaging the submarine. Although this is not applicable in most circumstances, there have been some very successful salvage operations whereby the boat is floated or mechanically towed to the surface – thus allowing the submariners to evacuate.

The range of medical conditions seen in survivors from a submarine accident varies depending on whether they have escaped or have been rescued.

SUBMARINE ESCAPE

Survivors who have escaped from a disabled submarine are likely to suffer from the following:

- Decompression sickness.
- Barotrauma – pulmonary, ear, sinus, gastric.
- Gas toxicities – chlorine, carbon monoxide, carbon dioxide.
- Hypothermia.
- Near drowning.
- Traumatic injuries and burns.

Decompression sickness

The internal pressure of the submarine is likely to rise with damage to the pressure hull (e.g. ingress of sea water, ruptured high-pressure air lines). The elevated partial pressure of nitrogen in the air complicates escape – first as the survivors may experience nitrogen narcosis and second as their tissues become saturated at the elevated inspired partial pressure. It has been shown that a survivor saturated in air can make a direct ascent from 1.7 ATA (equivalent to a depth of 7 metres) to the surface with a low risk of developing symptoms and signs of decompression sickness. For survivors saturated at deeper depths, the risk of life-threatening decompression sickness increases proportionately. On-site recompression facilities must be available to handle these casualties. First aid measures include the administration of 100 per cent oxygen and intravenous fluids.

Pulmonary barotrauma

The survivors wear a specially designed SEIS during an escape. This suit provides an air-filled space surrounding the head and supplying in-built buoyancy that assists their passage to the surface. The submariners are taught to breathe in and out normally as they make their ascent; however, panic may override their training, or, if the hood ruptures and they find their face in water, survivors may breath-hold. Pulmonary barotrauma (pulmonary tissue damage, pneumomediastinum, pneumothorax and cerebral arterial gas embolism) can all be expected in survivors as they surface. Urgent recompression may be lifesaving.

Other barotraumas

The SET rapidly pressurizes the escaping submariner from whatever the internal pressure of the submarine is to that of the external environment. For example, if the submarine is resting on the bottom at a depth of 180 metres of sea water (msw; internal atmosphere of 1 ATA), after entering the SET it will take approximately 20 seconds for the escaping submariner to be pressurized to 180 msw and the hatch to open. This rapid pressurization rate may take the escaping survivors by surprise, and middle and inner ear barotrauma is likely.

During a live training exercise, a British escaping submariner suffered a ruptured stomach during an escape from 150 msw in open water because of the rapid expansion of stomach gas.

Gas toxicities

Chlorine gas may be liberated from the submarine's main batteries if flooding occurs. Delayed bronchospasm and pulmonary oedema may result from intense, brief exposures that may also predispose the individual to pulmonary barotrauma during the escape.

If there has been a fire on board, the crew may be exposed to raised levels of carbon monoxide with resulting central nervous system depression.

Carbon dioxide toxicity is a major threat, and rising levels may well force the crew to escape before the rescue forces have arrived. Headache and dyspnoea are early warning signs.

Hypothermia and drowning

All survivors attempting escape should be wearing an SEIS that permits survival for a minimum of 6 hours in sub-Arctic water. This period can exceed 24 hours with water temperatures such as can be expected in more temperate climates. Problems

with localized frostbite can occur on exposed areas (e.g. hands and face). Dehydration and seasickness contribute to the effects of exposure. In adverse sea conditions, it is likely that survivors, particularly those who may be suffering other injuries, may aspirate sea water.

Traumatic injury

Significant injury occurring in the submarine before the escape is likely to prevent the individual from being able to enter and operate the SET successfully. Unconsciousness or major limb fracture precludes escape. However, where there is a will to survive, individuals can make superhuman efforts, and some survivors with lacerations, upper limb fractures, burns and other injuries can be expected on the surface. Survivors are likely to experience acute psychological stress reactions that may make initial assessment difficult.

SUBMARINE RESCUE

Once a submarine sinks beyond 180 msw, the only option normally available to the crew is to await rescue. Staying alive until the rescue forces arrive – which may take several days – becomes the primary focus. Regular monitoring of the internal atmosphere – the pressure, radiation levels, oxygen levels, and carbon dioxide levels – becomes essential. The medical problems experienced by the survivors are somewhat different from those experienced by survivors who make a successful escape.

Likely medical problems include the following:

- Hypoxia.
- Hyperoxia.
- Gas toxicities.
- Trauma and burns.
- Hypothermia.
- Decompression sickness.
- Radiation injury.

Pulmonary barotrauma should not complicate rescue because the ascent is controlled. However, the added complications of pulmonary gas toxicity, the lack of recompression facilities and the need to treat other injuries sustained in the accident indicate that management of such a rescue requires the involvement of an experienced underwater medicine physician.

Hypoxia

People usually do not lose consciousness from hypoxia if they are breathing an oxygen partial pressure of 0.10 ATA or greater. However, as oxygen partial pressures fall from 0.16 ATA, progressive symptoms of hypoxia may develop, including increased respiratory rate, clouded thought processes, decreased awareness of surroundings and, finally, unconsciousness. The crew should be monitoring the internal atmosphere and burning oxygen candles to alleviate this problem. If the internal pressure of the submarine rises, the percentage of atmospheric oxygen needed to maintain an adequate partial pressure will fall.

Hyperoxia

Oxygen is toxic in high concentrations. High partial pressures of oxygen can lead to central nervous system toxicity with grand mal seizures. The risk is increased if the survivors are also hypercapnoeic from rebreathing carbon dioxide. Breathing oxygen at lower partial pressures, but higher than 0.6 ATA, for prolonged periods leads to symptoms of pulmonary oxygen toxicity. The rapidity of onset of the relative symptoms increases as the partial pressure of oxygen is increased. Symptoms of pulmonary oxygen toxicity include chest tightness, cough, chest pain, shortness of breath and a fall in vital capacity. The severity of oxygen toxicity may be important when selecting a decompression schedule.

Gas toxicities, burns and trauma

Injuries resulting from trauma, burns and gas toxicities are similar to those seen in survivors who have completed an escape.

Hypothermia

At depth, the ocean temperatures may be only 5°C. Without power, the submarine cools to the temperature of the surrounding water, and the survivors may quickly develop hypothermia.

Decompression sickness

Most situations that lead to the disabling of a submarine involve some internal pressure increase in the submarine. This may be a result of flooding, high-pressure air leaks, salvage air and use of emergency breathing systems. If this increase in pressure is maintained for a sufficiently long period, the survivors will have accumulated a decompression obligation. Ideally, rescue vehicles are capable of transfer under pressure (TUP) – that is, the rescue vehicle is pressurized to the same pressure as that in the submarine, and the survivors are transferred at that pressure to the surface, where the rescue vehicle is mated to a recompression chamber. The survivors then transfer to the recompression chamber and undergo staged decompression. This process should therefore prevent the occurrence of decompression sickness; however, saturation decompression schedules may be required, and in the worst case up to 72 hours or so of decompression may be needed. Logistically, this is difficult to manage when submarine crew sizes may be as high as 180. Because the rescue process may take several days to extract the entire crew, it is likely that the pressure will continue to rise in the submarine. This means that the last-rescued survivors will have earned a greater decompression obligation than those rescued first.

Radiation injury

If a nuclear submarine suffers a major reactor accident, survivors may suffer from acute radiation injury. Radiation injury *per se* does not imply that the patient is a health hazard to medical staff, and treatment of life-threatening injuries takes precedence over decontamination procedures. Simple decontamination procedures include removing outer clothing and shoes, washing with soap and tepid water and irrigating open wounds and covering them with a sterile dressing.

SUBMARINE RESCUE VEHICLES

Rescue vehicles have been constructed by many nations including the United States, the United Kingdom, Sweden, Australia and Italy. Many of these vehicles are coming to the end of their working lives, and replacements are being sought. The US Deep Submergence Rescue Vehicle (DSRV) is aircraft transportable, but it requires a mother submarine (MOSUB) to transport it to the site of a disabled submarine. The DSRV can mate with specially modified MOSUBSs and can transfer survivors under pressure to the bow compartment pressurized up to 2 ATA. The distinct disadvantages of this system are the time it takes to transport the vehicle to the site and the likelihood of significant decompression sickness if the survivors are saturated at pressures greater than 2 ATA.

The British LR5 is not air transportable, and this therefore limits its range of operations to the UK area. It again is capable of transferring survivors to an MOSUB at 2 ATA, but currently it has no TUP ability with the surface.

The Australian Submarine Escape and Rescue Service (SERS) comprises the following:

- Surface recompression facilities for a maximum of 72 people.
- A rescue submersible *(Remora)* capable of operating in waters down to the crush depth of Australian submarines.
- A TUP facility (up to 5 ATA) with the surface recompression facility.
- An extension of life support capability (a means of resupplying the stricken submarine with oxygen candles, soda lime absorbent, food, water, medical supplies etc.) to provide time for the rescue service to be transported to the site.

The SERS has been exercised with TUP of crew from a Collins class submarine, and there is also a capability to transfer injured personnel from the submarine to the *Remora* and then to the recompression chamber facility by using a harness-pulley system.

FURTHER READING

Walker RM. A complete submarine escape and rescue organisation. *South Pacific Underwater Medicine Society Journal* 1998;**27**(2):95–101.

This chapter was reviewed for this fifth edition by Simon Mitchell.

65

Occupational groups

INTRODUCTION

This chapter deals with the specific problems encountered by various occupational groups. The type of diving performed by these groups is summarized, and some of the associated physiological effects and illnesses are mentioned in passing. Most of these effects and illnesses are more fully described elsewhere in this text.

Many of the traditional occupational diving groups have become extinct. The **Greek sponge divers** of Symi and Kalymnos have inspired many authors. In Symi, one diver in three was either dead or crippled from neurological decompression sickness (DCS) before he had reached marriageable age. Others were disabled at a later age from dysbaric osteonecrosis.

This chapter discusses the specialized diving groups other than those referred to elsewhere in the text, such as technical divers (see Chapter 62), deep and saturation divers (see Chapter 67) and submariners (see Chapter 64).

BREATH-HOLD DIVING

Breath-hold diving is readily available to all, without relying on complex equipment or facilities (see Chapter 61). It is employed by people living largely subsistence lives in developing areas and in remote locations and frequently permits diving to depths of 20 metres or so.

The major causes of death from this activity include drowning, often as a result of hypoxic blackout during ascent (see Chapter 3), cardiac problems and environmental hazards (hypothermia, marine animal injuries, ocean trauma and entrapment).

Because of the multiple and rapid ascents and descents, barotraumas are particularly frequent.

Ama

The **Ama** are the traditional female breath-hold divers of Japan and Korea, whose activities have been recorded for more than 2000 years. They dive repeatedly to depths as great as 18 to 20 metres, throughout the day, gathering shells, urchins and sea grasses. They dive throughout the year, and the interesting observations have centered on their adaptation to cold exposure, with various physiological modifications. They also have been noted to have an increased incidence of cardiac arrhythmias (especially during the winter months) and suffer some effects on foetal development.

Shell divers

Shell (pearl) divers from the Tuamotu Archipelago suffer from 'Taravana disease' – causing both death and disability. This disease was attributed to the extreme breath-hold diving exploits of these native fishers. The dives were to 30 to 40 metres, lasting around 2 to 5 minutes each, over a 7-hour period. The disease probably encompassed a variety of illnesses, including otological barotraumas, the drowning syndromes and possibly DCS.

Submarine escape tank trainers

Submarine escape tank trainers tend to dive to considerable depths, often 20 to 30 metres, to escort their submariners-under-training to the surface and ensure that an appropriate ascent rate and exhalation are achieved by these trainees. Because these divers are very experienced and well trained, barotraumas are not particularly frequent. Because the water is usually fresh, purified and warmed, many of the hazards of ocean diving are avoided. Unfortunately, the absorption of nitrogen with each dive does permit the occasional development of DCS, requiring recompression therapy.

Spear fishers

Spear fishers and other hunters tend to be less disciplined and more frequently hyperventilate before their dive. Because of the competitive nature of this activity, the diver may be motivated to exceed reasonable depths and durations. Under these conditions, the hypoxia that may develop with prolonged breath-holding

associated with exercise, as well as the hypoxia of ascent (see Chapter 3), may cause loss of consciousness during ascent, with subsequent drowning. This has been observed too frequently. These divers tend to be high risk takers, although they are often very competent in their aquatic skills. Other major problems include barotraumas of descent and marine animal injuries associated with hunting.

SURFACE SUPPLY DIVING

This equipment, using compressors or large storage cylinders, allows for prolonged durations at depth. The tethering of the surface supply increases the possibility of entanglement. Carbon monoxide toxicity from petrol-driven compressor exhaust contamination of the air intake is a recognized hazard.

Australian abalone divers

The Australian abalone divers, together with many others throughout the world, use a surface supply system because of their need to remain underwater for longer periods. The sea conditions are often treacherous, and the work is strenuous. The depths are usually less than 30 metres, and often less than 20. With the shallower depths, there is usually a greater effect of the sea state, with dangerous surge, and white water or rock formations. Marine and boating hazards are major contributors to accidents.

The diving is excessive, often 4 to 6 hours per day for more than 100 days per year. It is for this reason that the incidence of DCS and dysbaric osteonecrosis is increased. DCS is related to the excessive nitrogen load absorbed during these periods at significant depths and with inadequate decompression staging, and dysbaric osteonecrosis is related more to the duration underwater that causes a nitrogen load in the slower tissues. Treatments of DCS tend to be somewhat individualistic, varying from deep air to shallow or surface oxygen regimens, applied in an arbitrary manner.

Because of the equipment used, compressor problems (including carbon monoxide toxicity) are not infrequent.

Pearl divers

Pearl divers spend about the same time underwater as the abalone divers. They are much more regimented because they work as a team, usually exposed to similar depths and total durations, suspended from a drifting boat while collecting shells before surfacing and then performing more 'drifts'. Historical data clearly identify increasing depth to be associated with an increased risk of DCS. Current practice requires that exposure times and number of dives are reduced for the dives in the deeper range.

The problems are similar to those of abalone diving, mainly DCS and dysbaric necrosis. In more recent years, the introduction of oxygen decompressions following provocative diving has reduced risks. Similarly, the adoption of in-water recompression protocols using oxygen at 9 metres has probably improved outcomes when symptoms of DCS do occur. This prompt use of oxygen, at the earliest sign of any DCS symptom, has often allowed these divers to achieve excellent results with minimal treatment times.

Shallow construction and maintenance diving

Exponents of this type of diving are mostly ship and harbour divers, who often use surface supply equipment because it allows them greater duration underwater. Most of their maintenance and construction work is in relatively shallow depths, often less than 10 metres. These divers are less exposed to the risk of DCS and dysbaric osteonecrosis than are the shell divers. To avoid a complete loss of gas supply if the surface system fails, the diver should carry a reserve scuba cylinder on his or her back.

A rigid helmet gives an air space for clear communications and protection from head injury. It also reduces heat loss and decreases the risk of drowning should the diver lose consciousness. A light or welding shade can be fitted, as can a camera for video monitoring of activity by a surface operator.

Because the diver often works at a fixed site, it is common to wear heavy boots and extra weights. With this equipment, the diver may have to be lowered to the job and then hauled up. It is important that the weights be releasable so that the diver can ditch them in an emergency.

The rules for attendants, rescue (standby) divers and on-site recompression chambers vary with local protocols and are often influenced by depths and profiles. The presence of a recompression chamber at the site may be mandated by local standards if there is significant decompression time. Surface decompression, possibly on oxygen, may be a more acceptable and comfortable alternative to in-water decompression. This technique prescribes partial completion of decompression, usually to a depth of around 12 metres, in the water, followed by rapid ascent, removal of equipment and transfer into a chamber for recompression and completion of the decompression. This approach has the advantages of getting the diver out of the water earlier and completing the long 'shallow' decompression stops in a warm, dry environment on 100 per cent oxygen. The disadvantage is that the diver surfaces with dangerously supersaturated tissues and relies on expedited recompression in the chamber to avoid serious DCS. In reality, the technique has been widely used with few reports of problems. It seems to be successful.

Because these divers work in harbours and around ships, one of the major dangers is trauma from marine craft and underwater equipment (explosives, oxy-welding, high-pressure and suction appliances).

SCUBA DIVING

Self-contained underwater breathing apparatus (scuba) permits greater mobility than surface supply – at the cost of reduced duration underwater unless multiple cylinders are carried. It is thus usually used for shallow tasks of relatively short duration.

Scientific divers

Scientific divers often gather data and collect marine specimens in relatively shallow water, but for long periods of time. Not uncommonly, scientific divers are more skilled in their academic discipline than in diving. Thus, decisions are often based more on the needs of the former than on the limitations of the latter. Nevertheless, in recent years much work has been done in developing protocols for approaches to scientific diving, largely through the work of associative scientific diving groups. In the modern era, scientific divers are usually well-resourced and safe.

Dive instructors

Dive instructors conduct training dives in pools and open water for groups of recreational diver trainees who are often diving for the first time. Of all the occupational diving groups, dive instructors arguably bear the greatest responsibility for the safety of others during the course of their underwater work. Most training dives are conducted in relatively shallow water. Nevertheless, diving instructors have (over the years) been vulnerable to DCS based on their multiple repetitive exposures, and possibly because of multiple rapid ascents during training dives when completing skills such as emergency ascent training with students. In the modern context, at least some training organizations have permitted the conduct of these drills as 'simulated' ascents in a horizontal path across the bottom. This has ameliorated the risk to both instructors and trainees (trainees occasionally suffer pulmonary barotrauma during such exercises). The extra skills possessed by dive instructors to cope with both their own diving exposure and that of an inexperienced trainee are often sorely tested.

Fish farm divers

Aquaculture is established as an important industry in many countries such as Australia (tuna, salmon, pearl shell), New Zealand (salmon, mussels), Norway (salmon) and the United Kingdom (salmon).

With tuna, the fish are captured at sea and are then fattened and harvested within very large pens. Tuna divers have the added risks entailed in escorting the catch in ocean cages for days or weeks on the way back from the exposed ocean to sheltered bays. There, pens are used to feed, grow and add value to the fish for the lucrative Japanese sashimi market. Usually, scuba is used in the open sea and towing phases of the diving, with scuba or surface supply used for the diving at the actual farm (pen). Exposure to high seas, boating, underwater

construction equipment, high-pressure gas and suction pumps makes this a high-risk occupation.

Salmon farm divers also work with fish being grown in pens, but these pens are usually in sheltered waterways. The pens are frequently 10 to 30 metres deep and may hold as many as 5000 fish. The pen is usually surrounded by a protective heavier mesh, to deter predators, and the whole structure is tethered by mooring lines, sometimes extending to much greater depths than the pens themselves. The whole structure has to be cleaned and maintained by the divers, who use either scuba or surface supply breathing apparatus.

Although the conditions vary considerably, the task of these divers is usually to dive repeatedly to depths of 10 to 30 metres, often for a total of several hours each day, maintaining, cleaning and unsnagging nets and lines, conducting pontoon and jetty maintenance, feeding fish, removing dead fish and ensuring protection from other predators (e.g. seals and sharks).

Multiple ascents and descents increase the likelihood of dysbaric illness, both DCS and pulmonary barotrauma. The deeper dives, repetitive dives and multi-day diving probably also contribute to this risk. The presence of underwater lines increase the likelihood of entanglements, and predators do occasionally cause problems.

Aquaculture divers are another group that has substantially improved and standardized diving practice since the early days of the industry, and there are numerous examples of operations where previously poor safety records have been completely turned around. This has usually been achieved by the introduction of protocols prescribing acceptable limitations on diving activity and with the adoption of diving techniques that improve decompression (e.g. nitrox, oxygen), monitoring (e.g. computers) and thermal protection (e.g. drysuits).

Miskito Indians

The Miskito Indians of Honduras and Nicaragua have relied heavily on lobster fishing since the early 1960s. The free diving technique changed to scuba in the late 1970s, and the results of inadequate diver training, ambitious diving and the absence of reasonable medical and recompression facilities in these remote areas soon became apparent. Of the 5000 divers, most are employed on lobster boats that put to sea for periods of about 2 weeks. The divers descend to depths as great as 27 to 33 metres, 9 to 20 times a day. This extreme repetitive and multi-day diving exposure causes most of the divers to be affected by DCS, with a high incidence of neurological manifestations. Of great interest to the diving medicine community, this community of divers inevitably favours a self-selected population of survivors, some of whom appear able to undertake repetitive aggressive diving profiles with far less incidence of injury than would be expected. The reasons for the apparent 'resistance' of these divers to DCS is a subject of ongoing speculation and research.

The few recompression chambers available to this community are distant from the diving area, resulting in an average 5- to 7-day delay in treatment. Between 1991 and 1997, there were more than 200 divers treated in the local chamber, with 70 per cent having either paraplegia or quadriplegia as their presenting symptom. Despite the extreme delay, 65 per cent responded with good or excellent outcomes. Many of the others were left with significant residual symptoms, often being paraplegic and requiring self-catheterization for the remainder of their lives – which were frequently shortened by renal infections, bed sores and other disorders.

Other common problems encountered by this group include carbon monoxide toxicity (from incorrect positioning of the compressor intake), shark attack, air embolism and equipment failure. More recent attempts to reduce the mortality and morbidity of this group have centered on a more appropriate management of the marine resource (ensuring a greater supply of lobsters and thus obviating the need to dive deeper), reduction of alcohol and drug use, disability recompense and earlier treatments (surface oxygen, underwater oxygen and possibly even portable chambers).

Unfortunately, the Miskito Indians are typical of many poverty-stricken indigenous communities that have had to extend their diving activities to use marine resources and have then had to extend their diving activities deeper and longer as those marine resources become scarcer.

DEEP AND SATURATION DIVING

Deep occupational divers

Non-divers and many recreational divers think that the life and work of the professional diver are glamourous and exciting. This is not accurate. Occupational diving is often a tedious job with occasional catastrophic hazards. Usually, it is cold, wet and boring, but reasonably well paid.

People pay a diver to perform only a job that cannot be done in a less expensive manner. The most efficient diving firms survive. This situation creates high expectations and more stress on the workers. Some occupational divers derive little pleasure from diving and do not dive recreationally.

Almost every job that is required for surface construction is also conducted underwater. With steel work, for example, the diver can cut with flame cutters and mechanical saws, drill, rivet, use gas and electric welding equipment, bolt with normal and explosive bolts and apply protective coatings. The equivalent range of skills in concreting, carpentry or surveying can be applied. Often, a tradesman with a skill is trained as a diver, rather than teaching a diver a new skill.

Oil rig divers are exposed not only to extremely hazardous environmental conditions on the oil rigs at sea, but also to techniques and equipment that have small safety margins. The risks of DCS and dysbaric osteonecrosis are reflections of the large inert gas loading and also the lack of knowledge regarding dive exposures on the edge of our decompression experience. Deaths of the 1960 to 1970 'oil boom' divers in the North Sea were excessive, but they were reduced considerably when the deep bounce diving, often to 100 to 200 metres, gradually became replaced by saturation exposures.

For deep water tasks, the diver is generally kept at elevated pressure in a deck-mounted compression chamber and commutes to the work site in a submersible chamber. The diver normally operates with another diver, with one in the bell as attendant and the other at the work site. With a changeover in roles, the pair may work an 8-hour shift. The attendant's role is as communicator, tool passer, hose attendant and possibly gas recycler.

In deep water, the diver is normally breathing an oxygen-helium mixture from a system similar to that used in shallow water. Because of the cost of gas, there will probably be a return pipe system so exhaled gas is collected, purified and reused. The recycling from the diver is generally via the bell, to reduce the length of hose. The diver needs a source of heat to keep him or her warm. This source may be hot water from the surface via the bell or water heated in the bell. On-diver electrical heating is an increasingly common alternative. The bell is supplied with gas, power, communication and hot water from the surface and returns gas back to the surface for processing and reuse.

The use of different breathing gases and the complexities associated with delivering these gases at great depths and for long durations increase the likelihood of gas toxicities, hypoxia, DCS and dysbaric osteonecrosis (see Chapter 67).

The period between work shifts and for decompression back to 1 ATA is spent in a chamber mounted on the support ship or rig platform. It is equipped with inclusions such as bunks, table, shower and W.C. A communication system including television or video is now common.

Even in the relative comfort of saturation systems and decompression chambers, there are the continued problems of gas toxicities, contaminants and fire.

In pressure chambers, the high humidity and enclosed environment increase the likelihood of skin and ear infections. Ear infections can be particularly troublesome, and often prophylactic measures are indicated.

Caisson workers

Although not strictly applicable to a diving text, the experiences of caisson workers are of interest. These workers are exposed to relatively shallow 'depths', usually less than 20 metres, but occasionally in the 20- to 30-metre range. The work shifts last from 4 hours upward, and the slow compressions and decompressions make barotraumas much less likely. The major dysbaric problems are DCS, more frequently of the non-neurological type, and dysbaric osteonecrosis. Because of the long durations affecting the 'slow' tissues, dysbaric osteonecrosis is particularly prevalent and appears not to have been eliminated by the otherwise more conservative schedules imposed over the last few decades.

The high humidity and sometimes unhygienic conditions of the caissons and compression and decompression locks, may increase the likelihood of otological and dermatological infective disorders.

FURTHER READING

Blick G. Notes on diver's paralysis. *British Medical Journal* 1909;**2**:1796–1798.

Cross ER. Taravana: diving syndrome in the Tuamoto diver. In: Rahn H, Yokoyama T, eds. *Physiology of Breath-Hold Diving and the Ama of Japan*. National Academy of Sciences publication 1341. Washington, DC: National Academy Press; 1965:207–219.

Doolette D, Craig D. Tuna farm diving in South Australia. *South Pacific Underwater Medicine Society Journal* 1999;**29**(2):115–117.

Edmonds C. A study of Australian pearl diving 1988–91. *South Pacific Underwater Medicine Society Journal Pearl Diving Supplement* 1996;**26**(1):26–30.

Edmonds C. Pearl diving: the Australian story. *South Pacific Underwater Medicine Society Journal Pearl Diving Supplement* 1996;**26**(1):4–15.

Lepawsky M, Wong R, eds. *Empirical Diving Techniques of Commercial Sea Harvesters: The Proceedings of the Fiftieth Workshop of the Undersea and Hyperbaric Medicine Society, Vancouver, Canada*. Kensington Maryland: Underwater Hyperbaric Medical Society; 2001.

Millington T. "No-tech" technical diving: the lobster divers of La Mosquitia. *South Pacific Underwater Medicine Society Journal* 1997;**27**(3):147–148.

Smart D, McCartney P. High risk diving: Tasmania's aquaculture industry. *South Pacific Underwater Medicine Society Journal* 1990;**20**(3):159–165.

Wong R. Pearl diving from Broome. *South Pacific Underwater Medicine Society Journal Pearl Diving Supplement* 1996;**26**(1):15–26.

Wong R. Western Australian pearl divers drift diving. *South Pacific Underwater Medicine Society Journal Pearl Diving Supplement* 1996;**26**(1):30–36.

This chapter was reviewed for this fifth edition by Simon Mitchell.

Diving in contaminated water

INTRODUCTION

There is no need for the average amateur diver to enter contaminated water, but circumstances arise where a professional diver must do so. Often a medical officer with an interest in diving becomes involved as medical adviser to a professional diving squad. This brief chapter does not make the reader an expert on the subject. It aims to indicate the problems that should be considered. It is a summary of some of the points expounded in Barsky's text on the subject[1].

This question should always be asked: 'Is the dive really necessary?' Barsky mentions a case in which police dived in a sewage pond to recover a body. They found the body, and the task could be regarded as a success, but it was not necessary. The sewage plant had the capacity to drain the pond. If this had not been possible, then a search could have been conducted by dragging the pond with nets. The victim was seen to slip and fall into the pond, so there was no suggestion of foul play. The job was unnecessary and exposed the divers to a high-risk microbiological environment with inadequate protection.

If the dive is needed, then the following questions should be answered: What is the nature of the hazard or hazards? Can the diver be protected against them? Can the diver be recovered if he or she becomes incapacitated? Can the diver and the diving equipment be safely decontaminated?

HAZARDS

In general terms, hazards fall into four groups – chemical, biological, radioactive and thermal. Guidance on dealing with them should be sought from the local hazardous materials disposal organization. The members of this organization may not understand diving, but they will have the expertise necessary to advise on protection of attendants and how to decontaminate both attendants and divers.

Chemical hazards can be encountered through a need to dive in a processing plant or as a result of an accident where chemicals have been spilt. The first may be simpler because the composition of the materials will be known.

Biological hazards are generally caused by bacterial and/or viral contamination of the water. Normally, a laboratory can identify and quantify the bacterial contaminants. These may include *Aeromonas, Klebsiella* and *Salmonella*. Also of concern are amoebae such as *Naegleria fowleri* (see Chapter 29).

Diving in potentially radioactive water may be required if a carrier has an accident and containers need to be salvaged from water. This is often an overrated danger because most containers of radioactive material are damage resistant. In some countries, diving may be needed in nuclear reactors. This should be left to the expertise of a large company with experience in the work. In some cases, a remote-controlled vehicle can do the job. In others, a gas return line to the surface is needed to prevent gas pockets from forming in the reactor pipes. Sometimes, a diver in a 1-ATA rigid suit (which gives better shielding) can do the work. In all cases, there will be some radiation exposure.

Thermal hazards are discussed in Chapter 27. Heat stress can be a problem if a diver has to stand in the sun while the drysuit is decontaminated.

Diving in a contaminated environment requires good planning and calm implementation. There may be a claustrophobic element that some divers cannot tolerate because an immediate escape option may not be available. Previous work experience in a confined space is a good predictor of success in this field.

DIVING EQUIPMENT

The equipment used should be matched against the hazard and diving required. At a minimum, a second gas supply system is needed so that the diver can return on it if required. The diver needs protection from the substance in which he or she is diving. This protection normally requires a drysuit and helmet, which reduce or eliminate skin and eye contact with the hazard. It can be in a free-flow design such as a standard rig. This has the benefits that any helmet leak is likely to be outward and the helmet-to-suit join is well sealed.

A demand system such as the SuperLite (Kirby Morgan, Santa Maria, California) helmet can be used. The problem with these systems is that each inhalation normally creates a negative pressure in the helmet. This can cause the exhaust valve to leak a tiny amount of liquid into the demand valve. One solution in design of specialized contaminated environment equipment is to fit two exhaust valves in series to prevent leakage. The SuperLite (and similar) helmets allow attachment of a redundant gas supply to which the diver can 'bail out' if the primary gas supply (usually from the surface) fails. Also, a free-flow valve can be opened to supply gas to the helmet in the event of a flood or if the demand valve fails. The other major advantage of such helmets is that many occupational divers are familiar with them.

A drysuit can be connected to gloves so that the diver's hands are protected from contact with the toxic material. A possible problem with chemical pollution is that the suit must be resistant to attack from it. No suit material is resistant to all likely chemicals. A drysuit with a smooth surface is easier to decontaminate than a drysuit with fibre surface. It is also easier to patch to repair leaks.

Before the diver enters contaminated water, the system should be tested for leaks. This may involve a small pond (e.g. a play pool), which may also be part of the decontamination routine.

DECONTAMINATION

It must be possible to clean the diver and dispose of the washing liquid and other cleaning material safely. In many cases, a hose, a brush and a platform (so that the washings go back into the polluted environment) are adequate. Special care needs to be given to cleaning joins in the suit assembly. The helmet join is of concern because often any drips when it is opened fall inside the suit. A planned method of recovering and cleaning a disabled diver is needed.

Consideration should be given to the protection of the rest of the dive team. Of major concern are the persons cleaning the diver. In a civic matter, such as a police rescue squad, those responsible for cleaning up after land contamination may be available for this task. They will need training in the handling of the diver and the diving equipment.

Trials and exercises of the techniques before an emergency are useful methods of examining problems and testing solutions, and they provide insurance against adverse outcomes.

REFERENCE

1. Barsky SM. *Diving in High-Risk Environments.* 4th ed. Ventura, California: Hammerhead Press; 2007.

This chapter was reviewed for this fifth edition by Simon Mitchell.

67

Deep and saturation diving

HISTORY

Humans continue their efforts to reach even greater depths (see Chapter 1). Early in the nineteenth century, depth was limited by the capacity of the air pumps. After improvements to them, depth was limited by decompression sickness (DCS). The limited air supply also caused carbon dioxide accumulation in the helmet of the standard diver.

When decompression tables were introduced and compressors improved, humans could reach depths of about 70 to 80 metres before being seriously affected by nitrogen narcosis and no longer capable of useful work.

Problems

The introduction of helium as a diluting gas allowed the depth limit to be extended, and in 1937 a US diver reached 128 metres (420 feet). Dives to these depths require long decompression even for a short time at the working depth.

For example, a 70-metre air dive would require 100 to 150 minutes of decompression for a bottom time of 30 minutes. For the same bottom time at 100 metres, while breathing a mixture of 16 per cent oxygen in helium, nearly 3 hours of decompression

are required (about 100 minutes of this is spent breathing oxygen, with the risk of oxygen toxicity). Both these dives would involve a significant risk of DCS.

Deep diving is associated with a more rapid consumption of gas, increased respiratory resistance, thermal difficulties, voice distortion, sensory deprivation, inadequate information about decompression schedules and equipment problems. Other difficulties include a much greater risk of dysbaric osteonecrosis, inner ear disorders and a greater than usual danger from coincidental medical disorders.

Solutions

Three ways have been developed to cope with this problem of excessive decompression times. One is to avoid the excess pressure by operating from a submersible vehicle or a pressure-resistant suit at atmospheric pressure.

Hannes Keller demonstrated that decompression times could be reduced by **changing gas mixtures** to capitalize on maximum gas tension gradients. In 1962, his experiments culminated in a dive to 305 metres for 5 minutes of bottom time. The divers still required 270 minutes of decompression. Keller's companion died, and this approach did not become popular with commercial divers because of the short bottom time and the risk of severe DCS. The approach is being revived with the more serious forms of technical diving.

The total decompression requirements for a long task can be reduced by allowing the diver to stay at depth until the task is finished and then decompress slowly in a chamber. Thus, only one decompression is required. This is called **saturation diving,** and the first demonstration is attributed to Dr George Bond of the US Navy. Bond was exploiting a suggestion made by Behnke in 1942, as a method of increasing the duration of exposure in caisson workers. Although these men were instrumental in applying the concept of saturation diving, they were predated by Dr Orval Cunningham (Kansas City, Missouri in 1927), who used air under pressure for several days, followed by slow decompression, as a form of hyperbaric therapy.

The main value of saturation diving is that a diver needs the same decompression time for a dive lasting 2 days or 2 months. Once the body has equilibrated with the gases in the environment at any pressure, it will not take up any more gas, so the decompression time will not increase.

Bond tested this concept with animals and then with humans in compression chambers. In 1964, he had a group of four men in a cylindrical underwater house for 9 days at a depth of nearly 60 metres (Sea Lab I). Other early dives based on underwater houses, or habitats, were conducted by Link and Cousteau.

Instead of permanent underwater habitats, saturation dives can be conducted in transportable chambers. The first commercial work in saturation was conducted by Westinghouse Inc. The workers lived in a pressurized chamber on the surface called a **deck decompression chamber** (DDC), and they were lowered to work in a capsule called a **submersible decompression chamber** (SDC), often called a bell. This allowed their transfer to the working depth without any alteration in pressure. In 1965, this procedure was used for a series of dives to repair a dam in the United States. Four men at a time were pressurized, and they performed 800 hours of work in 12 weeks. With surface diving, the men could have performed only about 160 hours of work in the same period.

The main need for saturation diving is in the off-shore oil industry, which relies on saturation divers to carry out many tasks underwater. These include observations, welding joins in pipes, cleaning, anti-fouling and repairing damaged components. Military saturation dives have been conducted for a variety of purposes. Most have been for the recovery of valuable, dangerous or strategic items from the sea bed. Saturation diving techniques are also used for scientific purposes. One example is the Aquarius habitat located in about 20 metres of water off Key Largo in Florida. Aquarius, an undersea laboratory and home for scientists studying the marine environment, is owned by the National Oceanic and Atmospheric Administration (NOAA) and operated by Florida International University (Figure 67.1). Saturation diving techniques allow scientists to live and work underwater 24 hours per day for missions that typically last 10 days.

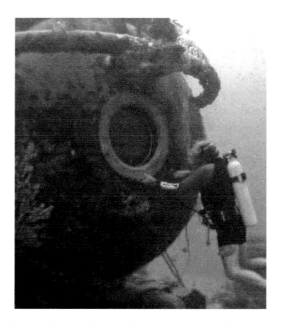

Figure 67.1 A diver working to maintain the outside of Aquarius by cleaning off marine growth. He is using a hookah rig that includes a typical second stage regulator attached to an air hose that leads to Aquarius and an air storage tank. A secondary 'bail-out' bottle is on his back for safety if problems develop with the hookah rig. (From National Oceanic and Atmospheric Administration. http://oceanexplorer.noaa.gov/technology/diving/aquarius/aquarius.html.)

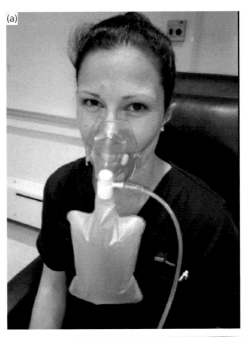

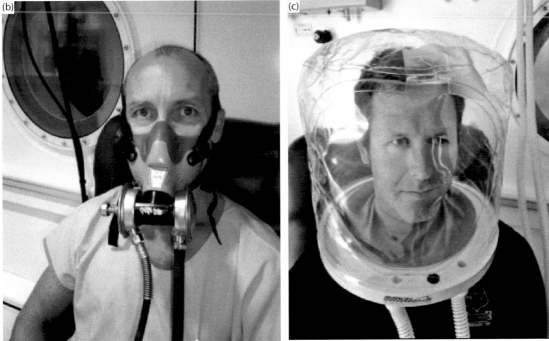

Plate 6, front. Hyperbaric medicine. **(a)** A reducer connects to a flow meter, with oxygen passing to an oro-nasal mask and bag. **(b)** For more comfort, oxygen can be supplied via a hood surrounding the patient's head. This arrangement also allows for vocal communication. **(c)** A demand valve and regulator analogous to scuba, often with an overboard dump system for exhaled gas.

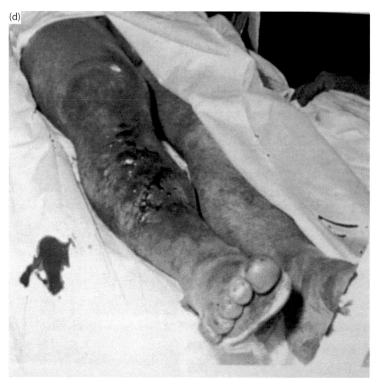

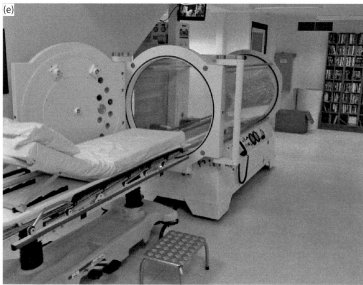

Plate 6, back. **(d)** Gas gangrene, showing a swollen leg with pallor, haemorrhagic bullae and necrosis. The condition responded to hyperbaric oxygen therapy. **(e)** A one-person hyperbaric chamber used for patients undergoing hyperbaric medical treatment.

SATURATION DIVE PROCEDURES

Many skills are needed to conduct a saturation dive. The facilities include a diving tender, compression chambers, large quantities of compressed gas and technical staff. There are also many logistical problems in navigation and nautical skills necessary to support such an operation. The details are beyond the scope of this book. The aim of the remainder of the chapter is to outline the more important aspects of conducting a dive using a DDC and SDC. First, the biomedical and habitability problems in conducting a saturation dive are considered, and then the conduct of a dive is outlined. More common medical problems are mentioned in Chapter 69.

ENVIRONMENT REQUIRED

The area occupied by the divers needs to have a controlled atmosphere. The loss of pressure or temperature control can be fatal. The environmental maintenance systems need to be reliable and be supplemented by alternative systems. Allowance must be made for a power failure. Evacuation proceedings to be used if the ship or oil rig has to be abandoned need consideration.

Contamination of the atmosphere also must be considered. Gas purity standards are discussed in Chapter 19, but more stringent standards are needed for deep saturation dives, given that small changes in gas composition result in large changes in inspired partial pressures. Prevention of contamination, with monitoring systems to measure and control oxygen and carbon dioxide levels, are needed. Alternative breathing gases must be supplied directly to the divers, for use if the chamber atmosphere becomes contaminated. For a deep dive, this can involve enormous reserves of gas.

In large chamber complexes, it may be possible to transfer the divers to another chamber if contamination occurs. Most groups conducting saturation dives have their own procedures and prescribed limits for certain contaminants. The limits specified reflect the attitudes of various authorities, as well as the operational performance of each diving system. Examples of such recommendations are as follows:

Oxygen – Partial pressures of 0.2 to 0.5 ATA have been used, and the most common is about 0.4 ATA. This gives a safety margin between risks of hypoxia and pulmonary oxygen toxicity. There has been a more recent tendency to increase the oxygen pressure to about 0.5 ATA during decompression. This assists in off-gassing and reduces the risk of DCS. Because of the fire risk associated with high oxygen concentrations, the chamber oxygen is generally kept below 21 per cent during about the last 10 metres of ascent. The reduction of oxygen pressure may require a slowing of the ascent rate. The alternative is to use periods of breathing high-oxygen mixtures from a mask with an overboard dump system.

Carbon dioxide – This is kept below a limit of 0.005 ATA, equivalent to 0.5 per cent at 1 ATA. For shorter periods, a higher limit, 0.015 to 0.02 ATA, is tolerable. A high carbon dioxide level leads to hypercapnoea and a reduced work capacity.

Diluting gas – This gas may be nitrogen for shallow dives, but for deeper dives helium, hydrogen and nitrogen mixtures with oxygen have been used. Each mixture requires a different decompression schedule. Addition of extra nitrogen to an oxygen-helium mixture is often used to reduce the high-pressure neurological syndrome (HPNS), but it increases the risks of DCS. If using nitrogen cannot be avoided, it may be necessary to use a slower decompression than the standard oxygen-helium schedule. Hydrogen has been trialed as a diluting gas, particularly by the French. It is like nitrogen in reducing some of the HPNS symptoms and has been added to the helium-oxygen mixture at depth. If used in the DDC atmosphere, hydrogen has to be removed during ascent so that there is none left when the oxygen concentration is high enough for there to be a risk of combustion. Hydrogen is very explosive when mixed with more than about 4 to 5 per cent oxygen (e.g. the oxygen found in breathing gas), but at depth, the oxygen is diluted by so much inert gas that a hydrogen fire will not burn. This limits use of hydrogen to deep dives. Like helium, hydrogen raises the timbre of the diver's voice. The hydrogen-oxygen mix when used as a diving gas is sometimes referred to as hydrox, whereas mixtures containing both hydrogen and helium as diluents are termed hydreliox.

Trace contaminants – Various authorities specify arbitrary limits for a variety of possible contaminants. The limits are extrapolations from occupational health advisory groups, adjusted for depth. Because the designated contaminant limits are not comprehensive, medical staff members need to consider the toxicology of many preparations they prescribe or wish to use, at depth. For example, solvents may pose a problem. Mercury thermometers or sphygmomanometers should be avoided because of the possible generation of mercury vapour and the possibility of the chamber's being condemned because of amalgam formation. Other common sources of toxic products include paints, welding, refrigeration leaks and cooking fumes. Activated carbon or molecular sieve compounds may be needed to control contamination.

Temperatures – The high thermal conductivity of helium and hydrogen mixtures requires an increase in the optimal working temperature and narrows the range for thermal comfort. This may increase from about 25°C to 33°C, with greater depths. Deviations from this range can cause hypothermia or hyperthermia and need to be avoided. Hyperthermia may be rapid and not easily detected at an early stage.

Humidity – Humidity levels need less strict control than the other parameters. When using soda lime to remove carbon dioxide, a relative humidity (RH) of more than 75 per cent gives better performance. Other absorbents may require different optimal percentages. Higher RH also reduces the risk of static sparks, a possible source of ignition in the fire risk zone. The problem with accepting a high RH is the increased risk of certain bacterial and fungal infections, which can be a problem in saturation dives – so the range chosen is a compromise. With water from wet gear and showering, it is often difficult to keep humidity down to the 60 to 75 per cent RH range recommended.

Fire hazards – If the oxygen pressure is kept at 0.4 ATA, there will be a fire hazard in the chamber at depths shallower than about 50 metres. This is called the fire risk zone. To reduce the hazard, the amount of combustible material is limited as a precaution. At greater depths, there will be insufficient oxygen concentrations present to support combustion.

ENVIRONMENTAL CONTROL SYSTEM

Processing and analytical equipment is needed to provide the required environmental conditions. Typically, the chamber gas is drawn through scrubbers to remove carbon dioxide, then past a cold water radiator to condense excess water vapour and then past a heater coil to rewarm the gas to provide a comfortable temperature. Other chemicals absorb the trace contaminants and odours. The scrubbing and temperature control units are normally in the chambers. In the case of the DDC, they can be outside the chamber with pipes connecting the purification system to the chamber. If the equipment is backed up and can be isolated from the chamber, it can be serviced during a dive. If it is in the chamber, the divers must do any servicing; having the equipment inside the chamber simplifies the piping design.

Gas analysis equipment is needed to keep a check on the composition of the atmosphere. At a minimum, the following measurements are needed:

- Oxygen, to show when oxygen should be added to replace metabolic consumption and when it should be removed to avoid toxicity or reduce the risk of fire.
- Carbon dioxide, to show that the scrubbers are working. If there is a rise in reading, it may indicate that the absorbent is exhausted.
- Temperature and humidity are needed to show that the divers are in a comfortable thermal environment.

These parameters should be measured continuously in each compartment. Other monitoring may be less frequent. For example, trace contaminants build up slowly, and so daily measurements may be adequate.

It is also normal to have television monitoring of the divers in each compartment so the supervisors can watch for problems and possibly advise on any problems that occur.

OTHER HABITABILITY REQUIREMENTS

The divers need toilet and washing facilities. These are usually provided in a small outer lock. This allows the space to be depressurized for cleaning without depressurizing the rest of the chamber. Eating and sleeping spaces are provided in the inner compartment or compartments. To minimize boredom, it is normal to provide amusements such as access to television and music.

Consideration needs to be given to things that can go wrong. This can range from a power or equipment failure to sinking of the ship carrying the DDC. Answers to most problems have evolved. In some systems, the occupants of the chamber move to a chamber built into a life boat that is connected to the DDC. If the vessel sinks or catches fire, the DDC occupants move into the chamber on the life boat. The boat is then launched with surface crew to operate the chamber.

Gas is used by several processes, and the diver in the water will probably be on open circuit. Any equipment failure in the gas purification systems or contamination of the chamber requires the divers in the DDC to use the built-in breathing system (BIBS). This gas is normally collected, purified and compressed back in to cylinders for re-use.

THE SATURATION DIVE

Compression phase

It is common to commence an oxygen-helium saturation dive by compressing the subjects to about 2 ATA on air, thus allowing the chamber seals and oxygen sensors to be checked without wasting helium. At that stage, the divers and operators can test systems before continuing the compression with helium. The other alternative is to compress with helium and then oxygen to create an atmosphere with 0.4 ATA of helium without creating a dangerous oxygen-rich mixture.

The compression can continue till the desired depth is reached or a depth at which problems of compression arthralgia or HPNS can be expected. From that depth, compression is slowed, and pauses are introduced.

Several mechanical problems can occur during compression. In chambers with poor gas mixing, the lighter diluting gases can float over the heavier nitrogen and oxygen, thereby giving a hypoxic layer and an oxygen-rich layer. This can be avoided at the design stage by injecting fresh gas where there is good gas circulation. Sensors that are influenced by pressure can give misleading indications of gas concentrations. These should be avoided by selecting more suitable sensors. Rapid compression can cause overheating and hyperthermia.

At maximum depth

Once the chamber reaches working depth, the divers start to use the SDC. In normal operation, two divers enter the SDC from the DDC and are lowered to the work site. One diver remains in the chamber, and the other enters the water from a door in the bottom of the SDC and goes to work in diving gear. The divers are both supplied with gas from the surface. The diver also obtains gas and hot water from a hose that leads back into the SDC. Electrical power for lighting, heating and any tools also comes from the surface. Television cameras and voice communications allow the surface crew to monitor and assist in the work by lowering tools and operating cranes and hoists as needed.

The diver in the chamber is there to assist the diver in the water and to rescue the diver in the water if he or she gets into difficulties. The normal work pattern is an 8-hour shift with the diver and the SDC operator swapping about half-way through the shift.

When pressurized, there is a depth range through which the divers can move without risking DCS. It is normal for the depths to be chosen so that the sea bottom is the lower limit of this depth range and DDC depth is at the upper limit of the range. A saturated diver can move through a range of depths from 100 metres to 129 metres and return without concern about DCS.

The diver commonly uses modified demand equipment such as a SuperLite helmet (Kirby Morgan Dive Systems, Santa Maria, California). It is fitted with a gas heater so the inhaled gas is warmed. The diver is warmed by a hot water suit. A back-mounted cylinder of gas is used to return to the SDC if there is a gas supply failure. Because of the gas density, the cylinder has a very short endurance. A cylinder that lasts an hour will last less than 2 minutes at 300 metres.

Decompression phase

The decompression phase is long because the rate of ascent is set by the gas elimination from the slowest tissues. The US Navy schedules take about 12 days to decompress divers from 300 metres of pressure. Boredom of the divers and chamber operators, with subsequent loss of concentration, may develop during the protracted decompression from a saturation dive.

A saturation dive is an expensive, complex operation, but it can be conducted with safety, provided everybody knows and does their job. What can go wrong is considered in Chapter 68.

FURTHER READING

Beyerstein G. Commercial diving: surface-mixed gas, Sur-D-O$_2$, bell bounce, saturation. In: Lang MA, Smith NE, eds. *Proceedings of Advanced Scientific Diving Workshop*. Washington, DC: Smithsonian Institution; 2006.

Davis RH. *Deep Diving and Submarine Operations: A manual for deep sea divers and compressed air workers*. 9th ed. London: Seibe Gorman & Company; 1999.

Haux G. *Subsea Manned Engineering*. London: Bailliere Tindall; 1982.

Sisman D, ed. *The Professional Diver's Handbook*. London: Submex; 1982.

This chapter was reviewed for this fifth edition by Michael Bennett.

Related Subjects

68

Hyperbaric equipment

INTRODUCTION

There are two main types of human occupied pressure vessels used in medicine and research. These are as follows:

- **Hyperbaric chambers,** where the ambient pressure can be increased from 1 ATA to many times atmospheric pressure depending on the structural capabilities of the vessel concerned. These chambers are used for diving, hyperbaric medicine and research and are built to withstand an explosive force (Plate 6).
- **Hypobaric chambers,** where the ambient pressure can be decreased from 1 ATA to sub-atmospheric pressure levels. These chambers are used for aviation, space medicine and research and are built to resist an implosive force.

Some chambers are capable of performing both functions, but these are not common and are mostly found in research centres. This chapter is concerned with the features of those hyperbaric chambers used in medicine.

Hyperbaric chambers have in common the single function of holding compressed gas, but they have been given various names – mainly deriving from the context in which they are used. Terms used for chambers used in diving include the following:

- The **recompression chamber** (RCC), where the major use of the hyperbaric chamber is for compressing a caisson worker or diver, usually as part of a therapeutic regimen. It may also be used in the training of divers, so that they may experience the effects of hyperbaria.
- The **decompression chamber,** where the major use is to decompress a subject already exposed to increased pressure. A **submersible decompression chamber** (SDC) is used to transport divers under pressure to and from the working depth (see Chapter 67). It usually allows transfer under pressure to a surface or **deck decompression chamber** (DDC). The DDC allows for the definitive decompression under controlled conditions. The diving bell, which is open at the bottom and exposed to ambient sea pressure, was the forerunner of the SDC.

The **hyperbaric chamber** is a term usually reserved for a therapeutic pressure vessel used in medicine. In the same context, **hyperbaric facility** is a term used to describe the chamber and supporting equipment, examination rooms and offices.

Only hyperbaric and recompression chambers are discussed in this section. These chambers consist of a strengthened vessel or hull that can be pressurized by compressed gas. The gas may be supplied from gas cylinders or direct from a compressor. Decompression is achieved by allowing the gas to escape.

Since the 1920s, numerous hyperbaric chambers have been designed for the treatment of divers and caisson workers. Many early chambers were also used for hyperbaric medicine and study of the effects of pressure change[1]. Initially consisting of a simple, single-compartment pressure vessel, chambers have become significantly more complex with the developing requirements of hyperbaric and diving medicine. The design of these structures requires the involvement of personnel ranging from the specialist diving physician and the diver to the design and construction engineer.

The initial consideration in designing a hyperbaric chamber concerns its expected use. There are several main types of recompression chambers[2]:

1. Large multi-compartment chambers used for research, as well as treatment of divers and caisson workers, and capable of compression to many atmospheres (greater than 5 ATA). These may incorporate a wet chamber where immersed and pressurized environments can be created for training, research and equipment testing activities.
2. Large multi-compartment chambers capable of moderate pressures (2 to 4 ATA). These chambers are used for treatment with hyperbaric oxygen.
3. Portable high-pressure multi-person chambers for treating divers and caisson workers on site as required.
4. Portable one-person, high- or low-pressure chambers. Initially designed for the surface decompression of divers, these are now more commonly found in hyperbaric medicine units, where several such units provide treatment

flexibility. These chambers have been used for the treatment of divers and caisson workers requiring recompression therapy[3].

Low-pressure units may be inadequate for the treatment of an emergency such as cerebral air embolism. Any properly designed high-pressure complex should be capable of treating both diving accident victims and hyperbaric medicine patients.

All chambers need a means of removing carbon dioxide. The alternatives are to install a scrubber, flushing with fresh gas or dumping the carbon dioxide overboard through the built-in breathing system. For a chamber that is routinely expected to be pressurized to more than 20 metres (3 ATA), the cost and noise of air flushing may make a scrubbing system preferable, but this introduces the need for more complex monitoring equipment. An engineer who is an expert in the field should be consulted.

Most countries have one or more codes that any chamber should comply with, and this coding includes a 'pressure vessel code' and usually a code defining appropriate plant, equipment and staffing for a hyperbaric facility. In Australia, reference is made to the US code series 'Pressure Vessels for Human Occupancy' (PVHO) and the Australian Standard series AS2299.2 – 'Work in compressed air facilities – Hyperbaric Facilities'[4,5]. There are complementary codes for scientific, caisson and industry operations. A ship-mounted chamber is normally guided by the code of the organization that classifies the ship (e.g. Lloyd's, American Bureau of Shipping or DNV).

Whatever the situation, strict attention must be paid to multiple standards and codes covering all aspects of the facility.

LARGE MULTI-COMPARTMENT RECOMPRESSION CHAMBER

This is a high-pressure chamber capable of accommodating several persons in each lock (internal compartment). It should be suitable for treating divers, caisson workers and patients requiring hyperbaric oxygen.

The recompression chamber may be composed of the following elements, the principles of which have medical implications. The finer technical details are not discussed.

Hull

The hull should consist of two or more interconnecting chambers or locks, some of which can be separately compressed or decompressed. The number of compartments depends on the purpose of the unit, but the simplest system usually consists of a large inner lock and a smaller outer lock. The inner lock is used for therapy and the outer lock for transfer of personnel.

The inner lock should have a medical lock to allow transfer of items such as food, excreta, drugs and equipment.

If constructed as a cylinder, the chamber diameter should be sufficient for an adult to stand erect in both locks, especially the inner lock, where most treatments are conducted. This requires an inner diameter of at least 2 metres. The length of the inner lock should be more than 3 metres to accommodate a prone patient on a stretcher and allow free movement of attendants around the patient.

A cylindrical shape has been the normal form for the hull since the early days. This shape efficiently distributes the stress of internal pressure and keeps the weight of steel required to a minimum. More recently, rectangular chambers have been developed using 'C-beams' of steel to provide sufficient strength to withstand the increased stress in the corners of the vessel. Pioneered by Fink Engineering in Melbourne, Australia, this design has become almost standard in hospital-based hyperbaric facilities. The great advantages of these chambers are that the maximum floor area and internal volume are given over to patient treatment and the space is less threatening to patients unfamiliar with pressure vessels. Large doors are usually fitted to facilitate access (see Figure 68.1).

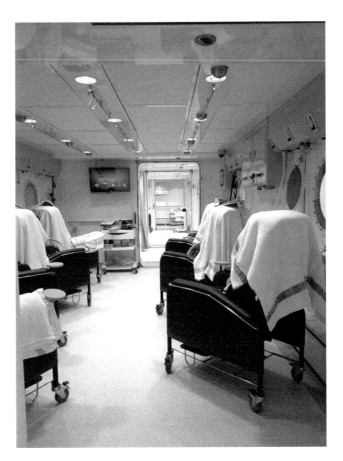

Figure 68.1 View of a large rectangular patient treatment chamber. (Photograph by M. Bennett.)

Pressure-sealed doors are needed both between the outer lock and the area outside the chamber and for the opening into the inner lock. Doorway dimensions and locations should allow easy entry and removal of persons and stretchers.

Observation ports should be fitted to all locks so that the entire compartment can be easily observed. All interior surfaces should be painted with light, easily cleaned, non-reflective, fire-retardant paint. The coating should minimize static electricity.

Furniture and fittings

Comfortable seating should be available for the anticipated number of occupants because decompression may be prolonged. Fold-away seating allows maximum use of space for different requirements. For hyperbaric therapy, the emphasis is usually on reclining seats made for comfort for patients who are often overweight or in some pain.

Both locks should have metal storage shelves or lockers for storage of medical instruments and other equipment.

Lighting can be either direct interior pressure-sealed and fire-safe lights, through hull fibreoptic lighting, or external lights separated from ceiling ports by heat filters or airflow cooling systems. Both locks should have shadow-free lighting.

Size and space should allow for one or two stretchers or trolleys to be used, at least in the inner lock. The trolley should be 1 metre high, with adjustable head and foot elevations and fitted with anti-static straps and lockable wheels. Because of the confined chamber space and door design, the trolley system may not be appropriate. In such cases, removable rails may be used to facilitate moving a stretcher into the inner lock.

Chamber plumbing

Intake openings into both locks should be muffled to keep sound levels below 90 dB at maximum compression rate. The inlets should be distant from the outlets to promote gas circulation and not adjacent to personnel or movable objects. Outlets should be placed in inaccessible positions on the ceilings and covered by grids. Outside the chamber, the pipe openings should be removed from the control panel to avoid a noise hazard. They should

not be near heating or electrical apparatus because of the danger of fire from possible high oxygen partial pressures in the exhaust gases.

Equalization valves may be needed between locks to allow doors to be opened and the transfer of people between compartments.

Breathing gas supply

Pressurization of both locks should be under the control of the panel supervisor or hyperbaric chamber supervisor. The chamber should be capable of a pressurization rate at least equal to that of diving and therapeutic tables. High-pressure air should be ducted into both locks from a large-capacity storage tank (receiver) after having passed through a filtration bank from an electrically driven compressor. A standby diesel or gasoline compressor is usually mandated.

Provision for breathing helium-oxygen or other gas mixtures may be required if divers are to be treated for decompression sickness (DCS). Most tables require the patient to breathe oxygen. A second storage bank of oxygen-nitrogen and oxygen-helium mixtures may also be needed for more advanced tables. Gas supplies also need to allow the attendant to breathe safe gas mixtures if the chamber atmosphere becomes contaminated.

Two systems of oxygen or mixture supply to patients and attendants are in common use, namely:

1. A reducer, flow meter, and an oronasal mask and bag. As an alternative, this may supply a hood surrounding the patient's head (see Chapter 49).
2. A demand valve and regulator analogous to scuba, often with an overboard dump system for exhaled gas. The exhaled gas is oxygen rich and, where possible, should be fed into such an overboard dump system to prevent high oxygen levels from developing in the chamber.

The breathing gas supply should be useable as an emergency air supply. It may be called a built-in breathing system (BIBS), and it should be fitted for all personnel in both compartments. These systems consist of demand valves connected by short, high-pressure hoses to spring-loaded bayonet mountings on a bulkhead. All hoses should be fire resistant. A breathing gas supply should be available that bypasses the main supply, coming from separate emergency bottles. This system ensures an air supply and prevents toxic fumes from overcoming the chamber occupants.

Communications

Communication facilities should include an intercom or two-way transmitter-receiver unit between all compartments and the control panel. A helium speech processor should be fitted if a helium-rich atmosphere is to be used. A sound-powered, electrically insulated, telephone from all locks to the control panel is a useful back-up in the event of a failure in the primary system.

Closed-circuit television coverage may be needed so all occupants can be monitored from the control panel. If electrically safe, or in a pressure housing, the cameras may be located inside the locks. If not electrically safe, they can be an observation port outside.

An auxiliary back-up electrical power source is needed for compressor, lighting and all ancillary equipment.

Transfer under pressure

If transfer to or from another chamber while under pressure is an operation requirement, the outer opening of the outer lock should be fitted with some system enabling a transfer under pressure from a portable chamber using a transfer sleeve. Such manoeuvres may require a sling and gantry or rails to support the mobile chamber. A stable system is needed to avoid pivoting at the connection between the chambers. In this regard, the NATO connection has become industry standard.

Fire

Sheffield and Desautels[6] reported that fires in 35 hyperbaric chambers have claimed 77 lives. Other incidents have involved experimental animals. The severity of these fires is indicated by the fact that in this series there were few survivors, none of whom were in a chamber that had an oxygen-rich atmosphere. Most recent fires have been

caused by occupants taking dangerous material into the chamber.

Any fire has three pre-requisites – a source to ignite it, fuel, and oxygen. Fire can be prevented by removing any of these elements. In a chamber, the hair on the diver's skin can provide fuel to spread the fire, and if the oxygen partial pressure is greater than about 1 ATA, hairless skin will burn. Oxygen must be available for the diver to breathe and is often present at high partial pressures, so two elements required for a fire are always present. Ignition sources must be rigorously sought and eliminated.

Further aggravating factors are the increased ease of ignition and combustibility that exist in some hyperbaric conditions. Substances that do not burn in air can burn if the oxygen partial pressure is elevated. This includes some substances treated with fire-retarding chemicals. Even static sparks generated by clothing could cause a fire as a result of the increased ease of ignition.

An apparent contradiction to these facts is that it is impossible to sustain a fire in some of the gas mixtures used in deep diving because of the low oxygen concentration. This cannot be used as an excuse to avoid precautions against fire because in these conditions there may be pockets of gas that can sustain combustion, and periods of high fire risk are encountered during compression and decompression.

The safety of the chamber occupants depends on the awareness of everyone involved of the fire hazards and on continuing vigilance to prevent any action that could increase the risk of fire. Risks must be appropriately identified, analyzed and minimized, and firefighting systems are mandatory.

All locks should be fitted with firefighting facilities using water as the extinguishing medium. A system of spray nozzles should be capable of wetting all surfaces thoroughly with a fine spray or mist within 2 to 3 seconds of the onset of any fire. Continuous spraying requires a compensatory air loss to avoid an increase in pressure as the locks partially flood. Activation of this system can occur automatically via ultraviolet, infrared and/or carbon dioxide sensors. Manual switches should be placed inside the locks and on the control panel. A secondary system of hand-operated hoses with spray nozzles should be fitted in each lock so that an attendant can direct water onto any source of fire or heat.

An oxygen elimination or exhaust dump system is a mandatory requirement for modern chambers when the subjects breathe from masks. It enables expired gases containing elevated oxygen and carbon dioxide pressures to be exhausted to the exterior. Techniques used include extraction from a reservoir bag using a Venturi system connected to the exhaust and the use of non-return valves.

Any padding allowed on stretcher or seats is best constructed of material that not only is fire resistant or non-combustible but also will not, if exposed to extreme temperatures, produce toxic fumes. The same applies to all clothing and bedclothes within the chamber, all of which should be specially treated to minimize the risk of static electricity build-up. High partial pressures and concentrations of oxygen increase the fire risk in a hyperbaric chamber.

Instrumentation and operation

Emphasis should be placed on obtaining rugged, reliable equipment in preference to sophisticated but delicate instruments.

Control panels should always be fitted with easily read instruments. They must be located in a manner that prevents confusion about the lock to which they refer. Colour codes are useful, with each lock having different coloured instruments.

Pressure and depth gauges should be sited in all locks and on the control panel. Two gauges may be coupled, one covering the low-pressure range and the other the high pressures. An independent pressure transducer connected to a chart recorder or logger is useful in providing a permanent dive profile record.

Ambient oxygen concentrations should be measured in both locks and displayed on gauges on the control panel. A warning system that is activated by the deviation of oxygen concentrations or partial pressures outside pre-set values should be incorporated. A similar system can be used to warn of a dangerous rise in carbon dioxide.

Clocks should be fitted so that elapsed time and individual compression and decompression times are easily recorded.

Flow meters that measure the ventilation rates on the exhaust lines from both locks allow adequate ventilation rates without air wastage and help minimize noise.

Temperature and humidity should be controlled and monitored.

Electrodiagnostic monitoring should be possible in each lock. Physiological parameters that may need recording include pulse rate, blood pressure, ventilation rates and volumes (if mechanically ventilated), electrocardiogram and end-tidal carbon dioxide. Some research facilities may also need an electroencephalogram, electronystagmogram or other monitors of interest for specific projects.

The foregoing is a broad guide to suitable design for a large treatment chamber. Interested readers are referred to the references and appropriate standards. Ideally, complex facilities should be situated near (or within) a major hospital to ensure optimal medical control, as well as expert maintenance. Ground-level locations are preferable because of transfer under pressure requirements with mobile chambers. In view of the high noise levels associated with these chambers, soundproofing is desirable.

PORTABLE RECOMPRESSION CHAMBER

These treatment chambers should be capable of being transported by air. Therefore, size and weight are important logistical concerns. The gas pressurization systems accompanying such units must be included in the size and weight allowances.

Most of these chambers are designed to accommodate two or three persons in the single or main lock. Apparatus is best kept to a minimum, providing only the essentials. These chambers are principally used for a diver suffering from DCS or air embolism. Once compression is achieved, the patient can be transferred while still under pressure for subsequent therapeutic decompression. The US Navy and the Royal Australian Navy have purchased small chambers that house a patient and attendant. If needed, a second chamber can be connected to it as an outer lock, or the chamber can be transferred if this is required. Figure 68.2 is a view of a pair of these chambers.

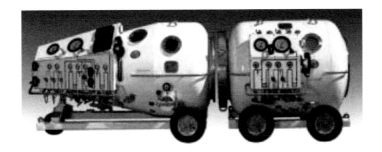

Figure 68.2 Portable, lock-on, two-person recompression chambers. A side view of the chamber system built by Cowan Manufacturing for the US Navy and the Royal Australian Navy. The cone-shape treatment chamber is shown next to the cylindrical transfer chamber. When the two chambers are joined together, they can be operated as a two-compartment chamber. (Courtesy of Cowan Manufacturing, Warners Bay, Australia.)

The minimum requirements for these chambers are as follows.

The hull should be of appropriate weight and dimensions to be loaded onto the transport aircraft. A maximum size would be about 2 to 3 metres in length, 1 to 1.5 metres in diameter and 600 kilograms in weight. Trolley or pallet mounting of the unit assists with later transport.

The door surround should have a transfer under pressure flange compatible with other systems.

A medical lock is valuable, as are observation ports. Adequate lighting and communication should be incorporated. A roll-in stretcher is of considerable advantage.

Soundproofing of inlets and protection of exhaust outlets similar to the large recompression chambers is essential. Temperature control may be needed in extreme climates and with rebreathing systems.

Oxygen or other breathing gas should be supplied independently of the chamber gas. An oxygen elimination system is advantageous. Rebreathing systems with carbon dioxide scrubbers may be used to reduce air consumption.

Compressed air supplies and compression facilities should be sufficient to provide for maximum pressurization and adequate ventilation of the chamber (main lock) for two occupants for a period during which transportation will occur.

Control panels for these types of chambers are usually located on the hull structure and include clocks, pressure gauges, communication facilities, flow metres, control valves and ancillary aids.

Electrophysiological monitoring connection plugs are advisable.

MEDICAL SUPPLIES

An emergency kit comprising examination and treatment instruments, drugs and dressings, should be available on site for both small and large recompression chambers. Some instruments and equipment that may be required in the chamber include the following:

- Stethoscope.
- Aneroid sphygmomanometer.
- Percussion hammer, pin, tuning forks.
- Urinary catheter, introducer, collecting bag.
- Sterile syringes and needles.
- Sterile intravenous cannulas and catheters.
- Intravenous transfusion sets, 'cut down' and suture sets.
- Intravenous fluids (e.g. Hartmann's solution, normal saline, plasma expanders).
- Thoracic trocar and cannula with sterile plastic tubing and underwater drain system or Heimlich valve.
- Endotracheal tubes and connections.
- Adhesive tape.
- Antiseptic solution and swabs.

- Sterile dressings.
- Automatic ventilator and connections.
- Ophthalmoscope, otoscope, laryngoscope (potential fire ignition sources and not to be taken into the chamber unless needed).
- Drugs that should be immediately available: frusemide, isoprenaline, lignocaine, aminophylline, phenytoin, diazepam, morphine, pethidine, prochlorperazine, promethazine, atropine, adrenaline, thiopentone, suxamethonium, a non-depolarizing muscle relaxant.

CONCLUSION

This chapter is included to introduce readers to some of the requirements of recompression chambers. New designs will be improved by the continued collaboration of doctors and engineers. One-person chambers have not been discussed because these are common only in hyperbaric therapy facilities. They would be used only rarely for treatment of DCS. If they are fitted with transfer under pressure facilities, there is a chance of transporting the patient to a better unit; if not, then the patient is committed to whatever treatment is available. Unfortunately, should an emergency arise within the recompression chamber, no help is possible directly to the occupant, and for this reason prolonged or deep treatment in a one-person chamber should be avoided if possible.

Finally, despite the excellent facilities that are available in most large chamber complexes, many diving accident victims are treated under primitive conditions in remote localities. Flexibility and improvisation are necessary and valuable qualities in the diving physician.

REFERENCES

1. Gill AL, Bell CNA. Hyperbaric oxygen: its uses, mechanisms of action and outcomes. *QJM* 2004;**97**(7):385–395.
2. Elliott DH, Vorosmarti J. An outline history of diving physiology and medicine. In: Brubakk AO, Neuman TS, eds. *Bennett and Elliott's Physiology and Medicine of Diving.* 5th ed. London: Saunders; 2003:4–16.
3. Pollock NW, ed. *Annual Diving Report.* 2007 ed. (based on 2005 data). Durham, North Carolina: Divers Alert Network; 2007.
4. Wolfe GK, Zeigler PL, Moino GE, *et al. Safety Standard for Pressure Vessels for Human Occupancy.* ASME PVHO-1-2007. New York: American Society of Mechanical Engineers; 2007.
5. AS 4774.2. *Work in Compressed Air and Hyperbaric Facilities.* Part 2. *Hyperbaric Oxygen Facilities.* Sydney: Standards Australia International; 2002.
6. Sheffield PJ, Desautels DA. Hyperbaric and hypobaric chamber fires: a 73-year analysis. *Undersea and Hyperbaric Medicine* 1999;**24**:153–164.

This chapter was reviewed for this fifth edition by Michael Bennett.

Hyperbaric medicine

INTRODUCTION

Hyperbaric medicine is the treatment of health disorders using whole body exposure to pressures greater than 101.3 kPa (1 ATA or 760 mm Hg). In practice, this almost always means the administration of *hyperbaric oxygen therapy* (HBOT). The administration of hyperbaric oxygen (HBO_2) involves the use of the equipment discussed in Chapter 68.

The treatment chamber is usually called a hyperbaric chamber, and it is often designed for both HBOT and the recompression of diving injuries. Such chambers may be capable of compressing a single patient (a mono-place chamber) or multiple patients and attendants as required (a multi-place chamber). For more details, see Chapter 68.

Despite increasing elucidation of therapeutic mechanisms and an improving evidence base, hyperbaric medicine still struggles to achieve widespread recognition as a 'legitimate' therapeutic measure. There are several contributing factors, but high among them are a poor grounding in general oxygen physiology and oxygen therapy at medical schools and a continuing tradition of charlatans advocating hyperbaric therapy (often using air) as a panacea. Funding for both basic and clinical research has been difficult in an environment where the pharmacological agent under study is abundant, inexpensive and unpatentable. More recently, however, there are signs of an improved appreciation of the potential importance of HBOT with significant US National Institutes of Health (NIH) funding for mechanisms research and from the US military for clinical investigation.

MECHANISMS OF HYPERBARIC OXYGEN

Oxygen breathing has a dose-dependent effect on oxygen transport, ranging from improvement in haemoglobin oxygen saturation when a few liters per minute are delivered by simple mask at 101.3 kPa (1 ATA) to raising the dissolved plasma oxygen sufficiently to sustain life without the need for haemoglobin at all when 100 per cent oxygen is breathed at 303.9 kPa (3 ATA). Most HBOT regimens involve oxygen breathing at between 202.6 and 283.6 kPa (2 and 2.8 ATA), and the resultant increase in arterial oxygen tensions to more than 133.3 kPa (1000 mm Hg) has widespread physiological and pharmacological consequences (Figure 69.1).

One direct consequence of such high intravascular tension is to increase greatly the effective capillary-tissue diffusion distance for oxygen such that oxygen-dependent cellular processes can resume in hypoxic tissues. Important as this may be, the mechanism of action is not limited to this restoration of oxygenation in hypoxic tissue. Indeed, there are pharmacological effects that are profound and long lasting. Although removal from the hyperbaric chamber results in a rapid return of poorly vascularized tissues to their hypoxic state,

even a single dose of HBO_2 produces changes in fibroblast, leucocyte, and angiogenic functions and antioxidant defences that persist many hours after oxygen tensions are returned to pre-treatment levels.

It is widely accepted that oxygen in high doses produces adverse effects as a result of the production of reactive oxygen species (ROS) such as superoxide (O_2^-) and hydrogen peroxide (H_2O_2). It has become increasingly clear since the early 2000s that both ROS and reactive nitrogen species (RNS) such as nitric oxide (NO) participate in a wide range of intracellular signalling pathways involved in the production of a range of cytokines, growth factors and other inflammatory and repair modulators[1]. Such mechanisms are complex and at times apparently paradoxical. For example, when used to treat chronic hypoxic wounds, HBOT has

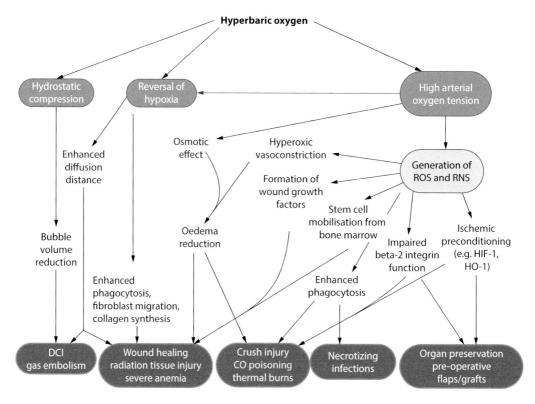

Figure 69.1 Summary of mechanisms of hyperbaric oxygen (HBO_2). There are many consequences of compression and oxygen breathing. The cell signalling effects of HBO_2 are the least understood but potentially most important. The relevance of these mechanisms is drawn to several example indications. CO, carbon monoxide; DCI, decompression illness; HIF-1, hypoxia inducible factor-1; HO-1, haemoxygenase-1; RNS, reactive nitrogen species; ROS, reactive oxygen species.

been shown to enhance the clearance of cellular debris and bacteria by providing the substrate for macrophage phagocytosis, to stimulate growth factor synthesis by increased production and stabilization of hypoxia-inducible factor 1 (HIF-1), to inhibit leucocyte activation and adherence to damaged endothelium and to mobilize stem cells from the bone marrow. The interactions among these mechanisms comprise a very active field of investigation[2].

One exciting development is the concept of *hyperoxic preconditioning* in which a short exposure to HBO_2 can induce tissue protection against future hypoxic or ischaemic insult – most likely through an inhibition of mitochondrial permeability and the release of cytochromes[3]. By targeting these mechanisms of cell death during reperfusion events, HBO_2 has potential applications in a variety of settings including organ transplantation. One randomized clinical trial suggested that HBOT before coronary artery bypass grafting reduces biochemical markers of ischemic stress and improves neurocognitive outcomes[4].

INDICATIONS FOR HYPERBARIC OXYGEN

The appropriate indications for HBOT are controversial and evolving. Practitioners in this area are in an unusual position. Unlike physicians in most branches of medicine, hyperbaric physicians do not deal with a range of disorders within a defined organ system (e.g. cardiology), nor are they masters of a therapy specifically designed for a single category of disorders (e.g. radiation oncology). Inevitably, the encroachment of hyperbaric physicians into other medical fields generates suspicion from specialist practitioners in those fields. At the same time, this relatively benign therapy, the prescription and delivery of which require no medical license in most jurisdictions (including Australia and the United States), attracts both charlatans and well-motivated proselytizers who tout the benefits of oxygen for a plethora of chronic incurable diseases. This battle on two fronts has meant that mainstream hyperbaric physicians have been particularly careful to claim effectiveness only for those conditions where there is a reasonable body of supporting evidence.

In 1977, the Undersea and Hyperbaric Medical Society (UHMS) systematically examined claims for the use of HBOT in more than 100 disorders and found sufficient evidence to support routine use in only 12. The Hyperbaric Oxygen Therapy Committee of that organization has continued to update this list periodically with an increasingly formalized system of appraisal for new indications and emerging evidence (Table 69.1)[5].

Table 69.1 Current list of indications for hyperbaric oxygen therapy

1. Air or gas embolism (includes diving-related, iatrogenic, and accidental causes)
2. Carbon monoxide poisoning (including poisoning complicated by cyanide poisoning)
3. Clostridial myositis and myonecrosis (gas gangrene)
4. Crush injury, compartment syndrome and acute traumatic ischemias
5. Decompression sickness
6. Arterial insufficiency (central retinal artery occlusion, enhancement of healing in selected problem wounds)
7. Exceptional blood loss (where transfusion is refused or impossible)
8. Intracranial abscess
9. Necrotizing soft tissue infections (e.g. Fournier's gangrene)
10. Osteomyelitis (refractory to other therapy)
11. Delayed radiation injury (soft tissue injury and bony necrosis)
12. Skin grafts and flaps (compromised)
13. Thermal burns
14. Sudden sensorineural hearing loss

Source: From Undersea and Hyperbaric Medical Society, 2014.

Around the world, other relevant medical organizations have generally taken a similar approach, although indications vary considerably–particularly those recommended by hyperbaric medical societies in Russia and China, where HBOT has gained much wider support than in the United States, Europe and Australasia. The Australia and New Zealand Hyperbaric Medicine Group (ANZHMG) publishes a list very similar to that of the UHMS, but in both the United States and Australia/New Zealand, the list of reimbursable indications is greatly restricted.

Beginning in 2004, several Cochrane reviews have examined the randomized trial evidence for many putative indications, including attempts to examine the cost-effectiveness of HBOT. Table 69.2 is a synthesis of these two approaches and lists the estimated cost of attaining health outcomes with the use of HBOT. Any savings associated with alternative treatment strategies avoided as a result of HBOT are not accounted for in these estimates (e.g. avoidance of lower leg amputation in diabetic foot ulcers).

This chapter is not the place for an exhaustive review of all indications for HBOT; rather, we summarize here three common indications as a representative sample. For a fuller discussion, see the text edited by Neuman and Thom[6].

LATE RADIATION TISSUE INJURY

Radiotherapy is a well-established treatment for suitable malignant diseases. In the United States alone, approximately 300 000 individuals annually become long-term survivors of cancer treated by irradiation. Serious radiation-related complications developing months or years after treatment (late radiation tissue injury [LRTI]) will significantly affect between 5 and 15 per cent of those long-term survivors, although incidence varies widely with dose, age and site. LRTI is most common in the head and neck, chest wall, breast and pelvis.

Pathology and clinical course

After an initial period of recovery from the acute damage associated with radiation therapy, the tissues undergo progressive deterioration characterized by a reduction in the density of small blood vessels (reduced vascularity), with subsequent hypoxia and the replacement of normal tissue with dense fibrous tissue (fibrosis). An alternative model of pathogenesis suggests that rather than primary hypoxia, the principal trigger is an overexpression of inflammatory cytokines that promote fibrosis – probably through oxidative stress and mitochondrial dysfunction – and secondary tissue hypoxia. Ultimately, and often triggered by a further physical insult such as surgery or infection, there may be insufficient oxygen to sustain normal function, and the tissue becomes necrotic (radiation necrosis). LRTI may be life-threatening and may significantly reduce quality of life. Historically, the management of these injuries has been unsatisfactory. Conservative treatment is usually restricted to symptom management, whereas definitive treatment traditionally entails surgery to remove the affected part and extensive repair. Surgical intervention in an irradiated field is often disfiguring and is associated with an increased incidence of delayed healing, breakdown of the surgical wound or infection. HBOT may act by several mechanisms to improve this situation, including edema reduction, vasculogenesis and enhancement of macrophage activity (see Figure 69.1). The intermittent application of HBO_2 is the only intervention shown to increase the microvascular density in irradiated tissue.

Clinical evidence

The typical course of HBOT consists of 30 once-daily compressions to 202.6 to 243.1 kPa (2 to 2.4 ATA) for 1.5 to 2 hours each session, often bracketed around surgical intervention if required. Although HBOT has been used for LRTI since at least 1975, most clinical studies have been limited to small case series or individual case reports. In a review, Feldmeier and Hampson[7] located 71 such reports involving a total of 1193 patients and 8 different tissues. There were clinically significant improvements in the majority of patients, and only 7 of 71 reports indicated a generally poor response to HBOT. A Cochrane systematic review with meta-analysis included 6 randomized trials published since 1985 and concluded that HBOT improves healing in radiation proctitis (relative

Table 69.2 Selected indications for which there is promising efficacy for the application of hyperbaric oxygen therapy

Diagnosis	Outcome (number of sessions)	NNT 95% CI	Estimated cost to produce one extra favorable outcome 95% CI (USD)	Comments and recommendations
Radiation tissue injury	More information is required on the subset of disease severity and affected tissue type that is most likely to benefit and the time over which benefit may persist.			
	Resolved proctitis (30)	3 2–12	22 392 14 928–89 536	Large multi-center trial ongoing.
	Healed mandible (30)	4 2–8	29 184 14 592–58 368	Based on one poorly reported study.
	Mucosal cover in ORN (30)	3 2–4	29 888 14 592–29 184	Based on one poorly reported study.
	Bony continuity in ORN (30)	4 2–8	29 184 14 592–58 368	Based on one poorly reported study.
	Prevention of ORN after dental extraction (30)	4 2–13	29 184 14 592–94 848	Based on a single study.
	Prevention of dehiscence (30)	5 3–8	36 480 21 888–58 368	Based on one poorly reported study.
Chronic wounds	More information is required on the subset of disease severity or classification most likely to benefit, the time over which benefit may persist and the most appropriate oxygen dose. Economic analysis is required.			
	Diabetic ulcer healed at 1 year (30)	2 1–5	14 928 7464–37 320	Based on one small study; more research required.
	Diabetic ulcer, major amputation avoided (30)	4 3–11	29 856 22 392–82 104	Three small studies; outcome over a longer time period required.
ISSNHL	No evidence of benefit more than 2 weeks after onset. More research is required to define the role (if any) of HBOT in routine therapy.			
	Improvement of 25% in hearing loss within 2 weeks of onset (15)	5 3–20	18 240 10 944–72 960	Some improvement in hearing, but functional significance unknown.

(Continued)

Table 69.2 (Continued) Selected indications for which there is promising efficacy for the application of hyperbaric oxygen therapy

Diagnosis	Outcome (number of sessions)	NNT 95% CI	Estimated cost to produce one extra favorable outcome 95% CI (USD)	Comments and recommendations
Acute coronary syndrome	**More information is required on the subset of disease severity and timing of therapy most likely to result in benefit. Given the potential of HBOT in modifying ischemia-reperfusion injury, attention should be given to the combination of HBOT and thrombolysis in early management and in the prevention of restenosis after stent placement.**			
	Episode of MACE (5)	4 3–10	4864 3648–12160	Based on a single small study; more research required.
	Incidence of significant dysrhythmia (5)	6 3–24	7296 3648–29184	Based on a single moderately powered study in the 1970s.
Traumatic brain injury	**Limited evidence indicates that for acute injury HBOT reduces mortality but not functional morbidity. Routine use is not yet justified.**			
	Mortality (15)	7 4–22	34104 19488–58464	Based on four heterogeneous studies.
Enhancement of radiotherapy	**There is some evidence that HBOT improves local tumor control and reduces mortality for cancers of the head and neck, as well as reducing the chance of local tumor recurrence in cancers of the head, neck and uterine cervix.**			
	Head and neck cancer	5	14592	Based on trials performed in the 1970s and 1980s. There may be some confounding by radiation fractionation schedule.
	5-year mortality (12)	5 3–14	14592 8755–40858	
	Local recurrence 1 year (12)	5 4–8	14592 11674–23347	May no longer be relevant to therapy.
	Cancer of uterine cervix:			
	Local recurrence at 2 years (20)	5 4–8	24,320 19456–38912	As above.

CI, confidence interval; HBOT, hyperbaric oxygen therapy; ISSNHL, idiopathic sudden sensorineural hearing loss; MACE, major adverse cardiac events; N/R, not remarkable; NNT, number needed to treat; NSAID, nonsteroidal anti-inflammatory drug; ORN, osteoradionecrosis; USD, US dollars.

Source: From Bennett M. The Evidence-Basis of Diving and Hyperbaric Medicine: A Synthesis of the High Level Evidence With Meta-analysis. 2006. http://unsworks.unsw.edu.au/vital/access/manager/Repository/unsworks:949

risk [RR] of healing with HBOT, 2.7; 95 per cent confidence interval [CI], 1.2 to 6), following hemi-mandibulectomy with reconstruction of the mandible (RR, 1.4; 95 per cent CI, 1.1 to 1.8) and the restoration of bony continuity with osteoradionecrosis (RR, 1.4; 95 per cent CI, 1.1 to 1.8). HBOT also prevents the development of osteoradionecrosis following tooth extraction from a radiation field (RR, 1.4; 95 per cent CI, 1.08 to 1.7) and reduces the risk of wound dehiscence following grafts and flaps in the head and neck (RR, 4.2; 95 per cent CI, 1.1 to 16.8)[8]. Conversely, there was no evidence of benefit in established radiation brachial plexus lesions or brain injury.

SELECTED PROBLEM WOUNDS

A problem wound is any cutaneous ulceration that requires a prolonged time to heal, does not heal or recurs. In general, wounds referred to hyperbaric facilities are those in which sustained attempts to heal by other means have failed. Problem wounds are common and constitute a significant health problem. It has been estimated that 1 per cent of the population of industrialized countries will experience a leg ulcer at some time. The global cost of chronic wound care may be as high as $25 billion US per year.

Pathology and clinical course

By definition, chronic wounds are indolent or progressive and resistant to the wide array of treatments applied. Although there are many contributing factors, most commonly these wounds arise in association with one or more comorbidities such as diabetes, peripheral venous or arterial disease or prolonged pressure (decubitus ulcers). First-line treatments are aimed at correction of the underlying disorder (e.g., vascular reconstruction, compression bandaging or normalization of blood glucose level), and HBOT is an adjunctive therapy to good general wound care practice to maximize the chance of healing.

For most indolent wounds, hypoxia is a major contributor to failure to heal. Many guidelines for patient selection for HBOT include the interpretation of transcutaneous oxygen tensions around the wound while the patient is breathing air and oxygen at pressure (Figure 69.2). Wound healing is a complex and incompletely understood process. Although it appears that in acute wounds healing is stimulated by the initial hypoxia, low pH and high lactate concentrations found in freshly injured tissue, some elements of tissue repair are extremely oxygen dependent, for example, collagen elaboration and deposition by fibroblasts and bacterial killing by macrophages. In this complicated interaction between wound hypoxia and peri-wound oxygenation, successful healing relies on adequate tissue oxygenation in the area surrounding the fresh wound. Certainly, wounds that lie in hypoxic tissue beds are those that most often display poor or absent healing. Some causes of tissue hypoxia are reversible with HBOT, whereas some are not (e.g., in the presence of severe large vessel disease). When tissue hypoxia can be overcome by a high driving pressure of oxygen in the arterial blood, this can be demonstrated by measuring the tissue partial pressure of oxygen with an implantable oxygen electrode or, more commonly, a modified transcutaneous Clarke electrode.

The intermittent presentation of oxygen to those hypoxic tissues facilitates resumption of healing. These short exposures to high oxygen tensions have long-lasting effects (at least 24 hours) on a wide range of healing processes (see Figure 69.1). The result is a gradual improvement in oxygen tension around the wound that reaches a plateau in experimental studies at about 20 treatments over 4 weeks. Improvements in oxygenation are associated with an eight- to ninefold increase in vascular density over both normobaric oxygen and air-breathing controls.

Clinical evidence

The typical course of HBOT consists of 20 to 30 once-daily compressions to 2 to 2.4 ATA for 1.5 to 2 hours each session, but it is highly dependent on the clinical response. There are many case series in the literature supporting the use of HBOT for a wide range of problem wounds. Both retrospective and prospective cohort studies suggest that 6 months after a course of therapy, about 70 per cent of indolent ulcers will be substantially improved or healed. Often, these ulcers had been present for many months or years, a finding suggesting that the application of HBOT has a profound effect, either primarily or as a facilitator

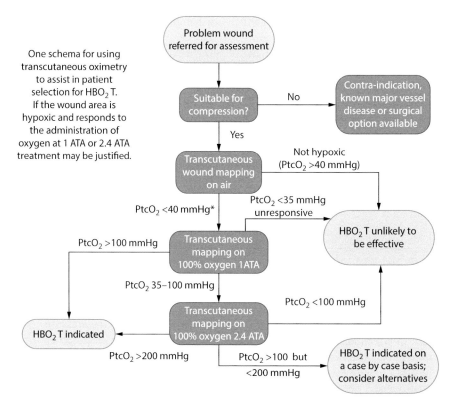

One schema for using transcutaneous oximetry to assist in patient selection for HBO₂T. If the wound area is hypoxic and responds to the administration of oxygen at 1 ATA or 2.4 ATA treatment may be justified.

Problem wound referred for assessment

Suitable for compression? — No → Contra-indication, known major vessel disease or surgical option available

Yes

Transcutaneous wound mapping on air

Not hypoxic (PtcO₂ >40 mmHg)

PtcO₂ <35 mmHg unresponsive

HBO₂T unlikely to be effective

PtcO₂ <40 mmHg*

PtcO₂ >100 mmHg

Transcutaneous mapping on 100% oxygen 1ATA

PtcO₂ 35–100 mmHg

PtcO₂ <100 mmHg

Transcutaneous mapping on 100% oxygen 2.4 ATA

HBO₂T indicated

PtcO₂ >200 mmHg

PtcO₂ >100 but <200 mmHg

HBO₂T indicated on a case by case basis; consider alternatives

Figure 69.2 Using transcutaneous oximetry to assess suitability for hyperbaric oxygen therapy (HBOT). *In diabetic patients, a value of less than 50 mm Hg may be more appropriate. PtcO₂, transcutaneous oxygen pressure.

of other strategies. A Cochrane review included nine randomized controlled trials and concluded that the chance of ulcer healing improved about fivefold with HBOT (RR, 5.20; 95 per cent CI, 1.25 to 21.66; $P = 0.02$). Although there was a trend to benefit with HBOT, there was no statistically significant difference in the rate of major amputations (RR, 0.36; 95 per cent CI, 0.11 to 1.18)[9].

CARBON MONOXIDE POISONING

Carbon monoxide (CO) is a colorless, odorless gas formed during incomplete hydrocarbon combustion. Even though CO is an essential endogenous neurotransmitter linked to NO metabolism and activity, it is also a leading cause of poisoning death, and in the United States alone it results in more than 50 000 emergency department visits per year and about 2000 deaths. Although there are large variations from country to country, about half of

non-lethal exposures are the result of self-harm. Accidental poisoning is commonly associated with defective or improperly installed heaters, house fires and industrial exposures. The motor vehicle is by far the most common source of intentional poisoning.

Pathology and clinical course

The pathophysiology of CO exposure is incompletely understood. CO binds to haemoglobin with an affinity more than 200 times that of oxygen, thus directly reducing the oxygen-carrying capacity of blood and further promoting tissue hypoxia by shifting the oxyhaemoglobin dissociation curve to the left. CO is also an anaesthetic agent that inhibits evoked responses and narcotizes experimental animals in a dose-dependent manner. The associated loss of airway patency, together with reduced oxygen carriage in blood, may cause death from acute arterial hypoxia in severe poisoning. CO may also cause harm by other mechanisms, including direct disruption of cellular oxidative processes, binding to myoglobin and hepatic cytochromes and peroxidation of brain lipids.

The brain and heart are the most sensitive target organs because of their high blood flow, poor tolerance of hypoxia and high oxygen requirements. Minor exposure may be asymptomatic or may manifest with vague constitutional symptoms such as headache, lethargy and nausea, whereas higher doses may cause poor concentration and cognition, short-term memory loss, confusion, seizures and loss of consciousness. Although carboxyhaemoglobin levels on hospital admission do not necessarily reflect the severity or the prognosis of CO poisoning, cardiorespiratory arrest carries a very poor prognosis. Over the longer term, surviving patients commonly have neuropsychological sequelae. Motor disturbances, peripheral neuropathy, hearing loss, vestibular abnormalities, dementia and psychosis have all been reported. Risk factors for poor outcome are age more than 35 years, exposure for more than 24 hours, acidosis and loss of consciousness.

Clinical evidence

The typical course of HBOT consists of one to three compressions to 2 to 2.8 ATA for 1.5 to 2 hours each session. It is common for the first two compressions to be delivered within 24 hours of the exposure. CO poisoning is one of the longest-standing indications for HBOT – based largely on the obvious connections among exposure, tissue hypoxia and the ability of HBOT to overcome this hypoxia rapidly. CO is eliminated rapidly via the lungs on application of HBOT, with a half-life of about 21 minutes at 2.0 ATA versus 5.5 hours breathing air and 71 minutes breathing oxygen at sea level. In practice, however, it seems unlikely that HBOT can be delivered in time to prevent either acute hypoxic death or irreversible global cerebral hypoxic injury. If HBOT is beneficial in CO poisoning, it must reduce the likelihood of persisting and/or delayed neurocognitive deficit through a mechanism other than the simple reversal of arterial hypoxia resulting from high levels of carboxyhaemoglobin. The difficulty in accurately assessing neurocognitive deficit has been one of the primary sources of controversy surrounding the clinical evidence in this area.

To date, there have been six randomized controlled trials of HBOT for CO poisoning, although only four have been reported in full. Whereas a Cochrane review suggested that overall there is insufficient evidence to confirm a beneficial effect of HBOT on the chance of persisting neurocognitive deficit following poisoning (34 per cent of patients treated with oxygen at 1 ATA versus 29 per cent of those treated with HBOT; odds ratio, 0.78; 95 per cent CI, 0.54 to 1.1)[10], this may have more to do with poor reporting and inadequate follow-up than with evidence that HBOT is not effective. The interpretation of the literature has much to do with how one defines neurocognitive deficit. In the most methodologically rigorous of these studies, by Weaver and colleagues[11], a professionally administered battery of validated neuropsychological tests and a definition based on the deviation of individual subtest scores from the age-adjusted normal values were employed. In this study, if the patient complained of memory, attention or concentration difficulties, the required decrement on neuropsychological testing was decreased. Using this approach, 6 weeks after poisoning, 46 per cent of patients treated with normobaric oxygen alone had cognitive sequelae compared with 25 per cent of those who received HBOT ($P = 0.007$; number needed to treat [NNT], 5; 95 per cent CI, 3 to 16). At 12 months, the difference remained significant (32 per cent versus 18 per cent; $P = 0.04$; NNT 7; 95 per cent CI, 4 to 124) despite considerable loss to follow-up.

On this basis, HBOT remains widely advocated for the routine treatment of patients with moderate to severe poisoning – in particular in those older than 35 years, presenting with metabolic acidosis on arterial blood gas analysis, exposed for lengthy periods or with a history of unconsciousness. Conversely, many toxicologists remain unconvinced about the place of HBOT in this situation and call for further well-designed studies.

ADVERSE EFFECTS OF THERAPY

HBOT is generally well tolerated and safe in clinical practice. Adverse effects are associated with both alterations in pressure (barotrauma) and the administration of oxygen.

Barotrauma

Barotrauma occurs when any noncompliant gas-filled space within the body does not equalize with environmental pressure during compression or decompression. About 10 per cent of patients complain of some difficulty equalizing middle ear pressure early in compression, and although most of these problems are minor and can be overcome with training, 2 to 5 per cent of conscious patients require middle ear ventilation tubes or formal grommets across the tympanic membrane. Unconscious patients cannot equalize their middle ear pressure and should have middle ear ventilation tubes placed before compression if possible. Other less common sites of barotrauma of compression include the respiratory sinuses and dental caries. The lungs are potentially vulnerable to barotrauma of decompression, as described in Chapter 6 in the context of diving medicine, but the decompression following HBOT is so slow that pulmonary gas trapping is extremely rare in the absence of an undrained pneumothorax or lesions such as bullae.

Oxygen toxicity

The practical limit to the dose of oxygen, either in a single treatment session or in a series of daily sessions, is oxygen toxicity. The most common acute manifestation is a seizure, often preceded by anxiety and agitation, during which time a switch from oxygen to air breathing may prevent the convulsion. Hyperoxic seizures are typically generalized tonic-clonic seizures followed by a variable post-ictal period. The cause is an over-whelming of the antioxidant defence systems within the brain. Although these seizures are clearly dose dependent, the onset is variable both among individuals and within the same individual on different days. In routine clinical hyperbaric practice, the incidence is about 1 in 1500 to 1 in 2000 compressions.

Chronic oxygen poisoning most commonly manifests as a myopic shift. This is caused by alterations in the refractive index of the lens following oxidative damage that reduces the solubility of lenticular proteins in a process similar to that associated with senescent cataract formation. Up to 75 per cent of patients show deterioration in visual acuity after a course of 30 treatments at 202.6 kPa (2 ATA). Although most patients return to pre-treatment visual acuity values 6 to 12 weeks after cessation of treatment, a few do not recover. A more rapid maturation of pre-existing cataracts has occasionally been associated with HBOT. Although a theoretical problem, the development of pulmonary oxygen toxicity over time does not seem to be problematic in practice – probably because of the intermittent nature of the exposure.

CONTRAINDICATIONS TO HYPERBARIC OXYGEN

There are few absolute contraindications to HBOT. The most commonly encountered is an untreated pneumothorax. A pneumothorax may expand rapidly on decompression and come under tension. Before any compression, patients with a pneumothorax should have a patent chest drain in place. The presence of other obvious risk factors for pulmonary gas trapping such as bullae should trigger a very cautious analysis of the risks of treatment versus benefit. Earlier bleomycin treatment deserves special mention because of its association with a partially dose-dependent pneumonitis in about 20 per cent of people. These individuals appear to be at particular risk for rapid deterioration of ventilatory function following exposure to high oxygen tensions. The relationship between distant bleomycin exposure and subsequent risk of pulmonary oxygen toxicity is uncertain; however, late pulmonary fibrosis is a potential complication of bleomycin therapy, and any patient with a history of receiving this drug should be carefully counseled before exposure to HBOT. For patients recently exposed to doses higher than 300 000 International Units (200 mg) and whose course was complicated by a respiratory reaction to bleomycin, compression should be avoided except in a life-threatening situation.

REFERENCES

1. Fosen KM, Thom SR. Hyperbaric oxygen, vascular stem cells and wound healing. *Antioxidant and Redox Signalling* 2014;**21**(11):1634–1647.
2. Thom S. Oxidative stress is fundamental to hyperbaric oxygen therapy. *Journal of Applied Physiology* 2009;**106**:988–995.
3. Yogaratnam JZ, Laden G, Guvendik L, Cowen M, Cale A, Griffin S. Pharmacological preconditioning with hyperbaric oxygen: can this therapy attenuate myocardial ischemic reperfusion injury and induce myocardial protection via nitric oxide? *Journal of Surgical Research* 2008;**146**(2):282–288.
4. Jeysen ZY, Gerard L, Levant G, Cowen M, Cale A, Griffin S. Research report: the effects of hyperbaric oxygen preconditioning on myocardial biomarkers of cardioprotection in patients having coronary artery bypass graft surgery. *Undersea and Hyperbaric Medicine* 2011;**38**(3):175–185.
5. Weaver L (ed). *Hyperbaric Oxygen Therapy Indications*, 13th ed. Undersea and Hyperbaric Medical Society, Bes Publishing: 2014.
6. Neuman T, Thom S, eds. *Physiology and Medicine of Hyperbaric Oxygen Therapy*. Philadelphia: Saunders; 2008.
7. Feldmeier JJ, Hampson NB. A systematic review of the literature reporting the application of hyperbaric oxygen prevention and treatment of delayed radiation injuries: an evidence based approach. *Undersea and Hyperbaric Medicine* 2002;**29**(1):4–30.
8. Bennett MH, Feldmeier J, Hampson N, Smee R, Milross C. Hyperbaric oxygen therapy for late radiation tissue injury. Cochrane Database of Systematic Reviews 2012; Issue 5, Art No.: CD005005.
9. Kranke P, Bennett MH, Martyn-St JamesM, Schnabel A, Debus SE. Hyperbaric oxygen therapy for chronic≈wounds. Cochrane Database of Systematic Reviews 2012, Issue 4. Art No.:CD004123.
10. Buckley NA, Juurlink DN, Isbister G, Bennett MH, Lavonas EJ. Hyperbaric oxygen for carbon monoxide poisoning. Cochrane Database of Systematic Reviews 2011, Issue 4. Art No.: CD002041.
11. Weaver LK, Hopkins RO, Chan KJ, *et al.* Hyperbaric oxygen for acute carbon monoxide poisoning. *New England Journal of Medicine* 2002;**347**:1057–1067.

This chapter was reviewed for this fifth edition by Michael Bennett and Simon Mitchell.

Appendix A: Decompression tables

US NAVY STANDARD AIR DECOMPRESSION TABLES, ABRIDGED

The air diving decompression tables in the *US Navy* (USN) *Diving Manual* are presented here together with the US National Oceanic and Atmospheric Administration (NOAA) version. The complete instructions for the USN are rather longer than the version presented here. **The full and most up-to-date version of the tables should be consulted by any reader intending to dive on the tables.** The version presented here is for use by a reader who wants to learn how these decompression tables are used. The accuracy of the figures in the tables cannot be guaranteed. Also, the authors have no method of recalling this book if an error is discovered. Or, as happened with the third edition, the USN may release a revised table after the text is printed.

Note that some popular recreational diving tables are based on the USN tables (e.g. Professional Association of Diving Instructors [PADI]).

The USN tables cover depths and times beyond the limits of sensible scuba diving. They are presented because there may be a call to use them for longer dives, for example, when a diver is trapped underwater.

How to use the US Navy tables

For many divers, the no-decompression limits table is all they need to consult. They enter the table knowing the depth to which they intend to dive (rounded up to the next depth listed) and can read off the maximum allowed duration of the intended dive. The time (bottom time) is measured from leaving the surface until leaving the bottom. The tables assume the diver will descend at a rate of 60 feet per minute or slower.

The first column in both tables is the depth. In the first table, the second column indicates the time a diver should take to reach the first stop during the ascent (the discussion will return to this). In the second table, the second column is the maximum bottom time allowed before the diver needs formal decompression stops (mandated pauses at nominated depths during the ascent). On this table, a diver going to 85 feet uses the 90-foot table (the next deeper depth is used because there is no 85-foot table) and has a maximum bottom time of 30 minutes. At the end of this time, the table makers expect the diver to ascend at a rate of 30 feet per minute to the surface. The diver is not allowed to prolong the ascent. The other entries in this table are used to modify the decompression of a second (or later) dive to allow for the elimination of any nitrogen load not yet cleared following preceding dives.

If the diver needs to spend more time at a depth than allowed for in this table, he or she will need to stop at nominated depths during the ascent (decompression stops). If the diver in the last paragraph wanted to dive to 90 feet for 60 minutes, he or she would take 2 minutes and 40 seconds (from column 2, Table 1) to ascend to 10 feet, stop there for 25 minutes, then ascend to the surface, taking another 20 seconds. The total ascent takes 28 minutes, and the diver is in repetitive dive group M (reading across Table 1).

For decompressing from a second and subsequent dives, a procedure called a repetitive dive calculation must be undertaken. The letters are used as an indication of the amount of nitrogen in the diver's body. In Table 2, these letters are listed across the page for the no-decompression dives. Examination of this table shows that the diver moves through the alphabet as he or she spends more time at a depth, the diver moves through the alphabet more quickly the deeper the dive. Thus, our diver in the first example spending 30 minutes at 90 feet was a group H diver. If that diver had ascended after 10 minutes, he or she would have been a group C diver.

To use the letters, the first step is to allow for the nitrogen that is lost from the body during the time the diver spends on the surface. The residual nitrogen is used for this purpose. Consulting Table 3, our diver enters from the left at the row starting with 'H' on the diagonal. The next step is to move along the row until the intended time to be spent on the surface is reached (the numbers here are a span of time – so the first box in this row is for any surface interval from 10 minutes to 36 minutes). In this table, the figures are in hours and minutes. From the intended surface interval time, the user reads up the table to select the new repetitive group. These move back toward the front of the alphabet as more time is spent on the surface.

Once the appropriate repetitive dive group is identified, the diver moves on to Table 4. Below the letters in this table are figures called the residual nitrogen times. They are listed against the depth of the next planned dive.

For example, our diver finishes the first dive as a group H diver and waits on the surface for 3 hours. This diver is now a group D diver. If the next dive is to 60 feet, a group D diver has a residual nitrogen time of 24 minutes. This can be used in two ways. If it is intended that the second dive should not require decompression stops, then the maximum permitted time for a 60-foot dive of 60 minutes needs to be reduced by 24 minutes to allow for the residual nitrogen. So the new maximum bottom time is 36 minutes. If the next dive is for 40 minutes, the residual nitrogen time is added, and the second dive is considered to be 40 + 24 minutes = 64 minutes; this time can be used in the standard air decompression tables to find that the diver needs to stop at 10 feet for 2 minutes and is a group K diver for the start of the next surface interval if there is to be a third dive.

Table 1 USN no decompression limit and standard air decompression table for a first dive

Depth (feet)	Bottom time (min)	Time to first stop (min:s)	Decompression stops (feet)					Total ascent (min:s)	Repetitive group
			50	40	30	20	10		
40	200	–	–	–	–	–	0	1:20	(*)
	210	1:00	–	–	–	–	2	3:20	N
	230	1:00	–	–	–	–	7	8:20	N
	250	1:00	–	–	–	–	11	12:20	O
	270	1:00	–	–	–	–	15	16:20	O
	300	1:00	–	–	–	–	19	20:20	Z
50	100	–	–	–	–	–	0	1:40	(*)
	110	1:20	–	–	–	–	3	4:40	L
	120	1:20	–	–	–	–	5	6:40	M
	140	1:20	–	–	–	–	10	11:40	M
	160	1:20	–	–	–	–	21	22:40	N
	180	1:20	–	–	–	–	29	30:40	O
	200	1:20	–	–	–	–	35	36:40	O
	220	1:20	–	–	–	–	40	41:40	Z
	240	1:20	–	–	–	–	47	48:40	Z
60	60	–	–	–	–	–	0	2:00	(*)
	70	1:40	–	–	–	–	2	4:00	K
	80	1:40	–	–	–	–	7	9:00	L
	100	1:40	–	–	–	–	14	16:00	M
	120	1:40	–	–	–	–	26	28:00	N
	140	1:40	–	–	–	–	39	41:00	O
	160	1:40	–	–	–	–	48	50:00	Z
	180	1:40	–	–	–	–	56	58:00	Z
	200	1:20	–	–	–	1	69	72:00	Z
70	50	–	–	–	–	–	0	2:20	(*)
	60	2:00	–	–	–	–	8	10:20	K
	70	2:00	–	–	–	–	14	16:20	L
	80	2:00	–	–	–	–	18	20:20	M
	90	2:00	–	–	–	–	23	25:20	N
	100	2:00	–	–	–	–	33	35:20	N
	110	1:40	–	–	–	2	41	45:20	O
	120	1:40	–	–	–	4	47	53:20	O
	130	1:40	–	–	–	6	52	60:20	O
	140	1:40	–	–	–	8	56	66:20	Z
	150	1:40	–	–	–	9	61	72:20	Z
	160	1:40	–	–	–	13	72	87:20	Z
	170	1:40	–	–	–	19	79	100:20	Z
80	40	–	–	–	–	–	0	2:40	(*)
	50	2:20	–	–	–	–	10	12:40	K
	60	2:20	–	–	–	–	17	19:40	L
	70	2:20	–	–	–	–	23	25:40	M
	80	2:00	–	–	–	2	31	35:40	N
	90	2:00	–	–	–	7	39	48:40	N
	100	2:00	–	–	–	11	46	59:40	O

(Continued)

Table 1 *(Continued)* USN no decompression limit and standard air decompression table for a first dive

Depth (feet)	Bottom time (min)	Time to first stop (min:s)	Decompression stop (feet)					Total ascent (min:s)	Repetitive group
			50	40	30	20	10		
	110	2:00	–	–	–	13	53	68:40	O
	120	2:00	–	–	–	17	56	75:40	Z
	130	2:00	–	–	–	19	63	84:40	Z
	140	2:00	–	–	–	26	69	97:40	Z
	150	2:00	–	–	–	32	77	111:40	Z
90	30	–	–	–	–		0	3:00	(*)
	40	2:40	–	–	–	–	7	10:00	J
	50	2:40	–	–	–	–	18	21:00	L
	60	2:40	–	–	–	–	25	28:00	M
	70	2:20	–	–	–	7	30	40:00	N
	80	2:20	–	–	–	13	40	56:00	N
	90	2:20	–	–	–	18	48	69:00	O
	100	2:20	–	–	–	21	54	78:00	Z
	110	2:20	–	–	–	24	61	88:00	Z
	120	2:20	–	–	–	32	68	103:00	Z
	130	2:00	–	–	5	36	74	118:00	Z
100	25	–	–	–	–	–	0	3:20	(*)
	30	3:00	–	–	–	–	3	6:20	I
	40	3:00	–	–	–	–	15	18:20	K
	50	2:40	–	–	–	2	24	29:20	L
	60	2:40	–	–	–	9	28	40:20	N
	70	2:40	–	–	–	17	39	59:20	O
	80	2:40	–	–	–	23	48	74:20	O
	90	2:20	–	–	3	23	57	86:20	Z
	100	2:20	–	–	7	23	66	99:20	Z
	110	2:20	–	–	10	34	72	119:20	Z
	120	2:20	–	–	12	41	78	134:20	Z
110	20	–	–	–	–	–	0	3:40	(*)
	25	3:20	–	–	–	–	3	6:40	H
	30	3:20	–	–	–	–	7	10:40	J
	40	3:00	–	–	–	2	21	26:40	L
	50	3:00	–	–	–	8	26	37:40	M
	60	3:00	–	–	–	18	36	57:40	N
	70	2:40	–	–	1	23	48	75:40	O
	80	2:40	–	–	7	23	57	90:40	Z
	90	2:40	–	–	12	30	64	109:40	Z
	100	2:40	–	–	15	37	72	127:40	Z
120	15	–	–	–	–	–	0	4:00	(*)
	20	3:40	–	–	–	–	2	6:00	H
	25	3:40	–	–	–	–	6	10:00	I
	30	3:40	–	–	–	–	14	18:00	J
	40	3:20	–	–	–	5	25	34:00	L
	50	3:20	–	–	–	15	31	50:00	N
	60	3:00	–	–	2	22	45	73:00	O

(Continued)

Table 1 *(Continued)* USN no decompression limit and standard air decompression table for a first dive

Depth (feet)	Bottom time (min)	Time to first stop (min:s)	Decompression stops (feet)					Total ascent (min:s)	Repetitive group
			50	40	30	20	10		
	70	3:00	–	–	9	23	55	91:00	O
	80	3:00	–	–	15	27	63	109:00	Z
	90	3:00	–	–	19	37	74	134:00	Z
	100	3:00	–	–	23	45	80	152:00	Z
130	10	–	–	–	–	–	0	4:20	(*)
	15	4:00	–	–	–	–	1	5:20	F
	20	4:00	–	–	–	–	4	8:20	H
	25	4:00	–	–	–	–	10	14:20	J
	30	3:40	–	–	–	3	18	25:20	M
	40	3:40	–	–	–	10	25	39:20	N
	50	3:20	–	–	3	21	37	65:20	O
	60	3:20	–	–	9	23	52	88:20	Z
	70	3:20	–	–	16	24	61	105:20	Z
	80	3:00	–	3	19	35	72	133:20	Z
	90	3:00	–	8	19	45	80	156:20	Z
140	10	–	–	–	–	–	0	4:40	(*)
	15	4:20	–	–	–	–	2	6:40	G
	20	4:20	–	–	–	–	6	10:40	I
	25	4:00	–	–	–	2	14	20:40	J
	30	4:00	–	–	–	5	21	30:40	K
	40	3:40	–	–	2	16	26	48:40	N
	50	3:40	–	–	6	24	44	78:40	O
	60	3:40	–	–	16	23	56	99:40	Z
	70	3:20	–	4	19	32	68	127:40	Z
	80	3:20	–	10	23	41	79	157:40	Z
150	5	–	–	–	–	–	0	5:00	C
	10	4:40	–	–	–	–	1	6:00	E
	15	4:40	–	–	–	–	3	8:00	G
	20	4:20	–	–	–	2	7	14:00	H
	25	4:20	–	–	–	4	17	26:00	K
	30	4:20	–	–	–	8	24	37:00	L
	40	4:00	–	–	5	19	33	62:00	N
	50	3:40	–	–	12	23	51	91:00	O
	60	3:40	–	3	19	26	62	115:00	Z
	70	3:40	–	11	19	39	75	149:00	Z
	80	3:20	1	17	19	50	84	176:00	Z
160	5	–	–	–	–	–	0	5:20	D
	10	5:00	–	–	–	–	1	6:20	F
	15	4:40	–	–	–	1	4	10:20	H
	20	4:40	–	–	–	3	11	19:20	J
	25	4:40	–	–	–	7	20	32:20	K
	30	4:40	–	–	2	11	25	43:20	M
	40	4:20	–	–	7	23	39	74:20	N
	50	4:00	–	2	16	23	55	101:20	Z
	60	4:00	–	9	19	33	69	135:20	Z

(Continued)

Table 1 *(Continued)* USN no decompression limit and standard air decompression table for a first dive

Depth (feet)	Bottom time (min)	Time of first stop (min:s)	Decompression stop (feet)					Total ascent (min:s)	Repetitive group
			50	40	30	20	10		
170	5	–	–	–	–	–	0	5:40	D
	10	5:20	–	–	–	–	2	7:40	F
	15	5:00	–	–	–	2	5	12:40	H
	20	5:00	–	–	–	4	15	24:40	J
	25	4:40	–	–	2	7	23	37:40	L
	30	4:40	–	–	4	13	26	48:40	M
	40	4:20	–	1	10	23	45	84:40	O
	50	4:20	–	5	18	23	61	112:40	Z
	60	4:00	2	15	22	37	74	155:40	Z
180	5	–	–	–	–	–	0	6:00	D
	10	5:40	–	–	–	–	3	9:00	F
	15	5:20	–	–	–	3	6	15:00	I
	20	5:00	–	–	1	5	17	29:00	K
	25	5:00	–	–	3	10	24	43:00	L
	30	5:00	–	–	6	17	27	56:00	N
	40	4:40	–	3	14	23	50	96:00	O
	50	4:20	2	9	19	30	65	131:00	Z
	60	4:20	5	16	19	44	81	171:00	Z
190	5	–	–	–	–	–	0	6:20	D
	10	5:40	–	–	–	1	3	10:20	G
	15	5:40	–	–	–	4	7	17:20	I
	20	5:20	–	–	2	6	20	34:20	K
	25	5:20	–	–	5	11	25	47:20	M
	30	5:00	–	1	8	19	32	66:20	N
	40	5:00	–	8	14	23	55	106:20	O

Source: From *US Navy Diving Manual Revision 6 SS521-AG-PRO-010 (2008)*. Washington, DC: Naval Sea Systems Command; 2008.

Instructions for use: Table 2

No-decompression limits: This column shows, at depths greater than 30 feet, the allowable diving times (in minutes) that permit surfacing directly at 60 feet/minute with no decompression stops. Longer exposure times require the use of the Standard Air Decompression Table.

Repetitive group designation table: The tabulated exposure times (or bottom times) are in minutes. The times at the various depths in each vertical column are the maximum exposures during which a diver will remain within the group listed at the head of the column. To find the repetitive group designation at surfacing for dives involving exposures up to and including the no-decompression limits, enter the table on the exact or next greater depth than that to which exposed, and select the listed exposure time exact or next greater than the actual exposure time. The repetitive group designation is indicated by the letter at the head of the vertical column where the selected exposure time is listed.

Example: A dive was to 32 feet for 45 minutes. Enter the table along the 35-foot-depth line because it is next greater than 32 feet. The table shows that because group D is left after 40 minutes' exposure and group E after 50 minutes, group E (at the head of the column where the 50-minute exposure is listed) is the proper selection. Exposure times for depths less than 40 feet are listed only up to approximately 5 hours because this is considered to be beyond field requirements for this table.

Table 2 USN table for calculation of repetitive dive group

Depth (feet)	No-decom-pression limits (min)	Repetitive groups (air dives)														
		A	B	C	D	E	F	G	H	I	J	K	L	M	N	O
10	–	60	120	210	300	–	–	–	–	–	–	–	–	–	–	–
15	–	35	70	110	160	225	350	–	–	–	–	–	–	–	–	–
20	–	25	50	75	100	135	180	240	325	–	–	–	–	–	–	–
25	–	20	35	55	75	100	125	160	195	245	315	–	–	–	–	–
30	–	15	30	45	60	75	95	120	145	170	205	250	310	–	–	–
35	310	5	15	25	40	50	60	80	100	120	140	160	190	220	270	310
40	200	5	15	25	30	40	50	70	80	100	110	130	150	170	200	–
50	100	–	10	15	25	30	40	50	60	70	80	90	100	–	–	–
60	60	–	10	15	20	25	30	40	50	55	60	–	–	–	–	–
70	50	–	5	10	15	20	30	35	40	45	50	–	–	–	–	–
80	40	–	5	10	15	20	25	30	35	40	–	–	–	–	–	–
90	30	–	5	10	12	15	20	25	30	–	–	–	–	–	–	–
100	25	–	5	7	10	15	20	22	25	–	–	–	–	–	–	–
110	20	–	–	5	10	13	15	20	–	–	–	–	–	–	–	–
120	15	–	–	5	10	12	15	–	–	–	–	–	–	–	–	–
130	10	–	–	5	8	10	–	–	–	–	–	–	–	–	–	–
140	10	–	–	5	7	10	–	–	–	–	–	–	–	–	–	–
150	5	–	–	5	–	–	–	–	–	–	–	–	–	–	–	–
160	5	–	–	–	5	–	–	–	–	–	–	–	–	–	–	–
170	5	–	–	–	5	–	–	–	–	–	–	–	–	–	–	–
180	5	–	–	–	5	–	–	–	–	–	–	–	–	–	–	–
190	5	–	–	–	5	–	–	–	–	–	–	–	–	–	–	–

Source: From *US Navy Diving Manual Revision 6 SS521-AG-PRO-010 (2008)*. Washington, DC: Naval Sea Systems Command; 2008.

Instructions for use: Table 3

Surface interval time in Table 3 is in *hours* and *minutes* (7:59 means 7 hours and 59 minutes). The surface interval must be at least 10 minutes. Find the *repetitive group designation letter* (from the previous dive schedule) on the diagonal slope. Enter the table horizontally to select the surface interval time that is exactly between the actual surface interval times shown. The repetitive group designation for the *end* of the surface interval is at the head of the vertical column where the selected surface interval time is listed. For example, a previous dive was to 110 feet for 30 minutes. The diver remains on the surface 1 hour and 30 minutes and wishes to find the new repetitive group designation. The repetitive group from the last column of the 110/30 schedule in the Standard Air Decompression Tables is 'J'. Enter the surface interval credit table along the horizontal line labelled 'J'. The 1-hour-30-minute surface interval lies between the times 1:20 and 1:47. Therefore, the diver has lost sufficient inert gas to place him or her in group 'G' (at the head of the vertical column selected).

Note: Dives following surface intervals of more than 12 hours are not considered repetitive dives. Actual bottom times in the Standard Air Decompression Tables may be used in computing decompression for such dives.

Table 3 USN surface interval credit table for calculation of repetitive dive group following the surface interval since previous dive

New group designation

	Z	O	N	M	L	K	J	I	H	G	F	E	D	C	B	A
Z	0:10 0:22	0:23 0:34	0:35 0:48	0:49 1:02	1:03 1:18	1:19 1:36	1:37 1:55	1:56 2:17	2:18 2:42	2:43 3:10	3:11 3:45	3:46 4:29	4:30 5:27	5:28 6:56	6:57 10:05	10:06 12:00
O		0:10 0:23	0:24 0:36	0:37 0:51	0:52 1:07	1:08 1:24	1:25 1:43	1:44 2:04	2:05 2:29	2:30 2:59	3:00 3:33	3:34 4:17	4:18 5:16	5:17 6:44	6:45 9:54	9:55 12:00
N			0:10 0:24	0:25 0:39	0:40 0:54	0:55 1:11	1:12 1:30	1:31 1:53	1:54 2:18	2:19 2:47	2:48 3:22	3:23 4:04	4:05 5:03	5:04 6:32	6:33 9:43	9:44 12:00
M				0:10 0:25	0:26 0:42	0:43 0:59	1:00 1:18	1:19 1:39	1:40 2:05	2:06 2:34	2:35 3:08	3:09 3:52	3:53 4:49	4:50 6:18	6:19 9:28	9:29 12:00
L					0:10 0:26	0:27 0:45	0:46 1:04	1:05 1:25	1:26 1:49	1:50 2:19	2:20 2:53	2:54 3:36	3:37 4:35	4:36 6:02	6:03 9:12	9:13 12:00
K						0:10 0:28	0:29 0:49	0:50 1:11	1:12 1:35	1:36 2:03	2:04 2:38	2:39 3:21	3:22 4:19	4:20 5:48	5:49 8:58	8:59 12:00
J							0:10 0:31	0:32 0:54	0:55 1:19	1:20 1:47	1:48 2:20	2:21 3:04	3:05 4:02	4:03 5:40	5:41 8:40	8:41 12:00
I								0:10 0:33	0:34 0:59	1:00 1:29	1:30 2:02	2:03 2:44	2:45 3:43	3:44 5:12	5:13 8:21	8:42 12:00
H									0:10 0:36	0:37 1:06	1:07 1:41	1:42 2:23	2:24 3:20	3:21 4:49	4:50 7:59	8:00 12:00
G										0:10 0:40	0:41 1:15	1:16 1:59	2:00 2:58	2:59 4:25	4:26 7:35	7:36 12:00
F											0:10 0:45	0:46 1:29	1:30 2:28	2:29 3:57	3:58 7:05	7:06 12:00
E												0:10 0:54	0:55 1:57	1:58 3:22	3:23 6:32	6:33 12:00
D													0:10 1:09	1:10 2:38	2:39 5:48	5:49 12:00
C														0:10 1:39	1:40 2:49	2:50 12:00
B															0:10 2:10	2:11 12:00
A																0:10 12:00

ENTER HERE → Repetitive group at the beginning of the surface interval from previous dive

Source: From *US Navy Diving Manual Revision 6 SS521-AG-PRO-010 (2008)*. Washington, DC: Naval Sea Systems Command; 2008.

Instructions for use: Table 4

The bottom times listed in Table 4 are called 'residual nitrogen times' and are the times a diver is to consider that he or she has already spent on the bottom when the diver starts a repetitive dive to a specific depth. These times are in minutes. Enter the table horizontally with the repetitive group designation from the Surface Interval Credit Table. The time in each vertical column is the number of minutes that would be required (at the depth listed at the head of the column) to saturate to the particular group.

Example: The final group designation from the Surface Interval Credit Table, on the basis of a previous dive and surface interval, is 'H'. To plan a dive to 110 feet, determine the residual nitrogen time for this depth required by the repetitive group designation: enter this table along the horizontal line labelled 'H'. The table shows that one must *start* a dive to 110 feet as though one had already been on the bottom for 27 minutes.

This information can then be applied to the Standard Air Decompression Table or No-decompression Table in a number of ways:

1. Assuming that a diver is going to finish a job and take whatever decompression is required, he or she must add 27 minutes to the actual bottom time and be prepared to

Table 4 USN residual nitrogen time table

Repetitive groups	Repetitive dive depth (ft) (air dives)															
	40	50	60	70	80	90	100	110	120	130	140	150	160	170	180	190
A	7	6	5	4	4	3	3	3	3	3	2	2	2	2	2	2
B	17	13	11	9	8	7	7	6	6	6	5	5	4	4	4	4
C	25	21	17	15	13	11	10	10	9	8	7	7	6	6	6	6
D	37	29	24	20	18	16	14	13	12	11	10	9	8	8	8	8
E	49	38	30	26	23	20	18	16	15	13	12	12	11	10	10	10
F	61	47	36	31	28	24	22	20	18	16	15	14	13	13	12	11
G	73	56	44	37	32	29	26	24	21	19	18	17	16	15	14	13
H	87	66	52	43	38	33	30	27	25	22	20	19	18	17	16	15
I	101	76	61	50	43	38	34	31	28	25	23	22	20	19	18	17
J	116	87	70	57	48	43	38	34	32	28	26	24	23	22	20	19
K	138	99	79	64	54	47	43	38	35	31	29	27	26	24	22	21
L	161	111	88	72	61	53	48	42	39	35	32	30	28	26	25	24
M	187	124	97	80	68	58	52	47	43	38	35	32	31	29	27	26
N	213	142	107	87	73	64	57	51	46	40	38	35	33	31	29	28
O	241	160	117	96	80	70	62	55	50	44	40	38	36	34	31	30
Z	257	169	122	100	84	73	64	57	52	46	42	40	37	35	32	31

Source: From *US Navy Diving Manual Revision 6 SS521-AG-PRO-010 (2008)*. Washington, DC: Naval Sea Systems Command; 2008.

take decompression according to the 110-foot schedules for the sum or equivalent single dive time.

2. Assuming that one wishes to make a quick inspection dive for the minimum decompression, the diver will decompress according to the 110/30 schedule for a dive of 3 minutes or less (27 + 3 = 30). For a dive of more than 3 minutes but less than 13, the diver will decompress according to the 110/40 schedule (27 + 13 = 40).

3. Assuming that one does not want to exceed the 110/50 schedule and the amount of decompression it requires, the diver will have to start ascent before 23 minutes of actual bottom time (50 − 27 = 23).

4. Assuming that a diver has air for approximately 45 minutes of bottom time and decompression stops, the possible dives can be computed: a dive of 13 minutes will require 23 minutes of decompression (110/40 schedule), for a total submerged time of 36 minutes. A dive of 13 to 23 minutes will require 34 minutes of decompression (110/50 schedule), for a total submerged time of 47 to 57 minutes. Therefore, to be safe, the diver will have to start ascent before 13 minutes, or a standby air source will have to be provided.

Recreational use

It is unsurprising that many recreational divers have found using these tables something of a challenge. Various authorities and training agencies have attempted to make tables that are simpler to use, although based on the same principles. Some of these tables are discussed in the following sections of this appendix.

It is also worth noting that our confidence in the ability of these and other tables to prevent decompression sickness (DCS) is reduced with each repetitive dive. The calculations behind the tables described earlier are theoretical and based on very little experimental evidence in actual divers – in some cases none at all.

USN divers (in common with military divers in general) have operational reasons to accept a risk of DCS that would not be reasonable for a recreational diver. Most diving physicians recommend recreational divers use the Canadian Defence and Civil Institute of Environmental Medicine (DCIEM) tables (see later). These tables are more conservative than the USN tables discussed earlier and have been tested in practice up to a point.

Finally, most recreational divers now use 'dive computers', or electronic depth and time recorders into which a decompression algorithm has been inserted. These devices inform the diver in real time about the time remaining to the no-decompression limit, as well as indicating any decompression stops required if that limit is breached. The relative risks of many of these algorithms are unknown, and most details are of significant commercial confidence.

Although the arguments are not fully settled, the introduction of these dive computers has run parallel with an apparent reduction in the incidence of DCS. This may well reflect the inability or unwillingness of many recreational divers to use manual dive planning tables, rather than directly reflecting a safer decompression algorithm.

BRITISH SUB-AQUA CLUB DECOMPRESSION TABLES

The complete version of the 1988 British Sub-Aqua Club (BSAC) tables consists of seven tables for diving at altitudes from sea level to 250 metres. The first three tables are printed here with the permission of BSAC and Dr Tom Hennessy, who developed them. These tables are from a copyright document. The information presented here is to assist the reader in assessing whether a diver has followed the tables. The complete tables are available in a waterproof booklet from BSAC (www.bsac.com).

For a first dive, the diver uses Table A. The table is entered on the left-hand side with the deepest depth planned for the dive. The diver then looks across to find the dive time. This is the time from leaving the surface to reaching 6 metres on the return to the surface (or reaching 9 metres if a 9-metre decompression stop is required). The time used should be the next longer tabulated if the exact time of the dive is not listed.

If the dive is to the left of the line that separates no-stop from decompression diving, the diver can surface at a rate of 15 metres/minute to 6 metres and 6 metres/minute for the last 6 metres. If the dive is on the decompression side of the table, then the decompression stops listed below the time are to be taken. The diver may then ascend to the surface at the stipulated rate.

At the foot of each table is a series of letters in a row titled 'Surfacing code'. This is an estimate of the nitrogen load at the end of the dive. To allow for any nitrogen remaining from previous dives, the diver uses the Surface Interval Table and enters on the line that starts with the surfacing code. For example, if the surfacing code was F, the diver would go to line F. The surface interval until the next dive is found, and another letter is found, called the current tissue code. For example, a diver who surfaced in group F and then spends between 90 minutes and 4 hours on the surface is in group C. This means that the diver should use Table C for the next dive.

Example: A diver wishes to make two dives to 18 metres with a surface interval of 2 hours. How long can each dive be without having to make decompression stops? What decompression stops are needed if the dive time for the second dive is to be 50 minutes?

Table A is used for the first dive. The longest time allowed before decompression is required is 51 minutes. The diver has to be back at 6 metres by that time. To get there, it would be necessary to leave the bottom 50 minutes after leaving the surface.

On returning to the surface, the diver is in surface code F. In the surface interval table for a diver who surfaces in group F, the diver is in group C after 2 hours. Table C is used for the second dive.

It will be found that the second dive can be for no longer than 15 minutes if decompression stops are to be avoided. If the dive time for the second dive is to be 50 minutes, then the decompression required is 21 minutes at 6 metres.

The complete BSAC tables also contain altitude tables and rules for flying after diving.

Table 5 BSAC Table A – no decompression limits, mandated decompression stops and repetitive dive codes. BSAC 88 Decompression Tables, London

Depth (metres)	Ascent time (min)	No-stop dives						Decompression stop dives							
3	(1)	–	166	∞											
6	(1)	–	36	166	593	∞									
9	1	–	17	67	167	203	243	311	328	336	348	356	363	370	376
12	1	–	10	37	87	104	122	156	169	177	183	188	192	197	201
15	1	–	6	24	54	64	74	98	109	116	121	125	129	133	136
18	1	–	–	17	37	44	51	68	78	84	88	92	95	98	101
Decompression stop (minutes) at **6 metres**								1	3	6	9	12	15	18	21
Surfacing code			B	C	D	E	F	G	G	G	G	G	G	G	G

Depth (metres)	Ascent time (min)	No-stop dives						Decompression stop dives						
21	1	–		13	28	32	37	51	59	65	68	72	75	77
24	2	–		11	22	26	30	41	49	53	56	59	62	64
27	2	–		8	18	21	24	34	41	45	47	50	52	55
30	2	–		7	15	17	20	29	35	39	41	43	45	47
33	2	–			13	15	17	25	30	34	36	38	40	42
36	2	–			11	12	14	22	27	30	32	34	36	37
39	3	–			10	12	13	20	25	29	30	32	33	35
Decompression stops (minutes) at **9 metres**										1	1	1	1	2
at **6 metres**								1	3	6	9	12	15	18
Surfacing code			B	C	D	E	F	G	G	G	G	G	G	G

Depth (metres)	Ascent time (min)	No-stop dives						Decompression stop dives						
42	3	–			9	10	12	21	23	26	28	29	31	32
45	3	–			8	9	10	19	22	24	26	27	28	30
48	3	–				8	9	18	21	23	24	25	26	28
51	3	–					8	17	19	21	22	24	25	26
Decompression stops (minutes) at **9 metres**									1	1	1	2	2	3
at **6 metres**								2	3	6	9	12	15	18
Surfacing code			B	C	D	E	F	G	G	G	G	G	G	G

Source: From British Sub-Aqua Club. Copyright British Sub-Aqua Club, 1988.

Table 6 BSAC Table B for calculation of repetitive dive from surface code after the first dive, and the surface interval

Dive time (minutes)

Depth (metres)	Ascent time (min)	No-stop dives					Decompression stop dives							
3	(1)	–	∞											
6	(1)	–	80	504	∞									
9	1	–	27	113	148	188	255	272	284	292	300	307	314	321
12	1	–	14	52	67	84	116	129	137	143	148	152	156	160
15	1	–	8	31	40	48	69	79	86	90	94	98	101	105
18	1	–		21	27	32	47	55	61	64	68	71	74	76
Decompression stop (minutes) at **6 metres**							1	3	6	9	12	15	18	21
Surfacing code		B	C	D	E	F	G	G	G	G	G	G	G	G

Depth (metres)	Ascent time (min)	No-stop dives					Decompression stop dives						
21	1	–		15	19	23	35	42	47	50	52	55	57
24	2	–		12	15	19	28	35	39	41	43	45	47
27	2	–		10	12	15	23	29	33	35	36	38	40
30	2	–		8	10	12	20	25	28	30	32	33	35
33	2	–			8	10	17	22	25	26	28	29	31
36	2	–			7	8	15	20	22	24	25	26	28
39	3	–				8	14	19	21	23	24	25	26
Decompression stops (minutes) at **9 metres**									1	1	1	1	2
at **6 metres**							1	3	6	9	12	15	18
Surfacing code		B	C	D	E	F	G	G	G	G	G	G	G

Depth (metres)	Ascent time (min)	No-stop dives					Decompression stop dives						
42	3					–	15	17	20	21	22	23	24
45	3					–	14	17	18	19	20	21	22
48	3					–	13	16	17	18	19	20	21
51	3					–	12	15	16	17	18	19	
Decompression stops (minutes) at **9 metres**								1	1	1	2	2	3
at **9 metres**							2	3	6	9	12	15	18
Surfacing code		B	C	D	E	F	G	G	G	G	G	G	G

Depth (metres)	Ascent time (min)	No-stop dives					Dive time (minutes) — Decompression stop dives							
3	(1)	–	∞											
6	(1)	–	359	∞										
9	1	–	49	79	116		182	199	211	220	227	234	241	248
12	1	–	20	31	44		71	83	90	95	100	104	108	112
15	1	–	11	17	24		40	48	54	57	61	64	67	70
18	1	–	7	11	15		27	34	38	40	43	45	47	50
Decompression stop (minutes) at **6 metres**							1	3	6	9	12	15	18	21
Surfacing code		B	C	D	E	F	G	G	G	G	G	G	G	G

(Continued)

Table 6 *(Continued)* BSAC Table B for calculation of repetitive dive from surface code after the first dive, and the surface interval

Depth (metres)	Ascent time (min)	No-stop dives					Dive time (minutes) — Decompression stop dives						
21	1			–	7	10	20	26	29	31	33	35	37
24	2				–	8	16	22	25	26	28	29	31
27	2					–	13	18	21	22	24	25	26
30	2					–	11	16	18	19	20	22	23
33	2					–	10	14	16	17	18	19	20
36	2					–	8	12	14	15	16	17	18
39	3					–	8	12	14	15	16	17	18
Decompression stops (minutes) **at 9 metres**									1	1	1	1	2
at 6 metres							1	3	6	9	12	15	18
Surfacing code		B	C	D	E	F	G	G	G	G	G	G	G

Depth (metres)	Ascent time (min)	No-stop dives					Decompression stop dives						
42	3					–	10	•	13	14	15	16	
45	3					–	9	•	12	•	14	•	15
48	3					–	8	•	12	•	13	14	
51	3					–	8	10	11	12	•	13	
Decompression stops (minutes) **at 9 metres**								1	1	1	2	2	3
at 6 metres							12	3	6	9	12	15	18
Surfacing code		B	C	D	E	F	G	G	G	G	G	G	G

Surface interval table

Last dive code		Minutes 15	30	60	90	Hours 2	3	4	6	10	12	14	15	16
G	G	F	E		D		C			B				A
F	F	E		D			C			B			A	
E	E		D		C				B				A	
D		D		C				B					A	
C			C				B					A		
B			B								A			
A					A									

Source: From British Sub-Aqua Club. Copyright British Sub-Aqua Club, 1988.

US NATIONAL OCEANIC AND ATMOSPHERIC ADMINISTRATION MODIFIED AIR TABLES

The NOAA version of the USN tables is an example of how tables can be condensed to a form that allows their use by a diver who is uncertain of the likely depth or duration when he or she enters the water.

Table 7 NOAA no decompression dive table. National Oceanic and Atmospheric Administration www.ndc.noaa.gov

NOAA NO-DECOMPRESSION AIR TABLE

WARNING:
EVEN STRICT COMPLIANCE WITH THESE CHARTS WILL NOT GUARANTEE AVOIDANCE OF DECOMPRESSION SICKNESS. CONSERVATIVE USAGE IS STRONGLY RECOMMENDED

ESDT RESIDUAL NITROGEN TIME
+ABT ACTUAL BOTTOM TIME
RNT EQUIVALENT SINGLE DIVE TIME

(USE ESDT TO DETERMINE END-OF-DIVE LETTER GROUP)

CHART 1 - DIVE TIMES WITH END-OF-DIVE GROUP LETTER

(00) MAXIMUM NO-STOP TIME

DEPTH MSW	DEPTH FEET	A	B	C	D	E	F	G	H	I	J	K	I	M	N
12	**40**	5	15	25	30	40	50	70	80	100	110	130	150	170	(170)
15	**50**		10	15	25	30	40	50	60	70	80	90	(100)	120 / 5	160 / 21
18	**60**		10	15	20	25	30	40	50	55	(60)	70 / 2	80 / 7	100 / 14	
22	**70**		5	10	15	20	30	35	40	45	(50)	60 / 8	70 / 14	80 / 18	
25	**80**		5	10	15	20	25	30	35	(40)		50 / 10	60 / 17	70 / 23	
28	**90**		5	10	12	15	20	25	(30)		40 / 7		50 / 18	60 / 25	
31	**100**		5	7	10	15	20	22	(25)	30 / 3		40 / 15			
34	**110**			5	10	13	15	(20)	25 / 3		30 / 17				
37	**120**			5	10	12	(15)		20 / 2	25 / 6	30 / 14				
40	**130**			5	8	(10)	15 / 1		20 / 4		25 / 10				

CHART 2 - SURFACE INTERVAL TIME

GROUP LETTER	A	B	C	D	E	F	G	H	I	J	K	I	M	N
A	12:00 / 0:10	12:00 / 3:21	12:00 / 4:50	12:00 / 5:49	12:00 / 6:35	12:00 / 7:06	12:00 / 7:36	12:00 / 8:00	12:00 / 8:22	12:00 / 8:51	12:00 / 8:59	12:00 / 9:13	12:00 / 9:29	12:00 / 9:44
B		3:20 / 0:10	4:49 / 1:40	5:48 / 2:39	6:34 / 3:25	7:05 / 3:58	7:35 / 4:26	7:59 / 4:50	8:21 / 5:13	8:50 / 5:41	8:58 / 5:49	9:12 / 6:03	9:28 / 6:19	9:43 / 6:33
C			1:39 / 0:10	2:38 / 1:10	3:24 / 1:58	3:57 / 2:29	4:25 / 2:59	4:49 / 3:21	5:12 / 3:44	5:40 / 4:03	5:48 / 4:20	6:02 / 4:36	6:18 / 4:50	6:32 / 5:04
D				1:09 / 0:10	1:57 / 0:55	2:28 / 1:30	2:58 / 2:00	3:20 / 2:24	3:43 / 2:45	4:02 / 3:05	4:19 / 3:22	4:35 / 3:37	4:49 / 3:53	5:03 / 4:05
E					0:54 / 0:10	1:29 / 0:46	1:59 / 1:16	2:23 / 1:42	2:44 / 2:03	3:04 / 2:21	3:21 / 2:39	3:36 / 2:54	3:52 / 3:09	4:04 / 3:23
F						0:45 / 0:10	1:15 / 0:41	1:41 / 1:07	2:02 / 1:30	2:20 / 1:48	2:38 / 2:04	2:53 / 2:20	3:08 / 2:35	3:22 / 2:48
G							0:40 / 0:10	1:06 / 0:37	1:29 / 1:00	1:47 / 1:20	2:03 / 1:36	2:19 / 1:50	2:34 / 2:06	2:47 / 2:19
H								0:36 / 0:10	0:59 / 8:34	1:19 / 0:55	1:35 / 1:12	1:49 / 1:26	2:05 / 1:36	2:18 / 1:54
I									0:33 / 0:10	0:54 / 0:32	1:11 / 0:50	1:25 / 1:05	1:35 / 1:19	1:53 / 1:31
J										0:31 / 0:10	0:49 / 0:29	1:04 / 0:46	1:18 / 1:00	1:30 / 1:12
K											0:28 / 8:10	0:45 / 0:27	0:59 / 0:43	1:11 / 0:55
L												0:26 / 0:10	0:42 / 0:26	0:54 / 0:40
M													0:25 / 0:10	0:39 / 0:25
N														0:24 / 0:10

CHART 3 - REPETITIVE DIVE TIME

msw	*12*	*15*	*18*	*22*	*25*	*28*	*31*	*34*	*37*	*40*	GROUP LETTER
fsw	40	50	60	70	80	90	100	110	120	130	
	7 / 193	6 / 94	5 / 55	4 / 46	4 / 36	3 / 27	3 / 22	3 / 17	13 / 12	3 / 7	**A**
	17 / 183	13 / 87	11 / 49	9 / 41	8 / 32	7 / 23	7 / 18	6 / 14	6 / 9	6 / 4	**B**
	25 / 175	21 / 79	17 / 43	15 / 35	13 / 27	11 / 19	10 / 15	10 / 10	9 / 6	8 / 2	**C**
	37 / 163	29 / 71	24 / 36	20 / 30	18 / 22	16 / 14	14 / 11	13 / 7	12 / 3		**D**
	49 / 151	38 / 62	30 / 30	26 / 24	23 / 17	20 / 10	18 / 7	16 / 4			**E**
	61 / 139	47 / 53	36 / 24	31 / 19	28 / 12	24 / 6	22 / 3				**F**
	73 / 127	56 / 44	44 / 16	37 / 13	32 / 2	29 / 1					**G**
	87 / 113	66 / 34	52 / 8	43 / 7	38 / 2						**H**
	101 / 99	76 / 24									**I**
	116 / 84	87 / 13									**J**
	138 / 62	99 / 1									**K**
	161 / 39										**L**
	187 / 13										**M**
											N

BLACK NUMBERS (TOP) ARE RESIDUAL NITROGEN TIMES (RNT)
GREY NUMBERS (BOTTOM) ARE ADJUSTED NON-STOP REPETITIVE DIVE TIMES.
ACTUAL DIVE TIME SHOULD NOT EXCEED THIS NUMBER

Source: From National Oceanic and Atmospheric Administration.

CANADIAN DEFENCE AND CIVIL INSTITUTE OF ENVIRONMENTAL MEDICINE TABLES

The complete DCIEM (now known as Defence Research and Development Canada [Toronto]) decompression publication contains tables for in-water and surface decompression with the diver breathing oxygen as well as a wider selection of depths and times for in-water decompression with the diver breathing air. The information in this appendix is from a short version of the tables for the sports diver marketed by Universal Dive Techtronics (UDT) Inc. and is presented with the permission of DCIEM and UDT. The tables, in a waterproof format, and an instruction book are available from UDT (2691 Viscount Way, Richmond, British Columbia, Canada). The complete DCIEM tables should be consulted for the other tables.

Table A: air decompression

This table gives no-decompression limits, repetitive group letters and decompression stops for dives that require stops. The group letters move from A through to M as the diver spends more time at

Table 8 DCIEM Table A for calculating no decompression limits, decompression stops and repetitive dive group. UDT Inc, Richmond

Depth (ft)	Depth (m)	No-decompression bottom times (minutes)				Decompression required bottom times			
20'	6 m	30 A	150 E	360 I	720 M				
		60 B	180 F	420 J	∞				
		90 C	240 G	480 K					
		120 D	300 H	600 L					
30'	9 m	30 A	100 E	190 I	300 M	360	400		
		45 B	120 F	210 J					
		60 C	150 G	240 K					
		90 D	180 H	270 L					
40'	12 m	22 A	60 D	90 G	150 J	160 K	180 M	200	215
		30 B	70 E	120 H		170 L	190		
		40 C	80 F	130 I					
50'	15 m	18 A	30 C	50 E		85 H	105 J	124 L	132 M
		25 B	40 D	60 F	75 G	95 I	115 K		
60'	18 m	14 A	25 C				70 H		
		20 B	30 D	40 E	50 F	60 G	80 I	85 J	92 K
Decompression stops in minutes				at 10	3 m	5	10	15	20
70'	21 m	12 A						60 H	
		15 B	20 C	25 D	35 E	40 F	50 G	63 I	66 J
80'	24 m	10 A							
		13 B	15 C	20 D	25 E	29 F	35 G	48 H	52 I
90'	27 m	9 A	12 B	15 D	20 D	23 E	27 G	35 G	40 H
									43 I
100'	30 m	7 A	10 B	12 C	15 D	18 D	21 E	25 F	36 H
								29 G	
110'	33 m		6 A	10 B	12 C	15 D	18 E	22 F	36 G
									30 H
120'	36 m		6 A	8 B	10 C	12 D	15 E	19 F	25 G
130'	39 m			5 A	8 B	10 C	13 D	16 F	21 G
140'	42 m			5 A	7 B	9 C	11 D	14 F	18 G
150'	45 m			4 A	6 B	8 C	10 D	12 E	15 F
Decompression stops in minutes				at 20	6 m	–	–	5	10
				AT 10	3 m	5	10	10	10

ASCENT RATE is 60' (18 m) plus or minus 10' (3 m) per minute
NO-DECOMPRESSION LIMITS are givin for first dives
DECOMPRESSION STOPS are taken at mid-chest level for the times indicated at the specified stop depths
→ Table B for Minimum Surface Intervals and Repetitive Factors
→ Table C for Repetitive Dive No-Decompression Limits
→ Table D for Depth Corrections required at Altitudes above 1000' (300 m)

Source: Courtesy of Defence Research and Development Canada, Toronto; and UDT Inc., Richmond, British Columbia, Canada.

depth. For example, for a dive to 60 feet (18 metres) for less than 14 minutes the diver is in group A, and at the maximum dive without stops (50 minutes) the diver is in group F. If the diver remains at depth for longer, he or she crosses onto the right-hand side of the tables and must make the decompression stops listed further down the tables. Note that there are two sets of decompression stops: the 3-metre (10-feet) stops for shallower dives and the schedules for dives deeper than 18 metres; these may require stops at 6 metres (20 feet).

Tables B and C: surface intervals and repetitive factors

Table B is used to allow for the elimination of nitrogen during intervals on the surface. The user enters the table on the line corresponding to his or her repetitive dive group at the end of the last dive and finds the number that is in the column headed by his or her surface interval. This factor can then be transferred to Table C to find the no-decompression stops limit for a second dive.

For example, a diver surfaces in group F and spends 2 hours 15 minutes on the surface. What is the longest dive he or she can make to

18 metres without stops? The diver enters Table B on row F. At the intersection of this row with the column from 2 hours to 2 hours 59 minutes, the diver finds 1.4. This is transferred to Table C. At the intersection of 1.4 and 18 metres is the no-stops limit for the second dive, 29 minutes.

The factor from Table B can also be used to calculate stops. If the task in the second dive considered in the previous paragraph took 50 minutes, the diver multiplies this by the factor obtained from the surface interval table and uses this time in Table A to obtain the decompression time. In this case, 1.4 × 50 = 70, so the stops for the second dive are for a 70-minute dive to 18 metres (10 minutes at 3 metres). The resulting repetitive group letter (H) can be transferred to Tables B and C for any later dive. The diver can use Table A without allowance for a previous dive when he or she has been on the surface for enough time for the factor to fall to 1.0. The depth, as in other tables, is the maximum depth reached during the dive. The bottom time is the time from leaving the surface until beginning the ascent to the stop or surface. The ascent rate should be 18 ± 3 metres/minute (60 ± 10 feet/minute). The stops times are the times to be spent at the nominated depths.

Table 9 DCIEM Table B for calculation of the repetitive dive factor from dive group and surface interval

Rep. groups	0:15 0:29	0:30 0:59	1:00 1:29	1:30 1:59	2:00 2:59	3:00 3:59	4:00 5:59	6:00 8:59	9:00 11:59	12:00 14:59	15:00 18:00
A	1.4	1.2	1.1	1.1	1.1	1.1	1.1	1.1	1.0	1.0	1.0
B	1.5	1.3	1.2	1.2	1.2	1.1	1.1	1.1	1.1	1.0	1.0
C	1.6	1.4	1.3	1.2	1.2	1.2	1.1	1.1	1.1	1.0	1.0
D	1.8	1.5	1.4	1.3	1.3	1.2	1.2	1.1	1.1	1.0	1.0
E	1.9	1.6	1.5	1.4	1.3	1.3	1.2	1.2	1.1	1.1	1.0
F	2.0	1.7	1.6	1.5	1.4	1.3	1.3	1.2	1.1	1.1	1.0
G	–	1.9	1.7	1.6	1.5	1.4	1.3	1.2	1.1	1.1	1.0
H	–	–	1.9	1.7	1.6	1.5	1.4	1.3	1.1	1.1	1.1
I	–	–	2.0	1.8	1.7	1.5	1.4	1.3	1.1	1.1	1.1
J	–	–	–	1.9	1.8	1.6	1.5	1.3	1.2	1.1	1.1
K	–	–	–	2.0	1.9	1.7	1.5	1.3	1.2	1.1	1.1
L	–	–	–	–	2.0	1.7	1.6	1.4	1.2	1.1	1.1
M	–	–	–	–	–	1.8	1.6	1.4	1.2	1.1	1.1

Repetitive factors (RF) given for surface intervals (h:min)

Source: Courtesy of Defence Research and Development Canada, Toronto; and UDT Inc., Richmond, British Columbia, Canada.

Table 10 DCIEM Table C for calculation of maximum dive time using the repetitive dive factor calculated from Table B

Depth		1.1	1.2	1.3	1.4	1.5	1.6	1.7	1.8	1.9	2.0
30'	9 m	272	250	230	214	200	187	176	166	157	150
40'	12 m	136	125	115	107	100	93	88	83	78	75
50'	15 m	60	55	50	45	41	38	36	34	32	31
60'	18 m	40	35	31	29	27	26	24	23	22	21
70'	21 m	30	25	21	19	18	17	16	15	14	13
80'	24 m	20	18	16	15	14	13	12	12	11	11
90'	27 m	16	14	12	11	11	10	9	9	8	8
100'	30 m	13	11	10	9	9	8	8	7	7	7
110'	33 m	10	9	8	8	7	7	6	6	6	6
120'	36 m	8	7	7	6	6	6	5	5	5	5
130'	39 m	7	6	6	5	5	5	4	4	4	4
140'	42 m	6	5	5	5	4	4	4	3	3	3
150'	45 m	5	5	4	4	4	3	3	3	3	3

Repetitive factors no-D limits given in minutes according to depth and RF

Source: Courtesy of Defence Research and Development Canada, Toronto; and UDT Inc., Richmond, British Columbia, Canada.

Table D: depth corrections

Table D is used to convert the depth of a dive at altitude to an effective depth that can be used in Table A and to find the correct depth for any decompression stops. The table is entered on the left-hand column in the row with the actual depth of the dive. A correction to be added to the depth obtained is obtained from the intersection of this row with the column that includes the altitude of the water surface at the dive site.

For example, a diver intends to conduct a 50-foot dive in water where the surface is at 4500 feet. What is the effective depth to be used for decompression? At the intersection of the actual depth 50 feet row and the 4000- to 5000-feet column is found 10 feet. This is to be added, so the diver should decompress for a 60-foot dive. The bottom of the column shows that any stops to be taken should be at 18 and 9 feet

instead of 20 and 10 feet. A further increase of one depth should be added if the diver has been at a lower altitude less than 12 hours before the dive. This corrects for the additional nitrogen remaining in the diver's body. For a diver to fly after a no-decompression stops dive, the DCIEM table instructions require that he or she should wait till the repetitive factor in Table B has decreased to 1. The diver should have a minimum surface interval of 24 hours after a decompression dive.* The complete instructions for the tables have much information that has been omitted here. This includes rules for omitted decompression and a multilevel dive decompression procedure, as well as rules for adjustments for multiple repetitive dives.

This appendix was reviewed for this fifth edition by Michael Bennett.

---

* Flying after diving guidelines have been the subject of a workshop organized by the Undersea and Hyperbaric Medicine Society. It is reported (Sheffield, PJ, Abstract 20, Supplement to Undersea Biomedical Research, Vol 17, 1990) that the consensus was for more stringent rules than the DCIEM rules. The workshop suggested a wait for 12 hours for divers who had less than 2 hours diving (surface to surface) in the last 2 days. Divers should wait at least 24 hours before flying after multiday unlimited dives. A delay of at least 24 hours, and preferably 48 hours, was suggested after any dives requiring decompression stops. It is not known whether DCIEM will change their rules in line with these guidelines.

Table 11 DCIEM Table D for calculation of dive times for diving at altitude

Actual depth ↓ ↓	1000 →1999 300 m →599		2000 →2999 600 m →899		3000 →3999 900 m →1199		4000 →4999 1200 m →1499		5000 →5999 1500 m →1799		6000 →6999 1800 m →2099		7000 →7999 2100 m →2399		8000 →10 000 2400 m →3000	
30' 9 m	10	3	10	3	10	3	10	3	10	3	10	3	20	6	20	6
40' 12 m	10	3	10	3	10	3	10	3	10	3	20	6	20	6	20	6
50' 15 m	10	3	10	3	10	3	10	3	20	6	20	6	20	6	20	6
60' 18 m	10	3	10	3	10	3	20	6	20	6	20	6	20	6	30	9
70' 21 m	10	3	10	3	10	3	20	6	20	6	20	6	30	9	30	9
80' 24 m	10	3	10	3	20	6	20	6	20	6	30	9	30	9	40	12
90' 27 m	10	3	10	3	20	6	20	6	20	6	30	9	30	9	40	12
100' 30 m	10	3	10	3	20	6	20	6	30	9	30	9	30	9	40	12
110' 33 m	10	3	20	6	20	6	20	6	30	9	30	9	40	12		
120' 36 m	10	3	20	6	20	6	30	9	30	9	30	9				
130' 39 m	10	3	20	6	20	6										
140' 42 m	10	3														

Add depth correction to actual depth of altitude dive

| 10' 3 m | 10 | 3.0 | 10 | 3.0 | 9 | 3.0 | 9 | 3.0 | 9 | 3.0 | 8 | 2.5 | 8 | 2.5 | 8 | 2.5 |
| 20' 6 m | 20 | 6.0 | 19 | 6.0 | 18 | 5.5 | 18 | 5.5 | 17 | 5.0 | 16 | 15.0 | 16 | 5.0 | 15 | 4.5 |

Actual decompression stop depths (feet/metres) at altitude

Source: Courtesy of Defence Research and Development Canada, Toronto; and UDT Inc., Richmond, British Columbia, Canada.

Appendix B: US Navy recompression therapy tables

INTRODUCTION

The US Navy (USN) 18-metre oxygen recompression table (USN Treatment Table 6 [TT6]) has become nearly universal therapy for recompression in decompression illness, although some physicians (particularly in the United Kingdom and Australia) call it the almost identical Royal Navy Table 62 (RN62).

To guide users in the selection of a decompression therapy table, the *US Navy Diving Manual* contains four flow charts. These are reproduced here (Figures 1 to 4). After the appropriate chart, the reader is guided to selecting an appropriate table. These tables are also presented here. Note that much of the text that contains advice on selecting and using the tables has been omitted. Any person using these tables, or any other therapy table, should have the complete original document. This presentation is offered as a teaching aid and not as an official guide.

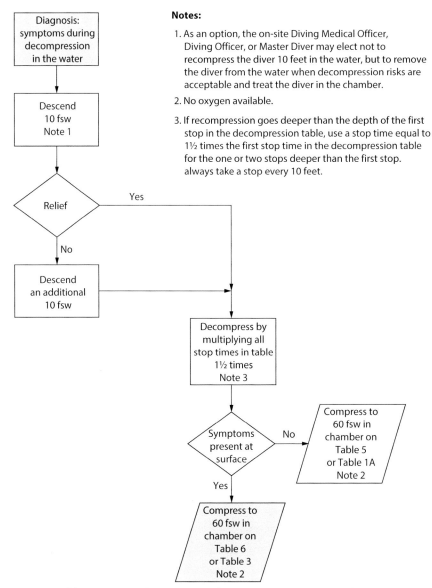

Notes:

1. As an option, the on-site Diving Medical Officer, Diving Officer, or Master Diver may elect not to recompress the diver 10 feet in the water, but to remove the diver from the water when decompression risks are acceptable and treat the diver in the chamber.

2. No oxygen available.

3. If recompression goes deeper than the depth of the first stop in the decompression table, use a stop time equal to 1½ times the first stop time in the decompression table for the one or two stops deeper than the first stop. always take a stop every 10 feet.

Treatment of decompression sickness accurring while at a decompression stop in the water

Figure 1 (From *US Navy Diving Manual Revision 6 SS521-AG-PRO-010 (2008)*. Washington, DC: Naval Sea Systems Command; 2008.)

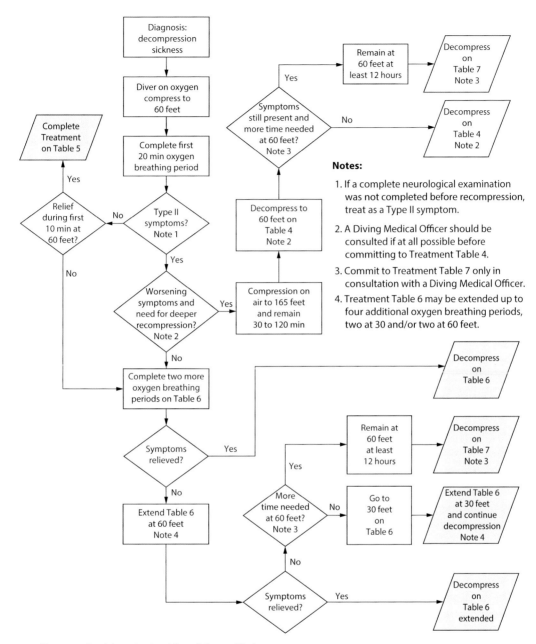

Decompression sickness treatment from diving or altitude exposures

Notes:

1. If a complete neurological examination was not completed before recompression, treat as a Type II symptom.

2. A Diving Medical Officer should be consulted if at all possible before committing to Treatment Table 4.

3. Commit to Treatment Table 7 only in consultation with a Diving Medical Officer.

4. Treatment Table 6 may be extended up to four additional oxygen breathing periods, two at 30 and/or two at 60 feet.

Figure 2 (From *US Navy Diving Manual Revision 6 SS521-AG-PRO-010 (2008)*. Washington, DC: Naval Sea Systems Command; 2008.)

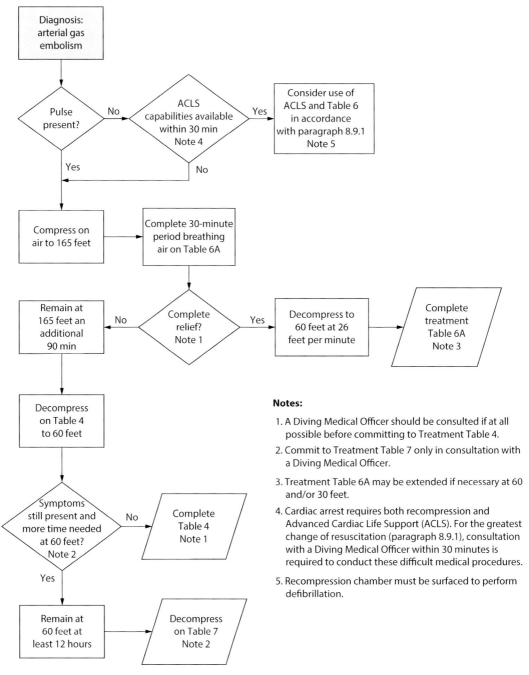

Treatment of arterial gas embolism

Figure 3 (From *US Navy Diving Manual Revision 6 SS521-AG-PRO-010 (2008)*. Washington, DC: Naval Sea Systems Command; 2008.)

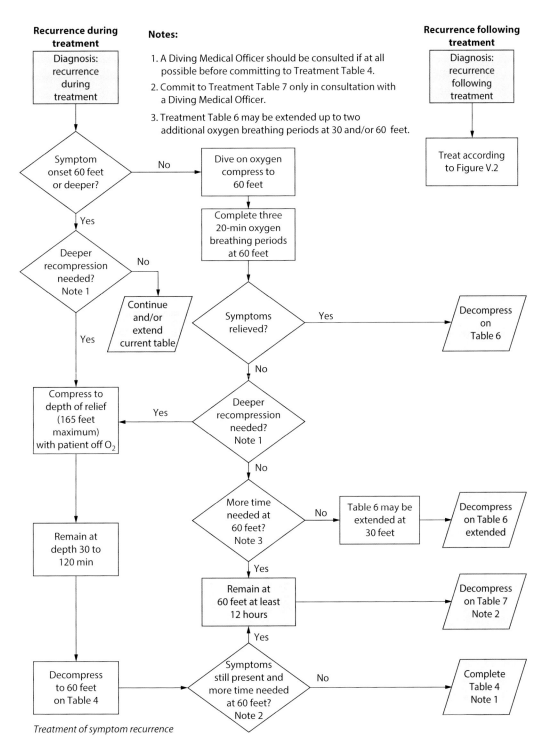

Treatment of symptom recurrence

Figure 4 (From *US Navy Diving Manual Revision 6 SS521-AG-PRO-010 (2008)*. Washington, DC: Naval Sea Systems Command; 2008.)

TREATMENT TABLE 5

Treatment Table 5 (TT5) was originally developed as a short 60-foot (18-metre) oxygen treatment for type I decompression sickness (DCS). It is now rarely used for this purpose, with the growing realization that isolated type I disease is rare in the recreational diving population and that TT5 was often applied inappropriately. TT5 is now more commonly used to prevent DCS when a diver has missed decompression (See Table 1).

Table 1 USN treatment Table 5

Depth (feet)	Time (minutes)	Breathing media	Total elapsed time (h: min)
60	20	Oxygen	0:20
60	5	Air	0:25
60	20	Oxygen	0:45
60–30	30	Oxygen	1:15
30	5	Air	1:20
30	20	Oxygen	1:40
30	5	Air	1:45
30–0	30	Oxygen	2:15

Source: From *US Navy Diving Manual Revision 6 SS521-AG-PRO-010 (2008).* Washington, DC: Naval Sea Systems Command; 2008.

TREATMENT TABLE 6

TT6 is the most commonly used table for the treatment of both DCS and cerebral arterial gas embolism (CAGE), although it was originally developed specifically for the treatment of type II DCS (see Figure 5).

The instructions for use in the *US Navy Diving Manual* are as follows:

1. This table is used for treatment of type II or type I DCS when symptoms are not relieved within 10 minutes at 60 feet.
2. The descent rate is 25 feet/minute.
3. The ascent rate is 1 foot/minute. Do not compensate for slower ascent rates. Compensate for faster rates by halting the ascent.
4. Time at 60 feet begins on arrival at 60 feet.
5. If oxygen breathing must be interrupted, allow 15 minutes after the reaction has entirely subsided and resume the schedule at the point of interruption.
6. The tender breathes air throughout unless the tender has had a hyperbaric exposure within the last 12 hours, in which case oxygen is

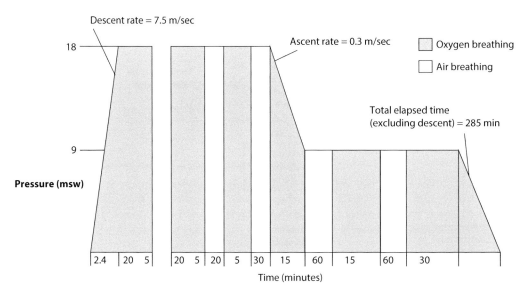

Figure 5 USN Treatment Table 6. US Navy Treatment Table 6 (or Royal Navy Table 62). Depths are expressed here as metres of sea water (msw). An initial period at 18 msw (60 feet) breathing 100 per cent oxygen with air breaks is followed by a slow ascent to 9 msw (30 feet). (From *US Navy Diving Manual Revision 6 SS521-AG-PRO-010 (2008)*. Washington, DC: Naval Sea Systems Command; 2008.)

breathed at 30 feet in accordance with paragraph 8.13.5.7.

7. TT6 can be lengthened up to two additional 25-minute periods at 60 feet (20 minutes on oxygen and 5 minutes on air) or up to two additional 75-minute periods at 30 feet (15 minutes on air and 60 minutes on oxygen), or both. If TT6 is extended only once at either 60 or 30 feet, the tender breathes oxygen during the ascent from 30 feet to the surface. If more than one extension is done, the tender begins oxygen breathing for the last hour at 30 feet and during ascent to the surface.

TREATMENT TABLE 6A

Treatment Table 6A (TT6A) was developed as a treatment for CAGE. This table begins with a 'spike' to 165 feet (50 metres) to 'crush' any bubbles and encourage the movement of gas through the cerebral circulation (See Table 2). After this spike, TT6A is identical to TT6. It is now very rarely used.

The *US Navy Diving Manual* suggests the following:

1. This table is used for treatment of arterial gas embolism where complete relief is obtained within 30 minutes at 165 feet.* Use also

Table 2 USN treatment Table 6A

Depth (feet)	Time (minutes)	Breathing media	Total elapsed time (h: min)
165	30	Air	0:30
165–60	4	Air	0:34
60	20	Oxygen	0:54
60	5	Air	0:59
60	20	Oxygen	1:19
60	5	Air	1:24
60	20	Oxygen	1:44
60	5	Air	1:49
60–30	30	Oxygen	2:19
30	15	Air	2:34
30	60	Oxygen	3:34
30	15	Air	3:49
30	60	Oxygen	4:49
30–0	30	Oxygen	5:19

Source: From *US Navy Diving Manual Revision 6 SS521-AG-PRO-010 (2008).* Washington, DC: Naval Sea Systems Command; 2008.

when one is unable to determine whether symptoms are caused by gas embolism or severe DCS.

2. The descent rate is as fast as possible.

3. The ascent rate is 1 foot/minute. Do not compensate for slower ascent rates. Compensate for faster rates by halting the ascent.

4. Time at 165 feet includes time from the surface.

5. If oxygen breathing must be interrupted, allow 15 minutes after the reaction has entirely subsided and resume the schedule at the point of interruption.

6. The tender breathes oxygen during ascent from 30 feet to the surface unless the tender has had a hyperbaric exposure within the last 12 hours, in which case oxygen is breathed at 30 feet in accordance with paragraph 8.13.5.7.

7. TT6A can be lengthened up to two additional 25-minute periods at 60 feet (20 minutes on oxygen and 5 minutes on air) or up to two additional 75-minute periods at 30 feet (60 minutes on oxygen and 15 minutes on air), or both. If TT6A is extended either at 60 or 30 feet, the tender breathes oxygen during the last 90 minutes of the treatment: 60 minutes at 30 feet and 30 minutes during ascent to the surface.

8. If complete relief is not obtained within 30 minutes at 165 feet, switch to Treatment Table 4 (TT4). Consult with a Diving Medical Officer before switching if possible.

* Note in point 8 the consequence of extending treatment at 50 metres. USN TT4 may take more than 30 hours to complete and is not to be entered into lightly.

TREATMENT TABLE 4

TT4 is an air or air and oxygen table designed for use in either serious type II DCS or CAGE. It is recommended for treatment of worsening symptoms during the first 20-minute oxygen breathing period at 60 feet on TT6, or when symptoms are not relieved within 30 minutes at 165 feet using air Treatment Table 3 or TT6A (See Table 3).

Table 3 USN treatment Table 4

Depth (feet)	Time	Breathing media	Total elapsed time (h: min)
165	½–2 h	Air	2:00
140	½ h	Air	2:31
120	½ h	Air	3:02
100	½ h	Air	3:33
80	½ h	Air	4:04
60	6 h	Air	10:05
50	6 h	Air	16:06
40	6 h	Air	22:07
30	12 h	Oxygen/Air	34:08
20	2 h	Oxygen/Air	36:09
10	2 h	Oxygen/Air	38:10
0	1 min	Oxygen	38:11

Source: From *US Navy Diving Manual Revision 6 SS521-AG-PRO-010 (2008).* Washington, DC: Naval Sea Systems Command; 2008.

These days it is very rarely used; the alternatives of repetitive TT6 or the use of heliox such as in the Comex tables (see Appendix C) are preferred because they are more practical and safer for the attendant.

Table 4 USN treatment Table 7

Depth (feet)	Time (hours) from leaving 60 feet	Ascent rate (free/hour)	Steps to get ascent rate
60	A minimum of 12 hours hold at 60 feet		
60	0	3	2 feet every 40 min
40	6	2	2 feet every 60 min
20	16	1	2 feet every 120 min
4	32	–	(4 hours hold and then surface 36 hours after leaving bottom)

Source: From *US Navy Diving Manual Revision 6 SS521-AG-PRO-010 (2008).* Washington, DC: Naval Sea Systems Command; 2008.

TREATMENT TABLE 7

This oxygen–air table is indicated for the treatment of unresolved or life-threatening symptoms of DCS or CAGE. It is used after initial treatment on TT6 or TT4 where serious symptoms remain (See Table 4).

This appendix was reviewed for this fifth edition by Michael Bennett.

Appendix C: Recompression therapy options

COMEX OXYGEN, AIR AND HELIOX THERAPY TABLES

This set of recompression tables was developed commercially in order to employ the theoretical advantages of breathing helium-oxygen mixtures (heliox). These mixtures allow increased nitrogen elimination without a high risk of oxygen toxicity. The most commonly used is the Comex 30 – a 30-metre maximum depth table employing heliox with 20 per cent oxygen (see Plate 3 (a) for these tables).

AUSTRALIAN SHALLOW IN-WATER OXYGEN TABLES

Table aust 9 (royal australian navy 82)

Short oxygen table

Table 1 Royal Australian Navy Table 9. Shallow in-water oxygen table

Depth (metres)	Elapsed time		Rate of ascent
	Mild	Serious	
9	0030–0100	0100–0130	12 minutes per metre (4 minutes per foot)
8	0042–0112	0112–0142	
7	0054–0124	0124–0154	
6	0106–0136	0136–0206	
5	0118–0148	0148–0218	
4	0130–0200	0200–0230	
3	0142–0212	0212–0242	
2	0154–0224	0224–0254	
1	0206–0236	0236–0306	

Source: From Royal Australian Navy.

Notes

1. This technique may be useful in treating cases of decompression sickness in localities remote from recompression facilities. It may also be of use while suitable transport to such a centre is being arranged.
2. In planning, it should be realized that the therapy may take up to 3 hours. The risk of cold, immersion and other environmental factors should be balanced against the beneficial effects. The diver must be accompanied by an attendant.

Equipment

The following equipment is essential before attempting this form of treatment:

1. Full-face mask with demand valve and surface supply system *or* helmet with free flow.
2. Adequate supply of 100 per cent oxygen for the patient and air for the attendant.
3. Wetsuit for thermal protection.
4. Shot with at least 10 metres of rope (a seat or harness may be rigged to the shot).
5. Some form of communication system among the patient, the attendant and the surface.

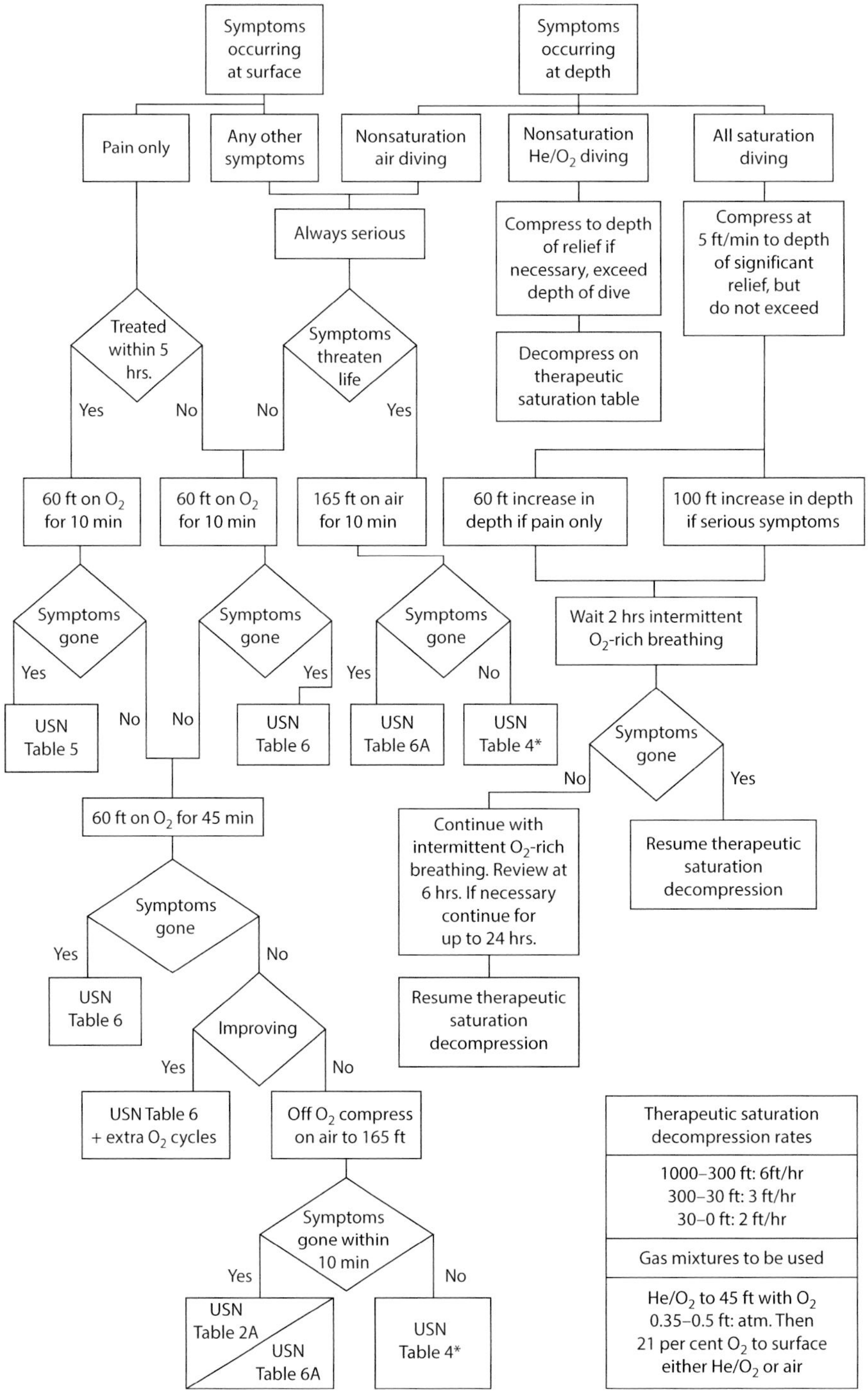

*Always use the oxygen version or USN Table 4, for both patient and attendant(s).

Figure 1 Duke university flow chart for the treatment of decompression illness. USN, United States Navy. (Courtesy of Duke University, Durham, North Carolina.)

Method

1. The patient is lowered on the shot rope to 9 metres while breathing 100 per cent oxygen.
2. Ascent is commenced after 30 minutes in mild cases, or 60 minutes in severe cases, if improvement has occurred. These times may be extended to 60 minutes and 90 minutes, respectively, if there is no improvement.
3. Ascent is at the rate of 1 metre every 12 minutes.
4. If symptoms recur, remain at depth a further 30 minutes before continuing ascent.
5. If the oxygen supply is exhausted, return to the surface, rather than breathe air.

6. After surfacing, the patient should be given 1 hour on oxygen, 1 hour off, for a further 12 hours.

DUKE UNIVERSITY FLOW CHART

This flow chart is used to guide the treatment of divers following the development of symptoms at the surface or at depth (See Figure 1).

This appendix was reviewed for this fifth edition by Michael Bennett.

Appendix D: Diving medical library

CLASSICS

Bert P. *La pression barométrique* [Barometric Pressure] (1878). The Hitchcock translation. Columbus, Ohio: Columbus Book Co.; 1943.

Davis RH. *Deep Diving and Submarine Operations*. 6th ed. London: Siebe, Gorman and Co.; 1955.

Fulton JF, ed. *Decompression Sickness*. London: Saunders; 1951.

Haldane JS, Priestley JG. *Respiration*. Oxford: Clarendon Press; 1935.

Hill L. *Caisson Sickness and the Physiology of Work in Compressed Air*. London: Edward Arnold; 1912.

Rahn H, Yokoyama T, eds. *Physiology of Breath-Hold Diving and the Ama of Japan*. Washington, DC: National Academy of Sciences; 1965.

Undersea Medical Society. *Key documents of the biomedical aspects of deep diving sleceted from the world's literature 1608–1982*. Vols 1–5. Bethesda, Maryland: Undersea Medical Society; 1983.

CURRENT MEDICAL TEXTS

Bennett PB, Cronjé FJ, Campbell ES. *Assessment of Diving Medical Fitness for Scuba Divers and Instructors*. Flagstaff, Arizona: Best Publishing; 2006. ISBN 978-1-930536-31-9.

Bookspan J. *Diving Physiology in Plain English* (reprinted 2006). Dunkirk, Maryland: Undersea and Hyperbaric Medical Society; 1995. ISBN 0-9304061-3-3.

Bove A, Davis J, eds. *Bove and Davis' Diving Medicine*. 4th ed. Philadelphia: Saunders; 2004. ISBN 0-7216-9424-1.

Chan G, Lippmann J. *Am I Fit to Dive*. Melbourne: Submariner Publications; 2013. ISBN 978-0-9586452-6-3.

Edmonds CE, Bennett M, Mitchell SJ, Lippmann J. *Diving and Subaquatic Medicine*. 5th ed. London: Arnold; 2014.

Elliott DH, ed. *Medical Assessment of Fitness to Dive*. Guilford, United Kingdom: University of Surrey Biomedical Seminars; 1995. ISBN 0-9525162-0-9.

Parker J. *The Sports Diving Medical*. Melbourne: Submariner Publications; 2002. ISBN 0-9587118-6-0.

Wendling J, Ehrsam R, Knessl P, Nussberger P, Uské A. *Medical Assessment of Fitness to Dive*. Biel, Switzerland: Hyperbaric Editions; 2001. ISBN 3-9522284-1-9.

FIRST AID

Divers Alert Network. *Dive and Travel Medical Guide*. Durham, North Carolina: Divers Alert Network; 2010.

Diving Diseases Research Centre (DDRC). The DDRC *Underwater Diving Accident Manual*. 6th ed. Plymouth, United Kingdom: DDRC; 2012. ISBN 978-1-905492-25-1.

Lippmann J, Bugg S. *The DAN Emergency Handbook*. 7th ed. Melbourne: Submariner Publications; 2013. ISBN 978-0-9752290-5-7.

Lippmann J. *Oxygen First Aid*. Melbourne: Submariner Publications; 2012. ISBN 0-646-23565-6.

SPECIALIST TEXTS

Bachrach AJ, Engstrom GH. *Stress and Performance in Diving.* San Pedro, California: Best Publishing; 1987. ISBN 0-941332-06-3.

Balestra C, Germonpré P, Marroni A, Cronjé FJ. *PFO and the Diver.* Flagstaff, Arizona: Best Publishing; 2007. ISBN 978-1-930536-39-5.

Brubakk AO, Neuman TS, eds. *Bennett and Elliot's Physiology and Medicine of Diving.* 5th ed. Philadelphia: Saunders; 2003. ISBN 0-7020-2571-2.

Donald K. *Oxygen and the Diver.* Hanley Swan, United Kingdom: The SPA Ltd; 1992.

Edmonds C. *Dangerous Marine Creatures.* Flagstaff, Arizona: Best Publishing; 1995. ISBN 0-941332-39-X.

Fife CE, St Leger Dowse M, eds. *Women and Pressure: Diving and Altitude.* Flagstaff, Arizona: Best Publishing; 2010. ISBN 978-1-930536-54-8.

Hope A, Lund T, Elliott DH, Halsey MJ, Wiig H, eds. *Long Term Health Effects of Diving.* Bergen: Norwegian Underwater Technology Centre; 1994.

Kindwall EP, Whelan HT. *Hyperbaric Medicine Practice.* 3rd ed. Flagstaff, Arizona: Best Publishing; 2008. ISBN 978-1-930536-49-4.

Lippmann J, Mitchell SJ. *Deeper Into Diving.* 2nd ed. Melbourne: Submariner Publications; 2005. ISBN 0-9752290-1-X.

Lundgren CEG, Miller JN, eds. *The Lung at Depth.* New York: Marcel Dekker; 1999. ISBN 0-8247-0158-5.

Williamson JA, Fenner PJ, Burnett JW, Rifkin JF. *Venomous and Poisonous Marine Animals.* Sydney: University of New South Wales Press; 1996. ISBN 0-86840-279-6.

JOURNALS

Aviation, Space and Environmental Medicine. Aerospace Medical Association. ISSN 0095-911X. https://www.asma.org/publications/asem-journal

Chinese Journal of Nautical Medicine and Hyperbaric Medicine. http://eng.med.wanfangdata.com.cn/JournalDetail.aspx?qid=zhhhyx#. ISSN 1009-6906

Diving and Hyperbaric Medicine. South Pacific Underwater Medicine Society and European Underwater and Baromedical Society. http://www.spums.org.au. ISSN 0833-3516.

Journal of Applied Physiology. American Physiological Society. ISSN 8750-7587 (print); ISSN 1522-1601 (online). http://jap.physiology.org/

Pressure. Undersea and Hyperbaric Medical Society. ISSN 0889-0242. http://www.uhms.org

Undersea and Hyperbaric Medicine. Undersea and Hyperbaric Medical Society. ISSN 1066-2936. http://www.uhms.org

ONLINE REFERENCES

DAN America: http://www.diversalertnetwork.org/medical/faq/

DAN Asia-Pacific: http://www.danasiapacific.org/main/diving_safety/DAN_Doc/main.html

DAN Europe: http://daneurope.org/web/guest/medicalquestions

DAN Southern Africa: http://dansa.org/

Edmonds C, Thomas R, McKenzie, Pennefather J. *Diving Medicine for Scuba Divers.* 2012 ed. http://www.divingmedicine.info/

Edmund Kay's Doc's Diving Medicine Home Page: http://staff.washington.edu/ekay/

Ernest S Campbell's Ten-Foot Stop: http://www.scuba-doc.com/tenfootstop/

UK Sports Diving Medical Committee: http://www.uksdmc.co.uk/

ONLINE RESEARCH DATABASES

EMBASE (subscriber only): http://www.elsevier.com/online-tools/embase

Google Scholar: http://scholar.google.com.au/schhp?hl = en

Medline (subscriber only): http://www.ebscohost.com/nursing/products/medline-databases

PubMed (US National Library of Medicine): http://www.ncbi.nlm.nih.gov/pubmed

Rubicon Research Repository: http://rubicon-foundation.org/

WORKSHOP PROCEEDINGS

Proceedings of UHMS and/or DAN Workshops: http://archive.rubicon-foundation.org/xmlui/search?order=DESC&rpp=10&sort_by=0&page=1&query=uhms+workshop&etal=0

DIVING MANUALS

National Oceanic and Atmospheric Administration. *NOAA Diving Manual.* 5th ed. Washington, DC: US Government Printing Office; 2013. 9781930536630.

US Navy Diving Manual Revision 6. SS521-AG-PRO-010 (2008). Washington, DC: Naval Sea Systems Command; 2008.

This appendix was reviewed for this fifth edition by John Lippmann.

Appendix E: Diving medical training

The Royal Navy, the United States Navy and the Royal Australian Navy have regular courses for their officers; on occasion places are made available to members of other navies. The British and Australian courses have sometimes been offered to civilian physicians who can demonstrate a need to attend. There are also courses offered by several other navies throughout the world, again predominantly to train their own medical officers.

Other courses are offered, or approved by, some of the societies or organizations mentioned in Appendix F. These include the Undersea and Hyperbaric Medical Society and Divers Alert Network (DAN) America. Some hospitals with hyperbaric units offer diving medical courses, often combined with training in hyperbaric medicine. Introductory courses in diving medicine are also available that concentrate on fitness to dive and diving accident management.

Courses are normally advertised in the journal or newsletter of the appropriate diving medical society.

This appendix was reviewed for this fifth edition by John Lippmann.

Appendix F: Diving medical organizations and contacts

PROFESSIONAL SOCIETIES

The Undersea and Hyperbaric Medical Society (UHMS) (http://uhms.org) is based in the United States. Its journal, *Undersea and Hyperbaric Medicine,* workshop reports, newsletters and abstracts are required reading for an interested physician. It has a worldwide membership. The UHMS holds an Annual Scientific Meeting and publishes the abstracts from these meetings. The UHMS also hosts workshops (often in partnership with Divers Alert Network [DAN]) on specialized topics and publishes these as reports.

The South Pacific Underwater Medicine Society (SPUMS) (http://spums.org.au) is based in Australia. Membership is mainly from Australia, New Zealand and South East Asia, but with increasing membership from Europe and the United States. SPUMS holds an annual scientific meeting, and the presented papers are published in *Diving and Hyperbaric Medicine,* which is a joint journal of SPUMS and the European Undersea Biomedical Society (EUBS).

The European Undersea Biomedical Society (EUBS) (http://eubs.org) has predominantly European-based subscribers, holds an annual scientific meeting and jointly publishes the journal *Diving and Hyperbaric Medicine* with SPUMS.

The Southern African Underwater and Hyperbaric Medical Society (SAUHMA) (http://sauhma.co.za) is based in South Africa.

The Asian Hyperbaric and Diving Medical Association (AHDMA) (http://ahdma.org) is based in Malaysia and has members from throughout Asia. It holds an annual conference.

Some other relevant societies and organizations include the following, although the list is not exhaustive:

Baromedical Nurses Association (BNA) (hyperbaricnurses.org).
British Hyperbaric Association (http://www.hyperbaric.org.uk).
Diving Medical Advisory Committee (DMAC) (http://www.dmac-diving.org).
Dutch Society of Hyperbaric Medicine (http://www.duikgeneeskunde.nl).
European Baromedical Association for Nurses, Operators and Technicians (EBAss) (http://www.ebass.org/).
Gesellschaft für Tach- und Überdruckmedizin (GTUEM) (http://www.gtuem.org).
Hyperbaric Technicians and Nurses Association (HTNA) (http://htna.com.au).
Italian Society for Underwater and Hyperbaric Medicine (SIMSI) (http://www.simsi.org/).
Japanese Society for Hyperbaric and Undersea Medicine (http://www.jshm.net).
National Baromedical Services (NBS) (http://www.baromedical.com).
Scott Haldane Foundation (http://www.scotthaldane.nl/en).

Société Belge de Médecine Hyperbare et Subaquatique (http://www.sbmhs-bvoog.be).

Société de Médecine et de Physiologie Subaquatiques et Hyperbares de langue Française (MEDSUBHYP) (http://www.med-subhyp.com/).

Swiss Underwater and Hyperbaric Medical Society (http://www.suhms.org).

DIVERS ALERT NETWORK

Internationally, the Divers Alert Network (DAN) consists of five membership-based associations, representing various regions. The common mission of improving recreational diving safety is mainly funded through the sale of dive accident insurance. DAN collates data on diving accidents and analyzes these data in regular reports. It also supplies emergency and routine health information to divers, diving physicians and others. It distributes diving safety texts and conducts a variety of training programs and seminars for divers, from lay divers to physicians.

DAN America (http://www.dan.org): Durham, North Carolina, United States. Tel: +1-919-684-2948; hotline: +1-919-684 9111.

DAN Asia-Pacific (http://www.danap.org): Ashburton, Victoria, Australia. Tel: +61-3-9886-9166; hotline: +61-8-8212 9242.

DAN Europe (http://www.daneurope.org): Roseto, Italy. Tel: +39-085-893-0333; hotline: +39-06-4211 8585.

DAN Japan (http://www.danjapan.gr.jp): Kagawa, Japan. Tel: +81-45-228-3066; hotline: +81-3-3812 4999.

DAN Southern Africa (http://www.dansa.org): Midrand, South Africa. Tel: +27-11-245-1991; hotline: +27-828-106010.

This appendix was reviewed for this fifth edition by John Lippmann.

Index

Pages followed by f indicate figures; those followed by t indicate tables.